1 MONTH OF
FREE
READING

at

www.ForgottenBooks.com

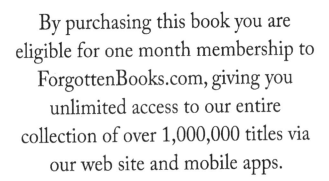

By purchasing this book you are
eligible for one month membership to
ForgottenBooks.com, giving you
unlimited access to our entire
collection of over 1,000,000 titles via
our web site and mobile apps.

To claim your free month visit:
www.forgottenbooks.com/free930943

ISBN 978-0-260-15113-1
PIBN 10930943

AMERICAN
PRACTICE OF SURGERY

A COMPLETE SYSTEM OF THE SCIENCE AND
ART OF SURGERY, BY REPRESENTATIVE SUR-
GEONS OF THE UNITED STATES AND CANADA

EDITORS:

JOSEPH D. BRYANT, M.D., LL.D.
ALBERT H. BUCK, M.D.

OF NEW YORK CITY

COMPLETE IN EIGHT VOLUMES

Profusely Illustrated

VOLUME EIGHT

NEW YORK
WILLIAM WOOD AND COMPANY
MDCCCCXI

V.

EDITORIAL NOTE.

THE completion of this, the last volume of the series, carries with it the duty of acknowledging frankly our indebtedness to those who have enabled us to bring this great undertaking to a successful issue. We desire, in the first place, to thank those who are the real constructors of the edifice—the authors of the one hundred and two articles of which these eight volumes are composed. We are the more pleased to make this acknowledgment as these gentlemen have at all times stood ready to accept our occasional suggestions, often yielding their own preferences in order that a more complete and harmonious whole might be secured. Our acknowledgments are also due the publishers, who have heartily co-operated with us by doing all in their power to make these volumes as attractive and instructive as possible. Not only have they permitted the very free use of pictorial illustrations, but, as soon as it became apparent that the number of pages specified in the original "Announcement"—viz., an average of about eight hundred pages to the volume—would not suffice for the accomplishment of the work in accordance with the plan which we had originally laid down, they authorized us to increase the average to about nine hundred pages.

The credit for the indexing is due to Dr. J. Haven Emerson, for the earlier volumes, and to Dr. R. J. E. Scott, for the later ones.

THE EDITORS.

CONTRIBUTORS TO VOLUME VIII.

JAMES BELL, M.D., Montreal, Canada.

Professor of Surgery and Clinical Surgery, McGill University; Surgeon, Royal Victoria Hospital, Montreal.

ALEXANDER HUGH FERGUSON, M.D., C.M., Chicago, Ill.

Professor of Surgery and Clinical Surgery, College of Medicine, University of Illinois; Surgeon, Cook County Hospitals at Dunning; Consulting Surgeon, The Mary Thompson Hospital, Chicago.

ALEXANDER ESSLEMONT GARROW, M.D., C.M. (McGill), Montreal, Canada.

Assistant Professor of Surgery and Clinical Surgery, McGill University; Assistant Surgeon, Royal Victoria Hospital, Montreal.

CHRISTIAN R. HOLMES, M.D., Cincinnati, Ohio.

Professor of Otology, Rhinology and Laryngology, Medical Department of the University of Cincinnati; Member of the Building Commission of the New General Hospital, Cincinnati.

JAMES ALEXANDER HUTCHISON, M.D., L.R.C.P. and S. (Edin.), Montreal, Canada.

Assistant Professor of Surgery and Clinical Surgery, McGill University; Attending Surgeon, Montreal General Hospital; Chief Medical Officer to the Grand Trunk Railway System and Grand Trunk Pacific Railway Company.

MAJOR CHARLES LYNCH, Medical Corps, United States Army.

FRANK W. LYNCH, M.D., Chicago, Ill.

Assistant Professor of Obstetrics and Gynæcology, Rush Medical College, University of Chicago; Attending Obstetrician and Gynæcologist, Presbyterian Hospital; Attending Obstetrician, St. Joseph Hospital.

LEWIS S. McMURTRY, M.D., LL.D., Louisville, Ky.

Professor of Gynæcology and Abdominal Surgery, Medical Department of the University of Louisville; Attending Surgeon, Louisville City Hospital, and the University Hospital.

JOHN B. MURPHY, M.Sc. (England), **M.D., LL.D.**, Chicago, Ill.

Professor of Surgery and Clinical Surgery, and Head of Surgical Department, Northwestern University; Chief Surgeon of Mercy Hospital; Attending Surgeon, Columbus and St. Joseph's Hospitals; Consulting Surgeon, Cook County and Alexian Brothers' Hospitals.

JOSEPH RANSOHOFF, M.D., F.R.C.S., Cincinnati, Ohio.

Professor of Surgery, Ohio-Miami Medical College, University of Cincinnati; Attending Surgeon, Cincinnati, Good Samaritan, and Jewish Hospitals.

J. LOUIS RANSOHOFF, M.D., Cincinnati, Ohio.

BENJAMIN R. SCHENCK, M.D., Detroit, Michigan.

Junior Attending Gynæcologist, Harper Hospital, Detroit; Associate Gynæcologist, Providence Hospital, Detroit; Consulting Obstetrician, The Woman's Hospital, Detroit.

SIDNEY SMITH, LL.B., New York City.

Member of the New York Bar.

STEPHEN SMITH, M.D., LL.D., New York City.

Consulting Surgeon, Bellevue, St. Vincent's, and Columbus Hospitals, New York.

GEORGE DAVID STEWART, M.D., New York City.

Professor of the Principles of Surgery, University and Bellevue Hospital Medical College; Visiting Surgeon, Bellevue Hospital and St. Vincent's Hospital, New York.

CHARLES F. STOKES, M.D.

Surgeon-General, United States Navy.

J. E. SWEET, M.D., Philadelphia, Pa.

Assistant Professor of Experimental Surgery, University of Pennsylvania, Philadelphia.

CONTENTS.

PART XVI.

REGIONAL SURGERY.
(Continued.)

PAGE

Intrathoracic Surgery, ... 3
(Heart and Œsophagus Excluded.)

I. Surgical Diseases of the Pleura, ... 3
II. Wounds of the Thoracic Cavity and its Contents, . . 16
III. Abscess and Gangrene of the Lung, ... 19
IV. Bronchiectasis and Pulmonary Emphysema, ... 23
V. Parasitic Affections of the Lungs, ... 25
VI. Pulmonary Tuberculosis, ... 28
VII. Neoplasms of the Lungs, ... 30
VIII. Surgical Affections of the Mediastinum, ... 31
IX. Operations on the Chest, ... 43

Surgery of the Spleen, ... 59

Anatomy, ... 59
Physiology, ... 60
Malformations and Anomalies, ... 61
Wandering Spleen, ... 61
Rupture of the Spleen, ... 64
Stab Wounds and Gunshot Wounds of the Spleen, . . . 66
Abscess of the Spleen, ... 67
Tumors of the Spleen, ... 69
Cysts of the Spleen, ... 70
Chronic Splenic Anæmia (Banti's Disease), ... 71
Operations on the Spleen, ... 74

Surgical Diseases and Wounds of the Kidneys and Ureters, . . . 78

I. Anatomy, Embryology, and Physiology, ... 78
II. Methods of Investigating the Condition of the Kidney, 81
III. Congenital Abnormalities of the Kidney and Ureter, . . 85
IV. Wounds of the Kidney and Ureter, ... 90

Surgical Diseases and Wounds of the Kidneys and Ureters (*Continued*). PAGE

V. ABNORMAL CONDITIONS AND DISEASES OF THE KIDNEYS (TUBER-
    CULOSIS AND TUMORS EXCEPTED), ... 96
VI. TUBERCULOSIS OF THE KIDNEY, ... 121
VII. ESSENTIAL HÆMATURIA, ... 131
VIII. TUMORS OF THE KIDNEY, ... 132
IX. WOUNDS AND DISEASES OF THE URETER, ... 141
X. OPERATIONS UPON THE KIDNEYS AND URETERS, ... 146

Surgery of the Pancreas, ... 159

I. ANATOMY AND PHYSIOLOGY, ... 159
II. PANCREATITIS, ... 162
III. CYSTS OF THE PANCREAS, ... 180
IV. WOUNDS OF THE PANCREAS, ... 187
V. TUMORS OF THE PANCREAS, ... 188
VI. PANCREOPTOSIS, ... 190
VII. PANCREATIC CALCULUS (PANCREATICO-LITHIASIS), ... 190

Surgery of the Liver, Gall-Bladder, and Biliary Passages, . . . 193

ANATOMY OF THE LIVER AND BILE-DUCTS, ... 193
PHYSIOLOGY OF THE LIVER AND BILE-DUCTS, ... 203
ABNORMALITIES OF THE LIVER AND BILE-DUCTS, ... 204
PERITONEAL POUCH; RUTHERFORD MORRISON'S SPACE, . . 206
TRAUMATIC AFFECTIONS OF THE LIVER, ... 206
SUPPURATION IN THE LIVER, ... 208
HYDATID CYSTS OF THE LIVER, ... 214
TUMORS OF THE LIVER, ... 219
ACTINOMYCOSIS OF THE LIVER, ... 225
SYPHILIS OF THE LIVER, ... 226
PORTAL CIRRHOSIS, ... 227
HEPAPTOSIS, ... 229
INFLAMMATORY AFFECTIONS OF THE GALL-BLADDER AND BILE-DUCTS, 229
TUBERCULOUS INFLAMMATION OF THE GALL-BLADDER, . . . 233
ACTINOMYCOSIS OF THE GALL-BLADDER, ... 233
GALL-STONES; CHOLELITHIASIS, ... 233
TUMORS OF THE BILIARY DUCTS, ... 252
SURGICAL TREATMENT IN DISEASES OF THE GALL-BLADDER AND
    BILE-DUCTS; GENERAL CONSIDERATIONS, ... 256
INDIVIDUAL OPERATIONS ON THE GALL-BLADDER AND THE CYSTIC
    DUCT, ... 262
OPERATIONS ON THE COMMON DUCT, ... 271
OPERATIONS ON THE HEPATIC DUCT, ... 275
OPERATIONS ON THE INTRAHEPATIC BILE-DUCTS, ... 275
AFTER-TREATMENT FOLLOWING THE DIFFERENT OPERATIONS UPON
    THE GALL-BLADDER AND BILE-DUCTS, ... 276
TREATMENT OF THE SEQUELÆ AND COMPLICATIONS, ... 277

Surgical Diseases, Wounds, and Malformations of the Urinary Bladder PAGE
and the Prostate, ... 279

I. ANATOMY AND PATHOLOGY OF THE URINARY BLADDER, .   .   . 279
II. OPERATIONS ON THE URINARY BLADDER, ... 321
III. ANATOMY AND PATHOLOGY OF THE PROSTATE, ... 337
IV. OPERATIONS ON THE PROSTATE, ... 370

Surgery of the Ovaries and Fallopian Tubes, ... 391

CONGENITAL ANOMALIES, ... 397
DISPLACEMENTS, ... 398
CIRCULATORY DISTURBANCES, ... 401
ATROPHY AND HYPERTROPHY OF THE OVARY, ... 401
RETENTION CYSTS OF THE OVARY, ... 402
PELVIC INFECTION, ... 403
TUBERCULOSIS OF THE TUBE AND OVARY, ... 420
OVARIAN NEOPLASMS, ... 422
PAROVARIAN CYSTS, ... 429
NEOPLASMS OF THE FALLOPIAN TUBE, ... 443

Surgery of the Uterus and its Ligaments, ... 444

I. MALFORMATIONS OF THE UTERUS, ... 444
II. DISPLACEMENTS OF THE UTERUS, ... 454
III. PROLAPSUS UTERI (PROCIDENTIA), ... 487
IV. INVERSION OF THE UTERUS, ... 510
V. FIBROIDS OF THE UTERUS, ... 515
VI. CARCINOMA OF THE UTERUS, ... 581
VII. OPERATIONS FOR UTERINE CANCER, ... 610
VIII. OTHER OPERATIONS FOR CANCER OF THE UTERUS,   .   .   . 645
IX. PALLIATIVE TREATMENT OF UTERINE CANCER; TREATMENT OF
RECURRENCES FOLLOWING OPERATON; GENERAL MEASURES
TO BE EMPLOYED IN CASES OF UTERINE CANCER, .   .   . 657
X. FURTHER DETAILS REGARDING UTERINE NEW-GROWTHS,   .   . 663
XI. METHOD OF COMPARING THE RESULTS OF OPERATIONS FOR
UTERINE CANCER, ... 678
XII. RESULTS OF RADICAL OPERATIONS UPON THE UTERUS,   .   . 683

Extra-Uterine Pregnancy, ... 690

The Cæsarean Section and its Substitutes, ... 701

PART XVII.

THE LAW IN ITS RELATIONS TO THE PRACTICE OF SURGERY.

The Civil Obligation of Surgeon and Patient in the Practice of American   PAGE
Surgery, ... 713
    I. THE CIVIL OBLIGATION, ... 713
   II. DEFINITION OF "SURGEON" AND THE "PRACTICE OF SURGERY," 715
  III. THE RELATION OF SURGEON AND PATIENT MUST EXIST TO CON-
        STITUTE THE OBLIGATION, ... 716
  IV. THE CIVIL OBLIGATION A CONTRACT, ... 721
   V. THE OBLIGATION OF SURGEON TO PATIENT, ... 723
  VI. THE OBLIGATION OF PATIENT TO SURGEON, ... 732
 VII. THE RECOGNIZED LEGAL REQUIREMENTS OF THE SURGEON, . 736
VIII. CONSENT TO SURGICAL OPERATIONS, ... 743
  IX. CONSENT TO USE OF ANÆSTHETICS AND TO MAKING AUTOPSIES, 753
   X. VIOLATION OF THE CIVIL OBLIGATION BY THE SURGEON CON-
        STITUTES MALPRACTICE, ... 756
  XI. ORDINARY PROCEDURE IN ACTIONS FOR MALPRACTICE, . . 765
 XII. THE SURGEON AS A WITNESS, ... 770
XIII. COMPULSORY PHYSICAL EXAMINATION OF PLAINTIFF, . . 779
XIV. ADMISSIBILITY IN EVIDENCE OF PICTURES, HOSPITAL RECORDS,
        AND SURGICAL TREATISES, ... 783
 XV. EXHIBITIONS IN EVIDENCE BEFORE JURIES, ... 790
XVI. WHAT CONSTITUTES PRIVILEGED COMMUNICATIONS, . . 795
XVII. WAIVER OF PRIVILEGE, ... 798
XVIII. THE AWARD OF DAMAGES, ... 807
XIX. EXPLANATORY REMARK; ATTITUDE OF THE COURTS; CONCLUDING
        SUGGESTIONS, ... 816

PART XVIII.

ADMINISTRATIVE SURGICAL WORK.

Hospitals and Hospital Management, More Particularly with Reference
    to the Surgical Needs of these Institutions, ... 823
  INTRODUCTORY REMARKS, ... 823
  THE MODERN METROPOLITAN HOSPITAL, ... 830
  THE PROPER LOCATION FOR A HOSPITAL, ... 835
  THE HOSPITAL UNIT, ... 840
  LIGHT, ... 850
  WINDOW SHADES, SCREENS, ETC., ... 853
  HEATING AND VENTILATING, ... 855
  THE ADMINISTRATION BUILDING, ... 861
  THE RECEIVING WARD, ... 863

Hospitals and Hospital Management, More Particularly with Reference
to the Surgical Needs of these Institutions (*Continued*).   PAGE

THE SURGICAL PAVILION, ... 867
THE MEDICAL PAVILION, ... 872
MEDICAL PHOTOGRAPHY, ... 876
THE ROENTGEN-RAY DEPARTMENT, ... 878
CHAPEL, MORGUE, AND PATHOLOGICAL LABORATORIES, . . . 879
THE KITCHEN AND SERVICE BUILDING, ... 881
THE MANAGEMENT OF HOSPITALS, ... 881
THE ORGANIZATION OF THE MEDICAL AND SURGICAL STAFF, . . 886
THE NURSING DEPARTMENT, ... 889
SPECIAL HOSPITALS, ... 893

Military Surgery, ... 895

ORGANIZATION OF THE LAND FORCES OF THE UNITED STATES, . 896
REWARDS IN THE ARMY MEDICAL SERVICE; PAY, ALLOWANCES, AND
PROMOTION, ... 905
DUTIES OF THE MEDICAL DEPARTMENT, ... 913
SUPPLIES, ... 922
ORGANIZATION IN TIME OF WAR, ... 923
HOME TERRITORY, ... 932
FIELD ARMY, ... 940
ADMINISTRATION OF THE MEDICAL DEPARTMENT, ... 944

Naval Surgery, ... 970

DUTIES OF MEDICAL CORPS, ... 970
ACCIDENTS AND WOUNDS IN TIME OF PEACE, ... 972
WOUNDS BY BITES AND STINGS, ... 974
SCALDS, ... 975
IRRESPIRABLE GASES, ... 976
ASPHYXIATION, ... 978
DAMAGE DONE TO THE EARS, ... 979
SPACE ALLOTTED THE MEDICAL DEPARTMENT ON A BATTLESHIP, . 981
ANÆSTHETICS, ... 984
GENERAL SURGICAL TECHNIQUE, ... 985
DUTIES OF THE MEDICAL CORPS WITH REFERENCE TO BATTLE, . 986
WOUNDS OF NAVAL WARFARE, ... 1013
HOSPITAL SHIPS, ... 1020
LANDING PARTIES, ... 1028

Administrative Railroad Surgery, ... 1030

INTRODUCTORY REMARKS, ... 1030
HISTORICAL NOTICE, ... 1031
ORGANIZATION OF THE RELIEF WORK, ... 1032
PERSONNEL OF A RAILROAD MEDICAL ORGANIZATION, . . . 1038
FIRST-AID AND EQUIPMENT, ... 1040

Administrative Railroad Surgery (*Continued*).

PAGE

THE HOSPITAL CAR, ... 1046
AMERICAN METHODS OF PROVIDING RELIEF FOR THE DIFFERENT
    KINDS OF RAILROAD INJURIES, ... 1047
THE CARE OF MEN ENGAGED IN RAILROAD CONSTRUCTION WORK, . 1052
THE MEDICAL CHEST, ... 1056
LEGISLATION, ... 1057
PHYSICAL EXAMINATION OF EMPLOYEES, ... 1057
MEDICO-LEGAL QUESTIONS, ... 1058
STATISTICS, ... 1059
RAILROAD SURGICAL ASSOCIATIONS, ... 1060
BIBLIOGRAPHY, ... 1060

APPENDIX

The Relation of Blood-Pressure to Surgery, ... 1063

General Index to Volumes I.-VIII., ... 1083

PART XVI.

REGIONAL SURGERY.
(Continued.)

INTRATHORACIC SURGERY.*

(Heart and Œsophagus Excluded.)

By *JOSEPH RANSOHOFF, M.D., F.R.C.S., and J. LOUIS RANSOHOFF,*
M.D., Cincinnati, Ohio.

I. SURGICAL DISEASES OF THE PLEURA.

Pneumothorax.—Pleural cavities, in the true sense of the word, do not exist under normal conditions. With the exception of residual spaces at each base, the lungs entirely fill the pleural sacs. It is only when the space is distended by air or fluid that a true pleural cavity exists. In the pleural space there exists at all times a negative pressure. An opening into this space, either from within or from without, gives rise to pneumothorax, the air entering under pressure. Pneumothorax is, as a rule, due to a penetrating wound of the thoracic wall caused either by a bullet or by a knife wound. In some cases pneumothorax results from a fracture of the ribs, which, by producing a penetrating wound of the lung, allows the air to enter from within, or, through an injury of the thoracic wall, permits it to enter from without. Pneumothorax may also be caused by a rupture of an abscess of the lung, or by a tuberculous or bronchiectatic cavity. In this class of cases the pneumothorax is of a very high grade, as the large amount of air forced into the pleural cavity causes an immediate collapse of the lung and gives rise to a complete pneumothorax. Cases of this nature, unless infection occurs, are amenable only to medical treatment.

The extent and rapidity of development of pneumothorax depend upon the size of the opening. When the aperture is large, the air rushes in with great velocity, the lung collapses, and a complete pneumothorax results. If the opening is smaller, the air enters but slowly and a part of it is forced out with each inspiration, as the lung, not being completely collapsed, still functionates. In case the perforation is small and runs in an oblique direction, a valve-like disposition of the soft tissues may take place and the further entrance of air thus be prevented.

In the more severe cases of pneumothorax, an effusion of blood takes place into the pleural cavity as a result of the injury of the thoracic wall or of the lung, and there is produced a hæmopneumothorax. Then if, in addition, infection occurs and pus forms, a pyopneumothorax is developed. In cases of severe pneumothorax, the distention of the thorax is extreme. The intercostal spaces

---

* This article belongs more appropriately in the early part of the preceding volume, but, as the authors were unexpectedly prevented from finishing their work at the time when the printers reached that point, it was thought advisable to transfer the article to its present position.— The Editors.

may protrude beyond the plane of the ribs, the diaphragm is forced down to a low level and is perhaps immobile, the heart and large vessels are forced over to the opposite side of the thorax. These severe cases may result from the rupture of a tuberculous or bronchiectatic cavity. With each inspiration a comparatively large amount of air in the cavity is forced into the pleural sac, and, should a valve-like disposition of the walls of the cavity prevent its return, air under great pressure may be present in the pleural cavity.

SYMPTOMS AND PROGNOSIS.—The symptoms and prognosis of pneumothorax depend largely on the presence or absence of infection, on the degree of its virulence when it is present, and on the complications. In slight cases there are practically no symptoms, and the patient recovers rapidly, as the air is promptly absorbed. In one of the author's cases, for example, an extensive unilateral pneumothorax was completely absorbed in forty-eight hours. In strong contrast with this are the cases in which a complete one-sided pneumothorax develops rapidly and perhaps produces prompt death. Such cases of death are due, it is thought by some, to an inhibition of the heart's action from excessive irritation of the vagus terminals in the pleural membrane. The heart's action is rapid, irregular, and weak, and the blood-pressure is low; the heart itself is displaced to the opposite side and its action is thereby further impeded. Respiration is seriously embarrassed, being rapid and shallow. Physical examination shows a marked tympany of the entire side. The lung, as it lies collapsed in the costovertebral groove, manifests no vesicular evidences whatever of its presence. In case infection occurs at a later stage, which is likely, symptoms of sepsis are added to the above-described symptom-complex. If effusion complicates pneumothorax, succussion sounds may be heard.

Pneumothorax due to the rupture of the wall of a cavity, tuberculous or otherwise, is usually ushered in by a sharp pain at the seat of rupture following a severe paroxysm of coughing. Collapse may take place, and, in many cases, for self-evident reasons, infection occurs. An x-ray examination, in these cases, is very instructive. (Fig. 1.) It shows the absence of the lung shadow in its usual position and the displacement of the organs of the mediastinum. It may also very clearly show the low level of the diaphragm and the displacement of the liver or spleen.

The very severe cases are often promptly fatal. If the immediate outcome is not bad, the patient has a good chance of recovery, provided infection does not occur and causal complications do not forbid.

Bilateral pneumothorax caused by a transverse gunshot wound of the thorax is nearly always immediately fatal. The mild cases usually recover unless accompanied by severe symptoms, so that the prognosis depends in great measure upon the agent that causes the pneumothorax. (Vide article on "Gunshot Wounds," Vol. II., page 719.)

TREATMENT.—The wound must, of course, be treated aseptically and made surgically clean. Antiseptics should not be used except externally, as they cause increased irritation of the exposed pleural surfaces and sometimes induce severe coughing. The wound should be sealed to prevent the further entrance of air and a large sterile dressing should be applied. If the enclosed air is not quickly absorbed, it may be aspirated. The lung promptly expands when the air is removed. Rehn has made very exhaustive researches into the causes of disturbances in respiration and circulation due to pneumothorax. He claims that the chief danger is due to displacement of the bronchi of the sound lung. The pulmonary ligament which extends from the hilus of the lung to the diaphragm is placed on a stretch and the bronchial veins and arteries are further displaced. These displacements and the bending of the arteries and bronchi result in a diminished supply of both air and blood to the sound lung. He suggests, as a de-

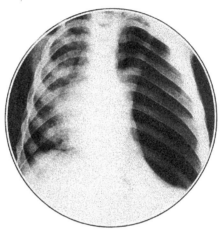

Fig. 1.—Radiogram Showing Complete Left Pneumothorax. Diaphragm concave; the septum is pushed to the right side. (From the x-Ray Laboratory of the Cincinnati Hospital.)

sirable therapeutic measure, the placing of the patient on the afflicted side, so that the bending of the arteries and bronchi may be relieved or lessened by the weight of the collapsed lung.

Hydrothorax, the effusion of clear fluid into the pleural spaces, is not of course due to inflammation. It occurs in the course of the general anasarca incident to the terminal stages of heart and kidney affections. If it is so excessive as to interfere with respiration, the fluid should be aspirated.

Pleurisy with Effusion.—A clear serous effusion into the pleural cavity is often the first stage of an empyema. It may be due to one of many causes. In some cases it is of undoubted tuberculous origin, although the tubercle bacillus can rarely be found in the exudate. Inoculation experiments, however, frequently show the tuberculous nature of the infection. It may also be metapneumonic, particularly in children. These cases are very prone to run by gradual stages into an empyema. The pneumococcus is usually the offending micro-organism. Pleurisy with effusion occurs, in some cases, in the course of acute articular rheumatism, or it may occur in the course of any of the acute infections. The cases in which the pleurisy follows one of the acute infections are the ones which most often terminate in empyema. In many instances it is impossible to determine the etiological factor. It seems as though, in a certain percentage of cases, cold and exposure are predisposing causes. These cases most frequently turn out in the end to be of tuberculous origin.

An effusion that takes place in an adult, without apparent cause, and without acute symptoms, should always be suspected as having a tuberculous origin. In the recognition of tuberculous pleurisy with effusion cyto-diagnosis deserves a foremost place. Musgrave analyzed seventy-two cases at the Massachusetts General Hospital and corroborated the rules formulated by Widal, viz.:—

1. A predominance of lymphocytes in the effusion indicates an early stage of pulmonary tuberculosis.

2. Predominance of polymorphonuclear cells indicates an acute inflammatory process.

3. A large number of endothelial cells occurring in sheets or plaques means mechanical effusion or a transudate.

PATHOLOGY AND PROGNOSIS.—In the simple cases the prognosis is mostly favorable, the effusion being spontaneously absorbed or the condition being entirely cured by a single tapping. Serous effusions due to the pneumococcus or the pyogenic cocci are merely preliminary stages of an empyema. An examination of the pathological conditions in these cases shows an acute inflammation of the pleural surfaces, the blood-vessels being injected and the surfaces more or less covered with plastic lymph. The fluid contains fibrin flakes in greater or less quantity. The microscopic examination of the fluid shows the presence of fibrin and of numerous leucocytes. As the process gradually merges into empyema, the lymphocytes and pus corpuscles become more numerous. The lung is, of course, more or less collapsed in accordance with the amount of the fluid.

TREATMENT.—The treatment may be either medical or surgical. Effusions of moderate degree may undergo absorption without surgical intervention. But if, after a reasonable attempt has been made to secure absorption, the fluid remains, aspiration is urgently indicated. It is particularly important, in cases in which the effusion has taken place after an attack of pneumonia, that aspiration be resorted to promptly, for the fluid, if allowed to remain, nearly always becomes purulent. When the exudate has reached such a bulk as seriously to hamper the respiration and the heart's action, immediate aspiration is indicated.

Empyema.—Empyema, or the accumulation of pus in the pleural cavity, very often constitutes a later stage in the course of pleurisy with effusion. Transition forms, between the simple clear effusion and one containing fetid pus, are occasionally met with. Empyema occurring as a primary affection, without the preceding serous effusion, is observed only when an abscess ruptures into the pleura or in the presence of pyæmia. This abscess may be either an abscess of the lung, or an abscess of the bronchiectatic variety, or a subphrenic abscess. An abscess of the liver, or even one of the kidney or the spleen, may rupture into the pleura. A primary empyema may also be due to rupture of a caseous lymph node or to an ulcerative process in connection with a carcinoma of the œsophagus. Then, again, in certain cases it may be due to penetrating injuries of the thoracic wall. The majority of empyemata are metapneumonic. According to Bergeat fifty per cent of all empyemata are of this character; of Morrison's one hundred cases, ninety-one were of pneumococcus origin. They occur most frequently in children. The pneumococcus is the offending micro-organism. The prognosis in these metapneumonic empyemata is usually favorable, if the pus is promptly evacuated and drainage instituted.

The septic empyemata due to the streptococcus and staphylococcus, constitute another class of cases of empyema. They are very malignant and demand active and radical therapy. The disease occurs most frequently during the course of one of the acute infections, particularly scarlet fever. At times a secondary infection of the pus with saprophytic bacteria occurs, making the prognosis all the more grave. In those cases in which empyema complicates subdiaphragmatic abscess, one may expect to find the colon bacillus in the pus, which in that event gives forth the characteristic odor of the germ. In some few cases the amœba of dysentery is found in empyemata secondary to liver abscess.

The tuberculous form of empyema has special characteristics. The effusion, for example, is often hemorrhagic, a symptom common to tuberculosis and malignant neoplasms of the pleura. These cases run a typical course. The fluid, at first serous, reaccumulates quickly after each tapping, and in the end becomes purulent. The pleural cavity itself is studded with miliary tubercles and tuberculous caseous foci. The adhesions and the thickening of the pleura are excessive. The process is of a progressive nature, and, unless surgical intervention is instituted, the patient nearly always succumbs. Even after a radical operation the outcome is, naturally, often fatal. In case the adhesions are dense, there will probably be formed a limited empyema which is often very difficult to diagnosticate and to locate.

SYMPTOMATOLOGY.—The symptoms of empyema are those of pleuritic effusion, together with manifestations which point to septic intoxication. These manifestations vary according to the nature of the infecting agent, being most severe in those cases in which the micro-organisms belong to one of the virulently septic varieties. In such cases the prostration is great. The signs common to pleural effusion are absolute flatness on percussion and absence of vocal and tactile fremitus and of the breath sounds. The diaphragm assumes a low level and is immobile, and the mediastinal organs are displaced to the opposite side. Unless the pus is evacuated, the patient, as a rule, succumbs. There are two ways, however, in which spontaneous recovery may take place; but both of them are uncommon. The pus may burrow to the outside, form a subcutaneous abscess, and rupture. This is called *empyema necessitatis* and is more common in children. The other form is the rupture into a bronchus and the discharge of pus through the bronchial tree. This rarely has a favorable outcome, as the prostration from the violent coughing is very great and a secondary aspiration pneumonia may prove fatal. However, in a certain number of cases, recovery has taken place in this manner. In another class of cases the accumulation of pus becomes encapsulated and the fluid absorbed, leaving merely a mass of cheesy material which may in time lose its virulence. This is, nevertheless, a comparatively unfavorable outcome, as the patient is never fully restored to health. The longer the pus accumulation is allowed to remain *in situ*, the more remote are the chances of permanent recovery. The lung, which was at the beginning merely collapsed, loses its expansile powers by reason of adhesions, and even if the fluid has been evacuated, the lung cannot expand. Both the parietal and the visceral layers of the pleura become tremendously thickened, so that the lung is bound by firm bands to the costo-vertebral gutter. The

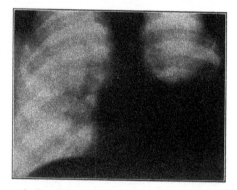

Fig. 2.—Radiogram of a Case of Empyema of the Left Side. Note the concave border. (From the x-Ray Laboratory of the Jewish Hospital, Cincinnati, Ohio.)

pleura forms a dense mass of elastic tissue, tough and resistant, which the Germans call "die Schwarte." It is these old-standing cases which are so difficult to bring to a successful termination. Even in recent cases of empyema, the purulent effusion is, technically speaking, encapsulated, since the parietal and visceral layers of the pleura are adherent along the limits of the pus-containing cavity. This is of importance, since, as Koenig first pointed out, it is impossible, either by aspiration or by open incision, to produce a complete collapse of the lung and consequent pneumothorax.

DIAGNOSIS.—The diagnosis of empyema is made by means of the physical signs, and must be substantiated by aspiration. There are some cases in which the fluid may be a trifle cloudy and, on examination, show many leucocytes. Shall these be considered as cases of empyema? It is well to consider them as ordinary serous effusions and give them an opportunity to recover with the aid of simple aspiration. In most cases, however, where the physical signs are associated with the systemic indications of sepsis (namely, high temperature and leucocytosis), the exploratory aspiration will reveal a creamy pus laden with virulent bacteria which vary according to the etiology, since empyema is practically never, except as a result of injury, a primary disease. In old-standing cases the pus may be sterile. In cases of lobar pneumonia, when, after the crisis, the temperature runs an irregular course and the symptoms of sepsis continue, empyema should always be suspected. The x-ray picture will, in many instances, clear up an obscure case, as the accumulation of fluid shows a distinct shadow. In some instances, owing to the fact that cheesy matter fills the abscess cavity, aspiration will fail to withdraw any fluid. It is in these cases that an x-ray picture is of particular value. (Figs. 2 and 3.)

In a differential diagnosis of the fluid accumulations within the chest, the x-ray is a most valuable adjunct, to be used in corroborating the results obtained by physical examination. The certainty with which, for example, an empyema

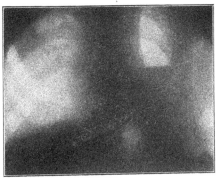

Fig. 3.—Radiogram of a Case of Pyopneumothorax, on the Left Side. (From the x-Ray Laboratory of the Cincinnati Hospital.)

can by this means be distinguished from a hydropericardium is shown by the comparison of radiograms of these two conditions. (Figs. 2 and 4.)

At the time of aspiration an etiological diagnosis should be made in every case by culture or by inoculation experiments, as the treatment may depend in a large measure on the nature of the infecting agent. In some instances it is particularly difficult to differentiate empyema from subphrenic abscess. The history of the case is, of course, valuable. In empyema the upper border of the fluid assumes a concave level, with the concavity upward, while in subphrenic abscess the border is convex. X-ray pictures are particularly valuable in this class of cases. Whenever there is a possible doubt as to the diagnosis, aspiration should always be practised.

TREATMENT.—The treatment, in every case of empyema, is early evacuation of the pus. The more desperate the case the more positive the indications. In cases apparently moribund, the patient must be given a chance and it is surprising to see how often these desperate cases do well after free drainage is instituted. The usual case demands a partial resection of one or more ribs. Simple thoracotomy does not give adequate drainage, as the space between the ribs is too small to admit an adequately large drainage tube. Contrary to the experience of most surgeons, Farquharson advises simple thoracotomy, and reports a series of cases successfully treated in this way. There is one class of cases in which simple thoracotomy, or, at times, even simple aspiration, may suffice; that is, cases of early metapneumonic empyema in children, in which cases aspiration may at least be tried once. (A valuable method of continuous drainage, recently devised by Thiersch, will be described farther on—see page 49.)

Injections of various antiseptics into the pleural cavity, after aspiration, have been repeatedly tried and given up. Murphy has recently recorded some excellent results from the injection of two-per-cent formalin, in glycerin, after

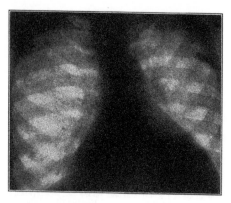

FIG. 4.—Radiogram of a Case of Hydropericardium. Note the clean outline of the shadow.
(From the x-Ray Laboratory of the Cincinnati Hospital.)

preliminary aspiration. It is to be hoped that this treatment will be successful, for, whereas it is an easy matter to open the chest, it is often very difficult to obliterate the cavity and so to cause the opening to close.

The incision into the pleura is followed by the insertion of a double-barrelled drainage tube of quite large calibre. It should be retained only as long as it may be required for the drainage and closure of the cavity. In some instances, especially in children, and when the affection is of an acute character, a prompt cure follows operation—as, for example, after one or two dressings. If retained for too long a time the tubes cause discharge and hinder a cure. In fact, they may have to be retained to eliminate the products which they themselves cause. They should be gradually shortened as the cavity fills up. As the opening has a tendency to close before full pulmonary expansion has taken place, recurrence of the empyema often happens unless this precaution is taken. In place of the tube a double-flanged hard-rubber tunnelled button has been devised by Wilson. In the experience of the writer it offers no advantage over the tube.

The after-treatment is simple. Except in cases of very foul pus, irrigation is contra-indicated, as it interferes with the expansion of the lung and may, by irritation of the pleura, cause paroxysmal coughing. Cases of sudden death have occurred from shock following extensive irrigation of the pleural cavities. The expansion of the lung takes place very promptly in early cases and occurs spontaneously. When the expansion does not take place promptly it must be encouraged by breathing exercises, by calisthenics, or by blowing into Woulfe's bottles. (See p. 52.) Aspiration of the air of the empyema cavity by means of a funnel placed over the opening and connected with an aspirator, or preferably by means of a large Bier vacuum cup, has a distinct tendency to cause the lung to expand by direct suction. The aspiration apparatus of Bryant (J. D.) * is simple and effective, bringing about a cure in from six to eight weeks, and lessening the duration of the treatment "at least one-third." (Abbe.)

It should be remembered that in cases of empyema, particularly in young individuals, there is subsequently a marked tendency to lateral curvature of the spine. As soon as the general condition of the patient permits, the deformity should be corrected by properly devised orthopedic exercises. In cases where the services of a well-equipped orthopedic establishment are not available, good results may be obtained by having the patient swing from a horizontal bar or preferably from hanging rings. The earlier the deformity is taken in hand, the greater is the probability that a complete correction of the deformity will be secured.

Decortication.—In old-standing cases—often called *empyema inveterata*—both the parietal and the visceral layers of the pleura become so thick that the cavity cannot fill up, and consequently the pus, however thoroughly evacuated, reaccumulates. Strange as it may seem, patients with large unopened empyemas may go about for a long time in comparative comfort. As a rule, however, they show evidence of chronic sepsis which, if unrelieved by operation, is likely to prove fatal within a year or two. In these chronic cases special operations must be devised to cure the condition. Until 1877 these cases were considered absolutely hopeless. At that time, after the introduction of the operation of multiple rib resections by Estlander, the ideas with regard to the curability of chronic empyema underwent a radical change. The various modifications of thoracoplasty by Schede, Quénu, and Jaboulay served only to make the mobilization of the chest wall more complete and less hazardous, and the contact of the flap with the retracted lung more extensive. These operations were all based on the erroneous idea of the permanent disability of the lung bound down by adhesions to expand. In 1893 Fowler and Delorme elucidated a new fact regarding the functional value of lung tissue long bound down by fibrous adhesions. It was that the power of expansion is not lost, and that, if freed from its fetters, the lung would again expand and functionate. The true originator of this idea was probably Cornil, though the first cases were published by Fowler and Delorme. The fundamental idea of the operation is the thorough freeing of the lung from the adhesions which bind it to the vertebral column. The

* Transactions of the American Surgical Association, vol. xiv., 1906, and Surgery, Gynæcology, and Obstetrics, 1908, vi., 179–188.

tremendously thickened pleura which the Germans call "Schwarte," must be dissected from the entire surface of. the lung. This is called "decortication." This must, of course, be preceded by a complete thoracoplasty after the manner of Estlander or Schede. All thickened pleural scar tissue must be carefully dissected away. A particular feature of the operation, which must not be neglected, is an incision cautiously carried through the length of the groove or angle of reflexion of the costal and pulmonary layers of the pleura. If the incision is limited to the costal part of the angle and carried downward toward the chest wall, there is no danger of wounding large vessels or of opening the sound pleura. It may be necessary to repeat these operations many times before a thorough cure is effected. However, with patience a successful termination may be expected in the majority of cases.

While, in children, empyemata as a rule heal promptly after simple opera-

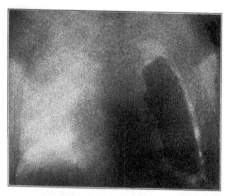

Fɪɢ. 5.—Radiogram of a Large Empyema after the Cavity had been Filled with Thirty-three-percent Bismuth Paste. (From the x-Ray Laboratory of the Jewish Hospital of Cincinnati, Ohio.)

tions, in older subjects and particularly in cases due to tuberculosis, there is often a tendency toward chronicity of the process. Fistulæ connected with a large suppurating empyema cavity continue to discharge for months and even years, with little tendency to heal. To prevent this, Beck has instituted the practice of injecting a subnitrate ·of bismuth vaseline paste (thirty-three per cent). From 120 to 800 grammes of the mixture may be used and the injections repeated as often as may be necessary. (Fig. 5.) Many successful cases have been recorded by a number of American and foreign surgeons,— cases in which the external wound healed promptly, after even a single injection. Many cases have likewise been reported in which closure was effected after thoracoplasty had failed. Nemanoff thus reports four cases from Katjari's clinic at St. Petersburg, in which one injection was sufficient in each case to effect a closure, whereas the same patients had been treated at the clinic for six months without success. Ochsner reported fourteen cases to the American

Surgical Association in 1909, in all of which operation had been performed without success. In twelve cases the wound healed completely.

Discission.—In 1903 the author published a new feature in these operations. It is evident that the hemorrhage and shock following a thorough decortication of the lung are of a serious character, and that the dissection of the thickened pleura is a tedious and hazardous undertaking. In considering how these drawbacks might be overcome the author observed that an incision carried through the thickened pleura until the lung tissue is reached, widens out rapidly; this widening continuing with each inspiration until the cut becomes a broad groove. This widening is due to the expansion of the lung and the tendency inherent in divided scar tissue to retract. Where one incision, carried to the lung tissue, widens into a groove, so will a second and a third and as many more

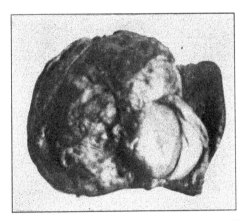

Fɪɢ. 6.—Photograph of an Endothelioma which Appeared in the Form of a Mediastinal Tumor. In size it was as large as the head of an adult. A radiogram of this tumor, taken during the patient's lifetime, is shown in Fig. 7.

as may be made. Acting upon these data the author devised what he calls discission of the pulmonary pleura as a substitute for the operation of decortication. The special feature consists of gridironing the pulmonary pleura with parallel and cross incisions made at distances of about a quarter of an inch the one from the other. Little islands of thickened pleura are thus left on the surface of the expanding lung. Even during the course of the operation great expansion of the lung is noticeable. The fundamental idea of the operation is to carry each cut completely through the thickened pleura.

Neoplasms of the Pleura.—The neoplasms of the pleural cavity are, in the majority of cases, secondary; either coming through metastasis or spreading through the thoracic wall. The most frequent of the latter are carcinomata, which spread, through direct progression, from the breast. In the majority of these cases the new-growth develops in the scar, as a recurrence, after the removal of the primary growth. Such recurrent growths are rarely amenable to surgical intervention. Sauerbruch, however, since the perfection of his chamber, has operated on several of these cases, but without results which warrant the general adoption of the operation.

Both carcinoma and sarcoma are observed in the pleura, their appearance here being secondary to metastatic growths of the lung from neoplasms in other regions of the body (notably the long bones and the kidney). The only primary neoplasm which is seen in the pleura with any frequency is endothelioma. This form of tumor was first described by E. Wagner. Lenhartz and Lochte have collected eighteen cases. The tumor begins as a diffuse thickening of the pleura which grows with great rapidity. When the endothelioma springs from the mediastinal pleura the tumor assumes the form and produces the

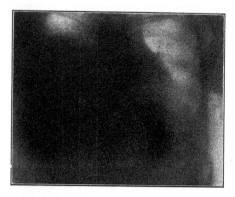

Fig. 7.—Radiogram of an Endothelioma of the Mediastinum. Only the apex of the right lung is visible; the left lung is less compressed. The patient was a woman forty years old. At the postmortem examination the superior vena cava was found to be completely occluded. The gross specimen, much reduced in size, is shown in Fig. 6. (From the x-Ray Laboratory of the Jewish Hospital of Cincinnati.)

symptoms of a mediastinal tumor. These tumors often grow to enormous size, filling one side of the chest and even encroaching on and compressing the other lung and the great vessels. (Figs. 6 and 7.) The breathing sounds, when the lung is thus compressed, entirely disappear. An exudation of fluid accompanies the process in every case, so that it is with difficulty that a diagnosis can be made. On tapping, the fluid is nearly always found to be blood-stained, and some small pieces of the tumor may come away. Here it may be well to state that a blood-stained fluid obtained by aspiration invariably indicates either tuberculosis or the presence of a malignant neoplasm. The diagnosis can partially be made by the rapid development of the process and the extreme cachexia—phenomena which are associated with very little if any fever. Of course, there is no leucocytosis, and this also helps in arriving at a diagnosis. The therapy is merely palliative, as no operative procedures are in order.

If the accumulation of fluid causes severe symptoms, tapping may be instituted as often as necessary.

Echinococcus of the Pleura.—Echinococcus of the pleura, even in localities where echinococcus is frequently observed, is seldom seen as a primary affection of the pleura. It may be secondary to echinococcus disease of either the liver or the lung. In the course of its growth, the echinococcus cyst compresses the lung, displaces the heart, and may even, in some instances, by causing absorption of the chest wall, reach the integument in its onward growth. The symptoms are those of a pleural tumor, as the disease runs its course without fever. The signs are usually those of circumscribed pleural effusion. On tapping, the characteristic fluid containing hooklets is obtained, and the diagnosis is easily

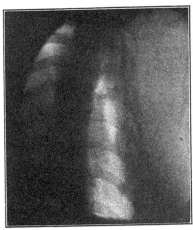

Fig. 8.—Radiogram of an Enormous Hæmangioma (Congenital) of the Chest Wall. The picture shows indentation of all the costal arches on that side. Death resulted from an escape of the tumor contents into the pleura. (From the x-Ray Laboratory of the Jewish Hospital of Cincinnati.)

made. The fluid contains no albumen, this fact distinguishing it from ordinary pleuritic effusions. The prognosis of pleural echinococcus is very unfavorable, a few recoveries having followed the emptying of the cyst through the bronchi or through an ulceration of the overlying integument. The treatment consists in aspiration, which, as in echinococcus cysts elsewhere, is occasionally followed by recovery. Injection of iodine and silver-nitrate preparations is often followed by recovery. In most cases, however, a recovery cannot be achieved without thoracotomy (with or without rib resection), which will permit the thorough evacuation of the fluid and the daughter cysts. The cyst wall should be treated with silver-nitrate solution.

Tumors of the ribs and costal cartilages and at times even of the overlying soft parts of the chest wall, by growing inward, involve the pleural cavities, and, by displacing the lung, cause more or less severe symptoms of compression or displacement of the lung. Fig. 8 illustrates this. It is a radiogram from a girl, seventeen years old, with an enormous congenital hæmangioma. The compression of the ribs and of the entire chest wall is clearly shown. The tumor extended over the whole left side of the chest, from the diaphragm quite to the axilla. Death resulted from rupture into the pleura.

II. WOUNDS OF THE THORACIC CAVITY AND ITS CONTENTS.

Wounds of the thoracic cavity and its contained structures form one of the interesting chapters of military and civil surgery. The injuries due to penetrating bullet wounds are particularly instructive. (See also Vol. II., p. 719.) The observations made during the Boer, Spanish-American, and Japanese wars have revolutionized the prevailing ideas with regard to the symptoms, gravity, and treatment of these injuries. This is largely if not entirely due to changes in the form and nature of the projectiles used. The wounds formerly seen were made by the soft lead bullet at comparatively close range. These terrible wounds were of common occurrence in the Civil and Franco-Prussian wars. The soft bullets flattened at the moment of impact and were deformed by any resisting tissue encountered. These flattened and deformed bullets often tore tremendous holes in the thorax, splintering the ribs, carrying fragments of bone with them into the chest cavity, and causing multiple injuries of the heart, lungs, and the mediastinal structures. These soft bullets literally tore and lacerated their way through the chest. The destruction of lung tissue was very great and the consequent hemorrhage speedily fatal. Wounds of the heart were practically fatal in every case. In addition, pieces of clothing were frequently carried into the chest cavity, thereby further complicating the condition by the severest forms of infection. This severe form of injury is to-day sometimes seen in civil practice, the result of attempted suicide or of a revolver fight, in which the same sort of soft bullet is used. Still more terrible wounds were made by the dum-dum or mushroom bullet, a steel jacketed bullet with a soft lead nose. This bullet, at the moment of impact, assumes a mushroom shape and is capable of causing enormous tissue destruction. Its use, however, has been interdicted by the International Peace Congress. The arms now in use by the armies of the entire civilized world throw a steel-jacketed missile of high velocity and long range. Its calibre is small. The effect of these projectiles is entirely different from that of the old style. The wounds of ingress and egress are of small size, that of egress being little larger than that of ingress. The velocity and hardness of this missile are such that it is practically never deformed or deflected from its course. Instead of causing comminuted fractures of a rib, the bullet usually bores a clean hole and splinters of bone are not often carried into the lung tissue. The old form of extensive laceration of the lung is not often seen; instead, the bullet bores a perfectly clean, smooth channel through the lung tissue, a channel which tends quickly to fill with blood clot and heal. Owing to the small destruction of lung tissue, the hemorrhage is much less severe and not often fatal, unless the perforation involves the root of the lung.

Another very interesting feature is the fate of the bullet. The old-time bullet usually spent its force in entering the thoracic cavity and often did not have sufficient impetus to regain the outside. The modern high-velocity projectile almost without exception forces its way entirely through the thorax. This, of course, makes a difference in the liability to infection; for the bullet which remains in the thorax is likely to be a carrier of pyogenic organisms.

The track of the bullet may assume any direction—frontal, sagittal, or oblique. Bullet wounds in the long axis of the lung may be seen, the bullet entering the supraclavicular or intraclavicular fossa. This is due to the prone position frequently assumed by the combatants. The symptoms are not at all constant. In many cases the injured soldier does not fall, and may even continue the fight. Occasionally, aside from slight pain and cough, the symptoms are practically nil. These cases are, however, the exception, as the symptoms are usually distressing, perhaps even out of proportion to the damage done. There are usually some dyspnœa and cyanosis. The latter may be absent and is dependent upon the amount of hemorrhage into the pleura and the consequent compression of the lung. In cases of severe hemorrhage the dyspnœa is intense. In these cases the patient is in a state of collapse and displays all the symptoms of severe hemorrhage. These symptoms, however, usually disappear in the course of from ten to fourteen days. Hæmoptysis is not a constant symptom. It appeared in about half of Kuettner's series of cases. This symptom is of little prognostic significance, as it is present in many mild cases and may be absent in the most severe, even the fatal ones. It may be evanescent or may last for several weeks. Hæmothorax is present in practically every case, though it may be of the most varying degree. As a rule, it reaches its height three or four days after the infliction of the injury and is then gradually absorbed. An injudicious movement or rough transportation may, however, cause a renewal of the hemorrhage as late as three weeks after the receipt of the injury. As may be seen, hæmothorax is the most constant complication of injury of the lung.

Pneumothorax, formerly an almost invariable complication of bullet wounds of the chest, was very rare during the late wars. Kuettner saw it only four times. At the moment of injury a variable amount of air escapes from the wounded lung into the pleural cavity. But, owing to the small size of the bullet wound, it is small in amount and soon becomes absorbed. The lung itself does not collapse and still fills the pleural space. The outside wound is usually so small that a valve-like action of the soft parts occurs and effectually prevents the entrance of air from the outside. Emphysema of the subcutaneous tissues is seen in about one-fifth of all cases. It is, however, usually of slight degree and of little clinical significance, except in so far as it aids in pointing conclusively to injury of the lung.

Empyema is one of the rare sequelæ of modern rifle-ball wounds of the lung. It is seen only after great neglect in cases in which operative interference has been attempted. Hernia of the lung is practically an unknown complication.

In some cases the patient is carried off by constantly recurring and increasing hemorrhages, due as a rule to extensive injury of the lung caused by rib splinters. Secondary hemorrhage may occur as late as three or four weeks after the injury. There is always some secondary infiltration of the lung around the bullet channel. This is usually insignificant and causes no symptoms. If excessive, the symptoms may resemble those of pneumonia. A true pneumonia, however, is unknown.

The prognosis of small-calibre rifle-ball wounds of the lung is most favorable. Very few succumb, usually those in whom injuries of the large vessels at or near the root of the lung have occurred. These injuries are nearly always fatal. The treatment should be ultraconservative. The chest should be enveloped in sterile dressings after the site of the injury has been made as aseptic as possible. Morphia should be given to control the restlessness. Aspiration, particularly in military practice, should not be used, as the bleeding quickly recurs; and, besides, there is a great liability to infection. Should empyema occur, free drainage should be promptly instituted. Absolute rest should be strictly enjoined for from four to six weeks after the injury.

The story of bullet wounds of the lung is quite different in civil practice, as the large-calibre, soft-lead bullet is used. In these cases the symptoms are severe, the hemorrhage is great owing to the extensive laceration of the lung, and infection is a common occurrence. The patient is usually brought into the hospital in a state of profound shock, with intense dyspnœa. Pneumothorax of large extent is common. The free air in the pleural cavity may even prove salutary, since, by causing complete collapse of the lung, occlusion of the visceral wound is furthered.

The prognosis of these cases is bad. Of twenty-one cases of gunshot wounds of the lung admitted to the Cincinnati Hospital in the years from 1903 to 1908, fifteen terminated fatally. Of these, many were brought into the institution in a moribund condition. In cases of this nature the treatment should be radical, as the only hope of recovery is in gaining control of the bleeding. This, of course, is best accomplished by an extensive thoracotomy, if possible, under increased pulmonary pressure. The lung should be grasped and drawn into the opening in the thoracic wall and tightly tied. In case one of the large vessels at the base is injured, an attempt should be made to suture it. If this is unsuccessful, the wound should be tamponed. Garre advises closure of the thoracic wound without drainage.

The symptoms of stab wounds of the chest are similar to those of bullet wounds. The prognosis is, however, not so grave, as the amount of tissue destruction is usually not so great. Of eighteen cases admitted to the Cincinnati Hospital during the same period, only five terminated fatally. In stab wounds the liability to infection and consequent empyema is very great. The treatment is the same as that of bullet wounds of the lungs. In the civil injuries of the chest occurring in his service at the Cincinnati Hospital, it has been the practice of the writer, after thorough sterilization of the wound, to seal it hermetically and then to immobilize the injured side as far as possible by strapping; thus decreasing the probability of further hemorrhage. In stab wounds, when the hemorrhage is profuse, thoracotomy should be made with a view to suturing or ligating the wounded lung. While sutures of the lung easily tear through the fragile tissue, little pressure is necessary to stop the bleeding. It must always be borne in mind that the blood pressure in the vessels of the lung is only one-third of that of the general circulation.

III. ABSCESS AND GANGRENE OF THE LUNG.

Abscess and gangrene of the lung are comparatively infrequent affections. Although considered by most authors as distinctly separate conditions, the separation of these diseases seems entirely artificial. The occurrence of acute abscess cavities in the lung is due in all cases to the destruction of tissue. If this leads to the formation of larger sequestra, a gangrene results; but if the tissue is destroyed in small particles, we have an abscess. This seems to be the only difference. Both Korte and Lenhartz hold this view. Abscess and gangrene of the lung occur, in by far the greater majority of cases, in males during middle life. This is perhaps due to their more irregular habits of life, their over-indulgence in alcohol, and their greater liability to exposure and consequent infection. The greater number of cases seem to follow pneumonia, either lobar or lobular; more frequently the latter. Of forty-nine cases reported by Tuffier, twenty-five complicated a pre-existing pneumonia. In some cases the abscess undoubtedly occurs as an acute secondary affection engrafted on a previously existing tuberculous cavity. A secondary form of abscess or of gangrene is that due to the rupture of an old bronchiectatic cavity. Abscesses due to aspiration into the bronchus or to the entrance of a foreign body are not so common as in former years. This is due to the perfection of bronchoscopic technique by Killian and Jackson, and to the power, which we now possess, to localize such bodies by aid of the x-ray. In this way foreign bodies are removed from the lower air passages before infection has a chance to occur. Even after foreign bodies are coughed up or removed, the abscess may persist. In one case, operated upon with recovery, the abscess persisted for four months after a peanut shell, which had caused it, had been expectorated.

Abscesses and gangrene of the lung are most apt to follow pneumonia in run-down and debilitated subjects and victims of Bright's disease, chronic alcoholism, and particularly diabetes. It seems that the more debilitated the subject, the greater the predisposition to gangrene and the less the likelihood of abscess. In some cases abscess and gangrene follow the acute infectious diseases. In such cases the lesions under consideration are probably due to infectious emboli. Embolic abscesses of the lung occurring during the course of septico-pyæmia, particularly in puerperal cases, do not often come under the surgeon's care, as their course is, as a rule, fatal, no matter what treatment may be adopted. When the physical examination, and particularly that by means of the x-ray, shows that the abscess or gangrene, even if metastatic, is limited to a part of the lung which is accessible, operation may be undertaken to save life.

In some instances abscess of the lung follows subphrenic suppuration—either abscess of the liver or typical subphrenic abscess. A not infrequent cause of abscess and gangrene is the aspiration, into the air passages, of pus or blood which has been drawn down from the upper air passages or from the pharynx. This is particularly likely to occur during operations (under anæsthesia) on the jaws, the tongue, the nose, or the throat. In order to prevent this it is wise to administer the anæsthetic through a tracheotomy tube, care being taken to pack the pharynx in such a manner as to preclude the entrance of blood and pus into the air passages. Korte has reported a case of abscess of the lung due to the aspiration of water. The infectious organisms of a lung abscess are usually the pneumococcus, the streptococcus, and the staphylococcus. When the abscess develops secondarily to subphrenic suppuration, the colon bacillus and, at times, the amœba of dysentery may be found. Occasionally the abscess is due to influenza.

In gangrene of the lung we have, superimposed on this infection, the presence of the saprophytic organisms of decomposition. A lung abscess in its full development is a regular cavity, filled, in most cases, with yellow odorless pus. The walls are covered with granulation tissue, and microscopically a zone of connective-tissue infiltration may be seen. When the abscess has persisted for some length of time the pus becomes very fetid. In the early stages of gangrene there may be seen a dark-brown mass of necrotic lung tissue in the centre of a large irregular cavity with ragged necrotic walls. The cavity is usually filled with a foul-smelling brown fluid containing similar particles of lung tissue. Microscopically, the contents of the abscess cavity are composed of pus cells, micro-organisms, and, above all, elastic tissue. In contradistinction the fluid found in gangrene contains little or no elastic tissue, as it disappears in the course of the decomposition of the lung tissue effected by the saprophytic bacteria. Crystals of leucin and tyrosin are nearly always present. Around the focus of gangrene or the abscess cavity is found a reactive inflammation and a hepatization of the lung tissue.

By far the greatest number of abscesses and foci of gangrene occur in the lower lobe. This is due in all probability to the poorer blood-supply and also to the natural results of gravity. Of thirty-seven cases observed by Korte, twenty-eight occurred in the lower lobe.

SYMPTOMS.—The most characteristic form of abscess or gangrene of the lung is that following pneumonia. The fever, which before has been regular or perhaps has fallen by crises, becomes irregular, higher, and intermittent. The leucocytosis is usually pronounced. The patient displays all the symptoms of the most profound septic intoxication. The prostration is great. The changes in fever are accompanied by chills and rigors. The coughing is distressing and enormous quantities of pus are usually expectorated. The sputa, in abscess and in gangrene, are different. That from the lung abscess is of great quantity and consists of an almost pure yellow pus. On microscopic examination it is found to contain micro-organisms, pus cells, and elastic-tissue fibres. The sputum of gangrene is even more characteristic. Its odor is strong and most offensive. It has a sweetish, sickening quality which is unmistakable. It is usually thin, of a dark greenish-brown color, and is expelled in large quantities. Under the microscope hæmatoidin, leucin, and tyrosin crystals may be found. As a rule, elastic-tissue fibres are not found. The pain is usually not marked. The most frequent complication of lung abscess and gangrene is the secondary involvement of the pleura. This occurs in a large majority of cases. In nearly all cases there are, over the site of the abscess, adhesions and an obliteration of the pleural cavity. These adhesions

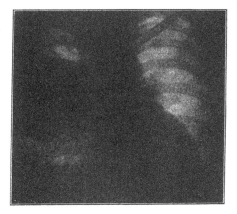

Fig. 9.—Radiogram of an Abscess of the Middle Lobe of the Right Lung. Note normal lung shadows above and below. Spontaneous recovery took place by (?) rupture into a bronchus. (From the x-Ray Laboratory of the Cincinnati Hospital.)

are salutary in their effect, as they prevent the general infection of the pleura. These form the most favorable cases for operation, as they may be drained without infecting the entire pleura. If these adhesions do not occur, the abscess may rupture into the pleura and so give rise to a putrid empyema.

The physical signs are not typical and are usually those of cavities in general; even these may be obscured and rendered uncertain by the presence of a layer of normal lung tissue over the lesion. The Roentgen ray is of the greatest value in diagnosticating and localizing these lesions. (Figs. 9 and 10.) Exploratory aspiration should not be done. It is unreliable at best and it entails a great risk of infecting the pleura. If done at all, it should be followed by immediate operation. The accurate localization of these lesions is of paramount importance, particularly where an operation is to be done. The success of the operative treatment of these cases depends largely on the rapid completion of the operation. Consequently, the more accurate the localization the better the prognosis.

PROGNOSIS.—The prognosis of these cases is very grave, and if they are allowed to run their course, death usually follows. According to McArthur, eighty per cent of cases of gangrene of the lung die, if left to themselves. Nearly seventy per cent recover after operation. The presence of adhesions makes the prognosis more favorable for operation. Their presence can be determined by the use of a fine aspirating needle introduced a short distance. The absence of movement of the needle with respiration shows that adhesions are present. In the absence of adhesions the movement of the pulmonary on the parietal pleura will give the needle a rocking movement. There are several ways in which recovery may take place without operation. For example, the abscess cavity may open into and discharge its contents through a bronchus; or it

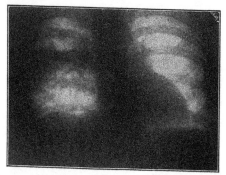

FIG. 10.—Radiogram of the Chest of a Patient who had Recently Recovered from an Abscess of the Right Lung. Note the presence of a transverse scar in the middle lobe. (From the x-Ray Laboratory of the Cincinnati Hospital.)

may break into the pleural cavity and form an empyema necessitatis and so drain to the outside. These relatively favorable results are so rare that they are never to be awaited.

TREATMENT.—The only rational treatment of gangrene and abscess of the lung is immediate operation—that is, an operation performed as soon as the morbid states can be accurately localized. The prognosis after operation is not so bad as it would seem. Korte had a mortality of only 28.5 per cent. The proper procedure is a radical evacuation of the abscess cavity. The patient is anæsthetized, if possible, in the Sauerbruch chamber (Fig. 170, on page 418 of Vol. VII.), or, in its place, a Brauer apparatus may be employed, although one can operate without it. In cases where the expectoration is profuse, there is danger of suffocation from aspiration of the pus into the bronchi. Under these circumstances the operation should be performed with the patient prone and the head properly supported and lower than the chest. In a patient recently operated upon by the writer the chloroform mask was twice greatly soiled with pus from the abscess, although the operation was of short duration.

As a first step, one or two ribs are resected over the site of the lesion. The further steps in the operation depend upon the presence or absence of pleural adhesions. If the lesion is adherent to the parietal pleura, the abscess or gangrene cavity may be immediately opened. An aspirator is thrust into the lung tissue to localize the site of the disease. This is followed by a grooved director. After this the abscess is widely opened, best by means of a thermocautery. If there are any loose sequestra of lung tissue, these too are removed. But any attempt to remove partially adherent sequestra is absolutely contraindicated, as copious and uncontrollable hemorrhage may result.

The operation is concluded by inserting a large drainage tube into the cavity. If the cavity is large a Mikulicz drain may be used. In case the pleura is not adherent, one of several procedures may be followed. Probably the best is to suture the two layers of the pleura tightly together with deep interlocking sutures and then to proceed with the opening of the abscess cavity. If the case is not one of great urgency, adhesions may be obtained by packing with iodoform gauze and opening the abscess a few days later. This is, however, not a very wise method, as the production of adhesions is extremely problematical and an extensive pneumothorax is likely to result. In case the abscess cavity cannot be absolutely localized, Tuffier has adopted a very ingenious idea. After resecting one or two ribs he peels the parietal pleura, without opening it, from the thoracic wall. The hand is then introduced between the pleura and the chest wall and the entire lung is palpated. The general feasibility of this procedure is open to question. A more detailed description of the operation of pneumotomy will be given later.

IV. BRONCHIECTASIS AND PULMONARY EMPHYSEMA.

Bronchiectasis.—Bronchiectasis is one of the end-results of chronic bronchitis or emphysema; it is characterized by paroxysms of severe coughing. Its etiology is rather complicated, being dependent on two factors which act together. The chronic inflammation destroys the elastic tissue of the bronchi, substituting in its place an inflammatory fibrous tissue, non-resilient and non-elastic. The paroxysms of coughing, which take place when the larynx is closed, exert a tremendous intra-alveolar pressure and cause the weakened walls of the bronchi, which are unable to regain their normal size, to dilate. In the cavities thus formed secretion collects and further dilates the cavity. These secretions, by irritating the mucous membrane, excite further coughing and further dilatation, and thus a vicious cycle is formed. The weight of the retained secretions also tends further to dilate the cavity. Perforation of the bronchiectatic wall may result in an acute abscess or in pulmonary gangrene.

There are two main forms of bronchiectasis: the cylindrical and the saccular. The cylindrical bronchiectasis is a more or less general process involving the middle and smaller bronchial branches. In the cut sections these dilatations are close together, largely obliterating the lung parenchyma. This process may be general throughout both lungs and may involve the entire bronchial tree. These are not surgical cases, as they are not in any way amenable to surgical intervention. Treated by inhalations and proper hygienic regulations, such bronchiectatic conditions are compatible with a long and fairly comfortable life.

The saccular bronchiectasis is the form which particularly interests us. Involving as it does a localized portion of the bronchial tree, it is amenable to surgical methods. It usually begins with a small saccular dilatation of the end of a medium-sized bronchus. This increases in size at the expense of the surrounding lung parenchyma, which becomes obliterated by a chronic interstitial pneumonia. There may be several of these cavities scattered through an entire lobe, and they may communicate with one another; or a number of small cavities may be grouped around a large central one. A further interesting form of bronchiectasis is that which follows the obliteration of the lung in consequence of a chronic interstitial pneumonia, usually of tuberculous origin. Here the sacculation is principally due to the pressure of the retained secretions. In still another form it may be due to atrophy of the lung following a long chronic empyema.

Symptoms.—The symptoms are characteristic. The coughing is most marked early in the morning, when the patient rises from the recumbent posture. It is distinctly paroxysmal, and is followed by the expulsion of quantities of secretion. After expelling the sputum the patient may be fairly comfortable until the advent of another paroxysm of coughing. The sputum is purulent, and, if a secondary infection occurs, it may possess a fetid and disgusting odor. The patient, suffering from the effects of constant coughing and of sepsis, gradually loses strength. In many cases gangrene supervenes.

Prognosis.—The prognosis is grave, as sooner or later the disease contributes to a fatal termination.

Treatment.—The treatment should be primarily medical and, only in extreme or otherwise hopeless cases, should surgical treatment be considered. In case the patient's life is a burden and he is continuously and steadily losing ground, operation is indicated. It must, however, be remembered that the prognosis is entirely different from that of primary abscess or of gangrene of the lung. Of fifteen cases operated on by Korte, eleven succumbed to the immediate effects of the operation. The cavity should be treated like any other abscess cavity of the lung,—that is, it should be opened and thoroughly drained.

There is a fair proportion of cases of intra-pulmonary suppurating cavities the result of abscess or of bronchiectasis which it may be impossible to localize or reach for drainage. In them the induction of an artificial pneumothorax with air or nitrogen gas may be attempted. As pneumothorax sometimes causes a wound of the lung to decrease, so the condition artificially produced tends to cause contraction of the pus cavity.

Pulmonary Emphysema.—Until recently pulmonary emphysema has been considered purely a medical affection and beyond the pale of surgical therapy. After exhaustive research Freund concluded that the dyspnœa incident to pulmonary emphysema is partly due to the inability of the thorax to keep pace with the great distention of the lungs. In autopsies of emphysematous subjects degenerative changes in the costal cartilages have long been observed. They are of a nature to impair the elasticity of the ribs. Whether the condition is primary or secondary seems immaterial. The dilated lungs completely fill the thorax, which does not allow their further expansion during inspiration. This throws the entire work of expansion on the diaphragm, which is unable to perform it, and the consequence is severe dyspnœa. It was Freund's idea to mobilize and increase the expansion of the chest by dividing the costal cartilages near the sternum, thus permitting the latter to be lifted in inspiration. A varying number of cartilages is divided—of course, symmetrically. If the relief is not sufficient, this division may be repeated until all the cartilages, from the second to the tenth inclusive have been divided. The pleural cavity, of course, should not be opened. A number of operators have resected portions (from one to two inches in length) of the upper costal cartilages, including a part of the first rib. The technique is simple and the operation not hazardous. It seems, however, that after simple removal of the costal cartilages regeneration may occur, and it has therefore been deemed necessary to remove the perichondrium with the cartilage. Goodman, in the first of his four cases, saw this regrowth of the part removed. He has reported four cases with improvement in each. Seidel has collected eight cases which were operated on for emphysema, and all with good results. In six cases the results were permanent, with great diminution in the dyspnœa and cyanosis. Though this operation is too recent to warrant a judgment of the results, it seems that it is a method which should be tried in cases in which the symptoms are very severe.

V. PARASITIC AFFECTIONS OF THE LUNGS.

Actinomycosis.—Actinomycosis of the lung is a rare condition in America, though somewhat more common in Central Europe. Even there, fortunately, it occurs very rarely. Like other forms of actinomycosis it is due to the ray fungus, and is particularly common among people working about grain and cattle. It may be either primary in the lung or secondary to actinomycosis of the mouth, tongue, and pharynx. This is perhaps the more common form. When primary in the lung the infection enters through inspiration of grain dust carrying the minute ray fungus. After it has made a lodgment it may follow one of two courses:—It may cause a general superficial ulceration of the entire bronchial tree, giving rise to general capillary bronchitis; or it may begin with a superficial ulceration of the mucosa of one or more of the small bronchial radicles. The first of these two courses is very rarely observed, and the conditions established are not such as could possibly be benefited by surgical interference. In the second course the ulcerative action is followed by a peribronchial inflammation of the surrounding lung parenchyma and the formation of bronchopneumonic consolidations. These lesions frequently merge, forming one or more larger masses. The centre of the mass breaks down, and thus an abscess cavity is formed. The periphery of the lesion presents the typical actinomycotic infiltration,—an infiltration of very dense fibrous tissue, containing, of course, the active ray fungus. One of two things may now occur. The abscess, breaking into a large bronchus, may discharge its contents through the bronchial tree. This is, however, liable to be followed by general aspiration pneumonia. Or, progressing further by new infiltration and then breaking down, the lesion reaches the pleura and there gives rise to certain changes. As a rule, there is first a pleural effusion with all its attendant signs. In other cases, however, very little effusion takes place, but instead the pleural cavity is obliterated by dense fibrous tissue. This dense fibrous tissue may cause a retraction of the whole side of the thorax. The further spread of the actinomycotic process spares neither ribs, soft tissues, nor mediastinal contents. It may ulcerate into a blood-vessel and so cause a generalization of the process by metastasis. In the final stage, when the chest wall is invaded, fistulæ form and discharge upon the outside. In this stage the picture is typical. The chest wall is retracted and is the seat of a typical actinomycotic induration. Large fistulæ discharge their contents containing the ray fungus.

Though the course of this disease may extend over a period of several years, the process is invariably fatal, unless surgical interference is resorted to. In the embolic form multiple lesions are found throughout both lungs, and the condition is, of course, beyond the reach of surgery. Surgical intervention is also of no avail in cases in which the pulmonary lesions are secondary to involvement of the mouth, pharynx, and upper air passages.

SYMPTOMS.—The symptoms are in no way pathognomonic. In the first stage the physical signs and the symptoms are very like those of incipient pulmonary tuberculosis, and that is the diagnosis which is usually made. The most common site of actinomycosis, however, is in the lower lobe, while that of tuberculosis is in the apex. If the sputum is carefully examined, the ray fungus will probably be found and the diagnosis may be made at an early stage. In the later stages the diagnosis is, of course, easily made. Before any operative interference is resorted to, the lesion should be accurately localized by means of the physical signs and the x-ray.

PROGNOSIS.—Even with operation the prognosis is extremely unfavorable. Karewski, in his dissertation in 1907, stated that only six successful cases had been reported. To these he added two more out of five on which he had operated. The prognosis, of course, depends on the earliness of the diagnosis and the thoroughness with which the disease is eradicated.

TREATMENT.—The treatment is entirely different from that of abscess, in which condition a simple opening is made and drainage established. In actinomycosis, on the other hand, all the diseased tissue must be thoroughly eradicated by the knife and thermo-cautery. If any vestige of diseased tissue remains, the process will continue. Potassium iodide should be administered in these cases (in conjunction with surgical procedures) for a long time, as by some it is considered effective in actinomycosis.

Echinococcus.—In America echinococcus of the lung is a very rare disease. It is perhaps most frequently encountered in Australia and in certain parts of Germany and the Tyrol, where the domestic animals live in close contact with the farmer. Echinococcus of the lung is second in frequency to echinococcus of the liver. As in other forms of lung disease due to aspiration, it is most frequently found in the lower right lobe. It usually begins as a small cyst in the interior of the lobe and grows rapidly at the expense of the lung tissue. Owing to its spongy structure, the lung is an ideal locality for the rapid growth of echinococcus; the lung tissue offering little resistance to its rapid progress. The capsule, usually very thin, is formed principally through degeneration of the lung tissue, and only in slight degree by newly formed scar tissue. The process itself excites very little inflammatory reaction. Advancing very rapidly, the process quickly invades the pleural cavity and gives rise to a pleural effusion. In this pleural effusion the echinococcus is found free. In other cases the contents of the cyst break into a large bronchus and are discharged through the bronchial tree to the outside. Often growing to an enormous size, the echinococcus cyst may completely fill one side of the chest, displacing the heart, mediastinal contents, the diaphragm, and the peritoneal organs.

SYMPTOMATOLOGY.—The symptoms, which depend entirely upon the seat and extent of the process, are, of course, variable. While still confined to the interior of the lung tissue the process may advance with practically no symptoms. When the tumor reaches a large size, the symptoms are those of pleural effusion. If careful examination is made, even in the early stages, a small area of dulness and absence of breathing sounds may be made out. The only occasion upon which an absolute diagnosis can be made is when the tumor ruptures through a large bronchus and the cysts are found in the sputum. Frequently these cases are tapped in the belief that the condition is simply an ordinary pleural effusion. A microscopic examination will easily reveal the presence of the echinococcus. An examination by means of the Roentgen ray will frequently reveal the site of an otherwise obscure lesion.

PROGNOSIS.—The prognosis depends entirely on the treatment. As soon as the diagnosis is made, operative interference is indicated. If the lesion is confined to a small area of the lung, resection of the lung may be made. This course, however, is rarely indicated. If possible, the sac should be dissected out. This is, however, not absolutely necessary and is frequently attended by profuse and even dangerous hemorrhage.

TREATMENT.—The treatment here may be the same as that employed in cases of echinococcus of the liver—that is, the sac, after being widely opened, should be thoroughly drained and its walls stitched to the parietal pleura. Daily irrigations with silver-nitrate solution will soon cause a shrinkage and obliteration of the sac.

VI. PULMONARY TUBERCULOSIS.

The question of surgical treatment of tuberculosis of the lungs has been agitated for many years and is still unsettled. The admirable results of medical, dietetic, and hygienic treatment of early tuberculosis preclude the general adoption of the perhaps more brilliant, but surely more dangerous, operative treatment. During the early stages the difficulty of accurately localizing an apical lesion and the surety that this lesion is solitary make the surgical treatment impossible at this stage. The treatment of abscess cavities which have become gangrenous or secondarily involved, is an entirely different matter. Even as early as the seventeenth century, Baglin attempted to treat these abscess cavities by tapping and injecting into them different substances. He met, however, with no success. Mosler was the first to put this treatment on a scientific basis. He treated a number of cases by injecting diluted solutions of both potassium permanganate and carbolic acid. His plan of treatment, however, met with no encouraging results and was given up.

With the discovery of the tubercle bacillus by Koch, the injection of tuberculous cavities was revived. An emulsion of iodoform was the favorite medicament. After some years this treatment also was abandoned. It has long been observed that the accidental occurrence of pneumothorax may have a favorable influence on tuberculosis of the lungs. Forlanini was the first to take advantage of this in a strictly scientific way, but it was Murphy, of Chicago, who first practised it extensively and gave the method wide circulation. In 1898 he published the report of a number of cases which had been treated by the induction of an artificial pneumothorax. His method was to inject nitrogen gas into the pleural cavity in varying amounts. Nitrogen was used because it is more slowly absorbed than any other gaseous substance. These injections were repeated as soon as the effect had disappeared,—that is, at intervals varying from three weeks to two months. This treatment met with little encouragement, and little has been heard of it for several years. Only last year, however, Schmidt revived this treatment, and he claims to have had brilliant results.

The radical, surgical treatment of apical tuberculosis by pneumotomy has been advocated in many instances and at various times for many decades. It would seem to have a place in the treatment of apical cavities in which secondary septic infection has taken place. The author has operated on three advanced cases with a view to drainage. All of the cases succumbed within a few months; the drainage proved to be insufficient. This has been the experience of almost all operators, so that incision and drainage for tuberculous cavities ought rarely if ever to be practised.

Tuffier has reported a case of pneumectomy in which he claims that there was no recurrence. Similarly favorable results have been reported by quite a number of operators. Thus Willard reports four recoveries out of six operations. The mortality of this method is necessarily so high that it should be discouraged by all surgeons. Even for the most radical surgeons it is too visionary a procedure. The patient is exposed to one of the most dangerous operations without any assurance that a permanent cure will be the result. Perhaps with the general use of the different means which we now possess of operating on the thorax under positive or negative pressure, this danger may be somewhat overcome. It has been shown experimentally that large portions of the lung may be resected without causing serious inconvenience to the animal. Murphy was the first to show this. Even then, however, the operation of pneumectomy for tuberculosis of the lung is an unjustifiable one. Its only possible use could be in the earliest stages of localized apical tuberculosis, and these cases are almost without exception cured by the modern medical methods.

Quite different is the operation advised and exploited by Quincke. He very accurately observed that one of the chief reasons of the rapid spread of tuberculosis of the lungs is to be found in the rigidity of the chest wall. Adhesions are early formed between the parietal and visceral pleuræ, and, as a result, there is provided a tissue which is unable to contract and which serves as an admirable nidus for the development and growth of a tuberculous focus. All cavities must heal by the filling in of the unoccupied space with granulation tissue and by the contraction of the surrounding tissues. It can be easily seen that in the lung, owing to the immobility of the chest wall, this becomes most difficult. After noticing the brilliant results obtained, in old chronic empyemata, from multiple rib resections, Quincke advised and practised the same procedure for tuberculosis of the lungs. His treatment met with brilliant results, particularly in cases of small isolated cavities. The last series of cases was reported this year by Professor Friedrich; the results which he obtained in these cases being admirable. Quincke's original idea was to confine the operation of rib resection to cases in which the apex of the lung was the seat of the perfectly formed cavity. Even in these advanced cases a considerable improvement was noticed in many instances; the fever becoming less and the process, although not cured, being brought to a standstill. This treatment has been undergoing development now for many years, and has been brought to its apotheosis by Professor Friedrich. He advocates its employment particularly in those cases which resist careful medical treatment. His procedure is, first, to make a wide flap as in the Estlander operation. The ribs of the entire affected side, from the second to the ninth inclusive, are then removed, as large a portion as possible of each rib being excised. The operation should be done with as great speed as is consistent with safety. Any opening of the chest cavity is contra-indicated, as it may vitiate the end-result by causing an infection of the pleural cavity. The immediate effect of the operation is early seen in the reduction of temperature, the lessening of the secretion, the decrease in cough, and the improvement in general condition.

Reasoning from the pathology of pulmonary tuberculosis one may deem this method of treatment the most rational one devised. As in tuberculosis of any part of the body, great improvement is seen after the part has been put at rest. This method of Friedrich's is the only way in which the rest treatment may be applied to the tuberculous lung. When one considers, however, as has already been intimated, how much may be done by the non-medical measures even for those with restricted means, by special treatment at home or in sanatoria, it seems improbable that any surgical treatment will find a wide application. Only in the event of a cavity failing to heal, does it seem proper to resort to surgical measures.

VII. NEOPLASMS OF THE LUNGS.

Primary neoplasms of the lung are, fortunately, of rather rare occurrence. They are, as a rule, beyond the realm of surgical interference. This is perhaps due to the insidious onset of the disease and the absence of symptoms during the early stages. When these patients at length come to the surgeon for advice and treatment, the new-growth is usually of such an enormous size as to make

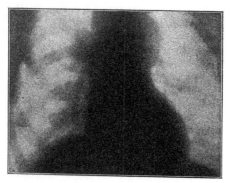

Fig. 11.—Radiogram of a Tumor of the Upper Lobe of the Right Lung. (From the x-Ray Laboratory of the Cincinnati Hospital.)

surgical interference impossible. (Fig. 11.) The most frequent of the tumors encountered in the lung is carcinoma, and among these the large medullary variety is the one usually observed. Occasionally one encounters an endothelioma, this form of cancer developing either from the superficial lymph tracts of the pleura or from the interalveolar lymph spaces.

In early cancer of the lung, the diagnosis is most difficult. X-ray examinations have recently revealed primary carcinoma of the lung in quite a number of instances. In the large material of the Eppendorf Hospital at Hamburg, Otten found nine cases in four years. Two cases were operated on with indifferent results. One of Lenhartz's cases was operated on after thoracotomy, and the patient is still living and well after one year and a half.

Secondary or metastatic tumors of the lung are of rather frequent occurrence. They are mostly of the sarcoma type and are particularly common after periosteal sarcoma of the long bones. The diagnosis may be made by the previous history, the dyspnœa and cough, and the blood-stained sputum. There are also the usual signs of secondary pleural effusion. As in carcinoma of the pleura, aspiration must occasionally be made to give relief. The aspirated fluid is almost always sanguineous, and the relief given is of short duration. The x-ray will often help us in locating a tumor of the lung.

In a few instances, primary tumors of the lung have been successfully removed. With the earlier diagnosis made possible by the x-ray and the greater safety of modern methods of operating on the thorax,—methods which make it possible to prevent a serious pneumothorax,—primary tumors of the lung will in the future be made the subject of operative interference, with at least a modicum of hope.

VIII. SURGICAL AFFECTIONS OF THE MEDIASTINUM.

In the septal space between the two pleural sacs are contained the heart within the pericardium, the large blood-vessels at its base, the division of the trachea, the thymus gland or what is left of it, the œsophagus, the descending aorta, and the thoracic duct. In addition, there are the many lymph nodes and the laryngeal nerves, particularly the left, which winds around the aortic arch. All of these structures have important anatomical relations. Within the mediastinum there is also a great deal of loose areolar tissue, the planes of which are continuous above with the structures beneath the deep fascia of the neck, while below they run to the intermuscular space of the diaphragm.

All affections of the mediastinum, whether the result of trauma, of infection, or in the broadest sense neoplastic, have many of the symptoms in common by reason of the fact that the mechanical pressure which they exert is, in a measure, independent of their nature. Thus, the effects caused by pressure on the trachea or a primary bronchus, or on the superior cava or the innominate veins, and the symptoms dependent upon irritation or paralysis of the muscles supplied by the recurrent laryngeal nerve, are common to many affections of the mediastinum, whatever their character.

Injuries and Emphysema.—Injuries of the tissues within the mediastinum, except those resulting from penetrating wounds of the heart and large blood-vessels, are uncommon. Fractures of the sternum and of the spine may give rise to hemorrhage into the loose cellular tissue, but this is insufficient to cause pressure symptoms and the extravasated blood is ordinarily absorbed. In severe crushes of the chest, a tear of the trachea or of a bronchus has been noted repeatedly, but the concomitant injuries have been so severe that speedy death has resulted. When the injury to the air passages is less extensive, mediastinal emphysema results. This often has been seen after subcutaneous injuries of the trachea in the neck and after tracheotomies, when an effort has been made to close the tracheal wound without provision for the escape of the air to the outside through drainage of the wound. Perforation of the trachea or bronchus by a foreign body may also be followed by mediastinal emphysema. After wounds of the lower part of the neck mediastinal emphysema sometimes results without involvement of the trachea.

Symptoms.—Emphysema of the mediastinum manifests itself by gradually increasing dyspnœa and cyanosis. The area of heart dulness diminishes and may entirely disappear. Emphysematous crackling can usually he heard. If the patient lives long enough, the emphysema spreads to the neck and on to the anterior abdominal wall. In grave cases, the patient usually succumbs before the effects of infection are made manifest. In perforations of the trachea or bronchus by a foreign body, mediastinitis as a rule develops.

Treatment.—The treatment of mediastinal emphysema is limited to the making of incisions in the neck or the thorax when the emphysema has extended so far. These incisions are palliative. The radical treatment consists of a low tracheotomy, if the primary source of the condition is in the upper trachea, and of the introduction of a long tracheal cannula or tube into the bronchus with the view of passing the point of leakage in the broncho-tracheal tree.

Mediastinitis.—Inflammation of the cellular tissue within the mediastinum is rather uncommon. Primary infections occur only from perforating wounds or as the result of the infection of a hæmatoma consequent on severe injury. Secondary infections are of more frequent occurrence and come from many causes. Suppuration within the bronchial lymph nodes, ulceration of foreign bodies through the œsophagus or trachea, ulceration of the œsophagus from malignant disease, extension of suppuration from disease of the sternum, ribs, or vertebra, and cellulitis of the neck are among the more common etiological factors. The condition occasionally follows infections of the subfascial tissues at the root of the neck, notably after tracheotomies in which the parts have become infected, perforation of the œsophagus, and operations on this organ.

Anatomically, the inflammation may manifest itself in a diffuse cellulitis or in an abscess that is more or less limited. In the cases in which the inflammation develops from infected lymph nodes or from some diseased condition of the sternum or one of the vertebræ, a limited abscess is likely to form. According to Hare, thirty out of thirty-six cases reported were located in the upper and anterior mediastinum.

Symptoms.—The symptoms of inflammations within the mediastinum vary much with the site of the focus of infection. All cases present the general symptoms of a severe toxæmia, namely, fever, chills, and rapid pulse. The local symptoms for the most part are severe pains, with a sense of great oppression in the chest. In abscesses of slow growth, particularly of tuberculous origin, the syndrome may be that of mediastinal tumor. Owing, however, to the adaptability of the contents of the abscess to contiguous structures, pressure symptoms are rarely as pronounced as in tumors or aneurysms.

Diagnosis.—The diagnosis is facilitated by the history of a preceding infection deep-seated within the neck, or of some primary disease in the sternum or costal cartilages or within the lymph nodes about the spot where the trachea divides. In the more fortunate cases, the abscess approaches the surface at the root of the neck on either side or below the sternum, thereby making the diagnosis relatively easy. In several instances (Heidenhain, Cavazzini, Rasumowski), an abscess of the posterior mediastinum has worked its way into the neck through a perforation of the œsophagus caused by a foreign body. In these cases the track along which the pus had travelled was followed by dissection from the neck down to the abscess and a cure was effected by the establishment of drainage. The x-ray will be found as helpful in localizing a mediastinal abscess in its early stage as it is in revealing the presence of a tumor or an aneurysm in this region.

PROGNOSIS.—The prognosis of suppuration within the mediastinum is always grave. In hyperacute cases, death comes from sepsis within a week or less. In the cases which are not so acute, death may result suddenly from perforation into a bronchus. Perforation into the pleura or the pericardium may likewise occur.

TREATMENT.—In the treatment of mediastinitis, prophylaxis must be considered. In operations on the lower part of the neck, and particularly on the œsophagus, a special effort to prevent infection should be made. Foreign bodies should be removed from the air passages and œsophagus before ulceration and perforation take place. The active treatment consists of securing effective drainage as early as possible after an abscess is located. Here the x-ray and exploratory aspiration are invaluable. It may be quite a difficult matter to establish drainage, and in certain cases it may be possible to do this only by trephining the sternum and resecting one or more of the costal cartilages. von Bergmann has repeatedly trephined the sternum as the first step in exploring for the abscess. The operation is simple enough, and when the general condition of the patient militates against the employment of ether or chloroform the operation may be done under cocaine. By means of subperiosteal cocaine infiltration, the writer was able, in one instance, to remove a disc of bone, one inch and a half in diameter, without pain. Trephining the sternum was resorted to successfully by Galen.

Access to an abscess of the posterior mediastinum may be obtained by the subperiosteal resection of one or more ribs posteriorly, or of a transverse process of a vertebra, and then displacing the pleura. Most of the operations have hitherto been performed for tuberculous abscesses connected with the lower cervical and upper dorsal vertebral bodies. In a few instances the removal of a foreign body from the thoracic portion of the œsophagus has been successful; and again, in a few cases, the œsophagus has been resected for carcinoma, but invariably with fatal results. Experimental operations under negative pressure, recently made on animals, give some promise that operations on the structures within the posterior mediastinum may in the near future yield better results.

In the case of an abscess in the upper part of the posterior mediastinum, access may be obtained from the root of the neck. In this way it is possible, on the left side, to reach the third and even the fourth vertebral body.

Tumors of the Mediastinum.—Tumors of the mediastinum, up to quite a recent date, possessed only a clinical and pathological interest. With the possibilities given by modern improvement of technique, they have become distinctly surgical. All tumors of the mediastinum present, within wide limits, similar symptoms, the severity of which depend upon the size, nature, and chiefly the situation of the growth. For practical purposes, aneurysm of the aortic arch may be considered in the same class with mediastinal tumors. These growths are either benign or malignant. The former, if one excludes aneurysms and enlargements of the lymph nodes of the tracheal bifurcation, are few in number as compared with malignant tumors. In infancy the enlargements of the thymus gland should likewise be considered as, in part at least, belonging to the mediastinum.

The benign affections include retrosternal goitres, dermoid and echinococcus cysts, aneurysms of the aorta and its primary branches, and fatty tumors, which latter are of slow growth.

Gussenbauer first described those lipomata which spring from the parietal pleura and grow into the mediastinum, occasionally perforating an intercostal space and enlarging under the superficial muscles of the thorax.

In adults the most common growth, next to aneurysms, is a dermoid, which, by reason of its small size, may produce no symptoms and be found only at autopsy. A dermoid, however, may grow sufficiently in size to assume clinical significance, and, like dermoids elsewhere in the body, it may become secondarily infected.

Hyperplasia of the bronchial lymph nodes often occurs in children and is, as a rule, tuberculous in character. These enlargements rarely produce pressure symptoms.

Malignant tumors include carcinomata and primary lymphosarcomata (Fig. 12), or endotheliomata. The carcinomata, as a rule, are secondary and develop in lymph nodes within the mediastinum and in the cellular tissue about the root of the lung. The endotheliomata are sometimes of slow growth, and assume enormous proportions. In the tumor represented in Fig. 6 the total mass exceeded that of an adult head, compressing both lungs and displacing the heart. In Hodgkin's disease the mediastinal lymph nodes are frequently involved toward the end, and may give rise to severe compression symptoms.

Enlargement of the Thymus.—Although Allen Burns, more than a century ago, described the condition known as thymic asthma and ascribed it as probably due to pressure from an enlarged thymus gland, it is only within the last ten years that pediatrists particularly, and more recently surgeons, have had their attention called to the condition. In young children, and more rarely in adults, an enlarged thymus gland may cause death from pressure exerted chiefly upon the trachea and to a less extent upon the great vessels. The situation and relations of this very vascular gland—lying, as it does, in front of the trachea, fixed between the vertebral column behind and the sternum in front, occupying the superior anterior mediastinum, extending to the thyroid in the neck, and in close relationship to the innominata vein and the superior vena cava—account for the symptom complex which one observes when the gland is enlarged. It is enclosed within a loose capsule from which it is easily shelled out. The arterial supply comes from the internal mammary and the inferior thyroids. The maximum of its development occurs between the first and the second years of life. As a part phenomenon of the condition (now recognized as "status lymphaticus," a term first introduced by Paltauf), enlargement of the thymus gland is important in infancy.

SYMPTOMS.—The symptoms which may make this condition a surgical one are, for the most part, the result of pressure on the trachea. The dyspnœa may come on gradually or may develop with great rapidity. In a number of instances the respiration has been comparatively normal between the attacks of dyspnœa. In still other instances there has been observed, in the dyspnœic crises and during expiration, a small dome-like tumor situated above the sternum, while during inspiration this tumor diminished in size or disappeared entirely. Unfortunately, the presence of this swelling is far from constant. Difficulty in deglutition has been observed in three cases. By means of radiography the diagnosis is now made reasonably sure.

PROGNOSIS AND TREATMENT.—The prognosis of enlargement of the thymus gland is very grave. While in some instances spontaneous cure has been noted,

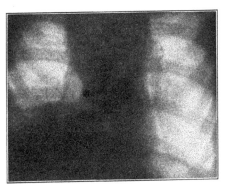

FIG. 12.—Radiogram of a Primary Sarcoma of the Mediastinum; Diagnosis Confirmed by Autopsy.
(From the x-Ray Laboratory of the Cincinnati Hospital.)

and the persistent use of the x-ray has been followed by marked improvement and often by a cure in many others, surgical intervention may at any time be demanded to relieve pressure. Intubation or tracheotomy may give temporary relief, although in every case thus far recorded a failure to give permanent relief has substantiated the diagnosis of pressure lower down. Out of eight cases Veau cites four in which tracheotomy or intubation failed, and these negative results made the diagnosis of thymic enlargement certain. As to the other surgical measures which may be employed in the condition which we are now considering, it is sufficient to mention only one, viz., the exposure, and possibly afterward the removal, of the thymus gland, an operation that was first performed by Rehn, in 1896. (*Berlin. klin. Wochensch.*, Siegel, 1896.) Since that date cases have been recorded by Koenig, Purrucker, Ehrhardt, Hinrichs, Boschardt, and Jackson. Altogether, nine cases have been reported, and in each the improvement was immediate. The operation is not so grave as one would at first imagine from the depth of the organ behind the sternum and from its relations to the great vessels. But, as Moizard (*Jour. de Méd. et de Chir.*, June 10th, 1909) properly states, "the thymus of the cadaver is not that of the living infant. It is movable, not adherent, and is lodged in a capsule from which it is easily displaced. Its capsule alone is closely adherent to contiguous structures. Therefore, as soon as the capsule is opened, the gland forces itself like a hernia through the incision during expiration. It is easily seized and enucleated. Furthermore, all the blood-vessels that run to the superior portions are easily tied. In cases where the operation cannot be prolonged the mere opening of the capsule above the sternum may, as it has in a number of instances, cause sufficient bulging of the gland toward the surface to give relief."

The operation for the relief of an enlarged thymus gland begins with a median incision extending from the cricoid cartilage to a point a little below the

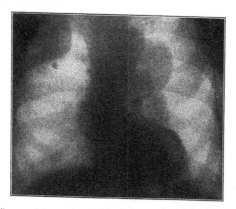

FIG. 13.—Radiogram of Multiple Aneurysms of the Aorta. Five separate aneurysms can be distinguished, and in this number is included one of the innominate artery. Correctness of diagnosis was verified by autopsy. (From the *x*-Ray Laboratory of the Cincinnati Hospital.)

sternal notch. The soft parts are divided by blunt dissection until the capsule of the gland is reached. In three of the cases operated on, the tumor itself, after the completion of the incision, projected at once into the wound. The capsule of the gland is next opened and the gland withdrawn from the interior. It may now be fixed by catgut sutures to the margins of the wound and left in this position without further interference. This exopexia of the gland was the operation performed by Rehn and two other operators, and proved sufficient to relieve all symptoms. Resection of the gland, if it is deemed advisable, is made by gently lifting the organ from its capsule and tying off the blood-vessels which enter the upper pole. The removal of the gland has not been followed by any untoward symptoms. Experiments on animals made by Swale Vincent (*Jour. of Physiology*, 1904), by Tarully (quoted by Ehrhardt), and by Fischl (*Muench. Wochensch.*, 1907, p. 45) have shown that no toxic symptoms follow thymectomy in young animals and that the gland possesses no functions essential to life and well-being.

Sarcomata and lymphosarcomata originating in the thymus gland have occasionally been observed in adults and, in a few instances, in early childhood. They present the physical evidences of neoplasms of the superior mediastinum. They are rarely subject to operation, although the writer, in 1906, saw a patient from whom Durante had successfully removed a sarcoma of the thymus. With the tumor was removed a portion, one inch in length, of the innominate artery.

Aneurysm of the Thoracic Aorta and of its Primary Branches.—Although aneurysms of the arch and of the thoracic aorta constitute nearly one-half of all aneurysms, they belong, for the most part, in the domain of medicine. Nevertheless, in some instances surgical intervention may become necessary. Any portion of the arch or of the thoracic aorta may be the site of an aneurysm, and radiography has shown that, in very many cases, two or more aneurysms may be present in the same subject. (Fig. 13.) Dahlen observed multiple aneurysms three times in twenty-seven cases. (*Zeitsch. f. klin. Med.*, 63, p. 163.)

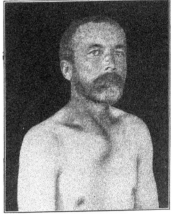

FIG. 14.—Aneurysm of the Ascending Portion of the Arch of the Aorta. The tumor occupies the first and second interspaces and extends into the neck; a portion of the sternum has undergone atrophy through pressure. (Case of Dr. John Musser, of Philadelphia)

DIAGNOSIS. — The diagnosis of aortic aneurysm, particularly in its beginning, is sometimes very difficult, and sudden death from rupture into the trachea, pericardium, or pleura may take place in a case in which the disease was not even suspected.

SYMPTOMS.—The symptoms are almost altogether due to pressure effects or to occlusion of one or other primary trunk, in both of which conditions variation in the radial pulse is produced. The pressure symptoms are those common to mediastinal tumors in general and vary with the site of the aneurysm.

An aneurysm of the ascending portion of the arch will, by pressure on the vena cava, cause distention of the veins of the head and upper extremities; or, in rare instances, the pressure, being confined to the innominata, will produce effects on one side alone. Such an aneurysm of the arch, as it grows, erodes as a rule the sternal ends of the second and third ribs and at times also the sternum itself. (Fig. 14.) Effects due to pressure on the trachea may be long delayed.

Aneurysms of the transverse arch, by pressure on the trachea and left recurrent laryngeal nerve, cause intense dyspnœa, paroxysmal cough, and paralysis of the left vocal cord, with aphonia. Pressure on the sympathetic may cause unevenness of the pupils, with unilateral hyperæmia of the integument of the face and sweating. Aneurysms of this part of the arch, even when small, may rupture into the trachea and quickly become fatal.

In two instances the writer saw temporary relief to the dyspnœa from the use of Koenig's tracheotomy tube. In these cases the aneurysm, though suspected, was not demonstrable. In both of them, however, the presence of

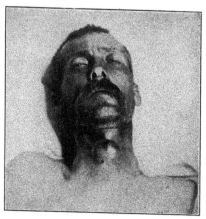

FIG. 15.—Front View of the Neck of a Patient with Aneurysm of the Transverse Arch of the Aorta.
(Case in the Cincinnati Hospital.)

the tracheal cannula seemed to hasten the extension of the ulcerative process to the trachea.

Aneurysms of the second portion of the arch erode the upper part of the sternum and frequently grow into the root of the neck. (Figs. 15 and 16.) Aneurysms of the posterior part of the arch and of the thoracic aorta produce, as a rule, less well-marked pressure effects on the trachea. In most cases, however, they are associated with severe pain from erosion of the vertebral bodies and involvement of the left intercostal nerves. The œsophagus and left bronchus are frequently pressed upon, and varicose dilatation of the intercostal veins is sometimes seen. If aneurysms of the thoracic aorta come to the surface, they, as a rule, erode the costal arches to the inner side of the scapular border.

The relations of an aortic aneurysm to the trachea are frequently manifested by the tracheal tugging of Oliver, which shows itself in a palpable upward and downward movement of the trachea in the neck when the patient holds his breath. In some instances, Cardarelli has observed, under like conditions, a lateral movement.

DIAGNOSIS.—While the diagnosis of the existence of a large thoracic aneurysm is frequently a simple affair, it is often difficult to determine its exact relations. An aneurysm of the arch of the aorta has frequently been mistaken for an aneurysm of the innominate artery, and in many cases it has been treated by distal ligation, on a mistaken diagnosis. The chief factor that makes the diagnosis difficult, is the frequency with which an aneurysm of the arch is associated with a dilatation of one of the primitive trunks, notably the innominate. Fortunately, radiography permits us accurately to locate an aneurysm of the aorta, and by means of the wavy outline or double contour of the shadow

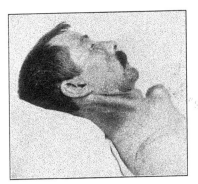

FIG. 16.—Profile View of the Patient Shown in Fig. 15.

to make the diagnosis positive. (Fig. 17.) There are exceptions to this, however, as witness the following case which was under the writer's observation:—

A patient, 43 years of age, was admitted to the Jewish Hospital with tracheal stenosis. An x-ray photograph (Fig. 18) showed a small lobulated tumor without the outline characteristic of pulsation. A deep-seated abscess was suspected. Bronchoscopic examination showed a tracheal stenosis without pulsation. Death from tracheal compression seeming imminent, a low tracheotomy was made and a long cannula inserted. Relief to the dyspnœa was immediate, but it lasted only two days. Four days later, under cocaine anæsthesia, the sternum was trephined with a view to exploring the mediastinum. Immediately after the button was removed, the aneurysm ruptured into the trachea and death resulted in a short time. The autopsy revealed a small sacculated aneurysm of the arch.

PROGNOSIS.—The prognosis of aortic aneurysms is, of course, very grave. While death usually ensues within two or three years from the time when the diagnosis is made, in very exceptional cases life has been prolonged for many years. This is an important fact to remember in considering surgical intervention. The latter must not be credited with prolonging life, unless an actual improvement in the patient's condition takes place and a demonstrable reduction in size and increase in hardness of the tumor are shown by physical examination or by radiography. Furthermore, the production of an organizable clot in one part of an aneurysmal sac may force its growth in another direction. In a case reported by the writer, in which silver wire had been introduced into the aneurysmal sac, the improvement, which was only temporary, was followed by rupture into the right pleura. It was found that a firm clot had formed about the wire.

TREATMENT.—Only sacculated and single aneurysms can under any conditions be considered fit for surgical intervention. This is limited to the distal ligation of the arteries at the root of the neck, on the one hand, and, on the other, to securing an organizable blood clot in the sac by means of foreign substances (such as silver wire, steel watch springs, etc.) introduced into it, or by the prolonged and repeated irritation of the wall of the sac by long needles introduced from without, after the method of Macewen. In 1879 Corradi combined

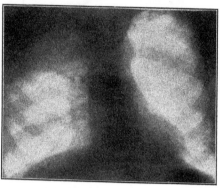

FIG. 17.—Radiogram of an Aneurysm of the Descending Part of the Thoracic Arch. The picture shows by double contour the existence of pulsation. (From the x-Ray Laboratory of the Cincinnati Hospital.)

the introduction of wire with galvanism, and in this way good results have been obtained in a large number of instances.

The technique of the operation is simple. It is fully described by Le Conte and Stewart on page 276 of Vol. VII. The clot formation under this method takes place immediately and is generally manifested before the end of the session through changes (apparent to the eye and hand) in the pulsation and consistence of the tumor. From time to time the changes become more marked, until, in the most favorable cases, a nodule, with only a communicated pulsation, replaces the previous expansible tumor. This was the history of four of the ten cases recorded by Stewart.

Macewen's Process of Needling.—The process of needling devised by Sir W. Macewen is based on the fact that by irritation of the arterial wall—*i.e.*, the sac wall—of an aneurysm, a reparative exudate is formed. The irritation is applied at as many points as possible, with the idea of thereby generating fibrinous clots in such number and so large as to occlude the sac. Macewen has reported a number of positive cures and Caselli one of an innominate aneurysm. In the original communication (*Lancet*, 1890, Vol. 2, p. 1086) Macewen fully describes the method of needling with pins of sufficient length completely to transfix the aneurysm and to permit of manipulation within it. The long pin, which ought to be as slender as possible and tapering to a fine point, is made to penetrate the sac and pass through its cavity, until it comes in touch with the opposite side. The point may then be manipulated from the distal wall, if the sac wall is dense, or the blood current itself may cause sufficient to-and-fro movement to produce the desired scratching of the sac wall. After the point of the pin has been left for ten minutes in one position, it may be shifted to another portion of the sac. If the aneurysm be very large, several pins may be introduced from several points, a considerable interval of space being allowed

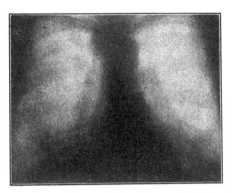

FIG. 18.—Radiogram of a Small Aneurysm of the Transverse Arch of the Aorta Simulating a Mediastinal Abscess. The mass appears lobulated and has a single contour. Rupture into the trachea. (From the x-Ray Laboratory of Jewish Hospital, Cincinnati.)

to exist between the individual pins. Repeated sessions, at intervals of a few days, are necessary to effect consolidation.

Ligation of the Common Carotid and Subclavian.—In well selected saccular aneurysms of the ascending arch or of the innominate, the simultaneous tying of the common carotid and the subclavian has been performed many times, since it was first done by Rossi in 1843. The writer has performed it in five cases, the first of which only was fatal from the operation. (*Amer. Jour. Med. Sciences*, 1880, p. 352.) Death resulted from septic pleurisy. In all of the other cases a marked improvement occurred, although a positive cure was not effected in any. In these four cases two of the number lived for two and a half to three years after the operation and one of them returned to his work as a fireman. (Figs. 19 and 20.)

The danger from the operation itself is not very great if one excludes the fatal effects of cerebral anæmia that occur in about ten per cent of the cases in which the common carotid is tied. Unless the left carotid is thoroughly-patulous, as shown by the temporal pulse, the operation is out of place. In very large aneurysms that are near to rupturing, it is likewise contra-indicated. It must be confessed that the results obtained by distal ligation, for aneurysms of the aorta and innominate, are far from encouraging. Jacobsthal, in 1903 (*Zeitsch. f. Chir.*, Vol. 78, p. 239), had critically considered 120 cases. The immediate mortality was over 12.9 per cent. Jacobsthal concedes that only three cases lived after three years. That the prognosis is better than one would infer from this statement is shown by the fact that the patients of Heath and

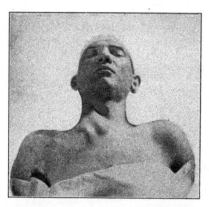

Fig. 19.—Photograph of the Neck and Upper Part of the Chest in a Patient Affected with Aneurysm of the Innominate Artery. The picture shows the appearance of the parts before the operation. (Case at the Cincinnati Hospital.)

Stimson who were living after three and four years, are not included among the cures. In Poivet's collection of ninety-four cases, seven per cent of cures are claimed. The largest individual experience is doubtless that of Guinard, who has had fifteen cases of aneurysm of the aorta and root of the neck in which distal ligation was performed. There was only one death due to operation. No details are given as to the end-results.

Aneurysms of the Innominate.—Until radiography rendered possible a differential diagnosis between an aneurysm of the aorta and one of the innominate, the two conditions, when they were not coexisting, were often confounded. It is now possible, not only to identify an aneurysm as belonging to·the innominate, but also to recognize the part of the trunk primarily involved. When an aneurysm of the innominate is not part of an aortic sacculation, it is, as a rule, sacculated. In its growth it first involves the structures of the superior mediastinum and then extends into the neck. The pressure symptoms result from its relationship to the innominate vein, the right recurrent laryngeal nerve, and the trachea.

TREATMENT.—The treatment of aneurysms of the innominate is much like that of aneurysms of the aorta. The best results have been obtained by distal simultaneous tying of the carotid and subclavian. When other intrathoracic aneurysms are present, operative interference is contra-indicated. A case of this kind, in which von Eiselsberg recently refused to operate, was so far benefited by the injection of gelatin that the visible tumor completely disappeared. (*Wiener klin. Wochensch.*, 1907, p. 188.) According to Imbert and Pons (quoted by Matas) one-fourth of the cases ought to be benefited by the distal operation. The danger that cerebral anæmia will follow the tying of the common carotid of one side may, according to Guinard (*Rev. de Chir.*, 1909, p. 229),

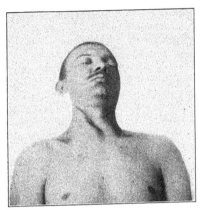

Fig. 20.—Photograph of the Same Patient (Fig. 19), taken One Month after Simultaneous Distal Deligation.

be disregarded provided the anastomotic circulation between the external carotids is intact. In all the fatal cases, according to this writer, the latter was interfered with by some grave operation, notably by operative work on the jaws.

IX. OPERATIONS ON THE CHEST.

The operations on the chest differ from those on the rest of the body in that they must be performed without interrupting the regular action of the heart and lungs, which action is necessary to the maintenance of life. Any interruption of the heart's action is likely to prove immediately fatal. For this reason it will be seen that the surgery of the thorax and its contents demands special care in the choice of the anæsthetic, in the position of the patient, and in the maintenance of intrathoracic pressure. The choice of the anæsthetic is most important, and so also is the manner in which it is given. In cases of empyema one-half of the breathing capacity may be lost, and for this reason great care should be taken not to give any anæsthetic that may interfere with the function of the remaining lung tissue. It is evident, therefore, that ether and nitrous oxide are thoroughly unsuited for this class of cases, as a part of the narcotic effect, in both of these agents, is due to partial asphyxia.

When possible, the lesser operations, such as thoracotomy or even the resection of one rib, should be done under local anæsthesia. The operation, however, cannot be made absolutely painless. When all is considered, it will be seen that chloroform is the best available anæsthetic. It must be given with unusual care and the heart's action carefully watched. The necessity of this will be seen when it is remembered that the heart is already working under an additional strain from the presence of increased intrathoracic pressure.

Lately, some of these operations have been done in the preliminary stage of ether anæsthesia, in the so-called *Ether Rausch* of the Germans. This is valuable only in the operations of short duration, as the entire operation must be completed in a very few minutes. One of the most important details, in operations on the thorax, is the posture of the patient.. In the text-books, almost without exception, the generally accepted procedure is to place the patient on the sound side with a sand bag under the ribs. While this position is most convenient to the operator, rendering the field of operation easy of access and widely separating the intercostal spaces, it may be—so far as the patient is concerned—unwise and even dangerous. The correctness of this statement becomes apparent when we consider that the only or the chiefly available lung capacity is thereby further compromised. This was strikingly borne out in two cases which came to the author's notice. They were cases of empyema in adult males. In both of them death occurred on the table with symptoms of dyspnœa, quick and shallow breathing, and cessation of the pulse. In neither of these cases were the surgical manipulations sufficient to warrant the sudden cessation of life. Nor was it apparently the fault of the anæsthetic, which was given in each case with great care. Hence we are perhaps justified in attributing these deaths to the faulty position in which the patient was placed. The supine position is the proper one to adopt. If it is necessary to make an incision on the posterior aspect of the thorax, this must be done by allowing the side of the thorax to project over the edge of the table. Recently Elsberg, in a series of experiments, has demonstrated that operations on the chest are best borne by the patient when lying flat on the abdomen. In this position it is claimed that the respiratory disturbances due to the opening of the chest cavity are the slightest. Elsberg, himself, induced a double pneumothorax without any alarming symptoms.

Operating in the Sauerbruch Chamber or with the Aid of the Brauer Apparatus.—The experiments of Sauerbruch and Brauer have revolutionized thoracic surgery. Sauerbruch first demonstrated his apparatus before the German Congress of Surgeons in 1902. His aim is to prevent operative pneumothorax by operating under negative pressure (a partial vacuum) in an air-tight chamber. For this purpose only 8 to 10 mm. of negative pressure is necessary. The surgeon himself undergoes no discomfort from this slight reduction of pressure, while it is sufficient absolutely to prevent the collapse of the lung and the subsequent pneumothorax. The patient's head projects from the chamber and the anæsthetic is thus given without difficulty. Either chloroform or ether may be used.

The Sauerbruch apparatus (Fig. 172, on page 418 of Vol. VII.) is based on the fact, known to physiologists, that the normal expansion of the lungs is due to the difference between the positive pressure in the bronchial tree and the negative pressure in the pleural spaces. As long as this negative pressure is continued the collapse of the lung and consequent pneumothorax cannot occur. The Sauerbruch operating chamber is an air-tight room of sufficient size to accommodate an operating table, seats for the operators and assistants, and instrument trays. On one side is an air-tight door, which may further be protected by a small air-tight vestibule, so that one may enter and leave the operating

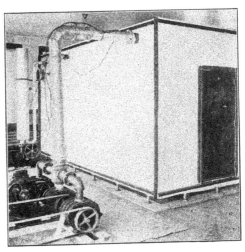

Fig. 21.—View of the Outside of the Universal Differential Pressure Chamber—First Experiment.
(After Meyer.)

room during the operation. On the opposite wall is a circular opening in the chamber partly closed by a collapsible rubber ring. Through this ring the patient's head projects, the rubber fitting closely around the neck. The rubber need not fit tightly, as it is kept firmly in place by the negative pressure within the chamber. On one side of the chamber is an opening connected with a vacuum pump run by an electric motor. On the opposite wall is an ordinary water valve connected with a mercury manometer. The valve is set at − 8 to 10 mm., a sufficient negative pressure to prevent the collapse of the lungs. The valve works automatically. When the pressure is below − 8 to 10 mm., the valve opens and allows a small amount of air to enter until the pressure again rises to − 8 to 10 mm. In this way the air within the chamber is constantly replaced by fresh air from the outside. The chamber may be further elaborated by lights, a telephone, and a small sterilizer.   The chamber in the clinic at Breslau (formerly Mikulicz's clinic) is a very elaborate affair, with all possible improvements. Figs. 21 and 22 represent an improved Sauerbruch chamber, devised at the Rockefeller Institute by Willy Meyer and in use at the German Hospital.   It has the advantage of permitting differential pressure by means of two chambers, one within the other.

The surgery done in the Sauerbruch chamber gives cause for encouragement. The most extensive thoracic resection for recurrent carcinoma of the breast has been done without any pneumothorax.   Of course, before the patient is re-

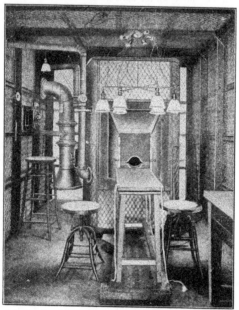

Fig. 22.—View of the Interior of the Universal Differential Pressure Chamber—First Experiment.
(After Meyer.)

moved from the chamber, the opening must be absolutely closed by a skin-muscle flap taken from the back.   The apparatus was originally devised for making the thoracic portion of the œsophagus accessible.   Several attempts at this operation have been made in the Mikulicz clinic since the installation of the Sauerbruch chamber, but none has been successful.   It serves admirably in all ordinary operations of the pleura and lung, where a wide opening of the pleural cavity is necessary.   It scarcely seems possible, however, that the thoracic portion of the œsophagus (as, for example, in a case of carcinoma) will ever come within the realms of surgical intervention, although experiments on animals have occasionally been successful

The Sauerbruch chamber can be used to great advantage in operating on stab and bullet wounds of the heart, as the opening into the pleural sac may be made as large as necessary. It should be remembered, however, that some elevation of pressure is of great advantage in operating on stab wounds of the heart, as hemorrhage is thereby decreased. Sauerbruch reports a very interesting case of this sort. During the suturing of the heart and pericardium, the pressure was merely reduced to − 3. A slight pneumothorax resulted, not enough, however, to bring the patient into any jeopardy. The sutures were passed with a great degree of ease, as there was no bleeding to inconvenience the operator. As soon as the suture was completed, the pressure was again lowered to − 8 mm., the pneumothorax thus being overcome before the flap was replaced.

Brauer devised a positive-pressure apparatus to take the place of the Sauerbruch chamber. His apparatus consists of a mask, which is closely applied to the face. To this is attached a compressed-air tank and an anæsthetic apparatus. A mercury manometer is also attached to the apparatus. In this way the administration of the anæsthetic and the positive air pressure are kept up at the same time, thus maintaining the air in the bronchial tree at a positive pressure and preventing collapse of the lung when the chest is opened. This apparatus is much simpler than the Sauerbruch chamber and is much more available for general use. Only a few of the largest clinics are able to afford the expense of a Sauerbruch chamber. The disadvantages of the Brauer apparatus are the sudden changes in the volume of the lung, the danger of interstitial emphysema, the rapid loss of heat, and the difficulty of maintaining anæsthesia. One of the greatest dangers is that due to the interference with the circulation from the establishment of a positive pressure in the pleural cavity. The apparatus has been used, however, with excellent results in many clinics.

Recently Dryer and Spanaus have endeavored to ascertain experimentally the comparative values of the Sauerbruch and the Brauer apparatus. They made two hundred and fourteen experiments, doing all sorts of operations. They determined that, so far as the practical value is concerned, there is no difference between the two methods of preventing pneumothorax. Kuettner has used both methods an equal number of times and his decision is that they are both of equal value. This being the case, it would seem that the Brauer apparatus is the more valuable of the two, as it is portable, less expensive, and therefore available for a greater number of surgeons. The cabinet of Janeway and Green and the positive pressure incident to the ether administration by the intubation method (Meltzer) are each worthy of the thoughtful consideration that bespeaks beneficent surgical advance.

Dr. Teske has done some experimental work on an entirely new method of avoiding operative pneumothorax by inducing an artificial hydrothorax. He claims that the simple adhesion of the two pleural surfaces is sufficient to prevent the collapsing of the lung. This adhesion he aims to establish by interposing a thin layer of water between the two pleural surfaces. At the beginning of the operation he injects a small amount of sterile salt solution into the pleural cavity. The chest is then opened and a continuous stream of salt water is kept flowing into the pleural spaces. He claims that, by this method, any operative procedures may be carried on easily and without any risk of collapse of the lung. If, on the other hand, the animal is turned on its belly and the water allowed to flow out, the lung immediately collapses. So far, this method has been tried in an experimental way only, but it looks as though it might offer a very safe, easy, and simple method of preventing pneumothorax in operations on the human subject.

The older methods of preventing the collapse of the lung, while not so sure as these newer ones, are, nevertheless, of great importance. Tuffier's original idea, which is still carried out and which the author has used many times, depends on the principle that pneumothorax cannot result without collapse of the lung.

The details of this method are as follows:—An incision is made over a rib and the bone is resected without opening the pleural cavity. Large needles, armed with heavy catgut, are now introduced through the unopened pleura into the lung itself; the number of sutures employed being sufficient to attach the lung firmly to the chest wall. The pleura is then opened. As the operation proceeds, more of the lung is grasped and fastened to the chest wall. In this manner the collapse of the lung is effectually prevented.

Aspiration.—Aspiration is the simplest of all operations on the chest. It rarely comes within the scope of the surgeon and is generally done by the medical practitioner. The chest should be prepared with all the aseptic precautions commonly employed in a major operation, the needle of the aspirator being carefully sterilized. Failure to do this accounts for the relative frequency with which serous effusions are, by repeated aspirations, given a purulent character. The operation is so simple that it is often performed by a physician who is either not conversant with the details of an aseptic technique or disregards them. Aspiration is usually done over the central point of the dulness. In cases where the entire chest is filled with fluid the puncture should be in the sixth or seventh interspace, in the midaxillary line, or in the eighth interspace in the posterior axillary line. If possible, the patient should be in the recumbent posture, with the side of the thorax projecting over the bed. The arm of the affected side should be bent over the head so that the intercostal space is made as wide as possible. Some prefer to do the operation with the patient in the sitting posture. This, however, is somewhat dangerous, as an attack of syncope is liable to occur. The index finger of the left hand having been placed over the centre of the interspace selected, the skin is stretched upward. The aspirating needle is grasped firmly in the right hand and entered with a quick stabbing motion at the lowermost part of the intercostal space. This will prevent any injury of the intercostal vessels. The direction of the needle should be slightly upward, and, if the operation is carried out correctly, the rib need not be touched. If desired, local anæsthesia by means of ethyl chloride may be employed. The operation, however, is so quickly done that it is practically painless.

The withdrawal of the fluid should be effected very slowly, in order that there may not be too rapid a change in the intrathoracic pressure. Most authorities agree that not all the fluid should be withdrawn at one sitting. As soon as the desired amount of fluid has been obtained, the needle is quickly removed and a small pledget of gauze is placed over the opening and fastened by adhesive plaster. It should be remembered that it is necessary to employ a needle of large calibre, one that cannot easily be blocked by flakes of fibrin. The chief danger of the operation is syncope, of which mention has been made above. Cases of sudden death from too rapid evacuation of the fluid have been reported. The danger of hemorrhage is very slight, as the wounding of the lung is effectually prevented by the interposition of the layer of fluid and, if the proper precautions are taken, the intercostal artery is rarely wounded, and then only when the puncture is made in the posterior quarter of the space between the angle of the rib and the spine. Here the intercostal artery runs in the centre of the space and is not protected by the overhanging flange of the rib.

Therapeutically, aspiration is used only in those cases of simple pleurisy with effusion, in which the fluid shows but little or no tendency to undergo absorption, and in certain other cases in which the object is to relieve the distressing symptoms of hydrothorax due to cardiac or renal disease or to an intrathoracic neoplasm. When pus is present, aspiration is of little value as a therapeutic measure, unless supplemented by the methods described in the section relating to the treatment of empyema.

Recently Thiersch has devised a method of continuous drainage for use in cases of empyema. The chest is aspirated through a large trocar and cannula. A large fenestrated Nélaton catheter is passed through the cannula and the latter instrument is then withdrawn. A piece of rubber tissue, provided with a small orifice, is slipped over the catheter and tied fast at the point where it emerges from the chest cavity. The rubber tissue is fastened firmly to the chest wall, thus providing a rather tight closure of the thoracic cavity at the site of puncture. The outer end of the Nélaton catheter is connected with a large soft-walled drainage tube, which fits into a bottle placed below the bed. (Fig. 23.) The large soft tube acts after the fashion of a vein, permitting the exudate to escape under increased internal pleural pressure, while it does not allow the entrance of air because of the coaptation of the walls in inspiration. The result is a reliable mechanism which effectively permits the drainage of the exudate and prevents the occurrence of pneumothorax. Many empyemas and practically all the metapneumonic cases are, according to Friedrich, completely healed by means of this apparatus without further surgical interference.

Thoracotomy.—Thoracotomy is the opening of the chest cavity through an intercostal space. The operation is very simple. As a rule, it may be done under infiltration anæsthesia, by means of the Schleich or other solutions. The site of the incision should be located in the same manner as that for exploratory aspiration. In fact, it is a good plan to precede the incision by exploratory puncture. The skin being pressed upward, an incision, 4 or 5 cm. long, is made over the centre of the interspace selected and the wound is cautiously deepened, layer for layer, until the internal intercostal fascia is reached. A dressing forceps is now introduced in close proximity to the needle and the blades are separated. In this manner the pleura is opened without any danger of hemorrhage. A tube is inserted into the cavity and firmly secured with a silkworm-gut suture and a safety pin. The pus is allowed slowly to escape. The tube should be as large as the interspace will permit and sufficiently firm not easily to collapse. Care should be taken to secure the tube firmly in its place, as it may easily be lost in the pleural cavity.

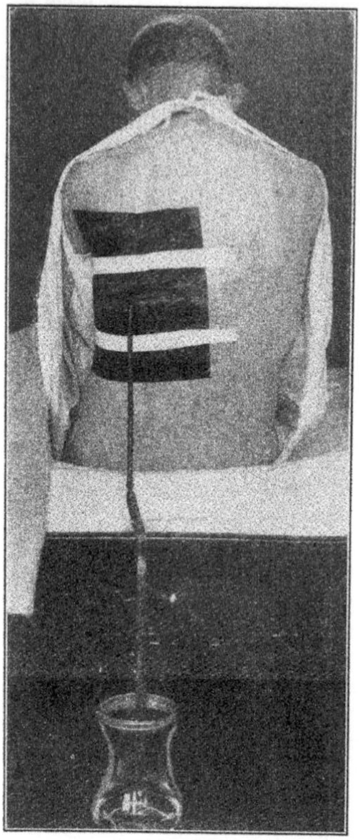

Just a word as to the direction of the tube. Its purpose is merely to keep the wound open and promote discharge, and for this purpose a short tube answers as well as a long one. A long tube is harmful for two reasons: In the first place, it interferes with the proper expansion of the lung; and, in the next place, and still more important, the long tube coming into contact with the visceral pleura is painful and, by its irritation, excites paroxysms of coughing. The operation is finished by placing a very large occlusive dressing around the thorax.

The indications for simple incision (thoracotomy) are not very frequently observed. The space is so small that adequate drainage is almost impossible to establish. The neighboring ribs are apt to compress the drainage tube. The opening does not permit the digital exploration of the cavity, nor does it allow the escape of clots, large masses of fibrin, or inspissated pus, which are almost sure to decompose and thus further to add to the septic symptoms.

Fig. 23.—Thiersch's Drainage.

Simple thoracotomy may, however, be tried in metapneumonic empyemas of very young children, in whom the ribs are elastic enough to permit separation.

Resection of Ribs.—The usual procedure, in the treatment of empyema, is thoracotomy with the resection of a portion of one or, in some cases, more ribs. Here, as in all other purulent accumulations, the desideratum is adequate drainage. The seventh rib, in the mid-axillary or post-axillary line, is usually selected for drainage. Lower ribs are not available for the reason that the diaphragm in its movements is apt to become engaged in and to obliterate the opening. The skin over the rib selected is first put on the stretch between the thumb and forefinger of the left hand and an incision about 4 or 5 cm. in length is made down to the rib. The periosteum is next sharply incised and, with a blunt periosteotome, separated from its outer aspect. The muscles inserted above and below are then, together with the attached periosteum, separated from the bone. Some trouble may be encountered at this point of the operation. Having freed the rib from its periosteum above, below, and in front, the surgeon should introduce a Doyen rib raspatory, and in his manipulations with this instrument he should always keep close to the rib. By moving it sharply backward and forward the rib is entirely freed from its attachments, the pleura being left intact. With the aid of the raspatory, used as a retractor, the soft tissues at the sternal end of the rib are next pushed out of the way, the rib shears introduced, and the rib sharply cut through. The raspatory is now forcibly pushed or pulled toward the dorsal portion of the rib and the soft tissues in this locality are held out of the way. The rib cutter is again introduced and the rib divided. As a rule, in ordinary cases, a piece of the rib, an inch and a half or two inches long, should be removed. If any bleeding is encountered, it is from the intercostal artery, which should be tied. As a rule, however, no hemorrhage is seen. The intercostal fascia and the parietal pleura are next divided by a small incision, thus opening the pleural cavity and allowing the pus to escape. By means of a dressing forceps, the incision is enlarged to the desired extent. When the wound is enlarged in this manner, no troublesome hemorrhage is encountered. If pus is present in large amount it should be evacuated slowly to prevent the possibility of collapse of the lung from sudden change in blood pressure. After the evacuation of the pus the pleural cavity may be thoroughly explored by the operator's finger, and any large masses of detritus removed. The exploration may determine the necessity of immediately making multiple resection. In case the exudation is very fetid, the cavity may be irrigated. As a rule, however, this step is unnecessary, and needlessly prolongs the period of anæsthesia. Furthermore, irrigation has, in a number of instances, been followed by sudden death, probably due to arrest of the heart's action from vagus irritation. As a last step a large drainage tube is inserted securely and a large sterile dressing applied.

Beck advises what he calls "pleurocostomy"—that is, stitching the costal pleura to the skin. This, however, is entirely unnecessary and may result in a permanent fistula.

The post-operative treatment is simple and consists merely in changing the dressing frequently and keeping the tube open. At each change of dressing it is important to make sure that the tube is firmly secured, as these tubes are very frequently lost after the operation. Unless the secretion becomes malodorous, no irrigation is necessary. In many of these acute cases the patient completely recovers in from three to five weeks, the length of time depending on the rapidity with which the lung expands. This expansion may be aided, after the lapse of a few days, by breathing exercises and by the use of the

Woulfe bottles * and markedly by the Bryant apparatus already mentioned. (See page 11.) In children recovery is particularly rapid, probably owing to the great elasticity of the ribs.

The cases offering the gravest prognosis are those of tuberculous origin, as, even after the most radical operation, long-standing suppurating sinuses are apt to result. It must be realized, however, that no patient affected with empyema, even if apparently moribund, is too far gone to be given the chance of recovery which this comparatively simple operation offers. A marked change for the better often occurs within a few hours after the operation.

Thoracoplasty.—When an empyema fails to be relieved by a resection of one or more ribs and drainage, it has a tendency to become inveterate. There then remains within the thorax a pus-secreting cavity, bounded by the chest wall on the one hand and the diaphragm and bound-down lung on the other. The dimensions and location of the cavity necessarily vary within wide limits. In these cases there is no tendency to spontaneous closure, and for the relief of the patient multiple rib resection becomes necessary. The number of ribs to be resected necessarily varies with the dimensions of the cavity. For the formal operation of multiple rib resection, the term "thoracoplasty" has been reserved. Its object is to permit the sinking in of the chest wall by removing the rigid ribs and by applying its soft parts directly to the lung, thus closing the dead space previously occupied by the empyema.

Estlander's Operation.—Estlander's operation consists of the removal of as many ribs as may be necessary through separate incisions made in the line of an intercostal space and of such length as may be necessary for the removal of rib sections of the required length. By making the incision in the intercostal space the sections of the upper and the lower ribs can easily be removed through one incision. Thus, through four separate incisions sections of at least eight ribs may easily be removed. In many cases that are not of too long standing, this operation permits very extensive sinking in of the chest wall; but, when the parietal pleura is very thick and inelastic, the result of changes which have been going on for many years, even very extensive rib resection will fail to produce the desired result.

Schede's Operation.—To overcome the difficulty mentioned in the preceding paragraph, Schede removes not only the ribs, but likewise the offending pleura. His operation is commenced with a large U-shaped incision which begins below the second rib, near its anterior attachment, and extends downward in an oblique direction as far, if necessary, as the tenth rib. Thence, it continues, in a gentle curve with upward concavity, backward to the posterior axillary border, where it gradually extends upward to the posterior border of the scapula as high up, if necessary, as the second rib. The huge flap thus outlined is made to include all of the soft parts down to the ribs and the intercostal muscles. It

---

* Woulfe's apparatus consists of two large wash bottles connected by a rubber tube. These bottles are half-filled with water. By blowing into one bottle, the patient is able to force the fluid, under considerable pressure, into the other bottle. This increases intratracheal pressure and promotes the expansion of the lungs.

is then reflected upward in such a manner that the scapula may be involved. All hemorrhage having been arrested, the ribs are next resected with heavy bone forceps, and with them are included the intercostal muscles and the thickened pleura. The operation is completed after the lung has been decorticated, or after Schede's method of discission of the pleura has been practised by pressing the large flap against the lung. This operation is very severe and is followed, if carried out in the way described, by a relatively high mortality. Therefore, if Schede's operation is to be performed, it may be well to do it in two sittings, the flap being prepared at the first and the rib resections made at the second.

In debilitated subjects the safety of the patient will often require that one or two ribs be resected at a time, beginning from below upward and thus gradually reducing the size of the cavity. In this way it may be that four, five, or even

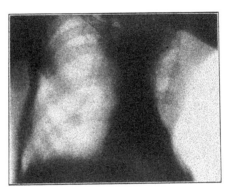

FIG. 24.—Radiogram Showing End-Result after Schede Operation. (Author's first case.)

more operations may be needed for completely closing the cavity. Although in this way more time will be required for effecting a cure, it is a safer course to pursue than that of performing this very extensive operation in one sitting.

It may here be remarked that the operations for empyema are becoming more and more atypical. Where a fistula is present, as it usually is, this is enlarged sufficiently to permit, as far as possible, the digital exploration of the cavity. Guided by the finger, the surgeon makes an incision upward and other incisions in one or two intercostal spaces, and then removes portions of the ribs. Digital exploration is then made, and, if this reveals an extension of the cavity still further upward, the removal of additional sections of ribs is undertaken. Step by step, at one or more operations, the necessary number of ribs is removed. The difficulty, of course, grows as the shorter ribs (especially the first) are reached. The end-results, in two cases of complete Schede operations done by the writers, are shown in the accompanying radiograms. (Figs. 24 and 25.)

Pulmonary Decortication.—Whatever method of thoracoplasty may be adopted, the treatment of the pulmonary pleura by decortication is to be made part of the operation. If one follows the method of Fowler, the thickened pulmonary pleura is removed by careful dissection. Delorme makes a temporary resection of the chest wall by reflecting a large flap consisting of the whole thickness. Decortication of the lung, by the use of knife and scissors, immediately follows. The flap is then replaced, as in the Schede procedure. Temporary resection, by means of a flap of the entire thickness of the chest wall, has had few followers. Decortication—or, preferably, discission of the lung, where practicable—limits the number of ribs to be resected. With the freeing of the lung, by one or the other of these procedures, expansion at once follows, and therefore little deformity results even after extensive rib resection. In many instances there is a tendency to re-formation of the costal arches.

In the rare cases of bilateral empyema, extensive operations on both sides

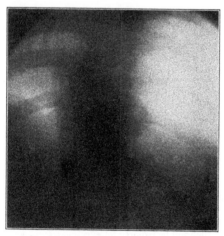

Fig. 25.—Radiogram Showing End-Result of Schede Operation. (Author's second case.)

are not feasible. Aspiration of one side and incision of the other constitute the best treatment available under the circumstances. Temporary improvement is all that can be looked for. At a later operation drainage of the second pleural sac may be established.

Friedrich's Multiple Rib Resection for the Treatment of Unilateral Pulmonary Tuberculosis.—The patient, who is usually in a debilitated condition, must be carefully prepared by a pre-operative course of forced feeding and stimulation. Friedrich recommends a preliminary course of treatment with digitalis for the purpose of toning up the heart. The operation may be begun under infiltration anæsthesia; but, as general anæsthesia is, as a rule, necessary before the operation is completed, it is as well to begin immediately with chloroform. The large U-shaped flap incision, spoken of in the description of the Schede operation, is the one to be employed. The incision should be begun at the point of origin

of the pectoralis major muscle on the second rib; it should next be carried
downward, with a slight anterior convexity, to the tenth rib; then it should
be continued along the upper border of the tenth rib nearly to the erector spinæ
muscle; and, finally, it should be continued upward to a point on the second
rib midway between the spine and the scapula.   The ribs, from the second to
the tenth inclusive, should be well exposed, and all the soft parts, together with
the scapula, should be reflected upward.   Beginning with the tenth rib each
rib is completely removed in the following manner:—An incision is made through
the periosteum of the entire exposed portion of the rib.   Then a Doyen rib
elevator is passed completely around the rib and pushed rapidly forward and
backward until it has completely separated the rib from the soft parts.   The
rib is next divided anteriorly as far forward as possible.   The surgeon, grasping the divided end of the rib and using the index finger to protect the underlying pleura, then removes the entire section of the rib by a twisting movement.
The intercostal muscles are now removed by blunt dissection and the intercostal
arteries are tied.   Great care should be taken to avoid any injury of the underlying pleura.   The flap is finally replaced, a small opening being left at the
lower posterior angle for drainage.   If the patient is in a condition unsuitable
for enduring the complete operation at one time, it may be performed in several
sittings.   The after-treatment is simply the resumption of the dietetic and
hygienic régime.

Pneumectomy.—*Partial Pneumectomy.*—Partial pneumectomy has occasionally been practised in cases of malignant disease, in severe lacerations, and
several times in isolated tuberculous lesions.   It is, however, an operation which
is rarely justifiable.   After the lesion has been located, the chest cavity is
opened by an intercostal incision and the ribs are widely separated by Friedrich's rib spreader.   (Fig. 26.)   It is rarely necessary to resect a rib.   The
diseased portion of the lung is grasped by the hand and delivered to the outside.
A heavy clamp is fastened securely over the base of the part to be resected.
By traction on this clamp as large a portion of the lung as is desired may be
delivered.   When the diseased portion has been completely delivered, its base
is compressed with an angeiotribe and the lung removed either with a knife or
with the thermocautery.   The hemorrhage is controlled by whipping over the
stump with a deep continuous interlocking suture.   A second layer of sutures
is now applied in much the same manner as the Lembert suture in intestinal
work.   (Fig. 27.)   It is usually necessary to drain the thoracic cavity after
pneumectomy.

Complete Pneumectomy.—Complete pneumectomy has been most carefully
worked out on dogs by Willy Meyer.   The chief difficulty of this operation—
complete closure of the bronchial lumen—has been most carefully elaborated.
The following description is quoted from Willy Meyer's article.   (*Jour. Amer.
Med. Ass'n*, Dec. 11th, 1909.)   "Through an intercostal incision the lung is pulled
forward with the left hand and its main bronchus palpated; with an anatomic
forceps the spaces between the accompanying vessels and bronchial wall are penetrated, one after the other, from the front backward; a silk thread is pushed

between the blades of the forceps by the assistant and pulled through by the operator. Then, traction being exerted on the first ligature, a second silk thread is pulled through and tied distally. The vessel is then divided. The vessels are tied, one after the other, close to the heart. This manner of securing the vessels in the depth of the thoracic cavity is preferable to using a Deschamps needle with a double thread. According to anatomic findings, which vary much according to the early or late division of the pulmonary vessels, from two to four such vessels have to be ligated. The bronchus is now entirely freed;

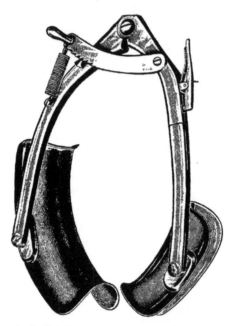

FIG. 26.—Rib-spreader, for Use in Operations on the Lungs. (After Mikulicz, modified according to Fr'edrich; about one-half actual size.)

the loose connective tissue is pushed off with a gauze mop, proximally and distally, in order to have the bronchial stump as long as possible. A bayonet clamp is placed on the bronchus near to its base, its blades being covered with rubber tubing. Above it the bronchus is crushed, usually with Doyen's large intestinal crusher. The remaining fibrous sheath is ligated with silk, a clamp is placed distally, and the bronchus is cut off. Before the bayonet clamp is removed, or after its removal, according to the ease of access, the bronchus is secured on both sides with a pointed forceps. In order to accomplish this safely, a branch of the vagus nerve must often be pushed aside with a blunt instrument. Care should be exercised to avoid injuring the nerve. The two clamps are pulled on and the crushed part is pushed back into the lumen of the bronchus with anatomic forceps or a tucker. Two or three top sutures (silk) draw the uncrushed part of the stump over the buried, crushed portion. The sutures should not include much tissue and they should not penetrate into the lumen of the bronchus. When they are tied, air-tight occlusion results. If material is lacking, the pericardium can be hooked by the needle on one side of the bronchial stump and thus used to advantage for closure." The operation, which

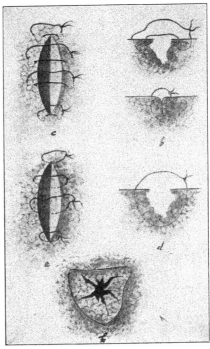

FIG. 27.—Diagram Showing Sutures in Lung Tissue and a Wound in the Lung. (After Friedrich.) *a–c*, Inverted sutures; *d* and *e*, penetrating sutures; *f*, excision of a wound of the lung.

must be done under some form of differential pressure, is completed by closing the thoracic wound and making it as air-tight as possible.

Operations on the Anterior Mediastinum.—Access to the anterior mediastinum is best obtained through the sternum. An incision is made down to the bone and the soft parts are retracted. The sternum may be removed in one of several ways. Probably the safest is to use the trephine, or, better still, the burrs recently devised by Hudson. Friedrich advises the transverse division of the sternum between the second and third ribs, with the ligation of the internal mammary arteries. A more serious method of procedure is that advised by Milton—the vertical splitting of the sternum with saw and chisel. After the bone has been removed in one of these ways, the incision is deepened by blunt dissection and the tissues of the anterior mediastinum are exposed. This operation is usually done for the relief of mediastinal abscess. In these cases the abscess should be opened, as far as possible, by means of blunt dissection. Dr. Christian has collected the reports of forty cases of dermoids and teratomata that were removed from the anterior mediastinum.

Operations on the Posterior Mediastinum.—The object of such an operation is to obtain access either to the œsophagus or to one of the bronchi. The patient is placed in a prone position. Beginning at a point on the third rib, three inches distant from the vertebral column, the surgeon carries an incision down to and a little beyond the sixth rib. From the ends of this incision he carries transverse incisions inward to the vertebral column. The exposed ribs are then resected subperiosteally. In order to obtain sufficiently free access, it is at times necessary to resect the transverse processes of the vertebræ. If it is desired to expose the œsophagus, a bougie should be introduced into it through the mouth. If this operation is carried on in the pneumatic cabinet, the pleura may be freely opened. If, however, the operation is done under ordinary conditions, the pleura must be carefully pushed away by blunt dissection. Great care should be taken not to injure the important nerves in the posterior mediastinum. If possible, these operations should be completed without drainage.

SURGERY OF THE SPLEEN.

By ALEXANDER ESSLEMONT GARROW, M.D., C.M. (McGill), Montreal, Canada.

Anatomy of the Spleen.—*Blood-Vessels, Lymphatics, Nerves.*—This duct-less gland, essentially a lymphatic structure, and classed among the accessory organs of nutrition (Piersol), lies far back in the left hypochondrium, between the fundus of the stomach and the diaphragm. It is very vascular and highly elastic, has a purplish color, and varies markedly in shape, size, and weight. Its long axis lies parallel with the back part of the tenth rib and it extends from the ninth to the eleventh ribs in the mid-axillary line.

The phrenic surface, convex and rarely fissured, is moulded to the diaphragm. The gastric and renal surfaces, directed to the right, are in relation with the stomach and left kidney. Lying between these visceral surfaces and the phrenic area is a triangular part, which rests upon the splenic flexure of the colon and the costo-colic ligament.

The anterior border separates the phrenic from the gastric surface; it is sharp, and presents the characteristic notches, which can be palpated in movable and enlarged spleens.

The splenic artery lies between the layers of the lieno-renal ligament, but before it enters the hilus, situated on the gastric surface, it divides into seven or eight branches. The splenic vein lies in the same fold of peritoneum and receives the blood from the inferior mesenteric vein.

While the splenic pulp has no lymphatic vessels, those from the capsule unite to form channels lying in the lieno-renal ligament.

The filaments of the splenic plexus of nerves accompany the ramifications of the artery into the organ.

Structure of the Spleen.—Beneath the serous coat there is a firm fibrous capsule containing elastic fibres and involuntary muscle cells. Numerous bands—trabeculæ—arising from the capsule divide the spleen into many lobes; these are further subdivided into smaller compartments by a fine recticular structure arising from the trabeculæ. Lymphoid tissue, in the form of cords, occupies the compartments. The terminal branches of the splenic artery penetrate the pulp-cords and open into the venous radicles which lie between the cords of lymphoid tissue. This anatomical structure explains the great difficulty in controlling hemorrhage in splenic wounds.

The Malpighian corpuscles are dense accumulations of lymphoid tissue in the adventitia of the splenic radicles.

The spleen is supported by three folds of peritoneum—the licno-renal, gastro-splenic, and costo-colic.

Physiology of the Spleen; Results Following Extirpation.—Our knowledge of the functions of the spleen is very imperfect. A ductless gland, it is supposed to possess an internal secretion which, judging from the effects of splenectomy, is not essential to health, or, if it is, can readily be supplied by other organs or tissues.

The spleen shares with the lymph nodes and bone marrow in the formation of white cells. In severe anæmias it is believed to revert to its fœtal function of forming red cells; in health and in disease, it destroys them. What useful purpose is served by its rhythmical contractions and dilatations, and by its engorgement after meals, we do not know. That it plays some part in metab-

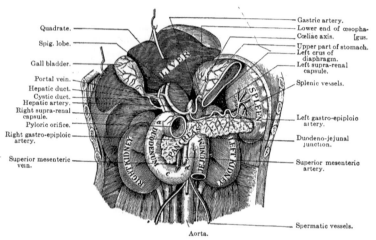

Quadrate.

Spig. lobe.

Gall bladder.

Portal vein.
Hepatic duct.
Cystic duct.
Hepatic artery.
Right supra-renal capsule.
Pyloric orifice.

Right gastro-epiploic artery.

Superior mesenteric vein.

Gastric artery.
Lower end of œsopha-
Cœliac axis.   [gus.
Upper part of stomach.
Left crus of diaphragm.
Left supra-renal capsule

Splenic vessels.

Left gastro-epiploic artery.

Duodeno-jejunal junction.

Superior mesenteric artery.

Spermatic vessels.

Aorta.

Fig. 28.—Semi-diagrammatic Representation of the Relations of the Spleen to the Neighboring Intra-Abdominal Organs. (After Testut.)

olism is suggested by the quantity and variety of nitrogenous compounds which are found in it.

The enlargement of the spleen in many infectious diseases and intoxications may indicate a reaction that is destined to assist that which takes place in lymphatic structures in general, providing a defensive mechanism against bacteria and their toxins.

Extirpation of the human spleen for injury and disease has become an event of frequent occurrence during the last decade. Post-operative studies, in these cases, while teaching us that an alteration in the blood is the most constant feature following splenectomy, have added little to our knowledge of splenic functions. In the main, Warthin's observations on splenectomized animals have been corroborated by these investigations. The loss of a normal spleen, as in the case of trauma, seems to be followed by more disturbance than occurs when the organ is diseased; in the latter, vicarious compensation may have existed for months or years. In a few instances very unusual symptoms have occurred, such as profound anæmia, marked emaciation, great muscular weakness, cardiac disturbances, high fever, abdominal pain, etc. Sepsis, thrombosis, and severe hemorrhage of pre-operative or operative origin may, in such cases, be responsible for these uncommon sequelæ.

A transitory hypertrophy of the thyroid gland, mental derangement, and epileptiform convulsions have occurred in a few cases. On the other hand, recovery has taken place without any appreciable disturbance.

The blood changes, on the whole, are common, and are as follows:—(1) A moderate fall in the number of red cells; (2) a genuine though transitory leucocytosis; (3) a primary fall in the percentage of hæmoglobin, which gradually rises to the normal; (4) in from four to eight weeks there develops a relative and actual lymphocytosis; (5) a moderate eosinophilia occurring later, possibly after months.

A persistent and very marked leucocytosis accompanied by fever indicates sepsis.

Enlargement of the lymph nodes, common in splenectomized animals, is seldom seen in the human being after extirpation of the spleen.

Pain in the long bones, particularly in the tibiæ, is due to compensatory changes in the medulla, which becomes more vascular, assumes the fœtal type, and is rich in nucleated red cells.

Malformations and Anomalies of the Spleen.—Congenital absence is usually associated with other errors of development.

Large spleens at, or soon after, birth are due as a rule to syphilis or rickets.

The single notch may be replaced by several. Deep fissures may partially or completely divide the organ into several parts constituting lobulated or multiple spleens.

The normal or undersized spleen may have associated with it numerous splenculi—accessory spleens or small portions of splenic tissue—scattered over the peritoneum, but chiefly in the gastro-splenic omentum.

The spleen at birth may occupy any part of the abdominal cavity, and occasionally even the chest, when the diaphragm is imperfect. Litten states that it has been found within the stomach.

No other organ exhibits such variations in shape.

Wandering Spleen.—The normal spleen has a limited range of movement due to the excursions of the diaphragm. No abdominal organ, however, can wander so far afield as this gland does when it becomes a vagrant. When a wandering spleen becomes fixed in a new situation by adhesions it is said to be dislocated. (Fig. 29.)

Movable spleen is more common in women who have borne children than in men.

ETIOLOGY.—Splenomegaly from splenic anæmia, leukæmia, etc., is not a frequent factor in producing mobility. Perisplenic adhesions and compensatory hypertrophy of its ligaments prevent displacement in these diseases. Acquired or congenital elongation, undue elasticity or weakness of the suspensory ligaments, seem to be the chief causes. The condition has been discovered in several members of a family.

Splenoptosis may exist alone or it may be associated with a movable kidney (very rare) or a general enteroptosis.

Rupture of the ligaments from violence is mentioned both by Litten and by Ssawiljew as a cause of acute displacement.

While more frequently found in the left iliac fossa, a movable spleen may occupy the pelvis, right iliac fossa, or the sac of an inguinal hernia; indeed, it may lie in any part of the abdominal cavity.

PATHOLOGY.—Occasionally but little change from the normal will be found. As a rule, however, owing to circulatory disturbances brought about by traction,

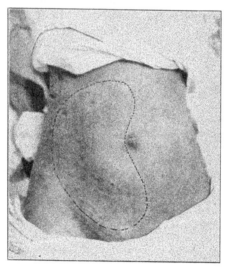

FIG. 29.—Wandering Spleen Compl cat ng a Pregnancy at the Fourth Month. (Case of Dr. Asa B. Davis, reported in the Bulletin of the Lying-in Hospital, New York City. The organ was successfully removed.)

pressure, and slow torsion, the organ is enlarged from venous congestion and parenchymatous hemorrhage, or diminished from sclerosis and atrophy. Adhe-sions to neighboring structures are very common.

When acute torsion of the pedicle induces strangulation the spleen becomes enlarged and congested, hemorrhagic infarcts and subcapsular hemorrhage occur, and in time the organ may become gangrenous, rupture, or be the seat of an abscess.

SYMPTOMS.—A movable spleen, like a movable kidney, may be discovered by accident; the condition having given rise to no symptoms. More frequently, however, it causes considerable distress and may jeopardize life from twisting of the pedicle or from obstruction of the bowels, either by traction on its adhesions or by pressure. A sense of weight and dragging, and pain of a dull aching character referred upward are common. Rectal and vesical tenesmus may occur when the spleen is impacted in the pelvis. Menstrual disturbances, chronic constipation, and digestive disturbances are due to pressure or traction. Sharp attacks of abdominal pain, associated with variations in the size of the gland, are believed to be due to disturbances in the circulation brought about by slow torsion or by thrombosis of the vessels of the pedicle.

When there is an associated general enteroptosis there will often be present the symptoms of general neurasthenia—headache, insomnia, nervousness, digestive disturbances, and constipation.

Hæmatemesis and melæna would indicate obstruction to the circulation induced by a spreading thrombosis or by traction on the vessels.

Jaundice and ascites may also occur.

Twisting of the pedicle gives rise to sudden and very alarming abdominal symptoms characterized by pain, vomiting, constipation, marked tenderness, and usually a distinct increase in the size of the spleen. Bland Sutton has drawn attention to the sudden diminution in the size of the organ at operation, when the torsion is untwisted.

DIAGNOSIS.—The diagnosis, in many cases, is very simple. A normal-sized soft spleniform mass exhibiting the characteristic notch or notches, and moving by posturing into the left hypochondrium, will not likely be mistaken for anything else; but an enlarged dislocated spleen, impacted in the pelvis, can readily be taken for an ovarian or uterine tumor. In the general abdominal cavity it has been mistaken for a tumor of the kidney, an appendicular abscess, a mass of impacted feces, a displaced kidney, and an ovarian tumor.

TREATMENT.—A simple wandering spleen causing no symptoms should be treated by the application of a suitable pad and an abdominal belt.

A painful wandering spleen, giving rise to repeated attacks of abdominal distress, especially when associated with variations in its size and marked tenderness, should be subjected to splenopexy, since in the majority of cases adhesions will have formed and there is besides the danger of twisting of the pedicle.

Twisting of the pedicle demands immediate operation. If the congestion rapidly subsides after untwisting, and there is no evidence of gangrene or necrosis, splenopexy should be done. If, on the other hand, the spleen is the seat of hemorrhagic infarction, rupture, or gangrene, or if the splenic vessels are thrombosed, splenectomy should be performed. (See Operations on the Spleen.) One should carefully examine the pedicle for the tail of the pancreas before applying the ligatures, and should note the condition of the mesenteric vessels and of those lying in the gastro-splenic fold.

Splenectomy for wandering spleen, complicating pregnancy, has been successfully performed. (Bulletin of the Lying-in Hospital of the City of New York, Asa B. Davis, 1908, V., 24.)

The examination of the spleen, following its removal, has revealed evidence of disease not previously suspected, viz., tuberculosis.

Rupture of the Spleen.—Rupture of a normal spleen is due to severe violence inflicted on the lower part of the thorax or upper part of the abdomen on the left side. It is usually associated with injury to the left kidney, left lobe of the liver, stomach, tail of the pancreas, intestines, or with fractured rib, lacerated lung and pleura; one or more of these may be involved. There may be no evidence of cutaneous injury.

Rupture of a diseased and especially an enlarged spleen, such as is present in malaria, leukæmia, and typhoid fever, may, on the other hand, follow slight injury, such as a push, or a simple muscular action as in bending, and it is said to occur spontaneously. Subcutaneous rupture is more common than an open wound of the spleen.

ETIOLOGY.—Kicks, blows, crushing injuries, falls from a height, being run over by cabs, automobiles, etc., and precipitate labor have produced rupture of the spleen.

In enlarged spleens the exposed position of the organ, the tense capsule, the friable condition of the hyperæmic tissue, and frequently the presence of infarcts, explain the liability to rupture.

Bryan (*Annals of Surgery*, 1909, 50, 856) has collected twenty-five cases of ruptured spleen that occurred during typhoid fever. In not a single instance was the diagnosis made prior to operation. This complication usually occurs about the beginning of the third week, and it may be the unsuspected cause of a sudden and fatal termination at this stage of the disease.

PATHOLOGY.—The lesion or lesions present will depend upon the pre-existing state of the spleen, whether normal or diseased, and upon the nature and severity of the accident. A slight injury to the normal spleen may merely occasion a small parenchymatous or subcapsular hemorrhage. Such hemorrhages may be completely absorbed or they may become encapsulated, giving rise to simple cysts.

Occasionally the capsule softens and ruptures, the effused blood exciting peritoneal irritation and, it may be, signs of severe internal hemorrhage, in an apparently convalescent case. .

Complete tears may be single or multiple; a part of the spleen or even the whole organ may be torn away, and come to lie with clots in any part of the peritoneal cavity.

Cantlie (*Journal of Tropical Medicine and Hygiene*, 1907–1908, X.–XI., 201) calls attention to the frequency of rupture on the visceral surface (internal), in malarial spleens. He reports six out of seven cases in which this lesion was produced by slight, external violence.

The effused blood may be clotted in the neighborhood of the spleen; elsewhere it is fluid. It may be found in the lesser cavity of the peritoneum, from associated injury.

SYMPTOMS.—In general, the symptoms are those of severe abdominal injury —symptoms and signs of shock and collapse, accompanied by those of internal hemorrhage.

Kelly compares the condition of a ruptured pathologic spleen with that of a ruptured tubal gestation. The early abdominal signs may be overlooked or masked in the presence of other associated injuries such as concussion of the brain, pulmonary injury, multiple fractures, etc.

The pain is referred to the upper left quadrant; it increases in severity and extent. There is tenderness over this area and usually there is also early rigidity. The pain is aggravated by respiration and especially by pressure on the last two ribs. (Eliot.) All of these signs gradually increase in severity and extent and are followed by meteorism.

Dulness, at first recognized in the left flank, spreads as the bleeding increases. Ballance and Pitt (Clin. Soc. Trans., 1896, XXIX., 77) called attention to the immovable character of the dulness of the left flank, in bleeding from ruptured spleen. In this locality the blood tends to clot early, whereas in the lower abdomen and right flank, the blood remains fluid, and hence the dulness is movable in these areas. This sign has been corroborated by numerous observations.

As a rule, there is marked evidence of shock and collapse. Pallor, restlessness, dizziness, and syncope are in proportion to the amount of blood lost. Signs and symptoms of hemorrhage may be delayed for hours or even for a day or two, when the primary hemorrhage is retained within the capsule.

A simple contusion of the spleen may give rise to all of the aforementioned symptoms, save those of severe hemorrhage.

PROGNOSIS.—The prognosis depends upon the extent of the injury and the amount of blood lost. Death may take place within half an hour, usually from hemorrhage and shock combined. Vincent (Revue de Chirurg., 1893, XIII., 449) says that seventy-five out of one hundred deaths from ruptured spleen are due to hemorrhage.

Ross (Annals of Surgery, 1908, XLVII., 66), quoting Berger's statistics, says that in ninety-two per cent of the unoperated cases of ruptured spleen the patient dies.

TREATMENT.—An early diagnosis and prompt surgical intervention may materially lessen the high mortality in those affected with hemorrhage from the spleen. A ruptured spleen or a suspected rupture of this organ demands immediate laparotomy. Open the abdomen through the left semilunar line. If the spleen or its pedicle be the source of the bleeding, control the hemorrhage by digital compression of the pedicle, until clots and blood are removed. The damaged organ is examined and, if only a single rent exists, an attempt to close it, by suture and an omental graft or gauze packing, should be made, provided the organ is normal and not enlarged. When a large part of the spleen is torn off, or if the organ is extensively lacerated, remove it. If it be widely adherent to surrounding parts from an old perisplenitis, splenectomy should not be attempted, but firm packing applied. Statistics show that the best results follow tamponade. Suturing alone is not safe.

Before the abdomen is closed care should be taken to explore thoroughly contiguous organs. Breaking this rule has been responsible for death from a continuation of the bleeding from renal, mesenteric, or other vessels, and from infective peritonitis due to an unrecognized ruptured bowel.

Combat shock and the effects of hemorrhage by all useful and well-tried means.

When gauze packing is used, it is well to employ a drainage tube in the loin. In aseptic cases of splenectomy the wound should be closed without drainage.

In complete avulsion, ligate every bleeding vessel in the pedicle; clamps may be employed in urgent cases.

For Senn's method of closing wounds in the spleen see "Operations." The cautery should not be used in splenic hemorrhage. The removal of gauze packing may be followed by hemorrhage.

Chaput (Bull. et Mém. de la Soc. de Chirurg., 1908, XXXIV., 1171) successfully removed both spleen and kidney for injury.

Stab Wounds and Gunshot Wounds of the Spleen.—Compared with rupture and contusion of the spleen, stab wounds and gunshot wounds are comparatively rare. The latter are more frequent than the former. Penetrating wounds of the upper left quadrant, left flank, or lower left thoracic region may be followed by partial or complete prolapse of the spleen.

Open wounds of the spleen are almost invariably complicated with injury to contiguous organs and structures. Legueu (Bull. et Mém. de la Soc. de Chirurg., Dec. 25th, 1906, 1084) collected thirty-three cases of stab wounds in which the pleura and diaphragm were involved in one hundred per cent; the stomach and liver in forty-two per cent; the kidney in twenty-four per cent; the intestines in fifteen per cent; and Lejars ("Chirurgie d'Urgence") refers to complicating pulmonary and pancreatic lesions.

Injury to the spleen is to be suspected, when the situation and direction of a penetrating wound or the points of entrance and exit of a perforating wound, with its intervening track, are so situated as to involve the splenic region.

SYMPTOMS.—There are none which are pathognomonic, but there will be evidence of an intra-abdominal lesion, as shown by local and general signs and symptoms,—viz.: shock, tenderness, local rigidity, etc.,—to which will be added those indicative of moderate or severe hemorrhage. A rapidly spreading peritonitis suggests involvement of a hollow viscus.

If the patient is seen early, a prolapsed spleen is readily recognized. This may occur through a comparatively small wound, which strangulates the protruding part, and in time may lead to gangrene.

The mortality is high, due largely to hemorrhage and to other visceral complications.

TREATMENT.—Immediate laparotomy is demanded in every case of suspected wound of the spleen. Every useful means of combating shock and counteracting the effects of hemorrhage should be employed while one is performing the operation. The site of the incision will depend upon the certainty of the diagnosis; it is preferably made through the outer border of the left rectus. Bleeding from the organ or from one of its vessels should be immediately controlled by digital compression of the pedicle, while the clots are removed and fluid blood is rapidly soaked up by pads. The further treatment will depend upon the condition of the patient and the character of the splenic injury.

Fragmentation or pulpification of the organ requires splenectomy. Extensive injury to the vessels in the pedicle necessitates removal of the organ. Clean cuts, whenever possible, should be closed by mattress sutures of catgut, introduced by a blunt needle, but an omental graft or a gauze tamponade should be added to give additional security.

In lacerated wounds with or without loss of substance an attempt should be made to control hemorrhage by tamponade, but, if this fails, splenectomy should be performed. In the majority of cases it is wise to use a rubber drainage tube in the loin. The mortality is greater for splenectomy than for suture and tamponade in treating gunshot and stab wounds of the spleen.

An uninjured prolapsed spleen should be carefully cleansed and replaced after the incision has been freely enlarged.

The gangrenous portion of a strangulated spleen has been removed with the Paquelin cautery, the resulting area being allowed to heal and retract (Burgess, in *Indian Medical Gazette*, Nov., 1906, 445). In the majority of cases, however, the infected organ will be best treated by splenectomy, either through a fresh incision or by an enlargement of the original one. Drainage should be employed.

Having dealt with the spleen the surgeon should make a careful examination of the stomach, intestines, liver, kidney, pancreas, etc., and any injuries found should be suitably treated.

Abscess of the Spleen.—Suppuration in the spleen is not of frequent occurrence. This may be explained on the assumption that it possesses strong bactericidal properties. (Adami and Nicholls.) An abscess may develop in the spleen without discoverable cause, the pus being sterile; or it may follow a subcutaneous injury, being then possibly due to hæmatogenous infection of a hæmatoma. The organ may become involved in suppuration, by the extension of an infective process in one of the neighboring organs or tissues, such as a perinephritic or subdiaphragmatic abscess, an empyema, a perforating duodenal or gastric ulcer, etc. In pyæmia it is—though less frequently than is the case in many other organs—the seat of multiple foci of pus.

Secondary infection is invariably due to septic embolic infarcts or to metastatic inflammation. The primary focus may be anywhere in the body, and may have perfectly healed. Secondary abscess in the spleen may, though rarely, be a complication of malaria, relapsing fever, or typhoid. Johnson ("Surgical Diagnosis," II.) reports an instance in which the abscess was due to putrid thrombosis of the splenic artery, there being at the same time suppuration in the head of the pancreas. Anderson (*Indian Medical Gazette*, June, 1906, 212) reports two cases of abscess in malarial fever. In both of these, the abscess, which contained much pus and necrotic tissue, was due, he thinks, to secondary infection of a hemorrhagic infarct.

The absœsses may be multiple or single, deep-seated or superficial, very small or very large. Litten reports one that contained 15 litres of pus, and Lyons, commenting on the case, says that such an abscess might simulate ascites. Numerous adhesions may bind the organ to the stomach, colon, diaphragm, or abdominal wall. The pus may be thin or thick, yellow or dark-brown, fetid from gangrenous or necrotic tissue, sterile and odorless, or teeming with micro-organisms.

SYMPTOMS AND CLINICAL COURSE.—A splenic abscess may be latent. In the fulminating form there will be the general and local signs of deep-seated suppuration. Fever is variable, but is apt to assume the hectic type; emaciation is pronounced, and gastro-intestinal disturbances are prominent; diarrhœa is frequently present, and there will be a leucocytosis. Pain, dull and aching or lancinating, often radiates to the left shoulder. Tenderness and local rigidity will be in proportion to the perisplenitis. Inflammatory œdema over the splenic area is suggestive of advancing suppuration.

It should be remembered, however, that simple enlargement of the spleen occurs in those diseases which are most often complicated by splenic abscess.

A small central splenic abscess may become encapsulated and its contents inspissated or infiltrated with lime salts.

Where the suppuration advances rapidly the abscess may rupture into the peritoneal cavity, one of the hollow viscera, or the pelvis of the kidney, or it may perforate the diaphragm, invade the pleura or lung, and be discharged through a bronchus.

Belloni and Moschini (Abstract in *Jour. Amer. Med. Assn.*, 1910, LIV., 1097) report two cases. In one a subphrenic abscess was suspected, but the autopsy showed the presence of a small splenic abscess with independent empyema.

The diagnosis of splenic abscess is difficult, for the condition may simulate subdiaphragmatic or perinephritic abscess, or even simple enlargement of the spleen.

The mortality is very high, whether the abscess be treated surgically or left alone, since it complicates an already serious condition, viz., pyæmia, grave typhoid, severe malaria, suppurating peritonitis, etc.

TREATMENT.—Abscess of the spleen has been successfully treated by repeated aspiration, incision, and drainage, and by splenectomy.

Aspiration is hazardous and not likely to be successful. The aspirating needle can be used safely only when the spleen is adherent to the abdominal wall.

The site of the incision will depend upon the size of the organ. It may be necessary to resect a portion of the ninth or tenth rib and then incise the abscess through the diaphragm, the operation being performed in one or two stages. An intraperitoneal incision will enable the operator to ascertain the size of the organ, the presence or absence of adhesions, and the possible existence of a suppurating perisplenitis. With such information he can then readily decide whether it is better to drain through the chest, the flank, or the anterior abdominal wall. A non-adherent suppurating spleen might better be removed in order to avoid peritoneal infection. Splenectomy should not be attempted when the spleen is extensively adherent.

Tuberculosis of the Spleen.—Primary tuberculosis of the spleen is rare. A few cases have been diagnosed prior to operation or autopsy. Secondary involvement is more common in children, less so in adults. In both forms the spleen is moderately enlarged; the parenchyma is soft, swollen, dark-red in color, and scattered over with minute, round, gray tubercles. In the chronic form cheesy nodules, as large as hempseeds or hazelnuts, may be rarely found, since death usually occurs before such changes have taken place.

Carle, Lannelongue, and others report successful splenectomies for supposed primary tuberculosis of the spleen. (Moynihan.)

Litten reminds us that amyloid spleen may coexist with tuberculous infiltration in the chronic varieties of tuberculosis.

Localized tenderness and pain usually indicate perisplenitis.

Splenectomy is indicated for tuberculous spleen provided the diagnosis can be made and that the disease does not exist elsewhere, at least in a severe or active form.

Tumors of the Spleen.—The relative immunity of the spleen from newgrowths has long been recognized, but no satisfactory explanation has been offered to account for this. Primary tumors in this organ are of such infrequent occurrence that they are classed among the curiosities of surgery and pathology. Even secondary growths are comparatively rare.

Fibroma, adenoma, and other varieties of benign tumors have been described by the pathologist, but they are of no surgical interest.

Sarcoma of the spleen, though rare, is the most common tumor met with. Jepson and Albert (*Annals of Surgery*, 1904, XL, p. 81) describe a fibrous, a lymphoid, and an endothelial form, according as the tumor originates in the capsule and trabeculæ, in the lymphoid tissue, or in the endothelial structure.

Pathologists are not agreed upon the nature of the endothelial overgrowths not infrequently met with in this organ.

The aforementioned authors report thirty-two cases of primary sarcoma, including one of their own. Twelve were operated upon by splenectomy.

The case which was reported by Heinricus, and which was treated by enucleation, under the assumption that it was benign, proved on microscopical examination to be a sarcoma.

DIAGNOSIS AND SYMPTOMS.—The diagnosis of sarcoma at an early stage is beset with difficulty. The spleen cannot be palpated and percussion is not to be relied upon. Pain may or may not be present at the beginning. As a rule a sarcoma grows rapidly.

In a displaced organ, or when the growth is large enough to project beyond the costal margin, the discovery of a hard, nodular, irregular mass in the spleen is strongly suggestive of sarcoma.

It should be kept in mind that in all other enlargements the outline of the spleen is more or less retained.

Pain radiating in character, tenderness on pressure, and cachexia are present in varying degrees. Examination of the blood throws no light on the condition.

TREATMENT.—If the diagnosis can be established before metastases take place, infiltrating adhesions form, or recognizable cachexia appears, then splenectomy should be performed. Otherwise operation is useless and unjustifiable.

Primary cancer, while theoretically possible from overgrowth of epithelial inclusions, is unknown; even secondary carcinomatous masses are rarely seen in the spleen.

Cysts of the Spleen.—*Simple Cyst.*—Simple cysts of the spleen may be large or small, unilocular or multilocular, subcapsular or deep-seated. Their sac wall varies in thickness, is usually lined with epithelium, and in old cysts may be infiltrated with lime salts. The color and specific gravity of the fluid vary. In serous cysts it is a clear, pale, or straw-colored fluid of low specific gravity. Hemorrhagic cysts contain blood or blood remnants in varying quantities. Lymph cysts have a clear transparent fluid rich in albumin. They may remain stationary or grow slowly in size. Rapid enlargement is usually due to hemorrhage. Cholesterin and hæmatin crystals, one or both, are invariably present in the fluid.

While the mode of origin of these cysts is obscure, it is believed that trauma plays an important rôle in their production. Some may arise from degeneration of pulp tissue.

Small deep-seated cysts are discovered only at autopsy. Large cysts cause splenomegaly, with or without displacement. A feeling of weight or fulness may lead to the discovery of a tumor. Marked enlargement in the upper pole may cause dyspnœa and palpitation of the heart. Nausea, vomiting, and constipation are due to pressure or traction of a rapidly growing cyst. Pain and tenderness are due either to rapid enlargement from hemorrhage, to stretching of the capsule, or to an associated perisplenitis. Fluctuation in a splenic growth is pathognomonic.

A simple cyst of the spleen may be mistaken for a pancreatic, a mesenteric, or an ovarian cyst, for cystic disease of the left kidney or left lobe of the liver, or for a left hydronephrosis.

A simple cyst of the spleen rarely ruptures or suppurates.

Dermoid Cyst.—But one dermoid cyst of the spleen has been reported, and that by Andral. (Johnston, *Annals of Surgery*, 1908, XLVIII., 50.)

Hydatid Cyst.—Hydatid disease of the spleen is rare in North America. Lyons found only nine cases recorded up to 1901. The cyst is usually unilocular and single. As in other organs, it may remain latent, shrivel up, grow rapidly and burst, or suppurate. The disease follows the same clinical course in the spleen that it does in other organs, and the prognosis is the same in either case. Rupture may occur into a contiguous organ, as, for example, the lung.

The diagnosis depends upon the discovery, in the spleen, of a cyst containing a colorless, slightly opalescent, non-albuminous neutral fluid, having a specific gravity of from 1002 to 1010. The fluid of a dead cyst will show hooklets and scolices, and a suppurating one may discharge portions of its beautifully laminated wall.

Puncture for diagnostic purposes is hazardous, since leakage has been followed by severe urticaria, by evidences of peritoneal irritation, and, in rare instances, by death preceded by convulsions and collapse. (Rolleston.)

TREATMENT.—When a simple cyst is adherent, incise and drain it or else enucleate it; if it is non-adherent, splenectomy is justifiable. Suspected hydatid cysts should not be aspirated; splenotomy with drainage or splenectomy yield satisfactory results.

Chronic Splenic Anæmia (Banti's Disease).—Professor Osler has given the above title to the disease, which is also known by the following names:—splenic anæmia, primary splenomegaly, splenic pseudoleukæmia, etc., and he has further defined it as "A chronic affection, probably an intoxication of unknown origin, characterized by a progressive enlargement of the spleen which cannot be correlated with any known cause, such as malaria, leukæmia, syphilis, cirrhosis of the liver, etc. (primary splenomegaly); anæmia of a secondary or chlorotic type (leucopenia); a marked tendency to hemorrhage, particularly from the stomach; and in many cases a terminal stage, with cirrhosis of the liver, jaundice, and ascites (Banti's disease). The conditions described as primitive splenomegaly and Banti's disease are initial and terminal stages respectively of this malady." (Fig. 30.)

The chief feature of this disease is the primary enlargement of the spleen, at first unaccompanied by blood changes or alterations in the liver, thus sharply distinguishing it from the various blood diseases associated with a secondary splenomegaly, such as leukæmia and pernicious anæmia; from cirrhotic changes in the liver with secondary or associated enlargement of the spleen, such as occur in atrophic hepatic cirrhosis, hypertrophic

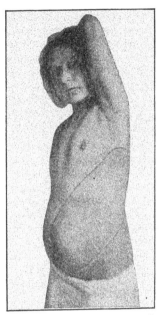

FIG. 30.—Enlarged Spleen in Banti's Disease. (From Zancan, in *Il Policlinico*, 1909, xvi., 5.)

cirrhosis of the liver, hæmochromatosis, and hepatic cirrhosis in infancy and early childhood. From Hodgkin's disease with splenomegaly it is distinguished by the absence of lymph-node involvement; from splenomegaly secondary to malaria, syphilis, tuberculosis, rickets, scurvy, etc., by the history and other corroborative evidences of these diseases. In this stage it cannot be distinguished from cases of splenomegaly of unknown origin, which are not associated with anæmia and which do not run the progressive downward course of splenic anæmia. It is distinguished from amyloid spleen by the evidence of this disease elsewhere and by the presence of syphilis, tuberculosis, or some chronic suppurating focus.

ETIOLOGY.—The cause is unknown. Barr believes that it arises from vasomotor paralysis of the splanchnic area. Since splenectomy may cure the disease, it is commonly believed to be due to some chronic intoxication, which is removed by the operation. There have been recorded a few cases having a symptom-complex and clinical course indistinguishable from the symptom-complex and clinical course of splenic anæmia,—cases in which it was discovered that the portal or the splenic vein was obstructed by thrombosis, sclerosis, or calcification, or by pressure from without, but whether primary or secondary to the splenomegaly is not known.

The disease now under consideration may attack the young or the old, but chiefly young male adults. A history of heredity has been occasionally noted.

PATHOLOGY.—The spleen may reach a colossal size. In Bovaird's case the organ weighed twelve and one-half pounds. Rolleston reports the average, in cases collected by him, to be sixty-one ounces (not quite four pounds). The enlarged organ retains its shape, and is smooth and firm. The enlargement is due to a hyperplastic fibrosis of the capsule, trabeculæ, and reticulum, with atrophy and sclerosis of the splenic pulp, often involving the Malpighian corpuscles. In a few cases with the clinical history of splenic anæmia there has been found a remarkable hyperplasia of the endothelial cells that line the sinuses and blood channels. As a result of this hyperplasia there are produced nodules and tumor-like masses, which were formerly described as endotheliomata or sarcomata, but are now regarded as simple products of a true hyperplasia of this tissue, even though similar masses have been found in the lymph nodes, liver, and elsewhere. Hemorrhagic infarcts have been observed, and perisplenitis with adhesions is common. The lymph nodes are not enlarged, but a reversion to the fœtal type of bone marrow has been occasionally noted.

CLINICAL COURSE AND SYMPTOMS.—The disease usually runs a protracted course—from ten to twelve years or even longer,—nevertheless death may occur within three and a half years. Remissions and periods of improvement are observed, but, on the whole, the tendency is progressively downward. Often the enlargement of the spleen is found accidentally, but a feeling of weight and tension in the left hypochondrium may lead to its discovery. Pain and tenderness may be prominent symptoms in the presence of perisplenitis or hemorrhagic infarcts. A souffle and friction rub have been occasionally heard.

The blood changes invariably follow the splenomegaly, and it may be years before they become pronounced. At first, there is only a diminution of the hæmoglobin, with some delay in coagulation; later on, there develops a gradually increasing corpuscular anæmia, aggravated very often by hemorrhage. The white cells remain normal or become diminished in number. In the later stages of the disease, or after severe hemorrhages, nucleated red cells may be found, and a polynuclear leucocytosis indicates some intercurrent affection. The poikilocytosis of essential anæmia is absent. Hemorrhages from various sources are of common occurrence. In Osler's cases hæmatemesis was a prominent symptom, recurring frequently, and was due, he believes, to diapedesis, gastric erosion, or œsophageal varices, or to mechanical obstruction from traction or pressure exerted by the enlarged spleen. Epistaxis, hæmaturia, menorrhagia, bleeding from the gums, retinal hemorrhages, and purpuric manifestations have also been observed.

The increasing anæmia, with or without hemorrhage, leads to a general deterioration of health and gives rise to nervous, cardio-vascular, and gastro-intestinal disturbances. Headache, vertigo, dyspnœa, and cardiac palpitation on muscular or mental exertion, syncopal attacks, œdema of the ankles, and effusion into serous cavities may be present. Loss of appetite, nausea, and diarrhœa soon produce emaciation. Pigmentation of a steel-gray or bronze hue, sometimes associated with leucoderma, is of common occurrence. The final stage, characterized by a gradually increasing cachexia and an aggravation of the previous symptoms, is often associated, as first pointed out by Banti, with cirrhosis of the liver, jaundice, and ascites. Fever is not a prominent symptom, but, during the last stages, a rise of temperature with or without chills frequently takes place in the evening. Death may occur in the second stage from sudden, severe, protracted, or recurrent hemorrhages. In the last stage of the disease, death may be due to exhaustion, hemorrhage, or some intercurrent affection.

DIAGNOSIS.—When an operation is contemplated, great care should be exercised to avoid a mistake in diagnosis. Especially is this true in the aleukæmic state of leukæmia (Osler and Lyon), in some cases of pernicious anæmia with markedly enlarged spleens, in splenomegaly secondary to cirrhosis of the liver, and in some forms of renal enlargement. (Lyon.) For a full account of this interesting disease the reader is referred to the classical papers of Banti,[1] Osler,[2] Sippy,[3] Bovaird,[4] Rolleston,[5] Gaucher,[6] * Senator, and others.

PROGNOSIS AND TREATMENT.—As a rule, unless the spleen is removed splenic anæmia terminates fatally, and this in spite of medical and general treatment, which may, however, temporarily improve the patient's condition. X-ray treatment has not yielded the beneficial results that its early employment promised.

Although we are ignorant of the cause of the splenic enlargement, there is good reason to believe that the subsequent course of the malady is intimately associated with the diseased organ, since splenectomy, even in the later stages, has been followed by a cure, or at least an arrest in the downward progress, with an amelioration of the prominent symptoms.

Splenectomy may be called for in the first stage to relieve distressing symptoms, but at this period a diagnosis cannot be made with certainty. When cirrhosis of the liver and ascites are present, successful results have followed epiplopexy and splenectomy. In the majority of cases reported the interval of time that has thus far elapsed is too short to enable us to judge of the permanency of the recovery. Death from hæmatemesis has followed splenectomy for supposed Banti's disease, and at the post-mortem examination it was discovered that in reality there was cirrhosis of the liver, with secondary enlarged spleen. Nor should it be forgotten that splenectomy for splenomegaly com-

* These numbers refer to the corresponding numbers in the bibliography at the end of this section.

plicating syphilis, malaria, etc., may be followed by marked improvement in health.

MORTALITY FOLLOWING SPLENECTOMY.—The death rate will manifestly depend upon the stage of the disease at the time of the operation and the severity of the symptoms, the presence or absence of adhesions, recent hemorrhages, the result of preparatory treatment, and the skill and experience of the operator. The chief dangers are hemorrhage and shock. The post-operative complications which have been recorded are, apart from sepsis: convulsive fits, tetany, and thrombosis of the mesenteric vessels causing gangrene and septic peritonitis.

Too much reliance should not be placed on statistics, since successful cases are more frequently reported than failures. Johnston (*Annals of Surgery*, 1908, XLVIII., 50) has collected sixty-one cases with twelve deaths—a mortality of but 19.6 per cent.

BIBLIOGRAPHY OF BANTI'S DISEASE OR CHRONIC SPLENIC ANÆMIA.—(1) Banti: *Archiv. della Scuola d'anat. patholog.*, 1883, II., 53. (*Beiträge zur path. Anat.*, 1898, XXIV., 21.)—(2) Osler: *Am. Jour. Med. Sci.*, 1900, CXIX., 54; 1902, CXXIV., 752.—(3) Sippy: *Am. Jour. Med. Sci.*, 1899, CXVIII., 428–570.—(4) Bovaird: *Am. Jour. Med. Sci.*, 1900, CXX., 377.—(5) Rolleston: *Clin. Journal*, 1902. —(6) Gaucher: Bull. et Mém. de la soc. méd. d'hôp. de Paris, 1892, IX., 35, 632; also *La France Méd.*, 1892, XXIX., 529.

Operations on the Spleen.—*Splenectomy.*—Extirpation of the spleen at the present moment is the operation of choice, and is perfectly justifiable in the following conditions:—

(1) Trauma from contusion, from gunshot or stab wounds, and from rupture, when the organ is so seriously damaged that suturing and packing with gauze cannot be relied upon to control hemorrhage.

(2) Prolapse with laceration and infection.

(3) Hypertrophied wandering spleen, which cannot be retained by splenopexy.

(4) Wandering spleen which is diseased.

(5) Torsion of the pedicle of a movable spleen the blood-supply of which has been seriously affected by strangulation.

(6) Simple hypertrophies of unknown origin, not associated with grave blood disturbances, but which give rise to distressing abdominal symptoms.

(7) Banti's disease. Here splenectomy offers the only hope of cure.

(8) Primary sarcoma of the spleen prior to metastases or evidences of marked cachexia.

(9) Cysts, primary tuberculosis, some forms of abscess of the spleen.

The operation should not be performed for leukæmia nor for hypertrophy, which is only a local symptom of grave constitutional disease, with the possible exception of malarial spleens which are uninfluenced by medical treatment. Even when the operation is justifiable, it may be impossible to perform it in the presence of dense and vascular adhesions.

The mortality is largely modified by the pathological condition requiring operation, the state of the patient, and the skill of the surgeon. Johnston's statistics (*Annals of Surgery*, 1908, XLVII., 50) show that, from 1900 to 1908, 355 splenectomies were performed, with a mortality of 18.5 per cent—or 13.2 per cent if the traumatic cases are excluded, and 11.5 per cent if, in addition, operations for leukæmia are excluded. One must keep in mind, however, that successful cases are more frequently reported than failures. Early diagnosis and prompt surgical treatment will lessen the death rate in traumatic cases.

Splenectomy is a simple operation when the spleen is of normal size, not adherent, and has a long pedicle. The most experienced operator, however, may be compelled to abandon the attempt to remove a large and densely adherent organ, in a stout individual.

The chief dangers are shock and hemorrhage.

Technique of the Operation.—The spleen may be exposed by a vertical or an oblique incision. A vertical incision in the mid-line is best for large spleens and for exploratory purposes in traumatic conditions; a vertical incision through the outer border of the left rectus, or an oblique one along the costal margin, for small spleens. A combination of a vertical and a lateral incision in the loin may be necessary to get sufficient exposure. The incision should be free and long enough to render the delivery of the spleen easy.

The pedicle should be clearly exposed and tied by interlocking ligatures of catgut or silk. Avoid including the tail of the pancreas or the branches of the splenic artery which go to the stomach, in the bight of the ligature. Clamp the pedicle close to the spleen before severing it. For safety, tie separately the vessels which project beyond the bight of the ligature.

When the spleen is densely adherent, deal with all adhesions first, tying and packing as may seem best. Avoid wounding the capsule of the spleen and close all raw surfaces on the hollow viscera. It is sometimes better to ligate the pedicle, if it can be exposed, before separating the adhesions.

In very large spleens, ligation may be made possible only by making the spleen "turn turtle" and by having the assistant depress the outer edge of the wound. Undue traction must never be made on the pedicle, because it induces severe shock. The writer was much impressed with the advantages of resection of the lower costal cartilages in dealing with a very large and adherent spleen removed by Willy Meyer. The use of suitable clamps (with perfect locks) to control the pedicle may be of service in cases of extreme urgency (chiefly traumatic). In clean cases close the abdomen with layered sutures and without drainage. In infected cases, in which gauze packing is not employed, drain through the loin, closing the abdominal incision. If the tail of the pancreas has been cut, drain through the loin.

Post-operative thrombosis involving the splenic vessels and extending to the mesenteric and portal trunks is a most serious complication and usually ends fatally.

Splenotomy.—Splenotomy is the incision of the spleen for the purpose of opening and draining an abscess. The same procedure may be used in treating simple and hydatid cysts. The operation may be performed in one or two sittings.

When the abscess or cyst is adherent to the abdominal wall or diaphragm it may be opened at once by an abdominal incision made over the most dependent area of fluctuation; if it is not adherent, the first operation consists in exposing the spleen and in packing the exposed area with sterile gauze to induce protective adhesions; the evacuation of the collection of fluid being postponed until two or three days later. In operating through the chest wall remove a portion of one or two ribs (ninth and tenth), displacing the pleura if possible. If this cannot be done, expose the diaphragm and pack with gauze. Wait until firm adhesions form, then open the abscess on the second or third day.

It is better in all cases to aspirate before incising the abscess wall and to drain the cavity by a rubber tube, with or without gauze packing.

Splenopexy.—Splenopexy is the fixation of a movable spleen to the abdominal wall in the upper left quadrant of the abdomen. Several methods have been devised.

Kouwer, in 1895, introduced the plan of replacing the spleen and packing around it with gauze, until firm adhesions anchored the organ. Halsted, as reported by Osler, has employed this method with success.

Rydygier retains the spleen in position by placing the lower pole in a retroperitoneal pocket. Expose the organ by a central or lateral incision. Cut through the peritoneum only, between the ninth and eleventh ribs, by a convex transverse incision, the convexity being upward. Strip up the peritoneum below the incision sufficiently far to hold the lower pole of the spleen. If possible, strip the peritoneum above the incision, in order to hold the upper pole. Place the spleen in the pocket thus formed. Close the peritoneal incision snugly around the pedicle of the spleen by silk or catgut sutures. When the lower pole alone is pocketed, suture the lower lip of the peritoneal incision to the gastrosplenic omentum and rub with gauze the phrenic surface of the upper pole and the diaphragmatic peritoneum, with the hope of inducing adhesive peritonitis. Introduce a few silk sutures through the peritoneal and subperitoneal tissues, immediately below the spleen, to prevent it slipping downward in its new situation.

This method cannot be employed when the hilum extends, as it may do, to the inferior pole of the spleen. The writer saw such a case in Pearce Gould's clinic. Possibly lateral pockets might be formed in such cases.

Bardenheuer's method consists in exposing the spleen from the flank, drawing it through an opening in the peritoneum, and then covering it with the muscles of this region. Basil Hall (*Annals of Surgery*, 1903, XXXVII., 481) modified this operation by drawing only the lower pole through the peritoneum, suturing the rent in this structure snugly around the lower half at the level of the notch, and covering this portion with the layers of the abdominal wall.

Bardenheuer makes an incision in the mid-axillary line from the tenth rib to the iliac crest. From the upper end a second incision of about equal length is made backward into the loin. Both incisions extend to, but not through, the peritoneum. The latter is stripped up in all directions sufficiently to provide a location for the spleen, which is then drawn through an opening made for that purpose.   The peritoneal rent is sutured snugly around the pedicle.   Several sutures unite the peritoneum and fascia, just below the spleen, to prevent further separation of this structure and displacement of the organ.   The rectangular wound is closed with layered suturing.

Direct fixation of the spleen by sutures passed through its substance or its capsule is dangerous and cannot be recommended.

Partial resection of the spleen and enucleation of cysts have also been performed, but the chief danger of these operations is hemorrhage.   The late Dr. Senn (*Jour. Amer. Med. Assn.*, 1903, XLI., 1241) describes a method of controlling hemorrhage from, and suturing wounds of, the spleen, which might be employed with advantage in these cases.   This consists in the use of an angiotribe (forcipressure) with broad blades.   The tissues are compressed slowly, the pulp being thus expelled and a band of trabecular and reticular tissue, containing occluded vessels, being left.   These bands are subsequently united by catgut sutures.

SURGICAL DISEASES AND WOUNDS OF THE KIDNEYS AND URETERS.

By JAMES BELL, M.D., Montreal, Canada.

I. ANATOMY, EMBRYOLOGY, AND PHYSIOLOGY.

THE kidneys occupy the upper portions of the lumbar fossæ on each side of the vertebral column, behind the peritoneum and the viscera contained within the peritoneal cavity.

Development.—There are three stages in the development of the kidney and ureter: first, the pronephros, which in the human subject is only transitory; second, the mesonephros, which comprises the Wolffian body and duct; third, the metanephros or permanent kidney. The mesonephros is fully developed at the end of the second month, and atrophies with the development of the metanephros or permanent kidney. The permanent kidney consists, developmentally, of two portions—the excretory and the secretory. The excretory portion consists of the ureter, pelvis, and collecting tubules, which arise from the Wolffian duct. The secretory portion consists of the glomeruli and convoluted tubules, which arise from the mesoderm.

Anatomical Relations.—On the abdomen the lower pole of the right kidney is 2.5 cm. above the umbilical line and 5 cm. from the mid-line. The upper pole lies at the level of the seventh costo-cartilaginous junction, 3 cm. from the mid-line. On the back, the right kidney extends from the eleventh dorsal spine to the second lumbar spine, the hilum being situated opposite the first lumbar spine. The left kidney is 1–2 cm. higher than the right.

In front of the right kidney are found a portion of the right lobe of the liver, the second portion of the duodenum, and the hepatic flexure of the colon. In front of the left kidney lie portions of the stomach, pancreas, splenic flexure of the colon, splenic vessels, spleen, and the small intestine. Both kidneys lie upon the diaphragm, the anterior layer of the lumbar aponeurosis, the external and internal arcuate ligaments, the psoas and transversalis muscles, the two upper lumbar arteries, and the last dorsal, the ilio-hypogastric, and the ilio-inguinal nerves. The twelfth rib lies behind the right kidney, while behind the left are found the eleventh and twelfth ribs. The suprarenal capsule is in relation to the upper pole of each kidney.

General Description of Structure.—The kidney (Fig. 31) has a characteristic bean-like shape; it is flattened from side to side and presents, on its internal border, a depression called the "hilum." At this point the vessels enter and leave the kidney. It measures about four inches in length, two and one-half inches in breadth, and one inch and a half in thickness. The weight of the organ is about four and a half ounces (140 grammes).

The coverings of the kidney are of considerable importance from a surgical view-point. Lying directly upon the kidney is a thin, but strong, fibrous coat, the "tunica fibrosa." This structure or capsule is easily stripped from the kidney and leaves, under normal conditions, a smooth surface. It passes into the hilum, forms a covering for the papillæ, and is reflected upon the outer surface of the pelvis. It also sends a fine process outward to cover the nerves and vessels that enter the hilum, and another one backward to be attached to the aortic sheath and lumbar fascia. This latter band is known as the "ligamentum

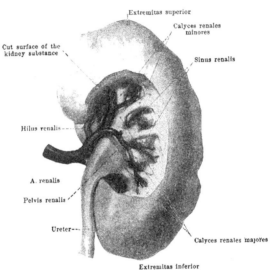

FIG. 31.—The Normal Kidney. (From Spalteholz.)

suspensorium renis." Outside this fibrous capsule, and loosely connected with it by bands of thin fibrous tissue, is the fatty capsule or "capsula adiposa." This acts as a protective casing or buffer for the kidney. In the new-born, the fat is absent; in fact, it does not appear, as a rule, until the tenth year. It varies much in amount, becomes altered in inflammatory conditions of the kidney, and diminishes rapidly in emaciation.

The fibrous tissue enclosing the fat presents certain thickenings. Thus, for example, on the posterior surface there is a thickening which is known as the "fascia retrorenalis." It is continuous with the fascia covering the psoas and quadratus lumborum muscles. Then, on the anterior surface, there is a band-like thickening the fibres of which extend to the subperitoneal tissue behind the colon. This thickening is always present on the left side, but is frequently absent on the right. These fascial attachments are naturally of great importance in the maintenance of the normal position of the kidney.

On longitudinal section, the kidney is seen to consist of a dark portion, the cortex, and a lighter portion, the medulla. The light portion is distributed in the form of pyramids. The dark portion covers the base of the pyramids and dips down between them. The apices of the pyramids, or papillæ, terminate in the calyces—small spaces which receive the urine from the papillæ; the latter, in turn, open up into the infundibula—three tubular sacs, one at each extremity and one in the middle of the kidney. The infundibula finally coalesce to form the pelvis, which again ends in the excreting duct, the ureter.

Blood Supply.—The renal artery, a branch of the abdominal aorta, enters the hilum of the kidney and divides into two or three branches before penetrating its substance. In this situation, small branches are given off to supply the ureter, suprarenal capsule, and surrounding cellular tissue.

At the beginning of the columns of Bertini—the spaces between the pyramids —the branches enter the substance of the kidney and run along beside the pyramids, at the base of which they turn at right angles. Along their whole course, they give off branches to the glomeruli, and at the base of each pyramid a set of branches passes downward to the papillæ. The glomerular vessels pass out of the glomeruli as the efferent vessels, and again break up around the tubules in the cortex, and from these the blood is collected by veins. There are three sources of venous collection, the above-mentioned being the first. The second one is formed just beneath the capsule, and the third is at the apex of each one of the pyramids. These veins join together to form the renal vein, which empties its blood into the inferior vena cava. The anterior and posterior portions of the kidney have separate arterial supplies, and the arteries do not communicate with each other. There is, therefore, between these two sources of blood supply, a line of separation which is located at or near the longitudinal mid-line of the kidney, usually 5 or 6 mm. posterior to it. In this line, therefore, the kidney may be split open with the least danger of hemorrhage.

The arterial supply to the fatty capsule comes from the renal artery and the first lumbar artery.

It must be borne in mind that occasionally a supernumerary renal artery arises independently from the aorta for the supply of one or other pole of the kidney.

Nerve Supply.—The nerve supply to the kidney comes from the renal plexus, which is made up of branches from the splanchnics, semilunar ganglion, aortic plexus, solar plexus, spermatic plexus, and vagus. The connection with the spermatic plexus accounts for the pain felt in the testicles in certain diseases of the kidney; and reflex anuria is produced by disturbances of the vasomotor functions of the renal plexus.

Lymphatics.—The lymphatic vessels of the kidney consist of a superficial and a deep set. These join together at the hilum and, after receiving lymphatic vessels from the ureter and suprarenal capsule, open into the lumbar lymph nodes.

Histology of the Kidney.—The cortex and medulla are made up of tubules, blood-vessels, and a connective-tissue framework. Each tubule commences in the cortex as a glomerulus, which consists of a tuft of blood-vessels invaginating its blind end. This glomerulus is lined by a syncytium, *i.e.*, a protoplasmic mass showing no cell-outlines in silver preparations. From the glomerulus proceeds a convoluted tubule lined by cubical epithelial cells which show distinct rods. This passes into a spiral tubule which has a similar lining and which, in turn, becomes straight. This straight portion is known as the descending limb of Henle's loop, and is lined by clear, flat cells. As it nears the apex of the pyramid, it turns on itself and proceeds upward again as the ascending limb of the loop. The lining cells of this portion become granular and cubical. When this limb reaches the cortex, it takes on a zigzag course and its cells become taller and distinctly rodded. Following this, it passes into the second convoluted tubule, having cells similar to the first. Next come the junctional tubules which have a larger lumen and more flattened epithelial cells. These junctional tubules pass into collecting tubules which have a still larger lumen lined by a columnar type of cell; and lastly, these collecting tubules join with others to form larger ducts which pass through the medullary substance, open at the apex of the papilla, and are known as the ducts of Bellini. They are lined by clear columnar cells.

The Ureters.—The ureter is a muscular tube about sixteen inches in length in the adult, and normally has about the diameter of a goose quill. It lies behind the peritoneum, and conveys the urine from the kidney to the bladder. It is not necessarily of uniform diameter and is very distensile, and usually it is found very considerably dilated on the proximal side of an obstruction. This is well shown in cases in which a calculus has lain for some time in the lower end of the tube near the bladder. The muscular coat of the ureter consists of two layers—an outer circular layer and an inner longitudinal one. The mucous lining consists of areolar tissue lined by transitional epithelium. It is a contractile tube. Its blood supply is derived from branches of the renal, spermatic, internal iliac, and inferior vesical arteries. The nerve supply is derived from the inferior mesenteric, spermatic, and pelvic plexuses.

Physiology.—The main function of the kidney is the excretion of urine, by which means the waste products are eliminated from the body. This function is vicarious and more or less complemental to the elimination of waste products by the skin, intestines, and other emunctories. The kidney is also thought to possess the function of internal secretion, by which an important product is manufactured, but which, up to the present time, is but little known. Without entering upon a discussion of the experimental work through which these conclusions have been arrived at, it may be said that the watery part of the urine, holding solids in solution, is filtered through the blood-vessels of the glomeruli, and that the function of secretion is performed by the epithelium of the tubules.

II. METHODS OF INVESTIGATING THE CONDITION OF THE KIDNEY.

The methods of investigating the kidney in cases in which a renal affection is suspected, may be classified, for surgical purposes, under four headings:—(1)

History and symptoms; (2) External examination of the patient; (3) Internal examination of the patient; (4) Examination of the urine.

(1) *History and Symptoms.*—The first symptom to be considered, and the one which most frequently calls the attention of the patient to his malady, is that of pain. Although this symptom is nearly always present to a greater or less extent in surgical diseases of the kidney, yet its form is rarely characteristic; for even "renal colic," which is looked upon generally as typical, may be simulated by conditions affecting the gall-bladder, stomach, vermiform appendix, or nervous system. Thus one sees, in the different kidney lesions, all degrees of pain, from the extreme severity of the most pronounced renal colic down to the merest sensation of an ache in the side or back. The situation and extent of the pain, however, are more characteristic. A pain in the loin which tends to radiate down the thigh or toward the scrotum or vulva, is suggestive of an origin in or about the kidney.

Pain which is aggravated by exertion or jarring of the body is suggestive of calculus. Frequency of micturition, which is usually indicative of a bladder lesion, would appear to be sometimes one of the earliest symptoms of renal tuberculosis; it is also a symptom of renal calculus.

Blood in the urine is a symptom which frequently calls the attention of the patient to the urinary system, and there are also the general symptoms which are due to kidney insufficiency. These are constitutional and consist of nausea, vomiting, headache, general malaise, etc.

The personal and family history should be looked into, more especially where tuberculosis is suspected. Heredity also plays an important part in renal calculus.

(2) *External Examination of the Patient.*—(*a*) Inspection.—On account of the depth at which the kidney is placed the cases in which information is obtained by inspection are somewhat limited. They comprise those cases in which a large swelling of the kidney or perirenal tissue exists or where an injury has occurred in that region. Where possible, one should view these patients, not only in the recumbent position, but also in the erect posture. They should also be viewed from the front, back, and side.

(*b*) Palpation.—The usual method employed in palpating the kidney is with the patient lying on his back and the knees drawn up in order to relax the abdominal muscles. The examiner stands on the side on which the kidney to be palpated is situated. One hand is then placed behind the level of the twelfth rib and the other in front, just below the costal margin. The patient is instructed to breathe normally, and, while he is doing so, both hands of the examiner are brought as near together as possible. Having obtained all the information possible by this means, the examiner should next instruct the patient to breathe deeply, in order that the kidney may be forced downward. Guyon* suggested "ballottement rénal," which consists in giving a quick push with the hand upon the loin in order to make the kidney strike against the hand which is placed on the abdomen. Israel recommends that palpation be done with the patient

---

* "Leçons cliniques sur les maladies des voies urinaires," Paris, 1894.

lying on the normal side, in order that the kidney shall fall toward the abdominal wall. Wuhrmann,* on the other hand, examines the patient in a standing posture, himself sitting on a stool in front of him. He claims that by this method the kidney reaches its maximum of descent, but, apparently, he overlooks the fact that the abdominal muscles are more rigid.

(c) Sudden Pressure.—Sudden pressure over the twelfth rib, posteriorly, elicits pain in many cases of renal calculus. This phenomenon has come to be considered by many as characteristic.

(d) Percussion.—Percussion is of value in establishing the relations of the kidney, or supposed kidney tumor, to the hollow viscera.

(3) Internal Examination.—Under this heading are comprised all the newer methods of investigation—skiagraphy, separation of the urines of the two kidneys, functional tests, cryoscopy of the blood, and cryoscopy of the urine.

(a) Skiagraphy.—By means of the Roentgen rays we are able, in most cases, to diagnose with certainty at least one condition, namely, "renal calculus." Shadows are also produced by large collections of pus and by tumors, as in other parts of the body. These shadows, however, are rarely confused with those produced by stone. Kuemmel, in his latest work,† states that every kidney stone produces a shadow, and that where no shadow is seen no stone exists. There must, however, be exceptions to this rule, as in the case of very stout patients, and in that of small stones and those containing little mineral matter, which are not very resistant to the Roentgen ray. Uric acid and urate calculi are the least resistant to the x-ray and therefore give the least distinct shadows.

(b) Separation of the Urines of the Two Kidneys.—This procedure is now almost invariably accomplished by means of cystoscopy and ureteral catheterization. The importance of determining whether both kidneys exist and are functioning normally, cannot be overestimated, and the examination of the separated urines gives the most exact and reliable information on these points.

Many forms of segregator have been employed for securing the urine separately from each kidney, those of Harris and Luys being the best known in this country.

With ordinary care and skill ureteral catheterization is neither difficult nor dangerous, and it enables us to determine whether or not two kidneys exist, and, if they do, whether the abnormal urine is coming from one kidney or from both. At most, an anæsthetic, either general or local, may be necessary.

(c) Tests of the Functional Activity of the Kidneys.—The theoretical test consists in the introduction, into the body, of substances which are rapidly excreted by the kidneys. Potassium iodide, sodium salicylate, sodium benzoate, and certain coloring substances have been used in this way. The test consists in a demonstration of the functional capacity of the kidney to excrete these

* von Bergmann und Bruns: "Handbuch der praktischen Chirurgie," 4ter Bd., dritte Auflage.

† "Die Grenzen erfolgreicher Nierenextirpation und die Diagnose der Nephritis nach kryoskopischen Erfahrungen," xxxi. Congress der Deutschen Chirurgen, 1901.

substances. The two substances now used in this way are indigo-carmine and phloridzin. Delayed excretion of the indigo-carmine shows diminished functional activity of the kidney, and, with the cystoscope in position, it demonstrates the situation of the ureteral openings in the bladder.

A solution of 0.04 gramme of indigo-carmine dissolved in 10 c.c. of distilled water is injected intramuscularly, and at the end of eight minutes the cystoscope is introduced and the ureteral orifices observed. Under normal conditions the blue should appear in from ten to fifteen minutes. Further delay in one or both kidneys indicates impaired function.

The phloridzin test is based upon the fact that a subcutaneous injection of phloridzin will, when the kidneys are normal, cause sugar to appear in the urine within ten or fifteen minutes. (The indigo-carmine test has this advantage over the phloridzin test, that ureteral catheterization is not necessary.)

The technical details of the phloridzin test are as follows:—Both ureters having been catheterized, a period of five minutes is allowed to elapse in order to obtain sufficient urine for the ordinary examination. Then 0.01 gramme of phloridzin, dissolved in 1 c.c. of warm distilled water, is injected subcutaneously. It must be borne in mind that phloridzin is only very slightly soluble in cold water, and therefore the solution must be used while warm; otherwise, only distilled water will be injected and the phloridzin will remain in the glass or syringe.

At the end of ten minutes the urine is collected in a number of test tubes, each containing a five-minutes' flow. Each of these specimens is tested as soon as the flow is completed, and, when the sugar appears, the examination may be concluded.

(d) Cryoscopy of the Blood.—A few years ago von Koranyi and Kuemmel * recommended this method as a means of testing the sufficiency or insufficiency of the kidneys. They reasoned that, if the kidneys were not functioning normally, they would not remove from the blood the metabolic products which under ordinary circumstances are excreted by these organs. They therefore concluded that the blood would have a greater molecular concentration, and thus a lower freezing-point, than normal. Practically all investigators place the normal freezing-point of the blood at a point between 0.56 and 0.60. It must be clearly understood that this method is not a means of determining whether an anatomical lesion of the kidney does or does not exist. On the other hand, we presuppose that such a lesion does exist and we employ this method merely to determine how near we are to a state of kidney insufficiency.

The ordinary tests of the urine are those employed for the purpose of determining the reaction and the specific gravity, the presence or absence of albumin, sugar, bacteria, salts, pus, blood, urea, etc., and, in certain cases, the physiological test—viz., the injection of some of the urine or its components into a guinea-pig. This is to be done both with the combined urine and also with the separated urines.

* "Untersuchungen ueber den osmotischen Druck tierischer Fluessigkeiten," Zeits. f. klin. Med., Bd. 33, 34, 1897.

(e) Cryoscopy of the Urine.—Cryoscopy of the urine is employed as a means of comparing the functioning power of the two kidneys; it is not in itself a test of great value.

A few years after Dresser * had applied this method to the testing of the combined urines, Casper and Richter † introduced it as a means of comparing the functioning powers of each kidney separately, and also for the purpose of obtaining an indication as to the safety of performing a nephrectomy. They placed the limit of safety at $-1°$ centigrade, and considered that any rise above that point indicated a dangerous degree of kidney insufficiency. No lengthy discussion of the subject is needed to warrant the statement that, in the majority of cases, reliable information is obtained by this means. There are, however, a few cases in which a polyuria is produced by ureteral catheterization, and thus an abnormally high freezing-point is obtained.

The technique of the procedure is as follows:—The apparatus usually employed is that of von Bechmann. It consists of a glass cylinder containing a freezing-mixture of ice and salt. Into this mixture is placed a smaller glass cylinder, within which is a still smaller one. This middle cylinder is merely an air mantle employed in order to obtain a uniformity of temperature in the innermost tube, which contains the urine and the mercurial end of the thermometer. A strong wire with a loop on the end is passed down into the urine for the purpose of stirring it. The stirring is kept up continuously in order to prevent the watery portions of the urine from crystallizing on the sides of the vessel and thus concentrating the remainder of the urine. About 10 c.c. of urine is poured into the innermost tube and as soon as the mercury begins to fall the stirring is commenced and kept up steadily until the test is completed. It will be noticed that, after falling for some time, the mercury will suddenly commence to rise, and when this ceases the reading is taken.

A very low excretion of urea (less than 0.75 gramme in two hours) from the presumably healthy kidney is an unfavorable condition for nephrectomy. This may, however, be due to a toxic nephritis, a condition from which recovery will take place.

III. CONGENITAL ABNORMALITIES OF THE KIDNEY AND URETER.

A great variety of congenital abnormalities of the kidney have been described. They are usually classified as: Abnormalities of form; Abnormalities of position; and Abnormalities of number. Abnormalities of the ureter are most frequently found associated with, and are more or less dependent upon, abnormalities of the kidney.

Abnormalities in the Form of the Kidney.—These are usually the result of more or less complete fusion of the two kidneys. This fusion varies from a

---

* "Ueber Diurese und ihre Beeinfluessung durch pharmakologische Mittel," Archiv f. experimentelle Pathologie und Pharmakologie, 29. Bd., 1892.

† "Functionelle Nierendiagnostik, mit besonderer Beruecksichtigung der Nierenchirurgie," Berlin-Wien, 1901.

mere fibrous connection to complete union, the resulting kidney mass being sometimes quite irregular; but, more frequently, the fusion assumes the form of an arch, the so-called horseshoe kidney being produced. In the commonest form of horseshoe kidney the lower extremities of the two kidneys are fused so as to form an arch with the concavity directed upward. The renal pelvis lies anteriorly and there are also usually abnormalities of the blood-vessels and the ureter. This form of kidney is found once in about 1,100 autopsies.* The superior extremities of the kidney are sometimes united in such a manner as to form a horseshoe kidney, with the concavity directed downward. This form

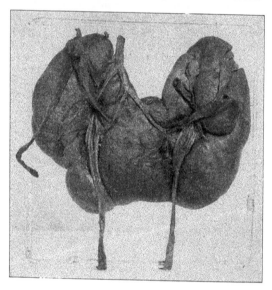

FIG. 32.—Horseshoe Kidney in Adult. (From a specimen in the Pathological Museum of McGill University, Montreal.)

is much rarer than the preceding, constituting about seven per cent of the horseshoe abnormalities of the kidney.† The isthmus may be behind the aorta, but it is usually in front of this vessel. Partial nephrectomy and other operations have been done upon the horseshoe kidney. A positive diagnosis, except by exploration, is impossible. (Figs. 32 and 33.)

The two kidneys may be found together on the same side, forming one elongated kidney from which the ureters pass to the opposite sides of the bladder as in the normal arrangement, or the pelves may be directed, one toward each side of the body. The fusion of the two kidneys sometimes takes another form, viz.,

* von Bergmann's "System of Practical Surgery," American edition.
† Robinson, Medical Fortnightly.

one in which the union is so complete that an irregular kidney mass is found lying upon the vertebral column in the middle line.

Abnormalities in the Position of the Kidney.—Abnormalities of position are of not infrequent occurrence and are of great importance to the surgeon.   Graser * collected two huudred instances of congenital misplacement.   (See Fig. 34, which shows a displacement of the right kidney.)   One or both of the kidneys may be misplaced, and sometimes the misplaced organ is solitary, perhaps the result of fusion.   The most common misplacement is probably downward, the

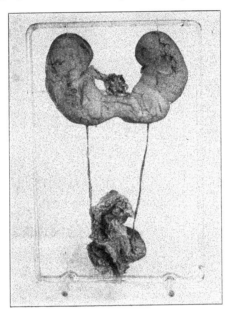

Fig. 33.—Horseshoe Kidney in a Child, with Ureters and Bladder attached. (From a specimen in the Pathological Museum of McGill University, Montreal.)
The fusion is less marked than in the adult kidney shown in Fig. 32.

kidney being generally found at the promontory of the sacrum or in the pelvis. In cases in which the organ occupied the latter situation operation has several times been undertaken for the removal of a pelvic tumor, the true nature of which was discovered only at or after operation.   One of the earliest and best known cases of this kind was that reported by Dr. William M. Polk, of New York, in 1882,† where he removed a pelvic tumor which proved to be a solitary kidney.   Dr. Cullen, of Baltimore,‡ has recently reported a similar case, in

* von Bergmann's "System of Practical Surgery," American edition.
† New York Medical Journal, 1883.
‡ Surgery, Gynæcology, and Obstetrics, July, 1910.

which the diagnosis was made by an exploratory operation, the kidney being left undisturbed. (Displacements have also been referred to under the heading of Abnormalities of Form.)

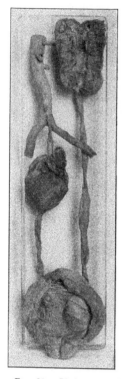

Abnormalities of Number.—Congenital absence or atrophy of one kidney is not very rare. Morris * estimated its frequency as 1 in 2,650 cases; and there have been reported many instances where the solitary kidney has been removed for disease, with (of course) a fatal result. Hence the importance of determining the existence and the condition of a second kidney before proceeding to a nephrectomy. At the present day this is easily done by means of the cystoscope and ureteral catheterization. Congenital absence of both kidneys is also an actual occurrence, but, as such a condition is incompatible with life, it is of no surgical interest.

Supernumerary kidneys are rare and of no surgical importance. Lobulation of the kidney (persistence of fœtal type) is not rare. This condition is important surgically, as it is thought to predispose to disease—tuberculosis, for example.

Abnormalities of the Ureters.—Abnormalities of one or both ureters are not rare. They occur as follows: as an absence of one ureter; as an increase in the number of ureters; as a double ureter; and as a fusion of the two parts of a ureter of double origin. (Fig. 35.)

The most important abnormalities are those which occur at the termination of the ureter—such, for example, as an irregular or incomplete opening into the bladder, which may result in hydronephrosis. In a man, fifty years of age, upon whom the

FIG. 34. — Displacement of Right Kidney, and Anomalous Distribution of Blood-vessels. (From a specimen in the Pathological Museum of McGill University, Montreal.) The right kidney lies low down at the level of the brim of the pelvis, and receives its blood-supply from an artery given off just above the bifurcation of the aorta. The left kidney is in its normal situation. There is hydronephrosis of both organs.

writer operated for a chronic hydronephrosis, of moderate size, the ureter was found to be obstructed at the bladder and dilated to a diameter of more than one inch and a half throughout its whole length. Its walls were thin and it contained the same clear fluid as did the kidney. The obstruction was probably congenital.

The ureter is also said to terminate sometimes in the urethra, the vagina, the seminal vesicle, or the rectum.† In such cases derangement of function would produce symptoms, and the diagnosis could generally be made positive by a direct exami-

* "Surgical Diseases of the Kidney and Ureter," vol. i.
† Watson and Cunningham's "Genito-Urinary Diseases."

nation (with the cystoscope, in most cases), while treatment would be determined by the individual conditions. Valvular, strictured, and distorted conditions of the ureter, of congenital origin, are occasionally found and may produce hydronephrosis. A diagnosis can usually be made by means of the cystoscope, and such conditions are sometimes amenable to operative treatment.

Abnormalities of the renal arteries are very common. They occur as often as three times out of seven cases. (Morris.*) There are frequently found two, three, four, and even as many as five arterial trunks to a kidney. (Figs. 36 and 37.) Abnormalities as regards the point where they enter the kidney, and also in respect of their point of origin, are common.

Extra arteries sometimes run into the kidney at unusual places, near the upper or the lower extremity. This abnormality is of course important, as it may seriously complicate a nephrotomy or a nephrectomy; and, in one case of injury to the kidney, in the author's experience, a fatal hemorrhage occurred, after nephrectomy, from an abnormally placed artery which had not been included in the ligature applied to the pedicle, and which bled into the peritoneal cavity through a rent in the peritoneum that had been produced by the traumatism. (Fig. 36 shows an unusually large variety of anomalies of the blood-vessels and, among others, supernumerary aberrant arteries.)

Of 1,590 autopsies performed in the Royal Victoria Hospital (Montreal) between the first of January, 1894, and the first of January, 1910, the following congenital abnormalities of the kidney and ureter were found:—Horseshoe kidney, 6; congenital absence of one kidney

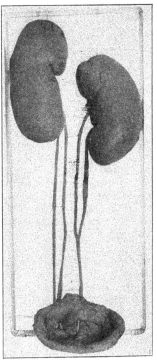

Fig. 35. — Complete and Partial Double Ureters. (From a specimen in the Pathological Museum of McGill University, Montreal.)
The right ureter is completely double and opens by two separate entrances into the bladder. The left ureter is double above and single below, and empties into the bladder by a single orifice.

and ureter, 7. (A small portion of one ureter was found in a case in which this tube did not open into the bladder.) In one of these cases, in which the left kidney and ureter were absent in a female, there was also absence of the following parts: the left cornu of the uterus, the left ovary, and the left Fallopian tube.

* "Surgical Diseases of the Kidney and Ureter."

In this same series of autopsies the following further abnormalities were found:—

Fœtal lobulation of kidney	17	Double pelvis and double ureters	20
Accessory arteries	19	Double ureters, complete	10
Accessory veins	7	Double ureters on the right side	2
Accessory artery in the upper pole	6	Double ureters on the left side	5
Accessory artery in the lower pole	2	Double ureters on both sides	3
Accessory artery (location not mentioned)	11	Double ureters, incomplete	10
Accessory artery in the right kidney	13	Incomplete double ureters on the right side	3
Accessory artery in the left kidney	6	Incomplete double ureters on the	
Accessory artery in both kidneys	5	left side	6 .
Double pelvis (above)	3	Incomplete double ureters on both sides	1

IV. WOUNDS OF THE KIDNEY AND URETER.

Injury to the Kidney and Ureter without open Wound.—The kidneys are deeply placed in the body, and apparently are thus most effectually protected from injury. Nevertheless, injuries to the kidneys are not very rare, and are very important. Kuester * is quoted by von Bergmann ("System of Practical Surgery") as having found, out of 30,000 cases which he examined in the Basle Clinic, only 10 instances of injury to the kidney, and in only one of these was there an open wound. General surgical experience, however, would seem to indicate that accidents of this nature occur much more frequently than the above report would lead one to believe. Thus, for example, in the Royal Victoria Hospital, in Montreal, 9,920 surgical cases were treated in the years 1903 to 1910, and among these there were seven cases of laceration of the kidney without open wound. Laceration of the kidney substance, injury of vessels, and detachment of the ureter, may all occur from blows and crushes upon the loin, back, or abdomen, without an external wound. Laceration of the kidney may also occur from muscular exertion. (Watson.†) The experiments made by Kuester upon animals ‡—experiments which consisted in throwing them violently against the floor or the wall—showed that when the kidneys were empty, with the ureter unobstructed, laceration did not take place nearly so rapidly as when the kidney contained blood or urine, with the ureter ligated. In many instances the kidney injury is only a part, and sometimes only a minor part, of the general injury produced by the accident. Such cases are not considered in the present article. Frequently, however, when the kidney is the organ mainly affected by a severe injury, there are also more or less serious injuries of adjacent structures (spleen, peritoneum, intestines, etc.)—injuries which are to be considered as complications of the kidney injury. The extent and the nature of the damage done to the kidney vary very much; in some cases there may be a simple tearing of the capsule or a slight laceration of the glandular substance, while in others the organ is completely crushed. Stellate lacerations on the surface of the kidney are the most common, and, in the

* Deutsche Chirurgie, Bd. lii.
† "Genito-Urinary Diseases," by Watson and Cunningham.
‡ Quoted by von Bergmann, in his "System of Practical Surgery."

more severe injuries, the kidney may be torn completely in two, transversely or longitudinally.* Injury to the blood-vessels and separation of the ureter may also occur in this form of accident. (See Uronephrosis.)

The most common cause of uncomplicated kidney laceration is direct violence to the loin, such as a kick from a horse or from the toe of a boot, a fall upon a stake, and so forth. Complicated injuries are more frequently produced by crushing accidents. The immediate results of these injuries are shock, hemorrhage, extravasation of urine, and sometimes uronephrosis. (See Uronephrosis.)

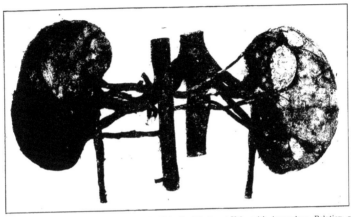

Fig. 36.—Double Renal Arteries, and Right Double Renal Vein, with Anomalous Relation of the Blood-vessels at the Hilum on the Right Side. (From a specimen in the Anatomical Museum of McGill University, Montreal.)

The main renal artery (*right side*) sends off a supernumerary branch of small size to the upper pole of the kidney, and enters the upper part of its hilum in two branches. An additional smaller arterial trunk rises from the aorta half an inch below the first, and enters the kidney at the lower part of its hilum. A supernumerary right renal vein passes from the back of the hilum behind the artery and enters the S. V. C. about half an inch below the main renal trunk. *On the left side* the renal artery bifurcates near the hilum, one branch entering the kidney anteriorly to the vein, while the other enters in the normal situation behind it. A supernumerary left renal artery rises from the aorta about one inch and a quarter below the main trunk, and enters the lower end of the kidney. A small vein rises from the back of the hilum behind the artery and the ureters, and joins the main left renal vein one inch and a half beyond.

The hemorrhage may be perirenal, subcapsular, into the kidney substance, intraperitoneal, etc., but, except in serious injuries to the vessels, spontaneous arrest of hemorrhage is the rule. The arrest, however, may be only temporary, and secondary hemorrhage may follow, and aneurysm of the renal artery of both the sacculated and the false varieties has been described by Morris.†

"A young man, 24 years of age, came under the care of the writer thirty-nine days after having been kicked in the loin by a horse, the result of which had been continuous but moderate hæmaturia, with two or three sharp attacks of hemorrhage. Six days later, or forty-five days after the accident, he had a fatal hemorrhage."

*Fig. 38. See also The Medical Record, New York, Nov. 5th, 1910; article by Dr. Henry G. Bugbee.
† "Surgical Diseases of the Kidney and Ureter."

The ultimate results, if the patient survives the immediate danger of shock and hemorrhage, are: absorption of the extravasate of blood and the complete repair of the kidney; or infection and suppuration; or gangrene of the kidney produced by the cutting off of all the circulation by a thrombus or by

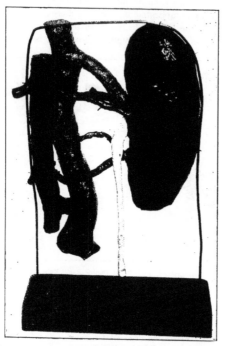

Fig. 37.—Double Renal Artery, the Right Kidney with Ureter and Blood-vessels, and the Aorta and Inferior Vena Cava. (From a specimen in the Anatomical Museum of McGill University, Montreal.) The renal artery bifurcates about an inch from the aorta, and enters the hilum of the kidney as two branches, one of which passes in front, and the other behind, the right renal vein. A large supernumerary trunk is given off about an inch above the bifurcation of the aorta, and enters the hilum of the kidney at its lower part.

occlusion of blood-vessels from crushing of tissue or other causes; or death from some other complication.

Extravasation of Urine.—The effects of a moderate extravasation of urine in the peritoneal cavity or in the perirenal tissue are not very serious for a short time; but ultimately the urine decomposes, and, if present in a large quantity, it produces gangrene of tissue and serious results, or, if the quantity extravasated is smaller, it paves the way for infection. Experiments upon animals and the results of accidental wounds of the ureter during operations have shown that the tissues possess a degree of tolerance of fresh urine that was formerly unsuspected.

Oliguria and anuria also occur, but these conditions are comparatively rare, and in cases in which there remains one kidney that is uninjured and is free from disease, diminution or suppression of urinary secretion can be explained only as a reflex phenomenon analogous to the reflex anuria which occurs so often in calculous disease of the kidney.

Infection and suppuration, perinephritis, pyonephrosis, pyelonephritis, and abscess may follow, and, when the peritoneum has been injured, suppurative peritonitis may develop. (See Suppurative Inflammations of the Kidney.)

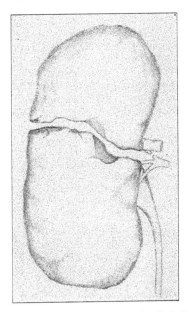

Fig. 38.—Rupture of Kidney by the Kick of a Horse in the Loin. (Author's collection.) Laceration of kidney extended into the pelvis, and there was a rupture of an abnormally placed arterial branch.

SYMPTOMS.—Shock is always present and out of proportion to the seriousness of the accident or the severity of the injury to the kidney. Hemorrhage is rarely so severe as to produce the characteristic signs of loss of blood, except in secondary hemorrhage, which may be fatal; and hæmaturia may be delayed for hours or days, and is often intermittent on account of the blocking of the ureter by blood clots, during the continuance of which condition normal urine from the other kidney only will be passed. Blocking of the ureter produces symptoms similar to those of renal colic, but milder in degree. The continued recurrence of attacks of hæmaturia is of serious significance, and is suggestive of possible secondary hemorrhage. Where recovery takes place, the kidney is susceptible of a wonderful degree of repair. This is also shown in kidneys which have been operated upon for the removal of calculus or have been subjected to exploratory incisions. (See Nephrolithotomy.)

DIAGNOSIS.—It is of the utmost importance that a diagnosis be made, not only of the fact that the kidney has been injured, but also of the nature of the lesion and of the presence or absence of complicating injuries, in order that, in suitable cases, operative treatment may not be unnecessarily delayed. At the moment of injury, and in the presence of shock, it is a very difficult matter to make such a diagnosis. Local pain and tenderness, muscular rigidity, and, later, hæmaturia, are the characteristic symptoms in uncomplicated cases; and these vary in intensity according to the severity of the injury. Extravasation of urine, extensive hemorrhage, and peritoneal complications are to be determined, each by its own special indications. A collection of fluid in the loin may consist either of blood or of urine, or of a mixture of both. A sample should be obtained by the use of an aspirator or by means of an exploratory incision, when the nature of the fluid may be determined. The most difficult injury to diagnose is one in which the main blood-vessels are involved, and where perhaps a moderate or intermittent hæmaturia may be the only sign.

A man, 45 years of age, was thrown from a sleigh, striking his right loin upon a stake. Hæmaturia, which was never severe,—in fact, it was only slight or moderate in degree,—persisted for two months, without pain or other symptoms, when the kidney was exposed for exploration. A copious hemorrhage occurred when the kidney was handled, and the patient died on the table. Post mortem it was found that the renal vein had been torn in the accident two months before, and had been bleeding into the pelvis.

In hæmaturia it is important to determine the origin of the bleeding, whether from the kidney or from the bladder. If the amount of blood from the kidney is slight, it will be more intimately mixed with the urine; if it comes from the kidney and is somewhat altered in appearance, washing out the bladder with a clear solution will show a moderately clear fluid immediately afterward; whereas, if the blood comes from the bladder itself, fresh bleeding will be produced by the washing. The cystoscope in such cases will make the diagnosis quite clear. In the more severe hemorrhages blood casts of the ureter will be passed with the urine, and, in the worst cases, the bladder may be filled with blood-clots, thus rendering it impossible to determine by any of these methods where the bleeding point is located.

PROGNOSIS.—In moderately severe injuries of the kidney the prognosis is good, and doubtless this organ is frequently the seat of an injury which is never diagnosed. Lesions of the blood-vessels and the ureter are the most serious, and a hemorrhage which persists for weeks is ominous. At first, the chief danger is either shock or hemorrhage, or the effect produced by both combined; later, anuria and, finally, the more remote dangers resulting from infection and suppuration, are to be feared.

TREATMENT.—In the earlier stages and until a diagnosis can be made, and also in the milder cases, palliative treatment is indicated, with—of course—treatment of shock in the more severe conditions. Rest in bed, cold applications locally, and the internal administration of morphia, with the treatment of the symptoms as they arise, are also commendable measures. Blocking of one of the ureters from blood-clots sometimes gives rise to considerable pain, especially if there is continued bleeding or if active urinary secretion within the kidney persists. Filling of the urinary bladder with blood-clots is a very distressing condition. Under ordinary circumstances, if the urethra is normal and will admit the passage of a large instrument, the blood-clots can usually be evacuated more or less satisfactorily by the Bigelow evacuator. In extreme cases, and under special circumstances, cystotomy may be required, and in long-continuing hemorrhage some blood-clot may remain in the bladder and stain the urine for days or weeks. In the most severe cases, especially if the hemorrhage continues, or if a large tumor has formed in the kidney region, operation is indicated. In any case of doubt, experience has shown that operative treatment is much safer than expectant treatment.

Technique.—The kidney may be exposed either by way of the loin or through the abdomen—preferably the former, except in cases in which there is reason to believe that there is a peritoneal or intraperitoneal lesion. An oblique incision is carried down to the kidney and exploration follows. This is a critical stage of the operation, as the landmarks will probably be obliterated by infiltration of blood, and as there may occur a serious hemorrhage the origin of which cannot be definitely located. The writer has lost two patients in this way. In one of these an aberrant artery, having been torn, retracted into the peritoneal cavity, and in the other case the renal vein was torn, and it was found impossible to clamp the proximal end of the vessel. Clamping of the pedicle temporarily with the fingers or by means of a clamp, where the vessels can be caught, will permit of an examination of the organ. The laceration of kidney substance may be treated by the use of a tampon or by suture. While the latter will certainly arrest hemorrhage, it is seldom necessary, as a very free hemorrhage, even from a large venous branch, may be arrested by the use of a tampon. Partial excision of the crushed portion of the kidney may be necessary, or even complete nephrectomy may be required. Serious injury to the renal artery necessitates nephrectomy.

It is important to see that the ureter is intact. If this structure is torn, it may be possible to anastomose or resect, or by other means to unite the torn ends at the time, or it may be necessary to bring the terminal end of the ureter out of the wound, and await a more favorable time or until it is quite clear that the kidney can be saved. (See also Operations on the Ureter.) In most cases it will be impossible to unite the torn ends of the tube. In all operations of this kind, the wound should be drained. A slowly developing tumor in the lumbar region indicates a collection of blood or urine, or a mixture of the two, either in the renal pelvis or within the fatty capsule.

According to various statistics about fifty per cent of the complicated cases are fatal, and thirty per cent of the uncomplicated ones. (von Bergmann's "System of Practical Surgery.")

Open Wounds of the Kidney.—Open wounds of the kidney are generally the result of either stab or gunshot wounds, and are comparatively rare. In cases of gunshot wounds, the kidney injury is generally complicated by injuries to other organs, or, more frequently, the kidney injury is only a part of a more serious result of the gunshot wound. An exception to this rule is found in the case of a direct wound by a spent bullet or a bullet from a toy weapon. In stab wounds, the injuries to the kidney vary very greatly. The wound may be a clean incised wound or a contused wound, large or small. In large wounds there may be prolapse of the kidney upon the loin. Gunshot wounds in the kidney, as in other organs, produce great laceration and destruction of tissue, though of course much depends upon the nature and velocity of the bullet traversing the kidney. In gunshot and stab wounds of the kidney, or of the parts in its neighborhood, the signs which indicate that this organ has been injured are hæmaturia and leakage of urine from the wound.

The prognosis and treatment depend upon the extent of the injury; but, as there is always the added risk of infection from without, operation of some form is always indicated, even if it be nothing more than to secure drainage. It is usually necessary, however, to expose the kidney and adopt measures for the arrest of the bleeding, and then to treat the wound on the general principles applicable to kidney injuries—viz., the application of a tampon, nephrotomy, partial or complete nephrectomy, etc. In some cases drainage alone may prove to be all that is required. Inasmuch as it is very probable, especially in gunshot wounds, that the peritoneum or some other intraperitoneal organs have been injured at the same time, a transperitoneal operation is most frequently indicated; and with it should usually be associated adequate provision for drainage through the loin. In case of injury to the ureter, the torn ends of this tube should be united, if possible, at the time, or—if this be not practicable—they may be brought out upon the loin, with a view to the making of a plastic operation later, for the purpose of restoring function. In any case, the indications are to save the kidney, if possible; but this can rarely be done, except in the milder and more superficial injuries.

V. ABNORMAL CONDITIONS AND DISEASES OF THE KIDNEYS.

(Tuberculosis and Tumors Excepted.)

Movable Kidney.—Normally, the kidney has a certain limited range of mobility, chiefly in the vertical direction. This is easily demonstrated in exploratory operations upon the abdomen, in which the kidney is manipulated. The normal range of movement has been estimated by Watson at from half an inch to an inch and a half. The terms "movable kidney" and "floating kidney" are applied to those conditions in which the kidney is abnormally movable, although the excessive mobility may not produce any symptoms. (This condition is often discovered accidentally, in the routine examination of a patient.) The terms "movable kidney" and "floating kidney" are often confused. Anatomically, a floating kidney is defined by Morris,* who mentions several cases, as one that is more or less completely invested by peritoneum, so disposed as to form a meso-nephron. This anatomical condition is rare and of course congenital, but it cannot be diagnosed except by exploration. Clinically, the terms are employed more or less interchangeably, the term floating kidney being used only where there is a wide range of movement. The term movable kidney is, however, the more suitable one and is applicable to all cases.

ETIOLOGY.—Among the predisposing causes the following have been described: shallowness of the fossa in which the kidney lies; emaciation, with atrophy of kidney fat; relaxation of the abdominal wall after pregnancy; pressure downward by the liver on the right side; and alteration in the ligamentous structures that lie in front of the kidney. Of all these the latter is probably the most important.

Movable kidney is often found as a part of a general enteroptosis, but, on the other hand, it more frequently occurs without any displacement of the other abdominal viscera. It is an acquired condition and is generally attributed to such exciting causes as falls, heavy lifting, and violent muscular exertion. An instructive case, illustrating the effect of a jar, is the following:—

A stout, middle-aged woman, with a very marked condition of movable kidney on the right side, was operated upon; and, on being returned to bed in a limp and helpless condition, she almost fell upon the floor and was put to bed in this way. As a probable result of the fall, the kidney was torn from its fresh attachments to the muscular wall of the abdomen. This fact was ascertained at the first dressing, forty-eight hours later, when it was discovered that the right kidney occupied an abnormal position and was freely movable.

Movable kidney is more frequent in women than in men (approximately ten times more frequent), and it occurs from ten to fifteen times more frequently upon the right than upon the left side.

Abnormal mobility of the kidney may result in hydronephrosis from kinking of the ureter and interference with the exit of the urinary secretion. It is also said to produce gangrene of the kidney—a condition which may occur from twisting of the pedicle to such a degree as to interfere with the circulation; but this could happen only when the mobility is great and when the vessels which form the pedicle are elongated. Sudden obstruction to the escape of urine produces urinary crises with symptoms resembling those of renal colic.

SYMPTOMS.—There are no characteristic symptoms of movable kidney. The symptoms generally complained of are usually referable to the abdominal viscera or the pelvic organs in women, and the diagnosis cannot be made definite except by palpation of the kidney and demonstration of its mobility in various directions. The most characteristic symptoms are those which refer to the kidney function. They are: pain resembling renal colic, polyuria, and urinary crises. Even these symptoms are not, as a rule, very well defined, and are often susceptible of some other explanation.

* "Surgical Diseases of the Kidney and Ureter."

Gastro-intestinal symptoms are perhaps the most common; they include pain or discomfort after food, with that indefinite group of symptoms called dyspepsia, which may even include jaundice.

The pelvic symptoms produced by movable kidney in the female have often been mistaken for the symptoms arising from uterine and ovarian lesions. Movable kidney is also frequently associated with the symptoms of general neurasthenia.

DIAGNOSIS.—The movable kidney may be mistaken for a distended gall-bladder, a retroperitoneal tumor, or a pancreatic cyst, for chronic or subacute appendicitis, for an ovarian tumor, a tumor of the colon, etc.

Where a movable kidney is suspected the patient should be examined, first, while lying upon the back. When the abdomen is carefully palpated the kidney may be found lying down toward the pelvis or over toward the middle line, and on gentle manipulation it will slip back into the loin with a perceptible jerky sensation. This is the most characteristic sign. Placing the patient carefully upon the side opposite to the supposed lesion, with the thighs flexed, and instructing him to cough and take long breaths, or placing him in a partial sitting position, may bring the kidney down within reach.

The patient may be examined for movable kidney on several occasions before it is finally discovered. At the time of the examination the organ may be in its normal situation, and it may not be possible to demonstrate its mobility.

PROGNOSIS.—There is no essential danger to life in a movable kidney. Hydronephrosis may be induced by the twisting or kinking of the ureter due to the displacement of the kidney, and such displacement may also be an important factor in the production of a general neurasthenia.

TREATMENT.—The treatment is hygienic, mechanical, and operative. Hygienic treatment, with rest in bed for a long period, and with a corresponding degree of improvement in the nervous condition, may effect a cure of the symptoms. The selection of suitable cases for operation or for mechanical treatment is most important. As a general rule, all pronounced cases, regardless of the cause, should be operated upon; the only exceptions being those in which the movable kidney is a part of a general enteroptosis in a neurasthenic patient. In such cases the result is most likely to be unsatisfactory, inasmuch as the patient will continue to complain of the symptoms notwithstanding the fact that the kidney remains fixed in the loin in its normal position.

In a general enteroptosis, where the patient's mind is fixed upon the kidney, and where in consequence he persists in keeping his bed, an operation upon the kidney, for the purpose of securing fixation in the normal position, will sometimes, in conjunction with medical and hygienic treatment, prove a very important step toward recovery from the nervous derangement.

In those cases in which the movable kidney is not associated with neurasthenia or enteroptosis, but is otherwise disturbing the health of the patient, operation is indicated and will generally effect a cure.

In neurasthenic patients, except as above stated, operation is likely to be disappointing, and should be undertaken only with great caution.

Mechanical treatment consists in the application of belts and abdominal supporters. It is difficult to see how the application of any mechanical support to the abdomen can do much good for a movable kidney, and it is quite clear that it cannot retain the organ in its place. However, in neurasthenia the abdominal supporter is often hailed by the patient as a great boon. The tendency to over-appreciate the treatment is as great as the tendency to overestimate the gravity of the lesion.

The results of operation are variously stated as in the neighborhood of 80 per cent of cures, from 5 to 10 per cent of failures, and 10 per cent of recurrences. There should be no mortality from the operation itself. Any mortality occurring from the operation is of course accidental.

Acute symptoms produced by kinking of the ureter and resembling renal colic are treated by putting the patient to bed and using manipulations to replace the kidney. Then, if such replacement cannot be effected by simple measures, operation is indicated. When the kidney is exposed for this purpose it should be fixed in its place by one or other of the operative methods to be hereafter described.

Nephrorrhaphy or Nephropexy.—The operation of nephrorrhaphy or nephropexy was first performed by Hahn in 1881;* he simply stitched the fatty capsule to the loin. This operation, as might be expected, was not always successful, and many modifications have been made in the operation since that time. The operative methods may be classified as follows:—(1) The removal or displacement of the fatty capsule and the suturing of the fibrous cpasule to the transversalis and oblique muscles in the posterior adominal wound. (2) The suturing of the kidney by means of sutures passed through the substance of the organ as well as through the enveloping fibrous capsule. (3) More or less complete decapsulation of the kidney, with sutures placed in such a way as to bring the bared surface of the organ in contact with the posterior abdominal wall. Scarification of the fibrous capsule and the employment of gauze packing to produce a granulating surface are measures that are resorted to with the same object in view. (4) Fixation of the kidney, by means of sutures, to the lower rib. This method is unnecessary, and not only is it more difficult and dangerous, but it is wrong in principle, as the object aimed at is to prevent displacement and not to obtain absolute immobility. Moreover, the firm fixation of the kidney to the freely movable chest wall would place it in a most unnatural position and subject it to severe strain. There have also been published descriptions of "sling operations" and "basket operations," in which the sutures are passed around the kidney instead of through its capsule or substance. In all these operations the incision is a loin incision, made either vertically along the outer border of the erector spinæ muscles or, more frequently, obliquely forward, in a direction parallel to the last rib and behind the peritoneum. Extensive or complete decortication is recommended by Edebohls.

Transperitoneal operation has been employed, but is not to be recommended.

* Centralblatt f. Chirurgie. 1881.

Secure fixation of the kidney to the posterior abdominal wall by sutures passed through both the fibrous capsule and the kidney substance, after displacement of the fat capsule, and either with or without partial or complete decapsulation, or one of the other methods mentioned as being employed for the purpose of securing closer union, can generally be relied upon to effect a cure of the abnormal mobility and, at the same time, in suitable cases, a cure of the symptoms also. The best suture material, in the writer's opinion, is chromicized catgut. Treves recommends kangaroo tendon. Silk and thread sutures are objectionable.

Uronephrosis or Hydronephrosis.—The terms "uronephrosis" and "hydronephrosis" are applied to conditions of the kidney in which there is distention caused by retained urine. Hence the name "uronephrosis," which is properly applied to recent cases in which the fluid possesses the chemical characters of urine. In old cases, in which the secreting structure of the kidney has been more or less completely destroyed, and in which the retained fluid no longer possesses the characters of urine, the term "hydronephrosis" is more appropriate. (Fig. 39.)

ETIOLOGY AND PATHOLOGY.—The conditions referred to above are due to some obstruction to the outflow of the urine. The effects of obstruction are first felt in the pelvis of the kidney, which becomes dilated. A continuance of the distention produces dilatation of the calyces, and it may entirely destroy the secreting substance of the kidney and convert it into a fibrous sac which is sometimes so large as to be mistaken for an ovarian or other abdominal tumor, or for a large cystic tumor of the kidney. Both kidneys are frequently the site of a hydronephrosis. Thus, Kuester * found this condition 32 times in 462 cases; Morris,† 274 times in 581 cases; and Newman, 448 times in 665 cases.

It is generally taught that the obstruction which causes hydronephrosis is usually an incomplete or intermittent one, and that sudden complete obstruction rarely produces hydronephrosis, but instead rapidly destroys the secreting structure of the kidney.

Recent experimental ligation of the ureter in dogs, by Dr. G. D. Scott,‡ would seem to show that sudden complete obstruction to the outflow of the urine does produce uronephrosis. The following are his conclusions, based upon the experiments made on twelve dogs which came to autopsy:—

"Without an exception, the twelve experiments support the following conclusions:—Contrary to the accepted theory, a sudden, complete, permanent obstruction of the ureter produces a hydronephrosis of a high degree.

"Hydronephrosis develops with greater rapidity after a sudden complete permanent obstruction of the ureter." § This view is also supported by the following case which came under the observation of the writer in October, 1903:—

* Quoted by von Bergmann in his "System of Practical Surgery."
† "Surgical Diseases of the Kidney and Ureter," vol. i.
‡ Journal of Surgery, Gynæcology, and Obstetrics, Aug., 1910.
§ Quoted from the Journal of Surgery, Gynæcology, and Obstetrics, Aug., 1910.

A boy, aged 12, while playing football, received a kick in the right loin about one o'clock in the afternoon. He was brought to the hospital twelve hours later with a tumor in the kidney region as large as the head of a new-born child and suffering great pain of a distensile character. The next morning, the mass was found to be much larger, and, about twenty hours from the time of the accident, the kidney was exposed in the loin. It was found to be greatly distended and, on incision of the pelvis, nearly a quart of blood-stained urine escaped. The ureter was found to be torn off about an inch from its origin in the pelvis of the kidney. Urine continued to discharge freely from the wound in the loin, and about three months later the kidney was removed and the boy made an uninterrupted recovery.

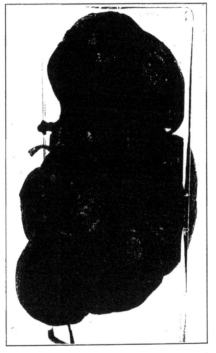

Fig. 39.—Hydronephrosis in Obstruction of the Pelvis of the Kidney by a Calculus. (From a specimen in the Pathological Museum of McGill University, Montreal.)

It seems probable, therefore, that too much stress has been laid upon the partial obstruction of the ureter as the sole cause of uronephrosis, although in most cases the causative conditions are, in the nature of things, produced more or less gradually.

The usual causes are ureteral obstruction, either congenital or acquired; and the obstruction may come from some outside influence or be located within the ureter. When it comes from without, it may be caused by the pressure of a new-growth or a collection of inflammatory products, or by some abnormality of a blood-vessel. (W. J. Mayo has recently reported a number of cases, in which he attributes the uronephrosis to this cause.*) Other causes are: twists, kinks, bends, abnormal positions of the kidney, movable kidney, etc. When the cause operates from within the ureter, it may consist of a stricture, a valvular condition, or the presence of a calculus, etc. It must also be borne in mind that a stricture or other internal obstruction is liable to aggravation at times from some alteration in the quantity and quality of the urine, as a result of which the mucous membrane becomes more or less swollen, just

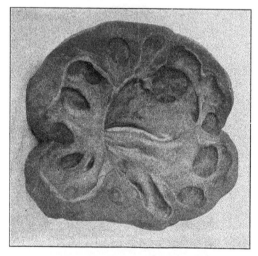

Fig. 40.—Pyonephrosis in Obstruction of the Ureter by a Carcinomatous Growth in the Pelvis of the Kidney. (From a specimen in the Pathological Museum of McGill University, Montreal.)

as occurs in stricture of the urethra, where similar changes in the urine are likely to produce retention of urine in the bladder. A slight ureteral stricture is thought to occur sometimes from an ascending gonorrhœa. It is remarkable how often calculi obstruct the ureter without producing an appreciable distensile effect upon the pelvis of the kidney. This is no doubt due to the fact that, while a calculus dilates the ureter above the point of obstruction, it also dilates it sufficiently at the point of obstruction to allow the urine to escape with a fair degree of freedom. It has been generally noted that the higher the obstruction the greater the probability of hydronephrosis, although it is said that stricture of the urethra, prostatic obstruction, and even phimosis may cause hydronephrosis, but the occurrence of this result from such a remote obstruction must be

* Journal of the American Medical Association. May 1st, 1909, lii.

extremely rare.* External pressure was found to be the cause in 142 cases examined by Morris from the records of the post-mortem examinations made at the Middlesex Hospital from 1873 to 1883. The details are as follows:— In 116 cases there was cancer of either the vagina, the uterus, the bladder, or the rectum, and in 2 others cancer of the ovary; in 4 the cause was cystitis; in 3 it was vesical calculus; in 1, tumor of the bladder; in 3, enlarged prostate; in 4, ovarian cysts; in 4, cancer of some abdominal organ; and in 3, constriction of the ureter.†

It is well known that the kidney substance, although greatly thinned from distention, may still possess secreting function, and some observers have thought that it is only in rare instances that the kidney function is entirely destroyed. There is no doubt, however, that in very advanced cases the kidney tissue is completely destroyed, the only structure remaining being a fibrous sac which is filled with fluid, and which—to all intents and purposes—constitutes a cystic tumor.

STATISTICS OF HYDRONEPHROSIS IN THE ROYAL VICTORIA HOSPITAL, FOR A PERIOD OF TWELVE YEARS (1898–1909).

Number of surgical cases treated in 11 years 14,503

Ages.

Cases of hydronephrosis................ 16	0 to 10	0
(Males, 3; females, 13.)	10 to 20	0
Cause, calculus 4	20 to 30	6
Cause, none found.................... 8	30 to 40	4
No data 4	40 to 50	1
Operated upon 12	50 to 60	1
Not operated upon................... 1	Over 60	1
Nephrectomy........................ 13		
Nephrotomy......................... 3		

Hydronephrosis, it is said, may involve only a part of the kidney, but it is not easy to understand how this can be possible.

SYMPTOMS.—Patients with a hydronephrosis of large dimensions often give no history of symptoms beyond those due to the mechanical effects of the intra-abdominal tumor—viz., a sense of pressure, weight, fulness, and interference with the function of those organs which are displaced or pressed upon; but a careful investigation will often elicit an antecedent history of renal symptoms which had occurred perhaps many years previously.

For example, an intelligent woman of 45, with a large hydronephrosis, gave a very clear history of having had, twenty-five years previously, symptoms which resembled those of renal colic, and which occurred occasionally during the space of one year, with also occasional hæmaturia. In this case the sac was removed, the ureter was found entirely unobstructed, and no cause could be discovered.

* The writer has had occasion to operate upon a man, fifty years of age, in whom an obstruction at the distal end of the ureter, probably congenital, produced a hydronephrosis with dilatation of the ureter to a diameter of an inch and a half or more.
† The writer has seen double hydronephrosis caused by a large fibromyoma of the uterus.

In the more acute obstructions pain and disturbance of urinary function may occur. Thus, for example, there may be a diminished flow of urine, alternating with polyuria; and the discovery of these facts may lead to early diagnosis and treatment directed toward saving the kidney.

DIAGNOSIS.—Hydronephrosis may be confounded with an ovarian, pancreatic, or hydatid cyst; with cystic disease of the kidney, pyonephrosis (into which it sometimes passes from infection of the fluid contents), or with nephritic. abscess; with a distended gall-bladder; or with a retroperitoneal tumor. A point which it is important to bear in mind in diagnosis is that kidney tumors of all kinds are laterally placed, and that, no matter how large they may become, they will always (except in anomalous congenital conditions) occupy a lateral position in the upper zone of the abdomen. Ureteral catheterization is valuable as a means of diagnosis, and—provided a metallic probe be first passed into the ureter—the x-ray will not only show, but will locate, any point of obstruction that may exist.

The fluid contents may be obtained for examination by aspiration, but, for obvious reasons, no great reliance can be placed upon the result, as in old cases the fluid may be so altered as to contain little or no urea or uric acid, while in some cystic conditions the fluid may contain urea.

TREATMENT.—Aspiration is said to have cured some cases. This, however, must be a very rare result, and, except for the purpose of securing fluid for examination, it is a very unsatisfactory procedure and not altogether devoid of danger, as it may be the means of introducing infection. Exploratory nephrotomy is safer and more satisfactory. Nephrotomy with drainage is rarely curative and generally results in the establishment of fistula, which is likely to become infected. In a large hydronephrosis of long standing, partial or complete removal of the sac, preferably the latter, is most satisfactory and is usually neither a difficult nor a dangerous operation. In earlier cases, it may be possible to remove the cause and preserve the kidney; and valvular conditions of the ureter may be dealt with in suitable cases by plastic operations. (See Operations upon the Ureter.) Drainage by means of the ureteral catheter has been recommended, but the procedure can hardly be looked upon as of practical application. Finally, a spontaneous cure may occur. It is possible that in some cases in which the disease was diagnosed as hydronephrosis, the real affection was a cystic degeneration of the kidney. (See Hypernephroma.)

Perinephritis.—Both the fibrous and the lipomatous forms of perinephritis often occur in connection with disease of the kidney (such, for example, as calculus, tuberculosis, etc.); the fibrous form producing condensation and hardening of the fibrous and fatty tissues of the renal capsule, and the lipomatous form causing an extensive growth of fatty tissue, which may invade the kidney itself. These processes are chronic and painless, and are of secondary importance as compared with the disease of the kidney itself; they do not require treatment and cannot be diagnosed, except by an exploratory operation.

Suppurative Perinephritis.—Suppurative perinephritis occurs as a result of the infection of the perirenal tissues, or is due to the extension of a suppurative process from the kidney or from some neighboring organ—the appendix, peritoneum, pleura, vertebræ, etc. Primary perinephritis—the term being used here in the sense of an infection independent of any similar process in the kidney itself—is rare. When the infection has not extended through the kidney from a calculous or tuberculous or inflammatory process, or from some neighboring organ, it is believed that bacteria, which are being eliminated by the urine, often find their way through the kidney and thus infect the perireneal tissues. In this way is to be explained the perinephritis which follows certain infectious fevers (such as scarlet fever), gonorrhœa, and other suppurative processes. The development of suppurative perinephritis is frequently the first indication of a chronic tuberculous lesion which has destroyed the kidney.

Infection may also take place through the blood current and through the lymphatic system, and it frequently follows trauma, the infection then spreading to the damaged tissue from without (in the case of an open wound) or through the blood current (in the case of an internal wound), just as happens in the case of an epiphyseal bone infection following a slight trauma of the bone with unbroken skin surface. The same explanation may be given in those cases of infection which seem to follow exposure to cold. An infective perinephritis may stop short of suppuration, developing only an acute or chronic inflammatory process, which may subside without producing an abscess. When suppuration occurs, it may do so in a fairly acute manner, but the process usually is of a more or less chronic character. The abscess may be diffuse or there may be multiple abscesses in the perirenal tissue, but most frequently the suppurative process finally develops into a single large abscess, which tends to point, generally, upon the loin, but which often opens into other organs or cavities—the peritoneal cavity or one of the pleural cavities, the bladder or the vagina, the spleen or the liver, etc. If not evacuated early, the abscess may burrow deeply. According to Morris,* in four or five out of every twelve cases which are allowed to pursue their course, the abscess opens into the pleura or the lung.

SYMPTOMS.—In acute suppurative perinephritis arising independently of previous disease in the kidney or its capsule, the symptoms are: pain, tenderness, and muscular rigidity, followed more or less rapidly by local signs of abscess (swelling, redness, heat, œdema, and tenderness) and accompanied by the usual constitutional symptoms (fever, chills, etc.). This primary form of perinephritis, however, is a rare affection. In the large majority of cases, suppurative perinephritis is developed upon a pre-existing disease of the kidney or its capsule,— such a disease, for example, as tuberculosis, calculus, etc.,—and is of a subacute or chronic character at the outset. Under these circumstances the symptoms develop less rapidly, and pain may be the only symptom for a considerable period of time. In the absence of other symptoms, this pain is difficult to explain, and often very puzzling. It may simulate the pain of hip-joint disease, spinal disease, pleurisy, and still other diseased conditions; and the constitutional symptoms may also develop gradually. Finally, however, an abscess of the acute form develops, and, if it happens to be located in

* "Surgical Diseases of the Kidney and Ureter," vol. i., 1901.

the upper pole of the kidney, the symptoms may simulate those of a pleurisy or a pneumonia.

DIAGNOSIS.—The diagnosis is difficult, and often impossible, until local signs develop. Cystoscopy and ureteral catheterization will often reveal an unsuspected absence of the function of one kidney, and it will ultimately be shown that this cessation of function is due to the destruction of the kidney by chronic tuberculosis.

PROGNOSIS.—Perinephritis in itself is not a serious condition, but if allowed to run its course it gives rise to complications which have been previously mentioned, and it is often a serious indication, on account of the primary cause. According to Kuester * there are thirty-four per cent of fatalities. In neglected cases, the abscess may open spontaneously upon the loin or burrow beneath the psoas muscle, producing contraction of this muscle. In such cases, fistulæ generally persist.

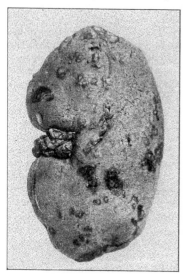

FIG. 41.—Acute Pyelonephritis; Free Surface of the Kidney showing the Cortex studded with Multiple small Abscesses, each one surrounded by a hemorrhagic zone. (From specimen No. 2860 in the Pathological Museum of McGill University Montreal.)

TREATMENT.—In the earlier stages of the disease, rest, soothing applications, and, when a diagnosis has been made, early operation, as soon as there are signs of suppuration, are the therapeutic measures indicated. The kidney is exposed by an incision in the loin. Careful exploration all around the organ, especially at its upper pole, may be necessary if the focus of the disease is to be discovered in its early development, but in many cases the kidney will be found to be destroyed, especially by tuberculosis, and nephrectomy will then be necessary. Should any other cause be discovered, it must, of course, be removed.

Suppurative Inflammations of the Kidney.—Apart from specific causes, such as calculus, tuberculosis, syphilis, actinomycosis, etc., suppurative inflammations of the kidney are classified according to the part involved. They are: pyelitis, pyonephrosis, pyelonephritis, and suppurative nephritis. Pyelitis is a suppurative inflammation of the pelvis of the kidney. Pyonephrosis is the term applied to the condition in which urine and the products of suppurative inflammation are pent up in the kidney. (Fig. 40.) This abscess-like collection of fluid often proceeds to destroy, by pressure, the

* von Bergmann's " System of Practical Surgery."

secreting structure of the kidney, finally converting the organ into a fibrous sac. Pyonephrosis is most frequently found as a late condition, secondary to calculus or an ascending gonorrhœal infection; or it may be due to the infection of a uronephrosis.

Pyelonephritis is the term employed when the suppurative process extends to the kidney substance. Surgical kidney is another, somewhat vague term that is applied to the same conditions. Then, finally, there is suppurative nephritis, also called diffuse suppuration of the kidney, in which multiple foci of infection and suppuration—usually of hæmatogenous origin—develop in the kidney substance. (Figs. 41 and 42.)

The conditions described above may be variously combined or they may pass one into the other; they all result from infection. The ordinary infecting micro-organisms are the staphylococcus, the streptococcus, the gonococcus, the pneumococcus, the typhoid bacillus, the colon bacillus, and the proteus vulgaris, as well as micro-organisms of other infectious diseases. Infection is usually secondary to some obstruction to the urinary outflow—such, for example, as stricture of the urethra, prostatic obstruction, etc. The part played by the colon bacillus, which is so generally found in inflammatory processes of the genito-urinary tract, is not well understood, and, although it is more uniformly found in kidney suppurations than are any of the other micro-organisms, it is rarely found alone, being usually associated

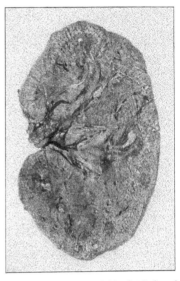

Fig. 42.—Acute Pyelonephritis. Cut Surface of the Kidney shown in Fig. 41.
There are multiple small abscesses located chiefly in the cortex.

with some of the other bacteria. The gonococci are thought to act in most cases by preparing the soil for the attacks of the other infective agents. (Watson.)

MODES OF INVASION.—There are two principal modes of invasion—that known as ascending infection, and that which takes place by way of the blood current. In the first of these methods the infection travels up along the ureter, and is generally due to the micro-organisms connected with a cystitis, a gonorrhœa, an enlargement of the prostate, or some other genito-urinary disorder. It is remarkable, however, when the frequency of gonorrhœa is considered, how seldom a clearly defined gonorrhœal infection of the kidney or its pelvis occurs. Infection by way of the blood current occurs much more frequently than was formerly supposed.   It is now an established fact that micro-organisms of infectious and suppurative diseases and of tuberculosis pass through the kidney in their elimination, and may thus become the means of infection.   Calculus, tuberculosis, and traumatism are often followed by suppuration of the kidney, and are to be considered as predisposing factors.   (See Renal Calculus and Renal Tuberculosis.)   Any form of kidney suppuration may occur as one of the phenomena of a general pyæmia.

In ascending infection the pelvis of the kidney is first involved.   The ureter shows generally only slight signs of inflammation.   From the view-point of diagnosis and operative treatment this is very important.   A pyelitis thus produced may, by extension, give rise to a pyelonephritis, a pyonephritic abscess, or even a suppurative nephritis.   In infection by way of the blood current foci form in the kidney substance and develop into small abscesses, which may, or may not, become fused into one or more larger abscesses which break into the pelvis and produce a pyelitis or a pyonephrosis by secondary involvement. Pyelonephritis and suppurative nephritis are in most instances secondary to cystitis, but it does not follow that these diseases are always the result of an ascending infection.   Micro-organisms may enter the blood from a diseased bladder or a septic phlebitis.   Indeed, from the fact that small foci of suppuration are found in the kidney substance before any evidence of infection is discovered in the pelvis of the kidney, it would seem that the infection must almost necessarily have occurred by way of the blood current.

The question is asked, whether, in suppurative nephritis, one or both kidneys are, as a rule, primarily infected.   This is a very important question from the view-point of early operative treatment, and yet it is almost impossible to furnish a trustworthy reply.   While it is recognized that, in cases which come to autopsy, both kidneys are by that time usually involved, there is reason to believe that at the outset, in a considerable number of cases, the infection is confined to one kidney.   There have been reported cases in which one kidney has been treated by operation, with an entirely satisfactory result, and this fact seems to show that the other had not been involved.   It is not safe, however, to conclude, from this evidence, that only one kidney has been infected, because it is possible that the second may have recovered spontaneously.   Experience shows that this is quite possible.   The use of the cystoscope and ureteral catheterization, when feasible, afford important aid in diagnosis, and so also does the x-ray, by means of which the presence of a stone in the kidney may be ascertained.

Pyonephrosis is often the result of an infected uronephrosis.

SYMPTOMS OF SUPPURATIVE INFLAMMATION OF THE KIDNEY.—The symptoms of such suppurative inflammation vary, of course, very much with the part and the extent of the organ involved, the mode of onset, and the virulence of the infection.   The essential symptoms are toxæmic in character, and these, with the local pain and tenderness, point to the character of the lesions, although the latter are often very slight.   In an ascending infection, the symptoms are likely to be less severe than when the infection takes place by way of the blood current.

It is impossible to diagnose one form from the other definitely until the local signs develop, but in suppurative nephritis there is a group of symptoms which invariably indicate a profound toxæmia.   In the more acute attacks, for example, there are chills, high fever, and profuse perspirations, with great prostration, anorexia, delirium, muscular pains, etc.   In such severe attacks micro-organisms (diplococci, etc.) may be found in the blood.   In another form of attack,— which is generally observed in old men who suffer from prostatic obstruction and bladder infection,—there are, instead of chills and fever, subnormal temperature, prostration, stupor, low muttering delirium, dry tongue, anorexia, and rapid emaciation.   Between these two groups of symptoms varying degrees of type and severity are found.   In suppurative nephritis the kidney is swollen and œdematous, but is not usually greatly enlarged.   In thin persons the organ may be palpable.   It is only in pyonephrosis that the kidney is usually enlarged to such a degree as to be easily palpable.   In pyelitis and pyelonephritis, the local signs of pain and tenderness, with toxæmia, are the most reliable indications upon which a diagnosis may be made.

The Urine.—Except in the case of a localized abscess or of a temporary obstruction in the ureter there is always pyuria; and, even when an abscess has formed, there are likely to be periodical discharges of large quantities of pus. In suppurative nephritis of an acute character there will be blood in the urine, although perhaps it may be recognizable only with the aid of the microscope. The urine is usually acid; it contains bacteria; and, unless the kidney substance is extensively diseased on both sides, the total quantity of urine passed is not materially diminished.   Albumin and casts are often, but not always, found. In pyonephrosis, intermittent attacks of pyuria are synchronous with corresponding alterations in the size of the kidney tumor and in the general symptoms; but, in chronic suppurative conditions, the symptoms may be very mild, indeed, unless the kidney structure has become so extensively diseased as to cause uræmia. These chronic forms of the disease are not infrequently seen in young men as a sequel to gonorrhœa.   This happened in the case of a young man twenty-three years of age, who was under the writer's care.   In this case an ascending gonorrhœal infection, without producing at any time very acute symptoms, ultimately caused death through a complete destruction of the kidney tissue, both of these organs being converted into pus sacs in the space of four years and nine months.

When, in a case of suppuration or inflammation of the lower genito-urinary organs, pain and tenderness develop in the kidney region and are accompanied by fever, an ascending lesion should be suspected.

PROGNOSIS.—The prognosis is very variable in any of the forms of suppurative disease of the kidney.   The process may be arrested before very serious harm has been done, or the lesions may be produced so gradually as to allow of spontaneous or operative relief.   In simple pyelitis all the symptoms may subside.   In pyonephrosis, if the cause is removed, as by the passage of a calculus or by the free escape of pus along the ureter, a complete subsidence of all symptoms may occur, at least for a time.   In pyelonephritis the prognosis is generally bad.   In ascending infections the symptoms may begin somewhat gradually, the probability being that only one kidney is involved, but, if operative treatment is not resorted to, the other kidney will soon become involved also; and, even if the kidney first involved be treated by operation, the other may become infected through the same source as the first, and the outlook will then be grave. In acute suppurative nephritis, the prognosis is generally, but not always, hopeless. The same may be said of the more chronic forms, in which only a limited number of foci occur and which may develop into abscesses that coalesce and break into the pelvis or that may be evacuated surgically. In such cases, recovery may take place. In suppurative nephritis of hæmatogenous origin the condition is almost always hopeless.

Renal Calculus; Nephrolithiasis.—For the formation of urinary calculi, which are produced mainly in the kidney and in the bladder, two conditions are requisite. These are: the precipitation of urinary salts, and the production of an albuminoid substance which binds the crystalline or amorphous solids together. This production of an albuminoid substance may be the result of a pre-existing inflammatory process, or it may be, as in primary stone formation, the result of the irritation caused by the deposition of urinary salts upon the epithelial lining of the part in which the stone is formed. It is believed by some investigators that an organic mould is produced by this colloid material, and that in this mould the urinary salts, generally in crystalline form, are deposited. However, while the organic mould may be demonstrated, after the removal of the mineral constituents of the stone, it does not follow that it was a pre-requisite to the stone formation. Generally speaking, it may be said that probably the production of colloid material in primary stone formation proceeds coincidently with the deposition of the mineral ingredients, and probably, as above stated, as a result of such deposit.

ETIOLOGY.—The causes of the formation of calculus in the kidney are of two classes—general and local. The general causes are chiefly those which produce faulty metabolism. Among these the most important are improper diet and deficient exercise; hence the frequent association of stone in the kidney with gouty conditions. Dietetic errors leading to stone formation in the kidney are: in children, overfeeding, improper and irregular feeding, unsuitable food, too much meat, too much sugar, and too little liquid. In the adult, in addition to the foregoing, the use of alcohol is believed to be a potent factor. There are also certain geographical influences which are not well undersood. It is a matter of observation that certain districts produce a greater number of calculi, even among people of the same race and nationality and of similar habits. This is sometimes attributed to the character of the drinking water of these localities, but it is difficult to understand how this could be an important factor in the causation of stone in the kidney. In Egypt, India, and certain tropical countries, where renal calculi are very prevalent, it is believed that their causation is often associated with certain parasitic diseases of the blood (Bilharzia hæmatobia, Filiaria sanguinis, etc.), in which diseases the ova or embryos may enter the kidney by way of the blood-vessels and form the nuclei of calculi.

Social condition, heredity, sex, and age all have an important bearing upon the formation of urinary calculi. The children of the poor, who are less carefully managed and are improperly fed, suffer more from calculi than do those in better circumstances, while in adults the well-fed and the self-indulgent probably suffer more frequently than the hard-working and abstemious.

Renal calculi are found at all ages. Some authors believe that they occur more frequently in early childhood and after forty years of age, while Morris' tables indicate a much greater prevalence in early adult life. It is a difficult matter to determine the correctness of such a statement, as it is not during the formative period of the stone that patients come under observation for its treatment, and, indeed, one often discovers at autopsy calculi which had never been suspected during life. Renal calculi are bilateral in as many as fifty per cent of the cases.

It is generally accepted that urinary calculi are found much more frequently in the male than in the female; the proportion is usually stated as about 95 to 5, in every hundred. The influence of heredity as a strong predisposing factor in the causation of urinary calculi, is well recognized.

Among local causes are the presence of a nucleus such as a foreign body, pus, blood, bacteria, necrotic tissue, etc. The presence of a nucleus can, however, rarely be demonstrated in renal calculi. Alteration in the character of the urine, although due to general causes such as retention from any cause, obstruction produced by adjacent spinal disease, toxæmia, etc., may be classed among the local causes.

Renal calculi vary very much in size, number, and shape, as well as in chemical composition. Fine particles like sand may clog the urinary passages and lodge in the pelvis of the kidney, or may form incrustations on the mucous membrane.

In a middle-aged man who recently came under the care of the writer for temporary anuria, the bladder wall was seen by the cystoscope to be coated with a sand-like substance, and, after this had been washed away, a fresh collection came down from the kidney. This substance consisted of uric acid in crystals and in little stones up to the size of a pin's head.

It is to conditions like this that the name "nephrolithiasis" is properly applied. Larger particles of more definite stone formation, and which are more or less readily passed with the urine, are known as "gravel," while those calculous formations which are not readily passed are called "stones" or "calculi," and may attain a very large size. At autopsy there have been removed from the kidney stones that weighed over two pounds, and there is one in St. Bartholomew's Hospital Museum, in London, which weighs thirty-six and one-half ounces. (Barrow.) Dr. David Barrow, of Lexington, Kentucky, brought before the American Surgical Association, in 1908, a stone which weighed one pound and two drachms, and which he had removed from the left kidney of a man aged forty-eight, with an entirely satisfactory result. The stone was not sectioned but was diagnosed as phosphatic.* The number of calculi varies from

* Transactions of the American Surgical Association, vol. xxvi., 1908.

a single stone to as many as a thousand found in a single kidney. (Watson.) As a rule, however, the number does not usually exceed half a dozen.

The shape of the stone varies with the position in which it is formed in the kidney. When formed in the kidney substance the calculus is usually small and round, and when formed in the pelvis or in one of the calyces it usually represents in a general way the shape of the cavity. In the pelvis it may reach a very considerable size, being elongated in the long direction of the kidney, with projections into the calyces, and the whole resembling a potato outgrowth When found in a calyx it is more or less pyramidal in shape, with the apex pointing down into the pelvis, or it may assume the form of a stag's horn.

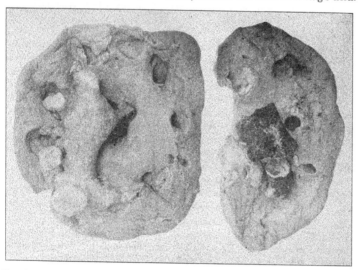

Fig. 43.—Stag-horn Calculi in the Pelvis of Both Kidneys belonging to the Same Patient. (From specimen presented to the Pathological Museum, McGill University, Montreal, by Dr. J. A. MacDonald.)

(Fig. 43.) When there are several stones lying in contact with one another, they are usually facetted.

In chemical composition renal calculi consist of uric acid and urates, of oxalates, and of phosphates. Calcium carbonate, cystin, and xanthin calculi are rare. The commonest forms of renal calculi are those composed of uric acid and urates.

Uric-acid calculi are brownish in color, hard, smooth, and round or oval in shape. They are heavy, they may reach a large size, and they are generally smooth on section, but sometimes they show a more or less concentric arrangement. This is especially seen when the stone has formed around a nucleus. They are often multiple. The urates of sodium, calcium, magnesium, and ammonium enter into the formation of calculi, but stones composed exclusively of urates are rare and found only in children. (Morris.) The oxalate-of-calcium calculus (the mulberry calculus) is the hardest and the heaviest of urinary calculi. It is brownish-yellow or black in color, rough, and nodular; hence the name "mulberry calculus." It is round or oval in shape and does not attain to a very large size. Phosphatic calculi are formed in alkaline urine and are therefore usually secondary to an inflammatory condition in the kidney. As a rule, they consist of the triple phosphate of ammonium, magnesium, and calcium. They are grayish in color, smooth or granular on the surface, and may reach a large size. They have a low specific gravity and are brittle; sometimes they are so soft as to crush when they are pressed between the fingers, but they are also sometimes of quite firm consistence.

Calculi of mixed composition are quite common; they probably occur much more frequently than published statistics would indicate, owing to the fact that usually only small portions of a calculus are analyzed. Thus, uric-acid calculi are sometimes mixed with urates, and oxalate-of-calcium calculi with carbonate of calcium, and any of the primary calculi may be encrusted or covered with phosphates, although this is less likely to occur in the kidney than in the bladder. In thirty-two of Watson's cases * the chemical composition of the calculi was as follows:—

Uricacid	9	Mixed calculi	4
Urates	4	Cystin	1
Oxalate of lime	7	Phosphates	3
Phosphatic masses	4		

In seventy-seven cases tabulated by Morris † the chemical composition is given as follows:—

Uric acid	17	Carbonate of lime	1
Oxalate of lime	34	Cystic oxide	2
Mixed calculi	10	Phosphates	13

Cystic-Oxide Calculi.—Cystic-oxide calculi are rare and are found in acid urine. They are small, smooth, round, and brittle, and have a pale whitish-yellow color and waxy appearance.

Xanthin Calculi.—Xanthin calculi are also rare and resemble cystin (or cystic-oxide) calculi except as regards their color, which is brownish.

The constitutional conditions, or diatheses, which predispose to calculi are described as the uric-acid diathesis, the oxalic-acid diathesis (or oxaluria), the phosphatic diathesis (phosphaturia), etc.

The following statistics have been compiled from the records of the Royal Victoria Hospital for fifteen years (1894–1909):—

Number of patients treated in the surgical wards in fifteen years			15,403
Number of cases of renal calculus			82
Number of cases operated on			28
Males	54	Right kidney	12
Females	64	Both kidneys	3
Left kidney	18		

* Watson and Cunningham's " Genito-Urinary Diseases," vol. ii.
† " Surgical Diseases of the Kidney and Ureter," vol. ii.

Ages of Patients affected with Renal Calculus.

0 to 10	0	40 to 50	12
10 to 20	3	50 to 60	15
20 to 30	25	Over 60	3
30 to 40	19		

Number of cases in which the calculus was located in the upper portion of the ureter.. 3
(These patients were operated upon through a loin incision after exploration of the kidney.)

Number of cases of ureteral calculi in lower end of ureter 12
(Of this number, 10 were operated upon, and 2 were not subjected to operation.)

Males	5	Left side	4
Females	7	Right side	4

(In 4 cases the records did not show on which side the calculus was located.)

Ages in the Ureteral Cases.

0 to 10	0	30 to 40	0
10 to 20	0	40 to 50	4
20 to 30	2		

Total number of post-mortem examinations in 15 years 1,482
Number of cases in which renal and ureteral calculi were found 30
(In 3 of these the calculus was in the ureter.)

Males	19	Both sides	5
Females	11	Cases of single stone	7
Left side	12	Cases of multiple calculi	23
Right side	13		

Composition of the Calculi.

Urates	8	Oxalates	5
Phosphates	4		

Ages of the Patients in the Calculus Cases.

0 to 10	0	40 to 50	7
10 to 20	1	50 to 60	7
20 to 30	3	Over 60	7
30 to 40	5		

EFFECTS OF RENAL CALCULUS UPON THE KIDNEY.—Calculi may form in the kidney substance or in the calyces or pelvis, and may remain quiescent through a lifetime, producing no symptoms. Such a course of events is probably quite exceptional, although long periods of quiescence may follow after an attack of pain or hæmaturia has occurred. The local effect of a calculus is to produce irritation, which prepares the way for infection and pyuria. 'Prior to the occurrence of infection the irritation produces lumbar pain or renal colic or hæmaturia, presumably when the stone becomes partially dislodged. Chronic inflammatory thickening of the surrounding tissues occurs when the stone is lodged in the pelvis, and obstruction of the ureteral outlet may lead to hydronephrosis or even to gradual destruction of the kidney tissue, until there remains only a fibrous sac enclosing the stone. Infection leads to pyonephrosis, and, more rarely, to pyelonephritis. When there are calculi in both kidneys, infection of one is apt to be speedily followed by infection of the other.

SYMPTOMS.—The cardinal symptoms and signs of renal calculus are pain, hæmaturia, frequency of micturition, pyuria, anuria, and tenderness on deep pressure, but none of these symptoms is characteristic of stone in the kidney, and they may all be produced by other pathological conditions of this organ.

Pain.—Pain may be absent altogether or may be referred, for example, to the foot, the external genitals, the groin, etc., and it is believed that it may even be felt upon the side opposite to that on which the lesion is located.   In large stones the pain is usually felt only as a dull indefinite ache in the lumbar region,

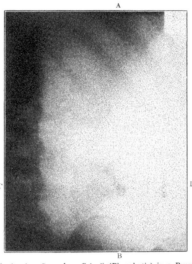

Fig. 44.—Skiagraph showing Secondary Calculi (Phosphatic) in a Pyonephrotic and Fistulous Kidney from which Stones had been Removed at a Previous Operation. (Author's case.)
Two straight lines drawn—the one from A to B, the other from C to D—will cross each other at exactly the spot where the shadow of the outermost one of the group of calculi is located.
This patient had double calculous pyonephrosis. The kidneys were operated upon (nephrolithotomy) on separate occasions, with a three-months interval between the operations. One kidney healed completely, but a fistula persisted and, as shown in the skiagraph, phosphatic calculi formed in the other.

this symptom being aggravated by exertion, jarring, lifting, etc.   In such cases the stone is not movable in the kidney.   On the other hand, renal colic—the pain which is generally considered most characteristic of renal calculus—is, in its worst form, among the most severe forms of pain which patients are called upon to endure.   The strongest men are often completely unnerved by it. The pain of renal colic begins suddenly, usually in the neighborhood of the kidney, in front or behind, and radiates down the line of the ureter to the groin, pelvis, or testicle.   It is produced by the movement of the calculus within the pelvis or in one of the calyces of the kidney, is spasmodic in character, and usually ceases suddenly when the stone has passed into the bladder or has fallen back into the pelvis of the kidney or away from the point of irritation.   When severe, the pain is accompanied by nausea and vomiting, by a frequent desire to micturate, and by a profuse perspiration and prostration. It may last for a varying length of time—from a few minutes to several hours. It varies much in severity as well as in duration, and may be produced by other causes than stone,—viz., by blood-clot, clumps of pus cells, etc. Another form of pain is observed when a calculus suddenly blocks the ureter, especially if the obstruction is located low down. The pain is then continuous and of a distensile character.

Hæmaturia.—Hæmaturia is a very constant symptom of renal calculus. In the majority of cases, especially as an early symptom, the blood is only microscopic in quantity, varying with the amount of exertion put forth by the patient;

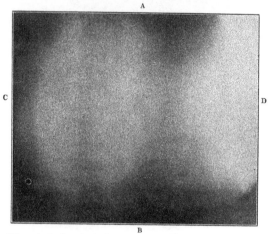

FIG. 45.—Skiagraph of a Stone in the Lower Part of the Kidney. (Author's case.)
Two straight lines drawn—the one from *A* to *B*, the other from *C* to *D*—will cross each other at exactly the spot where the shadow of the stone is located.
This patient had a large pyonephrosis, but the calculus was plainly shown in the skiagraph. It was found in the lowermost calyx of the kidney, and was removed through a vertical incision. The kidney was drained for a few days; complete and rapid recovery followed.

indeed, it may temporarily disappear when the patient remains in bed. Blood in macroscopic amount is also a common symptom, and even quite severe hemorrhages may take place, especially after infection has occurred and in the presence of rough stones which may cause ulceration through the walls of a blood-vessel. As might be expected, violent exertion, jarring from driving in a rough vehicle, etc., have the effect of producing or increasing hemorrhage from the kidney.

Anuria.—Anuria may occur from simultaneous or nearly simultaneous blocking of both ureters by stones, or by the blocking of the single ureter when only one kidney exists; or the blocking of one ureter may cause a reflex anuria in the other kidney. Partial or temporary anuria may occur during a severe attack of renal colic; and not infrequently, in a patient with a history of attacks of renal colic, hæmaturia, etc., it will be found that one kidney has ceased to secrete urine, and that blocking of the ureter that belongs to the functionating kidney is the cause of the anuria.

Pyuria.—Pyuria is found only after infection has taken place. This infection usually produces pyonephrosis, when the kidney will be large enough to be palpable, and, on close and continued observation, the organ will be found to vary in size, coincidently with absence of all discharge or with a free discharge of pus with the urine.

Frequency of Micturition.—Frequency of micturition is a well-established

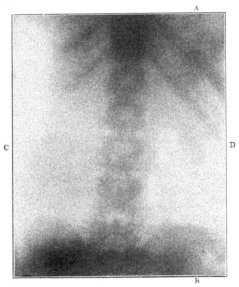

Fig. 46.—A Large Irregularly Shaped Stone in the Kidney, Giving, in the Skiagraph, a very Indistinct Shadow. (Author's case.)
Two straight lines drawn—the one from *A* to *B*, the other from *C* to *D*—will cross each other near the centre of the spot where the shadow of the stone is located.

but not easily explained symptom, which occasionally occurs in renal calculus, quite independently of any lesion of the urinary bladder.

Tenderness on Deep Pressure.—Tenderness on pressure may sometimes, even before infection has occurred, be elicited in thin people by pressing deeply into the loin.

DIAGNOSIS.—In addition to the symptoms and signs already enumerated, the heredity and personal habits of the patient must be considered, and the urine carefully examined. The continuous presence of urinary crystals is of some value as presumptive evidence (at least of a diathesis), and very few stones will escape detection by the *x*-ray. Some very large stones may be palpable, and in secondary stone formation particles of phosphate are passed from time to time. On the other hand, the diagnosis of stone from other diseases of the kidney,—tuberculosis, for example,—is not always easy, and, in the absence of hæmaturia or pyuria and skiagraphic demonstration, the diagnosis from disease of neighboring organs is also often difficult. When one has to depend upon symptoms alone, it must be remembered that diseases of the gall-bladder, appendix, and duodenum often closely simulate renal calculus in the right kidney. When blood or pus is present in the urine, cystoscopy and ureteral catheterization, with examination of the urine obtained from each side separately, will locate the lesion in the one or the other kidney, or possibly in both.

TREATMENT.—As patients do not consult a surgeon for renal calculus until a stone is suspected, prophylactic treatment—at least from the surgical point of view—is limited to the prevention of recurrence after removal of the stone. Under these circumstances a healthful mode of life, a simple diet of plain and easily digested food, carefully regulated so as to avoid the errors which are thought to be potent factors in producing stone, taken regularly and in moderation, and adapted to the needs and idiosyncrasies of the patient, and—in a general way—the avoidance of alcohol are the measures of greatest importance. The question of the use of alcohol and in what forms it may be taken, is one which must be decided for each individual case. Sufficient and suitable exercise, so as to secure perfect oxygenation of the blood and improved metabolism, completes the list of measures which embody the essential principles of prophylaxis. Lithia and other mineral waters may be given according to the indications furnished by the diathesis, but drugs are not required. The idea of dissolving a stone in the kidney or in the urinary passages by the internal administration of drugs has always had a strong hold on the lay but less on the medical mind. Among the plausible theories may be mentioned the following: that the administration of an acid will effect the solution of an alkaline stone; that, similarly, the administration of an alkali will act as a solvent of an acid stone; and that drugs like piperazin and the lithium salts, which dissolve urinary calculi outside the body, should exert a similar effect upon stones in the kidney. But experience does not support these theories; and it may be said at once that no drug is known which can be relied upon as a solvent for stone in the kidney. Nevertheless, treatment of this character is indicated, and may be very effectual in cases of nephrolithiasis,—cases in which the kidney pelvis, the ureter, and the urinary bladder are beset with urinary deposits in the form of "sand" or "gravel."

Urotropin, the important urinary antiseptic, may, by preventing or lessening urinary decomposition, be of use in phosphaturia. This drug is also said to dissolve stones composed of uric acid or of the urates. Turpentine is strongly recommended by Watson, and it is well known that, among its physiological effects, are stimulation of the kidney, producing an increased flow of urine or even—when the drug is administered in excessive amount or for too long a time—bloody urine. In any case, the use of plain distilled water or of water otherwise free from lime salts, and the taking of judiciously selected mineral waters, are always indicated, for the importance of keeping the urinary salts

in solution is obvious. But, even in such simple treatment, the good effect
may be nullified, or possibly harm may be done, by disturbing the digestion and
assimilation of food through the taking of large quantities of water at improper
times.

Operative Treatment.—The operative treatment of renal calculus is of comparatively recent origin, the first attempts to deal with a kidney containing a
calculus dating back to about 1870. In 1871 Simon removed a pyonephrotic
kidney for renal calculus, and in 1880 Morris introduced the operation of nephrolithotomy, which is now always selected as the operation of choice. Here,
as in many other surgical conditions, operative treatment, which at first was
ultra-conservative and restricted to cases in which serious damage had already
been done to the kidneys, is now universally employed, when possible, to arrest
such damage, as well as to deal radically and yet conservatively with the
more advanced cases. Thus, nephrotomy, nephrolithotomy, and nephrectomy
possess each their definite places and indications as therapeutic procedures.
The ability to make a positive diagnosis, rendered possible, in the great majority
of cases, by ureteral catheterization and by the employment of the Roentgen
ray, has contributed largely to this result. Accumulated experience has also
demonstrated the capacity of the kidney for repair and restoration of function.
As to what cases should be operated upon, the safest rule is to operate on all
cases unless there is a definite contra-indication to operation; for, although—
as has been pointed out—a patient may carry a stone in the kidney for a long
time without symptoms (and indeed most patients do this in the formative
period of the stone), nevertheless the general trend is toward irritation, obstruction of the ureter and anuria, and infection, with sepsis and disorganization of
the kidney tissue. In any case, therefore, when the presence of a stone in the
kidney has been demonstrated by the x-ray, or made reasonably certain by other
methods of investigation, an operation should be undertaken for its removal,
especially as it is highly improbable that such a diagnosis will be made until
after some symptoms have been produced by the stone. Under ordinary circumstances the operation of nephrolithotomy is neither difficult nor dangerous,
and generally yields very satisfactory results. Even where infection has taken
place, and where the pyonephrosis is both extensive and of long standing,
nephrolithotomy will generally be sufficient; although a fistula may remain
after operation in such cases. It is only in the most advanced conditions of
pyonephrosis, with destruction of the kidney tissue, that nephrectomy is necessary. In doubtful cases nephrolithotomy should be done first and nephrectomy
later, if found necessary. When both kidneys contain calculi, and more especially when infection has occurred in one or both, an important question arises
as to whether one should be operated upon first and the other later, or whether
both should be operated upon at the same time. The former plan would seem
to be the more conservative, but there is a growing tendency to operate upon
both at the same time. The important question to decide, in any case, of this
kind, is: Which course will be the least likely to arrest or impair the kidney
function temporarily, as anuria is the most serious result to be anticipated.

In acute obstruction caused by the passage of a stone into the ureter, if the obstruction is not speedily overcome by natural processes, immediate operation is indicated.

The treatment of calculous anuria is very important, and, while in many cases the patient recovers under expectant treatment, most observers agree that operative treatment in total anuria should not be delayed for more than forty-eight hours. When the pain has disappeared, or when it has been absent from the first, thus showing that there was no tension in the kidney, the indications are more serious; and in any case, when symptoms of uræmia appear, operation should not be delayed. It is a remarkable fact that uræmic symptoms are usually late in making their appearance in anuria, sometimes manifesting themselves as late as sixteen days after the establishment of this condition.* The object of operation in calculous anuria is, primarily, to allow of the escape of urine from the pelvis of the kidney, and to relieve the tension, so that the organ may resume its functions. A nephrotomy or pyelotomy is, therefore, the first indication, but, if a stone is found in the kidney or upper portion of the ureter, it will of course be removed at the same time, unless the patient's condition is such as to make any prolongation of the operation dangerous. When a stone is already known to be present in one or both kidneys, there will be no difficulty in determining the nature of the operation to be undertaken; but very frequently anuria occurs in a case in which no diagnosis has been made, and in which not even a useful history can be obtained. This may be due to the patient's condition or to the fact that, symptoms having occurred at intervals over a long period of time, accurate details have been forgotten. In such cases, whenever possible, a diagnosis should be made by means of an x-ray examination and by ureteral catheterization. Quite frequently, however, the patient's condition will not admit of such investigation, and yet the urgency of the situation calls for immediate interference. Under these circumstances an operation should be performed upon that one of the two kidneys which seems to have been most recently the seat of symptoms (pain, etc.); the latter fact warranting the inference that it, at least, has been recently a functionating organ. A further reason for operating may be found in the fear that the other kidney may have been previously disorganized by calculous disease, or indeed may never have existed. Should the kidney first exposed prove to be a functionless organ, it will be necessary immediately to operate upon the other. The great object is to tide the patient over his anuria, and then, if delay is necessary, the remaining calculus or fistula can be dealt with later.

When a calculus, having entered the ureter, fails to pass on into the bladder it usually becomes lodged either at the upper or at the lower extremity of the tube, or just above the brim of the pelvis. In the former situation it produces more acute symptoms and can also easily be removed through the lumbar incision made for the purpose of exposing the kidney; but, when it becomes lodged in the lower end of the ureter, the symptoms are less acute, the ureter becoming dilated above and around the calculus and allowing of the escape of

* Vol. ii. of Watson and Cunningham's "Genito-Urinary Diseases," 1908.

urine into the bladder, although the partial obstruction may lead to a hydrone-phrosis or pyonephrosis and ultimately to complete destruction of the kidney substance.   In this way it sometimes happens that conditions are established which, as referred to above, induce the surgeon to operate upon the kidney which has most recently been the seat of symptoms indicative of the presence of a calculus, rather than upon the kidney which seems to have been earlier and more seriously involved.

The following tables given by Watson * show the duration of anuria in 101 cases which were analyzed by him, and furnish a comparison between the results obtained in expectant treatment and those secured by operative treatment.   They also show a surprising degree of tolerance on the part of the tissues when subjected to these unfavorable conditions.   Patients recovered under both methods of treatment, even when the anuria had lasted as long as fifteen days.

(1) Duration of Anuria in 62 Cases Treated Expectantly.

(a) Twenty cases in which recovery took place.

Less than 48 hours	1	Between 5 and 7 days	8
To end of 48 hours	1	Between 7 and 10 days	3
To end of 4th day	1	Between 10 and 15 days	6

(b) Forty-two cases ending fatally.

4 days	1	12 to 16 days	11
5 to 8 days	15	23 days	1
8 to 12 days	14		

(2) Duration of Anuria in 39 Cases Treated by Operation.

(a) Duration of anuria in 26 cases ending in recovery.

1 day	2	5 days	2
2 days	2	5 to 8 days	9
3 days	2	8 to 11 days	2
4 days	2	11 to 15 days	5

(b) Duration of anuria in the 13 fatal cases.

2 days	2	Up to the 8th and 9th	2
Up to the 4th and 5th	2	Up to the 12th	1
Up to the 6th and 7th	4	Up to the 14th and 15th	2

VI. TUBERCULOSIS OF THE KIDNEY.

In general miliary tuberculosis the kidney may, and usually does, show numerous tubercles, and the urine may contain tubercle bacilli, but, as the kidney lesion is here a relatively small part of an eventually fatal systemic infec-tion, it has no special interest for the surgeon.

Rayer,† in 1841, showed that the kidneys might be the special site of a tuberculous process, and in 1872 Peters, of Toronto, removed a tuberculous kidney, but they, in common with other surgeons of that period, considered the renal tuberculosis to be always secondary to a focus of this disease in the bladder

* Op. cit.   † "Traité des maladies des reins," Paris, 1841.

or in the genital organs. Steinthal,* in 1885, showed this view to be erroneous by bringing forward instances where the kidneys manifested evidences of advanced tuberculosis without any involvement of the bladder or the genital organs.

Tuberculosis of the kidney is now known to be, at least in relation to the other surgical affections of this organ, a relatively frequent disease. Kronlein's statistics † show that in 29.8 per cent of all the surgical affections of the kidneys the lesion is tuberculous; and Israel ‡ states that one-third of all the purulent processes in the kidney are tuberculous in origin.

Tuberculosis of the kidney, with the exclusion of the general miliary form, usually affects at first only one of these organs, but, if the disease remains active or progresses in the one kidney, it will almost certainly extend to the second. Nevertheless, Kapsammer § points out that, of 191 cases in which death was due to kidney tuberculosis, there were 67 in which one of the kidneys was still free from the disease; and Israel § states that 88 per cent of all the renal tuberculosis that came under his observation had the disease still limited to one kidney; but many other surgeons put the frequency of one-sided tuberculosis at a much lower figure. As can be easily understood, the period of the disease at which the patient comes under observation determines almost wholly whether the disease is unilateral or bilateral.

Tuberculosis of one kidney is believed to be always secondary to a focus of this disease located elsewhere in the body, usually in a lymph node, the lung, or one of the bones. French surgeons, following the teaching of Guyon,|| have for a long time held that tuberculosis of the testicle and the urinary bladder was the most frequent, if not the only, source of tuberculous infection of the kidneys. From the anatomical position of these organs this method of infection has been termed "ascending or secondary kidney tuberculosis," and it has also been described as a urological infection. However, up to the present time no evidence has been brought forward to prove that tuberculosis of a testicle has a greater tendency than tuberculosis of a lung or one of the bones to produce tuberculosis of the kidney in the same subject.

Tuberculosis of the urinary bladder, as the only lesion of this disease in the genito-urinary system, has never yet been observed at a post-mortem examination, but at times, although rarely, there are seen cases where there is an extensive and advanced tuberculosis of the bladder and also of the ureter, and, to a lesser extent, of the pelvis of the kidney, with very slight tuberculous lesions of the calyces or of the apices of the pyramids, and those cases, it is maintained, demonstrate that the disease as regards the genito-urinary system was primary in the bladder and spread thence to the kidney, either along the walls of the

---

* Virchow's Archiv, Bd. c., 1885.

† XXXIII. Congress der Deutschen Gesellschaft fuer Chirurgie, 1904.

‡ Congress der Deutschen Chirurgen, 1905.

§ "Nierendiagnostik und Nierenchirurgie," Vienna, 1907.

|| "Tuberculose rénal," in Annales des maladies des voies génito-urinaires, 1888.

ureter or through its lumen. In the former case there may be a continuous growth of the disease, or the bacilli may be carried up by the lymph stream; while in the latter the bacilli are thought to be carried up the lumen by a backward flow of the urine. Possibly both methods of infection of the kidney may be active in the same case. There is, in addition, the possibility that infection is carried to the kidney by the blood from a tuberculous focus in the bladder, prostate, or testicle, just as from a focus in the lung. Baumgarten's experiments* show that an ascending infection of the kidney through the urine cannot take place with a normally functionating bladder or ureter. But, where there has been obstruction to the urinary outflow from the bladder, or a long-continued frequency of micturition with the resulting secondary changes in the ureter, a back flow of urine up the ureter is possible, and, therefore, an ascending infection of the kidney by means of the urinary stream.

French surgeons, as represented by Pousson † and Tuffier,‡ claim that this is the most frequent means by which the kidney is affected by tuberculosis; but, on the other hand, German surgeons, in agreement with English and American surgeons, although admitting that this ascending infection—the so-called secondary tuberculosis of the kidney—does exist, claim that it is a very rare occurrence. They hold—and in this they are strongly supported by clinical evidence and by pathological findings—that the kidneys are in the vast majority of cases the site of the first tuberculous lesion of the urinary tract and that later the ureter and the bladder may become affected either by a continuous advance of the bacilli along the ureteral walls to the bladder, or by the organ being infected by bacilli deposited on its mucous membrane from the infected urine, and they consider this latter method of bladder infection the more frequent of the two. Thus, the usual course of the disease is a primary tuberculosis of the kidney, with secondary infection of the bladder and therefore a descending infection. The kidney may also be infected by tubercle bacilli that happen to pass through it in their elimination from the circulation. When one kidney is affected by tuberculosis the urine from the other will frequently show a trace of albumin, slight turbidity, and a moderate number of pus cells. These may not be due to the disease having spread to the second organ, but may be only the result of a chronic nephritis which has been produced by the extra work required of the organ or by the irritation of the kidney from the tuberculous toxins in the circulating blood. But, if tuberculosis has been progressing for a considerable time in one organ, the transference of the disease from the one kidney to the other may take place through and by means of the general circulation, or through the anastomosing veins of the kidney capsule across the spine, behind the peritoneum, or on the under surface of the diaphragm. The disease may also ascend, as previously described, to the sound organ from a secondarily infected bladder, or both kidneys may at different periods be infected from a common focus.

* Berliner klin. Wochenschrift, 1905.
† Association Française d'urologie, 1904.
‡ "Traitement de la tuberculose du rein," Soc. de Chirurgie, Paris, 1900.

EXPLANATION OF PLATE LIV.

The upper figure shows a tuberculous kidney, laid open longitudinally, by the incision along its convex border. At its centre is seen a cavity, half filled with a caseous, myxomatous-looking mass. This cavity extends from the capsule to the pelvis, into which it empties, and replaces all the kidney tissue in this area. There is also seen at the upper part a small area of tuberculous matter which has not yet broken down. Sections from this area show tubercles and tubercle bacilli.

The lower figure shows the same kidney before being laid open. In the central portion, in which the kidney tissue has been destroyed by tuberculosis, is seen a yellowish constricting band which extends around the kidney. In the upper portion are seen several groups of tubercles lying beneath the capsule.

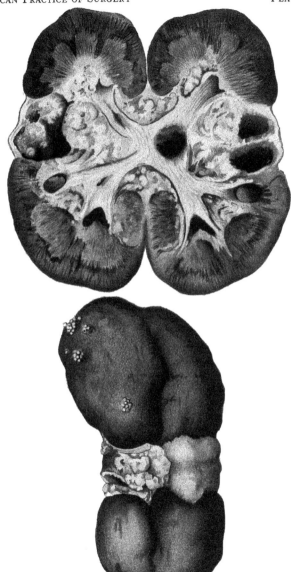

PRIMARY TUBERCULOSIS OF THE KIDNEY

(FROM THE COLLECTION OF DR. JAMES BELL)

tuberculous foci break down very early, giving rise to small areas lined by tuberculous granulation tissue which bleeds readily, and this explains how this form of the disease gives rise to early and severe hæmaturia. As the disease progresses the muscular wall of the pelvis is invaded and destroyed, with the result that it loses its power of expelling the urine, and then the destruction of the kidney tissue is followed in time, partly through the pressure of the retained fluid and also partly through the advancing tuberculosis, by the formation of a thin sac filled with tuberculous pus; but even here, although the ureter may have been blocked for a long time, a few kidney tubules capable of secreting a certain amount of urine may be found on the inner surface of the wall.

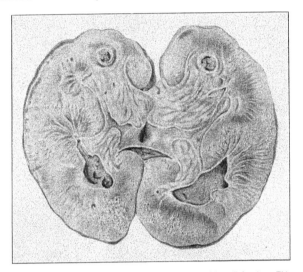

Fig. 47.—A General Seeding of the Kidney Parenchyma by Miliary Tubercles. This usually develops into a tuberculous pyonephrosis. (After Kapsammer.)

This pyonephrosis may also be produced by another and more common form of tuberculous infection of the kidney. In this form the tubercles are thickly deposited on one or more areas throughout the kidney substance, as a result of the bacilli being seeded there out of the blood stream. (Fig. 47.) The centres of these areas break down into caseous or purulent material, while at the same time the disease extends at the periphery by invading the surrounding tissue. This process continues, and the softened areas break through into the pelvis, where they empty themselves in whole or in part, producing a marked pyuria; and, as new foci of the disease are continually formed in the organ, and as the older ones continually extend, the kidney comes to be a sacculated mass lined by tuberculous granulation tissue and filled with caseous broken-down material. (Figs. 48 and 49.) At times the disease may extend through the kidney capsule and give rise to a perinephritic abscess. Then, again, in a pyonephrosis, where the ureter has become completely blocked for a considerable period, the contents may change from the usual thick caseous-looking pus into an almost clear straw-colored fluid.

Tuberculosis of the pelvis of the kidney or of the ureter has, up to the present time, never been found as the only focus of this disease in the urinary tract, so that, when present, it is looked upon as secondary to the same disease in the

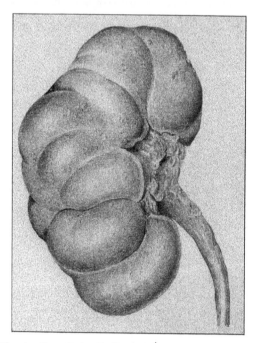

Fig. 48.—Tuberculous Pyonephrosis. The illustration shows lobulations and tubercles on the surface of the kidney. (After Kapsammer.)

kidney or in the bladder. The most usual method of infection of these structures is by tubercle bacilli from a diseased kidney being deposited upon and invading the mucous membrane of the pelvis or ureter and there producing foci of the disease. Occasionally, the walls of these structures may be invaded by a continuously advancing tuberculous growth from either the kidney or the bladder, but when, as occasionally happens, cases are found in which the mucous membrane of the pelvis or of the ureter shows very slight or even no tuberculous disease, while in the submucosa and the muscular coats it is advanced and extensive, they are considered as cases in which the infection has come through the lymph or blood channels. Occasionally, in tuberculosis of a kidney, there are seen, in its pelvis or in the ureter, inflammatory changes which, on microscopic examination, do not present evidences of tuberculosis; and Kapsammer thinks that these are the lesions which heal after the removal of the diseased organ, as he does not believe that removal of a tuberculous kidney would cause tuberculous lesions of the ureter to undergo healing. Tuberculosis of the pelvis as well as of the ureter may be found in all degrees, from a few

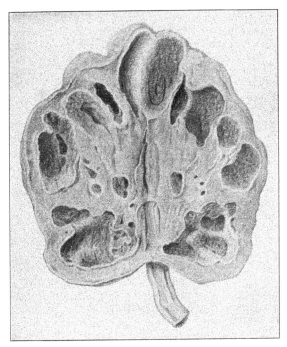

Fig. 49.—The Illustration Represents the Interior of the Same Kidney as that shown in Fig. 48. The organ has been laid open in such a manner as to show the numerous tuberculous cavities emptying into the pelvis. (After Kapsammer.)

tubercles in the mucosa to an extensive invasion of all the coats and even of the surrounding tissues. This disease may, and usually does, lead to a narrowing or even to complete obliteration of the lumen of the ureter, either by reason of the large amount of tuberculous tissue in its walls or by the contraction of the fibrous tissue in cases in which healing of a lesion has begun to take place. Ulceration of the ureteral walls also frequently occurs, and, where this is combined with the obstruction lower down, sac-like dilatations of the ureteral lumen may be found. Very occasionally, the tuberculous ureter is so thickened that it may be palpated through the abdominal wall; and also, as the inflammatory changes tend to shorten the ureter, its orifice in the bladder is drawn up, thus producing the crater-like appearance of this opening often observed through the cystoscope.

A kidney which is the subject of advanced and extensive tuberculosis, even when a large pyonephrosis has resulted, may not give rise to any local or subjective symptoms, and may not even be palpable, but usually tuberculous infection of the kidney of whatever type causes a feeling of dull pain in the lumbar region of the affected side, and this is often most marked when the patient is in bed, and in women it may be markedly increased during the menstrual period. The patient will often complain of a severe pain in the region of the affected kidney before the urine has come to show any abnormality. The pain caused by tuberculosis of the kidney may extend to the bladder, across to the other kidney, or upward toward the shoulder blade. Only in a few cases is the diseased organ palpable or tender, and, even when tuberculosis of the kidney is suspected, the palpable one must not immediately be judged to be the offender, as it may prove to be the sound organ which has undergone compensatory hypertrophy. The extension of tuberculosis to the ureter does not give rise to any special symptoms referable to this organ, save that it may be tender on pressure and, by reason of the thickening, as pointed out previously, it may come to be palpable. Gradual blocking of a ureter by tuberculosis escapes notice, but the sudden stoppage of a patent canal produces an acute pyonephrosis, with its accompanying symptoms.

Frequency of micturition has often been noticed in cases of tuberculosis of the kidney in which the bladder still remained free from any trace of this disease, and a satisfactory explanation of this symptom has not, up to the present, been forthcoming. Polyuria is almost always present, is often especially marked during the early stages, and is due chiefly to the accompanying interstitial nephritis, but also possibly to the fact that, where there is tuberculosis of the kidney proper, there is also likely to be more or less involvement of the pelvis of this organ or of the ureter, as described previously, with partial retention of the urine in the kidney pelvis—conditions which lead to pressure-atrophy of the tubules in the pyramids and ultimately to an interference with the water-absorbing portion of the kidney. This retention of the urine in the kidney pelvis may also be caused by the fact that the frequency of micturition interferes with the normal rhythmic contractions of the ureter.

Albumin is almost always present in the urine in cases of kidney tuberculosis, but is usually scanty in amount and does not in any way indicate the severity or the extent of the disease. Where only one organ is affected, the urine from the other may show a slight albuminuria, but this is comparable to that seen in cases of advanced tuberculosis in other parts of the system and usually disappears when the offending kidney is removed.

Pus is almost constantly present in the urine of patients who have tuberculous kidneys, except in the late stages of chronic cases, where the kidney has ceased to functionate. Sometimes the amount of pus is so scanty as to produce only a slight cloudiness; then again it may be so abundant as to form a large deposit, while in still other cases it varies greatly in amount from time to time.

Hæmaturia has been found in only one-third of all the cases of kidney tuberculosis, but it is sometimes so severe, even while there is only a very small area of disease in the organ, as to necessitate a nephrectomy; and Kapsammer thinks that the greater number of cases of the so-called essential renal hæmaturia are in reality instances of kidney tuberculosis. The reaction of the urine in the early stages of this disease is almost invariably acid, but, as the disease progresses, it may become alkaline, owing to an infection of the urine by other micro-organisms.

Very rarely, a phosphaturia is observed in kidney tuberculosis, and, even when it is present, it is probably safe to assume that the condition developed prior to this infection.

Fever is usually absent if there is not a mixed infection, and the heart does not tend to hypertrophy nor the blood-pressure to become increased.

At present, renal tuberculosis is a very frequently overlooked disease. Kapsammer points out that, during the ten years from 1897 to 1907, in the Vienna General Hospital, there came to post-mortem examination 191 cases of this disease, and, of these, only two were correctly diagnosed, and four partially so, while in 185 the disease was not even suspected, and, of these, 67 were still one-sided processes. Nearly all these cases had been under treatment for years, during which period of time they were looked upon as cases of simple chronic cystitis, and the question of their being of a tuberculous nature had not even been considered.

The final diagnosis of kidney tuberculosis must always rest on the demonstration of tubercle bacilli in the urine, and careful search of numerous slides of the urinary sediment, well stained, will almost always show them to be present. Smegma bacilli and acid-fast streptothrix are occasionally mistaken for tubercle bacilli. In women the urine to be examined should always be obtained by a catheter, and in men the glans should be carefully cleansed just previous to micturition and the first portion of the urine passed should be rejected. Even after these precautions the stained slides of the urinary sediment, after being competely decolorized by acid, should remain in alcohol for a short period.

After tubercle bacilli have been proved to be present in the urine, an endeavor should be made to determine the chief and probably also the primary site of the disease.. This is, from the clinical signs and symptoms, relatively easy in the advanced cases, but, where the disease has made only slight progress, it is often a matter of great difficulty. The bladder should first be carefully ex amined by the cystoscope to see if its lining shows any tubercles or tuberculous ulceration. The orifices of the ureters especially should be carefully examined, as their appearance will often indicate a kidney or a ureteral tuberculosis, as shown by marked congestion, by ulceration, or by the crater-like appearance previously described. Since it is now generally agreed that, in the vast majority of the cases of tuberculosis of the urinary tract, the primary lesion will be found in one or the other kidney, catheterization of both ureters is indicated. By this means one may not only determine whether one or both kidneys are involved, but may also, with the aid of a phlorizidin or an indigo-carmine test, or by cryoscopy, gain a fairly correct idea of the functional capacity of both kidneys. This knowledge of the functional condition of both organs is necessary in determining the future treatment of the case.

Up to the present time only very rare instances of the spontaneous healing of a tuberculous kidney have been brought forward, although healing processes —such as the formation of fibroid areas, the excessive growth of fatty tissue, or the calcification of a tuberculous mass—are frequently seen. It must therefore be admitted that, so far as one can judge, tuberculosis of a kidney, if untreated, usually leads ultimately to death. Since, as is well known, there is no drug the administration of which is certain to result in the healing of a tuberculous focus in the body, and since the therapeutic uses of the various forms of tuberculin are at present in the experimental stages, the only rational and effective method of treating one-sided kidney tuberculosis consists in removing the affected organ with, as far as possible, any surrounding diseased tissue. Before this procedure is carried out the other kidney must be proved to be capable of performing sufficient work for the needs of the body. The ideal condition for nephrectomy is that in which the disease affects only one kidney, the other and the remainder of the urinary tract being completely sound, and there being no marked tuberculous process in any part of the body. Ulceration of the bladder, with symptoms of a severe cystitis, is not a contra-indication to nephrectomy, as such ulcers are not always tuberculous, and, even if tuberculous, they may heal spontaneously after the diseased kidney has been removed. A slight albuminuria from the second kidney is frequently only a toxic manifestation, and disappears completely on removal of the offending organ. When a tuberculous pyonephrosis has become infected by other pyogenic organisms, as shown by the development of septic symptoms, the removal of such a focus of disease at once, or after draining for a short period, is demanded.

The extirpation of a tuberculous kidney should always be carried out by the lumbar route, and the ureter should, as far as possible, be removed and the cut end cauterized, when it may be permitted to drop back among the retroperitoneal tissues.

When both kidneys are affected by tuberculosis, in most cases no operative treatment is of any avail, except possibly to relieve symptoms, but under certain conditions and in certain cases it may be wise to remove the most seriously diseased kidney.

The following series of cases, which recently came under the writer's care, illustrate the chronic painless form of tuberculosis of the kidney:—

CASE 1.—An intelligent, educated young woman, an undergraduate nurse, 28 years of age, had never had any illness nor any disturbance of urinary function, nor—so far as she knew—any abnormality of the urine, until four weeks before operation, when signs of ureteral obstruction developed and the cystoscope showed that no urine came from the ureter of the affected side. At the operation (nephrectomy) the upper portion of the ureter was found to be almost completely obstructed by tuberculous disease and secondary fibroid degeneration. There was only a single tuberculous mass, about half an inch in diameter, in the lower pole of the kidney. In this case the disease in the ureter seemed to be farther advanced, and therefore of longer standing, than the focus in the kidney.

There was no family history of tuberculosis.

CASE 2.—Male, aged 24, had never had any illness (except syphilis two years previously), and never had any urinary symptoms nor urinary abnormality. He began to suffer from pain in the right loin eight weeks before operation, and a perinephritic abscess developed slowly. Cystoscopy showed absence of urine from the right ureter, and the urine found was normal in quantity and quality. At operation the shrunken kidney was found embedded in a dense fibrous tissue and was removed piecemeal (morcellement). It was definitely tuberculous. Paternal uncle died of pulmonary tuberculosis.

CASE 3.—Female, aged 40, domestic servant, had never had urinary symptoms nor urinary abnormality, although she had suffered from the grippe and from rheumatism within the past year and a half. About eight weeks before operation there was noticed in the left loin a small "lump," which proved to be a perinephritic abscess. The kidney, which was removed, was found embedded in a mass of very dense fibrous tissue. It was simply a fibrous sac, of about one-third the size of the normal kidney, and containing putty-like caseous matter. It was definitely tuberculous. There was a marked family history of tuberculosis.

VII. ESSENTIAL HÆMATURIA.

Essential hæmaturia is a term employed to designate a class of cases in which renal hæmaturia occurs without apparent organic lesion. The hemorrhage is free, sometimes profuse; continuous or intermittent; and lasts over long periods of time. It is usually unilateral, and frequently is accompanied by pain of such a character as to lead to a diagnosis of calculus or early tuberculosis, although it is often described as painless. Before exact diagnosis of calculus in the kidney had been made possible, in the great majority of cases, by the Roentgen ray and ureteral catheterization, many of these patients were submitted to an exploratory operation for stone, and yet no lesion was discovered; and, strangely enough, the operation was usually followed by complete and permanent cessation of the hemorrhage. But in some cases in which the operation failed to give relief or even seemed to increase the hemorrhage, and in which then the kidney was removed, no lesion could be discovered on the most careful examination.

The cause of this affection is obscure. After all the ordinary causes of renal hemorrhages have been excluded,—for example, traumatism, hæmophilia, toxæmia, and the local irritations produced by tuberculosis, inflammatory conditions, infections, neoplasms, calculus, etc.,—there remain many cases for which no cause can be found. Angioma, early tuberculosis, and obscure inflammatory changes in the kidney are among the causes to which, in such cases, the affection is usually attributed, and probably each one of them, as well as other conditions, operates in this way. At any rate, the clinical fact of the common association of pain and hæmaturia in many cases in which both of these symptoms are completely relieved by nephrotomy, points to renal congestion and tension, whatever the underlying cause may be.

Mr. Hurry Fenwick * reports two cases in which he demonstrated, by electric light, through an incision into the pelvis of the kidney, a bleeding papilla, which he removed, with the result that the hæmaturia was completely arrested. After a minute examination of both specimens, he thus described the part removed:— "There was no evidence of growth, but there was a congestion of the vessels, with extravasation of blood and an increase in the cellular stroma." In both cases the hemorrhage had been profuse and was not accompanied by pain. In this connection the history of the following case is instructive:—

A young woman, aged 32, during an attack of "grippe," had a troublesome, dull, aching pain across the loins for about one month. She recovered from this, but, whenever she caught cold, the pain would return for a day of two. Thirteen months later, she had a more severe attack, which persisted and caused her to abandon her course of training in the hospital training school, where she was an undergraduate nurse. This attack subsided in about three months, but one month later she had another attack of influenza, during which she began to have some frequency of micturition and passed urine which seemed to be composed of almost pure blood. The bleeding continued from September 19th until November 16th (1904), when she entered the hospital. She was anæmic and was passing large quantities of blood, intimately mixed with the urine, and some clots. She still complained of a dull pain across the loins and also of a definite pain which she referred to the region of the right kidney and which extended down along the course of the ureter. No evidence of stone or tuberculosis could be discovered. The kidney was exposed in the loin, delivered out of the wound, and incised along the cortex down to the pelvis, but nothing was found that might account for the hemorrhage. The bleeding into the bladder continued more or less intermittently and was at times so severe as to produce signs of syncope. Twenty-two days later, the kidney was removed and subjected to the closest pathological examination, but nothing abnormal was found except such changes as might fairly be attributed to the previous operation. She recovered promptly and, when seen six years later, was the picture of health. She reported that she had not had any trouble during this long period.

Although, so far as the writer is aware, there are no statistics relating to this subject, he has been impressed, in reading the reports of these cases, as well as in considering such cases as have come under his personal observation, by the large proportion of female patients among those who have been treated for this condition.

VIII. TUMORS OF THE KIDNEY.

The kidney is frequently the site of new-growths. They may spring from the organ itself or from the tissues immediately surrounding it, and, while a certain proportion of them are inflammatory, there remains a large class com-

* British Medical Journal, vol. i., 1900.

posed of the true tumors of this organ, besides those in which inflammation plays a doubtful rôle.

The true tumors of the kidney may have their origin in the parenchyma, in the pelvis, in the capsule, or in the tissues immediately surrounding it, whence they extend into the organ. This last class is often termed the perirenal or the pararenal group, but these growths are properly included with the kidney tumors. Renal tumors appear to be more frequent in men than in women, or, rather, the surgeon is more frequently consulted by the former for this condition, probably because the larger abdomen in the female permits a tumor to exist with less discomfort, and also because hæmaturia is earlier noted as an alarming symptom by the male. They are found most frequently in children and in adults over thirty years of age, while the period of adolescence—the period at which tuberculosis is most common—is relatively free. Occasionally tumors of the kidney develop during fœtal life, and then they may be so large as to hinder or prevent delivery.

PATHOLOGY.—Tumors of the kidney may, from a pathological point of view, be roughly divided into three groups. The first group comprises those which take their origin from the cells of the adult or fœtal kidney, and they are often referred to as the homologous new-growths of the kidney. The second group comprises those which take their origin from the cells or tissues which do not belong to the fœtal or adult kidney, but which have been included in this organ during its development. They are often therefore termed the heterologous new-growths of the kidney. The third group comprises those enlargements of the organ which are tumors in a clinical sense only, while, from a pathological view-point, they are retention cysts, due to a non-patency of the tubules.

Group 1.—The tumors of the first group may be subdivided into benign and malignant, and each of these subdivisions again into those of connective-tissue and those of epithelial origin.

The benign connective-tissue tumors are represented by small fibromata, which usually lie in or just beneath the capsule; by lipomata and fibro-lipomata or myo-lipomata, which also tend to be closely connected with the capsule; and by angiomata. The fibromata and lipomata and their mixed forms are usually very small, and give rise neither to subjective nor to objective signs nor to symptoms. At times, however, large tumors of similar structure are found in the kidneys, but these are generally thought to come from parts of the fatty or fibrous capsule which, through misplacement, have found their way into the kidney substance and are therefore heterologous tumors of this organ. The angiomata may develop on the inner wall of the pelvis, and under these conditions, even though they be small, they may give rise to such extensive and continuous bleeding as to necessitate a nephrectomy.

The benign epithelial tumors of the kidney are represented by the papillomata of the pelvis and the adenomata of the parenchyma. These true adenomata must be distinguished from the multiple small tumors of almost similar structure which are found in old fibroid kidneys, and which are to be looked upon as of the nature of a localized compensatory hypertrophy. The true adenomata are usually of small size, but may at times be as large as a closed fist, and they always possess a well-defined fibrous capsule. Their minute structure may be that of a tubular or of a papillary adenoma.

Under the malignant connective-tissue tumors are found the round-celled or the spindle-celled sarcomata, which are very rare. They constitute a group of tumors which are supposed to take their origin from endothelial cells, and are therefore termed endotheliomata or peritheliomata. An endothelioma is derived from cells that line capillaries, and in its minute structure it shows numerous small blood-filled spaces, surrounded by layers of large clear cubical to columnar cells, while a perithelioma is derived from the cells which line a perivascular lymph space, and which therefore shows in its minute structure numerous small capillaries provided with the usual flat endothelial wall, but having, immediately upon and outside this wall, numerous layers of cells similar to those found in the endotheliomata. However, both arrangements of cells in their relation to the capillaries may be found in the same tumor. These tumors, in their gross and minute structure, resemble the hypernephromata, and by some observers are thought to belong to this class.

The carcinomata constitute the malignant epithelial tumors, and appear in two forms. One is a rapidly growing tumor, which soon extends throughout the organ and leads to a marked increase in its size, while the other is a more slowly growing form, which apparently infiltrates the kidney, producing only small nodules, and often failing to cause any noticeable increase in the size of the organ.

Group 2.—The tumors of the second group cannot, as is feasible in the case of the first group, be subdivided into benign and malignant, for, if they are not all malignant from the first, they at least show a tendency to undergo malignant degeneration. The least malignant of these are the large fatty tumors of the kidney which develop in or just beneath the capsule. Besides the true fat cells these growths show developing fibrous-tissue cells, which may be of so embryonic a type as to cause them to be looked upon as sarcoma cells, and they almost always show a certain amount of smooth-muscle tissue, occasionally some myxomatous tissue. This admixture of cells in these growths is accounted for by their origin, which is, as shown by Mueller, from small portions of the true fatty capsule which have pushed their way, after the manner of a hernia, into the organ during its development; and thus the tumors show the fatty, fibrous, and smooth-muscle cells which exist in these small masses.

These tumors frequently show rapid growth and reach a large size, but they are always encapsuled and do not infiltrate, but merely destroy by compression the surrounding kidney tissue. They never give rise to metastases, but may be multiple, and are frequently found in kidneys which show some congenital abnormality of development; and they are termed lipomata, fibro-lipomata, myo-lipomata, etc., according to the types of cells that enter into their formation. They are to be distinguished from the small benign tumors which have already been described and which are known by similar names.

In 1883 Grawitz* pointed out that many of the small fatty-looking tumors that were frequently found in the cortex of the kidney during post-mortem examinations were small portions of the adrenal cortex which had apparently been included in this organ during its development, and he also showed that many of the large fatty-looking tumors of the kidney of hitherto unexplained origin were due to a growth of these small masses. He gave to these tumors the name "struma lipomatodes aberrata renis," which has been replaced at the present time by the more convenient name "hypernephroma," as suggested by Lubarch.† Stoerk ‡ has recently denied the adrenal origin of these tumors. (Plate LV.)

The hypernephromata, as indicated above, vary considerably. At one end of the scale we find tumors composed of a group of cells resembling exactly, in their morphology and in their relation to their blood-vessels, those of the adrenal cortex, and remaining latent throughout life; at the other, rapidly growing, very malignant tumors, the minute structure of which may still be similar to that of the adrenal, but may, especially at the rapidly growing border or in a metastasis, come to resemble that of a carcinoma or a sarcoma. Again, a rapidly growing hypernephroma may at any period of its growth become latent, and remain so throughout life, but, on the other hand, a hypernephroma, which is apparently latent, may give rise to a metastasis in a distant part of the body, without there being at any time clinical evidence of a tumor of the kidney.

The hypernephromata, even when rapidly growing, have a firm fibrous capsule which sends septa into the interior of the tumor, thus producing a lobulated appearance. The tumor, on section, shows a soft friable material, of a color varying from yellow to brown, which often exhibits large hemorrhages. In their minute structure these tumors show a network of fine capillaries, with the meshes between them filled with large clear cells, which contain, if examined in their fresh state, fat or glycogen globules. At times the tumor cells are columnar and stand on the capillaries at right angles to them, thus producing a perivascular or perithelial arrangement which has caused these tumors to be termed "peritheliomata."

All hypernephromata appear to have a capacity for malignant growth, although they may exist for years as benign tumors, and the microscopical picture shown by a hypernephroma which has taken on an active malignant growth may be identical with that shown by one which will remain a benign tumor throughout life. This adds to the difficulty of determining when a hypernephroma has become malignant, for the hæmaturia which some observers have taken to be the earliest sign of malignancy, is not a constant sign, and may be entirely absent where the tumor has infiltrated widely and has produced metastases. Degenerative changes, such as large areas of necrosis or large hemorrhages, are very frequently seen in these tumors, and sometimes almost all the growth may be discharged through the ureter, only a sac filled with blood being left be-

* Virchow's Archiv, Bd. 93, 1883.
† Virchow's Archiv, Bd. 135, 1894.
‡ Arch. f. klin. Chir., Bd. 87, S. 893, 1908.

hind. The wall of this sac is composed of fibrous tissue and upon its surface a few small tumor nodules may still be seen. In some cases, the wall of the tumor remaining intact, the degenerated material may become liquefied, and then the tumor will appear as a large cyst, which is often mistaken for a simple retention cyst of the kidney. Other malignant tumors of the kidney may show similar changes, but they are, beyond question, seen most frequently in these growths.

Hypernephromata are without doubt the most common of the malignant tumors of the kidney found in the adult, and hospital statistics generally correspond with those of the Royal Victoria Hospital, in which institution sixty-four per cent of all the malignant tumors of the kidney in adults under the writer's care have proved to be of this nature.

A third form of the heterologous tumors of the kidney is found almost exclusively in infants or young children. These tumors are composed chiefly of a very sarcoma-like mass of moderate-sized round cells, with irregularly scattered, small, gland-like structures, which consist at times of a solid double column of cells that are poorly differentiated from the surrounding sarcoma-like tissue, but which again may consist of a tube of cubical or columnar cells, with a definite lumen, and with a clear line of demarcation between it and the surrounding tissue. This latter condition is always best shown in the older portions of the tumor. The blood-vessels are numerous and thin-walled, but have no special relation to any group of the tumor cells. Very frequently these tumors contain smooth-muscular and myxomatous tissue, and occasionally striated muscle cells, cartilage, and bone, and it is owing to this admixture that they are considered mixed growths. They are also occasionally found in the fœtus, and there has been reported one instance in which it was found in a boy aged eighteen. Tumors of this variety are large, rapidly growing, and very malignant; they often appear to develop simultaneously in both kidneys, and usually beneath the capsule, as this structure is generally found stretched over the tumor and containing very numerous widely dilated veins. These tumors do not possess a well-defined fibrous capsule, but are surrounded by a rather thin layer of fibrous tissue that probably owes its origin to inflammatory changes in the surrounding kidney substance, which they destroy by compression rather than by infiltration. They very rarely, if ever, give rise to metastasis in the regionary lymph nodes, but show a great tendency to grow through the walls of the blood-vessels into their lumen, and small portions of these masses may be broken off and carried by the blood stream to the lungs, where secondary growths will then develop. If excised, these tumors recur rapidly in situ. Birch-Hirschfeld* has pointed out that these new-growths, which in their minute structure show the mixture of poorly formed glands and a very extensive sarcoma-like stroma or interglandular matrix, resemble very closely the early Wolffian body, and he therefore judges that they take their origin from rests of this structure which have been included in the kidney during its formation, just as happens in the case of portions of the adrenals which

* Beilage für allg. Path. und path. Anat., Bd. 24, 1898.

EXPLANATION OF PLATE LV.

The upper figure shows a kidney which has been laid open by an incision along the convex border in its long diameter. It will be seen that, in the upper two-thirds of the kidney, the normal structure has been replaced by a large, round, encapsuled mass. This mass, which measured about four inches in diameter, had a dry, grayish appearance on section. A microscopical examination showed it to be a typical hypernephroma,—that is, a tumor composed of cells markedly resembling those from the cortex of the adrenal.

The lower figure shows the same kidney unopened. The relations of the encapsuled mass of new-growth to the normal kidney substance are well shown.

PLATE LV

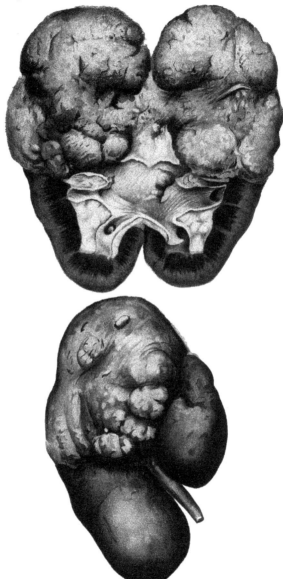

HYPERNEPHROMA OF THE KIDNEY

(FROM THE COLLECTION OF DR. JAMES BELL)

WALKER LITH & PUB CO. BOSTON,MASS

later give rise to hypernephromata. Muus,* however, thinks that these tumors resemble more closely the structure of an early fœtal kidney, and he thinks that they have their origin in rests of this organ, while Wilms † claims that all the cells and structures found in these tumors are the result of a special development of common mother cells, which he thinks are represented by the myxoma-like tissue. He then claims that this myxoma-like tissue represents mesodermal cells from a portion of a very early embryo which would later develop to form both the pronephron and the myotone, and that these cells, from some cause as yet unknown, have lost their organic connection with their surroundings and remain, for a certain length of time, as so-called "rests," and then later, owing to some stimulus, take on rapid independent growth and so produce a tumor which will contain the different types of tissue which they would have produced if they had remained in normal organic connection with the embryo. Thus, part of the cells develop along the lines of the Wolffian body, while others of the cells go to form muscle tissue, cartilage, and bone. The strongest support for this view is to be found in the fact that the metastases of these tumors often show the same admixture of different types of tissue as were found in the original tumor, but Birch-Hirschfeld's view—that these growths come from rests of the Wolffian body, and that the cartilage and bone are due to metaplasia of the connective tissue—has been the most widely accepted; and, as a convenient term, Birch-Hirschfeld has given to these growths the name "adenosarcoma." These tumors were often previously looked upon as forms of cancer, and this accounts for the statement, frequently met with in the older text books, that carcinomata of the kidney are frequently found in children.

Group 3.—The third and last group of kidney tumors might probably be better described as alterations in the form and structure of these organs due to disturbances of development, in which disturbances inflammatory processes may play a part. The group is composed of the true cysts of the kidney, that is, cysts not due, as has been shown above, to degenerative processes in the tumor. These true cysts may appear as a single large or small cyst in an otherwise unaltered organ. This form of cyst is lined by a single layer of flattened epithelium, and contains a weak albuminous fluid or colloid material. The cyst is probably produced by the gradual distention of a kidney tubule, the normal outlet of which has either never been open or has probably become secondarily closed by inflammatory processes. All the different stages are seen, from this solitary cyst to a condition in which the proper kidney tissue is almost completely replaced by a large number of cysts of varying size, lined with flattened epithelium and filled with a clear or blood-stained weakly albuminous fluid.

The condition of multiple cyst-formation is frequently found in the infant, and at times in the fœtus, and from this it has received the name of "congenital cystic kidney." (Fig. 50.) It almost always affects both kidneys, and although, as above stated, it is found mainly in infants and young children, it may first

* Virchow's Archiv, Bd. 155, 1899.
† "Die Mischgeschwuelste der Niere," Leipzig, 1899.

manifest itself in adult life by an enlargement of one or both organs. Here the condition was probably present at the time of birth, and the enlargement of the organ is due to an increase in the size of the individual cysts and not to new cyst-formation.

These multiple cysts, just as is believed to be true of the ordinary cyst, are generally thought to be dilated kidney tubules, the outlets of which were blocked during fœtal life. Other theories attribute this condition to inflammation of

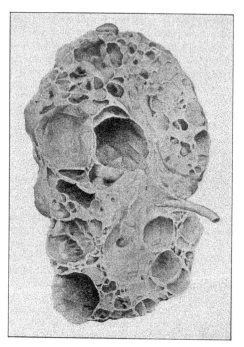

Fig. 50.—Congenital Cystic Kidney. The organ has been sectioned for the purpose of showing the distribution of the cysts. (From the Author's collection.)

the pelvis of the kidney or the papillæ during fœtal life, to failure—through some developmental error—of the convoluted and straight tubules to become normally joined, to multiple cystic adenomata, etc.

CHANGES PRODUCED IN THE KIDNEY PARENCHYMA BY THE NEW-GROWTHS.— Carcinoma is the only growth which, from the beginning, infiltrates and destroys the kidney parenchyma. Almost all the remaining growths are, in their early stages at least, surrounded by a more or less well-defined fibrous capsule, and do not infiltrate the surrounding tissue, but, if the tumor reaches any size, the kidney substance is compressed and shows inflammatory changes, which consist chiefly in an increased fibrosis of the interstitial tissue, with at times degeneration of the tubular epithelium. The free kidney also often shows slight inflammatory changes, which apparently first affect the stroma and later the secreting epithelium. The urine from the free kidney, therefore, as well as that from the one which is the seat of the new-growth, may show abnormalities due to this form of nephritis. These inflammatory changes in the unaffected organ, if not marked, often subside completely on removal of the diseased kidney with its tumor.

If the tumor interferes with the outflow from the pelvis of the kidney a secondary infection of the retained urine is apt to take place, and as a result there will be pyelitis or pyonephrosis. A compensatory hypertrophy of the unaffected kidney has not yet been observed.

METASTASES OF KIDNEY TUMORS.—Metastases of kidney tumors usually occur after the new-growth has reached considerable size. The only exception is to be found in the case of hypernephromata, which often, while still very small, give rise to new-growths in distant parts of the body, especially in the bones and lungs.

In the hypernephromata, the endotheliomata and peritheliomata, the sarcomata, and the so-called embryonal adenosarcomata, the transference of the growth almost always takes place by means of, or along, the blood stream, while in the carcinomata the growth spreads—as would be expected—along the lymph channels, and shows itself in the regionary lymph nodes. Very rarely, a portion of the growth carried by the urinary stream into the ureter or bladder, there becomes attached, and develops into a secondary growth.

Actinomycosis, syphilitic gummata, and echinococcus disease may also occur in the kidney.

SYMPTOMS OF KIDNEY TUMORS.—A tumor of the kidney frequently, but not always, produces a palpable mass in the kidney region, and, especially in children, this mass may be the sole evidence of the new-growth, for at times, and even when the tumor has given rise to extensive metastases, neither the affected kidney nor the tumor of the same may be palpable, especially if the latter is situated in the upper pole of the organ. Occasionally a tumor removed from some part of the body other than the abdomen proves to be a metastasis from a new-growth of the kidney which has given otherwise not the slightest evidence of its presence. Also, it must not be forgotten that a palpable mass in the kidney region may be produced by many other causes besides a tumor of neoplastic origin.

Spontaneous pain in the region of the kidney is only rarely noticed in the early stages, but later, when the new-growth, by reason of its size, comes to exercise pressure on the nerves of the part, pain is more common. Occasionally pain simulating renal colic is met with in kidney tumors, and this is probably caused by the passage of blood-clots or of small portions of the tumor along the ureter. With the lapse of time, especially in rapidly growing tumors, a constant pain, probably due to a stretching of the capsule, makes its appearance.

Hæmaturia is found with varying frequency in different tumors, but is much more frequent in adults than in children, as the adenosarcomata, which constitute the majority of the kidney tumors in childhood, are much less apt to give rise to bleeding than the hypernephromata, which certainly comprise the majority of the tumors of the kidney in the adult. Kuester* puts the frequency of hæmaturia in adults at 52 per cent and in children at 15 per cent. The hæmaturia may be caused by a breaking through of the growth into the kidney pelvis, but, as it occurs also in pararenal tumors, it may perhaps be due in some cases to congestion of the kidney or other disturbance of its circulation. Stoppage of the urinary outflow from the affected kidney is only rarely seen, and it is due to the presence of clots in the ureter.

Albarran and Imbert† have also noted the presence of incontinence of the urine in patients in whom there is a tumor of the kidney without involvement of the urinary bladder; but they have not furnished any explanation of this very unusual symptom.

French observers state that a varicocele on the same side as the affected kidney has been frequently seen, and that it is due to an interference with the return circulation in the spermatic vein, but a varicocele has not been found present in any of the cases in the Royal Victoria Hospital, Montreal. Hæmatonephrosis and subperitoneal hæmatomata have been found in cases in which there was a tumor of the kidney; and in cases in which the new-growth has produced thrombosis of the inferior vena cava, stasis of the blood in the lower extremities has taken place.

Icterus has been frequently observed in patients in whom a tumor had developed in one kidney, and this symptom is supposed to be due to a direct or indirect pressure on the common bile-duct, or possibly to an extensive hemorrhage. Occasionally, in a patient with a hypernephroma, a slight brownish pigmentation of the mucous membrane of the mouth is seen, and Chvostek has pointed out that kidney tumors appear to be associated with an abnormally low body temperature.

DIAGNOSIS OF KIDNEY TUMORS.—The demonstration of a new-growth of the kidney, even when it has reached a considerable size, is often very difficult and even at times impossible. However, tumors of the kidney of such a character as to require surgical intervention can usually be palpated, but rough manipulation should be avoided, as the hypernephromata and some of the other malignant tumors have their cells arranged in intimate relationship with very thin-walled blood-vessels, and pressure might force some of the tumor cells into the blood stream, thus producing emboli and metastases.

The urine in cases of kidney tumor, during the blood-free period, is wholly normal, save when, as pointed out previously, there is a secondary nephritis. This fluid affords a valuable means of distinguishing a case of kidney tumor from one of kidney stone or kidney tuberculosis, as the urine in the two latter conditions, during the blood-free interval, will contain a perceptible number of

* Congress der Deutschen Chirurgen, 1901.
† " Les tumeurs du rein," Paris, 1903. (Masson, éditeur.)

leucocytes. Essential hæmaturia and that due to a primary chronic interstitial nephritis must be carefully distinguished from a hæmaturia due to a tumor of the kidney, and here, unfortunately, the functional test is of no value. One must also remember that malignant growths of the kidney do not always cause hæmaturia, and also that hæmaturia can be found with benign tumors. Masses of the tumor cells, large enough to show the presence and the nature of the kidney tumor, have been occasionally found in the urine, but this happens only in rare instances. Catheterization of both ureters, in combination with the employment of the functional tests of the kidney, finds a wide range of application in determining not only the presence of a new-growth but also which one of the two kidneys is affected.

Previous to operation, and apart from the metastases, it is impossible to foretell with any degree of accuracy the nature of the kidney new-growth, and it must be remembered that a renal tumor may coexist with other pathological conditions of this organ, such as a renal stone or renal tuberculosis.

TREATMENT OF KIDNEY TUMORS.—The small tumors of the kidney, such as the fibromata, the myomata, the lipomata, and the adenomata, cannot be diagnosed, as they do not give rise to any signs or symptoms, and they do not require any treatment. The congenital cystic kidneys do not admit of any treatment, but the single large retention cyst of the kidney may be either completely excised or it may first be stitched to the skin surface and then opened and drained (marsupialation), when it will gradually undergo atrophy. In all other forms of kidney tumor complete removal of the organ with its tumor at the earliest possible moment is the only treatment, and in dealing with malignant tumors, or tumors suspected of malignancy, the surgeon must be guided by the same general principles which are applicable to the treatment of malignant growths in other parts of the body, and, as a general rule, when a malignant growth of the kidney has extended through the fibrous capsule or into the veins, recurrence after operation is inevitable. The fatty capsule should therefore always be removed, and, whenever possible, the lumbar route is to be preferred to the abdominal. The treatment of tumors of the kidney by the various serums or toxins recommended for the cure of malignant growths, or by the x-ray or by radium, has so far proved as valueless as it has in the treatment of other deep-seated malignant growths.

IX. WOUNDS AND DISEASES OF THE URETER.

Injuries of the Ureter.—Injuries of the ureter are somewhat rare, but may occur from contusion; in which case the ureter may be torn across, usually in its upper part, as in a case to which I have already referred. (See under Hydronephrosis.) This tube may also be ruptured or so contused as to cause obstruction to the flow of urine, or a localized death of tissue may permit of leakage of urine into the surrounding tissues. Gunshot and stab wounds, which are rarely uncomplicated, and accidental wounding or ligation of the ureter in surgical operations within the abdomen, especially upon the pelvic organs, must also be enumerated as causes. The ureter, furthermore, is sometimes injured in childbirth.

SYMPTOMS.—The symptoms of injury to the ureter are obscure and are due mainly to obstruction, when the symptoms are referable to the kidney; or they are due to the escape of the urine, which may produce in time a palpable fluctuating tumor. Extravasation of urine is followed by infection and death. of tissue, and finally by urinary fistula.

Lacerations and wounds of the ureter (except those made by the surgeon, as for removal of stones) manifest little or no tendency to heal, or, if the wound is of such a nature as to permit of healing, it is apt to be followed by stricture and more or less obstruction.

TREATMENT.—The treatment consists in providing drainage for the extravasated urine, and, except in the milder cases, a plastic operation will be required. Should the latter fail, the alternatives are nephrectomy or drainage through the loin.

Ureteral Calculus.—Except in rare instances, as when phosphates are deposited upon a foreign body, a tumor, or an ulcerated surface, calculi do not originate in the ureter but are arrested in their descent from the kidney. The lodgment of calculi in the ureter is much more common than is generally thought. It is stated by Leonard* that calculi are found twice as often in the ureter as in the kidney. Their arrest in the ureter may be temporary, the stone passing on into the bladder after a time, or a stone or stones may remain in the ureter for a long time without seriously impairing the health or usefulness of the patient. As already pointed out, the ureter dilates above and around the stone and thus accommodates itself to the presence of a foreign body, but ultimately hydronephrosis, with gradual destruction of the secreting tissue of the kidney, or infection and pyonephrosis and anuria, direct or reflex, are to be feared.

The favorite sites for the lodgment of calculi in the ureter are at the upper and lower extremities. They are also found at the brim of the pelvis, and may be distributed all along the ureter. In a certain type of frequently recurring or almost continuous renal colic, stones are apt to be found in the upper one or two inches of the ureter. When lodged in the lower portion of the ureter a stone may project partially into the bladder.

Ureteral calculi are either single or multiple,—most frequently single, especially when lodged in the lower end of the ureter. As small stones pass rapidly into the bladder and larger ones cannot enter the ureter, the size of the ureteral calculi varies within comparatively narrow limits. They are usually found from the size of a white bean to that of a walnut or even larger. In the case of the larger sizes it is safe to assume that the stone has increased in size during its stay in the ureter, as urinary calculi do in any part of the urinary tract. They are usually uric-acid or urate calculi, but oxalate calculi are also met with not infrequently.

SYMPTOMS AND DIAGNOSIS.—There are no characteristic symptoms. As already stated, the lodgment of calculi in the upper portion of the ureter is

* Lancet, 1905, vol. i.

usually preceded or accompanied by persisting or continuous renal colic, while calculi located in the lower portion of the ureter give little pain, and that of a vague and indefinite character. In acute obstruction by calculi the distensile pain felt in the kidney is apt to be very severe. The diagnosis can generally be made quite definitely by means of the x-ray (Figs. 51, 52, and 53; see also

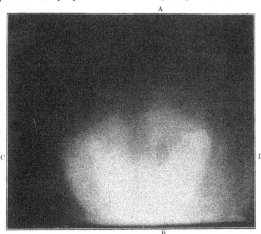

Fig. 51.—Skiagraph showing a Stone in the Lower End of the Ureter in a Young Man Twenty-six Years of Age. (Author's case.)

Two straight lines drawn—the one from A to B, the other from C to D—will cross each other near the centre of the spot where the shadow of the stone is located.

This patient had suffered for four years from dull pain in the pelvic and sacral regions and from pyuria. These symptoms had been preceded by renal colic and hæmaturia, and renal calculus had been diagnosed from these symptoms. The stone, which was as large as a walnut; was removed by the iliac-retroperitoneal operation. The proximal portion of the ureter was dilated to more than half an inch in diameter. The incision in the ureter was not sutured and the patient made an uninterrupted recovery.

Fig. 178 in Vol. I.), and when a stone is in the lower end of the ureter it can sometimes be felt through the rectum or vagina.

A wax-tipped ureteral catheter may be used for diagnosis, the calculus producing scratches upon the wax. (Kelly.*)

TREATMENT.—A surprisingly large stone may pass spontaneously after a long arrest in the ureter and even after pyonephrosis has existed for months or years; but when a stone has been lodged in the ureter for some time, or when it is producing active symptoms, or when it is of large size, it should be removed by operation. In acute conditions the administration of morphia or the use of a general anæsthetic, both of which are indicated for the relief of pain, may favor the passage of the stone; and when the latter is palpable through the rectum or vagina its passage into the bladder may be aided by gentle and discriminating massage. Copious water drinking may also facilitate the passage of a ureteral stone.

* American Journal of Obstetrics, vol. xliii, 1891.

Bransford Lewis * has introduced a forceps by means of which, and with the aid of the cystoscope, he grasps calculi that are lodged in the lower end of the ureter; and Kelly and others have dilated the ureteral orifice to allow of the easier passage of the stone. In most cases, however, the stone can be removed only by operation and incision in the wall of the ureter.

Ureteritis and Periureteritis.—Ureteritis and periureteritis are comparatively rare conditions. Inflammation of the ureter may be caused by infection introduced by instruments, or it may ascend from the bladder, as in gonorrhœa, or descend from the kidney, as in pyelitis and tuberculosis of the kidney; but, as

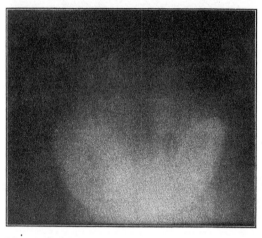

Fig. 52.—Skiagraph Showing a Stone in the Lower End of the Ureter in a very Stout Woman. The stone gives a very distinct shadow (oval in shape and placed vertically) at a point situated to the right of, and a short distance below, the centre of the photograph. (Author's case.)

This patient was a very stout woman who had not suffered from renal symptoms, but had been afflicted for years with indefinite pelvic pain and pyuria. The stone, almost as large as a walnut, was removed by the iliac-retroperitoneal operation. The ureter, which was moderately dilated, was ·not sutured after the removal of the stone, although the peritoneum had been torn in exposing the lower end of the ureter. The tear in the peritoneum was sutured and the patient made an uneventful and rapid recovery.

already pointed out, an ascending infection usually passes lightly over the ureter and attacks the pelvis of the kidney. The results of ureteritis are: stricture, irregularity of lumen, valvular conditions, etc., all of which may lead to uronephrosis.

Involvement of the ureter from neighboring organs, by contiguity, is very rare. Tumors of the ureter are also very rare, if we exclude ureteral growths which have extended from the pelvis of the kidney or the bladder. Papillomata, of a character similar to the papilloma which originates in the bladder, may develop in the ureter. The symptoms are hæmaturia, pain, and sometimes

* Personal communication.

a demonstrable tumor, but a diagnosis is difficult or often impossible. As in other parts of the body, such growths must be removed, but it will be necessary in this situation to remove the portion of the ureter involved, except when the growth is at the entrance to the ureter from the pelvis of the kidney or at its exit into the bladder.   In some cases, after the removal of the new-growth, the cut ends may be reunited (Fig. 54); or, if the part removed is in the lower portion of the ureter, the upper segment may be reimplanted into the bladder; and, finally, if the part removed is located high up in the ureter, the upper extremity of the lower portion may be implanted into the pelvis of the

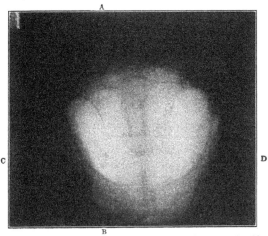

Fig. 53.—Skiagraph Showing Three Stones in the Lower End of the Ureter in a Man Forty-eight Years of Age.   These stones were palpable from the rectum.   (Author's case.)
The three stones are represented in the skiagraph by three small shadows (two of them quite distinct) which are located in close proximity to the point where the two imaginary straight lines—one drawn from A to B, and the other from C to D—cross each other.
This patient had suffered a great deal, first from renal colic and hæmaturia, and later from pain in the bladder, rectum, and pelvis.   Three stones could be distinctly felt by the fingers in the rectum, the smallest one being below and the largest above.   The lower end of the ureter was gently massaged and the patient, who was averse to operation, was instructed as to diet.   He went home and returned three months later with the largest stone in the bladder.   The others had been passed by the urethra. The stone remaining in the bladder was removed by median perineal cystotomy.   It was elongated and bean-shaped; it measured about three-quarters of an inch in length and three-eighths of an inch in diameter.

kidney.   In other cases the alternatives will be loin drainage or nephrectomy. A chronic cystic disease of the ureter, in which its mucous membrane is the seat of small cysts, sometimes very numerous, is described by Morris,* who cites several cases; and single cysts of the lower end of the ureter are reported by Fenwick.   (Any kind of new-growth may invade the ureter, and cases of carcinoma have been reported.)   In addition to the foregoing the ureter may be obstructed by kinks or twists (see under Movable Kidney), or congenital obstructions may lead to secondary changes in the ureter and kidney.

* " Surgical Diseases of the Kidney and Ureter," vol. i.

X. OPERATIONS UPON THE KIDNEYS AND URETERS.

A. OPERATIONS UPON THE KIDNEY.

Nephrectomy.—Nephrectomy, or complete removal of the kidney, is indicated in a variety of pathological conditions, among which are the following:— Tuberculosis, neoplasms, especially the malignant and semi-malignant newgrowths, severe injuries, hydronephrosis, pyonephrosis, and fistula. It may also be necessary to remove the kidney—in other words, to sacrifice a healthy kidney—for disease or injury of the ureter. The kidney may be approached through the abdomen (transperitoneal nephrectomy) or through the loin (lumbar nephrectomy), but, except in cases of large tumor or when for some reason it is considered advisable to explore the peritoneal cavity, lumbar nephrectomy is always to be preferred. Before the introduction and perfection of the cystoscope, which enables the surgeon to determine by ureteral catheterization, not only the existence but the functional condition of a second kidney, it was often considered safer and wiser to operate by the transperitoneal method in order to palpate the second kidney and thus secure some information about it, and at least to determine its existence, but at the present time this can hardly be considered an argument in favor of this form of operation. The more important advantages which may fairly be claimed for the transperitoneal method are: in operations upon large tumors it gives more room and enables the surgeon to ligate the pedicle with greater precision and safety. Its disadvantages are: the handling of the abdominal viscera and the exposure of the peritoneum to infection. The lumbar retroperitoneal operation is, therefore, generally employed in all but exceptional cases, and it is especially important to select the lumbar route when an infective condition of the kidney exists. Some surgeons operate only by the lumbar route (Israel) and remove the largest tumors in this way. The lumbar incision may be prolonged so as to give a great deal of room, retroperitoneally; or the peritoneum may be opened from the lumbar incision, thus facilitating the operation; or in some cases it may be necessary to remove a portion of the peritoneum, as, for example, when it is adherent to a malignant growth.

Lumbar Nephrectomy.—In lumbar nephrectomy the kidney is exposed either by a straight incision running vertically downward from the last rib to the middle of the crest of the ilium, along the outer border of the sheath of the erector spinæ muscles, or by an oblique incision which begins at the anterior border of the sheath of the erector spinæ muscles, about a finger's breadth below the twelfth rib, and is carried forward parallel with the rib to, or beyond, the crest of the ilium, according to the amount of space required. Many modifications of the oblique incision have been recommended. It may be continued down to Poupart's ligament or turned forward at the crest of the ilium and carried across to the border of the rectus muscle, as recommended by Koenig. The advantage claimed for the vertical incision is that there is less danger of hernia after operation; but, with our modern methods of closing a wound, this does not seem to be very important, and besides, this incision affords much less working room than does the oblique incision,—a matter of importance. In this, as in all other operations, it is much wiser to secure plenty of room than to subject an important organ to unnecessary manipulation. In nephrotomy, nephrolithotomy, nephrotresis, ureterectomy, and the removal of calculi from the upper part of the ureter, the kidney is exposed by the same oblique incision, and either the oblique or the straight incision may be employed for nephropexy.

Technique of the Operation.—The patient is placed upon the table lying upon his sound side, inclined slightly forward, with his knees flexed, and a sand or air pillow placed under the sound loin so as to extend the body and make the field of operation (the affected loin) more prominent. (Fig. 54.) After the oblique incision has been made (as above described) through the skin and superficial fascia, the latissimus dorsi, the external and internal oblique muscles, and the transversalis fascia are divided. The sheath of the erector spinæ muscles should not be injured, nor should the quadratus lumborum be cut except

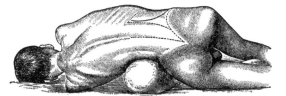

FIG. 54.—Position of Patient for Lumbar Nephrectomy. (From von Bergmann's " System of Practical Surgery.")

This figure is reproduced simply to show the position of the patient on the operating table. The incision usually employed begins at the anterior border of the sheath of the erector spinæ muscles, half an inch below the last rib, and is carried forward along a line parallel to the rib, or to a point beyond the crest of the ilium as far as may be necessary. The line of incision shown in the figure may be disregarded. The dotted line merely indicates certain landmarks—e.g., the crest of the ilium, the spinous processes of the vertebral column, etc.

to secure more room for delivery of the kidney, if necessary. Care should be taken not to wound the last dorsal nerve, the peritoneum, or the colon. If the peritoneum is accidentally wounded it should be immediately closed by suture. If more space is required to reach the upper pole of the kidney the eleventh and twelfth ribs may be excised subperiosteally, but this is seldom necessary. In this region care should be taken not to wound the pleura, which sometimes extends below the last rib, and, if it is accidentally wounded, the wound should be closed immediately, and probably no bad results will follow. The perirenal fat, protected by a thin layer of glistening fascia, will now bulge forward into the wound. When this is cut through, the kidney enclosed in its fibrous capsule may be separated by blunt dissection from the fatty capsule—a step which in most cases is not difficult to carry out. In old inflammatory conditions of the kidney, however, and in malignant neoplasms, it will sometimes be difficult or impossible to separate the kidney from the fatty capsule in this way; and, in the case of malignant growths, it should not be separated even if the procedure is possible, as it is most important to remove all the tissues which may have been infiltrated or which are simply in the immediate neighborhood of the growth. The stripping of the fatty capsule from the kidney should be carried out cautiously and systematically, care being taken to avoid tearing any of the aberrant blood-vessels which are not infrequently encountered. While an assistant presses the kidney up into the wound with a hand placed on the abdomen, the operator first separates the lower pole and anterior surface from the fatty capsule, thus exposing the most accessible part of the kidney and guarding against the danger of wounding the peritoneum. He next separates the posterior surface and upper pole and finally the pedicle, and then afterward carefully delivers the kidney out of the wound upon the loin and isolates the ureter from the remainder of the pedicle, which consists of the blood-vessels held together by fatty and cellular tissue. He then places a clamp on the pedicle in such a way as to leave room for ligation on the proximal side and yet clear of the kidney (the pelvis included) which is to be removed. This is the most critical part of the operation, as the pedicle is short, especially on the right side, where the renal vein is shorter than on the left, being only about an inch in length; and, in the case of a tumor or great enlargement of the kidney, the renal vein is difficult to reach, and besides, in malignant growths, especially hypernephromata, the tumor has a tendency to invade this vein. In hydronephrosis, pyonephrosis, and cystic disease the distended kidney may be reduced in size by aspiration or by puncture with a trocar. The pedicle should therefore be ligated as far as possible from the kidney and at the same time at a safe distance from the vena cava and aorta. At this stage a ligature should be passed through the pedicle with a blunt aneurysm needle, care being taken to avoid the vein. The clamp may now be relaxed, the ligature tied, and the tumor removed by cutting across the pedicle on the distal side with scissors; or, if the tumor is large, it may be necessary to remove it before tying the ligature, special care being taken to secure the pedicle by the application of the clamp. The pedicle having been thus ligated *en masse*, the ends of the vessels should be secured and ligated separately. Silk, linen thread, tendon, and catgut are all employed as ligature material for the pedicle, but strong pliable catgut is probably the best. Chromicized catgut is usually so hard that it is difficult to tie the pedicle securely with it. The ureter should not be cut until after the pedicle has been tied, as there is great danger of tearing the blood-vessels,—an accident which is, almost necessarily, at once fatal. It should be borne in mind that the ureter is strong and fully able to withstand the strain of the necessary manipulations, and therefore it should be left to safeguard the vessels up to the latest moment possible. The writer has to record a sad personal experience of an immediately fatal hemorrhage due to his having failed to appreciate the importance of this teaching.

The next steps in the operation are to place two ligatures around the ureter, then to divide the tube between these two ligatures, and finally to cauterize the cut ends. The distal end may be dropped back into the cavity or fixed by sutures into the lower angle of the wound. The latter is the safer course to adopt in most cases. When the ureter is diseased, as in tuberculosis, it should be removed, if possible, with the kidney; or, under special circumstances, by a later operation.   If the whole ureter is to be removed it will be necessary to extend the wound well down toward Poupart's ligament.   The wound is then closed and a drainage tube inserted, as the cavity remaining is large and in the operation there is much risk of infection, especially where the kidney has been the seat of an infective disease.   In very stout people lumbar nephrectomy it often a very difficult operation.   It may be impossible to deliver the kidney out of the wound without exerting dangerous traction on the pedicle, and it will then be necessary to secure more room by making an incision backward from the lower part of the original incision or by excising the eleventh and twelfth ribs to secure more space at the upper end of the wound, or an incision may be carried forward from the anterior border of the oblique incision without opening the peritoneum, which is stripped forward to expose the pedicle (para-peritoneal operation).   In old inflammatory conditions, especially chronic tuberculosis of the kidney, it may be impossible to separate the kidney from the condensed and altered fatty capsule.   In such cases the fibrous capsule may be incised and stripped off from the kidney and left behind with the pedicle.   Furthermore, when it is impossible to ligature the pedicle a clamp may be applied and left *in situ* for several days.   According to Treves, forty-eight hours may be considered sufficient, provided the clamp, at the end of that time, be removed gently.   In some of these cases the connective tissue of the pedicle will have become so sclerosed that there is practically no bleeding when the kidney is removed.   In any event bleeding points should be secured.   The adhesions about the kidney are sometimes so dense that it is impossible to isolate it wholly by any method, and in that case it may be removed *mor-cellement*.   (Tuffier.)   The lower pole is exposed and a clamp applied, and the part is then removed.   The upper pole is next to be dealt with in the same way, and finally the central portion; or the kidney may be removed in irregular masses beyond the clamp, and the pedicle then dealt with in the manner already described.   In dealing with large solid tumors it may be found impossible, after the kidney has been exposed, to secure the pedicle.   Under these circumstances it will be necessary to modify the operation in the following way:—Protect the lumbar wound, turn the patient upon his back, and then open the abdomen, thus converting the lumbar operation into a combined lumbo-abdominal nephrectomy.   After the pedicle has been secured by resorting to this supplementary step, the operation may be completed through the lumbar wound.

Abdominal Nephrectomy.—In this operation the incision is made either in the median line, which gives more room, or externally to the rectus abdominis muscle, which is more directly over the vessels of the kidney.   The patient is placed upon his back, the anterior surface of the body inclined slightly toward the sound side, and the abdomen is opened.   When the abdomen has been opened, if the existence and functional activity of a second kidney have not been already demonstrated by the cystoscope and ureteral catheter, the hand should be passed across to the other loin for the purpose of examining by palpation. This having been accomplished, the colon is pushed over toward the median line. The outer layer of the meso-colon is incised, either vertically or in a direction parallel with the colon, and the kidney is exposed. By incising only the outer layer of the meso-colon and carefully avoiding the inner layer, which contains the vessels, hemorrhage is averted. The incision in the outer layer should not be begun too close to the bowel, and, if carried vertically outward, the opening may be enlarged by adding transverse incisions at its outer extremity. In this way the blood-vessels of the colon and large blood-vessels found lying upon the surface of the kidney tumor may be avoided, and, by carefully packing away the intestines with gauze pads and controlling the cut edges of the wound in the meso-colon, the operation will be practically a retroperitoneal one. The kidney tumor is next carefully separated by blunt dissection and the pedicle and ureter are isolated. In this (transperitoneal) operation the pedicle is more easily managed than in the lumbar retroperitoneal operation. Its component parts can be isolated and the vessels tied separately, the artery being tied before the vein; or it may be tied after the tumor has been removed, as in the lumbar operation. A clamp or ligature should be placed upon the distal end of the pedicle to prevent the escape of blood, pus, or urine into the wound, when the pedicle is cut through. The ureter is ligated and cut off, and then the pedicle is cut across with scissors and the mass removed. The cut end of the ureter is cauterized and dropped back into the abdomen. It would be unwise to fix it into the lower angle of the abdominal wound, as it would be a source of danger in the peritoneal cavity i.e., would be liable to cause intestinal obstruction. The wound should now be thoroughly cleansed and all bleeding arrested, and, while it is undoubtedly not always necessary, it is generally a safe precaution to drain through the loin, for, by so doing, the opening in the peritoneum may usually be closed by suture, the wound cavity thus being converted into a retroperitoneal one. The abdominal wound will then be closed completely. The danger of wounding the vena cava in removing the right kidney should always be before the mind of the operator. This accident has been reported a number of times, generally with fatal results. Treves, Weir, and others report cases in which they arrested the hemorrhage and saved the patients by applying a lateral ligature to the wound in the vena cava. The physiological effect of the removal of a sound or partially useful kidney is not easily determined. The immediate effect is a diminution of the total secretion of urine, which, if the patient recovers, is soon restored to the normal quantity. The effects of purging and of cutting off the food, as a preparation for operation, the disturbances of nutrition due to the administration of the anæsthetic, and the post-operative disturbances must all be taken into account in considering the diminution of secretion which follows immediately upon operation. When the secreting structure of the kidney has become so disorganized by disease (whether neoplasm, inflammation, suppuration, or pressure) as to render it functionless, the other kidney has already taken on the burden of the secretion, and no effect should be produced upon it by the removal of the useless organ.

In any case, experience shows that the function of the urinary secretion is carried on perfectly well by one kidney after the other has been removed. Treves estimates the mortality attending nephrectomy at from fifteen to twenty per cent. Watson gives the following tables compiled from 1,118 nephrectomies which were performed between 1870 and 1900, and which were "collected and reported by Schmieden":—

Lumbar Operations.	Mortality Per Cent.	Abdominal Operations.	Mortality Per Cent.
First ten years	43.9	First ten years	55.0
Second ten years	26.9	Second ten years	48.0
Third ten years	17.0	Third ten years	19.4

With respect to the special conditions for which the operations were done the following data are given:

Hydronephrosis Operations.	Per Cent.	Pyelonephritis and Nephrolithiasis.	Per Cent.
Lumbar	10.8	Lumbar	32.2
Abdominal	27.0	Abdominal	41.0
Pyonephrosis Operations.	Per Cent.	Tuberculosis Operations.	Per Cent.
Lumbar	23.2	Lumbar	27.0
Abdominal	22.2	Abdominal	42.0

Operations for Malignant Tumors.	Per Cent.
Lumbar	28.0
Abdominal	38.0

There is little doubt that the statistics of the ten years following (1900–1910) will show similar and continuous diminutions in the mortality.

Partial Nephrectomy.—It has been satisfactorily demonstrated that portions of the kidney may be removed and that the operation will be followed by healing of the kidney wound. Benign tumors, cysts, fistulæ, and injured portions of the kidney may be removed in this way. Fenwick * reports two cases in which he removed angiomata of the kidney. Localized areas of tuberculosis have been removed in this way, but, with a better knowledge of the disease, surgeons have come to consider partial operations for tuberculosis as not sufficiently radical, but, in certain cases where both the kidneys are affected, it may have a field of usefulness as a palliative procedure. Partial nephrectomy for any malignant neoplasm, however small, is distinctly contra-indicated, and any new-growth which is not clearly benign calls for total extirpation of the affected kidney.

Technique of the Operation.—The kidney is exposed as for a lumbar nephrectomy. The diseased or injured area is removed in the shape of a wedge, with its base on the outer surface of the kidney. The wound is closed by sutures and usually no difficulty is experienced in controlling hemorrhage, and the kidney wound heals promptly.

Nephrotomy and Pyelotomy.—Nephrotomy or incision through the capsule or into the substance of the kidney is an operation performed for the relief of calculous anuria, suppurative nephritis, and abscess; it is also performed in pyonephrosis and hydronephrosis as a preliminary to more radical treatment,

* Brit. Med. Jour., vol. i., 1900.

and for exploratory purposes for the discovery of a calculus or the source of bleeding in hemorrhage from the kidney. It has also been employed to relieve tension in acute nephritis. The kidney is exposed by a lumbar incision. Where it is distended with fluid a puncture is made at any part and dilated to serve the purpose indicated. If a fluctuating point is discovered an opening is established at this point. In anuria and suppurative nephritis an incision may be made to relieve tension, and in the latter case to drain an abscess. One of the most important indications for nephrotomy is the exploration of the interior of the kidney and its pelvis. This operation will be described under the heading of Nephrolithotomy. Pyelotomy is practically the same operation, except that the incision is made into the fibrous structure of the pelvis instead of into the secreting structure of the kidney. It has one special indication, viz., the drainage of the pelvis in ascending infections such as gonorrhœa.

Nephrotriesis.—This is a term employed to designate an operation which is performed for the purpose of establishing a permanent discharge of the urine from the kidney upon the loin. It is indicated mainly in irremediable obstructions of the ureter in conjunction with a functionating kidney. Watson,* who has devised an apparatus for the collection of the urine as it flows from the loin, describes the essential conditions as follows:—

"The essential factors of long-continued or permanent drainage of the kidney or kidneys are: (1) That the channel of communication between the kidney and the surface of the body shall be kept free and sufficiently large to insure the unobstructed escape of urine from the organ through it. In order that this may be secured, it is absolutely necessary that a tube should be kept constantly, or the greater part of the time, in the fistulous tract, and that the end of the tube shall occupy a place in the kidney which will give free exit to the urine. (2) That the patient shall be kept dry. (3) That the contrivance, whatever it may be, which is worn for this purpose, shall be neither unsightly to others nor uncomfortable to the wearer."

In this operation the edges of the nephrotomy incision are sutured to the edge of the lumbar wound.

Nephrolithotomy and Pyelotomy.—In the early history of kidney surgery it was the rule to remove a kidney which contained calculi, especially if a pyonephrosis had developed secondarily to the irritation of the calculi. Experience has since shown that the kidney possesses remarkable reparative power, and the rule of the present day is to remove the calculi and save the kidney, in all except the worst cases or those in which serious complications have occurred. The following case not only illustrates the amount of repair which may take place in a kidney which is seriously damaged, but is also an evidence of the value of conservative operative treatment:—

More than twenty years ago a man, aged 27, came under the care of the writer with stricture of the urethra and double calculous pyonephrosis. The stricture was first treated and then a large calculus was removed from the right kidney, and several months later six calculi were removed from the left kidney. The

* " Genito-Urinary Diseases," in Watson and Cunningham's Treatise.

patient made an excellent recovery, after seventy-two hours of complete anuria following the second operation, but a fistula persisted in the left loin. He has been under observation ever since, as a hospital servant, and has been throughout, and still-is, in capital health, although he has had sixteen operations upon the fistulous kidney for secondary calculi, but none now for the last two and a half years.

In the great majority of cases which come to operation, the presence of calculi will have been shown, their size, position, and number demonstrated by the x-ray, and the condition of both kidneys determined by the cystoscope. Moreover, the history of the patient and the examination of the urine will have given valuable evidence as to the chemical composition of the calculi. Under these circumstances the operation is greatly simplified. It may be necessary in some cases, however, when only negative evidence has been obtained by the foregoing methods of investigation, to explore the kidney, after it has been exposed by the oblique lumbar retroperitoneal incision and first carefully palpated *in situ*. If no stone is discovered, the kidney should then, whenever possible, be enucleated from its fatty capsule and delivered upon the loin, where it is again carefully palpated, the examination not omitting the pelvis and the upper end of the ureter. If calculi have not been discovered by these methods, the next step will be an exploratory nephrotomy, which is carried out as follows:— The vessels being compressed by the fingers of the left hand or controlled by a padded clamp, an incision is made into the convexity of the kidney in its middle third, along a line about a quarter of an inch posterior to the lower border—the "bloodless line"—and well down into the pelvis. The finger can then be inserted into the pelvis and the calyces explored. In this way a stone of any considerable size can hardly be overlooked. A probe or ureteral catheter is also passed down the ureter to the bladder to make sure that a small stone has not escaped from the pelvis and become lodged in the ureter. The older method of exploration, known as "needling," has practically been abandoned, but may be employed as a *dernier ressort*. When a calculus has been found, it is easily removed by suitable forceps or a blunt scoop, aided by the fingers. The nephrotomy wound is then closed by catgut sutures and usually there is no serious hemorrhage, although in exceptional cases hemorrhage may be so severe as to necessitate a nephrectomy. When a calculus has been located by any method the kidney substance or the tissue of the pelvis is incised directly upon it and the calculus removed. It has been recommended that the kidney substance should be incised rather than the wall of the pelvis, as it has been thought that by so doing there would be less danger of a fistula persisting. If the ureter is unobstructed, there is little danger of fistula in either case, but, if the wound in either the kidney or the pelvis is large, it should be closed by a catgut suture. In pyonephrosis and suppurative conditions the various pus cavities within the kidney should be made to communicate freely and the kidney drained for a time. In aseptic cases the lumbar wound may be closed almost completely. Incisions should, as far as possible, be made radially in the direction of the vessels toward the pelvis and ureter. It is important that the calculi should be wholly removed, as any fragments left behind will serve as nuclei for further stone-formation. If the calculi are entirely removed in aseptic cases there is little danger of recurrence. When pyonephrosis has existed and a fistula remains, secondary calculi are likely to form and their presence necessitates further operation. Stones lodged in the upper portion of the ureter are removed through a longitudinal incision, which it is not necessary to suture.

Nephrorrhaphy or Nephropexy.—The indications for this operation and the principles upon which it is based have already been discussed. (See Movable Kidney.) So long as the principles are kept in mind the selection of the operation from among the great variety of methods proposed and employed by different surgeons, is largely a matter of individual preference. The operations most generally employed resolve themselves into two classes:—(1) Those in which, after the fatty capsule has been cleared away, the kidney is fixed, by sutures passed through the capsule and kidney substance, to the transversalis fascia and the lumbar muscles. The operation recommended by Morris* may be taken as the type of this class of operations. (2) Those in which a greater or less degree of decortication of the kidney is practised, and in which the attachment to the transversalis fascia and lumbar muscles is dependent mainly upon the everted capsule and the approximation of the opposite edges of the bared kidney substance. The kidney is exposed through either a vertical or an oblique incision, as has already been described, the fatty capsule is removed or displaced, and the kidney is brought out upon the loin and carefully examined. In the operation described by Morris three sutures are inserted into the posterior surface of the kidney in the following manner:—"Three sutures are passed deeply into the posterior surface of the kidney, one nearer the upper, the other nearer the lower end, and the third midway between the other two, but nearer the hilum. Each suture is buried for a length of three-quarters of an inch into the thickness of the organ. The upper suture passes through the upper edge of the shortened adipose capsule, the transversalis fascia, and the deep layer of muscles, and is tied to them; the lower suture is similarly passed through and tied to the lower edges of the same cut structures; and the intermediate suture is passed through both edges of the divided adipose capsule, fascia and muscles, and lashes all up together. The sutures are cut and buried in the wound." In the writer's experience this method of suturing the kidney has been very satisfactory, but the fatty capsule had better be eliminated from the line of sutures altogether and extra sutures may be added. The fibrous capsule may be rubbed by gauze or scarified, and a small piece of iodoform gauze may be inserted at the posterior angle of the wound behind the kidney, as recommended by Senn, to encourage granulation, or the wound may be closed completely, the muscular layers being sutured separately.

In Edebohls' operation, in which the most extensive decortication is practised and which may therefore be taken as a type of this class of operations, the fatty capsule is incised and the excess cut away, the fibrous capsule is incised along the course of the kidney in the middle line throughout its whole

* " Surgical Diseases of the Kidney and Ureter."

length and stripped back for some distance on each side along the whole length of the incision, leaving a large raw surface to be united to the lumbar muscles by sutures which are passed deeply into the kidney substance; and a drain is inserted, for the double purpose of carrying away the secretions and of producing irritation of the raw kidney surface and the deep muscles against which it is applied. This operation, modified in various ways, is extensively employed.

B. OPERATIONS UPON THE URETER.

Operations are performed upon the ureter for the relief of stricture, to restore continuity after an accidental wound or injury or partial resection for surgical lesions, and to direct the flow of urine into another viscus or out upon the loin, as in removal of the bladder, in implantation into the bladder, intestine, or pelvis of the kidney after resection, in partial or complete removal of the ureter (ureterectomy), and in removal of calculi (uretero-lithotomy). All these operations give good results and are very satisfactory, and, with the exception of the plastic operation for stricture and that of uretero-lithotomy, the general principle applied is the insertion of the ureter into the viscus, or one end of the ureter into the other (either end-to-end or laterally), so as to unite the external coats by suture and generally avoid, if possible, the inclusion of mucous membrane. End-to-end union of the divided ureter is also sometimes an exception to the inversion rule. A plastic operation for stricture (uretero-plasty) is carried out on the principle of the Heinecke-Mikulicz pyloroplasty. A longitudinal incision is made in the ureter through the stricture and the wound is sutured transversely. End-to-end union (uretero-ureteral anastomosis) has been found, both experimentally and in practice, to be frequently followed by stricture. To reduce the risk of stricture the ends are cut and sutured obliquely (Bovée's operation). (Fig. 55.) In Van Hook's operation the lower end of the ureter is ligated a quarter of an inch from its extremity and a longitudinal incision is made a quarter of an inch below the ligature, and through it the upper end, after having been slit up to the extent of a quarter of an inch from its extremity, is drawn by fine catgut sutures which are brought out about half an inch lower down and tied, thus inverting the outer walls which are reinforced with a couple of fine catgut sutures. For details of this operation, which is the one generally employed when there is sufficient length of ureter, the reader is referred to the article on "Surgery of the Ureter" by Christian Fenger in *Annals of Surgery*, Vol. XX., 1894.

For implantation into the bladder, intestine, or pelvis of the kidney, the end of the ureter is drawn into the cavity, the outer wall of which is first inverted, and fixed by sutures. In the latter situation W. J. Mayo recommends that the suture line in this and in plastic operations be reinforced by the application of a "fatty fascial flap" from the inner layer of the fatty capsule. In the *Journal of the American Medical Association*, May 1st, 1909, he describes this operation and reports a number of cases.

Removal of the ureter (ureterectomy) has already been referred to. It will seldom be necessary to remove the ureter when the kidney can be saved, and in such cases the method adopted for the discharge of the urine will depend upon the ingenuity and resourcefulness of the surgeon. In all these operations the ureter is generally exposed retroperitoneally, but it may also be approached transperitoneally.

Uretero-Lithotomy.—Calculi in the upper portion of the ureter are reached by an oblique incision which exposes the kidney. The incision may be carried forward, as far as necessary, extraperitoneally, and the stone removed through a longitudinal incision in the ureter. This incision, if long, may be sutured

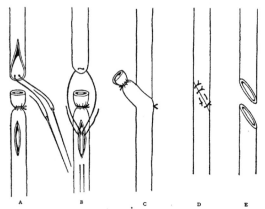

Fig. 55.—Methods Employed to Secure Union of the Divided Ends of the Ureter. (From Treves and Hutchinson, "Manual of Operative Surgery," 1909.)
A, B, C, Lateral union, Van Hook's method; *D, E*, oblique end-to-end union, method of Bovée.

or left unsutured. The wound should be drained. The calculus may sometimes be forced up into the pelvis of the kidney and removed by an incision into that structure. The following list of operations which have been employed for the removal of calculi from the lower end of the ureter, is given by Sinclair White in a recent article *:—1. The intravesical; 2. the perineal; 3. the parasacral; 4. the transsacral; 5. the vaginal; 6. the rectal; 7. the iliac extraperitoneal; 8. the combined intraperitoneal and extraperitoneal; and 9. the transperitoneal. He recommends the transperitoneal operation and reports two cases on which he had operated successfully in this way, although all the previous operations had been devised to avoid wounding the peritoneum. The advantages which he claims for the operation are that it enables the surgeon to clear up a doubtful diagnosis, and that it is less difficult and gives more room and light and thus enables the operator to carry out his operation with greater precision. While all these claims must be admitted, the fact remains that the retroperitoneal

* British Medical Journal, Jan. 8th, 1910.

operations are so satisfactory as to leave little to be desired.   Of the other operations the parasacral, introduced by Morris, the perineal by Fenwick, and the transsacral by Cabot, have been practically abandoned in favor of those by which the ureter is reached through the abdominal wall.   The intravesical operation may in some cases be considered the most suitable, as when the stone projects into the bladder, and Ballin* has recently reported a case in which he employed a combined transvesical and extraperitoneal method.   The vaginal method has been employed successfully, but the rectal route has nothing to recommend it, and much may be said against it.   The method which has been most commonly employed is the "iliac extraperitoneal."   It has also been employed in combination with intraperitoneal exploration (the combined intraperitoneal and extraperitoneal operation of White).   Gibson † has recommended and practised a modification of the iliac extraperitoneal method, by which more room and better exposure of the pelvis is secured.   The incision begins at the middle line, a finger's breadth above the pubes, and is carried outward in a direction parallel to Poupart's ligament and then extended vertically upward along the border of the rectus muscle.   When the peritoneum is reached it is drawn inward and the ureter dealt with in the usual way.   In all extraperitoneal operations, when the peritoneum is stripped inward toward the middle line, the ureter is carried with it.   When the ureter has been incised longitudinally and the stone removed, a probe should be passed on into the bladder from the incision, to make quite sure that the ureteral opening into the bladder is sufficiently free.   It is generally recommended that the incision in the ureter should be closed by a Lembert suture, but this is often difficult and sometimes impossible, and no harm seems to have arisen in cases where the incision was left unsutured.   Indeed, it is a question whether it is not better to leave it unsutured, as the slight narrowing of the lumen, which is unavoidable, and the extra manipulation, as well as the necessity of allowing the silk or thread sutures to remain behind, are all open to objection.   In any case, a drainage tube should be carried down to or near the opening in the ureter and left there for a few days.   The writer has never employed sutures in this operation and has never had any trouble from leakage of urine or in securing healing of the wound.

Operation of Uretero-Lithotomy.—For the removal of a calculus in the lower end of the ureter the procedure usually selected is the iliac extraperitoneal operation.   The patient lies upon his back, slightly inclined toward the sound side and with the head of the table somewhat low.   An incision is made along the outer half of Poupart's ligament and upward as high as the anterior iliac spine, or further if necessary.   The muscles and transversalis fascia are divided and the peritoneum pushed inward.   If the ureter is much dilated it may be easily found where it crosses the brim of the pelvis, or the stone, which has been located by the *x*-ray, will be felt through its walls.   When the ureter has been cleared and the site of the stone demon-

* Surgery, Gynæcology, and Obstetrics, March, 1910.
† Annals of Surgery, xlviii., 1908.

strated, it is steadied upon the finger and a longitudinal incision is made over the stone, which is pressed out and removed. It is rarely necessary to employ any instrument for the removal of the stone, but a small blunt scoop may sometimes be useful. A probe should then be passed downward into the bladder and upward into the pelvis of the kidney, to make sure that there are no more stones or other obstructive conditions. The modification of the incision for this operation recommended by Gibson has already been described. (See Ureteral Calculus.)

SURGERY OF THE PANCREAS.

By GEORGE DAVID STEWART, M.D., New York City.

I. ANATOMY AND PHYSIOLOGY.

ANATOMY.—The pancreas was, for a long time, held to present but little surgical interest, and it has only recently been brought forward into the domain of the operator. Surgical interference is restricted by the very close relations which exist between the pancreas and certain important organs, especially the large abdominal blood-vessels.

The position of the gland is entirely retroperitoneal; it lies behind the peritoneum of the lesser sac, which renders it unusually difficult of access. It is attached to the posterior abdominal wall, lies behind the stomach and transverse colon, in front of the first and second lumbar vertebræ, and extends behind the peritoneum across the upper part of the abdominal cavity, about three inches above the umbilicus. · (Fig. 56.) Between it and the vertebral column lie the vena cava, the abdominal aorta, and the superior mesenteric vessels. The large splenic vessels are closely connected with the pancreas, the artery running along its upper border, the vein at a slightly lower level behind the gland.

The long, flattened, lobulated gland is from five to six inches in length and weighs between two and three ounces. It is divided into four parts, which are named (from right to left) the head, neck, body, and tail. The head is lodged in the loop of the duodenum and is closely connected with the bowel. The left half of the head merges into the neck, which is rarely over an inch in length. The tortuous body lies behind the stomach, being attached to the posterior abdominal wall and the prevertebral tissue. The pointed tail lies in front of the kidney, terminating in contact with the gastric surface of the spleen; it follows the movements of the latter organ, and is the only movable part of the pancreas.

The common bile-duct grooves or tunnels the head of the pancreas; Helly found it to be completely surrounded by the substance of the gland in 62.5 per cent of the cases examined. The duct is, therefore, liable to become entirely obliterated in carcinoma of the head of the pancreas.

The duct of Wirsung, or the main pancreatic duct (Fig. 57), begins near the tail, runs through the middle of the organ toward the right, passes downward in the head, and empties into the duodenum; a variety of types has been distinguished.

159

The duct of Santorini (Fig. 57) is a short, usually subsidiary channel, but may constitute the chief outlet for the pancreatic juice. It opens independently into the duodenum in about fifty per cent of the cases. (Schirmer.)

The arterial supply of the pancreas consists of many small vessels derived from the splenic, hepatic, and superior mesenteric arteries. The solar plexus of nerves lies at the upper margin of the neck of the gland, and the branches which it sends into the pancreas follow the course of the arteries. The veins empty in part directly into the portal vein, and in part into the superior mesenteric veins. The pancreas is surrounded by a large number of lymphatics.

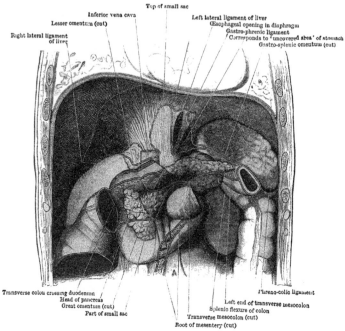

Fig. 56.—The Peritoneal Relations of the Duodenum, Pancreas, Spleen, Kidneys, etc. (From Cunningham's Anatomy.)

ANOMALIES.—The part of the head which is situated behind the mesenteric vessels may easily be detached, thus forming a separate lesser pancreas. The organ may be divided into two parts by a deep cleft, spanned by a thin layer of glandular tissue which also surrounds the duct of Wirsung. Sometimes the tail is split in two halves (bifid tail), each having a duct. The head of the pancreas may enclose the common bile-duct, or the superior mesenteric vessels may lie in the body. Occasionally there is an accessory duct. Again, there may be three ducts, each with an opening into the duodenum. The chief anomalies of the pancreatic duct concern its mode of termination in the duodenum.

ACCESSORY PANCREATIC BODIES.—Aberrant smaller glands have been found in the wall of the stomach and in the submucosa or the muscular layer of the duodenum, the jejunum, and the ileum, as far as the vicinity of the ileo-cæcal valve; sometimes they lie embedded in an intestinal diverticulum. A duct emptying into the bowel is invariably present. Such accessory glands may give rise to confusion with neoplasms.

Three forms of accessory pancreatic bodies have been distinguished by von Heinrich: (1) Masses of typical normal pancreatic tissue, with islands of Langerhans and centro-acinous cells; (2) masses of glandular tissue in which there are no islands of Langerhans; (3) aggregations of secretory cells among which no typical structures, no islands of Langerhans, are discoverable.

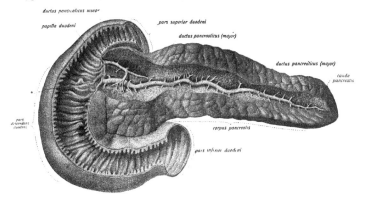

FIG. 57.—Dissection showing the Normal Gross Anatomy of the Pancreas and its Relations to the Duodenum. (From Sobotta.)

At * the location of the outlet the orifice of the major pancreatic duct may be seen.

Annular Pancreas.—In certain cases the pancreas clasps the duodenum after the fashion of a ring, usually surrounding the upper part of the second portion of the bowel. The constriction may lead to dilatation of the first portion of the duodenum and the stomach. An interesting case of annular constriction of the duodenum by pancreatic tissue is described by Ott, who attributes the presence of the ring to the persistence of the original embryonic *Anlage*, and points out the tendency of these fœtal remnants to undergo malignant degeneration.

STRUCTURE OF THE PANCREAS.—The pancreas in its general structure (Fig. 58) resembles other serous salivary glands, but is especially characterized by the presence of the islands of Langerhans, or interalveolar cell-areas—small collections of cells which are most numerous toward the tail. These islands of Langerhans are assumed to be concerned in the internal secretion of the pancreas.

The ducts of the pancreas are lined with a single layer of columnar epithelium, the cells decreasing in height from the chief duct toward the small ones. The tubular alveoli have a distinct membrana propria, which supports the secreting cells; these present a granular zone in their protoplasm. Intercellular secretion-capillaries have been demonstrated in the walls of the pancreas.

FUNCTION OF THE PANCREAS.—The pancreas, like several other glands, provides two secretions—an internal and an external, either of which may be impaired by disease. The internal secretion, which is concerned in control of sugar-assimilation, is provided by the islands of Langerhans. Changes involving these cell-areas do not interfere with the external secretion, which

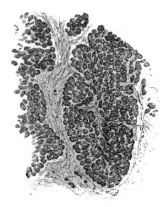

FIG. 58.—Histology of the Normal Pancreas. (Original.)
The magnification is too feeble to show the islands of Langerhans.

is the most important among all the digestive juices. It is poured into the duodenum at the diverticulum of Vater.

The two secretions are rarely interfered with at the same time, and then only in advanced pancreatic disease involving the entire organ.

II. PANCREATITIS.

The pancreas is subject to various types of inflammation, and it may be the seat of calculi, of cysts, and of the different forms of new-growths. Inflammation of the pancreas may affect chiefly the ducts, or the gland substance proper. A distinction is therefore made between two forms—the catarrhal and the parenchymatous, the latter being subdivided into acute hemorrhagic, subacute or purulent, and chronic pancreatitis or pancreatic cirrhosis. Gangrenous pancreatitis, which frequently follows the hemorrhagic form, is, like purulent pancreatitis, classified by many as subacute. The varieties will be considered separately in the following pages.

Catarrhal Pancreatitis.—This form of inflammation of the pancreas, due to an ascending infection of the duct of Wirsung, is seldom recognized, but presumably is often associated with infection of the lower part of the common bile-duct, such as occurs with impacted calculi. In other cases the infection may extend from an ulcerative process in the duodenum. According to the cause and its degree, catarrhal pancreatitis may be mild and transitory, or it may assume an acute character. In the latter case the inflammation may be followed by suppuration with abscess formation, or, in the graver cases, by symptoms of septicæmia and pyæmia.

The removal of the cause, such as biliary calculi, and the establishing of effective drainage of the biliary passages generally lead to the subsidence of the catarrhal pancreatitis; but the organ may remain in a state of chronic inflammation.

Acute Hemorrhagic Parenchymatous Pancreatitis.—Acute hemorrhagic pancreatitis (Fig. 59) is regarded by some as a secondary manifestation in different types of inflammation of the pancreas, whereas others hold that the hemorrhages themselves are the primary factor and the cause of the resulting inflammatory and necrotic processes. This is certainly true for a number of the cases.

It is exceptional for acute hemorrhagic pancreatitis to develop in an intact organ, free from lesions of any kind. A favorable soil is furnished by an inflamed, fatty, or sclerotic pancreas, or by biliary lithiasis. The pancreas in health is protected by the normal blood supply and by its immunity against its own secretions. The onset of the disease is rendered possible by circulatory changes and autodigestive processes.

Anatomically, the disease is characterized by an intra-pancreatic bloody extravasation, with more or less destruction of the glandular parenchyma.

ETIOLOGY.—Hemorrhagic pancreatitis occurs in both sexes and at all ages, but the period between thirty and forty-five years is most extensively represented. According to recent observations of European writers, the Latin races seem to be less susceptible than the Teuton and Anglo-Saxon. The intoxications and diatheses are important etiological factors. In most cases the disease is apparently referable to a general or local infection (general infectious diseases; pylephlebitis; gastric and duodenal ulcer and cancer). Gastro-intestinal affections and diseases of the liver, notably gall-stones, play a prominent part in the etiology of hemorrhagic pancreatitis. All these factors act by way of the vascular lesions to which they give rise. The circulation may be impeded by embolic obliteration of an arterial branch, or a septic embolus may give rise to intra-pancreatic suppuration with secondary hemorrhage. An obstruction of the venous return flow is equally injurious, and in certain cases venous thrombosis plays a leading part. The parenchyma is imperfectly nourished by the retarded blood supply, and auto-digestion then becomes possible.

Besides infection and circulatory disturbances, mechanical and chemical causes referable to gastro-intestinal and hepatic disease also enter into consideration. Infection of the liver usually terminates in lithiasis, which, in its turn, affects the pancreas. The seat of the calculi is more important ·than their number. When arrested in the ductus choledochus, they compress the head of the pancreas through the walls of the duct, giving rise to sclerosis. Virulent microbes from the stagnating bile may gain access to the organ, and thus give rise to suppurative or hemorrhagic pancreatitis. This is still more apt to follow upon the arrest of a gall-stone in the ductus choledochus in close proximity to the duct of Wirsung, as a result of which the pancreatic duct is compressed and the pancreatic juices are forced back into the glandular parenchyma, thus favoring auto-digestion and necrosis. A calculus in the ampulla of Vater is more likely than any other cause to give rise to hemorrhagic pancreatitis, through

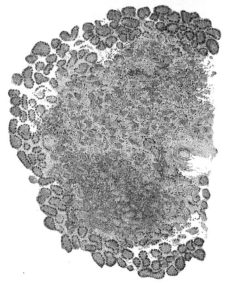

Fig. 59.—Acute Hemorrhagic Pancreatitis. At the periphery there is normal pancreatic tissue, but the central part is necrotic and shows extensive leucocytic infiltration. (Low magnification.)

penetration of bile into the pancreatic ducts. The pancreas in these cases has been found to be transformed literally into a blood-clot.

Hemorrhagic pancreatitis, while it may be produced experimentally by various micro-organisms or their toxins, is not strictly speaking a microbic disease. A specific pathogenic agent does not exist, and the action of microbes in this connection is usually secondary and contributory. The duct of Wirsung, under normal conditions, often harbors microbes, without any untoward results for the pancreas.

Pathological Anatomy.—In most cases the gland is covered in part, or entirely, with distinct extravasations of blood. Partial hemorrhages are usually confined to the head, but have also been noted in the body and even the tail of the organ. The reddish-brown lesions contrast with the grayish color of the normal portions. The entire pancreas is sometimes infiltrated with blood, and resembles a large blood-clot. The organ is considerably enlarged, even up to twice the normal size, softened, and easily indented. The symptoms indicative of compression of various adjacent structures—symptoms which are occasionally observed in the course of hemorrhagic pancreatitis—may be attributed to the enormous degree of hypertrophy which sometimes affects the pancreas. Peri-

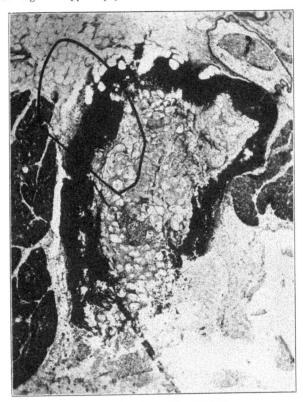

FIG. 60.—Acute Pancreatitis. (Original.)
The details of the oblong area surrounded by a heavy black boundary line may be seen in Fig. 61.

pancreatic hæmatomata are frequently present, and, as might naturally be expected from the anatomical relations, they are situated especially in front of the organ.

The microscopical findings consist in the combined lesions of necrosis and hemorrhage. (Figs. 59, 60, and 61.) Purely hemorrhagic types are rare. A number of intact acini and islands of Langerhans are usually present.

SYMPTOMS.—The patient is generally a stout, well-nourished individual, and is attacked in the midst of health. The onset of the disease varies with its cause. It may begin like hepatic colic, with pain in the region of the gall-bladder, the migration of a biliary calculus being actually the first stage of the hemorrhagic pancreatitis. In other cases the onset is abrupt, with extremely severe pain—of a neuralgic type—in the epigastrium, above or around the umbilicus. Sometimes the pain is described as above and to the left of the umbilicus, but it may be in the right hypochondrium or even in the lower abdominal region. (Opie.) The pain is more diffuse than that of chronic pancreatitis, which is confined to the entrance of the duct of Wirsung into the duodenum; it is distinctly aggravated by the slightest movement or by the mere weight

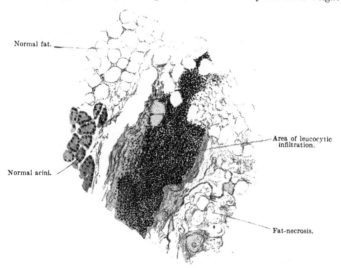

Normal fat.

Area of leucocytic infiltration.

Normal acini.

Fat-necrosis.

FIG. 61.—Acute Hemorrhagic Pancreatitis, characterized by leucocytic infiltration and fat-necrosis. (Original.) (Higher magnification of a limited part of the field shown in Fig. 60.)

of the bed clothes. In the further course of the attack the pain subsides to a certain extent, while signs of peritoneal reaction may manifest themselves in the form of moderate tympanites with rigid abdomen, particularly in the epigastric region. A peculiar type of painless, frequently repeated, vomiting occurs, in which bile or blood or both may be voided, but no fecal matter. This symptom is present only in the early stages. There is marked intestinal paresis. In a general way, it may be said that the clinical picture resembles both that of peritonitis and that of intestinal occlusion. The latter is never absolute, however, and there is no actual arrest of feces and gas. Certain cases are characterized by profuse diarrhœal discharges. That peritonitis does not exist is shown by the slow, full pulse, suggestive of great arterial hypertension.

Fever is rarely present in the early stages, and the temperature may, when symptoms of shock develop, become subnormal; leucocytosis is present in some cases, absent in others; jaundice, which occurred in ten per cent of the cases collected by Gessner, is probably due in most cases to coincident disease of the biliary passages.

The symptoms of hemorrhagic pancreatitis are not absolutely characteristic and are rarely all present in the same individual. The clinician must then look to certain signs that depend upon the relations of the pancreas to the neighboring organs, and upon the disturbed functions of the gland itself. The former, which are the result of irritation of the solar and cœliac plexuses, are expressed by pain, diarrhœa, vomiting, collapse, and vasomotor disturbances as evidenced by cyanosis. The changed character of the glandular secretions is ascertained by the examination of the urine and stools. The presence of glycosuria, which is more apt to be found at the beginning than at the end of the disease, possesses small diagnostic value; it occurs in only a small proportion of the cases and has no unfavorable bearing upon the prognosis. According to Leriche and Arnaud the glycosuria seems to be referable to a reflex action, instead of being dependent upon the destruction of the gland. The presence of fatty acids in the urine is more important, and useful information in this respect is likewise elicited from an examination of the stools. The discharge of necrotic fragments of pancreatic tissue is pathognomonic.

COURSE OF THE DISEASE.—The patient's general condition is very seriously impaired, and the emaciation which takes place within a few days may be very pronounced. The pulse becomes weak; signs of impending heart failure develop; the temperature may remain stationary, rise very high, or drop below normal. Death often takes place in the midst of a profuse attack of hæmatemesis.

Gangrenous Pancreatitis.—No sharp line of demarcation can be drawn between gangrenous pancreatitis and hemorrhagic pancreatitis, particularly when the former follows the hemorrhagic variety, as it does, according to Fitz, in at least one-half of the cases. Indeed, widespread necrosis is a constant sequel of the hemorrhagic lesion, and, in experimental cases, appears within a few hours. (Opie.) Subsequent changes in the extravasated blood are due to the invasion of bacteria, and the digestive action of the pancreatic juice brings about those changes in the gland which are described as gangrenous.

In cases of hemorrhagic pancreatitis that have survived the onset for about one week, the gland becomes dark or even black in color; a little later it is perceptibly soft and friable. It may be entirely separated from its attachments or remain connected to the surrounding structures by only a few shreds. The lesser peritoneal sac is filled with dark, bloody, foul-smelling fluid, and areas of fat necrosis may be found around the pancreas or behind the lesser peritoneal sac.

Infections by a variety of bacteria may occur, and frequently the abscess thus formed is limited to the lesser peritoneal sac, the foramen of Winslow being closed by adhesions. A general peritonitis rarely results. (Opie.) In some instances the abscess cavity may extend to the retroperitoneal tissues over the left kidney. Perforation may occur into the stomach or the duodenum, and in one of the cases reported a part of the pancreas was passed per rectum and identified. Gangrenous pancreatitis thus represents a later subacute stage of one of the acute forms of inflammation, particularly the hemorrhagic.

The symptoms of gangrenous pancreatitis appear at a later date in those who have survived the attack for a few days (from four days to one week). Usually the acute symptoms at the onset—viz., pain, tenderness, and vomiting—have subsided to some extent by the time the gangrenous changes take place. Constipation, if present, may give place to diarrhœa, and the stools often contain blood. Steatorrhœa is rarely present. Still later (about the end of the second week, according to Opie), owing to the invasion of the necrotic tissue by micro-organisms, fever, moderate in degree and irregular in course, may be present. For the same reason there are likely to be evidences of peritonitis, and a mass, in some cases well defined, in others vague, may appear, usually in the epigastric region. In the gangrenous cases glycosuria is rare. In twenty per cent of the cases collected by Fitz jaundice was present.

DIAGNOSIS.—In the early stages of the disease the diagnosis is based on the suddenness of the onset, the localization of the pain in the epigastrium, the vomiting, and the symptoms of collapse. Later, the appearance of a tumor in the epigastrium, usually between the stomach and the colon, suggests an exudate in the lesser sac of the peritoneum. This symptom is of the greatest value when it follows the acute symptoms, appearing in the gangrenous or suppurative stage. Evidences of disturbed metabolism, glycosuria, steatorrhœa, etc., are, according to Opie, rarely present; but, in both the early and the late stages, examination of the urine and feces may afford at least confirmatory evidence. (See also General Considerations, etc., page 175.)

Biliary colic often precedes and at times accompanies an attack of hemorrhagic pancreatitis. When the two are associated, differentiation may be exceedingly difficult; but pancreatitis is suggested by the facts that the symptoms are unusually severe and that the pain is perhaps located more to the left than to the right side. When the two coexist, as the result of a calculus lodged in the ampulla of Vater, differentiation may be impossible; but differentiation is not essential at this time, since the exploratory incision which completes the diagnosis, permits the proper treatment of both conditions. Perforation of the gall-bladder usually produces pain on the right side, but even this may be misleading. The writer recalls a case in which the patient had suffered from attacks of biliary colic for years. In the final attack the symptoms at first were not severe and were subsiding. Among other signs the medical attendant had noticed an enlarged gall-bladder. Suddenly the symptoms became severe and coincidentally the enlargement of the gall-bladder disappeared. A diagnosis of perforative cholecystitis was made, but at the operation there were found fat necrosis and other evidences of pancreatitis, while the gall-bladder was only moderately distended and not perforated. As an autopsy was not permitted, the exact pathological conditions could not be determined.

When an attack of pancreatitis is accompanied by severe constipation, the condition is often mistaken for intestinal obstruction. The suddenness of onset, the severity of the symptoms, and the limitation of the pain and distention to the epigastrium suggest pancreatitis; and, besides, the absence of stercoraceous vomiting and of marked peristalsis is against intestinal obstruction. Perforation of the stomach, duodenum, or other part of the alimentary canal may, in the early stage of the attack, while peritonitis is still localized, suggest hemorrhagic pancreatitis. Then again, in the later stages, if a localized peritoneal abscess is produced, particularly if the perforation has been in the lesser sac, the same difficulty may obtain. The history of a previous ulcer or malignant growth points to perforation; the history of a previous biliary infection to pancreatitis.

PHYSICAL EXAMINATION.—Palpation behind, at the level of the left costovertebral angle, is important, for, when this causes an exacerbation of the pain, it affords an excellent sign of the presence of acute pancreatic disease. Inspection of the abdominal wall often shows it to be splashed with livid, purplish spots, which give it a mottled appearance, and which, in conjunction with the cyanotic coloration of the face, should draw attention to the pancreas. Mayo-Robson's pressure point lies half-way between the end of the ninth rib and the umbilicus; tenderness or pressure at this point is considered by some as characteristic. Abdominal palpation may permit the demonstration of an abnormal resistance in the epigastric region, due to the marked enlargement of the pancreas; but, according to Opie, a tumor mass referable to the pancreas is rarely palpable in the early hemorrhagic stage.

TREATMENT.—There is some question, among writers on this subject, as to whether operation should be performed in the early or the later stages. Statistics published so far seem to indicate that a greater percentage of cures follows operation in the subacute stage—the stage of gangrene or suppuration—than in the early stages. Mikulicz, who published in 1903 the largest list of operations furnished up to that time, did not regard this showing of significance, because of the large number of unrecorded cases of patients who die in the early stage. Further, many of the operations have been undertaken in consequence of a mistaken diagnosis, and the long and tedious search for the lesion thus necessitated has added to the mortality. Mikulicz himself, in spite of his statistics, believed that early operation limited the necrosis and lessened the likelihood of such severe complications as venous thrombosis and pyæmia. Moynihan states that the affected pancreas and its surroundings form a phlegmon, which can be relieved only by free drainage. This author also says that, while in the less severe cases of pancreatitis the patient may live until an abscess forms or a slough separates, in the more severe ones he is likely to die unless surgical treatment is adopted early.

The surgical treatment of acute hemorrhagic pancreatitis consists in laparotomy, exposure of the pancreas, puncture or incision of the organ, drainage with tamponing, and, if necessary, drainage of the bile-passages. The operative procedures aim at: (1) prevention of the diffusion of pancreatic juice in the abdominal cavity: (2) correction of the harmful effects of the juice which has already escaped.

The degree of anæsthesia employed should be slight. Sometimes purely local anæsthesia (by ethyl chloride or by cocaine) suffices. The avenue of election for reaching the pancreas is through median laparotomy. The making of this incision is followed by division of the gastrocolic ligament and exposure of the pancreas, which should be punctured in several places or even incised freely, after which it should be thoroughly tamponed. Under all circumstances it is necessary to prevent the diffusion of the destructive secretion of the gland. To accomplish this, the liquid may be wiped out with compresses or aspirated. Wherever a retracted omentum, spattered with grease spots and on the verge of gangrene, is seen, it should be resected.

The cutting out of small portions (discission) and the tearing asunder of the lobes (dilaceration) of the pancreas—measures which are objected to by some on account of the danger of hemorrhage—are recommended by others (notably Leriche and Arnauld) in cases where the hemorrhagic and necrotic lesions are very pronounced. The procedures sometimes permit the withdrawal of necrotic fragments of pancreatic tissue and the opening of cavities, thus preventing the harmful absorption of toxic products, and have, moreover, the beneficial effect of lessening the volume of the organ.

The operation is completed by extensive tamponing of the pancreas, so as to separate it completely from the adjacent organs, and at the same time to insure the easy draining of the inflammatory and secretory products to the outside. One or two large drains should be inserted. Drainage is usually established by way of the gastrocolic, more rarely by way of the gastrohepatic omentum; sometimes both routes are adopted. Lumbar drainage may be indicated in the presence of a voluminous retropancreatic exudate. The tampons must be left in place for a long time, in order to guard against remote necrosis of the pancreatic tissue. During cicatrization, as long as the slightest secretion persists, the wound must be very carefully watched and autodigestion prevented by the local application of isolating fatty substances, such as lanolin ointment.

Concerning the statistics of the surgical treatment of acute hemorrhagic pancreatitis, Villar, at the Surgical Congress of 1905, reported five cures among twenty-one patients upon whom he had operated. Mikulicz's summary of all reported cases operated on up to May, 1903, includes 75 operations with 25 recoveries among 36 cases in which the pancreas was directly treated; whereas there were only four recoveries among 41 cases treated with free drainage, without interference with the organ itself. Dreesmann, in April, 1909, compiled from general medical literature 118 cases of acute hemorrhagic pancreatitis treated by operation.

Imfeld has recently (1910) reported a case of acute hemorrhagic pancreatitis, that occurred in a man thirty-six years old, who was successfully operated upon by Kocher, after a practically positive diagnosis had been made prior to the operation. The capsule of the pancreas was transversely incised for a distance of 3 or 4 centimetres; then the opening was tamponed with iodoform gauze, and drainage was effected by means of a large glass tube, around which peritoneum and fascia were sutured. The severe pain subsided almost completely after the operation; a fistula persisted for four months afterward.

When, as frequently happens, the biliary passages are involved either by obstruction or by infection, the obstruction should be removed, and—to overcome the infection—drainage should be established. Drainage may be required in the gall-bladder or in the common duct, or in both; the conditions present determining the appropriate treatment. Frequently the condition is so grave that only measures directed to the pancreas can be employed, the treatment of the biliary passages being left to a later date. When, however, a calculus is lodged at the duodenal orifice, this must be removed promptly, if possible, since without such removal pancreatic drainage will be inadequate.

The medical treatment is briefly as follows:—Pain should be controlled by morphine, but this must be given guardedly, since it obscures the symptoms and increases the distention; it should, indeed, be used only while the surgeon is waiting to make preparations for the operation. Sometimes the paroxysms are so severe as to require the administration of chloroform. Vomiting is best relieved by withholding food, by stomach lavage, and by introducing a saline solution into the rectum according to the method recommended by Murphy for use in the treatment of peritonitis. The absorption of fluid by the rectum takes place rapidly, supplies the place of that which has been lost by vomiting, and dilutes the toxins in the circulation. Collapse is treated by the injection of a saline solution into the rectum or the veins, or subcutaneously, and by appropriate heart stimulants. Nutrition, when the vomiting is severe, must be maintained by the measures recommended above and by rectal feeding.

Subacute Pancreatitis (Abscess of the Pancreas).—The suppurative type of pancreatic inflammation is characterized by multiple small abscesses which are scattered throughout the substance of the gland, and which, in their turn, may break down and coalesce into one large abscess. The disease may occur as a primary infection, or it may follow acute hemorrhagic pancreatitis, the germs in the latter instance finding a peculiarly favorable soil. (Opie.) The disease may originate (1) through the hæmatogenous route, the pus-producers reaching the pancreas by way of the blood, as in all metastatic suppurations; (2) through inflammation transmitted from the surroundings (gastric and duodenal ulcer and cancer); (3) through bacterial invasion of the ducts of a predisposed pancreas—one that is the seat of an acute hemorrhagic inflammation, of a chronic inflammation, of necrosis, of compression of the pancreatic duct, etc. Metastatic infections are not common; the most common are probably those which take place by way of the ducts.

Diffuse purulent infiltration of the gland and pancreatic gangrene represent the final stage of acute inflammation rather than a variety of subacute pancreatitis. When the two are combined a distinction between gangrene and suppuration is not possible. Depending upon the kind and severity of the infection, the gland may break down into a pulpy gangrenous mass, enclosed in a capsule of thickened connective tissue; or the abscess cavity may contain the hardened and contracted remains of the pancreas, which may be expelled through the stomach or the bowel.

SYMPTOMS.—In the suddenness of the onset and the character of the later symptoms, subacute pancreatitis resembles the acute form of the disease. The symptoms of the former, however, and especially the severity of the pain, are not so pronounced as they are in the acute form, and may subside by the third or fourth day, only to reappear about the eighth or ninth day, as the abscess continues to enlarge. The temperature at this stage may rise to 104° F. Chills and extreme weakness are present. Ileus is sometimes closely simulated. While the clinical picture may point to an involvement of the pancreas, a definite conclusion as to the type of the disease is extremely difficult to reach. In a smaller group of cases, particularly those following lithiasis or the development of a cyst or cancer, the onset may be gradual and there may be only abdominal pain or a sense of discomfort in the epigastric region, with gastric symptoms of varying intensity. (Opie.)

Favorable cases are characterized by the formation of a circumscribed abscess, surrounded by protective adhesions. The seat of predilection is the omental bursa, and the pus then becomes demonstrable on the right or the left of the middle line, either in the right renal region, or between the spleen and the colon, depending upon its origin from the head or the tail of the pancreas. Retroperitoneal suppuration may appear in the lumbar region. Pus burrowing above the lesser curvature of the stomach gives rise to the formation of a subphrenic abscess.

COURSE OF THE DISEASE.—The abscess, when left untreated, may empty itself by establishing an opening into the stomach or bowel, and thus spontaneous recovery may result. The pus may penetrate the diaphragm or force its way through the abdominal wall above or below the stomach. Rupture of the abscess into the free abdominal cavity usually terminates in fulminating peritonitis and death. Cases of chronic sepsis, with infarction of the spleen and the kidneys through infectious thrombosis, have been recorded.

TREATMENT.—Subacute pancreatitis is relatively amenable to surgical interference, which consists in incision of the abscess, after division of the gastrocolic ligament or the mesocolon, usually by way of a median laparotomy. The pus can also be evacuated through an incision in either the left or the right costovertebral angle. Abscesses situated at a great depth posteriorly may be operated upon through the lumbar region, or a counter-incision in that direction may be made. Subphrenic pancreatic abscess may be approached through the transpleural route, with costal resection. In all these procedures, the peritoneal cavity must be well protected with tampons against the destructive pancreatic secretion.

PROGNOSIS.—While the prognosis is more favorable than that of acute pancreatitis, the remote results are not always satisfactory, and the patients are exposed to a variety of complications. Diffuse purulent infiltration or multiple abscesses are, of course, less amenable to surgical treatment than is a single large abscess.

Chronic Interstitial Pancreatitis.—The chronic indurative form of pancreatitis (Fig. 62) is now conceded to be more common than was formerly assumed, but a pathognomonic symptom which positively indicates the existence of a chronic inflammation of the pancreas is not yet known.

Chronic pancreatitis is usually secondary, the interstitial inflammatory process being due to a variety of factors. Most cases can be traced to an ascending catarrh of the pancreatic ducts (sialangitis pancreaticus ascendens, Mayo-Robson). The catarrhal pancreatitis, in its turn, is mostly due to stagnation of the secretion, through mechanical or inflammatory obstruction of the pan-

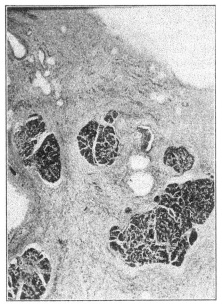

Fig. 62.—Chronic Interstitial Pancreatitis. The illustration shows extensive fibrosis and widely separated islands of pancreatic tissue. Magnified 75 diameters. (Original.)

creatic duct. The anatomical relations account for the likelihood of the occurrence of pancreatic involvement as the result of an occluded ductus choledochus. Stones blocking the duct of Wirsung or the biliary passages give rise to constant irritation and to inflammatory changes of the mucosa,—changes which prepare the ground for bacterial invasion.

Injurious agents travelling by the hæmatogenous or the lymphatic route are other important etiological factors. Arteriosclerosis—or, more accurately speaking, endarteritis obliterans—is responsible for a number of cases. Syphilis predisposes to these sclerotic processes, and some cases of chronic pancreatitis are doubtless of specific origin. The parts played by alcoholism and tuberculosis are not so well established. Inflammatory or neoplastic conditions of adjacent organs, especially the stomach or the duodenum, may lead to interstitial pancreatitis through direct extension. The entrance of micro-organisms is facilitated by the existence of intestinal tumors or biliary calculi.

Opie distinguishes between the interlobular and the interacinar types of chronic pancreatitis. In the former, the organ is traversed in all directions by broad bands of connective tissue, but the glandular parenchyma and the islands of Langerhans are preserved intact. In the interacinar type, on the other hand, the parenchyma itself disappears, and connective tissue takes its place; the islands of Langerhans are involved and usually present hyaline changes. As a result of the degenerative and destructive processes, the internal secretion of the pancreas is arrested, as shown by the onset of diabetes.

SYMPTOMS.—The clinical picture presented by cases of chronic interstitial pancreatitis is not sharply outlined, and the general symptoms are vague and indefinite, suggesting gastro-intestinal catarrh, or more commonly simulating an affection of the biliary passages. Biliary disorders may indeed be responsible for the pancreatitis, and their symptoms, notably icterus, may entirely mask those dependent upon the disease of the pancreas itself. Confusion may also arise in the case of a pancreatic neoplasm. Moynihan calls attention to the fact that the color of the jaundice, in chronic pancreatitis, is never so deep as that of malignant disease of the organ, and is more inclined to a pale golden yellow.

DIAGNOSIS.—It is only in the minority of the cases that a reliable guide is afforded by certain physical manifestations, such as the appearance of a tumor in the region of the pancreas. The enlargement of the organ does not often reach very large dimensions and, as the patient is usually a well-nourished, obese individual, it is not frequently palpable. Functional tests have their diagnostic uses, but their value is limited by the fact that the chronic indurative process does not necessarily involve the entire organ, while slight remnants of parenchyma are known to suffice for a fairly adequate secretion.

TREATMENT.—The treatment aims at arresting the inflammatory process and preventing its extension to the still intact segments of the pancreas. It is essentially the treatment of the causative cholelithiasis. Cholecystostomy may be performed, or one may resort to choledochotomy and cholecystectomy, perhaps combined with dilatation of the intrapancreatic portion of the ductus choledochus. (Czerny.) Cholecystenterostomy, on account of the danger of infection from the bowel, is not recommended. In certain cases of chronic pancreatitis, in which the pancreas causes an annular stenosis of the ductus choledochus, with obliteration of its lumen, Vautrin proposes freeing the duct by dividing the bridge of pancreatic tissue with the thermocautery. No matter which operative procedure is adopted, the biliary passages must be thoroughly inspected and a prolonged drainage (from two to three weeks) of the hepatic duct be instituted, with drainage of the subhepatic space.

The treatment of chronic pancreatitis, when it is not associated with disease oi the biliary system, may consist in simple laparotomy and drainage, or a posterior pancreatotomy may be performed. In long-standing cases of chronic pancreatitis, the treatment can be only palliative, on account of the impossibility of restoring the atrophic cells and islands of Langerhans which have undergone fibrous degeneration.

The list of operations recorded up to the present day includes 113 cases, with 8 deaths.

General Considerations in Regard to the Diagnosis of Pancreatic Diseases.

The clinical diagnosis of pancreatic disease is based upon the demonstration of certain disturbances of body metabolism, the result of partial or of complete loss of the internal and external secretions of the pancreas.

Disturbances of the Internal Secretion (changes in the urine).—The internal secretion of the pancreas is inaccessible, and the mutual relations between this gland and others having an internal secretion are very imperfectly known. Practical importance attaches to the connection of the pancreas with the sugar metabolism, and the feature of persistent or periodical glycosuria in the symptom-complex is always a strong support for the diagnosis of pancreatic disease. The urine must be repeatedly examined as to the presence of sugar, and any existing intolerance for carbohydrates, more particularly grape sugar, must be ascertained. In suspected cases, a positive outcome of the Kraus test for alimentary glycosuria is also suggestive. (In this method, 100 grammes of dextrose are added to the ordinary meal, and the urine is then examined for sugar.) It is not permissible, however, to base conclusions as to the existence of pancreatic disease solely upon the presence of diabetes or alimentary glycosuria, without demonstrable disturbances of the intestinal absorption.

Pentosuria and lipuria have been observed in diseases of the pancreas, but the evidence for the connection of these urinary changes with a disturbance of the internal secretion is still incomplete and indefinite.

Loewi recently suggests the identification of pancreatogenic diabetes by means of adrenalin instillations into the eye. These injections were found to cause mydriasis in the pupils of cats and dogs, after the pancreas had been extirpated; and this change is interpreted by him as due to the loss of pancreatic antagonism. Hagen regards the value of this test as extremely doubtful.

Cammidge Reaction.—The diagnostic value of this reaction of the urine is at present disputed, although up to a very recent date the majority of authors held that a positive outcome of the test is greatly in favor of pancreatic disease. Mayo Robson, who largely provided the clinical material for Cammidge's investigations, strenuously advocates the value of the method. Hess, who carried out the Cammidge reaction fifty times, including twenty-five clinical cases and twenty-five animal experiments, reaches the conclusion that it has only a corroborative value. From the detailed investigations of Schumm and Hegler, who examined the urine of seventy patients, in some of whom pancreatic disease was shown by operation to exist, it results that the Cammidge reaction cannot yet be ranked as a method free from clinical objections. These comments apply exclusively to the new so-called combined method, proposed by. Cammidge in 1906. It consists in subjecting the urine, which has first been freed from albumin and sugar, to acid hydrolysis, by boiling it with hydrochloric acid; the excess of acid is neutralized with lead carbonate; the glycuronic acids are precipitated from the filtrate by tri-basic lead acetate, the lead being removed by the introduction of hydrogen sulphide or simply by precipitation with sodium sulphate; and the remaining filtrate is subjected to the phenyl-hydrazin test. The outcome is positive when, at the end of a few hours, there is formed a light-yellow flaky precipitate, which is seen under the microscope to be made up of long, light-yellow, hair-like crystals, in the form of bundles. It is characteristic of these crystals to become promptly dissolved within from ten to fifteen seconds, at most a few minutes, after the addition of thirty-three per cent sulphuric acid. In order to exclude traces of sugar which have been overlooked in the reduction tests, Cammidge requires a control test in which the urine is treated in the same way, the acid hydrolysis, however, being omitted. The end-products of this combined Cammidge method are pure osazone-compounds (pentosazones), due to the liberation of pentose-like bodies, in the disintegration of the nucleoproteids of the pancreas.

It has been satisfactorily demonstrated that the Cammidge reaction is not based upon the presence of a uniform reaction-product, for this body in the urine of pancreatics may be either saccharose, dextrose, or dextrose and glycuronic acid. The unreliable character of the method is also illustrated by animal experiments.

According to Klieneberger's experience with nearly fifty cases, it is absolutely certain that a positive Cammidge reaction may occur, in exceptional cases, when pancreatic disease can be safely ruled out on the basis of the clinical findings and other functional methods. Hence, the test must always be controlled and confirmed by other more reliable procedures.

Disturbances of the External Secretion (changes in the stools).—Hypochylia or achylia of the pancreatic juice that is poured into the bowel is essentially expressed by the loss of the pancreatic ferments—tryptic (nuclease, trypsin), diastatic (especially diastase), lipolytic (steapsin), also the glucosid-splitting ferments. As pointed out by Klieneberger, the disturbances produced through loss of the pancreatic alkali, pancreatin, hæmolysin, etc., are relatively immaterial.

Quantitative and qualitative changes of the pancreatic ferments may be demonstrated either directly, in juice obtained from the duodenum or the stomach (Boldireff's oil-breakfast), or indirectly, by examining the stools. The disturbance of pancreatic function may also be traced indirectly through the effects of the loss of the important digestive ferments upon the assimilation of a diet of known composition. These findings are not entirely reliable, however, and are applicable only to chronic cases.

Absence or deterioration of the pancreatic ferments can also be shown through functional tests, in which there are introduced into the alimentary tract certain objects which resist the digestive juices of the upper passages and are normally digested in the duodenum. When the pancreatic juice is abnormal, the test substances are voided whole, or undigested, with the excreta. There are substances with which to test the action of trypsin, others for the action of the nuclease, and still others that aim at the glucosid-splitting property of the pancreatic juice (Sahli's glutoid test; Schmidt's nuclear test; Ferreira's salicin test). For practical purposes, changes in the stools furnish the most important indications; and the dejecta should always be examined as to the presence of fat and muscle fibres (steatorrhœa and azotorrhœa). The stools are often extremely abundant and characterized by a peculiar grayish discoloration.

Steatorrhœa.—Fat in the stools may be liquid or free, may be apparent to the naked eye, giving the stools an oily appearance, and, on cooling, may form a distinct layer. Sometimes, particularly in the stools that are colored a metallic gray, the fat is not macroscopically apparent, but can be better detected by chemical and microscopical examination. Undigested fat in the stools occurs in the form of neutral fat and split fat—that is, fatty acids and soaps. The relative proportions of these have also been considered of diagnostic value.

The digestion of fats is carried on by the pancreatic juice, the bile, the intestinal juice, and intestinal bacteria. Failure of any of these may cause fats to appear in the feces. (Moynihan.) Absorption and digestion are also diminished in diseases of the intestine or its lymphatic apparatus, namely in amyloid disease, in atrophy of the mucous membrane, in caseation of the mesenteric nodes, in tuberculous peritonitis, or when active peristalsis prevents the normal action of the digestive juices. (Nothnagel quoted by Opie, in Osler's "System of Medicine," Vol. V., p. 622.) Unabsorbed fat, when ingested in abnormal quantities, may also appear in the stools, but, as the capacity for absorption of fats varies widely in different individuals, no definite conclusions can be reached by observing the effect, on the feces, of the ingestion of a fixed amount of fats.

Azotorrhœa.—The presence of undigested proteids, particularly meat fibres, in the stools is also held to be evidence of pancreatic disease. According to Opie, it has not been so frequently observed as has the disturbed digestion of fats. Wientraud, on the other hand, suggests that the disturbance of proteid digestion is even greater than that of fat digestion. Fitz calls attention to the fact that this disturbance probably occurs only when there is extreme diminution of the pancreatic juice, and is significant only when the gastric digestion is normal, when there is no excess of meat in the diet, and when diarrhœa is not present.

The color of the stools, under normal conditions, is due to the presence of an insoluble pigment, the result of the action of the pancreatic juice on the soluble and absorbable bile pigments. Failure of either secretion, therefore, causes the stools to become light in color,—a tendency that is increased by the presence of steatorrhœa.

The quantity of feces passed is greatly increased in pancreatic disease, owing to the failure of digestion and absorption and to the presence in the feces of finely divided bubbles of gas.

The diagnostic value of the changes observable in the stools is summed up by Moynihan substantially as follows:—Steatorrhœa without jaundice, the bile passing into the intestine, suggests pancreatic disease. Steatorrhœa combined with azotorrhœa favors this diagnosis strongly. The two combined with glycosuria afford still stronger evidence; and, finally, if with these is found the pancreatic reaction (Cammidge's) in the urine, the diagnosis becomes almost a certainty. To this may be added Wientraud's opinion that azotorrhœa is stronger evidence in favor of pancreatic disease than is a steatorrhœa, for the former results from pancreatic failure alone, while the latter may be caused by the diseases of the intestine, tuberculous peritonitis, etc., as already mentioned.

A number of functional tests are based upon the fact that a considerable fraction of the specific ferments of the pancreas reappear unaltered in the feces, where they can be demonstrated after dilution or filtration. Hence, in anomalies of the pancreatic secretion, there will be a diminution or complete lack of the remnants of pancreatic ferments otherwise found in the stools. The ferments to be looked for are trypsin and amylase.

Fat-Necrosis.—The phenomenon of fat-necrosis (Fig. 63) is closely related to inflammatory conditions of the pancreas. It was first pointed out by Balser, in 1882, who interpreted the process as a proliferation of the fat cells at the expense of the parenchyma.

The appearance of the affected tissues is characteristic. When the abdomen is opened the fat in the neighborhood of the pancreas, or even at some distance, is seen to be studded with yellowish-white opaque spots, that contrast strongly with the surrounding normal yellow fat. Frequently the spots are surrounded by a hemorrhagic zone, and they may be close together or scattered. In the neighborhood of the pancreas, particularly, they may be large and confluent; scattered foci may be found in the meso-colon, in the omentum, in the perinephritic fat, and occasionally in the pericardium and the pleuræ, and even in the subcutaneous fat.

The minute changes which occur are the following: the neutral fat is split into fatty acids and glycerin, the crystals of fatty acid are deposited in the cells, of which the outlines remain, and the glycerin is absorbed. Later, the acids unite with calcium salts and may be demonstrated by micro-chemical reactions. Proliferation of the fixed tissue-cells occurs in the periphery of the necrotic areas. (Opie.)

That fat-necrosis occurring in separate foci is due to the escape of the pancreatic juice in the neighboring tissues and to a fat-splitting ferment which it contains, is strongly suggested both clinically and experimentally. Clinically, it has been observed that the necrosis occurs in its greatest intensity near the gland; further, that it occurs in connection with lesions which permit the escape of the secretion. Experimentally, Langerhans produced necrosis of the subcutaneous fat by injecting an emulsion of pancreatic tissue. By placing a ligature about the pancreas, one may produce fat-necrosis at a point distal to the obstruction; by cutting the gland and allowing its secretion to escape, one may produce foci of fat-necrosis in the immediate neighborhood; and Opie, by transplanting the duodenal end of the pancreas, with its severed ducts, into the subcutaneous tissue of animals, produced extensive necrosis of the subcutaneous fat. Further, Flexner has demonstrated the existence of a fat-splitting ferment in the necrotic areas so produced.

The fact that bile forms a favorable medium for the action of pancreatic ferments (particularly the fat-splitting ones), greatly increasing their activity, probably explains the frequent association of fat-necrosis with hemorrhagic pancreatitis, due to the entrance of bile into the pancreatic ducts. (Opie.)

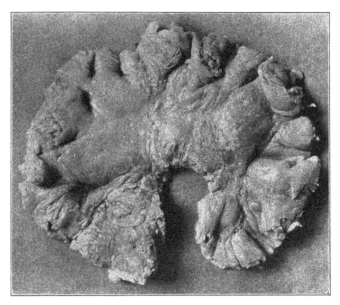

Fig. 63.—Fat Necrosis; Case of Acute Hemorrhagic Pancreatitis. (From the Museum of the New York University and Bellevue Hospital Medical College.)

The origin of fat-necrosis is, however, still a subject of controversy. There is no universal agreement in regard to the process being primary or secondary in character, and neither has the mode of distribution of the pancreatic juice or its effect upon the cells been definitely settled. Truhart, representing the fermentative theory, holds that the necrosis is produced through the excreted juice coming directly in contact with the fat. Lesions of the glandular parenchyma are very rarely responsible. In the great majority of cases, the cells themselves are diseased and their resistance is diminished, so that the juice is no longer poured into the excretory ducts, but escapes in all directions. This behavior explains the predominant involvement of the fat-tissue of the pancreas itself as compared with more distant areas. Bacterial infection is also claimed to be the cause of fat-necrosis of the pancreas; and Coste calls attention to the fact that the bacterial and fermentative theories may be reconciled by referring to microbic invasion the changes of the cells which give rise to the fermentative decomposition of fat.

Whatever the causation the diagnostic value is great. When the abdomen is opened, the characteristic opaque, yellowish areas call attention at once to the pancreas. Opie points out the fact that the lesion may be mistaken for caseous miliary tubercles or carcinomatous nodules that have undergone necrosis, but he states that the absence of elevation or other evidence of newly formed tissue shows that the necrosis is confined to the fat.

Hemorrhage.—All the other symptoms of pancreatic disease may be obscured by hemorrhage, which is sometimes fulminating in character, terminating in sudden collapse and death. This spontaneous bleeding into the substance of the gland may occur without later infection, constituting what is known as "apoplectic pancreas." It also occurs in acute hemorrhagic pancreatitis, which has already been considered on a previous page. According to Opie, increased knowledge of the pathology has led to a decrease in the number of reported cases of apoplexy of the pancreas.

Lesions of the pancreas are associated with a tendency to general hemorrhage, more particularly in the abdominal region. This pancreatic hæmophilia has been referred to the excretion of lime salts in the urine, as a result of which the blood is impoverished and the power of coagulation diminished.

III. CYSTS OF THE PANCREAS.

Cysts of the pancreas are divisible into true cysts and pseudo-cysts or cystoids.

(A) *True Cysts.*—True pancreatic cysts are sac-like swellings which have fluid or semifluid contents and which originate in the duct or in the substance of the organ. They may be either congenital or acquired. (A pure cystoma, probably derived from an accessory pancreas, has been recently reported by Hippel.) The following varieties may be described:—

(1) A few instances of congenital cystic pancreas have been recorded as pathological curiosities. The pancreas alone may contain cysts, or the same condition may prevail in another organ—for example, the kidney. The disease is not incompatible with life, the determining factor being the amount of functionating pancreatic tissue that remains.

(2) Retention cysts of the pancreas are the result of distention of the entire duct or of many of the finer ducts, or they may be due to obliteration of the main outlet; they may attain considerable dimensions. (Fig. 64.) The contents are usually semi-consistent and are composed of mucus and more or less altered blood. Gritty particles and fragments of stones are sometimes felt.

(3) Hemorrhagic Cysts. The pathology of this type of cyst is imperfectly understood. A distinction is made, by Hagenbach, between a hæmatoma, in which a pre-existing cyst becomes filled with blood, and an apoplectic cyst, due

to bloody extravasation into the softened and disintegrating parenchyma. Both the acute and the chronic forms of pancreatitis are known to give rise to hemorrhages into the substance of the organ, and such hemorrhages may give rise to cysts.

(4) Hydatid Cysts. This variety of cyst is assumed to be extremely rare, and in most cases the lesion has been discovered only at autopsy. Symptoms

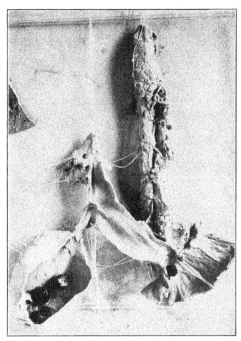

FIG. 64.—Specimen Showing Certain Lesions found Post Mortem in a Case of Cholelithiasis—viz., a stone in the common duct (which is dilated) and a d lated pancreatic duct. (From the Museum of the New York University and Bellevue Hospital Medical College.)

are not necessarily present in hydatid disease, unless a large portion of the gland is involved. Recovery is the rule after operative removal.

(5) Proliferation Cysts. Both benign and malignant cystic tumors of the pancreas have been reported. The distinction seems to be not only difficult, but largely arbitrary, and a study of the reported cases suggests that the so-called simple proliferation cyst represents in reality the transition to a cystomatous carcinoma. The interior of a proliferation cyst is often filled with polypoid masses, which always indicate malignancy.

(B) *Pseudo-cysts or Cystoids.*—A tumor with fluid contents, in the immediate vicinity of the pancreas, but not originating within this organ (peri-pancreatic cyst), is distinguished by the pathologist as a pseudo-cyst. A positive differentiation between genuine cysts and cystoids during life is always difficult and sometimes impossible, because a true pancreatic cyst may be very closely simulated by the entrance of secretion through a pancreatic injury which has occurred

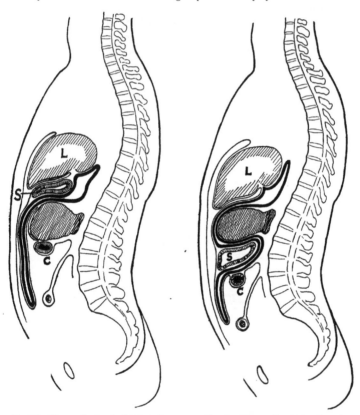

Fig. 65.—Diagram showing the Relations of a Cyst of the Pancreas to Various Neighboring Organs. The cyst is represented as projecting forward between the stomach (S) and the Colon (C). (After Oser, in Osler's "System of Medicine.")

Fig. 66.—Diagram in which a Cyst of the Pancreas is Represented as Projecting Forward between the Liver (L) and the Stomach (S). (After Oser.)

in connection with an injury inflicted upon the parts in the immediate neighborhood of the pancreas. Moynihan expresses himself as strongly inclined to believe that, in many cases of so-called pancreatic cyst, especially those of traumatic origin, the lesion is in reality located in the immediate vicinity of the pancreas, or represents a pseudo-cystic effusion into the lesser cavity of the peritoneum, or a localized extravasation of blood, etc. Hagen subdivides cystoids of the pancreas into endopancreatic and peripancreatic cysts, according to the fact whether a bloody extravasate has been poured into the pancreas itself or merely into the neighboring tissues. The extravasation, in the first of

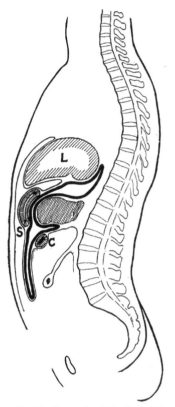
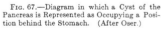
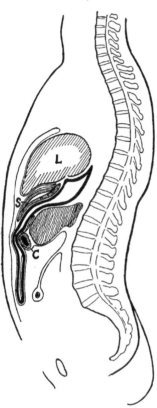

Fig. 67.—Diagram in which a Cyst of the Pancreas is Represented as Occupying a Position behind the Stomach. (After Oser.)

Fig. 68.—Diagram showing the Location of a Cyst of the Pancreas behind the Colon. (After Oser.)

these varieties, undergoes a secondary cystic transformation, through auto-digestion by the pancreatic juice; while the reactive inflammation in the vicinity leads to the formation of a capsule. Chronic pancreatitis may give rise to a similar series of changes through auto-digestion of retained secretion, softening of the parenchyma of the gland, and coalescence of individual lobules into cysts.

ETIOLOGY.—About thirty per cent of all cysts are referable to traumatism. Cysts may develop upon the soil of chronic pancreatitis. The distribution of pancreatic cysts among the sexes is about equal, and they have been observed at all ages between thirteen months and seventy-six years.

PATHOLOGICAL ANATOMY.—No part of the gland is exempt, but the head is less often affected than the body, the chances for complete retention being relatively slight near the outlet of the large excretory ducts. The usual starting point of pancreatic cysts is in the tail (seventy-one per cent of the cases, according to Lazarus). These cysts are usually more or less movable, following the normal slight movements of the pancreatic tail. As the weight of the cyst increases, its connections with its starting point or with the surroundings may become drawn out into a long strand or pedicle.

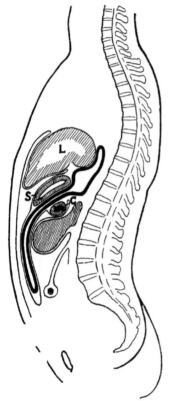

Pancreatic cysts are elastic, somewhat tense swellings, usually smooth and globular, and lined on the inside with cylindrical epithelium. Single and multiple, unilocular and multilocular cysts, divided into compartments by trabeculæ or rudimentary septa, have been reported. Occasionally a cyst is found to contain a set of smaller ones in the cyst walls. Blood in variable amounts is practically always present.

The anatomical foundation of retention cysts is essentially the result of chronic interstitial pancreatitis. The proliferation and subsequent contraction of the connective tissue lead to obstruction of the excretory ducts and retention of the secretion; the gland cells undergo fatty degeneration; the parenchyma is softened as the result of auto-digestion effected by the pancreatic juice; individual globules coalesce and form small cystic cavities, which in their turn become converted into larger cysts through

FIG. 69.—Diagram in which a Cyst of the Pancreas is Represented as Distending the Lower Layer of the Mesocolon and Presenting itself below the Transverse Colon. (After Oser.)

the breaking down of the septa. Further enlargement may occur as the result of accidental hemorrhage, through traumatism or erosion.

SYMPTOMS.—Cystic disease of the pancreas, in its early stages, before a tumor has developed, is unattended by definite symptoms. There is a history of epigastric pain and distress, vomiting, diarrhœa, and sometimes salivation.

Some cases are associated with marked weakness and emaciation. Pressure of a cystic growth on the bile-duct will naturally give rise to jaundice.

After the tumor has reached a sufficient size to be demonstrable, and especially when it presses upon the mesenteric plexus or the solar plexus of nerves, very severe pain is almost invariably complained of (cœliac neuralgia). According to the seat of the tumor, these pains are localized in the gastric region or in the right or left hypochondriac region. They are not often continuous and usually occur in attacks, sometimes under the picture of gastric crises. Further disturbances may arise through the relations of the cyst with neighboring organs, such as the stomach, the duodenum, the biliary passages, and the portal vein.

DIAGNOSIS.—Provided the possibility of a pancreatic cyst is kept in mind, its recognition does not meet with insuperable difficulties. A history of traumatism is suggestive; several years may have elapsed between the appearance of the cyst and the infliction of the injury. Cysts are characterized by their irregular, periodical increase in size, through hemorrhages due to the rupture or erosion of a blood-vessel. In certain cases, the diagnosis is facilitated by the periodical subsidence of the tumor, as the result of emptying of the cyst by way of the excretory ducts or through a fistula connecting with the bowel.

The behavior of the pancreatic secretion is not a reliable guide for the diagnosis, because in a large number of the cases a very small segment of the organ is involved, the larger part of the pancreas continuing to functionate. Even in cases of cystic disease secondary to interstitial pancreatitis, the functional diagnosis may afford no clue.

A very important aid in diagnosis is afforded by the retroperitoneal situation of the tumor. True intrapancreatic cysts lie behind the posterior layer of peritoneum which forms the lesser sac, and remain covered with this layer of the serous membrane, no matter in what direction they may extend. The relations of the cyst to the distended stomach contribute useful information. The stomach lies always in front of the tumor, but becomes gradually displaced as the cyst increases in size. In most cases, it is pushed upward and to the right, and the cyst emerges from under the greater curvature, pushing the transverse colon downward. The degree of pressure and displacement of the parts is determined by the size of the cyst; in extreme cases, the stomach is wedged under the liver, while the transverse colon may be pushed down as low as the symphysis pubis. The stomach may be pushed downward and the liver driven upward to the right, as the result of the cyst extending in a forward direction above the upper margin of the stomach. In other cases, the stomach, together with the transverse colon, may be pushed upward, as the result of a pancreatic cyst (originating at the inferior aspect of the gland) displacing downward the inferior layer of the transverse mesocolon. Cysts developing at the lower limit of the lesser peritoneal sac may also advance between the layers of the transverse mesocolon, with the result that the transverse colon passes directly across the front of the cyst. (See accompanying diagrams, Figs. 65–69.)

Differential Diagnosis.—Tumors of the gall-bladder and liver, notably echinococcus cysts, may give rise to confusion, but can generally be excluded by a careful examination.   Mesenteric cysts develop below the umbilicus, as a rule, and are more freely movable than those of the pancreas.   Renal or suprarenal tumors are not always easily distinguished from pancreatic cysts that extend into the hypochondrium, and Hagen points out that the demonstration of a kidney which has been crowded down by the cyst is sometimes helpful.   The differentiation of cysts of the pancreas from retro-peritoneal lymphatic cysts, on the basis of the clinical picture, is prac-tically impossible, whereas encapsulated retroperitoneal exudates should be recognized with the assistance of a detailed history.   Aneurysm of the abdominal aorta is identified by examination of the patient in the knee-chest position and by the pulsatory expansion on all sides, a phenomenon which is absent in cysts.

TREATMENT.—The treatment of pancreatic cysts is exclusively surgical, and may consist in:—

(a) Simple incision of the cyst after suturing it to the parietal peritoneum, with evacuation and drainage (Gussenbauer's method).   The object is to induce obliteration of the cavity through gradual shrinkage and agglutination of the cyst walls.   This method is the most generally applicable, but it involves the risk of a permanent fistula.

(b) Extirpation, partial or complete.

Technique of the Operation.—The abdomen is opened slightly to one side of the median line, above the umbilicus, and the cyst is exposed by dividing its peritoneal coverings.   In most cases it is reached and exposed by tearing through the great omentum, just below the stomach.   The abdominal cavity is protected by placing pads or tapes around the projecting part of the cyst.   The greater part of the cyst contents is withdrawn, a large aspirating needle being used for the purpose.   The puncture orifice in the cyst wall is then enlarged, and the cavity is temporarily packed with gauze, to prevent leakage of the contents. The edges of the opening are stitched to the parietal peritoneum.   Very large cysts may require trimming or excision of a part of the redundant walls.   A large drainage tube is introduced, and this, after two or three days, may be replaced by a Colt's suprapubic drainage apparatus.   (Moynihan.)

Formerly this operation was often done in two stages, and the cyst was left unopened until a few days after its wall had been stitched to the peritoneum. Some latitude is left the operator, in order that he may adapt the operation to the individual features of a given case.   Drainage has been secured through a stab wound in the loin (Pearce Gould); and the late Dr. Peters, of Toronto, in a case of hydatid cyst of the tail of the pancreas, operated entirely through a lumbar incision.

Total extirpation of the tumor is naturally the most certain and rapid, but at the same time a very serious, operation.   There are certain favorable cases of pancreatic cyst, with a small non-vascular pedicle, which are very easily excised. In the majority of the cases, however, extirpation meets with insuperable difficul-ties, in the shape of solid adhesions, profuse hemorrhage, and extreme liability to injure the pancreas.   This method must therefore be restricted—aside from the favorable cases above-mentioned—to those cysts which are suspected of malignancy.

Recamier's method, or aspiration of the cystic contents, is mentioned as of historical interest. The procedure has been abandoned as incompatible with the trend of modern surgery.

RESULTS OF TREATMENT.—According to Goebell's compilation, reported before the Surgical Congress of 1907, recovery followed in 183 of 190 cases of pancreatic cyst that were treated by incision and suture; whereas the mortality of total extirpation amounted to 10.7 per cent and that of incomplete extirpation to 55.5 per cent. The permanent results of incision are not so favorable, on account of the danger of an obstinate fistula, which may lead to death by a variety of complications.

Fistula.—After evacuation and drainage of a cyst, a fistula may persist for months, continuing to discharge pancreatic juice. In such cases, every possible effort should be made to dry up the secretion from the fistula, and Hagen recommends the antidiabetic dietetic treatment, inaugurated by Wohlgemuth. After all other measures have failed, nothing remains but to resort to a secondary extirpation or to divert the fistula into the stomach, as was successfully done by Doyen. Recurrence of the cyst has been noted after closure of a fistula.

IV. WOUNDS OF THE PANCREAS.

Isolated gunshot or stab wounds of the pancreas are extremely rare, owing to the deep and sheltered position of the gland in the abdominal cavity and also to the fact that it is partly protected by the costal arch. These cases are usually complicated by lesions of other organs, especially the stomach and liver. The most common cause of an injury to the pancreas, next to gunshot and stab wounds, is a violent blow upon the epigastrium—for example, by the kick of a horse. Severe subcutaneous injuries, through indirect violence, are relatively very rare, and may be caused by compression of the organ against the vertebral column, as happens in railroad or automobile accidents.

The symptoms are usually masked by the simultaneous lesion of some other important organ, such as the stomach, liver, or spleen. At the end of a few hours, the symptoms of peritonitis make their appearance, with tympanites, vomiting, and quickened pulse. Partial rupture and contusion of the pancreas give rise to the formation of a large epigastric hæmatoma. The pancreatic secretion in some cases leaks through a tear in the peritoneum into the lesser peritoneal cavity, where it may accumulate after the foramen of Winslow has been closed by an adhesive peritonitis (pseudo-cyst).

The diagnosis of pancreatic injury rests largely on circumstantial evidence, as afforded by a history of severe contusion of the entire trunk in a railroad or other accident.

Wounds of the pancreas, while necessarily grave, are not always fatal; the chief dangers are hemorrhage, infection, and fat-necrosis. There have been recorded instances of recovery even after complete transverse rupture of the organ. (Garré.) Untreated lesions are a menace to life, and it is therefore imperative that the entire gland be carefully inspected in all surgical interventions for traumatism in this region. Small, apparently insignificant wounds of the pancreas may give rise to inflammation several months after the infliction of the injury.

As regards the treatment it may be said that, in favorable cases of punctured or incised wounds, the torn edges of the pancreas can be brought accurately together, trimmed and repaired by strong catgut sutures passing through the capsule and the parenchyma, care being taken to avoid the duct of Wirsung. The peritoneum over the wound is then united by fine continuous or interrupted catgut sutures. In case of severe contusions of the organ, the hemorrhage must be thoroughly controlled, and provision for drainage made. The greatest danger for the patient is referable to fat-necrosis. The main feature of the treatment must therefore be open-wound treatment, with tamponing of the abdominal cavity and drainage of the secretion. The pancreas must be sutured carefully, so as to guard against necrotic changes, due to the operative traumatism.

V. TUMORS OF THE PANCREAS.

Carcinoma.—The pancreas is more often the seat of carcinoma than of any other neoplasm. Cancer of the pancreas (Fig. 70), although most common between the ages of forty and seventy, is not limited to maturity and old age, but may occur in youthful individuals and even in children. Among 121 cases reported by Kellermann, 75 were men and 46, women. Primary cancer of the pancreas is relatively rare, as compared to secondary invasion of the gland by a gastric cancer. The head of the pancreas is the part usually affected.

The following symptoms may be mentioned:—(1) Pain, either continuous or periodical, in the form of a severe cardialgia, which has been attributed to pressure or traction upon the cœliac ganglion; attacks of colic, usually the result of congestion through pressure upon the excretory duct; biliary colics, through pressure upon the ductus choledochus, in cancer of the pancreatic head; (2) icterus, in general slowly progressive, the result of pressure of the growing tumor upon the ductus choledochus, or of extension of the growth to the gall-bladder; (3) early onset of insidious cachexia, in strong contrast to the continued ingestion and assimilation of food, this function not being impaired until the end; (4) changes in the urine, which may be diminished or increased in quantity. The demonstration of sugar and fat is more important than that of albumin, which is sometimes present.

The symptoms depend to a great extent upon the direction in which the growth advances. Its extension upward and forward, involving the common duct and the pylorus, gives rise to pyloric obstruction. Ascites is character-istic of an extension toward the vena cava and the portal vein. When the growth extends to the right, it involves the common bile-duct and the pancre-atic duct, giving rise to chronic jaundice and distention of the gall-bladder, a sign which, since the days of Courvoisier, has been considered as virtually pathognomonic of cancer of the pancreatic head.

Palpation of the tumor is rendered difficult at first by the local tenderness, and later by the presence of ascites. Cancers of the pancreas have been described as smooth or irregular, often nodular or spherical. They lie in front of the spinal column, more on the right and toward the pylorus, or toward the cardiac orifice of the stomach, according as the growth is located in the head or the tail.

The differential diagnosis between cancer of the pancreas and chronic pancreatitis is very important, on account of the treatment to be adopted; the former disease being inoperable, or nearly so, whereas the latter is amenable to surgical interference.

Sarcoma of the Pancreas.—Sarcoma of the pancreas is much less common than carcinoma, and, like the latter, more often secondary than primary. In

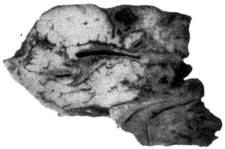

Fig. 70.—Primary Cancer of the Pancreas in a Woman Seventy Years of Age. The head of the organ is shown in cross section; the duct, which is of natural size, is cut obliquely. (From the Russell Sage Institute of Pathology.)

a few cases, secondary melanotic sarcomata have been successfully removed by operation. Martens recently operated upon a woman, thirty-four years of age, with cystic spindle-cell sarcoma of the pancreas; the patient lived in good health for a year after the operation.

Adenoma and Fibro-adenoma.—These forms of tumors are rare pancreatic neoplasms, sometimes accessible to surgical intervention.

A few cases of endothelioma have been reported, and syphiloma and tuberculoma are known to occur.

THE TREATMENT OF TUMORS OF THE PANCREAS.—Total extirpation of the pancreas for cancer has been successfully performed, the patient surviving the operation for five months (Francke's case); but this is a unique experience. The operation is possible only in a case in which the tumor is restricted to the pancreas. The technical difficulties of the operation are enormous on account of the deep position of the organ and the vicinity of many large blood-vessels, ligation of which is apt to induce necrosis of the parts supplied by them.

Among the palliative procedures the following may be mentioned: the formation of an anastomosis between the gall-bladder, the pancreatic duct, or the ductus choledochus, and the bowel, in order to divert the flow of the bile; and the making of a gastro-entero-anastomosis, or an entero-entero-anastomosis, for the control of ileus.

VI. PANCREOPTOSIS.   (MOVABLE PANCREAS.)

The pancreas is not exempt from displacements, and may fall forward or downward. In the latter case, it may be felt by palpation below the stomach. It has been found among the contents of a diaphragmatic hernia. Very exceptionally, the organ or an aberrant pancreas may be discovered in the sac of an umbilical hernia.

VII. PANCREATIC CALCULUS.   (PANCREATICO-LITHIASIS.)

The formation of a stone in the pancreas—pancreatico-lithiasis—is rare. It may follow upon cholelithiasis. Among two thousand autopsies in the Koenigsberg Medical Clinic, Rindfleisch found only three cases. In one instance, a large pancreatic calculus had compressed the ductus choledochus, and led to secondary infection of the biliary passages, stone-formation in the gall-bladder and ulceration of its walls, followed by peritonitis and death. Another case showed stone-formation in the pancreas in connection with chronic pancreatitis and atrophic changes of the glandular parenchyma. Jacobsthal refers to a case of ulcerative phthisis, with pancreatic calculi, which had caused dilatation of the duct and atrophy of the organ.

Pancreatico-lithiasis cannot occur without preliminary changes in the gland, because normal pancreatic juice dissolves the lime salts and the cholesterin, the forerunners of calculus. These are precipitated only as the result of epithelial disintegration and decomposition of the pancreatic juice. The predisposing factors consist in bacterial infection, by way of the bowel, and mechanico-anatomical obstructions, leading first to stagnation and then to decomposition of the pancreatic secretion.

The most important symptoms are pancreatic colics, swelling of the organ, and the passage of pancreatic calculi in the stools.

The treatment of an attack consists in the administration of narcotics and the application of warmth. Medicinal treatment aims at stimulating the secretion of the pancreas, so that the force of the current shall be sufficiently increased to overcome the resistance at the papilla.

Stones have been removed from the pancreas in the course of various operations. McBurney opened the duodenum, enlarged the papilla, and thus reached the duct of Wirsung. Pancreatomy, followed by exposure of the excretory duct, is recommended by Sonnenburg for calculi situated higher up in the organ.

BIBLIOGRAPHY.

Balser: Ueber Fettnekrose, in Virchow's Archiv, Vol. 90, 1882.—Cammidge:
(I) The pathology and surgery of certain diseases of the pancreas, in The Lancet,
March 19th, 1904. (II) An improved method of performing the pancreatic
reaction in the urine, in Brit. Med. Jour., May 19th, 1906. (III) The so-called
pancreatic reaction in the urine, in The Edinburgh Med. Jour., Vol. 21, 1907.—
Chiari: Die Sogenannte Fettnekrose, in Prager med. Wchschrft., No. 13, 1883.—
Dreesmann: Die Diagnose und Behandlung der Pankreatitis, in Münchener
med. Wchschr., No. 14, 1909.—Garre: Totaler Querriss des Pankreas durch
Naht geheilt, in Bruns' Beiträge z. klin. Chir., Vol. 46, 1905.—Hagen: (I)
Zur Bewertung der Cammidge-Reaktion, in Bruns' Beitr. z. klin. Chir., Vol.
61, 1908–9. (II) Ueber Pankreaserkrankungen, in Würzburger Abhandlungen,
IX., H. 12, 1909.—Helly: Zur Pankreasentwickelung der Säugetiere, in Archiv
f. mikroskop. Anatomie, Vol. 57, 1901.—Hess: (I) Experimentelle Beiträge zur
Aetiologie der Pankreas und Fettgewebsnekrose, in Münch. med. Wchschrft.,
No. 44, 1903. (II) Pankrc snekrose und chronische Pankreatitis, in Mittlg.
a. d. Grenzgeb. d. Med. u. Chir., 1908–9.—Hippel: Zur Diagnose der Pankreascysten, in Inaugural Dissertation, Greifswald, 1908.—Jacobsthal: Pan-
kreassteine, Münchener med. Wchschrft., No. 17, 1908.—Imfeld: Akute hæmor-
rhagische Pankreatitis durch Frühoperation geheilt, in Dtsch. Zeitschrft. f. Chir.,
Vol. 104, H. 1–2, 1910.—Klieneberger: Diagnostik der Pankreaserkrankungen,
in Medizin. Klinik, No. 3, 1910.—Langerhans: Fettgewebsnekrose, in Fest-
schrift für Virchow, 1891.—Leriche et Arnauld: Sur la pancréatite aiguë hémor-
rhagique, in Revue de Gynécol. et de Chirurg. abdom., Sept., Oct., 1909.—
Lazarus: Beiträge zur Pathologie und Therapie der Pankreaserkrankungen,
in Lehrbuch f. klin. Med., Nos. 51–52, 1904.—Loewi: Ueber eine neue Funk-
tion des Pankreas und ihre Beziehung zum Diabetes mellitus, in Archiv f. exper.
Pathol., Vol. 59, 1908.—Martens: Zur Chirurgie der Pankreascysten, in Dtsch.
Zeitschrft. f. Chir., Vol. 100, 1909.—Mayo: The surgical treatment of pancreatitis, in Surg., Gyn., and Obs., Vol. VII., No. 6, Dec., 1908.—Mayo
Robson and Moynihan: Diseases of the pancreas and their surgical treatment,
—a Monograph, Phila. and London, 1902.—Mayo Robson and Cammidge:
The pancreas, its surgery and pathology,—a Monograph, Phila. and London,
1907.—Mayo Robson: The clinical and pathological importance of chronic
pancreatitis, in Edinburgh Med. Jour., Dec., 1905.—Opie: (I) The anatomy of
the pancreas, in Am. Medicine, June 20th, 1903. (II) Lesions peculiar to the
pancreas, in Med. News, May 21st, 1904.—Opie and Meakins: Data concerning
the etiology and pathology of hemorrhagic necrosis of the pancreas, in Jour.
Exper. Medicine, Vol. XI., 1909.—Ott: Ueber die ringförmige Umschnürung des
Duodenum durch Pankreasgewebe,—an Inaugural Dissertation, Münich, 1909.—
Peters (Geo. A.): Hydatid cyst of the tail of the pancreas, in Canadian Pract.
and Rev., Feb., 1901.—Pearce: Cancer of the pancreas and glycosuria, in Am.
Jour. Med. Sciences, Sept., 1904.—Rindfleisch: Steinbildung im Pankreas, in
Mittlg. a. d. Grenzgeb. d. Med. u. Chir., Vol. 18, 1908–9.—Sahli: Ueber die

diagnostische und therapeutische Verwertbarkeit der Glutoidkapseln, in Dtsch. Archiv f. klin. Med., Vol. 61, 1898.—Schirmer: Beitrag zur Geschichte und Anatomie des Pankreas,—an Inaugural Dissertation, Basel, 1893.—Schumm und Hegler: Ueber die Brauchbarkeit der sogenannten Pankreasreaktion nach Cammidge, in Mittlg. a. d. Hamburgischen Staatskranken-Anstalten, Vol. X., H. 9. 1910.—Truhart: Ueber die akuten Erkrankungsformen der Bauchspeicheldrüse, in Petersburger med. Wchschrft., No. 7, 1909.—Villar: Chirurgie du pancréas,— a Monograph, Paris, 1906.—Vautrin: Traitement de la pancréatite chronique, in Revue de Chirurgie, No. 5, 1908.—Wohlgemuth: Untersuchungen ueber das Pankreas des Menschen, in Berliner klin. Wchschrft., No. 2, 1907.—Welko: Erkennung und Behandlung der Erkrankungen des Pankreas, in Prager medizin. Wchschrft., No. 11, 1909.

SURGERY OF THE LIVER, GALL-BLADDER, AND BILIARY PASSAGES.

By GEORGE DAVID STEWART, M.D., New York City.

Anatomy of the Liver and Bile-Ducts.—*The Liver.*—The liver belongs to the digestive system, both from the developmental and from the functional points of view. It is the largest gland in the body, weighing from forty-eight to fifty ounces in the male, not quite so much in the female. More important is its relative weight in the sexes and at different periods of life. Thus, in the adult male it is one-fortieth of the body weight, in the female one-thirty-sixth, and in children about one-twentieth.

The liver is situated in the upper part of the abdominal cavity, the greater part of its mass occupying the right hypochondriac region; the left lobe, however, extends across the epigastric region to or near the mammary line, sometimes projecting into the left hypochondriac region.

The outline of the liver (Fig. 71) varies with the variations in size and position of the organ, but is mapped out on the surface with sufficient accuracy in the following manner:—Select three points—one, half an inch below the tip of the tenth rib; a second, half an inch below the right nipple; and a third, one inch below the left nipple. These points are joined by lines slightly convex outward; the lower line, representing the corresponding border of the liver, is the most important from a practical point of view.

When the liver is normal in size and location, its inferior border in the right hypochondriac region lies under cover of the margin of the thorax and cannot be felt except in thin people and during deep inspiration. Where the liver is displaced downward, either by relaxation of its supports or by enlargement of its bulk, this border may be palpated even in stout people with thick abdominal parietes. In the epigastric region the inferior border may be felt crossing from the ninth costal cartilage on the right to the eighth on the left, and a considerable area of the parietal surface may be explored above this.

Variations in size, position, and shape are frequent. They may be physiological or pathological, depending on the conditions of the surrounding organs. Tight lacing occasionally forces the liver up, causing it to extend toward the left side of the abdomen; it constricts the liver, forcing the upper part more tightly into the dome of the diaphragm and pressing the lower into the abdominal cavity. In addition, the liver ascends and descends with every respiration, its range of motion being greater than that of the corresponding kidney,—a fact which helps to differentiate tumors of the liver, gall-bladder, etc., from kidney displacement. The liver also descends slightly when the upright posture is assumed.

The relations of the pleura to the liver are important surgically. On the right side the pleura is reflected from the chest wall to the diaphragm along a line extending from the back of the ensiform cartilage downward and outward along the ascending part of the seventh costal cartilage. In the nipple line this reflection is at the level of the eighth costo-chondral articulation; in the mid-axillary line it is beneath the tenth intercostal space; while

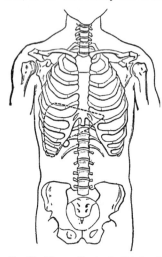

FIG. 71.—Diagram Showing the Relation of the Gall-Bladder and Liver to the Surface of the Abdomen. (From Mayo-Robson, on "The Surgery of the Gall-Bladder.") See also Fig. 81.

near the spine it is at the level of the eleventh rib, or slightly below. The lowest point of the pleural reflection is, therefore, in the mid-axillary line, where it corresponds to the tenth rib or the tenth intercostal space, and this level is normally about two inches from the lower border of the liver. (The only point where the pleural reflection may be below the level of the lower border of the thoracic wall, is at the spinal end of the twelfth rib; the surgical importance of this fact, however, relates rather to the kidney than to the liver.)

When the liver is enlarged upward it narrows the costo-phrenic sinus and brings the parietal in contact with the diaphragmatic pleura, this contact reaching higher and higher according as the enlargement increases. If, at the same time, the pleura is inflamed, the two layers may become adherent; and frequently, particularly in liver abscess, it is possible to approach and drain the abscess through the pleura without opening the pleural cavity.

The peritoneum covers the liver entirely, except that portion of the posterior surface of the right lobe which lies between the layers of the coronary ligament. Double folds of the peritoneum, like mesenteries, unite the liver to the diaphragm and anterior abdominal wall. Of these, the falciform ligament is of the greatest importance from a surgical point of view. It attaches the liver to the diaphragm and anterior abdominal wall as low down as the umbilicus, and encloses in its lower border a fibrous cord, the ligamentum teres, which represents the obliterated umbilical vein. The attachment of this ligament to the anterior abdominal wall does not correspond with the median line of the body, except for a short distance, an inch or two above the umbilicus. Above this level it is placed one inch or more to the right of the median line, a fact which should not be forgotten. Incisions in this region should be so placed as to avoid this ligament, because to open on the wrong side of it sometimes hampers the operation, and to open between the layers, particularly in those cases in which there is portal obstruction and dilatation of the veins, is often followed by annoying bleeding, difficult of control.

The fixation of the liver is effected by (a) the attachment of the hepatic veins to the inferior vena cava; (b) the coronary ligaments and the cellulo-vascular tissue between its layers; (c) the fibrous tissue near the vena cava and on the non-peritoneal surface of the right lobe; (d) the muscular walls of the abdomen; and (e) the lateral and suspensory ligaments.   (Piersol.)

The Bile Passages and Excretory Ducts of the Liver.—The excretory ducts of the liver may be divided into intrahepatic and extrahepatic. The intrahepatic ducts begin in the liver as minute channels located between the cells; apposing

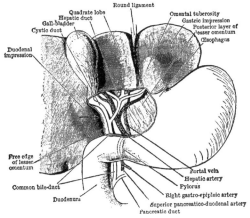

Fig. 72.—Structures Between the Layers of the Lesser Omentum. (From Cunningham's Anatomy.) The liver has been raised up, and the anterior layer of the omentum removed.   (Semi-diagrammatic.)

grooves on the latter forming at first their sole boundaries. These channels, known as bile canaliculi, unite outside the lobules to form larger ducts, the interlobular, and these, by further union, increase in size and are reduced in number until there emerge from the liver substance, at the bottom of the portal fissure, usually only two ducts—the right and the left.

The Extrahepatic Ducts (Fig. 72).—The extrahepatic ducts are the right and left bile-ducts, the hepatic duct proper, and the common duct; with these must be considered a diverticulum of the bile passages, the gall-bladder, together with its duct. The right bile-duct emerges from the liver at the bottom of the portal fissure, or is formed, soon after its emergence, by the union of several ducts. It drains the right lobe and is, therefore, the larger of the two ducts; and it runs downward, taking a more direct course than the left. The left bile-duct, formed just before or promptly after emerging from the liver, drains the left lobe, takes a more or less oblique course, and unites with the right at an angle of varying degree. Both right and left bile-ducts run their course in the portal fissure. Because of its greater diameter and more direct course the right duct is more liable to contain calculi than the left.

The hepatic duct (Fig. 73) is formed, in the right extremity of the transverse fissure, by the union of the right and left bile-ducts; occasionally by the junction of several terminal biliary ducts. It runs downward and slightly to the left in the right edge of the gastro-hepatic omentum. Above, near its origin, it lies in front of the right branch of the hepatic artery and the portal vein; below, it is in front and to the right of the portal vein; at the hilum of the liver, it is in intimate relation with the lymphatic and nerve supplies. Its length varies, within normal limits, from three-quarters of an inch to an inch and a half (25–31 mm.). Its diameter averages one-quarter of an inch (4–6 mm.), but the duct may become dilated, by the presence of an obstruction, sufficiently to admit the finger. Outside the portal fissure it is joined by the cystic duct, the union forming the common duct.

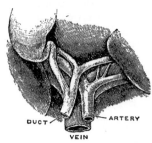

DUCT   ARTERY

VEIN

Fig. 73.—The Relations of the Bile-Ducts, Portal Vein, and Hepatic Artery at the Porta Hepatica. (From Bland Sutton.)

The apparently contradictory statements made by different authors— *e.g.*, by one, that the whole course of this duct lies in the portal fissure, by another, that it lies in the right edge of the gastro-hepatic omentum—are due to the following facts: (1) The length of the duct varies normally within relatively wide limits; (2) the duct may be formed at a high or at a low level; (3) its junction with the cystic duct takes place at varying levels. Besides, one observer sees it in the dead house, relaxed and stretched; another, in the dissecting-room, hardened *in situ;* still another, at the operating table, the liver pulled up and rotated, the duodenum and pylorus retracted downward. Further, the point from which the gastro-hepatic omentum leaves the liver, and the direction of its right edge can not be stated with mathematical precision.

The gall-bladder (Fig. 74), with its duct, the cystic, may be regarded as a diverticulum from the bile passages proper. It lies obliquely on the inferior or visceral surface of the liver, its direction being from before upward, backward, and to the left. It is divided into fundus, body, and neck, the latter merging, without definite external line of demarcation, into the cystic duct. The fundus, the anterior inferior extremity, usually reaches the inferior border of the liver, the latter being notched to receive it, and comes in contact with the anterior abdominal wall, but cannot be felt unless it is enlarged. The body occupies an excavation in the liver substance called "the fossa of the gall-bladder." As it approaches the portal fissure, it merges into the neck. The neck bends abruptly to the left, and where it merges into the cystic duct there is a second bend in the opposite direction. These curves are made permanent by the disposition of the peritoneal coat and surrounding connective tissue. Internally, they are marked by two folds of mucous membrane, crescentic in outline, which act—in the case of stones, at least—as partial valves. One of these valves divides the neck from the cystic duct. The space between—often referred to as the pelvis of the gall-bladder, or Hartman's pouch—is frequently the seat of a calculus which more or less effectively blocks the entrance to the cystic duct.

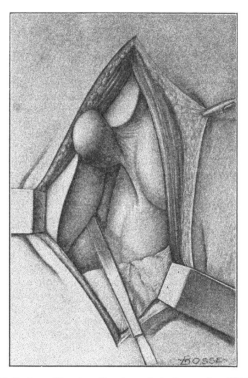

Fig. 74.—Gall-Bladder from a Dissection. There is an adhesion between the gall-bladder and the descending duodenum; the handle of the scalpel is placed between the kidney and the liver. (Original.)

The size and capacity of the gall-bladder vary. Its average length is about three inches (75 mm.); its diameter varies from one inch to an inch and a quarter (25–31 mm.); and it has a capacity of 30 to 45 c.c. (one to one and a half fluid-ounces). It distends readily, and when moderately stretched it holds 50 to 60 c.c.; under pressure, however, it may be made to hold 250 c.c., without rupture. (Mayo-Robson.) Cases have been recorded in which the gall-bladder was so distended as to be mistaken for an ovarian cyst.

The fundus of the gall-bladder is covered entirely by peritoneum, except in those cases where it is empty and retracted above the inferior border of the liver. The body, as a rule, is only partially covered; its upper portion, for a varying fraction of its circumference up to one-third, resting directly on the liver substance, to which it is bound by areolar tissue and small blood-vessels. Occasionally the covering of the body is complete, and there may even be a short peritoneal ligament that, after the manner of a mesentery, unites it to the liver tissue. The inferior, visceral, surface of the body and neck is free, as a rule, except for adhesions; occasionally, however, the right edge of the gastro-hepatic omentum is extended to the right, making a ligament of varying width, which attaches this surface to the first portion of the duodenum. (Fig. 74.)

The fundus usually lies in contact with the anterior abdominal wall, in the angle between the outer border of the rectus and the costal margin; occasionally, particularly when contracted, it does not even reach the inferior border of the liver. Distention of the gall-bladder carries the fundus downward and inward along a line extending from the ninth and tenth cartilages, on the right, to the umbilicus. Contraction and atrophy of the gall-bladder carry it up beneath the liver to the neighborhood of the portal fissure. The gall-bladder may be in contact with the first portion of the duodenum, the pylorus, or the body of the stomach, or it may be depressed downward and in contact with the transverse colon or the anterior surface of the right kidney. The variations are due to causes already mentioned, and also to the following: distention of the colon, which pushes the gall-bladder upward; enlargement of the liver; hepatoptosis and tight lacing, which carry it downward and to the left; distention of the stomach and enlargements of the left lobe of the liver, carrying it to the right.

The cystic duct (Fig. 75) begins at the neck of the gall-bladder, runs a somewhat irregular course backward and inward, and ends near the portal fissure, by joining the hepatic duct, the union forming the common duct; sometimes it joins the right bile-duct. Its length varies from an inch and a quarter to an inch and a half (31–38 mm.). Its diameter is one-half the size of the hepatic, viz., about 3 or 4 mm. On its inner aspect there are crescentic folds of mucous membrane, somewhat spirally arranged. They resemble and are a continuation of the folds already referred to in the neck of the gall-bladder, and are responsible for the convoluted appearance, externally, of both the neck and the cystic duct.

The cystic duct leaves the neck of the gall-bladder at its inner side, above its lowest point. Mayo points out that this is the case in all hollow organs having storage function, the purpose being to prevent the pressure of the contents from falling on the sphincter muscles. It is difficult to see the application of the principle here, however, since the direction of the organ is such that the pressure due to gravity, at least, is more particularly exerted on the fundus.

The common duct (Fig. 75), formed by the union of the cystic and hepatic ducts, begins near the mouth of the portal fissure and passes downward and in front of the foramen of Winslow, between the layers of the gastro-hepatic omentum, with the hepatic artery to the left and the portal vein behind and between the two.   Next, it descends behind the first part of the duodenum to the level of the upper border of the pancreas, then it runs between the pancreas and the second portion of the duodenum, and finally it perforates the wall of the second portion of the duodenum very obliquely, opening at the papilla on the posterior and internal wall, three and one-half to four inches (7 to 10 cm.) beyond

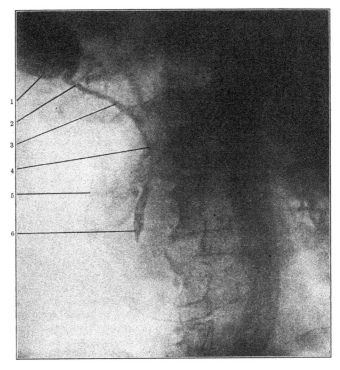

FIG. 75.—Radiograph Showing the Relations of the Cystic and Common Bile-Ducts to the Duodenum, and also the Abrupt Curve at the Neck of the Gall-Bladder.   (The radiograph was made by opening the abdomen, in a cadaver, placing a piece of flexible wire along the right border of the duodenum, and then injecting the cystic duct, the common duct, and the ampulla with an emulsion of bismuth.) (Original.)

1, Gall-Bladder ; 2, Cystic Duct ; 3, Supraduodenal Portion of the Common Duct ; 4, Retro-duodenal Portion of the Common Duct ; 5, Right Edge of Duodenum ; 6, Ampulla of Vater (common opening of the common bile-duct and pancreatic ducts).

the pylorus.   The dimensions of the entire canal are: diameter, one-quarter inch (6–7 mm.); length, three to three and one-half inches (7–9 cm.).   In average cases of common-duct obstruction, however, the finger can be introduced into an opening in the common duct, perhaps into and through the hepatic duct, sometimes even entering the right or the left bile-duct.

The common bile-duct (Fig. 76) may be divided into the following subdivisions: supraduodenal, retroduodenal, pancreatic, and parietal.

The supraduodenal division is an inch and a quarter long (25–31 mm.). It lies in the right edge of the gastro-hepatic omentum, in front and somewhat to the right of the portal vein and to the right of the hepatic artery. Neither of these vessels is near enough, however, to be harmed if reasonable care is observed. This part is the point of election for the removal of stones from the common duct. A small branch of the pancreatic-duodenal artery crosses the duct just above the duodenum, and three or four lymph nodes are in intimate contact with it.

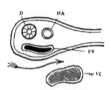

Fig. 76.—Section of the Free Border of the Lesser Omentum, Showing the Relations of the Common Bile-Duct.

HA, Hepatic artery; *D*, bile-duct; *PV*, portal vein; *VC*, vena cava. The arrow indicates the foramen of Winslow. (From Mayo-Robson, on "The Surgery of the Gall-Bladder.")

The second or retroduodenal division, about one inch (25 mm.) in length, lies behind the first portion of the duodenum, the portal vein lying behind and to the left, the vena cava directly behind.

The pancreatic or third portion, one inch (20–25 mm.) in length, lies between the head of the pancreas and the second portion of the duodenum. In some cases it occupies a groove behind the pancreas; in others it is completely surrounded by this gland. When the duct occupies a tunnel, it is more likely to be obstructed by swelling of the pancreas, and the difficulty of removing a stone by either the transduodenal or the retroduodenal route is increased. This portion of the duct is also in close relation with the inferior vena cava.

The intraparietal or terminal portion, after passing obliquely through the muscular coat of the duodenum, accompanied by the pancreatic duct, enters into a dilatation beneath the mucous membrane. This dilated portion, which is called the "ampulla of Vater" (6 or 7 mm. long by 4 or 5 mm. wide), receives the termination of the pancreatic duct (canal of Wirsung) as well, and is surrounded by a thin layer of unstriped muscular tissue. It opens on the mucous membrane through a small aperture at the summit of a papilla, the "caruncula major" of Santorini, which is placed on the posterior and internal wall of the duodenum, three and one-half or four inches (8–10 cm.) beyond the pylorus. (Mayo-Robson.)

The papilla just mentioned is at the upper end of a little ridge—called the "frenum carunculæ"—which may be seen projecting beneath the mucous membrane. Above the caruncle is quite constantly found a transverse fold of mucous membrane, which must be raised if one wishes to see the opening. Mayo states that this is the first normal valvula connivens and a guide to the opening of the duct. The escape of biliary secretions affords, however, a more certain means of identifying the opening.

The inner or mucous coat of the gall-bladder, covered by a single layer of columnar epithelium, is raised into ridges which bound irregular polygonal spaces about 5 mm. in diameter. These ridges may give a roughened surface to a stone tightly embraced by the gall-bladder. Tubular glands, lined with cells continuous with those found on the surface, are, according to some (Robson), abundant, while according to others (Piersol) they are few or are even wanting. They secrete mucus, and are the origin of the glairy fluid which is found to fill the gall-bladder in cases of obstruction of the cystic duct.

Blood-vessels of the Liver and its Ducts.—The liver tissue is nourished by the hepatic artery, a branch of the cœliac axis (Fig. 77), which runs to the right along the upper border of the pancreas, then turns upward behind the first portion of the duodenum, above the level of which it is carried still higher in the right edge of the gastro-hepatic omentum. This artery gives off certain branches from the horizontal or first part of its course, and in the transverse fissure divides into two terminal branches, right and left. The right branch passes in front of or behind the hepatic duct, and behind the cystic duct, to the right end of the

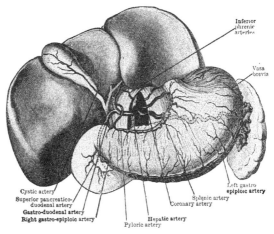

FIG. 77.—The Cœliac Axis and its Branches.   (From Cunningham's Anatomy.)

transverse fissure, where it divides and enters the substance of the liver. The left branch runs to the left end of the fissure and enters the left lobe.

The gall-bladder and cystic duct are supplied by a branch—the cystic artery derived from the right branch of the hepatic just after it has crossed above the junction of the cystic and hepatic ducts. The cystic artery runs downward and forward along the cystic duct to the gall-bladder, usually dividing into two branches—a right and a left. The latter, the more important of the two, courses along to the left of the duct, and is distributed between the gall-bladder and the liver. Occasionally the cystic artery arises from the pancreatico-duodenal, in which case it is liable to injury as it runs along the common duct.

The hepatic duct and the common ducts are supplied directly by short and small branches from the hepatic, the superior pancreatico-duodenal, and other contiguous vessels; in neither is there a special artery.

The portal vein, carrying blood to the liver for further elaboration, passes upward in the right edge of the gastro-hepatic omentum, behind and between the duct and artery, until it reaches the portal fissure, where these three struetures are rearranged, the duct being in front, the artery in the middle, and the portal vein behind. (Fig. 73.) At the portal fissure the portal vein, like the duct and artery, subdivides into two main branches and enters the liver substance.

Within the liver the three vessels run and divide together so that every branch of the portal vein is accompanied by a branch of the hepatic artery and one of the hepatic ducts, and the three, surrounded by a prolongation of the fibrous capsule and accompanied by branches of the lymphatics and nerves, run in special channels of liver substance called portal canals. (Fig. 78.)

The hepatic veins return the blood from the hepatic artery and the portal vein, carrying it by several branches into the inferior vena cava. Veins from all the extrahepatic ducts empty into the portal system, those from the gallbladder first passing through a named vessel, the cystic vein. This explains how infection derived from these ducts might be carried to the liver by portal

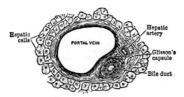

FIG. 78.—The Figure Represents a Section of a Portal Canal, showing its contained branches of the portal vein, hepatic artery, and bile-duct, surrounded by a prolongation of Glisson's capsule. (From Cunningham's Anatomy.)

radicles. According to Sappey, a few small veins leave the gall-bladder to enter the liver, directly joining the portal system.

Certain facts with reference to the vessels should be emphasized. The hepatic veins are intimately attached to liver tissue, do not collapse when cut, and bleeding from them is more severe and less easily controlled. Portal branches are surrounded by loose areolar tissue which permits their walls to fall together when cut. Mayo calls attention to a short transverse vein which may be found on the free anterior surface of the common duct, and which, when injured, is liable to be mistaken for the portal vein.

The Lymphatics of the Liver and its Ducts.—The lymphatics from the visceral surface of the liver empty chiefly into the gastro-hepatic lymph nodes that lie between the layers of the lesser omentum. A few vessels from the posterior part of this surface on the right lobe go to the lumbar lymph nodes, and a few from the corresponding part of the left surface pass to the cœliac nodes. From the parietal, upper, surface, the superficial vessels pass as follows: (a) from adjacent parts of the right and left lobes through the falciform ligament and the diaphragm to the anterior mediastinum, and thence to the right lymphatic duct; (b) from the anterior part of this surface to the gastro-hepatic nodes. From the posterior aspect of the right lobe, some vessels pass to nodes around the upper end of the inferior vena cava, others to the anterior mediastinal lymph nodes, while still others turn downward to join the cœliac group of nodes.

The deep lymphatics of the liver are divided into two sets: one accompanies the branches of the portal vein and ends in the gastro-hepatic nodes; the other accompanies the hepatic veins and passes with the vena cava through the diaphragm.

The lymphatic vessels of the gall-bladder are scanty, and this structure has no lymph nodes; to which anatomical peculiarity, as well as to the fact that the organ is elastic and therefore does not soon assume a tense condition, Mayo attributes the circumstance that infections of the gall-bladder, even when fairly severe, are not followed by a great elevation of temperature. One node, described as constant, is found in the angle formed by the junction of the cystic and hepatic ducts; another, mentioned by Quénu as constant, is found just to the outer side of the common duct at its commencement. Four or five nodes are found along the common duct, and, when enlarged, particularly by malignant deposits, they are liable to be mistaken for calculi. A few nodes are also found in the portal fissure beside the hepatic duct, and one is sometimes present at the neck of the gall-bladder.

Nerves of the Liver and its Ducts.—The liver, the gall-bladder, and the extra-hepatic ducts are supplied from the sympathetic through the hepatic plexus, a derivative of the cœliac plexus, which represents the upper element of the solar plexus. Pneumogastric filaments join the cœliac plexus, and branches from the left pneumogastric pass from the anterior wall of the stomach upward to the liver, accompanying the hepatic artery. None of these filaments, however, has been positively traced to the ducts. According to Jonas, filaments of the eleventh and twelfth dorsal and the first lumbar nerves are distributed to the diaphragm, reaching the common and cystic ducts and the neck of the gall-bladder,—facts which explain the characteristic gall-bladder spasm and the grunting respiration which follow manipulation, even under deep anæsthesia. (Kast and Meltzer, *Medical Record*, New York, Dec. 29th, 1906.) (The writer, in experiments on dogs, has observed that, when a ligature is tightened around the portal vein, there follows always an interruption in the respiratory rhythm. This change occurs so suddenly as to suggest direct interference with the pneumogastric.) Pain referred to the right shoulder is a common symptom of liver abscess, cholecystitis, and other affections of the liver, and it is supposed to be explained on anatomical grounds, by the fact that the phrenic nerve has part of its origin from the fourth cervical, which also gives rise to the supra-acromial. It is the experience of the writer, however, that the pain is more frequently scapular or is located even lower down. This scapular pain and hypochondriac rigidity are probably explained in great part by the irritation of the intercostals through their diaphragmatic filaments.

Physiology of the Liver and Bile-Ducts.—*The Liver.*—The secretion of bile, although one of the minor functions of the liver, is the chief one of surgical importance. The bile formed by the liver cells passes into minute canaliculi and thence flows down the hepatic and common bile-ducts into the duodenum. Under normal conditions bile is excreted daily to the amount of from twenty to thirty ounces, and this amount is modified very little by the action of drugs, as shown by Mayo-Robson.*

Bile is, for the most part, an excrementitious product, but it markedly aids pancreatic digestion and has some solvent action on fats, thereby promoting their absorption; it is also said to be a stimulant to the peristaltic movement of the intestines. It is not, however, absolutely essential to the economy, for a person may be quite healthy with all of the bile escaping externally. When, from any obstruction in the excretory ducts, bile cannot pass into the duodenum, it is absorbed by the circulation, giving rise to jaundice. Life is possible for months with complete retention of bile. The secretion of bile is independent of nerve influence, but, according to Starling, is stimulated by the action of secretin upon the liver cells.

The Gall-Bladder.—The gall-bladder is a diverticulum from the biliary passages, and is, by some, regarded as a reservoir for bile. It is maintained by them that, during the processes of digestion, when the acid chyme in the stomach passes over the papilla in the duodenum, the bile is expelled from the gall-bladder, but that, when the digestion is quiescent, this fluid is stored in its appropriate receptacle. The storage function of the gall-bladder, as pointed out by Mayo-Robson, cannot be important, since its capacity is only about one ounce, while twenty or thirty ounces represent the total daily output of bile. Murphy suggests that it may, like the bulb of a syringe, serve to produce, at times, a continuous flow. By many it is viewed as an obsolete organ, since patients get along perfectly well without it.

Abnormalities of the Liver and the Bile-Ducts.—*Abnormalities of the Liver.*— What might be termed normal variations in the size, shape, and position of the liver have already been referred to; hypertrophy and atrophy will also change, more or less, the relations of this organ. A linguiform process, called "Riedel's lobe" (Fig. 79), may extend downward, a greater or lesser distance, from the right lobe; it may overlie the gall-bladder or be placed to the right of that viscus. In the former case it adds to the difficulty of certain operations; in both it may obscure diagnosis, having been mistaken for a tumor of the gall-bladder, liver, or kidney, for movable kidney, and for other abdominal conditions. This tongue-like process has been regarded by some as the result of tight lacing, but it occurs in men and may grow from the left lobe (Cunningham); by others it is held to be uniformly associated with gall-stones. This latter statement, however, is not confirmed by the experience of all operators. (Robson.) Other abnormalities are :—(1) Transposition of the liver, occurring with transposition of other viscera; the large lobe being turned to the left. Several such cases, complicated with gall-stones, have been reported. (2) The liver may assume an almost vertical

* "Surgery of the Gall Bladder and Bile Ducts," 3d edit.

position. (Robson.) (3) Displacements downward are caused by pleural effusions and by other thoracic conditions; displacements upward, by ascites and by abdominal growths. (4) There may be an unusual amount of mobility. (See page 193.)

Abnormalities of the Gall-Bladder.—The following abnormalities have been recorded: (1) Complete absence, with absence of bile-ducts; (2) absence, the common duct being dilated; (3) double gall-bladder, each with a separate cystic duct; (4) double gall-bladder, with a single cystic duct; (5) gall-bladder completely surrounded with liver substance; (6) gall-bladder situated in a fossa under the left lobe; (7) ectopy of the gall-bladder, usually occurring in transposition of the viscera; (8) the gall-bladder may be bent on itself, the fundus directed toward the left; (9) hour-glass gall-bladder, probably the result of

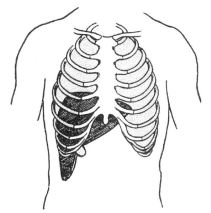

Fig. 79.—Linguiform Process of the Liver (" Riedel's lobe "). (From Mayo-Robson, on "The Surgery of the Gall-Bladder.")

inflammation. Further, the gall-bladder may be placed so low that, when the structure is inflamed, the resulting condition simulates appendicitis, particularly if the liver itself happens to have a linguiform lobe. Again, it may be retracted enough to be difficult to locate, or distended enough to invade the inguinal region.

Abnormalities of the Bile-Ducts.—(1) There may be complete obliteration of the bile-ducts, probably due to antenatal inflammation, and life has been possible in this condition for as long a period as six months. (Robson.) (2) Various degrees of obliteration may occur in the common duct, the duct behind such obliteration becoming enormously dilated. (3) The cystic and hepatic ducts may open separately into the duodenum, there being no common duct; or, in the absence of the gall-bladder, many ducts may extend from the liver to the duodenum. (4) Abnormal terminations of the common bile-duct have been reported, as follows:—(a) The duct of Wirsung may join the common duct higher up than normal, the ampulla being absent, and the common duct opening into the duodenum by a flat oval orifice. (b) The common duct and the duct of Wirsung may open separately into the duodenum, the ampulla and papilla both being absent. (c) The ducts may open separately at the apex of a normal papilla, the ampulla being absent.

Peritoneal Pouch.—The liver occupies and helps to bound a definite peritoneal space, which has been described by Morrison.* This space or pouch is bounded above by the right lobe of the liver, and below by the upper layer of the transverse mesocolon, which also forms its posterior boundary, where it is prolonged upward in front of the right kidney and suprarenal body, and its left, where it clothes the spine and the duodenum. On the right it is limited by the parietal peritoneum. It is irregular in outline and is prolonged upward both in front and behind the liver. To the right of the ascending colon, it extends downward toward the iliac region; through the foramen of Winslow it connects with the lesser sac of the peritoneum; while in front of the transverse colon it communicates with the greater sac. This space holds about one pint before overflow into the general cavity takes place, and its surgical importance lies in the fact that it may thus tend to limit extravasations or suppuration. It can be drained from in front, but much more efficiently from behind. It is also important to remember its limits in placing pads to prevent soiling during operations.

Traumatic Affections of the Liver.—*Contusions.*—Contusions are caused by blows or run-over accidents, which are not sufficiently severe to produce rupture. There may be some laceration of the liver tissue with ecchymosis, but, as the capsule is not torn, there is no intraperitoneal extravasation of blood or bile. If the injury is severe enough to produce hæmatoma, this may persist, or later become a cyst. Such a lesion may be followed by an abscess. The symptoms are: shock of varying degree and pain and tenderness over the hepatic region, with the absence of signs of extravasation of blood or bile into the peritoneal cavity. Rest in bed, fluid diet, and cold applied over the liver region for twenty-four hours or longer constitute the proper treatment. If the contusions are severe, the patient should be kept quiet and on a light diet for a week, to lessen the possibility of abscess formation.

Ruptures.—Ruptures are always serious and sometimes fatal. In the majority of cases they are caused by run-over accidents, severe kicks or blows, or by the ends of a broken rib. The peritoneal covering and capsule being broken, there is more or less extravasation of blood, which may be limited to the peritoneal pouch described by Morrison (see above) or, in severe cases, may extend rapidly to the whole peritoneal cavity. Should the patient survive the immediate effects of the injury without operation, general peritonitis or a subphrenic abscess may subsequently develop, or a hæmatoma may persist for some time.

The symptoms are severe shock, which is always present, and pain, which is located over the liver and is also referred to the umbilicus and right shoulder. Vomiting may be present, and, if the patient survives beyond twenty-four hours,

* Brit. Med. Journal, May 3d, 1894.

jaundice is likely to develop.   The local signs are: increased liver dulness and, in severe cases, abdominal rigidity, with increasing distention and other signs of peritonitis.

In any case of severe injury in the region of the liver, especially if complicated by broken ribs in that situation, rupture of the liver should always be suspected and the case carefully watched.   If, in addition to shock, severe pain and tenderness or signs of extravasation follow, with symptoms of internal hemorrhage, it is quite certain that rupture has occurred.   Jaundice coming on after twenty-four hours may be due to rupture of the gall-bladder or bile-ducts, but it is usually associated with some laceration of the liver substance.

In mild cases expectant treatment may be adopted.   The patient should be put to bed, the thighs flexed to relax the abdominal muscles, cold applied over the injured region, and fluid diet given.   Shock should, of course, be treated, and vomiting arrested if present.   If hemorrhage continues, or if signs of peritonitis arise, a laparotomy should be performed.   In severe cases operation should be undertaken immediately.   The abdomen is opened over the probable seat of rupture by an incision—median, subcostal, or in the right semilunar line.   Lannelongue resects the eighth, ninth, tenth, and eleventh costal cartilages and draws the ribs outward.   A free exposure of the injured area must be made.   Clots are rapidly cleared away and the extent of the injury determined.   If possible, the injured surfaces should be brought together by deep sutures inserted at some distance from the edges and including a considerable portion of liver substance.   The capsule should be sewn with fine catgut.   If hemorrhage cannot be controlled in this way, the larger vessels may be surrounded by a mass ligature of catgut, or packing with gauze will have to be resorted to.   The latter may be made more effective by using it in conjunction with mattress sutures.   Profuse hemorrhage from the liver may be temporarily controlled by pressing the portal vein and hepatic artery between the finger and the thumb, or by applying a temporary ligature of tape.

Da Costa says that the liver should be sutured to the belly wall; * Cheyne and Burghard suggest soaking the gauze which is to be placed in immediate contact with the bleeding surface, in adrenalin or hydrogen peroxide.†   Shallow breaks in the surface of the liver may be treated by the cautery, to control hemorrhage.

After the wound of the liver has received proper attention, the peritoneal cavity should be wiped out and the abdominal wound partially closed, room being left, however, for a drainage tube, which should always be placed, and, if gauze packing was used for controlling the bleeding in the liver, the free end of this should also be brought out of the abdominal wound.

In cases of a stab or a gunshot wound, and in those in which a rupture of the organ is complicated by compound fracture of the ribs, the relation of the liver to the abdominal parietes should be carefully considered.   A knife or bullet entering below the costal margin and passing horizontally backward

* "Modern Surgery," edition vi., page 1014.
† Vol. vii., page 109.

in a direction parallel with the sagittal plane, would not, in normal cases, wound the liver, except for the triangular area in the epigastrium. (See page 194.) Should the bullet be directed to the right, however, even though it maintained its horizontal course, the liver would be involved. Horizontal knife thrusts in the fourth intercostal space in front, or in the sixth. laterally, and anywhere between the sixth and tenth spaces posteriorly, would penetrate four layers of pleura, the edge of the lung, and the diaphragm, before wounding the liver. (Piersol.) Lower down, the lung might escape, but the two layers of pleura of the costophrenic sinus and the diaphragm would be involved. Alterations in the position of the liver, as modified by inspiration and expiration and by the horizontal or vertical position of the body, should also be regarded.

A wound of the liver complicated by a wound of the abdominal parietes should be treated by prompt operation, particularly directed to the control of hemorrhage. Afterward, the cavity should be cleansed and drainage established. The bleeding is usually best managed by gauze packing, which may also serve as a drain. In several cases of gunshot wounds, the writer has used through-and-through gauze packing, inserting several strands and removing these, one at a time; thus making sure that the strands were not acting as a plug, rather than as a drain, and, at the same time, avoiding the hemorrhage which might follow if all were removed too early. Sometimes a rubber tube can be effectively combined with the gauze.

Suppuration in the Liver.—Abscesses of the liver follow infection by staphylococcus, streptococcus, the colon and typhoid bacilli, and one protozoan organism—the Amoeba coli. Abscesses caused by pyogenic bacilli may be multiple or single; those resulting from the amoeba are usually single and are known as tropical abscesses. Mixed infections, are, of course, frequent.

Multiple Abscesses.—In multiple abscesses the infective agents reach the liver in different ways. (a) They may be carried to it through radicles of the portal vein, producing emboli in branches of these vessels in the liver, and resulting in a suppurating pylephlebitis. Such infections most commonly follow appendicitis, but they may also originate from an ulceration or infection at any point in the alimentary canal from stomach to anus. (b) Multiple abscesses may develop in the course of pyæmia, in which case the infective emboli are carried by the hepatic artery. (c) Abscesses may be located in the branches of the intrahepatic bile passages, the infection spreading to these from the gall-bladder or intestines. Such abscesses are commonly associated with obstruction of the common duct. (d) Lymphatic infection may follow various inflammatory conditions, particularly appendicitis. Suprahepatic abscesses in the cellular tissue between the liver and the diaphragm are usually due to a lymphogenous infection.

The onset is sudden, the symptoms acute. There are pain and tenderness over the liver, with slight regular enlargement of the organ. Chills and rigors occur, the body temperature rises rapidly, and sweating, diarrhœa, and rapid emaciation follow. In the later stages leucocytosis and jaundice, rarely marked, are present; the pus, when the condition is prolonged, may be found sterile.

The symptoms are those of pyæmia, to which are added pain, tenderness, and enlargement of the liver. The existence and site of a primary focus should be investigated. Frequently a perihepatitis may be present, giving rise to a friction rub which may be heard on auscultation. The development and disappearance of this rub furnish hints both as to the existence of inflammation and as to the establishment of subsequent adhesions. Rigors in a pyæmia may occur several times in the twenty-four hours, and more than one rigor in this space of time, accompanied by a sudden abrupt rise of temperature, is suggestive of pyæmia.

Little can be hoped for from surgical treatment. If evidence can be obtained that a single large collection of pus exists, this should be opened and drained. Other abscesses may be located by the finger and opened at the time of operation, or they may subsequently open spontaneously. In the early stages of suppurative cholangitis (see page 231) the gall-bladder or the common duct should be opened and drainage effected thereby, the obstruction being removed at the same time or subsequently. When the infection has progressed far enough to produce an abscess, it is manifest that little good can be effected by such drainage.

Localized Abscesses.—A localized abscess of the liver may follow fusion of a number of small abscesses, or sometimes a contusion, the extravasated blood having become infected. Two instances of the latter are mentioned by Osler.* A localized abscess may also form by extension from a contiguous inflammation—as, for example, from a subphrenic abscess or an empyema of the gallbladder. It is sometimes associated with head injuries; it may also develop around a foreign body, which has, through ulcerative action, found its way from the stomach or the intestines, or around one or more parasites, such as the round worm, the fluke, or a cluster of ray fungi. Tuberculosis is often associated with abscess, and suppuration frequently occurs in a hydatid cyst.

Tropical Abscess. (Fig. 80.)—By far the most common form of single abscess of the liver is that associated with tropical dysentery. According to Kieffer, these are single in seventy per cent of cases, and are found in the right lobe in from seventy to eighty per cent of cases.† They are undoubtedly due to Amœba coli, which can practically always be found in the walls of the abscess. The pus, in the tropical abscess, is a thick mucoid substance, reddish-brown in color, which has been compared to anchovy sauce. It contains broken-down liver tissue, with very few leucocytes. In Kieffer's experience, dysentery was an antecedent factor in every case; others have not found the relation so constant. The amœba may be found in the colon without abscess. This variety of abscess may develop weeks, months, or as long as two years after the attack of dysentery and after all ulcerative action has ceased. Amœbic abscesses are not confined to the tropics, but patients in whom they occur will usually be found to have, at some previous time, visited tropical or subtropical countries.

* Third edition, page 557.
† Phil. Med. Journ., Feb. 21st, 1903.

Left alone, an abscess may remain local or latent for a long time, presenting few symptoms, and perhaps unsuspected until a sudden complication ensues—such, for example, as rupture into a lung, with expectoration of pus; or the abscess may enlarge and make its way to the surface of the liver. In about twenty-eight per cent of the cases rupture occurs spontaneously, and in more than one-half of these it takes place in an upward direction. (Mayo.) The abscess may also open into the stomach, duodenum, or transverse colon, the contents being discharged *per rectum* or into the peritoneum or pleura, in which case immediate operation is demanded. The abscess may point externally through the abdominal wall, between the ribs or into the loin. Finally, in some

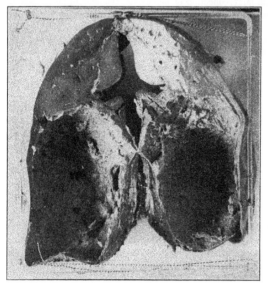

FIG. 80.—Section of the Liver through the Centre of a Large Abscess Occupying Most of the Right Lobe.
(From the Museum of the New York University and Bellevue Hospital Medical College.)

instances, it may open into the gall-bladder and bile-ducts, and Flexner has reported two cases of rupture into the inferior vena cava.

There is usually, at some time in the twenty-four hours, more or less elevation of temperature, but the fever curve is not typical, ranging indeed from subnormal to several degrees above; it is often accompanied by sweating preceded by a slight chill, which recurs more frequently at night. In the pyogenic infections the fever is higher than in amœbic abscess. In the latter, the fever is not high, nor is leucocytosis marked, unless there is a mixed infection. In the other forms a varying leucocytosis is found, the variation depending on the virulence and quantity of the germs. In cases of complete encapsulation, or where the germs are dead, both fever and leucocytosis may be absent. The other symptoms of sepsis will vary, the variation depending on the same factors as those which control the fever; they will be more marked in the pyogenic cases and in those in which the tropical abscess is complicated by a mixed infection. The existence of sepsis will be indicated by fever, weakness, emaciation, and loss of appetite—in the later stages, perhaps by diarrhœa; in tropical and in old encapsulated cases, sepsis will not be a prominent feature. Pain of a dull aching character is present at first, and is due to tension of the capsule, but, as the abscess nears the surface, this changes to the sharp lancinating pain of peritoneal or pleural involvement. Pain may be directly over the liver or it may be referred to the shoulder. Often the patient inclines to the right side, keeping the right thigh flexed, and there is considerable rigidity of the right rectus.

Jaundice may occur, and is due to blocking of the bile-ducts. The obstruction may affect only the smaller bile radicles, and in that case the jaundice is slight; but, if the obstruction is due to pressure on the common or hepatic duct, by an abscess projecting from the infected surface, the jaundice will be much more marked. Enlargements of the liver, if present, can be found on palpation as well as by percussion. Very rarely can fluctuation be elicited.

The diagnosis, particularly in tropical abscess, is difficult. Ill-health, with gradual emaciation and slight tenderness over the liver, coming on subsequently to an attack of dysentery, should excite suspicion, particularly if the patient has recently resided in a tropical or subtropical region. The temperature curve may suggest an infective cholangitis, but in the latter the presence of a varying degree of jaundice and the history of previous gall-stones would help to differentiate. The temperature curve may also resemble that of malaria, but an examination of the blood and the taking of quinine will settle the question. It may be extremely difficult, even impossible, to differentiate a tropical abscess of the liver from multiple abscesses. In the latter the history may point to a focus of infection, thus furnishing a clue of the utmost importance. In multiple abscesses the symptoms—the temperature curve and the leucocytosis—are more pronounced; indeed, this statement is true of pyogenic abscesses generally, either single or multiple, as compared with those caused by amœba. An abscess of the lung or a local empyema on the right side may simulate abscess of the liver. Close observation of the mode of onset, supplemented by aspiration through the chest wall and an examination of the pus, will help in differentiating the one from the other. A subphrenic abscess originating from an appendicular focus, an empyema of the gall-bladder with rupture, a perinephritic abscess, an ulcerative process extending from the stomach or the duodenum, may also cause difficulties in diagnosis. When the abscess involves the abdominal wall and discharges externally, it may be mistaken for an infection of the soft tissues. In all of these cases a careful weighing of the history, examination of the pus, and a thorough exploration of the region involved, if an operation is undertaken, will aid. In hepatic abscess the spleen is small,—a condition obtaining in few other infections. If it should be enlarged, this circumstance points to pylephlebitis. (Mayo.)

When the diagnosis has been established, operative treatment should follow. In suspicious cases an exploratory incision is allowable. Aspiration, as a curative measure, combined with siphon drainage, has been recommended by some. (Cantlie and Manson; Mayo, in " Keen's System of Surgery.") It is unsurgical, and, even as a diagnostic procedure, should not be resorted to until one is quite ready to proceed with the operation. Puncture of the liver for the purpose of locating pus should not be made until after the abdomen or the thorax has been opened. If the puncture is made through adhesions, there will be no danger of contaminating the peritoneum; if no adhesions exist, gauze should be carefully packed around the point to be punctured. Exploratory puncture without preliminary opening might be justifiable if it could be made certain that adhesions existed at the site selected; but this is a refinement in diagnosis attainable only in cases that have been under close observation. If the needle is used before or after an opening has been made and pus discovered, it should be left *in situ* as a guide.

To expose the liver three routes are available: (1) the abdominal (peritoneal); (2) the transpleural; (3) the combined.

(1) The Abdominal Route.—The abdominal incision is selected when the enlargement is downward; it should be placed over the most prominent part and at the site of adhesions when possible. If the liver is adherent one may aspirate at once; if it is not, gauze packing should be placed, the abscess should be located by the needle, which is left *in situ*, and the opening should be enlarged with dressing forceps, fingers, a grooved director, or other blunt instrument. Drainage should then be placed, and two tubes, as a rule, are better than one, as they permit the introduction of irrigation later. Irrigation should, however, never be employed at once, and, when used at a later stage, it should be carried out most gently and under little pressure. As cicatrization progresses the tubes are gradually withdrawn. The use of a vacuum cup assists in the drainage and collapse of the cavity. At first it may cause too much bleeding; when this occurs, early or late, the suction should be lessened or discontinued. If the cavity is large, a gauze tampon may be necessary to control oozing and to prevent the escape of septic material into the peritoneal cavity, if the latter has been opened.

(2) The Transpleural Operation.—Since a large percentage of liver abscesses point upward, this route will be utilized frequently. Under proper precautions, it is safe and easy, and affords the best drainage. (See Fig. 81.) By inspection, palpation, percussion, etc., the point of greatest prominence is ascertained, and this is the point to be selected—particularly if at this spot a friction rub has been heard and has subsequently disappeared, for it is then probable that adhesions exist. Portions of one or two ribs are now excised, care being taken not to injure or open the pleura. After the opening has been made, the parietal pleura should be carefully observed to ascertain whether or not the diaphragmatic pleura is adherent: when no adhesions are present the diaphragm may be seen gliding to and fro. When the latter structure is not adherent, or when one is in doubt, a curved needle armed

with a ligature may be inserted above and also below the proposed incision. An incision is then made through parietal pleura and diaphragm and it is noted whether or not the diaphragm and liver are adherent. Even if they are not, it is unnecessary to attempt to stitch them together, because they are in such close proximity—practically in contact—that a gauze packing, small in amount and placed just beneath the edges of the diaphragmatic opening, can be applied so as effectually to close the peritoneal cavity. Indeed, it is doubtful whether this step is needed, particularly when the incision is placed well posteriorly, since the weight of the liver and the intra-abdominal pressure keep the liver in contact with the diaphragm, and the pus, having free exit, has no tendency to enter the peritoneal cavity.

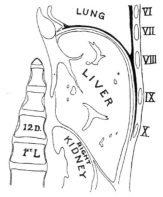

The operation just described can well be performed under local anæsthesia, and the writer has practised it many times. It is particularly useful in cases of great prostration, and where rupture of the abscess is feared from the vomiting that may follow the use of a general anæsthetic. When the abscess has already ruptured into the lung, and quantities of pus are being expectorated, a general anæsthetic is contra-indicated and local anæsthesia must be used.

FIG. 81.—Diagrammatic Antero-Posterior Vertical Section through the Trunk of the Human Body, Showing the Relations of the Liver to Surrounding Structures and Organs. (After Sabatta.)

It has been recommended to perform this operation in two stages—that is, first carrying the incision down to the pleura, then packing the wound, and waiting until adhesions shall have formed; or, if there are already adhesions here, but none between the peritoneal surfaces, packing the latter and waiting. If a general anæsthetic is used, the two-stage operation is usually unnecessary. When cocaine is used the two-stage operation is probably unnecessary, but may be adopted at much less cost to the patient.

(3) Combined Abdominal and Thoracic Operation.—A straight vertical incision in the abdomen is carried upward over the ribs, a sufficient number of these are excised, and the pleura is then pushed upward before the diaphragm is incised (subpleural operation). If the subpleural operation is found to be impracticable, the two layers of pleura—if not already adherent—are stitched together and the incision is deepened through pleura and diaphragm. The operation is finished by protecting the abdominal cavity, evacuating the pus, draining, and stitching together the edges of that part of the opening which is not needed, particularly the lower end. Such an operation, it seems to the writer, is usually unnecessary; indeed, the cases in which a combined operation is indicated are those where an exploratory abdominal incision is needed.

If, after the exploratory opening has been made, it is found that the abscess points upward, and that to drain downward would be difficult and would expose the peritoneum needlessly, a separate transpleural opening may be made as above described. If there are no adhesions between the liver and the diaphragm over the pointing abscess, the surgeon should introduce his fingers beneath the diaphragm, and should press the latter into the cavity left by the excised rib; after which the pleura, diaphragm, and diaphragmatic peritoneum may be stitched together and an opening made, in the centre of the stitched area, through all three structures. Then the wound may be packed and the liver opened, or the packing alone may be done and the remainder of the operation deferred until adhesions form between the diaphragm and the liver. If adhesions are already present, the operation is simplified.

The mortality of liver abscess, once as high as eighty per cent, is now between twenty and thirty per cent, and is still decreasing.

Hydatid Cysts of the Liver.—Hydatids of the liver (Fig. 82) are the larval or cystic stage of a tapeworm, the Tænia echinococcus, which in its adult life inhabits the intestine of the dog and other animals. The adult worm, about 4 mm. long (one-sixth of an inch), consists of four segments, the terminal one being larger than the others combined and containing about five hundred ova. When the terminal segment breaks off, it is carried along in the feces of the dog, the ova are liberated, and, leaving the intestine, are scattered widely, finding their way into the stomach of man through drinking-water, watercress, lettuce, and other articles of food. In the stomach the envelopes are dissolved and the embryo is set free. These embryos are oval and from one of their poles spines are directed backward, enabling the organism to burrow into the tissues, but pre-venting its return. Because so many reach the liver, it is supposed that they enter the radicles of the portal vein; but it is also probable that the liver is especially adapted for their development, as are the striated muscles for the development of trichinæ. (Rolleston.)

When the embryo reaches the liver, its hooklets disappear, its contents undergo liquefaction, and it enlarges, becoming transformed into a cyst or hydatid. It now consists of two walls—an outer, laminated, the ectocyst, and an inner, granular, the endocyst. The outer layer is elastic and contains char-acteristic wavy bands of homogeneous material, by means of which it is easily identified. The endocyst contains crystals of carbonate of sodium. Outside of these a third or adventitious coat is formed from the tissues of the host by compression and irritation. This coat is fibrous and is called the pseudo-cyst.

The fluid in a living cyst is clear, opalescent, of a low specific gravity (1002 to 1010), neutral in reaction, and contains no albumen but a considerable amount of chloride of sodium and other substances which may help to identify it. When the parasite dies the fluid becomes turbid and albuminous; when suppuration occurs the albumen increases and the fluid resembles pus.

Reproductive changes in the parasite result in the production of daughter cysts, grand-daughter cysts, and scolices. Daughter cysts begin as buds which project from the true walls into the cyst. Fluid develops in the interior of these buds, converting them into cysts, and they soon become detached, floating about in the fluid of the parent cyst.   In like manner grand-daughter cysts are developed from the walls of the daughter cysts.   Scolices, an early stage of the head of the future worm, develop inside the daughter cysts.   These are armed with suckers and a row of hooklets, and, if fed to the dog at this stage, will develop into the adult worm, by lengthening and transverse segmentation.   Scolices and hooklets are not found free in the fluid of the living cyst, being liberated only by rupture of the daughter cyst, which may be brought about by tapping or opening, or by death of the organism.   When present they serve, particularly the hooklets, as a certain means of identification.

The endogenous method of reproduction just described may go on until the parasite weighs from 10 to 15 kilograms (twenty-two to thirty-three pounds) and contains daughter cysts to the number of twenty-five, or even thousands.

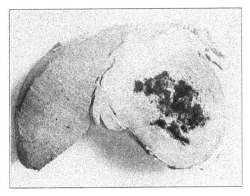

FIG. 82.—Hydatid Cyst of the Liver.   (From the Museum of the New York University and Bellevue Hospital Medical College.)

(Stiles, in Osler, Vol. I., p. 578.)   Exogenous reproduction, in which the buds grow outward into the tissues of the host, occurs in ruminants frequently, but only occasionally in man.   This method of reproduction is held by some to furnish one explanation of the occurrence of the rare condition known as multilocular cyst; another being the coincident growth of two distinct parasites. If no reproductive changes occur the cyst is said to be sterile; the fluid contains neither daughter cysts nor scolices, and its character can be determined only by microscopic examination of its walls.

A cyst may last for many years, the exact time being obviously hard to determine.   If not terminated by operation, the cyst may end in spontaneous death and cure, in rupture, or in suppuration.   Spontaneous death has been attributed to lack of vitality on the part of the parasite and to various other causes, none of which seems to be adequate.   Following the death of the cyst, the fluid becomes turbid and albuminous, absorption goes on, and concentration of what remains reaches such a high degree that the whole content is converted into a substance almost completely solid. The outer fibrous coat, in contracting, compels a shrinking and infolding of the true cyst wall, which may be infiltrated with lime salts; such a cyst may give no further trouble and may be regarded as spontaneously cured. Suppuration is a dangerous complication, which may occur in a growing or a quiescent cyst without manifest cause, more rarely in a spontaneously cured cyst. When this takes place, the symptoms of sepsis are added to the physical signs, and a differentiation cannot be made between it and tropical abscess, except by the microscope. When suppuration has occurred, rupture becomes more imminent and more dangerous. Rupture may occur spontaneously or be precipitated by trauma. It threatens the large and growing cyst, but may take place in the quiescent and small, particularly in one projecting from the liver surface; it may occur on the surface of the body, into the pleural or the peritoneal cavity, into one of the hollow viscera of the abdomen —the intestinal canal, the bile-ducts, etc., or into the lung or a bronchus. It may also take place into the inferior vena cava, the pericardium, the pelvis of the kidney, or into a blood-vessel. The most favorable situation, so far as the patient is concerned, is on the surface of the body; the next, into one of the hollow viscera. If rupture occur in a serous cavity, it is likely to set up a severe, even fatal inflammation; in the bile-ducts it causes pain and jaundice. It is not necessarily fatal, even when the rupture is into the inferior vena cava. (Deve-Rolleston.)

The prognosis will depend on the above factors and on the fact whether an operation is performed or not. When the cyst is large enough to be suspected, particularly if increasing in size, operation should be undertaken; if the cyst is decreasing in size, a spontaneous cure is probable, and a close watch may be kept upon it; but even then it is threatened with suppuration and rupture, and operation is therefore the safest procedure.

The general symptoms are not marked, as a rule, and may be absent even in a growing cyst. Frequently the condition is discovered at the autopsy or in the course of an examination for some other disease. Sometimes there is a sense of weight or dragging. Occasionally, when a perihepatitis develops, there is pain. Most of the symptoms are due to pressure or to complications introduced by suppuration or rupture. Pressure symptoms, as a rule, are rarely present, because of the slow growth of the cyst; their character will depend on the direction taken by the growth and on the particular viscus encroached upon. Ascites from pressure on the portal vein, or jaundice from pressure on the common duct may occur, but these symptoms are rare. Jaundice, however, is constant when a hydatid ruptures into the biliary ducts. Slow leakage into the peritoneum may also cause ascites. When rupture, into the lung, the stomach, or the intestine, occurs, hooklets and scolices may be recovered from the feces or the expectoration.

The local signs are more pronounced than the symptoms. There is painless enlargement of the liver, which may be general when the cyst is deeply embedded in the substance of the organ, or the enlargement may take the form of a distinctly localized, even pedunculated, tumor growing from one of the surfaces of the liver. Fluctuation is occasionally present, but frequently the cyst lies at such a depth and the tension is so great that it appears solid. Hydatid thrill elicited on percussion or on stroking the cyst, and supposed to be due to the impact of daughter cysts, is found in many cases; it is not constant, however, and may be found in cysts of other kinds.

Percussion gives a dull note except in those rare cases in which the cyst communicates with one of the hollow organs, and in those still rarer cases in which gas has developed from a gas-producing bacillus. Urticaria is said frequently to develop after rupture of the cyst.

An absolutely certain diagnosis can be made only by microscopical recognition of the scolices, daughter cysts, hooklets, or fragments of the cyst wall, which have been obtained through the occurrence of rupture or by exploration. Without these aids the diagnosis will be tentative and largely influenced by the location of the cyst. When the cyst is central it may be mistaken for cancer, gumma, cirrhotic enlargement, or a tropical abscess. Cancer is frequently secondary in the liver; it is also often multiple, and the primary lesion may be discovered elsewhere. It is irregular in outline and the cachexia is marked. In gumma the history, the Wasserman reaction, and the therapeutic tests will serve to differentiate. In cirrhosis the surface is irregular, the enlargement uniform. In tropical abscess there may be a history of tropical residence or previous dysentery, and there will be evidence of sepsis—fever, leucocytosis, etc., while, in the hydatid, eosinophilia is said to occur. Suppuration occurring in a hydatid produces symptoms like those of a tropical abscess, and differentiation is impossible, except by the microscope. When a hydatid projects upward, the area of liver dulness is increased, encroaching on the pleural cavity, although there may be no displacement downward of the liver. It is then necessary to differentiate the condition from pleural effusion and localized empyema. From pleural effusion it may be distinguished by the mode of onset, by the cyst moving with respiration, and by the fact that the area of the dulness does not alter on change of the patient's position. Skiagraphy, by revealing the upward increase in the size of the liver, is the best aid short of exploration. (Rolleston.) In localized empyema the disease is more acute, the previous history is suggestive, and there is evidence of septic infection. When the growth projects from the anterior or inferior surface, particularly the latter, it may be confused with a dilated gall-bladder, and this mistake is most likely when the gall-bladder is surrounded by dense adhesions. The gall-bladder, however, is pear-shaped, more movable, and occupies its own fossa, and there will usually be a history of gall-stone colic and perhaps of jaundice, both of which symptoms may occur when a hydatid ruptures into a bile-duct. Tumors or displacements of the kidney may give rise to confusion when tne growth is from the inferior surface. In most cases, however, the diagnostic points are evident. Malignant tumors in any part of the liver may be easily confused with hydatid cysts, particularly when the latter are multiple, such mistakes having occurred even after the abdomen has been opened. A deep location of the tumor in the substance of the liver renders more difficult both diagnosis and operation. Multiple cysts too are difficult to diagnose, and occasionally at operation some of them have been overlooked.

The treatment is entirely surgical; the following methods being available: enucleation of the cyst; incision and drainage; and tapping.

(a) Enucleation of the cyst, as recommended by Knowsley Thornton,* or some minor modification of this, is the best procedure. The liver is thoroughly exposed by an incision over the most prominent part of the tumor; if there are no adhesions, gauze packing is placed to protect the peritoneal or pleural cavity. A trocar is then inserted, the fluid contents are evacuated, and their nature determined if possible. The cyst is now opened by an incision made through the substance of the liver by a blunt instrument, or by a cautery following the needle, which has been left as a guide. The cut surfaces of the liver are also protected by gauze. The contents of the cyst are now removed as far as possible, and then the true walls are separated from the pseudo-cyst by blunt dissection, the fingers armed with gauze, or a dissector, being used for this purpose. As the contents and walls are removed, the liver substance and the pseudo-cyst contract and the hemorrhage is not severe. When everything has been removed, the cavity is obliterated by suturing with catgut, and the wounds in the liver substance and abdominal walls are closed without drains. It is sometimes difficult, however, and often impossible, to effect a complete removal, and it is therefore often necessary to provide drainage after the cut edge of the liver has first been stitched to the parietal peritoneum. As suppuration has occurred in a number of cases, and as bile-stained fluid frequently escapes for several days, Mayo considers it wise to depart from this ideal method and always to provide drainage, rubber tissue being preferred for this purpose to tubing.

Some prefer, if no adhesions exist, to pack with gauze and wait for adhesions, completing the operation at a second stage. This restricts the field of operation, and, if there is no other indication for waiting, the operation should be completed at one sitting.

If the cyst is in the upper part of the liver it may be necessary to attack it by the transpleural route, parts of two or three ribs being resected for this purpose. In this event, the two layers of the pleura bounding the costophrenic sinus should be sutured together, if not already adherent, above and below the site of the proposed opening in the diaphragm.

When the cyst is small, both sac and contents might be enucleated in their entirety by cautiously opening the pseudo-cyst. (Stiles, in Osler, Vol. I.)

(b) Incision with drainage is perhaps the operative method most frequently employed. The steps are the same as those already described, up to the moment of opening the cyst; after the cyst has been opened the contents (daughter cysts and endo-cysts) are removed as far as possible, and the cavity is flushed out with normal saline solution. A drainage tube is inserted and around this the cavity is packed with gauze. The margins of the incision in the liver are then

* Med. Times and Gazette, 1883.

united to the parietal peritoneum.   If all the cyst has not been removed, sub-sequent irrigation may be necessary.

When the contents are thick and caseous, a scoop or forceps may be needed for their removal. When suppuration has occurred the treatment is that of abscess, but even here partial or complete enucleation of the wall may be possible.

(c) Tapping by trocar or aspirator has been followed by cure. There is, however, a danger of leakage, and this danger is aggravated when suppuration exists; and the needle should never be used until after adequate exposure of the liver tumor.

Rupture into the peritoneum should be followed by immediate laparotomy, the removal of the cyst, and abundant drainage.

All raw surfaces, both in the abdominal wall and in the liver, should be pro-tected from the hydatid fluid during operation, as there is danger of infecting these surfaces.

Tumors of the Liver.—Primary tumors of the liver are uncommon, their pathology is not well understood, nor have they been clearly classified. Second-ary tumors are much more common and much better understood.

Benign Tumors.—The benign tumors found in the liver are endothelioma, fibroma, myoma, angioma, and adenoma; the teratoma occurs rarely; lipoma perhaps never. Angiomata, composed of dilated blood-vessels, grow to the size of a walnut, and occasionally are somewhat larger. They are discovered accidentally, give no symptoms, require no treatment, and are of interest only because of the bleeding which may occur during operations in their vicinity. Adenomata are also rare; they may be single or multiple. The single tumors may be derived (a) from liver cells; (b) from the intrahepatic bile-ducts; (c) from adrenal rests in the liver. Adenomata, particularly of bile-duct origin, may become cystic and may attain a large size. Those derived from liver cells may contain tubules lined with cubical epithelium, thus resembling primary carcinoma with cirrhosis. Multiple adenomata are most frequently found in connection with cirrhosis. By some (Cornil and Ranvier, "Man. d'Histologie Path.," Vol. II., page 438) they are regarded as complications of cirrhosis—that is, as a compensatory hypertrophy. Others (Dieulafoy and Engelhardt, quoted by Rolleston) believe them to be due to the same cause,—viz., an irritant,— which produces on the one hand fibrous hyperplasia (cirrhosis), on the other proliferation of the liver cells (adenoma). Brissand * believes the adenoma to be a stage between cirrhosis and cancer. Whether this view is correct or not, it appears that cirrhosis sometimes passes into adenoma and then into primary carcinoma.

Single adenomata, when small, produce no symptoms and demand no treat-ment. When large, they may produce jaundice, ascites, and other pressure symptoms. The solid tumors are treated by excision, the cystic by drainage. Multiple growths obviously do not come within the scope of surgical therapeutics.

Cysts of the Liver. (Figs. 83, 84, and 85.)—General cystic disease of the liver, analogous to that found in the kidney, has been reported, and the two

* Archives de Médecine, 1883, tome ii.

may be associated. The cause is not known and the condition is usually recognized *post mortem.* Simple cysts also occur. They may be multiple and small or solitary and large. They are surrounded by a thin wall closely adherent to the liver tissue, and the fluid may be clear or stained with bile or blood. Bland Sutton describes the removal of such a cyst and considers dilatation and fusion of bile-ducts as a probable cause. In two cases operated on by Mayo,* the cyst contained from one to two pints of clear fluid.

Multiple cysts are not amenable to surgical treatment. The solitary cyst can be treated by enucleation of its wall, as recommended for hydatids; such

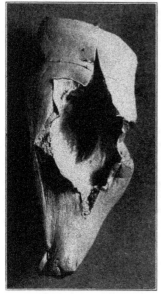

Fig. 83.—Cyst of the Liver. (From the Museum of the New York University and Bellevue Hospital Medical College.)

enucleation, however, is difficult and hemorrhage is apt to be severe. Simple drainage is said to be adequate in most of these cases.

Malignant Tumors.—Primary forms of malignant tumors are rare; secondary carcinoma and sarcoma are much more common, forming, according to Da Costa,† ninety-six per cent of all liver tumors.

Primary carcinoma (Fig. 86) may appear in several forms, as follows:— (1) as a massive tumor with rather distinct delimitation, often occupying an entire lobe; (2) as a nodular mass,—that is, one primary and many secondary nodules (the nodules are grayish, white, or opaque, grow rapidly, become necrotic, and as a result are umbilicated) (Fig. 87); (3) as an infiltrating or diffuse new-growth. A carcinoma of the last variety may invade the whole of a major lobe or the entire organ; there is a considerable production of new fibrous tissue, and the disease resembles, and may be mistaken for, portal cirrhosis. Indeed, many French writers maintain that the association of cirrhosis with adenoma and carcinoma is the rule rather than the exception. Writers of other nationalities, while admitting the occasional association of these benign and malignant processes, still contend that such association is not nearly so frequent as maintained by the French school.

Secondary carcinoma (Fig. 87) is the most common form of liver tumor. It usually follows a primary focus in the intestinal tract, but may be secondary to cancer of the ovary, rectum, breast, or other part of the body. It appears

* Keen's System, vol. iii., page 983.
† "Modern Surgery," page 876.

in the form of grayish or yellowish-white nodules, which soften in the centre and become umbilicated.

The general symptoms are: an insidious onset characterized by marked cachexia; jaundice is present in one-half the cases; ascites is rare, unless the growth presses on the portal vein; pain is present, but is usually not severe and may be absent; fever is also present in some cases. According to the Mayos embolic malignant metastases of the liver exhibit peculiar symptoms—a sudden

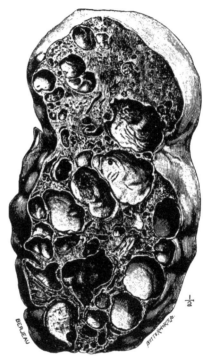

FIG. 84.—A Liver in Section; the Spaces on the Cut Surface are Dilated Bile-Canals. Specimen removed from a woman aged forty-six years and preserved in the Museum of the Royal College of Surgeons, London, England. (After Bland Sutton.)

pain in the liver, usually a chill followed by elevation of temperature, and slight jaundice. The local signs are: enlargement of the liver, sometimes great, often irregular; the liver is hardened, and in the nodular forms the nodules may be felt, or even in some cases seen.

In the earlier stages cancer of the liver usually escapes recognition; in the later, the diagnosis is based on the local signs and the cachexia. The tumor can be considered primary only after exhaustive research has failed to locate a primary lesion; usually the latter is discoverable, but in some cases, particularly in sarcoma, it escapes notice until the secondary lesions are extensive.

So far as treatment is concerned, excision may be resorted to in the nodular form of primary cancer of the liver, if the disease is recognized early enough, and particularly if it is confined to the left, the quadrate, or the so-called corset lobe. If the tumor is very small it may be removed by the cautery; for larger growths various methods have been adopted. Keen uses the cautery; in addition, he underruns the large veins with catgut, and packs with iodoform gauze which he removes in a few days. Frank advises cutting out the tumor together with a wedge-shaped portion of liver, so that the bleeding surfaces may be

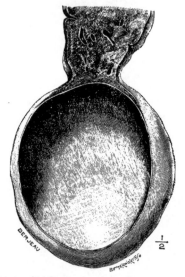

Fig. 85.—A Cyst (non-parasitic) Growing from the Free Border of the Liver. The specimen, which was obtained post mortem from a woman aged thirty-eight years, is preserved in the Museum of the Royal College of Surgeons, London, England. (After Bland Sutton.)

brought in apposition with sutures. Others, instead of using the knife, crush the liver with forceps. When only a thin portion of the organ is to be removed, Mayo recommends that it be first crushed with forceps and then cut away with the knife, the bleeding being temporarily controlled by means of compresses. Afterward the raw surfaces are brought in apposition, as far as possible, by means of quilted sutures. This method is valuable and may be applied to resection of a portion of the liver for any cause. Hemorrhage from surfaces which cannot be apposed for lack of tissue, or which bleed too much to warrant one in assuming the risk attending such apposition, can be controlled by packing gauze between them and holding it in place with interlocking sutures. In the vast majority of cases, however, the treatment is purely palliative.

Secondary cancer of the liver is not amenable to operation, but is of great importance as contra-indicating any attempt at removal of the primary growth. Cancer of the liver secondary to cancer of the gall-bladder, in which the infiltration is confined to a tongue-shaped lobe, forms an exception to the rule, and may be removed.*

Sarcoma of the liver (Fig. 88), either primary or secondary, is very rare. It is usually massive and diffuse, and may be mistaken for a manifestation of congenital syphilis. Secondary forms are softer than carcinoma, sometimes feel cystic,

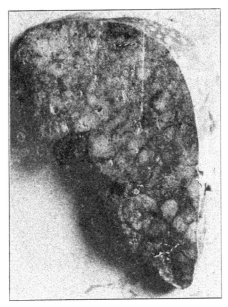

Fig. 86.—Primary Carcinoma of the Liver. (From the Museum of the New York University and Bellevue Hospital Medical College.)

and are much more rapid in growth. The latter statement is particularly true of the melanotic variety. Clinically, however, sarcoma of the liver cannot be differentiated from carcinoma, except that, when the disease occurs in an infant, the diagnosis is suggested by the age.

Tuberculosis of the Liver.—There are only two forms of tuberculosis of the liver that are amenable to surgical treatment—the so-called solitary tubercle and the tuberculous abscess. Solitary tubercle is the term applied to the large caseating masses; tuberculous abscess designates the condition which follows when these masses have been secondarily infected by pyogenic germs. Both

* Keen's "System of Surgery," vol. iii., page 984.

processes may be and frequently are multiple, which removes them from the field of surgery; but either may be single.

There are, as a rule, no definite clinical data that may be separated from the general signs. There may, of course, be some enlargement of the liver, and, when the process is situated near the surface of the organ, perihepatitis and a friction sound may develop. The solitary abscess secondarily infected with pyogenic germs will give the signs and some of the symptoms of a tropical abscess.

The proper treatment of a tuberculous abscess is to evacuate the pus through an incision, then to mop the abscess walls with iodine solution or carbolic acid, and afterward to apply alcohol; or one may introduce into the cavity two drachms

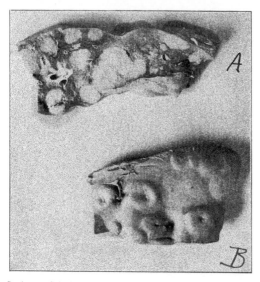

Fig. 87.—Carcinoma of the Liver, Secondary. The specimen at *A* shows the cancerous nodules in section; that at *B* shows umbilication of several of the nodules on the uncut surface of the organ. (From the Museum of the New York University and Bellevue Hospital Medical College.)

of a ten-per-cent mixture of iodoform in glycerin. Closure without drainage, after either of the manœuvres first mentioned, is recommended by some authors. A small pack should be introduced into the parietal wound and carried down to the liver, in order that, through the formation of adhesions, there may be provided ready access to the cavity, should it quickly refill, without involving the peritoneum.

If the pus is not too thick it may be evacuated and the iodoform emulsion introduced through a needle of large calibre.

When secondary infection develops in such an abscess and is severe, drainage should be the treatment adopted. precisely as in the case of a tropical abscess.

To induce hyperæmia, promote collapse of the abscess walls, and favor drainage, the Bier vacuum cup may be used.

The solitary tubercle is sometimes discovered in the course of an operation for some other condition, such as a tuberculous peritonitis; and under these circumstances, if there is actually only one such tubercle and if it is accessible, that part of the liver which is the seat of the lesion may with propriety be excised.

Actinomycosis of the Liver.—Actinomycosis is rarely found in the liver and may arise from a primary focus in the intestine, or it may spread to the liver from the gall-bladder. The disease produces numerous loculi of broken-down caseous material and pus, the latter probably due to secondary infection, and

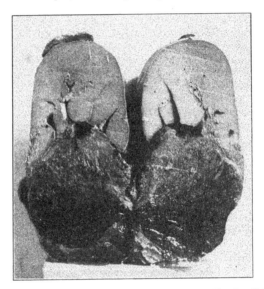

Fig. 88.—Melanotic Sarcoma of the Liver.   (From the Museum of the New York University and Bellevue Hospital Medical College.)

large areas may become involved, although it is usually somewhat definitely localized, with perhaps a few outlying loculi. The liver becomes adherent and the disease may spread to contiguous tissues, such as the diaphragm, lung, etc. The symptoms are those of abscess or tumor, or both, and the diagnosis is not made until after operation, when an examination of the tissue or the pus will reveal the ray fungus. The treatment consists in giving large doses of potassium iodide, which affects this disease as specifically, though not as rapidly, as it does syphilis. If abscesses form they should be evacuated. For irrigation of these Bevan recommends a one-per-cent solution of cupric sulphate, the same drug being administered internally in doses of from one-quarter to one grain, three times a day. Iodoform and carbolic acid have also been employed locally.

Syphilis of the Liver.—Tertiary lesions of the liver, gumma and cicatrices, are the only syphilitic lesions of surgical importance, and these chiefly from a diagnostic point of view. The gumma, in the early stages, consists of granulation tissue, pinkish in color and strongly contrasted with the surrounding liver; later, because of an endarteritis and perhaps also through the action of toxins, necrosis and caseation occur, and the mass, yellowish-white in color, becomes surrounded by a fibrous capsule. Softening may then occur preparatory to absorption, particularly under the influence of the iodides; or a secondary pyogenic infection may take place, converting it into a chronic abscess. Cicatrices represent the final stage of gumma, the result of organization. They may be linear, stellate, etc., are depressed, and divide the surface into nodules which resemble the "hobnails" of portal cirrhosis, but are larger and more irregular. Lardaceous areas often surround the gummata, but rarely occur in general portal cirrhosis.

If the gumma is large there is evidence of the presence of a tumor, which may be single or nodular; and, as such gummata frequently occur on the surface of the liver, there are perihepatitis and consequent pain, which latter symptom is often referred to the shoulder. Anæmia is also present, but the cachexia is not nearly so marked as in cancer. Fever may be present, and, depending on the situation of the gummata, they may cause pressure on the portal vessels or bile-ducts and so give rise to jaundice or ascites. They may also, when situated in the region of the gall-bladder, even cause attacks of pain resembling gall-stone colic. If small, the gummata may easily be overlooked.

As is true of this disease in other parts of the body, the manifestations of syphilis are protean. Rolleston says that, in the liver, such syphilitic lesions may simulate the following conditions: (1) Portal cirrhosis; (2) widespread lardaceous disease; (3) tumor of the liver—malignant, hydatid cyst, or enlarged gall-bladder; (4) suppuration in the liver; (5) cholelithiasis; (6) chronic splenic anæmia; (7) hypertrophic biliary cirrhosis. The condition most likely to be mistaken for gumma is carcinoma, and it may not be possible to decide the question even after the abdomen has been opened. Operations have been frequently performed and portions of the liver removed under the impression that the gumma was a localized cancer. In obscure enlargements, therefore, all means of diagnosis should be adopted: a careful history should be taken and search made for other evidences of the disease. The Wasserman and therapeutic tests may also be employed, and the patient put upon a course of iodides. After the abdomen has been opened, the finding of cicatrices in the liver—that is, evidence of absorbed gummata—would militate strongly against the diagnosis of carcinoma.

Operation on a gumma of the liver should never be undertaken until after the patient has been subjected to a course of the iodides or other specific treatment; but when this lesion has been exposed during an exploration, or under a mistaken diagnosis, it is permissible to remove it, if localized, and such removal may facilitate a cure of the disease. The writer once undertook such an operation after opening the abdomen in the belief that there was a tumor of the gall-bladder. The standing and reputation of the patient almost forbade even the suspicion of syphilis. When the abdomen was opened, a tumor resembling a carcinoma was found involving almost the whole of the quadrate lobe. This was removed without great difficulty and the wound healed promptly. On microscopic section the tumor was found to be a gumma about to break down. A course of the iodides was subsequently given with complete success. When a gumma is breaking down and ulcerating through the abdominal wall, it may be scraped out and drained to prevent or limit secondary infection.

Portal Cirrhosis.—Portal or atrophic vascular cirrhosis is not of surgical interest *per se*, but on account of the ascites which develops, and which in some cases is relieved by the operation of epiplopexy. This variety of cirrhosis is usually caused by alcohol; other poisons introduced into the stomach from without and certain poisons manufactured in the stomach, the result of faulty digestion, may also be causative factors. These, by increasing and prolonging the physiological congestion of the liver, may bring about a proliferation of the fine connective tissue which closely invests the intrahepatic vessels and ducts. When this contracts it produces portal obstruction, which alone, or aided by certain toxæmias (see page 237), results in catarrhal congestion of the stomach and intestines, in congestion and enlargement of the pancreas and spleen, and later in ascites.

As the change goes on, routes of collateral circulation develop in the following situations:—(*a*) Between the accessory portal veins in the falciform ligament and the diaphragmatic para-umbilical and epigastric veins (the distended para-umbilical veins forming the caput Medusæ); (*b*) the veins of Retzius and the retroperitoneal veins; (*c*) between the inferior mesenteric and the hemorrhoidal; and (*d*) between the gastric and the œsophageal veins. (Piersol.) By following these routes the portal blood, impeded in its course through the liver, passes to one side of the latter and enters the systemic veins.

Acting on the supposition that the ascites is due wholly or largely to the obstruction, and that the collateral circulation is compensatory, certain authorities have devised operations for increasing the capacity of the collateral channels by forming adhesions between various abdominal organs and the parietes. The principle underlying this method was suggested by Drummond, the actual operation was carried out by Morrison; and by these gentlemen the method was introduced into England and America. (Rolleston.) It had, however, previously been suggested by Talma, and the various operations are therefore accredited to Talma, or to Talma and Morrison conjointly.

Epiplopexy.—Because of the numerous venous radicles which it contains, and also because of its motility and the facility with which it may be attached to the parietes, the great omentum is the part selected by preference. Morrison firmly attaches this structure to the peritoneum of the anterior wall by numerous fine sutures. Schiassi places the omentum between the parietal peritoneum and the abdominal muscles. Mayo does the same in the following way:—A vertical incision is made on the right side over the liver and in a direction corresponding to a line drawn through the internal mammary and the deep epigastric vessels. Through this incision the liver can be explored and the diagnosis of cirrhosis confirmed. Then a second incision is made, four inches lower down, to, but not through, the posterior sheath of the rectus. This sheath is then extensively separated from the back of the muscle, and the omentum, drawn through the upper wound, is placed in the pocket thus formed and fastened with sutures. This may be repeated on the opposite side,—the exploratory or upper part being omitted,—and the segment of omentum between the two pockets may then be united to the peritoneum by stitches. The upper incision on the right side should be so placed as to avoid the attachment of the falciform ligament (see page 194), both because of the bleeding likely to be encountered, and of the damage which may occur to an important collateral circulation. For the same reason stitches in the round or falciform ligament should be omitted or placed with great care. The upper and lower incisions on the right side may be continuous as far as the posterior sheath of the rectus.

Other and earlier operations recommended had for their object to encourage the formation of adhesions between the liver and the diaphragm, by scraping, curetting, or rubbing with gauze the apposed peritoneal surfaces, and then holding these in apposition by means of stitches in the round ligament. The spleen has been treated in the same way. These operations, if performed to-day, should be supplemental to epiplopexy. In performing them the surgeon must keep in mind the danger of bleeding from too vigorous irritation of the peritoneum.

It has been recommended—to prevent the reaccumulation of fluid which might separate the apposed peritoneal surfaces and thus prevent union—that, immediately after the supplemental procedures described above, drainage be supplied and that the patient maintain for some time a sitting posture. Following epiplopexy the measures named are not necessary; continued drainage may invite suppuration, and, besides, if fluid re-accumulates rapidly it may safely be removed by tapping.

The theory that ascites is due to obstruction and hence that relief follows the establishment of new routes of collateral circulation, has been doubted by many. To account for the improvement Rolleston and Turner have advanced the theory that vascular adhesions furnish relief to the venous engorgement, and that this relief, in turn, permits a richer arterial supply and regeneration of the liver cells. Others believe that a part of the improvement is due to increased capacity of the lymphatic circulation. If either of the above theories is correct, then the operations tending to produce adhesions between the liver and the parietes would seem to be of more importance than those performed on the omentum, which operations relieve merely obstruction.

Aged patients, those suffering from vascular lesions (cardiac or arteriosclerotic), with advanced kidney changes, and patients affected with tuberculosis are not good subjects for operations upon the liver. According to Mayo the cases most suitable for such operations are those occurring in young individuals without alcoholic history—a very limited number. White,* in 227 cases, showed thirty-seven per cent cured and thirteen per cent improved. Other statistics

* British Med. Jour., Nov. 10th, 1906.

vary, but most authors agree with Rolleston that a cure is effected in only a small minority of cases.

For cases of hypertrophic or biliary cirrhosis, or for the secondary cirrhosis which follows splenomegaly, drainage of the gall-bladder has been resorted to. The results have not been satisfactory.

Hepaptosis.—Hepaptosis, abnormal mobility of the liver, usually occurs in women, especially those with abdominal walls rendered lax by repeated pregnancies, or it may be associated with Glenard's disease. (See below.)

Various degrees of hepaptosis are observed. In extreme cases the whole liver may be palpated below the costal margin, or it may even descend into the pelvis. With this descent there is usually a rotation, which brings the diaphragmatic surface in contact with the anterior abdominal wall.

As the condition is frequently a part of general abdominal ptosis (Glenard's disease) measures directed to the liver alone are usually of little value. Occasionally, in extreme cases, operation may be advised; this consisting in shortening the suspensory ligaments and fastening the edge of the liver to the abdominal wall by sutures. Other measures are the following: irritation of the peritoneum on the superior and external surface, to promote adhesions; fastening of the gall-bladder in the upper angle of the wound; plastic operations on the anterior abdominal wall, either alone or combined with hepatopexy; and overlapping of fascia, etc.

Inflammatory Affections of the Gall-Bladder and Bile-Ducts.—Inflammation of the gall-bladder and bile-ducts is caused in all cases by bacteria which have gained access either directly from the duodenum or by way of the blood stream. That the latter is possible has been shown by Welch, who found bacteria in the bile five days after an intravenous injection.* In the majority of cases, however, the infection probably travels up the common duct from the duodenum.

The bacteria usually found are the bacillus coli, the staphylococci, streptococci, typhoid bacilli, and pneumococci, either alone or in mixed infection. The most common predisposing cause is undoubtedly gall-stones, but anything causing obstruction to the bile-passages acts in the same way—*e.g.*, carcinoma, chronic pancreatitis, hydatids, round worms in the common duct, or a catarrhal condition of the duodenum affecting the terminal portion of the common duct. Kinking of the duct may be mentioned as a rare cause, and typhoid fever, pneumonia, influenza, and other acute infections may be complicated by inflammation of some part of the biliary apparatus.

The variety of inflammation depends upon the variety and virulence of the causative organism and the condition previously present. A mild inflammation may pass readily into one of severe type. Thus, a mild catarrhal affection of the mucous membrane may so obstruct the flow of bile that it acts as a strongly predisposing factor in the production of a suppurative form. The symptoms vary according to the particular part of the biliary passages involved. The following varieties have been described: (1) Catarrhal; (2) suppurative; (3) gangrenous or phlegmonous; (4) ulcerative; and (5) membranous.

* Bulletin of Johns Hopkins Hospital, 1801, ii., page 121.

(1) *Catarrhal Inflammations.*—(a) Catarrhal Inflammation of the Gall-Bladder; Catarrhal Cholecystitis.—This form of inflammation is due to a mild infection, which causes the mucous membrane to secrete a thick mucus. This mucus, in being forced through the bile-ducts, produces attacks which resemble closely those of biliary colic. Such a disorder may develop independently of or in connection with gall-stones. In chronic cases the gall-bladder undergoes enlargement and its walls become thickened and pouched; or the inflammatory process may go on to form fibrous tissue, with gradual obliteration of the gall-bladder.

The symptoms are very similar to those of cholelithiasis, and the two affections may often be associated. As a rule, however, the colic attacks are not so severe, the tenderness over the gall-bladder is not so marked, and jaundice, if present, is very mild and due to involvement of the common duct. The diagnosis may remain in doubt for some time, but the facts that no gall-stones are discovered in the feces, that the attacks are not severe, and that the condition yields to medical treatment, as it usually will, establish the nature of the disorder.

General medical treatment is usually satisfactory, but if the disorder persists and if there is any doubt as to the presence of gall-stones, cholecystostomy should be performed. (See page 262.) This operation is quite as effective in curing the trouble when gall-stones are not present as when they are, the free drainage soon restoring the diseased mucous membrane to its normal condition.

(b) Catarrhal Inflammation of the Bile-Ducts; Catarrhal Cholangitis.—The acute form of catarrhal inflammation is usually associated with gastro-intestinal catarrh and produces the transient jaundice commonly found in young adults who are otherwise healthy. The mucous membrane of the bile-ducts is affected to a varying extent; the swelling causing partial closure of the ducts. The material dammed up consists of a mixture of bile and mucus. The disorder may be associated with one of the specific fevers; it is also frequently present when calculi are lodged in the gall-bladder or cystic duct, and is then due to an extension of the inflammation along the mucous membrane. When stones are lodged in the common duct, catarrhal inflammation is present, frequently passing into a more severe inflammation, with pus formation. The acute form is the clinical entity known as "jaundice" by the laity.

In addition to the discoloration of the skin, there are nausea, vomiting, constipation, and marked depression of spirits. The chronic form is usually associated with some other disorder, but in some cases it represents merely a persistence of the symptoms which were present in the acute variety, without any concomitant organic lesion.

Medical treatment is sufficient to effect a cure in those cases in which catarrh is the only condition present, but, where other factors prevail, some kind of an operation, in accordance with the nature of the disorder, will be found necessary.

(2) *Suppurative Inflammations.*—(a) Suppurative Inflammation of the Gall-Bladder; Suppurative Cholecystitis; Vesical Empyema.—This disorder is usu-

ally due to calculi, especially when impacted in the cystic duct. It may also be found in association with tumors, typhoid fever, and other acute infections, even when no stones are present. The abscess, when formed, may rupture into the peritoneal cavity or into one of the neighboring viscera; it may also discharge externally or into the pleura or lung.

The symptoms depend on the cause, which is usually gall-stones. The constitutional symptoms are not as a rule severe, but, in some cases, rigors, chills, high temperature, and sweating are present. · (Mayo Robson attributes these phenomena to associated ulceration.) There are loss of appetite and emaciation, and a tumor can usually be felt. It is tender and moves freely with respiration. Jaundice may be present as a result of associated catarrh of the bile-ducts. If the condition is left alone the abscess may point in any one of various directions and a new set of symptoms arise; or a suppurative cholangitis may be present and obscure the symptoms which point more directly to the condition of the gall-bladder.

The treatment is cholecystostomy or cholecystectomy, the choice between these two depending upon the conditions present in the individual case. Thus, if the disorder is entirely confined to the gall-bladder, while the ducts remain free, cholecystectomy is indicated. If there is any obstruction in the common duct, it should be opened and the obstruction removed. If the cystic duct is not surely patulous, drainage of the common duct should be instituted. (See page 261.) Rarely, when choledochotomy has been performed, the gall-bladder should not be removed, but a cholecystostomy should be added.

(b) Suppurative Cholangitis of the Bile-Ducts.—This form of inflammation is found in cases of obstruction of the common duct, impacted stones being the most common cause, but malignant disease, hydatids, pancreatitis, and round worms frequently produce the disorder. It also occurs in the course of typhoid fever, and Mayo Robson mentions (page 105) influenza as a cause in some cases. As a rule, there is extensive involvement of the ducts, they are dilated at many points and filled with a mixture of bile and pus, and sometimes several of them fuse together to form one large abscess.

The symptoms observed in these cases are dependent on two factors—the obstruction and the infection. The obstruction may be of any degree, the infection of any grade of virulence. In some cases there is a history of previous colics. Occasionally an attack is characterized by chills, fever, and jaundice. The infection ceases and the jaundice subsides, but does not wholly disappear. These attacks may be repeated again and again; if the obstruction is removed, however, they cease. The disorder was first described by Charcot under the term "intermittent hepatic fever"; it is more properly an infective cholangitis. The disease may become aggravated at any time during its course by an increase in the obstruction, but more particularly by an increased virulence of the germs. The symptoms then become aggravated, the intrahepatic bile-ducts become dilated and filled with pus at many points, and the condition becomes one of the greatest gravity.

The proper treatment is drainage, with removal of the obstruction. Drainage may be instituted by means of a cholecystostomy, or, if the cystic duct is not patent, by means of a choledochostomy, or even by both. If the patient's condition is very serious, the simplest operation which will effectively provide drainage should be adopted; the removal of the cause being deferred to another time.

The more important complications of suppurative inflammation of the biliary ducts are the following: (1) Perforation, with general peritonitis; (2) a fistulous communication, either external or internal; (3) localized abscess formation; (4) formation of extensive adhesions; (5) obliteration of the gall-bladder or bile-ducts; (6) hour-glass contraction of the gall-bladder or stricture of the ducts; (7) calcification of the gall-bladder; (8) aneurysm of the hepatic artery as a result of ulceration from the bile-ducts; (9) hemorrhage from ulceration; (10) liver abscess. Empyema, pneumonia, and endocarditis may also complicate suppuration in the biliary passages.

(3) *Phlegmonous and Gangrenous Inflammations.*—Phlegmonous and gangrenous inflammations are confined to the gall-bladder. The walls of this viscus are rapidly invaded by the suppurative process and become œdematous, dark-green in color, or even black if gangrene has occurred. The peritoneum and the intestine in the neighborhood are quickly involved and soon become covered with lymph; or, if perforation has occurred, a general peritonitis rapidly ensues. The affection is rare, but has been found as a complication of typhoid and other acute fevers, or in association with gall-stones. When the angrenous process predominates, there is actual sloughing of an entire segment of the mucous membrane alone, or of all the layers of the bladder wall, with development of general peritonitis. Bland Sutton records a case in which a slough of the whole mucous membrane had formed, together with two perforations—one into the transverse colon and another into the general peritoneal cavity.

The symptoms are those of acute peritonitis, the signs at first being localized about the gall-bladder. Thus, there are severe pain, tenderness, abdominal rigidity, rapid and feeble pulse, quickened respiration, vomiting, and a rise of temperature; later, marked distention and tympanites occur.

The diagnosis is made only with great difficulty, but the true state of affairs may be suspected if a previous history of gall-stones is present. The existence of a circumscribed point of tenderness between the ninth cartilage and the umbilicus may help to distinguish the disorder from an appendicitis associated with a localized tenderness over McBurney's point.

Immediate laparotomy and cholecystostomy, or, if the walls are gangrenous in their entire thickness, a cholecystectomy, complete or partial, should be performed. A general involvement of the peritoneum should be treated by free drainage, by keeping the patient in the Fowler position, and by adopting other appropriate treatment.

(4) *Ulcerative Inflammation.*—Ulcerative inflammation may be found in the gall-bladder or bile-ducts, and is usually associated with calculi. In typhoid fever the ulcerative process is sometimes limited to the gall-bladder, the ulcer varying in depth in different cases. In some it extends only through the mucous

membrane, while in others it involves all the coats. The ultimate result may be a perforation or fistula, an hour-glass contraction of the gall-bladder, or an extensive formation of adhesions.

(5) *Membranous Cholecystitis.*—Membranous cholecystitis is a somewhat rare affection, but several cases have been described. The membrane may form on only a part of the mucous surface of the gall-bladder or bile-ducts, or it may involve the whole, thus causing the formation of a complete cast. The affection is usually associated with calculi, and the passage of the membrane produces severe pain like an attack of biliary colic. These casts may be found in the feces at operation. Such a case is reported in the *British Medical Journal* of April 23d, 1898, by Dr. Fenwick of New Zealand. In this case a complete cast of the gall-bladder was found in the feces after a severe attack of pain.

Tuberculous Inflammation of the Gall-Bladder.—Tuberculous inflammation of the gall-bladder is a rare affection; it occurs in association with tuberculosis elsewhere. It may be either a primary or a secondary process in the gall-bladder. Korte has described one case and has found the records of six others.

Actinomycosis of the Gall-Bladder.—Actinomycosis of the gall-bladder is a curiosity. A case of this nature is recorded by Mayo-Robson. In this instance the gall-bladder was enlarged and tender; the patient had suffered for eighteen months with pain in the right hypochondrium and general loss of weight. The gall-bladder was cleared out by operation, potassium iodide was administered, and the patient made a good recovery.

Gall-Stones; Cholelithiasis.—The chief constituents of gall-stones are cholesterin and bilirubin calcium; next in importance to these, Bland Sutton places calcium carbonate. Other bile pigments, bile salts, lime, desquamated epithelium, mucus, and sometimes foreign bodies, may also enter into their composition. According to Mayo-Robson, margarate, stearate, and palmitate of lime form the cement which binds the various ingredients together. Gall-stones formed almost entirely of bile pigment may be found; they are soft in consistence and may occupy the intrahepatic or the extrahepatic ducts. (Mayo-Robson.)

Cholesterin, the most important ingredient of gall-stones, is a monatomic alcohol, found in the blood and in various organs of the body. Since it is not excreted by the liver from the blood, and since it is found in other channels lined with mucous membrane and not connected with the bile, the conclusion is warranted that it is formed by the epithelium of the gall-bladder and bile-ducts. Why the cholesterin ordinarily present should form gall-stones in some cases and not in others, is difficult of explanation. Clinically, however, it is known that catarrh increases the amount of cholesterin, and that the longer the bile remains in the gall-bladder, the greater the amount of cholesterin. The former fact suggests the etiological importance of inflammation, the latter that of obstruction.

ETIOLOGY AND MODE OF FORMATION.—The etiological importance of germs was first suggested by Bernheim, who, in 1880, called attention to the frequent connection between typhoid and cholelithiasis. (Mayo-Robson.) Since then, both by clinical observation and by experimental evidence, the relationship has

been definitely established.   In Halsted's clinic it was found that one-third of
all cases of cholelithiasis gave a previous history of typhoid, and similar observations have been made by Robson and others.   Gilbert Dominice and Fournier,
in seventy cases of cholelithiasis, found colon bacilli, living or dead, in one-
third of the cases.

Cushing * noted, in several cases, the relation of cholelithiasis to typhoid.
In one case of cholelithiasis, although there was no history of typhoid, the bacillus of this disease was grown in pure culture from material taken from the
gall-bladder.   In other cases of cholelithiasis, in which there was a history of
preceding typhoid, the colon bacillus was found.   Cushing concludes that, during
the course of typhoid, the bacilli quite constantly invade the gall-bladder, there
retaining their vitality for a long time; that, in the course of time, they become
clumped, which suggests an agglutinative action; that these clumps serve as
nuclei on which are deposited biliary salts; that the micro-organisms may usually
be demonstrated in the centre of recent stones; and that, owing to the fact
that infective agents are present in such gall-stones, an inflammatory reaction
of varying intensity may be produced in these cases at any subsequent time.   The
frequency with which typhoid germs invade the gall-bladder and their persistency have quite recently been fully confirmed in a number of instances of
typhoid carriers.   Dowd has recently removed gall-stones containing typhoid
germs from patients in some of whom the attack of typhoid preceded the
operation by as long a time as thirty years.

Experimentally it has been shown in animals that micro-organisms not only
set up a cholecystitis, but also a tendency to cholelithiasis.   In two cases Gilbert
Dominice and Fournier succeeded in bringing about the formation of
a perfect stone.†   In order to produce stones experimentally by germs,
it was necessary to use cultures so attenuated that they were not pathogenic when introduced into the tissue of animals.   Virulent germs introduced caused sediment mixed with pus, but they showed no tendency to
cohere.   Attenuated germs, on the other hand, when injected into the gall-
bladder, were usually washed out, but occasionally they caused a stone to form.
If a foreign body was introduced at the same time, almost invariably the
formation of a stone followed.‡

The typhoid bacillus and the colon bacillus are the organisms which are
most frequently connected with cholelithiasis, but calculi have been produced
experimentally with staphylococci and streptococci, and even with non-patho-
genic germs.

The Routes of Infection.—The routes of infection are: (a) from the duodenum,
directly through the common duct; (b) from the blood, through the portal circulation.   It is doubtful whether the infective agent can pass up the common
duct directly while the flow of bile remains normal.   If, however, any obstruction
arises, the germs are then able to gain access.   Experimentally, in animals,

* Johns Hopkins Hosp. Bulletin No. 86, May, 1898.
† Arch. gén. de Méd., Sept., 1898.
‡ Mignot. in Arch. gén., Sept., 1898; and Brit. Med. Journal Supplement, 1898.

micro-organisms can be found in the bile after they have been injected into the portal circulation. In man, however, this is not a very common route of infection, but is probably the direction taken by infective agents in cholecystitis following appendicitis and other similar causes.

The Influence of Obstruction.—The second factor in the production of calculi —viz., obstruction—always, in some degree, accompanies infection; it may be increased by various other influences such as sedentary habits and lessened secretion of bile. Under the conditions of inefficient drainage and outflow, the organisms find not only easier access, but a more suitable medium for growth. Catarrhal or ulcerative affections of the duodenum may interfere with the secretion of the bile and hence diminish its outflow.

The time needed for the formation of biliary calculi cannot exactly be determined. They may begin to form as early as a few days after the establishment of an inflammatory condition, appearing at first as small particles on the mucous membrane and then continuing to grow by the deposit of cholesterin or bilirubin calcium, or of both. Once formed they do not tend to disappear except by escape through the common duct or through a fistulous communication, or by removal at operation. In Cushing's report, one case of empyema with numerous calculi was operated on three and a half months after an attack of uncomplicated typhoid.

Other factors in the etiology are: age, sex, diet, etc. Biliary calculi are rare before the age of thirty, common in middle life, and most common after the age of sixty, although many of those observed at this age, perhaps all, date their formation from an earlier period. Calculi also occur in the very young. Still * collected twenty cases in children, ten of which were in infants, and seven of these showed jaundice. Biliary calculi must, therefore, be considered a possible cause of icterus neonatorum. In some of the cases referred to, the stones were in the ducts, while in others they were in the gall-bladder. Still attributes the formation of calculi at this age to the viscosity of the bile.

Gall-stones occur more frequently in women than in men. According to the Mayo brothers, of eighteen hundred cases operated on, seventy-six per cent were in women, twenty-four per cent in men—a proportion which German and British statistics confirm. The disproportion is accounted for by several facts. Thus, sedentary habits are more common among women and constipation is more frequent; pregnancy, which throws additional work on the liver, has undoubtedly some predisposing influence; and tight lacing distorts the liver, lowers the fundus of the gall-bladder, may modify the circulation, and surely interferes with the flow of bile.

There is no doubt that diet has considerable influence on the production of gall-stones. As pointed out by Mayo-Robson, sodium glycocholate and sodium taurocholate, the normal salts of the bile, are produced by the metabolism of nitrogenous food. These salts hold cholesterin in solution, and, when they are diminished in amount, which may occur from a lessened ingestion of nitrogenous food, the cholesterin is precipitated. To this lessened consumption of nitrogen-

* Brit. Med. Jour., April 8th, 1899.

ous foods, Robson attributes the great prevalence of gall-stones in Germany. He further states that gall-stones are infrequent in diabetics, since their diet is mainly nitrogenous; while in the gouty, who limit nitrogenous ingestion, they are common.

The drinking of hard water has been suggested as an etiological factor in the production of gall-stones containing lime, but the relation has not been proven. A lessened amount of fluid intake may be a probable cause. (Mayo-Robson.)

The influence of a previous illness on the development of gall-stone disease is marked, and, as will be easily understood, the disease which most frequently precedes such a development is typhoid fever. The most striking statistics are those of Moynihan, who operated for gall-stone disease on seven individuals, all of them under twenty-one years of age and all of them giving a history of having previously had typhoid fever.

CLASSIFICATION.—Naunyn (quoted by Bland Sutton) has arranged gall-stones, according to their composition, in the following classes: (1) Pure cholesterin stones; (2) laminated cholesterin stones; (3) the common gall-bladder stones; (4) mixed bilirubin calcium stones; (5) pure bilirubin calcium stones, which occur in the form of small, black, waxy concretions, or as small, gray, pebble-like structures, with a metallic lustre; (6) rarer forms, among which should be included: (a) whitish concretions resembling pearls and consisting of a nucleus of bilirubin calcium coated with cholesterin; (b) calcium carbonate calculi—small chalk-like bodies which are very rare; (c) concretions formed around foreign bodies; (d) casts of bile-ducts, consisting of bilirubin calcium. These last are rare in man.

The size of gall-stones varies greatly. The largest calculus mentioned in the literature is described by Hutchinson and depicted by Mayo-Robson. It weighed three ounces and five drachms, and was nearly the size of a goose egg. The smallest gall-stones are very minute, and a quantity of these small stones is referred to as biliary sand. The average size of gall-stones is difficult to determine, but it may be stated that the cystic and even the common duct is often blocked by a concretion no larger than a cherry stone. The shape varies in accordance with a variety of factors. Thus, when there are several of them, the stones are facetted, and these facets are smooth. A single stone embraced closely by the gall-bladder may be rough and tuberculated, the tubercles corresponding to the foveola of the mucous membrane. A stone in one of the ducts, with companion stones at either end, may be barrel- or drum-shaped. Stones in the early stages are soft; those from the intrahepatic ducts are often curiously shaped, corresponding to the spaces in which they lodge. In number, stones vary from one to several thousand. Otto records an instance in which there were 7,802, Naunyn one in which there were 5,000 stones. As will be readily understood, the number will depend largely on the minimum of size to which one assigns the rank of a calculus and the patience with which one counts the small concretions usually called biliary sand.

PATHOLOGY, COMPLICATIONS, AND SYMPTOMS.—The pathology and symptomatology are all modified in great degree by the part of the excretory apparatus most affected, also by the degree of obstruction which exists and the virulence of the infection. They may, therefore, very well be considered together.

Gall-stones are produced in the gall-bladder more frequently than elsewhere, because of the more favorable conditions, viz., the relatively stagnant condition of the bile, the presence of micro-organisms, and, as pointed out by Naunyn, the presence of bilirubin calcium, which cements together the cholesterin crystals. In the gall-bladder too, the stones remain and grow, undisturbed by the currents in the bile-ducts. (Fig. 89.)

Gall-stones may exist in the gall-bladder under the following different conditions:—

(a) Without obstruction and with entire absence of infection.—Under these conditions there are no symptoms, and the presence of stones is unsuspected and often discovered only at autopsy.

(b) In the presence of a sudden temporary obstruction at the neck of the gall-bladder.—This may be due to the fact that a stone blocks the entrance, or that the latter is swollen through the influence of infection, or both. Under these conditions the gall-bladder becomes rapidly filled with a thin mucous fluid and spasm is produced. When relaxation takes place, the bladder empties itself and the attack ceases. The symptoms of this condition are: sudden colics, which last for only a few moments or may continue for several

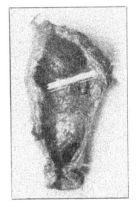

FIG. 89.—Gall-Bladder Containing a Gall-Stone at the Fundus and Another at the Neck. (From the Museum of the New York University and Bellevue Hospital Medical College.)

hours, and cease as suddenly as they began. Relief is frequently accompanied by vomiting; indeed, the latter may produce the necessary relaxation, and a dose of morphine frequently causes the same effect. There is little or no elevation of temperature or acceleration of pulse, owing to the facts that the infection is mild, that the lymphatics of the bladder are scanty and consequently absorption takes place only feebly, and that, as the organ is distensible, the infected material is not under great tension. (Mayo.) There is no jaundice. The pain is in or near the median line and radiates through to the back, and upward rather than downward. The condition is often mistaken for gastralgia. The attacks are intermittent and may not reappear for years, giving rise to the impression that they have been corrected by specific medication.

(c) Gall-Stones impacted in the Pelvis of the Gall-Bladder. (Fig. 90.)— In this condition the attack begins as in the former, but is more severe, lasts longer, and is accompanied by tenderness and rigidity. Frequently the gall-bladder becomes distended with clear fluid, with no admixture of bile (the so-called cystic bladder, *hydrops vesicæ felleæ*) and forms an apparent tumor. This condition may terminate in several ways:—(1) Drainage may be re-established and the tumor may disappear rather rapidly; (2) the tumor may disappear slowly by absorption; (3) the contents of the gall-bladder may become infected, producing an empyema; (4) the stone may be forced on, into or through the cystic duct, and, if it lodges in the cystic or the common duct, it will introduce new symptoms; (5) the gall-bladder may shrink on the stone, and typical colics. may not reappear.

The symptoms are as follows: there is colic, the pain lasting longer than it does in the ordinary attacks, and with it there are tenderness and rigidity; in some cases there is a recognizable swelling due to enlargement of the gall-bladder; the temperature is not high, for the reasons already stated; even in empyema it rises only to 101° or 102° F.; and the pulse is not much accelerated. The symptoms of the contracted gall-bladder are those of a chronic and persistent dyspepsia.

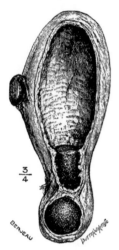

Fig. 90.—Gall-Bladder with Gall-Stone Impacted in the Cystic Duct. The small body on the gall-bladder is an accessory liver. (From Bland Sutton.)

Multiple calculi may exist in the gall-bladder under one of the following conditions:—(1) When the gall-bladder is filled with fluid, one of the stones occluding the duct permanently or temporarily, and causing continuous or intermittent distention. Sometimes in emaciated people a fremitus produced by the floating stones may be elicited. (2) Multiple stones may be found embedded in inspissated mucus. (3) The gall-bladder may contract on several stones, producing a loculus for each; this is called encapsulation. A solitary stone may occupy the gall-bladder, floating about in fluid, occasionally blocking the exit, and causing intermittent hydrops; or it may be firmly clasped by the contracted wall of the gall-bladder, as a result of which the stone assumes a tuberculated surface. Two stones in a gall-bladder which is contracted may produce the so-called hour-glass bladder. Sometimes a gall-stone may ulcerate through the mucous membrane and come to lie between the mucous and the muscular coats. The passage of communication between this pocket and the gall-bladder may later be obliterated, thereby producing a puzzling situation, spoken of as gall-stones in diverticula. (Bland Sutton.)

Among the interesting but rare pathological changes may be mentioned axial rotation of a gall-bladder and spontaneous fracture of gall-stones. (Bland Sutton.)

Gall-stones in the Cystic Duct.—When the cystic duct is occluded by a calculus, the part behind is often so dilated that it is difficult to delimit this duct with any precision. The size of a calculus necessary to block this duct depends on many conditions and cannot be exactly stated. Bland Sutton says he has often found the channel obstructed by a stone no larger than a cherry pit. Calculi in the cystic duct may be single or multiple. According to Bland

Sutton, they may occur in sets of three, the middle one facetted. These stones. are often bile-stained, showing that bile has trickled past and that the obstruction is not or has not always been complete; the stones are usually large, and must, therefore, have grown after entering the duct.

Stones impacted in the cystic duct give rise to the following lesions and symptoms: (1) A distended gall-bladder. According to Bland Sutton the largest gall-bladders are the result of distention caused in this manner, and they may be mistaken for a cystic kidney or an ovarian cyst. (Lawson Tait.) In the large gall-bladders, in which the bile is discharged intermittently, there may be an invasion by germs, usually the colon bacilli, and these may cause cholangitis with chills, fever, and sweating, or the pancreatic ducts may be invaded, as a result of which pancreatitis is set up and fat necrosis follows. (2) The gall-bladder may be contracted and thick-walled, containing a thin muco-purulent fluid. Under these conditions the patient, at irregular intervals, has chills, fever, and sweating, with a high temperature. The symptoms may be acute, but they subside rapidly. The digestion is disordered, the food taken causes distress, and there is loss of weight, but there is no jaundice. The elevation of temperature is explained by the grade of infection and by the fact that the duct is non-distensible and is fairly supplied with absorbents.

The marked gastric symptoms, with severe emaciation, which accompany contracted gall-bladder, may suggest gastric ulcer.

Gall-stones in the Common Duct.—Stones found in the common duct may have formed there or in the hepatic duct, but usually they come from the gall-bladder. The point at which a stone is arrested varies; the upper part of the common duct is the widest portion of the canal, but at any stage the irregularly acting elements of infection may cause a degree of swelling that will disturb the anatomical relations.

There may be only one stone, but frequently there are several. Sometimes the spaces between the stones are filled with biliary gravel, and occasionally the canal is filled with a soft, putty-like mass of cholesterin and inspissated bile. The degree of the blockade will then vary and is rarely absolute. When a single stone lodges, the duct behind dilates and gradually the bile forces its way around the stone. From time to time the stone is forced firmly into the undilated part of the duct and then complete obstruction is temporarily produced. The variations in the degree of the obstruction are expressed clinically by changes in the jaundice. A gall-stone lodged in this manner has been called by Fenger the ball-valve stone.*

The duct behind the stone often dilates until it is large enough to admit the finger, and this distention extends back to both the extrahepatic and intrahepatic ducts. Sometimes the dilatation of the common duct is so great that it has been mistaken for the gall-bladder. The gall-bladder, however, contrary to what would be expected, is usually contracted—a condition which is due, as pointed out by Courvoisier, to the greater degree of cholecystitis that has. existed.

* Amer. Journ. Medical Sciences, 1896, cxi.

A stone impacted in the common duct may produce ulceration, and rarely it opens into the abdominal cavity; more frequently, adhesions form and a fistulous communication is established with one of the hollow viscera, particularly the duodenum. In not a few cases this.ulceration occurs near the termination of the duct and is mistaken for a dilatation of the duodenal ostium, and sometimes through ulceration the stone comes to occupy a diverticulum. (J. D. Bryant.)

Infection often finds its way from the duodenum into the bile-ducts, there setting up cholangitis; and, when the latter is associated with ulceration, a general peritonitis or a local or subphrenic abscess is likely to develop. It would appear that an empyema is rarely established. Sometimes infection of the common duct extends to the neighboring veins, causing a septic pylephlebitis; if the portal veins are involved, multiple hepatic abscesses will result; if the azygos veins are involved, septic infarction of the lung may occur. The results of thrombosis of the vena cava are obvious; fortunately, these complications are rare.

When the dilated intrahepatic ducts become infected, multiple biliary abscesses are formed,—a condition which it is difficult to diagnose, and which is usually indicated by an exacerbation of the general symptoms and by well-marked jaundice due to complete obstruction of the ducts. These abscesses may ulcerate into the contiguous branches of the portal vein.

The symptoms, as will be easily understood, depend, not only on the degree of obstruction and the virulence and extent of the infection, but also on the location of the stone. Clinically, the following symptoms may be described:—(1) Temporary attacks of jaundice.—A stone which passes the cystic duct usually produces its symptoms while this object is in transit through that duct, and jaundice is not one of these. When, through infection and swelling of the mucous membrane, the stone is temporarily arrested in the common duct, the symptoms will be pain, local tenderness, increased rapidity of pulse, some elevation of temperature, jaundice more or less severe, but usually mild and always temporary, a rather sudden cessation of the symptoms, and the recovery of the stone from the stools. (2) Symptoms indicative of the presence of a ball-valve stone.— Here all the symptoms are remittent or even intermittent, and the intervals are irregular. When obstruction is complete, the pain, tenderness, etc., increase and jaundice deepens; the stools become light in color; and there is bile in the urine. The temperature, depending as it does on the grade and extent of the cholangitis, may be very high. When the bile begins to pass through the duct all the symptoms decrease and the jaundice fades. Jaundice, as has been pointed out, changes from time to time in the case of the single stone. It may become well-marked when the duct is completely obstructed, but very rarely indeed is it so pronounced and of such a deep shade as it is in the case of cancer of the gall-bladder, of the extrahepatic ducts, or of the head of the pancreas. (Courvoisier's law.) (3) Symptoms observed in multiple biliary abscesses.— The symptoms are those of severe infection; the liver is enlarged and tender, and the jaundice is that indicative of obstruction. This condition is rarely diagnosed, and once the diagnosis is established the outlook must be considered utterly hopeless. (4) Symptoms observed when .the ·obstruction is in the ampulla. (Fig. 91.)—The pancreatic ducts may then be infected, and the result will depend on the degree of infection, and also on the fact whether or not the accessory pancreatic duct is occluded. (5) Symptoms observed when stones ulcerate their way through from the common bile-duct to the duodenum.— When this event occurs there are usually marked symptoms of local peritonitis and obstruction. Sometimes, when the ulcer is located near the termination of the duct, a complete spontaneous cure follows. In some cases, however, the fistulous opening is sufficiently large to allow the fluid, but not the stones, or only a part of the stones, to escape. (6) Symptoms observed when the conditions are quiescent.—Stones may remain in the common duct or in a diver-

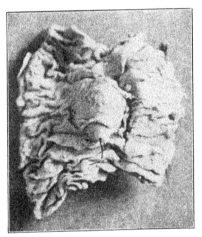

FIG. 91.—Mucous Membrane of the Duodenum; the specimen shows a stone in the ampulla of Vater.
(From the Museum of the New York University and Bellevue Hospital Medical College.)

ticulum for years without causing any symptoms. Usually, however, there are evidences of dyspepsia, with loss of flesh.

Gall-Stones in the Hepatic Duct.—Gall-stones in the hepatic duct are a not infrequent accompaniment of gall-stones in the other extrahepatic or intrahepatic ducts. It is unusual for them to occur independently of such association, although they may, of course, be formed in the hepatic ducts. When the common duct is obstructed by a gall-stone and all the ducts behind this are dilated, stones escaping from the gall-bladder may easily enter the hepatic ducts. Sometimes during operation a stone may escape in this way and elude capture.

Clinically, hepatic-duct stones may be classed with common-duct stones. The attacks which characterize their becoming impacted are much the same; infection is liable to occur, abscesses may form behind the stone or in the intrahepatic ducts, and jaundice is a constant symptom.

Stones in the Intrahepatic Ducts. (Fig. 92.)—Stones in the intrahepatic ducts are rare. · They are usually small and of the bilirubin calcium variety; they are soft and take the shape of the bile-ducts when the latter are dilated. There are frequently many stones in adjoining ducts, and when this is the case they are likely to be facetted. As a rule, the presence of these intra-hepatic calculi gives rise to no symptoms. The condition, furthermore, is not

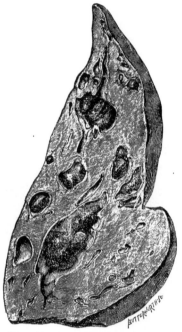

FIG. 92.—A Section of the Liver with Dilated Ducts Containing Gall-Stones. The illustration was engraved from a photograph supplied to the author by Dr. Mitchell Stevens. (From Bland Sutton.)

amenable to surgical treatment. Infection, however, may induce cholangitis, obstructive jaundice, and even abscess.

COMPLICATIONS.—The more important complications are the following:— (1) acute perforation of the gall-bladder; (2) biliary fistula; (3) intestinal obstruction; (4) adhesions; (5) stricture of the ducts; (6) involvement of the pancreas.

(1) *Acute Perforation of the Gall-Bladder*, with escape of its contents into the peritoneal cavity, is followed by a peritoneal crisis, the same as that which occurs after perforation of one of the other abdominal viscera. The history of the disease, in any given case, will help to establish the differentiation.

(2) *Biliary Fistula.*—In biliary fistula, where a communication is established between the gall-bladder or the dilated bile-ducts and some hollow viscus, the occurrence is usually preceded by severe symptoms. When the terminal portion of the common duct sloughs into the duodenum, causing an increase in the size of the ostium, the occurrence may be followed by permanent relief. Before the perforation occurs there are often marked symptoms of obstruction, and this is particularly apt to be the case when the fistula is located near the pylorus. Occasionally the opening, while permitting the discharge of the retained fluid, does not allow the stones, or at most only a few of them, to escape. Frequently the opening closes spontaneously, and often, while the more severe disorders are ameliorated, chronic digestive symptoms persist. In all cases where there are adhesions, and where the history suggests even remotely the existence of a biliary fistula, the separation of the parts at the time of the operation should be made with the greatest care, for fear of leaving undiscovered, in some rough and bleeding area, a minute communication with the bowel.

An external biliary fistula (the discharge of gall-stones on the surface of the body) occurs, but infrequently. The opening, in such cases, usually is near the umbilicus, the escaping contents being guided, no doubt, by the falciform ligament.

(3) *Intestinal Obstruction from Gall-Stones.*—A gall-stone large enough to block the intestine rarely finds its way into the latter, and, when it does, it probably reaches the intestine by way of a biliary fistula. The signs would be those of intestinal obstruction with a preceding history of gall-stones. Indeed, there may have been obvious swelling of the gall-bladder, which has disappeared only to be followed by signs of intestinal obstruction. (Bland Sutton.) In rare instances the stone may be felt in its course from the small to the large intestine. (Maclagan.) Prompt treatment is necessary.

(4) *Adhesions.*—Adhesions may interfere with the drainage and function of the gall-bladder, producing marked symptoms, whether stones be present or not. In most cases of gall-bladder disease, extensive adhesions are present, and their separation, during the progress of an operation, requires patient persistence.

The treatment of adhesions is the same as that for gall-stones. The gall-bladder, with the calculi contained in it, is to be removed; any bands that may obstruct the remaining common duct are to be divided; and afterward the great omentum and the transverse colon are to be transplanted upward in such a manner as to cover any existing raw surfaces and thus prevent adhesions between the stomach and duodenum—organs the normal performance of whose functions depends on unrestricted mobility.

(5) *Strictures of the Ducts.*—Strictures of the ducts result from the irritation caused by stones, and may develop after surgical removal of the latter or after they have escaped spontaneously. Strictures of the cystic duct should be treated by removal of the gall-bladder; those in the common duct by a plastic operation, by reimplantation into the duodenum, or by cholecystenterostomy.

(6) *Involvement of the Pancreas.*—Involvement of the pancreas is a common complication of impaction of gall-stones in the common duct, particularly in the

lower part. (See article on "Surgery of the Pancreas.") When the stone is in the ampulla the interference with drainage invites infection and pancreatitis. The obstruction may be complete, but even then, in a certain proportion of the cases, the accessory duct of Santorini permits the discharge of the pancreatic secretion. On the other hand, sclerosis of the head of the pancreas and cancer of that portion of the organ may obstruct the common bile-duct.

Other complications are: abscess of the liver, usually multiple; subphrenic abscess; peritonitis, localized when it complicates cholecystitis, more or less general when rupture has occurred; and pyelitis, which may result from rupture into the pelvis of the kidney. Cancer, which is a frequent complication, will be dealt with elsewhere.

ANALYSIS OF SYMPTOMS.—The signs and symptoms have already been considered to some extent in connection with the pathology and localization of gall-stones, but, for the purpose of diagnosis, it will be instructive to restate them in a general way. These symptoms are pain, nausea and vomiting, jaundice, fever, hemorrhage, enlargement of the gall-bladder, and perhaps enlargement of the liver.

Pain.—Pain is variable, its severity depending on the degree of obstruction, on the degree and extent of the inflammation, and on the fact whether the latter is limited to the ducts or has already invaded the contiguous peritoneum. Paroxysmal pain—biliary colic—is the most typical expression of the symptom. It occurs when a stone is impacted in the neck of the gall-bladder, or is being forced through the cystic or the common duct. It usually begins suddenly, lasts for a varying period of time (from a few hours to a few days), and ends suddenly, being frequently accompanied or preceded by vomiting. A sudden ending of the pain occurs when a stone impacted at the neck of the gall-bladder drops back, or when one impacted in the common duct is extruded into the duodenum. A more gradual cessation of the pain will follow when, although impaction remains, gradual dilatation of the duct permits the retained fluid to escape more or less freely. The same thing occurs when, in the case of a distended gall-bladder, the mild character of the infection permits a gradual absorption of the retained fluid to take place. A stone, passing from the cystic to the common duct, may clear the latter rapidly, slowly, or not at all, the result depending on the infection and the degree of the swelling. Pain is considered by some to be due to inflammation, by others to be the result of spasm; both, no doubt, are factors, and the character of the pain will depend on which predominates. The agonizing colic, resembling nephritic colic and accompanied by little or no increase of temperature, is strongly characteristic. The passage of tenacious mucus, or of pieces of the wall of a hydatid cyst, is also said to excite these colicky pains. The pain of associated peritonitis is often lancinating in character, and is further modified by the extent and severity of the peritoneal involvement.

Atypical pain occurs in almost endless variety. For example, pain may come on after the ingestion of food; it may be severe or be only a sense of discomfort; it is often a midline pain (Mayo), and suggests gastralgia or some form of dyspepsia. The pain caused by adhesions (gall-stones being present or having already passed) is also accompanied by gastric symptoms and may be severe, but is often dull or burning in character.

Pain and other symptoms suggesting dyspepsia are probably more common than the typical colicky pain. The pain accompanying stone in the gall-bladder and associated with a mild degree of inflammation is often of a dull, aching character, and is increased by pressure. Gradual distention of the gall-bladder causes pain of the same character. Severe pain accompanies the passage of a stone through a fistula and perforative cholecystitis. In the latter case, however, it is diffuse, resembling that which accompanies perforation of the stomach or the appendix.

Pain is usually localized in the right hypochondrium, but it may, particularly in the colics and infections, be limited to the ducts, gall-bladder, and liver, or be referred to the back and upward toward the right subscapular region. Sometimes the pain is transferred to the right suprascapular region and down the arm—a phenomenon which is explained by the connection between the phrenic and the suprascapular nerves. It is believed by the writer, however, that the pain does not commonly extend above the level of the scapular region, that it travels through the lower intercostals, and that it is reflected upward rather than downward.

Pain may be on the left side of the stomach, indicating the presence of adhesions (Mayo-Robson); it may simulate ulcer of the stomach; it may be reflected downward into the loin, suggesting kidney colic; or it may be exhibited over the precardium, suggesting cardiac difficulty. Peritonitis may produce pain in any part of the abdomen.

Tenderness.—In cholecystitis tenderness is found, according to Mayo-Robson, at the junction of the middle and lower thirds of a line drawn from the ninth costal cartilage to the umbilicus. Others locate it just beneath the outer border of the right rectus. The gall-bladder being a movable organ and liable to great variations in position, it is doubtful whether the area of tenderness can always be so definitely located. According to Boas, another point of tenderness is found two or three finger-breadths to the right of the spine of the twelfth dorsal vertebra. Tenderness over a distended gall-bladder may be very slight, and it is increased by inflammation, particularly of the peritoneum.

Nausea and Vomiting.—Nausea and vomiting are almost constant accompaniments of an attack of gall-stone colic; the vomiting usually subsides with relief of the colic, but in some cases it may persist. The vomitus at first consists of the contents of the stomach, but later it may become bilious, feculent, or even stercoraceous. Vomiting often determines the cessation of the colic, especially in those cases in which a stone blocks the orifice of the cystic duct only temporarily, afterward falling back into the gall-bladder. Nausea and vomiting due to reflex irritation frequently occur apart from colic, and are particularly common in cases of impaction of stone in the cystic duct or of obstruction at the neck of the gall-bladder, either from stone, from kinking, or from stricture. Vomiting may be either periodical or continuous, and is sometimes persistent even after relief of the obstruction by operation. Vomiting and pain without jaundice often lead patients to seek relief from supposed stomach or digestive trouble.

Jaundice.—Jaundice is present in a variable number of cases of cholelithiasis. It is said, by Murphy, to have been present in only fourteen per cent of his cases. Fuerbringer found it in twenty-five per cent, while Wolff states that in his experience it was present in one-half of the cases. It is due to obstruction of the flow of bile, and this in turn may be caused in a variety of ways:—It may be due (a) to obstruction of the common or hepatic duct by calculus; (b) to obstruction of the common duct by pressure of a stone in the cystic duct; or (c) to infection of the ducts, with swelling of the mucous membrane to such a degree as to produce occlusion, the infection extending from the gall-bladder (the seat of gall-stones, with cholecystitis) or from the duodenum. (See page 229.) The obstruction may also be caused (d) by stricture of the duct and by cancer or other tumor pressing on the duct.

The character of the jaundice varies; as a rule, it is not severe. Even in cases of impaction of a stone in the common duct, the jaundice is usually intermittent in character,—a phenomenon that is explained by the assumption that the accumulating bile escapes by passing between the stone and the wall of the duct—the so-called "Ball-valve action" of the stone. Thus the remittent nature of the jaundice becomes quite characteristic of the condition; it may vary from morning to night, or the variation may extend over a day. It never becomes so intense nor so persistent as the jaundice seen in cases of malignant disease of the head of the pancreas. It often deepens after a renewed attack of pain.

In stricture of the common duct the jaundice is, of course, continuous and does not vary at intervals. In the cases in which the jaundice appears subsequently to the colic, and after the stone has completely passed, it is only slight and disappears in a few days. Stone in the ampulla usually produces a deep jaundice.

Elevation of Temperature.—Gall-stones of themselves can cause no rise of temperature. The chill which occurs in biliary colic, and which is accompanied by a slight fever (100°–102° F.), is said by some to be due to nervous influence, by others to be always due to the inflammation present. As a matter of fact, probably both influences prevail. The degree of infection and its localization are the determining factors in the production of fever in cholelithiasis. Infection limited to the gall-bladder does not, as already noted, produce much fever; the scanty lymphatic supply preventing absorption of toxins to any great extent. The temperature in these cases does not often rise above 101° or 102° F. On the other hand, some authors say that a stone impacted in the cystic duct, and associated with purulent infection of the gall-bladder and duct, may produce irregular attacks of chills and a high temperature (from 105° to 107° Fahr.)— manifestations which are due to the excellent facilities for absorption afforded by the presence of lymph nodes on each side of the duct, and to the fact that the inflammatory products are under great tension. If suppuration supervenes the fever becomes continuous; but, if the obstruction is not permanent, attacks of cholecystitis produce a temperature which subsides as soon as the obstruction is relieved.

The classical temperature phenomena associated with cholelithiasis occur when there is obstruction in the common duct with infection extending more or less deeply into the intrahepatic ducts. This combination of pathological factors produces the disease known as infective cholangitis, which is characterized by an intermittent or remittent type of fever. The temperature curve is remarkably septic in type. There are periodical attacks of chills and a rise of temperature from 101° to 104° F., followed by sweating,—"the intermittent biliary fever" of Charcot,—and during the intervals the temperature may return to normal. Such an abrupt rise of temperature produces a characteristic appearance on a temperature chart. Moynihan calls such a chart the "steeple chart." When a chronic cholangitis is present the temperature is more remittent in type, the normal point not being reached between separate attacks; or it may remain persistently high, showing an extensive intrahepatic infection of the bile-ducts, or, in some cases, the existence of single or multiple hepatic abscesses.

Hemorrhage.—In deeply jaundiced cases the coagulation time of the blood is increased from the normal (viz., three or four minutes) to ten or twelve minutes or even a longer time; and there is a tendency to hemorrhage from both gastric and intestinal mucous membranes. A hemorrhage of this nature may be severe enough to cause death. Hemorrhage may also occur from ulceration either of the gall-bladder or of the ducts. During or following operation the same tendency is noted and sometimes is persistent; uncontrollable fatal oozing from the wound may occur. This is most liable to happen in the deep jaundice of cancer, in which disease all reparative tendencies are reduced; but it may follow prolonged and deep jaundice from any cause, and should be seriously considered before any operation is undertaken. Just why the blood shows this lack of a tendency to coagulate is not understood, and coagulation tests undertaken before operation give very little knowledge of practical surgical worth. However, when there is deep jaundice with purpuric spots, when the patient's vitality is at a low ebb, and when the coagulation time of the blood is increased, operation should not be attempted at all, or imperative operations should be limited to the least manipulation possible. For the relief of this hemorrhagic tendency, calcium chloride, calcium lactate, and adrenalin have been recommended; but each of these drugs has more opponents than advocates.

Enlargement of the Gall-Bladder.—Enlargement of the gall-bladder is caused by blocking of the cystic duct, which may be effected by the presence of a stone, by cancer of the head of the pancreas, or by cancer of the gall-bladder itself, and also by stricture of the common duct. In all of these, obstruction is the predominant factor. Impaction of a stone in the common duct, on the other hand, is usually associated with contraction of the gall-bladder, due to the facts that the obstruction is not complete and that repeated attacks of cholecystitis have produced in the gall-bladder a stronger tendency to contract than to expand.

In empyema there is, of course, inflammation, but not sufficient to overcome the enlargement.

The size to which the gall-bladder may be distended varies. There is on record a case in which the distended viscus was mistaken for an ovarian cyst. In another case the gall-bladder occupied the sac of a hernia. Ordinarily the enlargement forms a pear-shaped tumor situated just below the costal margin (unless displaced) and to the right of the rectus muscle. It moves with respiration, may be displaced from side to side, and can often be seen.

As a rule, the enlargement is accompanied by tenderness, which is due in part to the tension; but still more to the inflammation present. It is elicited by pressure over the enlarged organ, or, where the enlargement is not great, by pressure exerted beneath the ribs while the patient makes deep inspiratory efforts. An enlarged gall-bladder, without pain or tenderness, is usually cancerous.

When the gall-bladder is large enough to be recognizable by means of palpation, the organ contains mucus' (with or without bile, with or without gallstones) and pus, or it is the seat of cancer. When it is appreciably enlarged it oftens drags down the linguiform process or lobe of the liver, and the association of the two conditions is so frequent that Riedel (quoted by Bland Sutton) regards the presence of such a lobe, with other signs of cholecystitis, as evidence of the existence of an enlarged gall-bladder beneath. When the enlarged viscus is removed the linguiform lobe disappears. (Bland Sutton.)

Cancer in the gall-bladder forms a well-defined enlargement; cancer infiltrating the walls of this organ soon becomes apparent in the adjacent liver tissue.

Enlargement of the liver, with tenderness, is commonly present in an attack of colic, but it subsides when drainage has been restored by removal of the obstruction. In extensive cholangitis this enlargement and tenderness are well-marked and persistent.

The Urine.—In cases of obstructive jaundice the urine will show the presence of bilirubin and biliverdin (oxidation products of the bile) even before jaundice is apparent in the skin or in the sclera. Gmelin's test for the detection of bilirubin is performed by adding fuming nitric acid to the suspected urine in such a way that that the acid underlies the urine. At the junction of the two liquids there is formed a circular disk, with green above and a succession of colors—blue, violet, red, reddish-yellow—below. The presence of albumin which is precipitated, obscures the colors, and indican, by giving a blue, which, with the yellow of the urine, produces a green, also tends to mislead. (Mayo-Robson.) There are many other tests for bile in the urine. Ordinarily, a yellowish-green tint recognizable in the froth of shaken urine, or a similar stain given to filter paper, is sufficient to determine the presence of bile pigments.* In later stages of jaundice, albumin and renal casts may occur, and the latter may contain pigment granules and pigmented cells. (Bland Sutton.)

The Feces.—In obstructive jaundice there is usually constipation, and

* Kelly, in Osler, vol. v., page 695.

the stools become clay-colored and offensive in odor. The change in color is due to the absence of urobilin. The normal color of the stools is due, not to bile pigments which are absorbable, but to an insoluble, non-absorbable pigment which results from the action of the pancreatic juice on some of the bile pigments. The absence of either bile or pancreatic juice, therefore, produces this change in the color of the stools. (Keen's "Syst. of Surgery," Vol. III.) The color is also due, in part, to the presence of fat (steatorrhœa) and bubbles of gas. The digestion of fat is carried on by the bile and the pancreatic secretion, more particularly the latter. Hence steatorrhœa is even more marked in pancreatic failure. In pancreatic obstruction, unassociated with jaundice, the stools may be light or whitish from the large amount of fat present, and yet contain a considerable amount of biliary derivatives. "It is not always warrantable, therefore, to base, on the color of the stools, an opinion of the amount of bile that enters the intestines or the degree of biliary stasis." (Kelly, in Osler's System, Vol. V., page 698.)

Gall-stones in the feces constitute a most valuable piece of diagnostic evidence. To discover them the excreta should be carefully watched for a week or more after the attack of colic. The simplest and least offensive way is to mix carbolic acid with the evacuations and then to pour them on gauze stretched over the mouth of a suitable vessel. There are many small solid bodies which may in this way be separated from the feces, and which are often mistaken for gall-stones. Thus, the writer has in mind a recent case in which the patient brought a large number, fifty or sixty, of supposed stones. Under a magnifying glass these proved to be fruit seeds, although the patient insisted that he had eaten no fruit in over a week. Bland Sutton and others point out that small globular bodies are frequently found in the feces after the administration of olive oil, and that the laity and even careless physicians are thereby led to the erroneous conclusion that these bodies are extruded gall-stones.

The circulating blood also contains bile pigments which may be detected by filling a small capillary tube with blood from a puncture in the lobe of the ear, sealing both ends of the tube, and allowing it to stand vertically for a few hours, until the clot separates from the serum. Normal serum is colorless; a yellowish tinge indicates the presence of bile, and the depth of the color indicates the amount. (Hamil, quoted by Mayo-Robson.)

Skiagraphy is seldom of much value, because cholesterin stones, the common variety, produce no more shadow than does the liver substance. Calcium stones give a deeper shadow, but these stones are rare. The evidence afforded by the Roentgen rays is, therefore, not trustworthy.

For the purpose of detecting enlargements of the gall-bladder, some have advised the administration of a light chloroform anæsthesia or a dose of morphine. The administration of chloroform, because of its destructive action on the liver, should not be lightly undertaken.

DIAGNOSIS.—The diagnosis of cholelithiasis, based on intermittent attacks of biliary colic and the occurrence of jaundice, with the recovery of stones from the feces, is not difficult. On the other hand, there may be only vague symptoms of what appears to be a chronic and incurable dyspepsia, associated with a dull aching in the right hypochondrium, slight tenderness over the gall-bladder, and possibly some other symptoms. In such cases the diagnosis may be exceedingly difficult.

The history should always be taken with great care. By questioning the patient very closely one may elicit such facts as that he has had previous attacks of pain or a yellowish discoloration of the sclera, and thus a connection with some disorder of the biliary passages may be established. Due consideration should also be given to such etiological factors as the patient's diet and his habits as to the use of alcoholic drinks; he should also be asked whether he has previously suffered from typhoid or other abdominal infection. The history, however, may sometimes be misleading, as is well illustrated by the case reported by Bland Sutton, viz., that of a young woman who was suddenly seized with a violent pain in the abdomen. One physician diagnosed a twisted ovarian pedicle; her regular attendant considered the case one of biliary colic; Bland Sutton rather attributed the pain to appendicitis. Operation revealed a ruptured ectopic pregnancy, but calculi were also found in the gall-bladder and there was a chronic cholecystitis.

Differential Diagnosis.—The differential diagnosis will have to be made from the following list of diseases, which has been compiled from Mayo-Robson and others: hysteria; locomotor ataxia; acute dyspepsia with flatulence; chronic dyspepsia; appendicitis; right renal colic; pancreatitis, acute and chronic, and pancreatic calculus; ulcers, gastric, pyloric, or duodenal; peritoneal adhesions and pericholecystitis; intercostal neuralgia; malignant growth in the liver, gall-bladder, bile ducts, or head of the pancreas; pyloric stenosis; intestinal colic; angina pectoris; pneumonia and pleurisy; abdominal enlargements due to hydronephrosis, to tumors of the colon or the pylorus, and to ovarian or mesenteric cysts; and all conditions causing jaundice.

In the case of most of these diseases the differentiation should not be difficult.

A few of the more important diseases mentioned above will be considered in detail. In acute dyspepsia with flatulence, the pain is over the stomach and is relieved by simple treatment. In a case of chronic dyspepsia that has not been benefited by several months of intelligent treatment, there is usually found some anatomical basis for the disease. (Kelly, in Osler's System, Vol. V.)— In right renal colic the pain is usually in the back, loin, or groin; it is reflected down the ureter into the testicle or along the inner side of the thigh. The tenderness is over the kidney, posteriorly as well as anteriorly; the urine contains blood, in either macroscopical or microscopical amounts, a proportionate amount of albumin, perhaps crystals or even a calculus, pus, and epithelial cells, but no bile.—Lead colic will give a history of exposure, and there will be a blue line on the gums; the stomach or abdominal discomfort will be continuous; constipation is present; there are also anæmia, a basophilic degeneration of the red cells, and perhaps wrist-drop. The result of treatment will be convincing.—Intestinal colic has often an obvious cause; the pain radiates from the umbilicus, is intermittent, and disappears with the removal of the cause; tympanites is present, with eructation of gas or a discharge of gas and feces.—Pyloric stenosis with adhesions often gives symptoms closely resembling those of cholelithiasis; indeed, they are often associated, the pericholecystitis and perigastritis of gall-stones being a frequent cause of pyloric obstruction.   Pyloric stenosis without biliary disease may show a dilated stomach, visible peristalsis, and the characteristic vomitus; the pain is over the stomach and left side of the abdomen, and the characteristic gall-bladder pain is absent.—In ulcer (gastric, pyloric, or duodenal) pain is associated with the ingestion of food, there are nausea and vomiting, and the tenderness may be in the median line; all of these symptoms may occur, it is true, in cholelithiasis.   In ulcer, however, the pain recurs regularly; there may be tenderness posteriorly on the left side near the vertebra; there are hæmatemesis and hyperchlorhydria; jaundice and hepatic fever are absent.—Acute pancreatitis exhibits the symptoms of peritonitis and might be mistaken for acute cholecystitis were it not that the symptoms are more severe.   Exploratory operation is indicated in both cases.   Chronic pancreatitis is frequently associated with cholelithiasis, and, as drainage is called for, the differentiation between the two is not so essential.   The same is true of cancer of the pancreas. In pancreatitis the pain and tenderness are epigastric; the pain radiates to the scapula or to the left; there are rapid loss of flesh and fatty stools, and the Cammidge crystals may be found in the urine.   If jaundice occurs it depends on involvement of the bile-ducts.—In malignant disease pain is absent in the early, but continuous in the later stages.   There is gradual loss of flesh and the failure in strength is more marked; jaundice, once it has begun, is deep, persistent, and continuous.   A hard enlargement of the gall-bladder, followed by secondary nodules in the liver or a marked hardening of this organ, is often apparent.   Gall-stones and malignant disease are frequently associated.

Cholecystitis without stones may give the same symptoms as cholelithiasis with inflammation; differentiation is not very important, as the same treatment applies to both.   Appendicitis, as a rule, can be differentiated easily.   It is most difficult, however, to make the distinction in severe cases with peritoneal involvement, or where there is non-descent of the cæcum.   (Mayo-Robson.) The two diseases frequently coexist, a fact which, as Ochsner suggests, may be explained by infection of the gall-bladder from the appendix.

The localization of gall-stones in the excretory apparatus of the liver is also a part of diagnosis, and has been considered in detail under the heading of Pathology, Complications, etc.   It may here be briefly repeated that enlargement of the gall-bladder occurs when the cystic duct is blocked, and, when the common duct is obstructed by cancer of the head of the pancreas, it is liable to be contracted when a gall-stone blocks the common duct and there have been repeated attacks of inflammation.—Jaundice is absent in cases in which the stones are confined to the gall-bladder or the cystic duct, except occasionally when inflammation extends from these to the common and hepatic ducts. Jaundice due to stone in the common duct varies in intensity.   In cancer of the head of the pancreas, the jaundice comes late, persists, and is deeper in color. Further, it must be noted that jaundice is by no means pathognomonic of cholelithiasis, that it is present in a minority of the cases, and that it may be caused by other conditions—*e.g.*, tumors pressing on ducts, adhesions, floating spleen, movable kidney. (Bland Sutton.)—Stricture in any of the ducts is the result of ulceration, worms or hepatic cysts, fever, and various toxæmic conditions.

Tumors of the Biliary Ducts.—*Benign Tumors.*—The most common form of benign tumor of the biliary ducts is the adenoma. Tumors of this variety may be found in the intrahepatic canals where they appear in the form of en-capsuled masses, imitating the tubular arrangement of the canals. Structurally, they consist of tubules lined with a single layer of columnar epithelium, the tubules becoming solid columns of cells toward the periphery and suggesting cancer. In fact, according to Bland Sutton, it is hard to differentiate between adenoma and cancer, because in all cancers arising in the ducts, intrahepatic or extrahepatic, the underlying structure is tubular. Adenomata may be single or multiple, and some are dark-green in color, due to retained bile. Adenoma of the mucous membrane of the gall-bladder also occurs, and the Mayos and Mayo-Robson report cases of this sort, in which the tumor acted as a ball valve, causing intermittent obstruction. There is no treatment for intrahepatic adenoma, but, where the growth occurs in the gall-bladder, it can be removed.— Papilloma has also been found in the gall-bladder and common bile-duct. In the former locality it is rare, exists with or without gall-stones, and gives no special signs; in the latter it might cause obstruction.—Cysts—multiple, single, and echinococcus cysts—may also be found in the bile-ducts. The multiple cysts arise in the bile canals, but are not associated with obstruction. While they cause absorption of the liver tissue, they give rise at the same time to an enormous increase in the bulk of the organ. The cause of these tumors is not known; they are generally associated with cystic disease of the kidneys. There is no jaundice, nor is there any pain or other symptom except great enlargement of the liver. These tumors are never diagnosed and are of no surgical interest. (Bland Sutton.) Solitary cysts growing from the free margin of the liver, have been observed in women. (Fig. 93.) In one of these Bland Sutton found in the wall loculi lined with epithelium, and in certain parts of the wall he found liver tissue. He believes that these cysts are due to dilatation and fusion of bile-ducts, but he gives no explanation as to the cause which led to their production. The treatment is evacuation and drainage, or excision.

Echinococcus cysts in rare cases press on the ducts and produce obstructive symptoms. Occasionally they open into the ducts, and the vesicles and mem-brane are forced into the duodenum, where they produce obstructive and colicky symptoms. Sometimes echinococcus cysts rupture into the gall-bladder, or they may appear primarily in this organ.

Malignant Tumors.—The most common malignant tumor is cancer; sar-coma is rare. Cancer may affect the gall-bladder or the bile-ducts. In 1,800 operations performed on the gall-bladder and ducts, Mayo found malignant disease in 4 per cent of the cases. In 75 per cent of the malignant cases the gall-bladder was the part affected, and in only 5 per cent the ducts. Other authorities estimate that in from 14 to 15 per cent of the malignant cases the ducts are affected. The proportion of primary cases of cancer in the gall-bladder that are associated with cholelithiasis is given by Courvoisier as 88 per cent, by Siegert as 95 per cent, and by Beadle and Musser as 100 per cent. The last two observers agree that, in secondary liver cancers, no gall stones are present. All of these observations point strongly to cholelithiasis as a precancerous con-

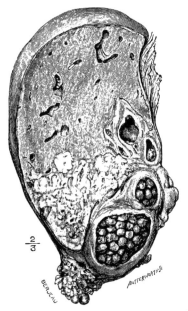

Fig. 93.—Section of a Gall-Bladder Affected with Cancer and Containing Calculi. The illustration shows at the same time the manner in which the liver is infiltrated. The specimen is preserved in the Museum of St. Bartholomew's Hospital, London, England. (From Bland Sutton.)

dition, and this is further borne out by the fact that 75 per cent of the cancer cases occur in women in whom cholelithiasis is more frequent. (See also page 248.)

Seventy-five per cent of cases of malignancy, as already stated, are in the gall-bladder. The process usually begins near the fundus, but may begin anywhere, even in the cystic duct. The tumor may project into the cavity as a fungating growth, or it may infiltrate the walls of the bladder and spread to the contiguous hepatic tissue. Often it is difficult to tell whether the tumor is primary in the liver or in the gall-bladder; when confined to the fundus, it may grow outward and produce peritoneal grafts. Sometimes the thickened, roughened walls of the gall-bladder embrace a group of stones, sometimes a single stone. Bland Sutton reports a case in which the tumor was primary in the neck of the gall-bladder and embraced a single stone. (Fig. 94.) Infrequently these thickened and contracted gall-bladders are free from adhesions. Jaundice begins when the growth spreads to the hepatic and common ducts, and ascites is a late manifestation of the disease. Involvement of the lymph nodes in the portal fissure occurs early.

The diagnosis may be easy or difficult. Usually there is a history of cholelithiasis, but frequently the symptoms of this disease have long been held in abeyance. Usually there is an easily recognizable tumor in the gall-bladder region. It is hard and painless, and frequently the adjacent part of the liver may feel

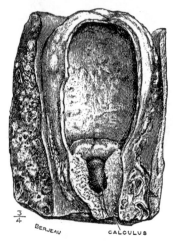

Fig. 94.—A Gall-Bladder with Primary Cancer of its Neck Extending into the Cystic Duct; a gall-stone is embedded in the growth. Specimen taken from a man aged seventy years, and preserved in the Museum of the Charing Cross Hospital, London, England. (From Bland Sutton.)

hard and sometimes nodular. Jaundice comes on late, at the time when the hepatic or common duct is involved; it is persistent, unchanging, and deeper in color than the jaundice seen in gall-stones. In addition, there is loss of weight and strength—an evident cachexia. Bland Sutton divides these cases into two classes: in one there is observed, clinically, a tumor of the gall-bladder, without any acute signs of cholecystitis, but with obvious cachexia; in the second, the symptoms in part suggest serious disease of the gall-bladder, in part cancer of the liver. In the latter class it may be impossible to make a diagnosis without exploration. He also calls attention to the fact that all hard growths of the gall-bladder are not of a cancerous nature, and should not be looked upon as incurable until after a thorough exploration has been made and the behavior of the growth has been watched for some time,—an observation which is confirmed by Mayo-Robson, Abbe, and others who have had to do with these growths.

As a rule, when a cancer of the gall-bladder has been diagnosed, it is already beyond surgical relief. When the growth is confined to the gall-bladder it should be excised along with any portion of contiguous liver tissue which has a suspicious appearance. Mayo states that, in several cases where the gall-bladder was removed for thickening supposed to be inflammatory, and which afterward turned out to be of a malignant nature, the patients were found to be well after the lapse of three years, while none of the individuals in whom the diagnosis of cancer was made at the time of operation survived more than one year; all of which strongly suggests the precancerous influence of gall-stones, the value of an early diagnosis, and the importance of cholecystectomy in any case in which suspicious circumstances exist. Contra-indications to a radical operation are: involvement of the hepatic or the common duct, with jaundice; metastasis in lymph nodes or liver; and ascites or peritoneal involvement.

Cancer of the common and the hepatic ducts is rare. It affects the common duct most frequently, but is also found at the junction of the hepatic, cystic, and common ducts. It may be found in association with gall-stones, but usually is not. Robson, however, believes that the irritation caused by stones which have been extruded is a common etiological factor. The growth is small, but the obstruction is usually complete, producing a dilatation of the intrahepatic ducts, which at first are filled with bile, later with a mucous fluid, clear or bile-stained. The growth is hard and feels and cuts like tough fibrous tissue. Under the microscope the tissue appears to be composed of columnar or spheroidal-celled epithelium, and in some specimens the tubular arrangement characteristic of adenocarcinoma is apparent. When located at the ampulla and arising from the epithelium of this part of the duct, the tumor must be distinguished both from a cancer of the duct just above the ampulla and from one that is seated in the duodenal mucous membrane in close proximity to the ampulla. (Bland Sutton.)

The symptoms are jaundice, cachexia, and occasionally dilatation of the gall-bladder. Jaundice comes early, at first is often intermittent, but later is constant. Pain is a varying symptom. In some cases it is absent, in others there are attacks resembling those of biliary colic. Evidences of infection are usually absent; sometimes, however, there are chills and fever.

When the ampulla is involved the pancreatic secretion may be blocked, the symptoms then being identical with those of primary carcinoma of the head of the pancreas. Other conditions with which it might be confounded are: cancer of the duodenum or stomach, involving the terminations of the ducts; a gall-stone impacted in the ampulla; or indeed any obstruction associated with jaundice.

The treatment is difficult to carry out and the results are not satisfactory. (See Surgical Treatment.) Radical measures are: excision, with reimplantation of the duct; or end-to-end anastomosis, if the growth is supraduodenal; or closure of the duct and a cholecystenterostomy. When the common duct has been dilated above an irremovable tumor, the dilated duct and the duodenum may be united—choledochoduodenostomy. When the hepatic duct is obliterated and the gall-bladder is too contracted, a portion of the liver surface may then be denuded so as to lay open a certain number of bile-ducts, and to the edges of this exposed area the borders of a wound in the jejunum may be stitched— intrahepatic cholangeo-enterostomy. (Bland Sutton.)

Sarcoma of the gall-bladder is rare and of comparatively little surgical importance. In 1889 Musser found but three reported cases. Since then others have been reported—one of the spindle-celled variety by Rolleston, and one specimen of melanotic sarcoma in the Hunterian Museum, referred to by Robson.

Surgical Treatment in Diseases of the Gall-Bladder and Bile-Ducts; General Considerations.—The indications for surgical interference in diseases of the gall-bladder and bile passages are fairly definite. In certain conditions—*e.g.*, acute cholecystitis (calculous or otherwise), empyema of the gall-bladder, atrophied gall-bladder contracted on stones, external biliary fistula, enlarged gall-bladder due to obstruction, and acute cholangitis—no doubt exists as to what should be done. Chronic pancreatitis the result of a stone impacted in the ampulla cannot reasonably be aided by anything short of operative measures.

Frequently recurring attacks of biliary colic are held by some to be sufficient reason for resorting to operation. Others think that in mild cases no harm can be done by waiting. It must be remembered that, in certain cases, the first evidence of gall-stone disease will be a severe attack characterized by fulminating symptoms that end in peritonitis and often in death. In other cases a mild attack may be followed by one of great severity. The conditions have by many been aptly compared to those observed in appendicitis. Mayo says that in gall-stone disease surgical interference should be instituted as soon as the diagnosis is certain, and that nearly every argument used for early operation in appendicitis applies with equal force to biliary calculi. The greatest difficulty will be experienced in deciding whether or not to operate on those patients who show vague symptoms, usually supposed to be gastric; but this is more a question of diagnosis than of treatment. This comparison with appendicitis and the brilliant results of operation in the hands of experienced surgeons may lead the inexperienced to conclude that operations on the gall-bladder and ducts are not more difficult than those ordinarily performed on the appendix—a conclusion, however, not justified by the facts; the anatomical difficulties alone making the problem one of much greater complexity.

The contra-indications are the same as for other severe operations; special contra-indications being found in the liability to hemorrhage, which occurs in deep jaundice, particularly when the jaundice is due to cancer. In the latter disease, even were there no jaundice, the reparative processes are so impaired and the tendency to healing so slight that operations should be undertaken only with the greatest care, and frequently not at all. (See page 255.) Where this liability to hemorrhage exists, chloride of calcium, lactate of calcium, thyroid extract, gelatin, and various other drugs have been recommended, but their reputed good effects are doubtful or at least not certain. Coagulability tests also are not to be wholly depended upon, for there are cases in which the coagulation takes place slowly, and yet in these oozing may not follow division of the smaller blood-vessels. Mayo says that in deep jaundice, accompanied by purpuric spots,—conditions which show that the blood cannot be maintained in the uninjured vessels,—operations should not, generally speaking, be undertaken.

Technique of the Operation.—Preparation of the Patient.—The patient should be prepared as for any severe abdominal operation. Special mention, however, may be made of the following details:—(1) As regards the choice of a cathartic to be administered as a preliminary measure, many prefer castor oil to other laxatives, because its use is attended with less tendency to the drainage of large amounts of serum. (2) Because of the special tendency to parotitis, Bland Sutton advises thorough cleansing of the mouth before operation. (3) Vomiting should be treated by thorough gastric lavage. (4) The skin should be prepared in the usual way, but with exceptional care. If any pustules are present, or if, as is frequently the case, the skin has been damaged by heat, cold, or other local irritant, it should be thoroughly painted with tincture of iodine.

Position of the Patient. (Fig. 95.)—The patient should be placed on the back and the lower chest should be raised in such a way as to permit the intestines to fall away from the visceral aspect of the liver. This was first recommended by Elliot, of Boston.* It may be accomplished by the use of a sandbag (twenty-four inches long and from sixteen to eighteen inches in circumference), by an air cushion, like the Edebohls kidney cushion and of similar dimensions, or by a table with a narrow, adjustable bridge like the kidney bridge, but placed nearer the head of the table. The sand bag is uncomfortable if put in place before the anæsthetic is administered; if placed or changed afterward, it disturbs the arrangements for asepsis and cannot be reduced in size to such a degree as to permit the placing of the final sutures. The air cushion is not so uncomfortable; its level may be changed by pulling the patient up or down, and it may readily be emptied to a degree sufficient to permit suturing. The adjustable table (Fig. 95), if at hand, meets all requirements. The arms should be placed on the table beside the trunk and not folded on the chest, where the elbows interfere with the field of operation.

Choice of an Anæsthetic.—Mayo prefers the open-drop method of ether anæsthesia; Bland Sutton begins with nitrous oxide, continues with ether, and then judiciously maintains the anæsthesia with chloroform. Many operators begin with nitrous oxide and continue with ether. Whatever method is decided upon, an experienced anæsthetist should be employed. Mayo cautions against attempting to force the anæsthetic to the point of suppressing the respiratory grunt due to spasm of the diaphragm.

Local anæsthesia may be employed with great satisfaction for simply exposing and opening the gall-bladder. In our work at St. Vincent's Hospital, cases of

* Annals of Surgery, 1895, vol. 22.

cholecystitis, with or without cholelithiasis, are frequently admitted in a condition which prohibits the employment of a general anæsthetic.

Instruments Required.—Only a few special instruments are necessary.
For retraction of the margins of the wound, the hand of a trained assistant is
best; but where this takes up too much room, and especially in exposure of the
deep ducts, a right-angled retractor, with adjustable blades of different lengths
and widths, will be found useful. Artery clamps with long handles, and at
least two or three with curved blades like the Carmalt clamp, should also be at
hand. A slight shoulder on the convex side of the blades near the point, for
the purpose of holding the ligature while the first knot is being tightened, adds
to the efficiency of the clamp. For aspirating the gall-bladder, an aspirator
with a large needle and a two-way stopcock is essential. Several full-curved,

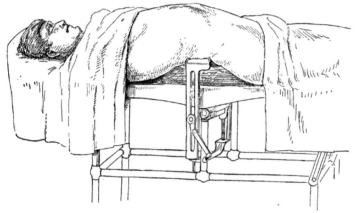

Fig. 95.—Adjustable Operating Table, with a Mechanical Contrivance for Causing the Abdominal
Portion of the Trunk to Arch Upward in Varying Degrees. (After the Mayos.)

small but strong needles, with a long-handled needle-holder, gall-stone forceps
and scoops, probes, and grooved directors are also necessary.

Incisions.—The vertical incision through the right rectus is the most useful.
Ordinarily it is made at the junction of the inner and outer thirds of the muscle,
but this should be determined to some extent by the location of the gall-bladder
—that is, by its distance from the mesial line, which should be determined as
nearly as possible beforehand. Thus, where a large Riedel's lobe is present,
the gall-bladder may be much nearer than normal to the median line. The
vertical position and the length of the incision will vary in different cases. Thus,
under the impression that a hardened rounded part of the liver is the gall-bladder,
one may place the vertical incision with its centre over the latter, and then later
find the upper part of this incision to be useless. In doubtful cases it is
wiser to make only a part of the vertical incision at first, as it is easy to extend
it up or down after the true level of the gall-bladder has been ascertained. Its

length too will vary with the requirements of each case. Ordinarily it should measure about four inches. If the deep ducts are to be explored, it must be long enough to admit the hand; if it is too long, it will give trouble by permitting the intestines to crowd out at its lower end. If, after the vertical incision is made, it is found that more room is needed in an upward and inward direction, this may be obtained by cutting the muscle obliquely, in a direction parallel with the costal margin (Fig. 96),—a modification recommended by Bevan and Mayo-Robson. In making this the operator should cut the fascia far enough away from the cartilages to permit of easy suturing. If the additional room is needed in a downward and outward direction, a similar incision may be carried outward from the lower end of the vertical portion. (Fig. 97.) Weir has

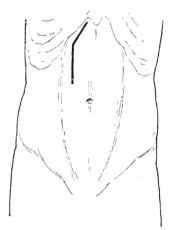 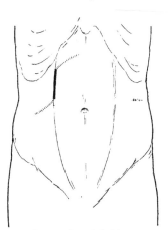

Fig. 96.—Mayo-Robson's Incision.   Fig. 97.—Bevan's Incision.

suggested * that this room may be gained by cutting the sheath of the rectus, while leaving the fibres intact.

Kocher's incision lies parallel with the costal margin. (Fig. 98.) It may, in a few cases, permit free access to the gall-bladder, but it does not expose the ducts as well as do the incisions described. Besides, because of the free division of the muscular fibres, it is more likely to be followed by hernia.

Kehr's incision, a vertical one, is unnecessarily long; its lower part being of little advantage.

Packing.—After the edges of the incision have been pulled apart sufficiently, the operative field should be carefully walled off by pads with tapes attached, one or more being placed deeply behind the liver and in front of the kidney, and another at the lower angle to prevent escape of the colon and small intestines. Frequently a third is needed at the outer part of Morrison's space and sometimes

* Med. News, Feb. 17th, 1900.

a fourth on the mesial aspect of the wound, to restrain the stomach. This latter pad may have to be removed during the operation. After exploration has been finished, additional pads may be placed in the depths of the wound to absorb the blood or other fluids which may escape; they may be so arranged as to close the foramen of Winslow.

Adhesions and Fistula.—Before the gall-bladder and ducts can be thoroughly exposed, it is often necessary to separate adhesions, and sometimes these are so dense as almost to discourage the operator. Careful, persistent effort, however, will usually overcome the difficulty. In making this separation, the surgeon should keep in mind the possible existence of a fistula, and if one is found it should be properly closed. Minute fistulæ have escaped the attention of operators and have caused death. Further, if a severe infection exists, the separation of adhesions may set up a peritonitis; in these cases, therefore, it is wise to drain the gall-bladder with the least possible trauma, the completion of the operation being deferred until the inflammation subsides. Serious bleeding is seldom encountered during the separation of adhesions; but if it is, the more conspicuous points should be caught and tied. Oozing is controlled by packing during the operation, and the field should again be inspected before the final steps are taken.

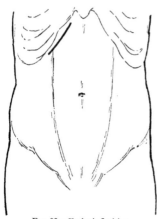

FIG. 98.—Kocher's Incision.

Exploring.—When adhesions, if any exist, have been removed, the biliary passages should be carefully explored. The size and degree of tension of the gall-bladder should be noted, and an attempt made to ascertain whether or not it contains stones. Often the gall-bladder is so enlarged as to interfere with further exploration, and in that event its contents must be aspirated before the examination may proceed. (See page 262.) The cystic duct should next be explored, and, if it contains a stone, gentle efforts should be made to press it back into the gall-bladder before an opening is made in the latter. Care should also be taken at all stages of the exploration or operation not to permit a stone to escape into the hepatic duct, where it may elude further attempts at capture, and thus, to some extent, mar the completeness of the operation. In exploring the hepatic duct and the upper part of the common duct, the finger should, and usually can, be passed into the foramen of Winslow, and the ducts grasped between the finger and thumb. The remainder of the common duct must be investigated by grasping the duodenum and duct at the same time. When adhesions interfere with exploration of the terminal segment of the common duct, Bland Sutton recommends tearing through the gastro-hepatic omentum and entering the lesser sac of the peritoneum. This procedure, however, is not often necessary. Attention should be also given to the head of the pancreas, to the pylorus, and to the liver itself. Enlarged lymph nodes will sometimes convey the sensation of soft stones, and, in order to differentiate between the two, it is necessary to consider the obstructive symptoms which have existed, or even to expose the nodes. It must also be remembered that enlarged lymph nodes have caused obstruction.

Rotating the Liver.—This manipulation, recommended by Robson, should sometimes be performed before exploration and always before operating. It is accomplished by pulling down the right lobe of the liver, the organ being held with gauze pads and rotated so that the visceral surface is turned forward and the ducts brought much nearer the surface. This procedure is one of great importance, as it adds materially to the ease and safety of subsequent manipulations. It is perhaps not putting it too strongly to say that not a single vessel should be divided, unless it is so accessible as to be easily controlled, —a condition often not possible without this preliminary rotation.

Drainage.—For draining the gall-bladder a stiff rubber tube, one-quarter of an inch in diameter, wrapped in four thicknesses of iodoform gauze, and covered with rubber tissue in the manner suggested by the Mayos, is the best. It is secured in the fundus of the gall-bladder by a purse-string suture of catgut, which passes through its gauze wrappings and may be drawn tight enough to prevent bile leakage without constricting the lumen of the tube. If the patient is restless, the tube may be further secured by a stitch in the skin, which —to prevent leakage at this point—should be placed with care, a suture larger than the needle being used for the purpose. (Fig. 99.)

Drainage of the common duct may be managed by cutting two holes opposite each other near the end of the tube, and sewing the latter into the opening of the duct by a purse-string suture, which also passes, at one point at least, through the tube. This permits bile to flow into the duodenum while at the same time it prevents tension. It may be removed after a few days, by which time the catgut will have been absorbed and adhesions will have formed a sinus. Drainage may be continued, as long thereafter as necessary, by a wick or a smaller tube passed into the sinus.

Drainage from the patulous stump of a cystic duct after cholecystectomy may be managed in the same way (i.e., securing the tube by a purse-string suture), but sometimes the stump is long enough to permit the use of a circular ligature; a single suture being passed afterward through the tube and the cut edge of the duct. These drains are needed only in septic conditions of the ducts.

For draining the adjacent area of blood and serum and providing against possible leakage, a split rubber tube with a wick of iodoform gauze, a cigarette drain, or a rubber tube with lateral openings may be used. Their presence does not interfere in any way with the subsequent healing. All tubes so placed should be secured by an absorbable suture, which prevents their immediate displacement, but later permits their removal.

Gauze packing may sometimes be required for controlling oozing; it should be placed with care, particularly in the bottom of Rutherford Morrison's space, and should be so arranged as to close the foramen of Winslow and not to ob_struct the colon or the duodenum.   It is wisest to place a rubber drain at the same time. When drainage is provided for bile, the dressings may be kept clean by interposing a short glass tube between the drain and a second piece of tubing, through which the fluid may be carried out through the dressings to a bottle at the side of the bed, or to a flask properly arranged in the dressings.

Preventing Adhesions.—Before the abdominal cavity is closed, the viscera should be rearranged in their natural position. Adhesions of the stomach and duodenum to the denuded surfaces should be prevented by placing the colon and upper edge of the great omentum between these surfaces and the viscera in question, and maintaining them there if necessary by sutures. (The Mayos.) In wide denudations the lower edge of the great omentum might be thus utilized.

Suturing.—Before any sutures are applied, the support should be removed from the patient's back to relax the abdominal wall. Layer suturing is probably the best, but it is difficult to secure the peritoneum independently, because of its friability and its intimate attachment to the posterior sheath of the rectus. These two layers, therefore, are taken together with a running suture of catgut, and this suture must be applied with care, because, owing to the fact that the fibres of the sheath are mostly horizontal, it tears out easily. The anterior layer of the rectus sheath is next closed in the same way. Silkworm-gut or silk sutures are finally used for the skin, all the layers being closed up to the tube. If the tube does not emerge at the upper angle of the wound, closure must be made above and below the tube.

Some operators supplement this layer suture by figure-of-eight sutures passed through the skin and the anterior layer of the rectus; others close the opening by a single layer of sutures passing through the entire thickness of the abdominal wall.

Individual Operations on the Gall-Bladder and the Cystic Duct.—The operations here referred to bear the following names: Cholecystostomy—the making and maintaining of an opening in the gall-bladder; cholecystectomy—the complete operative removal of the gall-bladder; cholecystendysis—incision of the gall-bladder, removal of any stones that may be present, closure of the opening, return of the viscus to the abdominal cavity, and closure of the outside wound without drainage; cholecystenterostomy—the making of an anastomosis between the gall-bladder and some part of the alimentary canal; and cholecyst-duodenostomy—the making of an anastomosis between the gall-bladder and the duodenum.

Cholecystostomy.—This operation (Figs. 99 and 100) is performed by the Mayos in the following manner:—The fundus of the gall-bladder is well exposed (care being exercised in separating adhesions and in detecting fistulæ, as already described on page 212) and is brought into the wound. If stones are found lodged in the pelvis of the organ or in the cystic duct, an attempt is made to force them gently back into the bladder before the latter is opened. Then the bladder is aspirated, a syringe with a large needle and a two-way stopcock being used for this purpose. Care is taken to prevent leakage beside the needle and to protect the neighboring parts against such an occurrence by gauze packing. After the bladder has been evacuated as completely as possible, it is opened, the remaining fluid is wiped out with small wipes or strips of narrow gauze, and the stones are removed by forceps or with the scoop. For removal of the cholesterin paste, the scoop or spoon is necessary. To make sure that all of the stones have been removed, the finger should be passed into the gall-bladder. It is also essential to make certain that the cystic duct is free from obstruction, a fact which will be made evident by the free flow of freshly secreted bile. The drainage tube wrapped with gauze and rubber tissue is now placed in the opening in the gall-bladder, and a purse-string suture is inserted at a distance of one-third of an inch from the edge of the opening in the

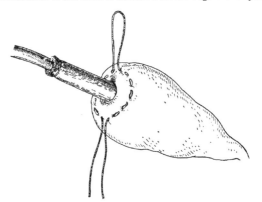

FIG. 99.—Placing the Drain in Cholecystostomy. (After Mayo.)

fundus. (Fig. 99.) This suture includes the entire thickness of the gall-bladder and also transfixes the gauze wrapping of the tube at one or more points. The edges of the wound are then inverted and, when the suture is tightened, the serous surfaces are in opposition to the rubber tissue. A second suture, inverting more of the gall-bladder, may be placed in a similar manner, but it is not essential that this shall transfix the gauze wrappings. The gall-bladder is then fixed to the peritoneum at the upper angle of the wound by about two stitches on each side; in some cases it is convenient to anchor the gall-bladder at a lower point in the wound. The purse-string sutures in the gall-bladder become absorbed in a few days, early enough to permit the removal of the drain, which may be done at the end of eight or ten days. Following this removal the peritoneal surfaces come in contact with one another and the sinus soon closes, unless stones have been left in the gall-bladder or unless there is occlusion of the cystic duct.

When a stone in the neck of the gall-bladder has resisted removal by manipulation, it may be extracted through an incision made over the stone, which incision may afterward be closed by sutures or left open. In either event, if it is necessary to save the gall-bladder, gauze may be packed around the tube in such a manner as to prevent all soiling of the peritoneum. (See page 212.) Usually such a tightly impacted stone will be found to occupy a loculus of a contracted gall-bladder, and the walls of the viscus are then in such a seriously damaged state that cholecystectomy is the only proper procedure. The same is true of a stone held firmly in the cystic duct; it should never be crushed for fear that the débris will serve as nuclei for further stones, but it may be removed through an incision—cysticotomy—followed by suturing and cholecystostomy. Usually, however, cholecystectomy is indicated.

There are several variations from the course here described. (a) If it is necessary to save a short shrunken gall-bladder, the tube may be held by a purse-string suture, which does not attempt to invert the gall-bladder; then four pieces of gauze (two inches wide) are attached to the gall-bladder on its four sides, each by a suture which catches the gauze one inch from its end and the

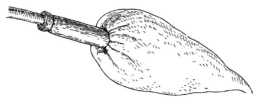

FIG. 100.--Placing of the Drain in Cholecystostomy Completed. (After Mayo.)

gall-bladder close to its cut edge. The free portions of the deep ends of the gauze are then packed carefully around the tube and bladder, and the other extremities are brought out of the abdominal incision and arranged in such a manner as to surround the tube. This manœuvre, as described by the Mayos, is valuable, and may be applied to drains elsewhere in the biliary canals, or indeed in any part of the abdomen.

(b) If the gall-bladder is adherent to the abdominal wall, it may be opened and drained through the adherent area without invading the peritoneal cavity.

(c) If the gall-bladder is located at some point away from its normal position, it may be drained through the loin. Some surgeons believe that this affords much more effective drainage, and they frequently adopt this route.

(d) When a doubt exists as to the extent and degree of virulence of the infection, the gall-bladder may be fixed to the external layer of the rectus sheath; this wound closes less rapidly and, if further trouble occurs, the infection will be guided to the surface.

Cholecystectomy. (Figs. 101 and 102.)—The incision, the separation of adhesions, the rotation of the liver, the protection of the peritoneum, and the exposure of the gall-bladder and ducts are the same in this as in the preceding operation.   When these steps have been taken a ring forceps is placed on the fundus of the gall-bladder, so as to straighten out this viscus and the cystic duct and thus definitely expose the latter.   (If the gall-bladder is distended its contents should be evacuated; if there is a stone in the pelvis or the cystic duct, it should if possible, be gently pressed back into the gall-bladder.)   When the cystic duct is exposed, a ring forceps is placed on the pelvis, the peritoneum around the cystic

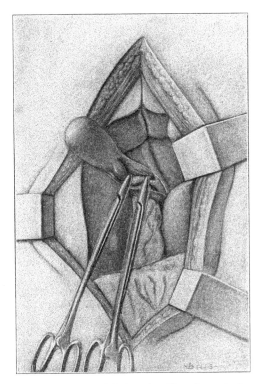

Fig. 101.—Cholecystectomy; First Stage of the Operation.   The peritoneum has been separated from the cystic duct and two clamps have been applied, preparatory to dividing the duct.   (Original.)

duct is divided, and by blunt dissection the duct is thoroughly exposed.   Two clamps are then placed on the duct, both of them beyond the impacted stone, if one is present, and the duct is divided between the two.   The peritoneum is now cut on both sides of the gall-bladder from the severed end of the duct to the fundus, so as to leave flaps, and, by gentle retraction on the forceps placed on the gall-bladder end of the duct, the artery is exposed and secured.   Continued traction, combined with blunt dissection by means of the finger, further separates the gall-bladder from the liver. When this separation has been carried to a point near the fundus, the vessel may be left as a tractor for steadying the liver. The deep end of the duct is then secured by a catgut ligature. The two peritoneal flaps are stitched together from below upward, the separation of the gall-bladder is continued in the same way until completed, and then the stitching of the peritoneal flaps is finished, the denuded surface of the liver thus being completely covered. A tube drain is stitched to the duct in the vicinity

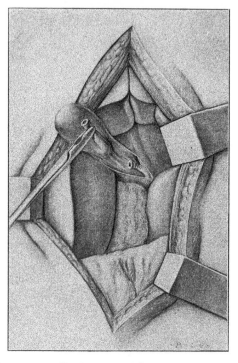

Fig. 102.—Cholecystectomy. The distal portion of the cystic duct is tied, the proximal portion together with the gall-bladder being lifted out of its peritoneal coat. Gauze is placed at the lower angle of the wound, for the purpose of restraining the intestines, and in the bottom of the wound between the liver and the duodenum. This figure also shows the pouch of Rutherford Morrison. (Original.)

of its cut end by passing a stitch through the peritoneum. Some surgeons omit the placing of this drain, but leakage has occured from the cut end of the cystic duct after several days. The tube, however, may be removed at the end of from six to eight days, for by that time there will have been formed a peritoneal sinus which will serve, for several days longer, to conduct any leakage to the surface.

Modifications of the Steps of the Operation.—The gall-bladder may be freed from its connections by beginning the work of separation at the fundus and continuing it inward to the point where the viscus contracts into the duct, the finger being placed in the opened gall-bladder as a guide. This is particularly necessary when the cystic duct is dilated, and may help the surgeon to avoid transfixing a dilated duct when the ligature is passed around it. This method is also advisable in cases in which dense adhesions around the neck of the gall-bladder make it difficult of recognition.

Splitting the peritoneal coat and removing only the mucous coat of the gall-bladder is a refinement that adds to the difficulty without accomplishing anything else.

When it seems wise, after cholecystectomy, to provide bile drainage, a tube may be stitched into the open end of the cystic duct; or, if the stump of the duct is long enough, it may be secured by a ligature and stitch; if leakage is likely to occur, it may be provided for by a gauze packing properly arranged. (See page 212.) In the course of ten or twelve days the tube may be removed, and, if the common duct is free, bile soon ceases to flow and the sinus closes.

The Mayos split the end of the cystic duct and secure the tube in position by stitches placed one on each side. Others introduce the tube directly, dilating the duct for this purpose if necessary.

The control of hemorrhage is not difficult, as a rule. The essential feature is to expose the parts so freely that clamping and ligature of all bleeding points may readily be accomplished. The cystic artery, secured in the manner already described, is the only vessel that is likely to bleed. Sometimes the tissues are so friable that it is difficult to render the artery secure. In these cases clamps should be placed on the duct and artery and left in place for forty-eight hours. They should be unlocked six hours before removal, for fear of tearing off that portion of the tissues which is embedded in their grasp. By surrounding their shanks with gauze, excellent drainage is afforded. The gauze should not be removed for several days after the removal of the forceps. (The Mayos.) The venous oozing of the liver is rarely difficult of control, and, as a rule, yields to pressure of small pads of gauze wrung out of hot saline solution. If this fails, deep stitches may be inserted into the liver with a non-cutting needle, and the two cut surfaces of the organ brought together; or, in severe cases, gauze properly arranged for later removal, may be compressed against the bleeding surface by these sutures.

In cholecystectomy for cancer of the gall-bladder, a V-shaped piece of the liver should be removed with the gall-bladder (cholecystectomy with partial hepatectomy) and the bleeding controlled as after cholecystectomy.

In hydrops of the gall-bladder Bland Sutton advises removing in the same way the thin strip of liver which spreads over the gall-bladder.

Indications for and against Cholecystostomy and Cholecystectomy.— Surgeons are not all agreed as to what shall be the choice between these two operations in every case. For cholecystostomy it may be urged that it is the simpler of the two, and that it may be performed (under local anæsthesia, if thought best) in urgent cases,—cases in which immediate drainage is: necessary. In the hands of the Mayos it has a mortality of one and a half per cent, and, according to them, is indicated in the following conditions: (a) in all cases of infection where the gall-bladder does not show serious. changes and the cystic duct is free; (b) in all cases of infection of the intrahepatic ducts where the cystic duct is free, as the best method of securing: drainage; (c) in gall-stones of the common duct where there is a strong probability that the stones will re-form (the gall-bladder being left as a guide to the deep ducts in possible future operations); (d) in permanent obstruction of the common duct—e.g., by cancer of the head of the pancreas,—for permanent bile drainage; (e) in benign stenosis of the common duct (present or prospective), in preference to cholecystenterostomy; (f) in urgent cases as a temporary expedient, which may, however, prove to be permanent; and (g) in cases of external biliary fistula, in which the opening is enlarged and the surgeon merely improves the cholecystostomy already performed by Nature.

Against the operation (cholecystostomy) the following objections have been urged: (a) liability to persistent fistula (this is likely to arise only when a stone in the cystic or the common duct has been overlooked, or when one or the other of these ducts is obstructed through the operation of some other cause); (b) the recurrence of gall-stones in the gall-bladder (this occurred in only one of twelve hundred cases operated on by the Mayos); and (c) the occurrence of carcinoma in the diseased gall-bladder (this is unlikely, and close inspection should enable one to decide). Minor arguments against it are the occurrence of a troublesome sinus due to the sutures used in fixing the gall-bladder, and of dragging pain due to strain on the adherent gall-bladder. The latter is not˙likely to give trouble; the former may be avoided by using: absorbable sutures.

Cholecystectomy is a more difficult operation and requires more time. Its. mortality, while less than two per cent, is still somewhat higher than that of cholecystostomy. It is indicated in injuries of the gall-bladder, in marked disease of this organ, in contracted gall-bladder with or without stones, in primary cancer of the gall-bladder, often also in cases in which a stone is impacted in the cystic duct, and in all cases in which the cystic duct does not provide efficient drainage.

Cholecystendysis.—In this operation the gall-bladder is opened, the stones are extracted, the opening is closed, the viscus is returned to the abdomen, and the abdominal incision is entirely closed. The operation does not provide drainage, is never to be used where any infection exists, and its application should be limited to cases of gall-stone disease, accidentally discovered during the course of other operations, where the gall-bladder is apparently normal. Kocher suggested, in such cases, that; because of the possibility of latent infection, the closed fundus should be fixed to a point in the deep part of the incision, and that a drain should be carried through the layers of the abdominal wall down to this point. Subsequent leakage and infection would thus be provided for.

Cholecystenterostomy.—Cholecystenterostomy (Figs. 103 and 104) is the making of an anastomosis between the gall-bladder and some portion of the alimentary canal. This operation is useful when there exists an inoperable stricture or an irremovable obstruction of the common duct, such as cancer of the head of the pancreas, of the duodenum (involving the papillæ), or of the common duct itself. In cases of cancer the mortality is so high that Mayo-Robson regards the justifiability of the operation as questionable. There is no doubt, however, that in properly selected cases the establishment of bile drainage in this way gives relief. It has been utilized in cases of irremovable stones in the common duct, but improved technique has markedly limited the number of stones that may be termed "irremovable." A frequent indication is persistent biliary fistula, the result of inflammatory processes or following cholecystostomy.

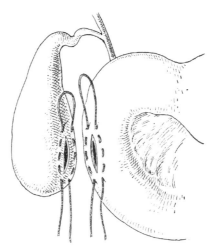

FIG. 103.—Cholecystenterostomy; First Step. (After Mayo.)

Various portions of the alimentary canal have been recommended for this anastomosis, as, for example: (*a*) The stomach near the pylorus; (*b*) the duodenum, two or three inches below the pylorus; (*c*) the jejunum; and (*d*) the hepatic flexure of the colon. The choice lies between the duodenum and the colon. The former is accessible and bile enters at the proper place to take its part in the processes of digestion; on the other hand, the duodenum may be so bound down by adhesions as to be inaccessible, and the anastomosis may interfere with its motility. Facts which favor the selection of the colon are: its easier accessibility, the simplicity of the operation, and the circumstance that, where broad adhesions exist, the operation may sometimes be performed extraperitoneally. Against the choice of the colon are: the possibility of infection of the ducts, the interference with digestion caused by the procedure, and the occurrence of biliary diarrhœa. The first two objections are theoretical and do not seem to have occurred in practice; biliary diarrhœa does not always follow, and, when it occurs, is to be preferred to continued jaundice, or—as Bland Sutton remarks—to persistent biliary fistula. Many experienced surgeons, among them the Mayos, strongly recommend the duodenum as first choice, the colon as second, stating, however, that their results following anastomosis with the colon have been satisfactory. Mayo-Robson, Bland Sutton, and others recommend the colon as first choice. If, for any reason, the jejunum is selected, a loop of this part of the bowel must be brought up over the transverse colon, and Mikulicz considered it wise to make an entero-anastomosis between the two arms of the loop.

Anastomosis between the gall-bladder and the duodenum, cholecyst-duode-

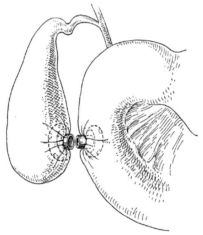

Fig. 104.—Cholecystenterostomy; the Murphy Button *in situ.* (After Mayo.)

nostomy, may be performed in exactly the same way as an anastomosis between the two loops of intestine. Some prefer to use the Murphy button or some other mechanical contrivance, others make a simple suture anastomosis. When the Murphy button is used the smaller male portion of the button should be placed in the gall-bladder. If an opening already exists in this viscus, the button may be passed through this opening into the cavity and its stem made to emerge through a smaller opening in the side of the fundus, one which fits the stem so snugly that the usual purse-string suture may be dispensed with. The larger opening in the fundus is then properly closed and a few reinforcing sutures should be placed around the button. Union with the colon may be effected by the same methods.

If the colon is utilized the great omentum may be attached in such a manner as to cover the line of anastomosis, and the same manœuvre is applicable in cases of cholecyst-duodenostomy where friability of the tissues on both sides leads to a suspicion that there is a lack of sufficient healing power. A cigarette drain should be anchored by a catgut suture close to, but not impinging on, the line of anastomosis. The abdominal wound is then closed.

There is a tendency for the anastomotic opening to contract, particularly when the obstruction is partial. Robson has reported such a case. The Mayos

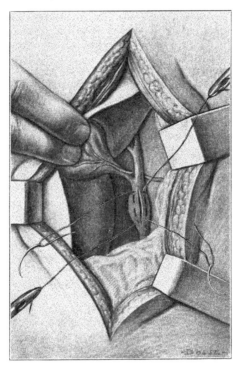

Fig. 105.—Choledochotomy. (Original.)

believe it probable that,. should the obstruction disappear and the bile resume its normal channel, the opening would likewise disappear.

Operations on the Common Duct.—*Choledochotomy.*—Choledochotomy (Fig. 105) signifies the opening of the common duct, usually for the extraction of gall-stones.

Complete exposure is even more necessary here than in operations on the gall-bladder. It is obtained by carefully arranging the patient's position, by rotating the liver to the farthest limit, and by making, high up, an oblique division, as complete as possible, of that portion of the rectus which is mesial to the vertical incision. The preparation of the patient, the protection of the peritoneum, etc., are the same as for cholecystostomy, and have already been described. Depending on the portion of the duct invaded, choledochotomy is divided into supraduodenal, retroduodenal, and transduodenal.

Supraduodenal Choledochotomy.—The gall-bladder should be emptied of its contents, whether fluid or stones, and to do this it is necessary to open the fundus. After evacuation is complete and the patency of the cystic duct has been established by noting the flow of bile, the gall-bladder is packed with gauze and the opening temporarily closed by a clamp or a ligature of tape,—preferably the latter, because it damages the tissues less,—to prevent the escape of bile.

The duct is now examined for stone, great care being taken not to dislodge any from the common into the hepatic, where they may elude further efforts to remove them. If a stone is found in the supraduodenal portion the operation may be proceeded with; if the stone is above or below this portion, an attempt is made to force it into the supraduodenal division; once in this division the stone is grasped between the thumb and forefinger and a longitudinal incision is made over it large enough to permit its removal without crushing.

Traction sutures placed on both sides of the opening will help in the further exploration of the duct, or long forceps may be used for grasping the sides of the incision. If other stones are apparent in the duct, they should be removed, and then a more thorough investigation should be made. Beginning above, the hepatic duct should be searched and emptied, a probe or a scoop being used for the purpose, or, if the duct is sufficiently dilated, the finger may be employed. Hidden stones may also be brought to the surface by gently milking or stripping the duct from above downward. The relief of obstruction located higher up will be indicated by a flow of bile; but such flow does not preclude the possibility of stones being lodged in either the right or the left bile-duct. The lower portions of the duct are investigated in turn, the finger being introduced for the purpose, if possible. For the removal of any stones that may be present, the scoop is the best instrument; to determine whether or not the canal is free, the best plan is to employ the probe or the finger.

The fish-tail tube is next inserted into the opening of the common duct and anchored in position by a catgut suture which unites the tube and cut edge of the duct. A cigarette drain may be placed beside this and a second one in Morrison's pouch, both of them being anchored by catgut sutures. The gauze packing arranged in the manner already described, or some modification, may occasionally be necessary, either for drainage, for the control of oozing, or for the absorption of fluids. The tube in the common duct should be connected with a flask placed in the dressings. The gall-bladder is, at the same time, drained and treated as in cholecystostomy.

The drains may be removed at the end of a week; occasionally it may be found necessary to let them remain longer. When they are removed a gauze wick may be introduced to prevent too rapid closure of the superficial wound.

Hemorrhage is rarely severe and may be controlled by the use of ligatures or by suturing; packing will suffice for slow oozing. The recommendation that no vessel should be severed unless it is accessible to proper treatment, cannot be repeated too often.

Variations in the Steps of the Operation.—If the cystic duct is dilated sufficiently a drain may be carried through the gall-bladder and this duct into the common duct, and the opening in the supraduodenal portion may then be closed with sutures. (Bland Sutton never closes the opening under any circumstances, stating that the incision heals quickly, often with scarcely any escape of bile.) Other reasons for adopting the course suggested by this author are that drainage is secure in this way, that an overlooked stone may be later recovered, and, finally, that a tedious operation, likely at best to be imperfect, is avoided. Even if the opening in the duct is sutured, a cigarette drain could, without detriment, be anchored in the neighborhood of the sutures.

If the gall-bladder is apparently normal and can easily be emptied by pressure, it is not necessary to add a cholecystostomy to the choledochotomy. This ideal condition, however, will seldom obtain.

The gall-bladder may be and frequently is contracted, suggesting cholecystectomy; but, because of the tendency to the re-formation of stones in the common duct, the gall-bladder should not be sacrificed. Instead, a drain may be inserted and some arrangement of gauze provided, as described on a previous page.

If dense adhesions exist, it may be impossible thoroughly to expose the duct. In this event the stone should be made as prominent as possible and the tissues covering it incised, care being taken to avoid other important structures, and no tissue being incised that cannot readily be controlled. Traction sutures or forceps can be placed on the sides of the incisions, and, if the case is urgent, the forceps may be left in place and surrounded by gauze for drainage, as already described.

Retroduodenal Choledochotomy.—This operation is advised for cases of stone impacted in that segment of the duct which lies behind the second portion of the duodenum. Kocher, who first described this operation,* advised cutting the peritoneum along the right margin of the duodenum, raising the latter by careful blunt dissection, so as to expose the duct, and then carrying out the rest of the operation as in the supraduodenal removal. The objections to this operation are: that the bowel may be so damaged as to lead to the formation of a fistula, and that there is danger of wounding the pancreas, which often surrounds this portion of the duct. Instead, an attempt should be made to move the stone up to the supraduodenal portion or down into the ampulla, in which latter location it can be removed by the transduodenal route, next to be described.

Duodeno-choledochotomy (Kocher's transduodenal choledochotomy).—This is the operation to be preferred when a stone, firmly impacted in a terminal segment or in the ampulla, resists all efforts to carry it upward into the supraduodenal part.

* "Operative Surgery," 1903.

The stone is made prominent and a longitudinal incision is made through the anterior wall of the duodenum over the stone. Precautions are taken to prevent soiling from an escape of the duodenal contents. The edges of the incision are now grasped with forceps and pulled apart, or traction sutures are used for this purpose. The stone will then appear beneath the tense mucous membrane of the posterior wall. This membrane is incised and the stone is extracted. If other stones exist above this, an attempt should be made to force them down. The posterior incision need not be sutured unless it is of some length. The incision in the anterior wall of the duodenum should be closed by suturing, in the same manner as that which is employed in closing the bowel elsewhere. If no soiling has occurred, the abdomen may be closed without drainage; if there is any suspicion of soiling, a cigarette drain may be anchored close to the site of the incision; such drainage indeed can do no harm in any case, and does not materially delay primary union.

If stones exist in the gall-bladder, or if there is thickening or some other sign of infection, this viscus should also be opened; or the presence of stone in the supraduodenal portion may demand removal at the same time; in which case both these operations should precede the duodeno-choledochotomy. When, preceding a transduodenal operation, a supraduodenal opening has been made, the scoop should be passed from one opening to the other to make sure that all stones have been removed, or a piece of gauze may be drawn through from the upper to the lower opening. (The Mayos.) One advantage of the operation just described is the fact that the obstruction may be found to be due to an unsuspected cancer of the duodenum or the papillæ.

Choledodectomy.—Choledodectomy, or excision of the common duct, is demanded very infrequently in cases of cancer, and more rarely still for stricture of the duct, congenital or acquired. According partly to the conditions present, and still more to the portion of the duct involved, the following methods of procedure may be employed:—(*a*) When the terminal portion of the duct and the papillæ are involved the excision should be performed by the transduodenal method, that is, through a longitudinal incision in the anterior wall of the duodenum, the growth being attacked from the side of the mucous membrane. (*b*) When the duct is involved higher up, complete excision, with end-to-end anastomosis, may be performed. A defect in the line of suturing is left, through this drainage is introduced, and the operation is then completed as in choledochotomy. A few successful cases have been reported. (*c*) When the excision leaves the duct too short for anastomosis, the upper portion may be reimplanted into the duodenum. The method employed by the Mayos is to make an incision, one inch long, in the duodenum, and through this incision to introduce forceps, by means of which the wall of the intestine is pushed outward at the site of the proposed implantation. A small cut is made here, the forceps is passed through, and the duct is caught and drawn into the small duodenal opening. Two stitches are placed in such a manner as to unite the outer surfaces of the duct and duodenum; continued traction invaginates more of the duct and duodenal wall and permits the placing of a second row of sutures. The incision in the anterior wall of the duodenum is then closed, drains are anchored in position, and the abdominal incision is closed. Halsted and others have reported cases.

Choledochenterostomy.—This operation, which has for its object the union of the common bile-duct with the duodenum, is only rarely called for, and can be performed only when the duct is greatly dilated. The union may be effected by means of a Murphy button, by bone bobbins, or simply by suture. Cases are reported by Robson, and the Mayos have treated a dilated hepatic duct in this way.

Choledochostomy.—This operation, which consists in attaching the dilated duct to the surface of the body and establishing permanent drainage, has been performed, but is seldom, perhaps never, demanded; its place is much better filled by choledochenterostomy.

If the gall-bladder is present and the cystic duct patulous, a cholecystenterostomy or a cholecystostomy may in most cases be substituted for the operations just described.

Plastic operations for filling in defects in the common duct have been devised by Steudenrach,* who has recorded a successful case.

For the treatment of cancer or stricture of the common duct there is thus a rather wide choice of operations.

Operations on the Hepatic Duct.—Gall-stones in the hepatic duct are not common. When present, they are usually associated with stones in the common duct, and should, with these, be removed through the opening made by a supraduodenal choledochotomy. After all discoverable stones have been removed in this way, provision should be made for the future escape of stones that may be washed down from above. This may be done either by dilating with forceps that portion of the duct which lies between the choledochotomy wound and the papillæ, or by making a large opening in the duct, leaving it entirely open, and providing ample drainage.

Hepaticotomy.—Only rarely has a solitary gall-stone been found impacted in the hepatic duct. When this occurs and the stone cannot be forced into the common duct, an incision may be made directly over the stone, or the stone may be crushed, or the incision in the supraduodenal portion of the duct may be carried up into the hepatic.

Hepaticostomy.—This operation is performed on a dilated hepatic duct. It consists in opening the duct and securing it to an opening in the abdominal wall. The operation has been performed under the impression that the duct was the gall-bladder. Under such conditions an anastomosis between the duct and the duodenum would be much more serviceable. (See page 269.)

Operations on the Intrahepatic Bile-Ducts.—Operations on the intrahepatic ducts are of casual and usually only of academic interest. Forbes Hawkes has reported a case in which stones were felt through the dome of the liver. In this case packing was arranged to produce adhesions, and several days later the stones were removed through an incision of the liver. The patient recovered.

* Trans. Ger. Surg. Cong., 1906.

To this operation, Bland Sutton applies the term "hepato-hepaticotomy." Where the gall-bladder is atrophied and the common or hepatic ducts strictured or obliterated, attempts have been made to relieve the jaundice by making an incision and suturing the obstructed ducts to an opening in the jejunum. This operation was first successfully performed by Kehr (quoted by Bland Sutton). It would seem, from the reports of others, that no infection follows such an anastomosis. This operation is labelled "hepato-cholangioenterostomy."

After-Treatment Following the Different Operations upon the Gall-Bladder and Bile-Ducts.—The after-treatment of these cases does not differ materially from that followed after other abdominal operations. The routine treatment is to return the patient to bed, place a pillow under the knees, elevate the head moderately, and enjoin absolute quiet. If the pulse is weak or is not recovering its tone rapidly enough, a hot saline enema may be given; and some advise adding to the enema from half an ounce to an ounce of brandy.

The bodily position just mentioned is the usual one, but, if one fears some lung complication, it is well to raise the patient's head and shoulders soon after he has recovered consciousness. On the other hand, if peritonitis or an escape of fluid is feared, it is well to keep the patient's shoulders low, as thereby any peritonitic effusion that may be present will be retained in Morrison's space, just as the Fowler position confines peritonitic effusions to the cavity of the pelvis. The patient may also be turned on the right side without interfering with this retention of fluids in Morrison's space. This position, furthermore, sometimes relieves vomiting and adds to the patient's comfort.

After a prolonged operation on the bile-ducts shock is a frequent occurrence and often severe. As a rule, there is little hemorrhage, and consequently the shock is not due to loss of blood; it probably results from the trauma inflicted on important viscera and on the nerve plexuses which are so abundant in that vicinity. It should, of course, be treated in the same manner as when it follows other abdominal operations, viz., by stimulants and by intravenous or intra-arterial injections of saline solution in combination with suprarenal extract, according to the method of Crile. (See the article on " Surgical Shock," in Vol. I.) A very effective plan of treatment is to introduce normal salt solution into the rectum according to the method of Murphy. This allays thirst, relieves the necessity for gastric ingestion of water, particularly where vomiting is present, and stimulates the kidneys. Morphia should practically never be administered, yet there are certain cases in which, administered soon after the operation, it promptly relieves the pain and wretchedness which accompany returning consciousness. After this single administration the drug should be withheld. In certain cases one may substitute, for the morphia, codeine phosphate, administered hypodermically; the constipating and other unpleasant effects of the former remedy being thus avoided. Even codeine, however, should be dispensed with, if possible.

Vomiting sometimes precedes and frequently follows these operations. It is due in part to conditions (adhesions, etc.) that preceded the operation, in part to the paralysis of the duodenum and stomach which follows the infliction of the trauma incidental to operation. Frequently the vomitus is great in quantity, and contains fresh or old bile. When, by its frequency or persistence, it is sapping the strength of the patient, resort should be had to gastric lavage. The introduction of saline solution *per rectum* slowly and in large quantities, according to the method of Murphy, is also extremely valuable. Morphia, in these cases of vomiting, should be very strictly avoided. The Mayos say that the retention of poisonous products—and in some cases even acute dilatation of the stomach—is prone to follow cholecystectomy.

The Feeding of the Patient after the Operation.—In the average case the patient is allowed nothing by mouth except a little cracked ice for the first twelve to eighteen or even twenty-four hours. During this time he is permitted to rinse the mouth with cold water, and after eighteen hours, if there is no vomiting, hot water is permitted—at first in half-ounce doses and afterward in gradually increasing quantities. Later, cool and then cold (not iced) water, depending on the behavior of the stomach, may be taken. Food is not given until after the lapse of from eighteen to twenty-four hours; then a little clear broth or peptonized milk is given, the quantity and frequency being gradually increased. Solid food should not be allowed until after the bowels have moved, which usually occurs on the third day; even then caution must be observed. When the ingestion of water, or liquid or solid food, excites vomiting, it should be withdrawn and recourse had to the rectum.

A cathartic may be administered by the mouth on the second day following the operation, but, if this proves to be too disturbing, enemas should be resorted to.

In those cases in which morphia must be administered it is wise to give calomel or other cathartic soon afterward; the stomach is then quiescent and the calomel helps to overcome the paralyzing effects of the morphia.

Treatment of the Sequelæ and Complications.—*Hemorrhage.*—Hemorrhage should be avoided by a proper selection of cases and by preliminary treatment with gelatin, lactate of calcium, etc. During operation the most scrupulous care should be exercised in controlling the bleeding, particularly the parenchymatous oozing. It would seem justifiable to abandon an operation which, in its early stages, exhibits an uncontrollable oozing. If hemorrhage follows an operation, a renewal of the packing, infusion of a saline solution, or, better, direct blood transfusion, may be tried.

Sepsis.—Sepsis should be avoided by proper drainage, and should be treated, if it follows operation, by surgical measures.

Adhesions.—Adhesions,—both those which existed before the operation and those which develop subsequently,—if they give rise to obstruction of the ducts or of the intestine, should be divided and their recurrence prevented by fixing the colon or great omentum over the denuded surfaces.

Acute Perforation of the Gall-Bladder or Biliary Passages.—This event should be treated in the same manner as perforative appendicitis, viz., by laparotomy, closure of the opening, and drainage. If the inflammatory products are free, the patient's head and shoulders should be elevated (Fowler) and pelvic drainage established; if they are confined to Morrison's space, the head should be kept low and drainage established in the loin.

Fistulæ.—Fistulæ may be internal or external. An internal fistula, if it causes symptoms of obstruction, demands laparotomy, with the adoption of suitable measures for closing the fistula and re-establishing the carrying function of the intestinal canal. Care must also be taken not to interfere with bile drainage.

An external fistula may be of either the mucous or the biliary variety. A mucous fistula discharges no bile, frequently follows cholecystostomy, and is due to obstruction of the cystic duct, usually from an overlooked stone, or from a stricture following stone; this form is best treated by cholecystectomy. A biliary fistula is accompanied, as a rule, by a moderate discharge of bile. Fistulæ of this nature may develop spontaneously or may follow cholecystostomy; the latter are usually due to a failure on the part of the surgeon to remove all the stones and should be treated by enlarging the opening and completely removing all foreign material, and then, if this fails, by cholecystectomy. Spontaneous biliary fistulæ are not frequent, but do occur, the opening being found near the umbilicus, in the loin, or indeed in almost any part of the abdomen. The opening in these spontaneous fistulæ is rarely adequate and should be enlarged. Ferguson recommends the injection of methylene blue, previous to operation, as a means of enabling one to follow the divisions of the cavity and remove all foreign material. Should this fail, cholecystectomy is indicated. According to the Mayos, an external biliary fistula may follow the fixation of the gall-bladder, in cholecystostomy, to the skin or the lower angle of the wound, thus permitting bile to escape in certain attitudes of the body. The treatment is to detach the fundus and then to place it properly.

Hernia.—Hernia rarely follows a short incision placed high; it is more likely to follow a long low incision. The treatment follows the lines laid down elsewhere. (See the article an "Abdominal Hernia," in Vol. VII.)

The recrudescence of gall-stones or the occurrence of cancer following operation for gall-stones will also require appropriate treatment.

A certain number of cases operated on for the relief of disturbances of the gall-bladder and common duct are not followed by a cure; instead, they become neurotic. Usually such patients have had many operations and have become intensely despondent. The chief symptoms are a painful dragging in the scar and a sense of discomfort—sensations which are generally constant, and which serve to differentiate the condition from mechanical interference due to adhesions, in which the attacks are more or less distinct. (The Mayos.)

The treatment is that of neurasthenia, care being taken to avoid the folly of adding another operation to the already long list.

SURGICAL DISEASES, WOUNDS, AND MALFORMA-TIONS OF THE URINARY BLADDER AND THE PROSTATE.

By *ALEXANDER HUGH FERGUSON, M.D., C.M., Chicago, Illinois.*

I. ANATOMY AND PATHOLOGY OF THE URINARY BLADDER.

ANATOMICAL CONSIDERATIONS.—The urinary bladder varies in size, shape, and position with the volume of its contents. Normally, it is entirely below the plane of the inlet of the pelvis.

The shape of the viscus is usually described as pyriform, except in the flaccid, empty condition. When the bladder is strongly contracted, the antero-inferior and superior surfaces are approximated until the cavity appears, in sagittal section, as a mere cleft, bounded by the thick walls of the organ. Below, this cleft is continuous with the urethra. In the distended condition, the borders and surfaces become gradually effaced and the viscus becomes almost ovoid in shape. As the bladder fills with urine, the first parts affected are the postero-lateral surfaces, expansion occurring more rapidly in the transverse than in the horizontal direction. The expanding viscus invades the perivesical spaces and presses downward and backward against the second part of the rectum and the vesiculæ seminales. Only when distention is marked, does the antero-inferior surface lengthen and the apex rise above the pubis. With extreme distention the bladder rises out of the pelvis and encroaches decidedly on the abdominal cavity.

The physiological capacity of the urinary bladder varies with different individuals, but may be stated approximately at from six to nine ounces. The maximum capacity is about twenty-four ounces.

The bladder presents for examination the following surfaces: (*a*) antero-inferior, or pubic; (*b*) posterior, or rectal; (*c*) superior, or intestinal; (*d*) two lateral, or obturator. (Fig. 106.)

The anterior, posterior, and obturator surfaces meet at the apex of the organ, where the urachus (the relic of the communication of the bladder with the allantois) is attached.

The anterior and inferior surface looks downward toward the symphysis. It is not covered by the peritoneum and is separated from the pubic bones by a space (cavum Retzii) containing areolar tissue, which is directly continuous with the subperitoneal fat.

Each obturator surface is covered by peritoneum as far as a line drawn from the urachus to the summit of the vesiculæ seminales. Below this line the

279

bladder is separated from the levator ani muscle by subperitoneal fatty tissue, in the meshes of which course the vessels and nerves. Just above this line of peritoneal reflection lie the remains of the hypogastric arteries. This surface is also crossed by the vas deferens.

The posterior surface is divided into two parts by the reflection of the peritoneum from the rectum in the male, and from the uterus in the female. The distance of this line of reflection from the base of the prostate varies from

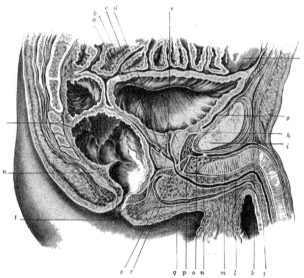

Fig. 106.—Median Sagittal Section of the Pelvis, Showing the General Relation of the Bladder and Prostate. (After Deaver.)

a, Ejaculatory duct in prostatic fissure; b, sinus pocularis; c, middle lobe of prostate; d, urinary bladder; e, prostate; f, sigmoid flexure; g, prevesical fat in space of Retzius; h, vesico-pubic muscle, i, symphysis pubis; j, suspensory ligament of penis; k, angle of penis; l, corpus spongiosum; m, corpus cavernosum; n, spongy portion of urethra; o, dorsal vein of penis; p, vesico-prostatic plexus of veins; q, accelerator urinæ muscle; r, bulb of penis; s, compressor urethræ muscle; t, sphincter ani muscles; u, raphe of levator ani muscle; v, rectum.

half an inch to two inches, according to the distention of the viscus. The ureters open into the bladder at the junction of the lateral and posterior surfaces.

The superior surface is entirely covered with peritoneum and lies in contact with the small intestines or the sigmoid flexure of the colon.

The appearance of the mucous membrane of the urinary bladder varies with the amount of distention. The mucosa is connected with the muscular tissue by a loose muscularis mucosæ. In consequence, the mucous membrane is formed into longitudinal folds in contraction; in distention it is more or less smooth; in extreme distention the muscular fibres are frequently separated and the mucosa puffs out into these interstices as diverticuli.

The trigonum vesicæ, bounded by the urethral opening and the ureteral orifices, is smooth in all conditions of the bladder. No muscularis mucosæ is present in this situation; the mucous membrane rests upon a compact muscular stratum, enforced by prolongations from the sheath of the ureters. The ureteral orifices are united by a band-like elevation, the plica ureterica. This is formed by the mucosa and muscularis in consequence of the oblique course of the ureters through the bladder wall. The orificium urethræ internum is at the apex of the trigonum and is usually crescentic in outline because of the projection of its lower border forward. This is due to a thickening of the mucosa enclosing bundles of muscle tissue, which not infrequently undergoes hyper-

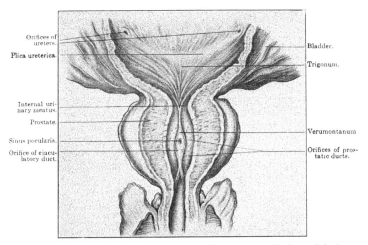

FIG. 107.—The Trigonum of the Human Urinary Bladder, the Prostatic Urethra, and the Prostate Gland. (After Deaver.)

trophy and becomes of surgical importance. It is called the uvula vesicæ and is continuous with the urethral crest in the prostatic portion of the urethra. (Fig. 107.)

The ureteral orifices are slit-like and are about 4 or 5 mm. long. The lateral borders are guarded by a projection which acts as a valve. This is known as the valvula ureteris and forms part of the thickening of the ureteral wall. Behind the trigonum vesicæ is the retrotrigonal fossa (fossa retro-ureterica), which corresponds to the "bas fond" of the French writers.

Structural Details.—Over the trigonum the mucosa is very thin and comparatively smooth. Elsewhere its thickness varies with distention, reaching sometimes 2 mm. The basement epithelium is of the columnar type, which gradually changes into an irregular polygonal cell. At the surface, the cells are plate-like in character. Few glands, if any, are found in the bladder.

The submucosa is composed of fibrous tissue, interwoven with elastic tissue.

It allows free movement of the mucosa and supports the blood-vessels and nerves. It is replaced beneath the trigonum by muscular tissue. The muscular structure is divided into three parts. The outer layer is longitudinal, and is thin and variable, being interspersed with areolar tissue. The inner circular layer is strong and robust; from a physiological standpoint, it is the most important layer. It is very weak until it reaches the level of the ureters. The innermost layer is connected with the muscularis mucosæ, and is important because it becomes condensed in the area of the trigonum and passes forward to form part of the internal sphincter of the urethra.

The blood-supply of the bladder is derived from the superior and inferior branches of the internal iliac artery; also from the middle hemorrhoidal, obturator, and internal pubic arteries. The veins form a submucous plexus which drains the mucosa and empties into an intramuscular plexus. These veins pass into an extraperitoneal plexus which empties into the prostatico-vesical plexus, at the sides of the prostate and bladder, and finally into the internal iliac veins.

Anomalies of the Urinary Bladder.—Anomalies of the urinary bladder are few; the chief one is exstrophy.

Exstrophy.—The bladder has been known to be entirely absent. (Gould and Pyle.) It has also been found in the form of multiple organs. (Scibelli, of Naples.) Diverticula, dilated ureters, and a patent urachus should not be mistaken for exstrophy. When the urachus is open, urine escapes from the umbilicus. This condition is due to the failure of the line of union between the allantois and the bladder to undergo obliteration. Sometimes the urachus forms a cyst.

Another anomaly is fusion of the bladder with other structures.

Ectopia Vesicæ.—In ectopia vesicæ not only is the bladder deficient, but so also are the bones, muscles, fat, and skin in front of it. The anatomical picture is here represented by a deficient bladder without an anterior abdominal wall; only the trigonum, bearing the ureteral openings and more or less of the posterior wall, is present. The suprapubic abdominal wall (hypogastrium) is absent. The penis is rudimentary and often presents complete epispadias. The symphysis is usually deficient; sometimes it is absent. Double congenital hernia of the inguinal variety is present in most cases. The umbilicus is not always recognizable. There is a constant dribbling of urine from the ureteral openings and, in consequence of this exposure, the mucous membrane and, secondarily, the surrounding skin are likely to become chronically inflamed. Eventually an ascending pyelonephritis terminates life. In some of these cases the patient, even without surgical aid, lives to a considerable age. For a complete and most instructive thesis on ectopia vesicæ, the reader is referred to a paper by F. Gregory Connell, which was awarded the Senn Medal at the fifty-first annual meeting of the American Medical Association, June 6th, 1900.

Treatment of Ectopia Vesicæ.—To overcome this disagreeable condition, operative procedures are well worth while. Palliative means, such as the use of urinals, vulcanite cups, etc., for the purpose of collecting the urine, are not to be recommended when there is no contra-indication to operation. The age at which surgical interference is advisable depends entirely upon the general health of the patient. The most desirable time, according to some surgeons, is between the ages of two and eight years. All things being equal, the sooner relief is given the better for all concerned. Infants bear operations of this character badly. The youngest infant to survive an operation (uretero-rectal) for ectopia was ten months old. The operation was performed by Dr. J. J. Buchanan, of Pittsburg, on Feb. 1st, 1908. (*Surgery, Gynæcology, and Obstetrics*, Feb., 1909.) The operation was a complete success. Inasmuch as ascending infection cuts short so many of these unfortunate cases, the surgeon, bearing in mind that, without surgical aid, sixty-nine per cent of the patients die before the age of twenty-one years, should advise operation before infection takes place. On the other hand, a locus minoris resistentiæ is established by an operation which predisposes to infection. One should rather run this risk, however, than attempt an operation after the ureters and kidneys have become infected. The writer would refuse to operate upon a case of ectopia if pyelonephritis were already present. It is true that patients with ectopia vesicæ have reached old age without any treatment. The first case of this kind known to have occurred in America was, according to Connell, reported in 1827 by Hamilton. The patient was a woman, aged forty years, who was then delivered of a child and afterward lived to be eighty.

In presenting the literature up to 1900, F. Gregory Connell furnished the following excellent classification of the different methods of treatment, palliative or radical:—

A.—Palliative Measures.

I. Apparatus.

II. (1) Flap of skin; (*a*) epidermis in (reversed); (*b*) epidermis out. (2) Flap of mucous membrane: (*a*) remaining bladder wall of patient; (*b*) intestinal wall of patient; (*c*) bladder of lower animals.

III. Suture of edges of fissure: (1) by direct suture: (2) preceded by preliminary suture.

IV. Miscellaneous:—(1) Dilatation of ureters; (2) plaster bandage; (3) catheters in the ureters; (4) fistula in perineum; (5) ureters inserted into the urethra. Nephrectomy on one side and lumbar ureteral fistula on the other.

B.—Radical Measures.

I. Axial implantation: (1) by sutures; (2) by apparatus.

II. Vesico-rectal anastomosis.

III. Implantation of trigonum vesicæ.

IV. Implantation in a manner imitating normal insertion into the bladder; or an attempt to make a valve.

V. Miscellaneous: (1) vesico-vagino-rectal fistula, with colpocleisis; (2) artificial anus, with ureters inserted into rectum; (3) artificial bladder, (*a*) opening into the urethra, (*b*) opening into the intestinal tract.

Palliative Measures.—There are two objections to palliative treatment: (*a*) no sphincter is provided; (*b*) no suitable receptacle is formed to hold the

urine. Even when the skin flaps are made and aided by osteoplastic approximation of the deficient bones and edges of the exstrophy (Trendelenburg),
sloughing and spreading infection are liable to occur. The best that is obtainable is to provide a spout over which a rubber urinal is attached to prevent the
urine from constantly bathing the surrounding skin. In one of my cases hair
grew in the pouch obtained by Wood's operation. In all, I performed three
operations, viz.: (a) a double inguinal herniotomy; (b) the turning down of
large skin flaps to form the anterior wall of the bladder; (c) the utilization of
the rudimentary penis as a permanent spout and the adjustment of flaps thereto.
Neither this operation nor any modifications of it (Thiersch) need any longer
be attempted. However, should any surgeon be disposed to select this procedure, he may derive some assistance from the following brief statement of
the steps which I adopted. The deficient bladder was filled with glass marbles,
which served by their weight to press the posterior wall and trigonum downward and backward, while the boy was kept constantly on his back. Three
or four times a day a pitcherful of boric-acid solution (saturated) was poured
into the bladder to produce as aseptic a field as possible. The inflammation
subsided in the course of a week. When I operated the marbles prevented
the raw surfaces of the flaps from coming in contact with the mucous membrane,
and, to my delight, union occurred by first intention. The marbles were not
removed until the third operation.

Should the conditions be favorable for Sonnenberg's operation, I should
be tempted to recommend it because of its less dangerous character. It
is true that neither a sphincter nor a receptacle is formed in this procedure; but a simple urinal can be worn with comfort. In this operation
the ureters are dissected up from their normal positions, and sutured into the
dorsal groove of the penis between the edges of a skin flap. Dr. J. Rilus Eastman,
of Indianapolis, has successfully operated by this method. The rest of the
bladder may be extirpated and the raw surface covered by skin flaps or grafts.
Let me suggest that, after a reasonable time, if no sepsis has occurred, there
could be no objection to making an anastomosis of the little penis with the
rectum, extraperitoneally. This procedure would no doubt form an additional
safeguard to ascending infection. It must be remembered that partial failure
is the rule after any of the palliative operations, and that, even in the most
successful cases, the urinal must be worn. Multiple operations for exstrophy
are usually necessary. Billroth performed nineteen operations on one patient
in the course of twenty-two months.

Transplantation of the bladder from one of the lower animals has not yet
been successfully performed.

Radical Measures.—Radical operations may be defined as those which aim
at diverting the urine into the large bowel or the rectum. Since the days of
Simon, of London (1851), and of Roux, of Paris, no material success was obtained
until Maydl (1892) implanted the trigonum of the bladder, with the distal
ends of the ureters, into the rectum. This trigonum-sigmoid implantation
was the logical sequence of the conclusions of Tuffier (1890), arrived at from

clinical observations, viz., that the implantation of cut ureters into the bowel fails because, in these cases, ascending renal infection is present. Maydl's operation soon became the one of choice. At least eighty patients (Buchanan) have been operated upon by this method with wonderful results as compared with those obtained by the old methods. The success of this operation is due to the preservation of the ureteral orifices, which fact renders ascending infection more difficult. Still, even here the mortality amounted to 28.7 per cent. This was due principally to obstruction of the ureters through twisting or kinking. The fact that the abdomen had to be opened was a serious objection to Maydl's operation, for peritonitis was not infrequent. Maydl thought it important to save the trigonum because it furnished the blood-supply to the ureter. This was soon demonstrated to be incorrect by Margarucci (International Congress at Rome, 1894), who showed that the ureter was nourished by independent blood-vessels descending along with it. These vessels supplied not only the ureter but also the mucous membrane above the ureteral orifices. Thus the contention that sloughing would occur if the continuity of the trigonum were disturbed, was disproved. The knowledge of the ureteral blood-supply justifies the surgeon in dissecting out each ureter separately,—due respect, of course, being shown the accompanying vessels,—and implanting them separately into the bowel, without considering the trigonum as essential to success. A practical recognition of the vascular supply of the ureter contra-indicates the operation of Maydl, or any modification of it. In short, all intraperitoneal operations that have been performed for the cure of ectopia of the bladder are no longer to be recommended. Experitoneal implantation of the intact ureters, with a button of bladder attached, by separate openings into the rectum, is easier to perform and has a lower mortality than Maydl's operation. This operation was first performed by Bergenhem, of Sweden, in 1894, as published in *Eira*, a Swedish journal. The second operation by this method was performed by Pozzi, of Italy, in 1897; the third, by Franklin H. Martin, of Chicago, in 1898; the fourth, by Capelle, of Rome, in 1898; the fifth, by Lenden, of Australia; and the sixth by the late George A. Peters, of Toronto, in 1899.

Another radical measure is the separate and extraperitoneal implantation of the ureters in the rectum. This procedure, which is known as Bergenhem's operation (Fig. 108), is carried out in the following manner:—Catheterize the ureters; cut through the mucous membrane of the ureters in a circular manner, around each ureteral orifice; leave a rosette of bladder attached to the terminal end of each ureter; and then dissect the ureter up liberally but without injuring the peritoneum and ureteral blood-vessels. Next, pass the finger into the rectum and locate the side of the bowel opposite the trigonum of the bladder; then substitute a blunt, curved forceps for the finger and push it through a small incision in the antero-lateral wall of the rectum. Remove the catheters, seize the mucous membrane of the rosette, and draw it and the ureter into the rectum; release the forceps and allow the rosetted ureter to recede into the rectum. Carry out the same procedure on the other side, and the operation is then

practically completed. The ureters must not be subjected to any tension, to
secure which result the wall of the rectum should be pierced high up. No
stitches are required to hold the ureters in the rectum. The forceps used must
not be too large. It is a mistake to leave the catheters in the ureters for a
few days, for this favors ascending infection. At least two deaths have followed
this procedure. The bladder may be subsequently extirpated and the defect
closed by a plastic operation.

Bergenhem's operation—which is known in America and England as Peters'
operation—is, in the writer's opinion, the best surgical procedure for the treatment of ectopia vesicæ. Buchanan (1909) gives a table of 98 patients who

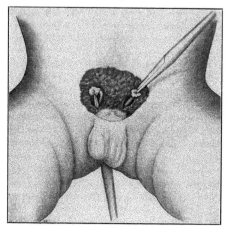

Fig. 108.—Separate and Extraperitoneal Implantation, Uretero-rectal: Bergenhem's Operation. (After Buchanan.)

survived the operation after intact ureters had been implanted into the bowel.
He states that only eleven are known to have developed ascending infection.
This statement, of course, includes Maydl's operation and modifications thereof.
The immediate mortality of Bergenhem's operation is but eleven per cent.
The patients are comparatively comfortable; they are able to hold the urine
in the rectum for three or four hours without leakage.

Injuries of the Bladder.—Traumatic injuries of the bladder, in which the
force is applied from the outside, the impact being on the abdominal wall,
occur, as a rule, only when the viscus is distended, inasmuch as the fundus then
rises above the symphysis pubis. Unless the injury involves only a part of
the bladder wall, and only a small part at that, the result is likely to be fatal.
The condition demands immediate surgical intervention. Other injuries, such
as those caused by fracture of the pelvis, by labor, or by instrumental manipulation inside the bladder, will be considered elsewhere. (See pages 287–289.)

Rupture of the Urinary Bladder.—Rupture of the bladder is comparatively infrequent; it occurs usually in men, as a direct result of a fracture of the pelvis, although overdistention may lead to rupture. Cases of the latter description, however, occur more frequently in women than in men.

The causes of rupture are predisposing and exciting. Among the predisposing causes may be mentioned distention of the viscus, alcoholism, urethral stricture, enlarged prostate, disease of the bladder wall, advanced age, etc. The exciting causes are traumatic and idiopathic in nature. How great a rôle in the production of a rupture of the bladder overdistention plays, cannot be determined definitely, but it is certain that mere overdistention of a normal bladder does not, *per se*, lead to rupture, except in very rare instances. In such cases there is usually an hypertrophy of the muscle. Guyon, for instance, believes that overdistention of the bladder causes the hypertrophied muscle to contract with such force that the viscus is ruptured. Dittel found, by experimentation, that if the bladder of a cadaver is filled with air, to the point of rupture, the rent always occurs in the posterior wall and intraperitoneally; whereas, if water is injected, the rent occurs intraperitoneally in about one-half the cases, and extraperitoneally in the other half. Of eight cases of rupture due to overdistention, in my practice, the rent was extraperitoneal seven times, and intraperitoneal only once. In most cases of rupture due to overdistention, trauma is the exciting cause.

Acute alcoholism lessens the elasticity of the bladder wall, increases the secretion of urine, and leads to overdistention by lessening the sensitiveness of the patient. Chronic alcoholism leads to the formation of diverticula by frequent overdistention and weakening of the bladder wall. Stricture of the urethra is operative, as a cause of rupture, by producing, at first, an hypertrophy and, later, an atrophy of the bladder wall. The cystitis which so frequently occurs in these cases must also be taken into account. The same is true when there is an hypertrophy of the prostate.

The diseases of the bladder wall that act as predisposing causes are cystitis, from any cause, tuberculous ulcers, and new-growths, either benign or malignant.

Rupture may occur at any age, but is most frequent between the twentieth and the fortieth years. In 23 cases, reported by Besley, 1 patient was a child three years of age, 5 were between twenty and thirty, 7 between thirty and forty, 6 between forty and fifty, and in 2 the age was not given.

The usual cause of rupture is traumatism, such as severe blows upon the abdomen, crushing injuries of the pelvis by a heavy weight, or the passing of some heavy object over the abdomen or downward into the pelvis.

Among the idiopathic causes of rupture may be mentioned muscular action upon an overdistended bladder due to urethral stricture, to an enlarged prostate, or to an imperforate urethra, as in a case reported by King; also retroversion of a gravid uterus, and labor pains.

The site of the rupture varies. The summit of the bladder and the posterior wall are the most frequent sites for intraperitoneal rupture. As a rule, the rupture is a clean tear, though occasionally it may be extremely ragged. Generally, the rupture resembles a perforation and rarely measures more than two or three inches in length. In intraperitoneal ruptures the bladder contents are thrown into the peritoneal cavity and peritonitis results, not infrequently ending in death. If the rent is a small one, only a portion of the urine escapes into the tissues, where it may become encapsulated and give rise to no further trouble. Usually, however, untreated rupture of the bladder is a fatal accident.

Incomplete ruptures occur only when the tear is extraperitoneal, and then little, if any, urine escapes, although the bladder wall may become infiltrated with urine. Necrosis then occurs, with extension upward to the ureters and kidneys.

Out of the 169 cases of rupture of the bladder collected from the literature, only 49 were extraperitoneal. According to Bartels, rupture of the bladder occurred 109 times in 179 cases as the result of fracture of the pelvic bones. This accident, no matter what its etiology, is always a serious affair and should be given prompt attention.

Just how these ruptures occur is difficult to explain. No one theory will explain all cases. Trauma, by producing a fracture of one or more of the pelvic bones, naturally would produce lesions which vary in degree and location. It is generally conceded that, in order that rupture may occur, the bladder must contain some fluid,—a condition which lessens the elasticity of the organ. The contents, owing to their fluid nature, are non-compressible, and the rupture takes place at the weakest part of the bladder wall. Most frequently the tears take place at the postero-superior aspect and in an antero-posterior direction. The rupture usually takes place from within outward, and the extent of the tear depends on the disposition of the muscle fibres rather than on the direction or force of the trauma.

When the bladder is filled with urine it extends above the symphysis pubis. The direction of a blow upon the abdomen is toward the back; hence, an intraperitoneal rupture will occur. If the bladder is distended slightly, the force of the blow is downward toward the lower and posterior wall, and an extraperitoneal rupture will occur at that site.

Besley concludes, as the result of experiments on the cadaver, that there is no particular order in which the coats of the bladder give way when a rupture occurs. Sometimes it is the mucous coat and sometimes the peritoneal coat which is the first to tear. When pressure is applied equally, the tear is at the weakest point, which is not always the same anatomically. Besley agrees with Stubenrauch that the coats tear from within outward.

As to the site of the tears, Bartels gives the following order as to frequency: (a) usually in the anterior wall, to the right or the left of the median line; (b) in the postero-superior wall; (c) in the postero-inferior wall; (d) in the superior aspect or junction of the neck and body, rarely. He believes that the anterior ruptures are never intraperitoneal, and in these cases, therefore, the urine spreads through the cellular tissues of the pelvis.

The most frequent complication occurring with rupture of the bladder is fracture of the pelvis. Laceration of the soft parts and severe traumatism of the other organs of the body have also been observed. Peritonitis and sloughing of tissue are the direct result of extravasation of urine and can be prevented only by prompt surgical intervention. Cystitis, pyelitis, and abscess of the kidney are seen occasionally as complications. Obstruction of the ureter by cicatricial contraction may cause an hypernephrosis. Cicatricial contraction about the urethra is a rather common occurrence following intraperitoneal rupture where there has been an extravasation of urine into the periureteral tissues.

Symptoms.—The first symptom of rupture of the bladder is severe pain in the lower abdomen, speedily followed by shock, although the nature of the case may be such that the patient loses consciousness at once and death may occur without return of consciousness. When shock is not so severe, the patient first complains of pain and then of an irresistible desire to urinate, although no urine can be voided unless the rupture be incomplete. There may be some nausea and vomiting, accompanied by early symptoms of acute peritonitis, especially if the urine be infected. In cases in which the urethra is uninjured, a catheter may be passed into the bladder, which will be found empty, or containing a small amount of bloody urine. By moving the catheter from side to side one may easily pass it through the rent, and then a variable quantity of bloody urine is withdrawn. When this occurs it is evident that the catheter has reached extravasated urine which may be in the free pelvis or in the extraperitoneal tissues.

If the catheter passes easily into the bladder, and a bloody urine free from clots is withdrawn, it is very probable that the kidney has been ruptured. If no urine, or a very small amount, is obtained, the case is probably one of rupture of the bladder. If the kidney is ruptured, pressure in the lumbar region is very painful. This is not evident when the tear is in the bladder. A free flow of blood from the urethra signifies that this channel has been ruptured.

With the lapse of time the various complications mentioned above occur. Usually, on the second or third day symptoms of peritonitis are manifested, and the case speedily terminates fatally. If the rupture is intraperitoneal, the peritonitis usually develops at once; if it is of the extraperitoneal variety, the course is not so rapid, but little less certain, finally, from cellulitis.

Diagnosis.—The diagnosis of ruptured bladder is of prime importance and should be made without delay; for, if rupture has occurred, then immediate operation is imperative, even though the patient be otherwise severely injured. The means of reaching a diagnosis are as follows:—

(1) History of the occurrence of an injury when the bladder was distended, accompanied by a sudden, painful, bursting sensation, and followed by shock.

(2) Hæmaturia; blood is present in the little urine that is voided.

(3) A great desire to urinate and inability to pass more than a drachm or two of urine that contains blood.

(4) Bimanual examination. A rectal examination of the bladder is of some importance. If the bladder is ruptured, the neck of the viscus feels soft

and flabby. This is made more apparent if the free hand exerts at the same time firm pressure above the pubic bone. The earlier this examination is made the more valuable it is. Later on, the extravasation of urine, in the extraperitoneal cases, and the accumulation of urine in the peritoneal cavity in the intraperitoneal cases, make it more difficult to palpate the bladder. Again, should local infection or peritonitis ensue, this examination of the bladder is useless.

(5) Extravesical tumor. If, several hours after the accident, a suprapubic or perineal tumor appears, the case is one of extraperitoneal rupture. When the rupture is intraperitoneal no tumor appears, but evidence of free fluid (urine) in the peritoneal cavity gradually becomes more and more manifest.

(6) Catheterization. In cases of rupture of the bladder the organ is found to be practically empty; blood is present in the little urine that is withdrawn. If, when the catheter is pushed with some force, it enters through the rent in the bladder into the peritoneal cavity, a large quantity of urine escapes at once. The instrument should be a large-sized silver catheter with a prostatic curve; its end encounters no resistance and may be palpated through the abdominal wall. Should water be forced into the catheter the quantity which returns when the viscus is ruptured is less than that originally injected.

(7) Air test. If the bladder is torn, the air forced into it through a catheter does not distend the bladder at all, but enlarges the abdominal tumor, palpable above the pubis; the air does not return through the catheter. No harm can be done by this test and it is infallible. So much do I rely upon it, that, in all cases of suspected rupture of the bladder, I pass a soft-rubber catheter and, with a Politzer air bag, use the air test and depend upon its findings as already stated. Then no time is lost in instituting a rational line of treatment.

(8) Cystoscope. This instrument is not of much value in diagnosing a ruptured bladder and should not be used. The effusion of blood is so profuse, even when constant irrigation is employed, that it is impossible accurately to observe the seat of the injury.

(9) Exploratory laparotomy. For diagnostic purposes laparotomy is not called for. I claim that the diagnosis of rupture of the bladder may be made by less severe methods. In considering the diagnosis, one must bear in mind other conditions that cause hæmaturia—such, for example, as diseases of the kidney, ureter, and bladder. Simple contusion of the bladder, caused by a blow upon the abdominal wall over a distended bladder, may result in hæmaturia.

Prognosis.—Surgical experience covers both the expectant and the operative treatment of rupture of the bladder, and it leaves no room to doubt the harmfulness of the former and the beneficial results obtainable by the latter. The expectant plan shows a death rate of 88.7 per cent in 365 cases; only 3 patients lived out of 237 cases when the rupture was of the intraperitoneal variety. Operative procedures, on the other hand, present a mortality of 42.2 per cent in 210 cases. (Watson and Cunningham, Vol. I., p. 450, ed. of 1909.) When we consider that eighty per cent of the cases are intraperitoneal ruptures (Watson) and that usually considerable time elapses before an operation can be performed, it is remarkable that the results of operative treatment have been as good as statistics show them to be. In view of our present prompt and efficient treatment of ruptures of the urinary bladder, the prognosis is as favorable as that of any other grave injury of a similar nature. The recovery of the patient depends upon (a) prompt operation, (b) having and maintaining an aseptic condition of the urine, and (c) the nature and extent of the complications, such as fractures of the pelvic bones, etc.

Treatment in Extraperitoneal Rupture.—In the majority of these cases the rupture is situated in the anterior wall or neck of the bladder. Ruptures situated on the lateral or posterior wall nearly always include the peritoneum. Immediately after the injury, the patient may be able to pass his urine, or a portion of it, before extravasation occurs into the peritoneum or into Retzius' space. Free incision into the dusky swelling, followed by drainage, is the only treatment of any avail. The bladder may be drained by several routes: (a) via the urethra, by means of a catheter passed in the usual way; (b) through a median perineal urethrotomy; (c) suprapubically, through a rent in the bladder; or (d), in cases in which there is any difficulty in establishing free drainage, a suprapubic cystotomy should be immediately performed, and a catheter passed into the urethra through its internal orifice. The four methods of draining the bladder are here mentioned in their order of efficiency. Do not lose time, do not sew the bladder, except when the tear is easily accessible; the partial suturing is best. For gaining an entrance into the bladder one long incision in that part of the perineum which involves the urethra, is, in my opinion, preferable. A simple incision into the scrotum, or into the root of the penis, or through the tissues above the pubis, is not always sufficient. The suprapubic incisions should be multiple; one of them should be large enough to allow of inspection of the rent in the bladder, and to enable the surgeon to insert, when necessary, a few sutures of chromicized catgut. The material for drainage should be iodoform gauze soaked in glycerin and surrounded by a fair-sized rubber tube split longitudinally. The hygroscopic action of the glycerin aids drainage. It is seldom necessary to wash out the bladder or the tissues bathed in urine, even after suppuration has occurred. If the urine is septic, prompt and efficient drainage is the only safeguard against a rapidly spreading infection.

Treatment in Intraperitoneal Rupture.—The steps in the operative measures are as follows: (a) Make an abdominal section; (b) sponge out the urine; (c) suture the rent in the bladder; (d) drain the pouch of Douglas, suprapubically in the male; (e) drain the bladder through the penis with a large catheter; (f) close the abdominal wall. The abdominal incision is usually made low down in the median line, in the instance of rupture of the bladder, and utilized for determining the site and extent of the rupture, whether it be intraperitoneal or extraperitoneal. In the former instance, however, it is extended into the peritoneal cavity, the rupture located, the borders cleansed and if necessary trimmed . . . and closed with . . . bent sutures; a superimposed row being placed if needful. Some operators employ the mattress suture of Cushing. In either instance, however, the borders should be so inverted as accurately to approximate the surfaces of the serous membrane immediately contiguous to the wound. When the rupture is low down sutures are more difficult to apply and the act will be facilitated by placing the uppermost first and using them as traction agents in exposing and suturing the lower part of the rupture.

In removing the urine from the peritoneal cavity, wiping should be avoided and careful cleansing should be practised, especially if the urine be unhealthy for any reason related to the bladder or the kidneys. The extravasated urine can be quickly, efficiently, and safely removed by the agency of sponge absorption, without danger of the traumatic friction incident to wiping.

The remaining steps above enumerated are carried out in a manner similar to that adopted in other operative instances.

If peritonitis is present, drain the retrovesical space through a punctured wound in the abdomen and pass a large, soft catheter through the urethra to carry off the urine in the bladder. In this stage it is needless to attempt any repair of the bladder, and unwise to wash out the peritoneal cavity. The peritonitis must be treated according to modern methods, viz., by free drainage, by means of multiple incisions if necessary; by the Fowler position; by proctoclysis (Murphy); and by leaving the healing of the wound in the bladder to nature or to a subsequent operation.

Cystitis.—Cystitis is inflammation of the urinary bladder. The symptoms of cystitis vary with the intensity of the inflammation and the virulence of the infection. Suffice it to mention the chief symptoms when the attack is violent. Pain in the bladder, when of a spasmodic character, is excruciating. It is ushered in with rigors and is followed by a high fever, ranging from 103° to 105° Fahr. Pain of a constant character radiates to the perineum, rectum, penis, groin, and hypogastrium. It sometimes shoots down the thighs. Suprapubic pressure causes increased pain and tenderness. Rectal examination reveals a tender perineum and bladder. Vesical tenesmus and forcing out of red blood at the end of urination are somewhat characteristic features of all the marked forms of acute cystitis. The urination becomes more and more frequent, more and more painful, and does not give relief; and finally the act is completed only by constant straining and bearing down, for the bladder does not contract at all. The urine contains blood, shreds, casts, and even sloughs. Pus is in abundance and ammoniacal changes in the urine add to the anguish of the patient. In a few days he sinks into a typhoid apathy, with dry furred tongue, hot skin, swollen abdomen, and delirium. Death may occur from general sepsis, from septic peritonitis, or from ascending pyelonephritis, which latter complication is manifested by uræmic coma. Fortunately, however, in the vast majority of cases of cystitis the symptoms are much less severe than those just described, as will appear under the proper headings, and thay terminate in resolution or in chronic cystitis. Cystitis may be classified in different ways, as follows: (1) according to the appearances presented; (2) according to the etiology; and (3) according to clinical features—as, for example, (a) acute, (b) chronic. The latter is the preferable plan.

Bacteriology of Cystitis.—In cystitis with acid urine, the following germs are found: Bacillus coli communis, alone; bacillus tuberculosis, alone; bacillus typhosus (Eberth's bacillus), alone; gonococcus, alone; pneumococcus, alone; streptococcus, alone. In cystitis with alkaline urine, the following germs are found: Bacillus coli communis, combined with bacillus proteus; diplococcus ureæ; staphylococcus; streptococcus.

Invasions of the urinary bladder by the various infections take place along four well-known routes, viz.: (1) from the posterior urethra (as, *e.g.*, in gonorrhœal infection); (2) from the kidney (as, *e.g.*, in tuberculosis of that organ); (3) from the adjacent structures (as, *e.g.*, in infectious prostatitis, metritis, salpingitis, and appendicitis); and (4) through the general circulation.

Acute Cystitis.—Acute cystitis comes on suddenly and soon involves the mucous membrane of the fundus and body of the bladder. Exposure to wet and cold plays an important rôle in persons who are diabetic, alcoholic, gouty, or rheumatic, or who harbor a latent infection. The bladder and surrounding structures are seldom free from bacteria. The exposure lessens the normal resistance of the bladder and the bacteria are then able to penetrate the mucous membrane, and inflammation is the result. The most frequent cause of acute cystitis is gonorrhœal infection (*vide* Gonorrhœal Cystitis, page 745, Vol. II.). Acute prostatitis and posterior urethritis must not be mistaken for inflammation of the bladder. Mixed infections of the bladder, induced by maltreatment of gonorrhœa, are quite common even in the most skilful hands. Cystitis may follow the passing of a catheter for the relief of retention of urine from gonorrhœa. Asepsis and antisepsis will not invariably prevent cystitis following instrumentation even in the female. It must be remembered that a catheter should never be used without the strictest surgical cleanliness and the employment of aseptic lubricants. Great injury to the pelvic bones often involves the bladder, and in many cases acute cystitis ensues. Here, again, latent infection plays its part in the etiology. When the bladder is the seat of a chronic infection, it is not surprising that acute infection follows instrumentation.

Pathology.—Acute cystitis may involve the mucosa alone, the mucosa and the muscular coat, and the perivesical tissues in addition to the mucous and muscular coats. The reddened and swollen mucous membrane, with its enlarged vessels, may be inspected through the cystoscope. Some parts appear more œdematous than others, and extravasations of blood are seen here and there. Plaques of lymph may be distributed over the mucosa. If the inflammation deepens, these plaques may coalesce and form a complete coating over the mucous membrane of the bladder. Eventually they separate and come away with the urine, leaving a raw surface behind which not infrequently ulcerates. Membranous cystitis is most frequently met with in women, in whom an entire cast of the bladder may be voided with the urine. It is associated with uterine disease. The colon bacillus is the principal organism found in these cases, although mixed infection is always present. In acute septic cystitis the mucous surface and the muscular tissue beneath become gangrenous, and within a few days this process of sphacelation may extend to and involve the peritoneum and perivesical tissues.

Symptoms.—Acute inflammation of the bladder develops somewhat suddenly. It may begin with an uncomfortable and frequent irritation in the region of the bladder, with or without chilly sensations. The patient complains of a hot scalding sensation at the neck of the bladder during urination, and he states that ease is obtained when the bladder is emptied. Pain, while always present, may not be a prominent symptom in mild cystitis. The urine is high-colored and cloudy. This mild form often passes off spontaneously. The body temperature may not be disturbed at all. Usually it ranges from 99° to 100° Fahr.

Subacute Catarrhal Cystitis.—Subacute catarrhal cystitis appears to be of a very superficial nature. The predisposing causes are: congestions following exposure to cold or the ingestion of turpentine, cantharides, arsenic, alcohol, or corrosive sublimate; or a congestion such as occurs in persons of the uric-acid diathesis. The exciting cause, of course, is infection by bacteria. Again, slight irritations following vesical irrigations, catheterization, descent of a stone from the kidney, retention of urine from any cause, result in congestion of the bladder and predispose to subacute catarrhal cystitis. This predisposition is also manifested after operations upon the bladder or upon surrounding structures, *i.e.,* operations upon the vagina and rectum. This form of cystitis usually subsides after the employment of vesical irrigations with a saturated solution of boric acid, or after the acidity of the urine has been neutralized by the internal administration of potassium acetate (gr. xx. t. i. d.), with or without the boric-acid irrigations.

The clinical characteristics are sudden onset, short duration, mild behavior. The attack passes off either spontaneously or with a minimum of local or constitutional treatment.

Acute Septic or Suppurative Cystitis.—This is a more severe type of cystitis; it lasts longer than the catarrhal variety and is either due to some virulent type of infection, following upon a gonorrhœa or a septic wound, or to an extension from a suppurating focus elsewhere in the tract. It is not unusual for the subacute catarrhal type to become more and more septic, and finally to result in chronic inflammation of the viscus or in the development of ulcerations.

Chronic Cystitis.—This type is so called because of its insidious approach, slow development, persistency, and the difficulty of effecting a cure.

The causes of chronic cystitis are identical with those of the acute form of the disease; the commonest one being catheterization without surgical cleanliness. A septic instrument passed clumsily into the bladder furnishes both the traumatism and the infection. It is true that organisms may engraft themselves upon the pabulum furnished by slight abrasions and congestion, and may then cause the catarrhal and the non-suppurative types of cystitis; or, again, these germs may not attack the bladder first, but may infect the urine, the cystitis then developing secondarily. It may be laid down as a certainty that suppuration is the most frequent condition in chronic cystitis. The urine is usually alkaline, seldom acid. The colon bacillus is present in company with many other germs.

If the urine is acid, one should suspect tuberculosis at once. The micro-organisms find their way into the bladder by way of the urethra, or in a descending direction from the kidney, or, finally, by way of the blood stream. The colon bacillus is ubiquitous and may find its way into the bladder after an attack of prostatitis. Lydston claims that hyperacidity of the urine never *per se* causes cystitis and that irritation produced by such urine is due to the crystals of uric acid, oxalate of lime, and the urates that it contains, and not to an excess of sodium diphosphate—the salt upon which the normal acidity of the urine depends.

The infection remains until the gross cause is removed, and among such causes may be mentioned: stone in the bladder, a vesical tumor, hypertrophied prostate, stricture of the urethra, kidney tuberculosis, or some affection of the spinal cord (injuries, paralysis from various causes, etc.). The presence of ulceration, encysted stone, papilloma, etc., formerly mistaken for cystitis, is eliminated by a cystoscopic examination.

Œdema Bullosum Cystitis.—This form of the disease, so called from the lesions which characterize it, is a rare type of cystitis, one in which the inflammation produces vesicles which, according to Bierhoff, Albarran, and others, are circumscribed and vary in size from a millet seed to a pea. They are produced by localized accumulations of serum beneath the epithelium. The bullæ have been observed in cases of catarrhal cystitis, septic cystitis, and the cystitis which is dependent upon gonorrhœa, carcinoma, cystocele, and pyosalpinx.

Membranous or Exfoliative Cystitis.—This form of cystitis follows parturition and is no doubt caused by the pressure of the fœtal head. It is characterized by the exfoliation of the mucous membrane of the bladder, either in particles or in one complete piece. Patches of lymph also form on the mucous membrane and are carried off by the urine.

Gangrenous Cystitis.—Gangrenous cystitis is sometimes called phlegmon of the bladder, and occurs when the infection is particularly virulent and the cystitis extremely severe and extensive. The entire mucous membrane may be destroyed, and perforation of the muscular coats has been observed. In a fatal case of puerperal infection, I observed the above-mentioned gangrenous condition of the mucous membrane. In this case, impaction of the fœtal head, with retention of urine, was present for three days before the physician saw her. He applied the forceps, delivered a dead child, and then catheterized the woman. On the sixth day after delivery I saw her; she was then in a moribund condition. The gangrenous condition was not limited to the bladder alone (as seen post mortem), but the vulva, urethra, and portions of the vagina, uterus, and left Fallopian tube were involved. The infectious agent was the streptococcus.

Diphtheritic Cystitis.—When the Klebs-Loeffler bacillus infects the bladder, the cystitis is accompanied by the formation of a false membrane, similar to that found in the trachea, the nose, and the throat of patients affected with diphtheria. In this form of cystitis the urine is extremely ammoniacal.

Chronic cystitis occurs in the following conditions, some of which are dealt with in other articles in this work:—

(a) Urethral stricture, abscess, calculus, foreign body, and injury.

(b) Prostatic abscess, calculus, tumor, tuberculosis, hypertrophy.

(c) Vesical abscess, calculus, tumor, foreign body, paralysis, or atony.

(d) Ureteral calculus.

(e) Nephrolithiasis, pyelonephritis, tuberculous kidney.

(f) Perivesical abscess, which may perforate into the bladder and cause cystitis.

Pathological Changes.—The bladder is very much altered in size, shape, color, and structure. Chronic congestion produces a bluish tinge; in some localities the mucosa is paler than normal, while in others it is congested and red. Small red petechial capillary hemorrhages are scattered here and there throughout the mucosa. The muscular structure becomes thickened and trabeculation ensues, and in some rare cases sacculations or diverticula develop. Retention cysts of the terminal ends of the ureters may occasionally be observed. In some cases, leucoplakia vesicæ is produced. The cylindrical epithelium becomes squamous (Heymann); the bladder wall may be an inch thick, from proliferation of the subepithelial muscularis, the new tissue forming large alveoli. (Halle.) The entire bladder becomes contracted by reason of the increase in the fibrous tissue, which may extend to the subperitoneal structures. Vesicles, bullæ, and cysts are rare conditions. (Bierhoff.) Many of the contributing factors, such as stone in the bladder, may still be active, and, until these are radically dealt with, the cystitis will continue.

Symptoms.—Chronic cystitis is not revealed by any pathognomonic symptoms. The act of urination occurs frequently and is uncontrollable. Pain is the most persistent symptom and pyuria the most constant sign. The pain is always in the bladder and is intermittent in character. It is the most intense when the bladder is full. If a stone is in the bladder, the pain is not relieved as soon as the urine is expelled, because the bladder always tries to expel the stone also. The same is true of intravesical growths and protrusions which obstruct the flow. (See farther on, under Prostatic Diseases.)

In pyuria the urine is scanty and cloudy, owing to the presence of pus, blood (sometimes), mucus, bladder epithelium, and occasionally fibrin. Bacteria are present in large numbers.

In hæmaturia the blood courses through the congested and inflamed mucosa. The bladder contracts to expel the urine; the detrusor muscle acts just too late and the sphincter is still on guard. The counter-action between the two results in a rupture of the vessels in the congested mucosa, and blood is expelled at the completion of urination. The vesical tenesmus may not be severe.

Diagnosis and Prognosis.—While the primary condition upon which the chronic cystitis depends may be difficult to discover, still the diagnosis is easily made. A simple cystoscopic examination reveals at once the characteristic appearance of an inflamed bladder. The remote cause should then be sought. A history of the case is a great help in making a diagnosis. One infection may subside and another, due to a different germ, take its place. The gonococci often leave the field and the inflammation will be continued through the agency of another bacillus—the bacillus coli communis. In this instance the history of the case is valuable. In all cases the urine should be examined in order to determine whether a diseased condition of the kidneys is a factor in the bladder condition. The patient should be subjected to a thorough examination, especially with reference to the spine, the rectum, and the genito-urinary organs. Catheterization of the ureters may be necessary before a diagnosis can be made. This, however, is not imperative as a means of ascertaining the condition of the bladder. The prognosis of a chronic cystitis depends upon its stage and cause.

A bladder that has been inflamed once, is liable to become infected again, although an apparent cure was obtained in the first instance. When, however, the cystitis is perpetuated by the presence of a stone in the bladder, kidney, or prostate, and the condition is successfully dealt with, cystitis is not likely to return. The same is true if an enlarged prostate keeps up the cystitis after the prostatic disorder has been cured. The cure of the cystitis in these cases is permanent unless the bladder or kidneys are permanently damaged. Atonic dilatation, extreme contraction, trabeculation, formation of diverticula, are conditions which are likely to persist more or less after the predisposing causes have been removed. Procrastination is generally answerable for these bladder conditions which torment and greatly incapacitate a person for life, and it is also accountable for the graver conditions—e.g., dilated and infected ureters and kidneys—that shorten so many lives.

Treatment.—Recurrent attacks of chronic cystitis may be materially diminished by the adoption of certain prophylactic measures—such, for example, as the regulation of one's mode of living, the selection of a proper place of residence, and the careful observance of dietetic rules. Attention should be paid to the asepsis and antisepsis of the patient as a whole. Indigestion, exposure, over-exertion, and fatigue of the genital organs must be avoided. Cystitis is apt to occur after horseback riding, cycling, or motoring. The patient who has a chronic cystitis should avoid as much as possible the passing of a catheter, sound, or cystoscope. The curative treatment of cystitis is both constitutional and local.

So far as constitutional measures are concerned, internal antiseptics are valuable remedies for inflamed bladders. Those of the formaldehyd-salicylic group are preferable. If it is found that formaldehyd irritates the kidneys it should be discontinued. Salol may be administered in doses of from ten to twenty grains three times a day, with or without the use of uva ursi; boric acid, in doses of ten to fifteen grains a day, is also useful. It is a drug which sometimes produces albumin in the urine and toxic symptoms, accompanied with great weakness and a rash, exanthematous in character. Benzoic acid, in doses of five grains, deodorizes the ammoniacal urine very materially. However, it is liable to distress the stomach. Urotropin, in seven-grain doses, is an excellent urinary antiseptic. It clears up the cystitis of typhoid in a few days. It has no effect on gonorrhœal or tuberculous cystitis. Formaldehyd, its active principle, is liberated from urotropin only when the urine is acid in the renal pelvis. It may be given for months to advantage. Care must be taken, however, lest it produce toxic symptoms. It may cause nausea, diarrhœa, albuminuria, intestinal colic, tinnitus aurium, hæmaturia, and even strangury. Should the urine at any time become scanty, the drug should be withdrawn at once, to avoid untoward effects. Before internal medication is begun, the reaction of the urine is somewhat suggestive of what conditions require to be corrected. If the urine is markedly acid, and of high specific gravity, potassium acetate, gr. xx. every four hours, accompanied by small doses of tincture of hyoscyamus, should render the urine alkaline and lessen the suffering.

In the presence of undoubted phosphaturia, the antiseptics already mentioned, together with boric acid, urotropin, and cystogen, are indicated. In rheumatic patients, salicylic acid counteracts both the phosphaturia (by rendering the urine acid) and the rheumatism. When gonorrhœa plays a part in the etiology, —and it often does,—balsam of copaiba, cubebs, santal oil, santyl, and buchu, all have a sedative effect, to say the least. The medical treatment of chronic cystitis is more or less contradictory, the infection in the mean time running its course locally or ascending to the kidney; the local treatment is the only really curative procedure. Pain and increased functional activity of the bladder must be relieved. Morphine is the chief drug for this purpose. If a patient dreads the use of the hypodermic needle, then it may be administered per os or per rectum. While the normal bladder does not absorb very much, the raw, granular mucosa does so with avidity; therefore one should be careful in using anodynes as injections into the bladder. Whatever the drugs may be they should be given well diluted with plain water, or with some of the alkaline or neutral mineral waters. Lydston says that the water of Garrod Spa is the best.

So far as the local treatment of chronic cystitis is concerned it may be said that, during the acute recurrent attacks, all local interference had better be omitted unless the patient is under the influence of an anæsthetic, when any local application may be administered that seems to be indicated from the cystoscopic appearance of the bladder. Up to a recent date, most of the treatment recommended for cystitis was empirical. We now formulate our attacks in accordance with the bacteriological findings and the exact conditions ascertained by aid of the cystoscope. Not long since, a case was referred to me because of bladder symptoms. A cystoscopic examination showed that the bladder mucosa was normal, and on further inquiry it was learned that the real lesion was an interstitial nephritis of the right kidney. The kidney was decapsulated and punctured, and this procedure relieved all the bladder symptoms. Kelly mentions an instance of "an enormous stone in the left kidney" of an old lady who was accused of having cystitis instead. These are only two of many instances that might be quoted in support of the importance of resorting to the use of a cystoscope before one can be sure of employing a rational treatment in chronic cystitis.

Irrigations with medicated solutions constitute a local measure of great value. The simplest apparatus is a glass funnel with a rubber tube attached and a catheter fastened to the distal end of the tube. The fluid is run into the bladder until a regurgitation occurs which shows that the bladder is full. Then the funnel is lowered and the fluid is siphoned out. This act is repeated until the fluid comes away absolutely clear. In chronic cases of cystitis it is a good plan to leave a few ounces of fluid in the bladder; distention should be avoided unless ulcer is positively excluded. In mild cases one irrigation a day may suffice: the frequency, however, depends clinically upon the relief obtained when the bladder is washed out. Sometimes the patient requests a repetition of the irrigation every two or three hours. In these cases continuous irrigation with a return-flow catheter is advisable, so that no urine whatever shall be retained in the bladder. Continual irrigation acts very well when residual urine is the cause which perpetuates the irritability. If a self-retaining catheter is well borne, continuous irrigation is not necessary. The strength of the solutions used for cleansing the bladder varies according to the drug employed and the condition of the bladder. The following solutions are safe and effective in the strengths mentioned:

Boric acid—fifty per cent of a saturated solution or one fully saturated.

Chinosol—1 in 4,000.

Salicylic acid—1 in 3,000 (saturation)—is useful in dissolving crusts formed of phosphates, and neutralizes the alkaline urine.

Alcohol—well diluted (1 in 50 or 100) does not usually irritate, and acts as an astringent, antiseptic, and deodorant.

Bichloride of mercury—1 in from 20,000 to 50,000.

Silver nitrate—1 in 20,000. Twenty years ago the writer was in the habit of injecting two ounces of a silver-nitrate solution, in the strength of ℥ ij. to the ounce of water, in cases of obstinate chronic cystitis, with excellent results. They were most likely cases of ulceration. If the cystitis is of tuberculous origin the silver nitrate does harm.

Collargol—one-per-cent solution is a favorite remedial solution for purpose of irrigation.

Potassium permanganate 1 in 5,000, is strong enough for the bladder.

Benatol (the glycerite of phenol)—is a recent antiseptic germicide and is non-irritating. It may be used in the same strength as lysol,—viz., one drachm to a quart,—and has no unpleasant odor.

Irrigations for chronic cystitis have their limitations. If, at the end of twenty days, the improvement has not been satisfactory, instillations or, better still, local applications of caustic solutions, should be used.

Instillations of strong bichloride solutions (Guyon) are excellent, especially in tuberculosis of the bladder. In this connection Kelly says: "I have not been able to use the bichloride in a solution stronger than 1 to 5,000, and yet in one case I was forced to use for some weeks a solution of 1 to 4,000."

Preliminary to instillation local anæsthesia should be produced by the application of cocaine (one-per-cent solution) and by the administration of morphia hypodermically. In the majority of cases, a silver-nitrate solution, of the strength of from one to twenty-five per cent, is most serviceable. The quantity injected into the bladder varies with the strength of the silver solution. Instillation of one of the strong solutions should not be repeated oftener than every four or five days.

Topical applications constitute the most effective method of treatment. A silver-nitrate solution (of twenty-five-per-cent strength), applied by means of an applicator through a cystoscope, is more suitable in the treatment of the female bladder. The solid caustic stick is easily applied to an ulcer through the Kelly cystoscope. Bransford Lewis, of St. Louis, Missouri, has devised an operating cystoscope for male cases. Long, slender applicators, curettes, biting forceps, etc. (Fig. 117), are used through this instrument, and the conditions are treated while under actual observation. Operating cystoscopes have been devised by others, but I think that the Lewis instrument is the best.

In chronic cystitis (cystitis dolorosa) local applications by the aid of the cystoscope and drainage afford the best means of putting the bladder at rest. While perineal section and suprapubic section may be necessary in the male, these measures should not be employed in the female. Forcible dilatation of the urethra and neck of the bladder secure capital drainage, and thus a vesico-vaginal fistula is averted. I have on several occasions dilated the female urethra to such an extent that it would admit my index finger into the bladder and would also permit the introduction of a large curette. In two cases, after curettage, I repeatedly packed the bladder (through Kelly's cystoscope) with iodoform gauze soaked in a ten-per-cent emulsion of iodoform in glycerin, and cured my patients without resorting to a vesico-vaginal cystotomy.

Ulcer of the Bladder.—Simple ulcer of the bladder is rare. It has been observed and described by Fenwick, Le Fur, Castaigne, Walker, and others. It may be defined as a non-inflammatory ulcer, chronic or acute, which sometimes penetrates the entire bladder wall. Although the ulcer may become infected and inflamed, it is claimed that infection of the bladder never produces it. It presents the same appearance as a gastric ulcer, and, indeed, may have a similar etiology—viz., a blocking of the terminal arteries or an interference with the trophic nerves.

Dr. George Walker, of Johns Hopkins University, Baltimore, reports two cases of ulcer of the bladder.

The first case was that of a man, aged 54 years, who had contracted gonorrhœa eight years previously. Eight months before he presented himself for treatment, frequent urination set in. He also complained of painful sensations which were felt deep in the perineum and which occurred during the day independently of micturition. He was compelled to empty the bladder every three hours during the day, but not so frequently at night. There was great discomfort from pain and burning in the urethra during urination. Physical examination of the rectum and genitalia revealed nothing abnormal. The urine was slightly turbid and contained a number of fine granules. Microscopic examination showed pus cells, bladder epithelium, a few bacilli and cocci, and no tubercle bacilli. Endoscopic examination disclosed a normal urethra. With the cystoscope there was found a small round ulcer on the left lateral wall of the bladder, about 2 cm.

behind the orifice of the left ureter. It was sharply punched out; the immediate edges were smooth and regular; the base was made up of a red, fairly firm-looking granulation tissue, over which was a thin coating of a fibrous exudate. The ulcer extended to the submucous tissue but not beyond it. The adjacent mucous membrane was slightly injected, but otherwise presented no change. The remaining mucosa was entirely normal; there was not the slightest evidence of a tuberculous process. The ureteral orifices looked healthy and emitted a clear fluid. The capacity of the bladder was normal.

In the second case, that of a man 27 years old, the patient gave a history of a remote attack of gonorrhœa. Blood began to appear in the urine three years previously; later, increased frequency of urination, with more or less pain, disturbed him greatly. The pain was described as a burning sensation referred to the perineum and hypogastrium. These signs and symptoms increased in severity up to about six months previously, when improvement began. The bleeding became less frequent and profuse. The general health of the patient did not deteriorate at any time. Examination of the entire body was negative. The urine was practically normal, save for some mucus, leucocytes, and bladder epithelium. The cystoscope revealed an ulcer on the right lateral bladder wall, slightly behind the ureteral orifice. It was as large as a dime, irregular in shape, and extended here and there in fine projections. The base presented a granulating surface, nearly level with the surrounding mucosa. It was bluish in color and most of the surface was covered with a smooth epithelium. The pathological appearances were those of a healing ulcer.

PATHOLOGY.—Three types of ulcer of the bladder have been described: (1) The acute perforating ulcer; (2) the simple ulcer, which becomes chronic; and (3) the exuberant ulcer.

The first and second types are usually found on the postero-lateral walls of the bladder. They present circular, clean-cut edges, with a base covered with red, non-exuberant granulation tissue, throughout which particles of fibrin are scattered.

The exuberant ulcer is usually solitary. The edges are slightly indurated and feebly injected. The mucosa of the bladder is elsewhere entirely normal. At the margin of the ulcer exuberant granulation tissue rises above the mucosa and bleeds very readily. This ulcer has no inflammatory surrounding halo. In a case of this nature which came under my observation, the ulcer was engrafted upon a tear of the bladder mucosa. This was produced during dilatation of a congenitally contracted bladder. There were, in this case, three of these exuberant ulcers.

Castaigne made a careful histological examination of the simple ulcer of the bladder. He found that, in the first stage, it showed a layer of necrotic tissue over the surface of the ulcer, and that, beneath this, ordinary granulation tissue was present. Immediately outside this zone, thrombosis of the smaller blood-vessels was found to exist. A bacteriological examination of stained smears and sections failed to reveal the presence of any micro-organisms. When cystitis arises, pyogenic organisms are found in great abundance; the simple ulcer is then converted into an infected ulcer with cystitis.

In the acute perforating ulcer, the perforation usually occurs before cystitis sets in. For a description of this ulcer, one must rely upon post-mortem findings. In an autopsy made by Castaigne, the perforation was found to be located at the posterior part of the bladder. The ulcer was 2 cm. in width, and it was the base of this ulcer that had given way. There were 3 litres of blood in the peritoneal cavity. The remainder of the genito-urinary tract was normal. In 1876, Bartlett described a perforating ulcer of the bladder which resembled very closely gastric ulcer. Johnston reports a case of an ulcer of the bladder which measured three inches in diameter. In the case reported by Chaufford in 1900 the ulcer of the bladder closely simulated a gastric ulcer and was situated in the upper posterior wall.

ETIOLOGY.—The etiology of simple ulcer of the bladder is an enigma. It appears to have no connection with infection or cystitis. It probably depends upon a local disturbance in the vessels of the mucosa or else is due to some trophic nerve lesion. Le Fur was able, experimentally, to produce ulcers of the bladder in rabbits. He injected organisms into the blood of the animals and then produced traumatisms in the bladder wall. Of course, a lesion of this nature would be described as an infected ulcer. Such ulcers really occur in scarlet fever, typhoid fever, diphtheria, etc.

Ulcer of the bladder is occasionally observed in cases of locomotor ataxia and can then be explained only upon the supposition that the trophic nerves are interfered with.

The simple healing ulcer is converted into the exuberant ulcer by the irritation of the urine, which prevents the formation of an epithelial covering.

SYMPTOMS.—Three prominent symptoms have been ascribed to simple ulcer of the bladder. They are: frequent urination, pain in the penile portion of the urethra, and hemorrhage. If the ulcer is of the perforating variety, symptoms of perforation of the bladder develop with astonishing rapidity.

In all the cases there is no attendant depreciation in the general health of the patient. While the frequent urination, pain, and hemorrhage are disagreeable, the patients are able to endure their malady until cystitis begins. No doubt, in a considerable number of instances the ulcer heals without the development of cystitis. When infection occurs, then all the signs and symptoms are those of cystitis. Micturition is now more painful and the urine becomes putrid. Phosphatic deposits irritate the raw surface of the ulcer and often lead to the formation of calculi. Microscopic examination of the urine reveals, not only the presence of blood, but also that of pus and of bacteria.

In the simple exuberant ulcer, there is certainly no infection at an early stage. The chief disturbances here are frequent urination and hæmaturia.

In the perforating ulcer, the patient may die from hemorrhage before peritonitis sets in. Such cases have been reported by Chaufford, Bartlett, Reeves, Pousson, Burgess, Castaigne, and others. The first symptom of the occurrence of a perforation is great and severe pain in the region of the bladder and groin.

The hæmaturia rapidly increases. Castaigne reports the following interesting case:—

The patient, a man of about 36, who was apparently in perfect health, was attacked one morning with a very acute pain in the right lumbar region. The pain extended to the glans penis, and was so severe that he could not walk. Urination was difficult, and gradually hæmaturia became very pronounced. The pain persisted, the hæmaturia continued, and the abdomen became tense and tender. The patient died in five days. The autopsy disclosed a perforation of the bladder, with blood and urine in the abdominal cavity and evidences of peritonitis.

DIAGNOSIS.—The diagnosis of simple ulcer of the bladder is impossible without the aid of the cystoscope. The ulcer appears as a circular, punched-out abrasion, with clean-cut, slightly indurated edges. The remaining mucosa is normal. After cystitis and infection have set in, it is impossible to tell whether the ulcer owed its origin to infection or whether it began as a simple ulcer and then afterward became infected.

It is necessary to distinguish the lesion from a tuberculous ulcer. The latter is usually irregular in shape; the edges are not clean-cut and they are indurated; the margins are undermined. The tuberculous ulcers are often multiple, and numerous tubercles may be seen in the surrounding mucosa. In addition, tuberculosis is found in other parts of the body, and the tubercle bacillus is identified in the urine.

Carcinomatous and other forms of ulceration of the bladder need only be mentioned, as they are readily differentiated from the simple ulcer.

PROGNOSIS.—Spontaneous cure of the simple ulcer not infrequently takes place. Occasionally one meets with a single linear scar in the bladder, with a history of cystic disturbance which was controlled by internal medication. In these instances the original lesion was doubtless a simple ulcer.

When cystitis is present the prognosis is grave, owing to the tendency to ascending pyelitis. Once kidney complications have occurred, there is very little chance for the ulcer to heal.

In the case of a perforating ulcer the prognosis depends upon an early diagnosis and prompt operative interference. Harrison, in one of his cases, recognized the fact that a perforation had taken place and saved his patient by operation.

TREATMENT.—The treatment of simple ulcer is both general and local. The administration of urotropin and alkalies internally renders the urine as aseptic as possible, and lessens the amount of irritation. Irrigation should be practised. Solutions of chinosol (1 in 15,000), silver nitrate (1 in 10,000), and protargol (1 in 10,000) are very useful. If these measures do not suffice, then the ulcer should be cauterized through the cystoscope.

When cystitis occurs these methods should be tried for a certain length of time, but drainage of the bladder is a *sine qua non* to success. The bladder may be drained subpubically or suprapubically; the ulcer is then cauterized or cut out entirely. Cystotomy for ulcer in the female bladder should not be found necessary, except in very rare cases.

Tuberculosis of the Bladder.—Tuberculosis of the urinary bladder occurs with extreme rarity and is almost always a secondary infection, the primary focus being either a general tuberculosis or a tuberculosis of one or more of the neighboring organs, especially those of the genito-urinary tract. If a primary focus cannot be found, it must by no means be accepted that such a one does not exist, but rather that it has been overlooked. The infection may extend from above, as from the kidney, or from below, as from the prostate, the seminal vesicles, or the urethra. In women, tubo-ovarian disease may extend into the bladder, but the fact that clinically such an extension is seen but seldom, speaks for the rarity of this mode of involvement. Women, as a rule, are not subject to genito-urinary tuberculosis; not nearly so often, at any rate, as are men.

The bacillus tuberculosis is prone to find a nidus in a region where a slight injury has been inflicted or where there has been a pre-existing inflammation. The bladder that has been slightly injured or inflamed is no exception, but, at the same time, it is far less vulnerable than are other organs of the body.

Descending infections also occur more frequently than ascending ones, although the bladder, kidneys, and prostate may be infected simultaneously.

When tuberculosis extends from the genito-urinary tract, the bladder presents evidences of an inflammatory action, usually about the ureteral openings and in the region of the trigonum. Ulceration is quite likely to occur early, often extending deeply, undermining the mucosa, and occasionally perforating into the perivesical tissues or into the rectum. At times there is either a deposit of very large tubercles throughout the entire mucosa, or there are present many miliary tubercles not limited to any particular area.

Cystitis and hypertrophy of the bladder are generally associated with tuberculosis; often the cystoscopic appearance of the bladder suggests a chronic infiltrating cystitis, non-tuberculous in origin.

SYMPTOMS.—The symptoms of tuberculosis of the urinary bladder are exceedingly deceptive. Frequent and painful micturition, some hæmaturia, occasionally pyuria, loss in weight, and the other constitutional symptoms usually met with in chronic infection, are some of the signs which should direct attention to a possibility of tuberculosis of the bladder. In the severe or advanced cases, the tubercle bacillus may be found in the urine, although this is to be considered by no means a symptom of any value, because, even in the very worst cases, no bacilli may be found. Again, this symptom, in a given case, may be referable to a cystitis which, on cystoscopic examination, proves to be of a tuberculous origin. Thus it will be seen that the symptoms vary with the character of the local conditions, their location, and the stage of development which they have reached. Some clinicians are of the opinion that many apparently mild cases of catarrh of the genito-urinary tract are in reality cases of tuberculosis of the bladder. It is well known that, in many cases, tuberculosis of the genito-urinary tract may exist for a long time without causing any appreciable symptoms, and that, even in severe cases, the symptoms are not indicative of the nature or extent of the lesion.

The discovery of tubercle bacilli in the urine and the effective inoculation of animals with the urinary sediment, may be accepted as positive evidence of tuberculosis. But, as stated above, such evidence cannot be obtained in every case. If tuberculosis is discoverable elsewhere, as in the lungs, intestines, prostate, kidney, or seminal vesicles, a cystoscopic examination of the bladder should be made at once. Even when bacilli are present in the urine, they can be found only with difficulty. Repeated examinations should be made in these cases, and not only a few slides but dozens of them should be examined for the bacillus. If bacilli are not found, the urinary sediment should be injected into a guinea-pig. If bacilli are present a general infection of the animal will occur within three or four weeks.

As observed through the cystoscope, the appearance presented by a localized tuberculous infection varies according to the stage of the process. One or more congested and red areas appear before the nodules are formed; these latter assume a grayish hue and break down to form round ulcers, surrounded by an inflamed mucous membrane. The ulcers have a tendency to coalesce and their margins become undermined. In time the ulcerated surfaces present a ragged, irregular appearance, with a dirty-gray base, and they bleed easily from sprouts of granulation tissue which spring up here and there. Sometimes the bladder is covered with yellowish-gray membrane which, when disturbed, leaves a bleeding surface. As a rule, mixed infection occurs soon after the ulcers form, and this new development adds to the suffering of the patient and also plays a part in the destruction of the mucous membrane of the bladder. Eventually the bladder becomes contracted and thickened, and loses all its normal elasticity, capacity, and contractility.

TREATMENT.—The treatment of tuberculosis of the urinary bladder resolves itself into general and local measures. The general measures are the same as those employed in the treatment of tuberculosis elsewhere in the body. The patient is advised to lead an outdoor life, strictly to observe the rules of hygiene, both personal and of a general nature, and to partake of the most nutritious and easily digested foods only. Tonics, such as cod-liver oil, iron, syrup of the hypophosphites, etc., may be given if necessary.

The administration of santal oil for two or three weeks reduces the swelling of the bladder. This may be followed by hexamethylen tetramine (gr. v. three times daily), which renders the urine acid and more or less aseptic.

The local treatment of tuberculosis of the bladder is, on the whole, followed by very satisfactory results, but the greatest perseverance and persistence on the part of both patient and physician are necessary. In not a few cases only a certain measure of relief can be afforded, and much depends upon the general treatment, which is administered in the hope that, with the raising of the patient's bodily resistance, a cure may be effected.

Irrigations of a tuberculous bladder do little or no good. A cystitis that is not very much benefited by irrigations with one of the usual medicated solutions (boric acid, silver nitrate, oxychlorine, chinosol, etc.) is, in all probability, tuberculous in character. It is a matter of experience that a ten-per-cent emulsion of iodoform in olive oil is soothing and to a certain degree curative; from one to three drachms may be injected into the bladder through a catheter once a day. This viscus should be washed out as long as a mixed infection is present. Boric acid is a very useful and favorite drug for this purpose. Personally, I prefer chinosol, gr. xv. to a pint of water.

Since the use of the cystoscope has become general, the treatment of tuberculosis of the bladder has become revolutionized. The individual ulcer or tubercle is directly attacked through the cystoscope with a spear, curette, injection needle, or the solid stick of silver nitrate; or concentrated solutions of a corrosive nature are applied on a cotton applicator. In women this treatment is easily carried on through Kelly's open cystoscope. The infected area is located and fixed in the distal end of the instrument; local applications are then applied accurately without burning the surrounding mucous membrane. It is more difficult to treat the male bladder through the cystoscope, but, with a suitable instrument, such as that devised by Bransford Lewis, topical applications can be successfully made. In very stubborn or aggravated cases, Guyon recommends curetting the bladder through an artificial opening established above the pubis. It is not good surgery to apply the curette to multiple and coalesced ulcers. In the male a solitary tuberculous ulcer may be attacked with a curette through a small speculum (caisson) introduced by way of the suprapubic opening. The ulcer should be burned and then packed with iodoform powder.

When the primary focus is in the kidney and is removed by a surgical operation, the disease of the bladder often clears up spontaneously. Cystotomy should hardly ever be resorted to in the female, and only as a last resort in the male. Through a perineal opening it is just as easy to employ advantageously the Kelly cystoscope in the male as it is in the female bladder.

Vesical Calculus.—Stone in the bladder may be primary or secondary: primary, when the calculus forms in a bladder which is the seat of a chronic cystitis, with alkaline urine; secondary, when the stone has descended from the kidney or one of the ureters.

The varieties of renal calculi are the same as those of vesical calculi, but, inasmuch as ammoniacal decomposition is more likely to occur in the bladder than in the kidney, the phosphatic stone is more often met with in the bladder than in the kidney. It is also a much softer and more friable stone when it has descended from the kidney. The form of the vesical calculus is usually rounded, unlike the renal stone which conforms to the shape of that portion of the kidney in which it is located. When there are many stones in the bladder their surfaces may be facetted; the surface of a vesical calculus may show markings of the bladder, or a groove or an hour-glass constriction, depending on the particular part of the bladder in which it happens to lie. A long stone suggests the likelihood that it has formed about a foreign body as a nucleus.

It may be stated with considerable emphasis that most, or all, of the stones found in the bladder have come originally from the kidney. If the bladder has been the seat of a chronic cystitis, and if there has been considerable ammoniacal decomposition of the urine for a fairly long period of time, the stone is quite likely to take its origin in the bladder by precipitation of phosphates, and in this case an inspissated mucus often forms the nucleus. In fact, given a nucleus, a calculus is very likely to form. Therefore, foreign bodies are very often found in the calculi; they become encrusted with phosphates and in due course of time there results a calculus.

As a rule, the position of the stone varies according to the position of the patient. However, it is not uncommon for a stone, especially one of considerable size, to stimulate contraction of the bladder, which eventually forces the stone into a pocket; it is then said to be encysted. The bladder may be sacculated; in which case the stone may be held firmly in one of these natural pockets. It is in these cases that the searcher often fails to detect the presence of a stone; and then, besides, no symptoms of stone in the bladder may be manifested. These facts must be borne in mind when one makes an examination of the bladder.

Vesical calculus is far more common in the male than in the female. The short urethra in the female allows many stones to pass out of the bladder, and, besides, cystitis is more common in the male. Even young boys are not exempt from vesical calculus. It will be remembered that, in the case of renal stone, both sexes are about equally affected.

Stone in the bladder, as already stated, may cause no symptoms, and it is safe to say that a large number are never detected during life. Symptoms are caused by a freely movable stone or when cystitis is set up. Therefore a small, rough stone, which is freely movable, is more likely to cause symptoms than a large, smooth stone.

SYMPTOMS.—The pathognomonic symptoms of this condition are painful and frequent micturition and hæmaturia. The signs are made apparent by exercise and are quieted by absolute rest. The pain is referred either to the perineum or to the glans penis, and is most severe at the end of urination, because it is then that the stone is forced against the neck of the bladder. Sometimes the stream of urine is suddenly arrested; often a change in the position of the patient will start the flow again. This is caused by the stone being forced against the urethral opening. The calculus may enter the prostatic urethra and completely close the canal, or it may produce only a partial obstruction of the duct with a consequent incontinence.

Hæmaturia is not nearly so prominent a symptom in vesical calculus as it is in tumor of the bladder or in renal stone. Only rarely is there a free flow of blood; as a rule, when hæmaturia is present, there is only a slight amount of blood mixed with the urine, or merely red corpuscles are found upon microscopic examination. Rest in bed is followed by a speedy cessation of the hæmaturia.

Sooner or later the condition of the patient becomes worse. The constant irritation caused by the movable stone, the ammoniacal decomposition of the urine, and the precipitation of phosphates, lead to cystitis, which, in time, becomes chronic or septic in character. The pain, which is almost continuous, becomes more severe and is not relieved by physiological rest. Blood is more often mixed with the urine and micturition becomes more painful. Constitutional symptoms, due to sepsis, now make their appearance, and the patient is no longer able to continue his work. He is invalided. Eventually, if the infection spreads from the bladder to the ureters and kidneys, a fatal suppurative pyelonephritis ensues.

DIAGNOSIS.—Whenever there is occasion to examine the urinary bladder, a careful search should be instituted for calculus, it being borne in mind that one may be present and not manifest any symptoms. If the stone is large and the patient thin, it may be possible to palpate the calculus on vaginoabdominal or recto-abdominal examination. However, the sound and the cystoscope afford the most satisfactory means of locating a stone. Latterly the Roentgen ray has also come to the fore as a means of locating calculi in the bladder. The radiograph not only shows the stone, but gives us an excellent idea as to its location, size, and shape, thus facilitating its removal. As a rule, however, the sound is used more often than the other methods of searching mentioned. It may be used conveniently, quickly, and by one not necessarily experienced, although the examination in this instance may not always be satisfactory. The patient is placed in the Trendelenburg or in the lithotomy position, or in the ordinary recumbent position. The bladder is first emptied with a catheter and then filled with sterile water or sterile boric-acid solution, or simply with air. Then either the ordinary metal sound, a Thompson's sound (Fig. 109), or a wax-tipped bougie is passed and a careful search is made for the stone; the patient's position being changed from time to time during the progress of the examination and all the recesses of the bladder being explored. The sound is moved back and forth, and rotated from side to side, so that no part of the bladder escapes exploration. If no stone is found, the bladder is emptied and another search is made with the patient in the extra-lithotomy position. Often the sudden release of the fluid will carry the stone toward the urethral orifice. The contact of the stone with the metal instrument is often not only palpable but also audible. If the wax-tipped bougie is used, the imprint of the stone on the wax is diagnostic. With the catheter it is also possible to gain an approximate idea of the size, shape, and consistency of the stone, the click being more pronounced in the hard than in the soft stones. The location of the stone may also be determined by means of the catheter.

The lithotrite is used by some operators for detecting stone, but the employment of this instrument is attended by greater difficulties than is the use of the catheter or the sound. It is a fact, however, that it often reveals the presence of a calculus that would escape detection by any other means but the x-ray or the cystoscope.

A cystoscopic examination has the additional advantage of making a visual inspection of the interior of the bladder possible, but the use of the cystoscope requires greater skill than is necessary for the successful employment of the catheter or the sound. It is well to emphasize the value of the Roentgen examination, and it should be taken advantage of wherever possible.

TREATMENT.—The treatment of this condition resolves itself into removal of the stone. This is accomplished either by litholapaxy or by lithotomy, perineal or suprapubic. The former operation, litholapaxy, is still preferred by many continental surgeons, but American operators prefer lithotomy because of the greater accuracy of procedure and the greater safety of the patient from infection. It should be remembered that this operation should be per-

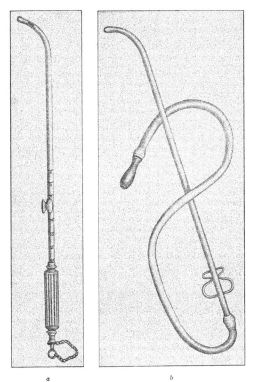

a *b*

FIG. 109.—Thompson's Sound (*a*) and Andrews' (*b*) Stone Searcher.

formed only by the professional surgeon and never by the occasional operator. Litholapaxy was introduced by the American surgeon, Bigelow, of Boston, in 1873, and is the ideal operation in certain cases. (For a detailed description of this procedure and lithotomy, see the section on Operations on the Bladder.)

Tumors of the Bladder.—Fortunately, tumors of the bladder, either benign or malignant, are rather uncommon. However, the surgeon is occasionally called upon to diagnose and treat cases of this nature.

Papilloma.—The most common variety is the papilloma, a benign tumor, which represents the overgrowth of the mucous membrane of the viscus. The papilloma is usually pedunculated and projects into the bladder like a cauliflower. The usual situation for these tumors is at, or near, the trigonum, and, as in the case of multiple papillomata of the skin, more than one tumor may be present. In fact, cases are on record where nearly the whole mucosa of the bladder was the seat of small pedunculated masses of this nature. Not infrequently the tumor may be broad, flat, and sessile, but this form is more rare than the pedunculated variety. It is, however, more likely to become malignant than the former.

The most common symptom of vesical papilloma is hæmaturia, not continuous, but remittent or intermittent. Without any apparent cause there is a free discharge of blood with the urine, and this phenomenon disappears as rapidly as it came. As a rule, the blood is admixed freely with the urine, but in some cases it is passed only at the end of urination. The periods between the attacks may be weeks, months, or years, and may lessen with the duration of the disease, although the patient may have the hæmaturia for many years without being aware of his condition. Unless the new-growth becomes malignant or the hemorrhage severe, the patient is not very likely to suffer from any constitutional disturbance.

There is rarely any pain or difficult urination unless the tumor is situated at or near the urethral opening and thus presents a mechanical obstruction to the free outflow of urine.

The diagnosis is readily made from the very suggestive history and the cystoscopic findings. Occasionally, especially in the case of very large pedunculated tumors, fragments of tumor masses may be found in the urine. In the case of females, visual inspection through Kelly's speculum may be of value. Bimanual examination is of very little assistance in these cases.

The treatment consists in the removal of the tumor, an undertaking which is usually accomplished through a suprapubic incision. The new-growth is excised freely after the cavity of the bladder has been made accessible according to the customary method of performing a suprapubic cystotomy. The raw surfaces are closed over, the edges of the mucous membrane being united by catgut sutures. Very small masses may be curetted and cauterized. In the female these new-growths may be operated upon through the urethra. Nitze performs the operation, in both the male and the female, through his operating cystoscope.

Hemorrhage is arrested by irrigating freely with a solution of adrenalin (1 in 5,000) or by pressure. It seems superfluous to call attention to the very great importance of observing the strictest antiseptic precautions in these cases. The other varieties of non-malignant tumors met with in the bladder are myxoma, fibroma, and angioma, the latter involving the veins. Mixed tumors are, of course, also seen.

Carcinoma and Sarcoma.—Of the malignant tumors the one oftenest seen is the squamous-cell variety of carcinoma, which occurs both as a primary and as a secondary manifestation, being either engrafted upon a pre-existing papilloma or on the site of one that has been removed. This form of tumor follows the usual course of a carcinoma involving some other part of the body, and leads to speedy dissolution. The secondary form may exist as a metastasis of a prostatic carcinoma or of a carcinoma located in some other part of the body. A tumor which develops primarily in the bladder rarely spreads to other organs, because of its exceedingly rapid course. Death occurs from exhaustion, hemorrhage, or infection.

The clinical symptoms of carcinoma of the bladder are, at first, similar to those of the benign tumors, although the hæmaturia is usually less abundant but more continuous. In fact, hemorrhage from the bladder is always suggestive of either carcinoma or tuberculosis. Cystitis is an early complication and is followed by painful and frequent micturition. The final stages of the disease are attended by a clinical picture not easily forgotten; the condition of the patient is deplorable, the pain being intense and almost unbearable. After the cystitis there follow in succession pyelonephritis, uræmia, and death.

The particular symptoms and findings readily suggest the diagnosis. The continuous hæmaturia, the emaciation of the patient, the pain, and, finally, the cystoscopic findings, are too significant to be overlooked. Bimanual examination may disclose the existence of a mass in the region of the bladder.

The treatment leaves much to be wished for, and rarely is productive of more than temporary relief. When the case is seen early and the growth is distinctly localized, its removal may be attempted, but not with the promise of a cure. The operation must be a radical one, as in the case of carcinoma elsewhere in the body. Therefore, when the tumor is located in or near the trigonum, the case is inoperable.

Tumors in the anterior wall of the bladder are those which are the most amenable to treatment and promise the strongest possibility of a cure. If the ureters are involved in the growth the removal of the affected portion is indicated, but the remainder of the ureters must be transplanted into the bladder higher up.

When radical removal is out of the question, the treatment resolves itself into giving the patient as much relief from pain as possible. Arrest of hemorrhage is expedient; suprapubic drainage may do much; vesical irrigations often give relief and should be employed whenever possible. Pithing of the spinal cord is not recommended.

Extirpation of the bladder need scarcely be considered in this connection, because, when such a procedure is indicated, the disease has assumed proportions which are entirely beyond the control of any operation, no matter how radical. When it is attempted, however, the ureters are preferably transplanted into the colon.

Sarcoma of the bladder occurs only very rarely. It is the tumor usually met with in children, although adults are by no means exempt. The symptoms are very similar to those of carcinoma, although there is considerable variation in individual cases. The diagnosis is made as in the case of carcinoma. The treatment is most unsatisfactory, because removal is not usually considered in any case. The most that can be done is to provide suprapubic drainage and make the patient as comfortable as possible by palliative measures.

Hernia of the Bladder.—This comparatively rare condition occurs in about one per cent of the cases of inguinal hernia and largely predominates in men. It manifests itself in a more or less extensive protrusion of a part of the bladder wall from the abdominal cavity. There is much variation in regard to the extent of this protrusion, cases being on record where the whole bladder, and in some instances even the prostate, has been discovered outside the abdominal wall. Whether such a thing as true vesical hernia exists, is extremely doubtful. Karewski states that no case of congenital hernia of the bladder has ever been reported. No matter whether or not hernia of the bladder is a genuine hernia, the fact that serious injury is extremely liable to happen to it during the performance of herniotomy, gives it great importance.

VARIETIES.—There are several varieties of vesical hernia. Undoubtedly the most common form is that associated with inguinal hernia, where the urinary bladder protrudes through Hesselbach's triangle alone or together with other abdominal contents, forming a direct hernia. There have been recorded a considerable number of instances in which a diverticulum or pouch of the bladder formed the whole or a part of the contents of the hernial sac. A more rare form is that in which the whole bladder is found within the sac of a large inguinal hernia. A variety seldom encountered is that in which the bladder forms the hernia without any peritoneal covering whatever. There are many instances on record which confirm the fact that cystocele is a possible complication of such various hernias as inguinal, ventral, obturator, rectal, etc. I have seen one case in which the bladder protruded like a hernial mass into the rectum. In ventral hernias the bladder occasionally has been found to protrude immediately above the pubic bone, a position in which it is extremely likely to be injured during the operation.

It is my belief that hernia of the bladder in the inguinal or femoral region is exceedingly rare, and that many of the cases which have been reported as such instances are really instances of the dragging of the bladder into the field of operation. It is a fact that surgeons who have had the greatest experience in this work meet with fewer hernias of the bladder than do those whose experience is limited.

COMPLICATIONS.—Aside from hernia of the bladder, complications affecting the viscus are liable to arise in the course of, or following, operations for the cure of inguinal, femoral, and ventral hernia. Retention of urine is a very frequent complication following any operation done in the vicinity of the bladder. This is easily corrected by means of the catheter and by altering the reaction of the urine,—i.e., by giving alkalies, as is usually indicated. A urinary fistula may result from an injury to the bladder wall inflicted during an operation for hernia. I have had occasion to close two such fistulas—one in the suprapubic and the other in the inguinal region. Cystitis may follow an operation for hernia. When it occurs, the treatment usually employed for this condition should be carried out.   Calculus is another complication to which hernia of the bladder may give rise.

The following cases will serve as illustrations:—

Charles Adams (*Clinical Review*, Vol. 12, No. 4) reports a case of inguinal hernia where the tumor was quite distinct from the testicle, was easily reducible, and presented all the indications of hernia without any vesical symptoms. On incising what was supposed to be the sac, he encountered and opened, inadvertently, a diverticulum of the bladder. This diverticulum, which was firmly adherent to the cord and canal, was cut away, its walls being too thin to suture, and the opening into the bladder was closed by a continuous suture.

S. C. Plummer (*Jour. Am. Med. Ass'n*, July 22d, 1905) reported a hernia of the bladder complicating an inguinal hernia, with an undescended testicle, on the left side. While operating for the hernia, he discovered a second sac. He opened it and much to his surprise found it to be the bladder. The wound in the bladder was sutured and primary union took place.

Harrington (*Annals of Surgery*, Sept., 1900) cites a case of hernia of the bladder (through the pelvic outlet) which had been caused by the traction of a large subperitoneal fibroma of the uterus. The bladder was restored to the pelvis, the tumor was removed, and the uterus was utilized to occlude the opening, its appendages having first been removed.

A rather unique case was reported by Collier (*Lancet*, June 6th, 1903). The patient was being treated for a double reducible congenital hernia. A truss failing to retain the hernia, an operation became necessary. On the right side the sac was found to contain the urinary bladder, and on the left side it contained the cæcum and appendix.

In another instance, reported by C. E. Ingbert (*Jour. Amer. Med. Ass'n*, Aug. 4th, 1906), the patient had a right inguinal hernia for seven years, but kept it in place with a truss. It finally became irreducible. The tumor mass was three inches long, two inches wide, and one inch in diameter ventro-dorsally. It was rather painful when pressed on or moved. In the hernial sac was found a hard mass about the size of an egg, which proved to be continuous with the bladder. It was pushed back and the canal closed.

C. B. Lockwood (Trans. Lond. Clin. Soc., Vol. XXXI.) reports a case of incomplete inguinal hernia on the left side. Four months previously, while operating on the opposite side for hernia, another surgeon had opened a finger-like extension of the bladder and had then closed the wound with sutures. Later, two phosphatic stones which had formed on the sutures were removed by lithotrity.

Verhoef (*Jour. de Chir. et Annales de la Soc. Belge de Chir.*, No. 2, 1903) reported two cases of accidental wounding of the bladder during operations for hernia. In one of the cases a portion of the bladder was in the sac, in the other it was not.

J. B. Harvie (*American Medicine*, April 4th, 1903) reported a case in which the entire bladder was found in the hernial sac. Before operation it was thought that the condition was one of strangulated hernia complicated by hydrocele. The upper part of the mass was very tender to the touch. The patient had had a reducible hernia for ten years, but had never worn a truss. The hernia became irreducible during an unsuccessful attempt to evacuate the bowel. Attempts at urination were frequent from this time on, but only a few drops of urine were passed at a time.

Subsequently, all the symptoms of a strangulated hernia appeared. When the sac was opened a portion of the intestine, about seven inches in length, was found to be gangrenous and was resected, the anastomosis between the divided ends of the organ being made by means of a Murphy button, reinforced with mattress sutures of very fine silk. "The hernial sac was clamped with a pair of ordinary artery forceps after reduction of the bowel, and an investigation was made of the remaining mass, which evidently contained fluid. A rather close examination failing to determine its exact identity, a small incision, 1 centimetre in length, was made, permitting the escape of between five and six ounces of clear urine. The moment the incision was made, and not until then, I suspected that we were dealing with the urinary bladder; and, in order to satisfy myself that it was actually the bladder, I explored its interior with my finger and found that the bladder had escaped into the scrotum in its entirety." Considerable difficulty was experienced in reducing the bladder, but it was finally accomplished.

CAUSATION.—There is a great deal of uncertainty as to the cause of hern.a of the bladder, but it would seem that thin, dilated bladders, urinary obstruction of some kind, senility, chronicity on the part of a pre-existing intestinal hernia, and general debility associated with the loss of much abdominal fat, are favoring factors.

Displacement of the bladder leading to a hernia of that viscus may be brought about by exaggerated intravesical pressure, due to the existence of some agency which serves to obstruct vesical drainage. An enlarged prostate or a stricture may cause not only hypertrophy of the muscular tissue of the wall of the bladder, but also considerable dilatation of the vesical cavity through over-distention. Displacement of the bladder, possibly laterally, may be brought about by this dilated condition, causing the wall of that organ to become located at or near the inguinal ring. Under these circumstances, any straining efforts which the patient may be forced to make, will push out a part of the bladder wall along with an inguinal hernia. In other cases the bladder may be pulled down into an inguinal sac through the adherence of part of the contents of the sac to that portion of the bladder wall which is covered by the peritoneum. Again, in still other instances, perivesical fat may drag upon the lateral wall of the bladder and thus form a hernia.

Personally, I have always felt that it is only by accident that the bladder is found in the canal, either because of careless manipulation on the part of the operator, or because of the formation of adhesions which draw upon the bladder.

DIAGNOSIS.—To make a diagnosis of vesical hernia is not an easy matter. In fact, unless the patient exhibit symptoms of cystitis or of distress referable to the bladder, it is an almost impossible task. Usually a vesical hernia is not discovered until the operator discloses the viscus in its abnormal position during the performance of herniotomy.

F. Karewski (*Archiv f. klin. Chir.*, Vol. 75) reports five cases, in one of which he succeeded in making a clinical diagnosis. In two cases the diagnosis was confirmed by the use of the cystoscope. In one case the condition was not recognized until the sac was opened; and in the remaining case the bladder was injured accidentally, its presence in the canal not having been suspected. Three of the cases were instances of crural hernia in women.

The presence of the following signs and symptoms should lead the surgeon to suspect hernia of the bladder:—This condition usually presents itself as a smooth, soft, partially reducible, fluctuating swelling which varies in size at different times. It can be emptied by pressure, a dough-like lump, dull on percussion, being left. A tendency on the part of the swelling to change its size rapidly and spontaneously is a characteristic sign. The essential points to be borne in mind are: (1) that the patient is capable of emptying the tumor by the act of micturition; and (2) that pressure applied to the swelling causes an imperative desire to urinate.

Two conditions—viz., (1) hydrocele of the tunica vaginalis testis, and (2) hydrocele of a hernial sac—may in some respects resemble vesical hernia and occasion error in diagnosis. Instances are on record in which a hernia of the bladder into the scrotum has been tapped under the supposition that the swelling was a hydrocele. Differentiation between hernia of the bladder and a hydrocele becomes clear, however, when we remember that the former can be reduced in size under pressure which gives rise to a desire to urinate, while the latter condition shows no connection with the urinary apparatus and is irreducible.

PROGNOSIS.—Accidental injury to the bladder during operation is the chief danger attendant upon vesical hernia. Serious results may follow such an accident. In addition to this, various grave complications may affect the bladder. Such are, for example: a cystitis due to inflammation, a calculus formed by the deposition of urinary salts, or a urinary fistula resulting from tapping. In the larger number of cases, however, the prognosis is good, a radical operation usually effecting a cure.

TREATMENT.—Palliative treatment of hernia of the bladder is exceedingly unsatisfactory. On the other hand, there is no special operative treatment for vesical hernia because this condition is usually encountered with the direct form of inguinal hernia. When the bladder is reached, it must be separated from the sac, and any bleeding vessels encountered should be ligated. The rotundity of the bladder should be restored by pressing it toward the region in which it belongs and fastening the perivesical tissue snugly around it. A few ligatures of fine catgut will suffice to do this and will at the same time take care of the dead spaces that have been formed during the dissection. Great care must be taken not to injure the bladder wall, especially the mucosa; for, if it is caught up in a suture or tied in a ligature, a urinary fistula is sure to result, and this may prove fatal. It was my misfortune to see such a case in consultation with a general practitioner who five days previously had attempted to perform Alexander's operation on the round ligaments of a young woman twenty-four years of age. Upon opening the wound I found that the bladder had been sutured in the inguinal canal, that infiltration of urine had taken place extensively, and that general peritonitis was in full swing. Two days later she died.

If the bladder has one or more finger-like processes protruding as in hernia, they should—according to their length, breadth, and shape—either be inverted into that organ or cut off. The short, broad, and funnel-shaped processes can easily be inverted into the bladder and held there by a stitch or two applied on the external surface of the viscus. In a case of suprapubic hernia of the bladder no special instructions are called for; it is simply necessary to liberate the injured parts carefully and then to secure coaptation of the torn halves of the recti in front of the organ. Occasionally it will be found necessary to do some plastic work upon the abdominal wall in this region in order to secure a sufficiently strong covering for the hernial site. In very fleshy persons the abdominal wall may be so deficient as to preclude plastic procedures. It is under these conditions that some surgeons use silver filigree. Obscure forms of hernia of the bladder, such as those in which the organ protrudes into the rectum, peritoneum, obturator foramen, and so on, are treated on general surgical principles according to the symptoms and signs which they manifest.

Hernia of the bladder in females—a condition known as cystocele—is dealt with elsewhere in this work.

Incontinence of Urine.—Two forms of incontinence of urine are recognized, viz.: true incontinence and false incontinence.

True incontinence is characterized by conditions which permit of the escape of urine from the bladder when it enters the organ, and a continuous onward flow.

False incontinence (overflow of urine) depends on conditions which interfere with the flow of urine from the bladder (retention) until the accumulation of pressure causes the escape.

One of the sequelæ of prostatectomy is incontinence of urine, which varies in degree from an occasional involuntary escape to a constant leakage from the bladder. In these cases of troublesome and continual dribbling, a urinal is essential to the patient's comfort. The popularity of prostatectomy —which may be attributed in part to the successful results obtained and in part to the low mortality experienced, in competent hands—has enticed men of little experience in any branch of surgery to attempt its performance.

The following may be mentioned as among the more important causes of incontinence:—(1) Incomplete prostatectomy; an undiscovered stone or the tissue that protrudes into the bladder being left. (2) Injury to the sphincter of the bladder—(a) by the operator; (b) by irritation of the neck of the bladder (irrepressible urination), after the operation, by purulent or acid urine; (c) by the size and shape of the enlarged prostate; (d) by atony or paralysis of the detrusor muscle, which condition may be present at the time of the operation; (e) by reflex irritation of the neck of the bladder from continuous or remote conditions—as, for example, rectal diseases, vesical calculus, rupture, local tuberculosis, congenital and constitutional conditions, new-growths, and diseases of the spinal cord. (3) Fistula, which may be suprapubic, perineal, or urethrorectal. The writer agrees with Greene (vide Greene-Brooks textbook, 1907, p. 22) that incontinence more frequently follows a fistula in the suprapubic region or a urethrorectal fistula than one in the perineal region, for it is common for the incontinence to cease when the fistula is healed. (4) Diverticula and cystitis. (5) Spinal paralysis.

TREATMENT.—In cases of incomplete prostatectomy, a second operation is necessary to relieve the conditions. The unremoved prostatic tissue must be eradicated, or the stone extracted, as the case may be. A second operation through the perineum is very difficult to perform. When the primary operation was perineal, the second operation should be performed suprapubically, and *vice versa*.

When cystitis fails to subside under proper treatment, and some degree of incontinence is present, which is common, a sacculated bladder or the existence of diverticula may be suspected. Under such conditions the writer prefers the suprapubic route for this operation. This route enables one to remove the offending portion of the prostate, extract the stone, or amputate the diverticula. In one instance, I encountered a troublesome suprapubic fistula, but it promptly closed as soon as perineal drainage had been established. Incontinence due to local or reflex irritation soon subsides when the cause is removed by proper treatment—such, for example, as vesical irrigations, administration of alkalies internally, removal of hemorrhoids, and cure of the hernia. Complete destruction of the vesical sphincter is irreparable. Hence incontinence dependent upon such a condition must be complete and permanent. Fortunately, however, this condition is rare indeed.

In clinical work one encounters many degrees of the patient's inability to retain the urine, these variations being due in some measure to the stamina of the sufferer and also in part to the amount of injury that has been done to the urogenital sphincter. Some men make no effort to hold the urine, but give way to the least desire to urinate. This is not to be wondered at when we consider their age, their enfeebled condition, their long-continued suffering, and, above all, the disappointment which these patients feel after they have passed through a trying operation upon the results of which they may have based strong hopes. They bemoan their lot and lament that they ever consented to the operation. They seem to forget the agonizing struggles which they experienced before the operation, and it is difficult to convince them of their comparative comfort since the prostatectomy. Even though, before the operation, the incontinence of urine, *per vias naturales*, was complete and permanent, necessitating the use of a urinal so long as the patient lived, the operation rarely fails to effect an unmistakable degree of relief. At least partial control of the urine is secured in the majority of cases. The patient, for example, may hold from two to five ounces before leakage occurs; the involuntary escape is often intermittent; the bladder holds more when the patient is asleep or is recumbent than when he is awake or standing up. In the erect posture the urine escapes in spite of him. In other cases a decided dribbling occurs after irritation, or when the patient is excited or fatigued. In the majority of cases there is hope of a cure, and in all cases some degree of improvement may be looked for. Dr. Samuel Alexander pointed out "that the hearty and intelligent co-operation of the individual patient must be enlisted to effect an improvement."

He says: "I have adopted the plan of treating several patients together in the hospital; so that those who are beginning to be taught to gain urinal control may be encouraged by those who have been taught, or who are at least further advanced toward a cure than they themselves are. The principle is to make the patient learn by practice to exercise voluntary control over 'what remains of the urogenital sphincter, thus preventing the escape of urine. If this can be done, anatomic control follows as a physiologic necessity." In cases of such loss of control in comparatively healthy men, the writer has brought the mucous membrane down over the perineal structures and caused it to unite with the skin. When a fistula of any kind is present, it should be treated locally with antiseptics, and, if these fail, by operation. The urethro-rectal fistula is always susceptible of relief by a surgical operation.

Retention of Urine.—Retention of urine is due to some form of obstruction to the outflow of urine from the bladder. It is met with in every-day practice and should be clearly understood by every physician.

ETIOLOGY.—There are three principal causes of retention of the urine, viz., obstruction, paralysis, and atony.

(a) Obstruction.—The flow of urine may be prevented by some condition in the penis itself. Phimosis, rings or bands placed around the organ, and tumors may be the cause of the retention. Carcinoma of the penis rarely causes retention. Cicatrization of the end of the urethra is especially apt to occur after amputation, and particularly after the circular variety of the operation. Three such cases have come under the care of the writer.

The injudicious use of nitric acid in the treatment of soft chancres may result in retention. I have seen one case of this kind.

Stricture is the most common cause of obstruction in the urethra. Stones, coming originally from either the bladder or the kidneys, may also become impacted in the urethra and thus obstruct the flow of urine. Whatever the source from which the calculus came, there is a history of urinary lithiasis.

Spasm of the detrusor muscle is a common cause of retention and calls for immediate attention on the part of the physician.

Acute retention after exposure to cold, after rather free wining and dining, is occasionally serious; and this is especially true when there is a stricture of the urethra or an hypertrophy of the prostate. Anything that produces congestion at the neck of the bladder, will cause spasm and, eventually, retention.

Obstruction in the prostatic portion of the urethra, a common cause of retention, is usually due to a new-growth, a stone, or chronic inflammation. Age, habits, and a history of gradually increasing urinary disturbances, will materially aid in determining that the cause of the retention is prostatic in character. (*Vide* Prostate.)

In the bladder itself, a neoplasm or a stone may cause a blocking of the internal urinary orifice and result in more or less complete retention. A papilloma may be forced into the inner end of the urethra and cause complete obstruction; a stone may become impacted in the same locality.

Besides these intrinsic causes, there are other conditions which are located in the neighboring structures and which play a part in the production of retention. Fibroids of the uterus, retroversion of the gravid uterus, and cysts or abscesses of the perineal structures, may, by the exertion of pressure, result in retention of the urine.

After severe injuries to the bladder, such as rupture, the urine is retained either in the peritoneal cavity or in the perivesical cellular tissues. (*Vide* Injuries to the Bladder.)

(b) Paralysis.—Under the heading of paralysis belong diseases of the spinal cord, especially tabes dorsalis and myelitis. Injury to the brain, the spinal cord, or the third sacral nerve, results in retention because of the interference with the innervation of the bladder. Functional disturbances, as in hysteria and following certain operations in the region of the bladder, occasionally result in retention.

(c) Atony.—When a bladder becomes overdistended, the muscles, from overstretching, lose their power to contract, and are incapable of emptying the viscus. At first, the vesical orifice of the urethra becomes closed, and then the urine follows the line of least resistance, later backs up in the direction of the ureters and kidneys, and often distends these structures enormously. This distention takes place slowly and the bladder does not rupture; finally, the sphincter of the neck of the bladder gives way and a certain amount of urine escapes. However, the bladder still remains overdistended, because the muscular coating is too weak to complete the evacuation of this cavity. This condition is found most frequently in old men with enlarged prostates.

Acute atony of the bladder is a very distressing and dangerous condition. Rupture is very liable to occur. Acute uræmia may also follow acute distention of the bladder. While chronic atony of the bladder may continue for years without endangering the life of the patient, still, sooner or later, infection occurs and ascending pyonephrosis follows, which usually causes death.

SYMPTOMS.—In acute retention the patient complains of great and constant pain in the lower abdomen. The bladder presents itself as a tense, hypogastric swelling, which is round and firm. In the paralytic cases, pain is absent. The distended bladder, in chronic cases, presents an appearance very closely resembling that of an ovarian cyst in a woman. On several occasions, in the last twenty-five years, patients who have been referred to me for abdominal section have been relieved by the use of the catheter.

Retention of urine is followed by rupture of either the bladder or the urethra, or by distention with overflow, which latter condition results in "false incontinence."

In acute cases, complete distention and overflow are the most favorable result pathologically. This safety-valve action of the bladder is necessary, or uræmia would develop. These cases get completely well if the obstruction is benign and the treatment suitable.

In chronic cases both the bladder and the kidneys suffer pathological changes. The former becomes hypertrophied and sacculated; the latter develops hydronephrosis, pyonephrosis, and pyelonephritis.

DIAGNOSIS.—Retention must be diagnosed from (a) suppression of urine. (b) calculous anuria, and (c) rupture.

(a) Suppression of urine occurs suddenly as a result of some severe shock or excitement or in consequence of an acute nephritis. The bladder is contracted and empty. Occasionally the secretion becomes less and less, the specific gravity and the percentage of albumin increase steadily, until, in spite of aid, the kidneys refuse to secrete at all.

(b) In calculous anuria, there is always a history of stone, with accompanying lumbar pains and the presence of blood in the urine. The bladder is empty.

(c) After a rupture of the bladder, the viscus is empty, but a little bloody urine can always be obtained by the catheter. The history of the case is that of injury or ulcer. (Vide Injuries of the Bladder.)

TREATMENT.—The acute spasm may be relieved by hot baths and by the administration of morphia and belladonna. If these fail, an attempt should be made to pass a soft-rubber catheter. If it is found that there is no permanent obstruction, a full-sized silver catheter, carefully and properly guided, will almost always relieve the retention. When a definite obstruction exists, the means of treatment vary with the acuteness of the retention. If the bladder is in danger of rupture, suprapubic aspiration must be done if one has failed to pass a catheter. When the obstruction is prostatic, catheters of different sizes and shapes, and of varying degrees of stiffness, should be tried before one resorts to the aspirator or the trocar. If the patient is in grave danger, suprapubic or perineal section should not be delayed. A good working rule to follow is: "Relieve the bladder temporarily, then prepare for a radical operation later, when the condition of the bladder, kidneys, and patient, is decidedly better."

In cases of retention due to stricture of the urethra, much time is often employed by good surgeons in the use of filiform bougies and like instruments. The operation of external urethrotomy is so curative that the writer does not hesitate to give these patients relief at one sitting, even with or without a suitable guide to the operation.

The prostatic cases demand prostatectomy sooner or later; the urgency depends more upon the general condition of the patient than upon the local findings. The reason for this is that the kidneys, ureters, and bladder have become gradually accustomed to the increased tension before complete stoppage takes place.

The danger of cystitis and ascending infection is not so great in the chronic cases as in the acute.

In dealing with the paralytic cases of retention, one should take great care not to produce infection of the bladder.

Bacteriuria.—This is a recent term; it signifies an infection of the urine with bacteria alone. Little or no pus is present and the bladder may be normal. In bacteriuria, the urine is turbid, yellowish in color, and has a bad odor, resembling that of stale fish or fecal matter. A microscopic examination of a centrifuged specimen shows the presence of the colon bacillus in great numbers. A few pus corpuscles and some epithelium may be observed in the field. It is not known how the urine becomes infected in all cases. A history of catheterization, of hæmaturia, of stricture, of recent gonorrhœal infection, and, in women, of pelvic inflammation, may be obtained in most cases.

It is agreed that bacteriuria may occur (a) through the urethra, (b) from the kidneys, (c) by way of the general blood current, and (d) through the lymphatics of neighboring organs. It is reasonable to suppose that the infection may occur through a collateral circulation of blood as well as by way of the lymphatics.

The course of disease is sometimes brief, lasting only a few days; it may end in death. But it is liable to recur and it is not infrequently protracted through many years. In spite of a foul-smelling urine, the organs remain apparently healthy and the general health of the individual may not appreciably suffer.

The diagnosis is made by an examination of the urine and of the bladder. The treatment is both general and local. Internally the most effective medications are urotropin (gr. v.–x.), salol, and preparations of methylene blue. Before local treatment is effective, the hiding-place of the germs must be located. If prostatic disease or a diverticulated bladder is present, then irrigations will only alleviate and not cure the condition. To effect a complete cure, prostatectomy or diverticulectomy must be performed. Should there be infection of the urethra, ureters, or kidneys, this must be controlled before the colon bacilli can be destroyed. (For further information on this topic the special treatises should be consulted.)

II. OPERATIONS ON THE URINARY BLADDER.

Suprapubic Aspiration.—The aspirator is one of the oldest and best instruments with which to empty the bladder. For temporary purposes, the smaller the needle the better, for, after the needle is withdrawn, the bladder wall closes the puncture immediately. In this procedure there is no danger of leakage of urine and very little opportunity for infection, if the tube is clamped close to the needle when it is withdrawn. Aspiration is indicated in cases of retention, no matter what the cause, and especially when the surgeon is without means of otherwise removing the obstruction. It is suited to many cases of temporary retention. For instance, when other means have failed to relieve the retention caused by gonorrhœa, it is perfectly proper to aspirate. In cases in which the bladder is incapable of emptying itself, as after a recent stricture of the urethra, where hot baths, morphine, etc., have proved unavailing and catheterization is impossible, the aspirator is indicated. It must not be lost sight of that great skill has been attained by some surgeons in the technique of catheterization, and therefore the fact that others have failed should not deter one from making the attempt. Not infrequently success is thus obtained, to the relief of all concerned. In prostatic retention the aspirator may be used when other instruments, such as properly shaped catheters, are not available. The operation may be repeated many times without danger, provided the cause of the retention and the surroundings of the patient do not contra-indicate such a course. I have known as many as twenty-five suprapubic punctures to have been experienced without complication. Repeated aspirations, however, are not to be recommended; before one resorts to such repetition rational treatment directed to the removal of the cause of the condition, should, if at all possible, be instituted. Some surgeons give this advice: "Never puncture a bladder, for surely the sphincter vesicæ will give way and afford relief by overflow." The adoption of such a course, however, is dangerous to the welfare of the bladder, ureters, and kidneys, and also to the life of the patient, and no good surgeon will commend it.

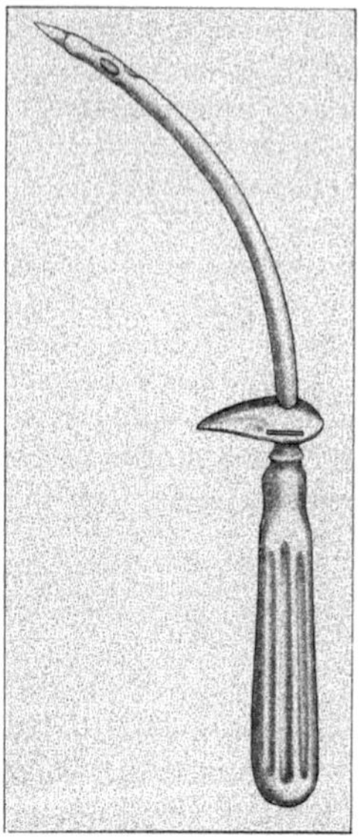

Operative Technique.—Cleanse the skin and then, with a sterile needle, puncture the bladder about an inch above the symphysis pubis, in the middle line of the body. The prevesical space (Retzius) must be traversed. If a few drops of one of the local anæsthetics is previously injected into the skin of that locality the patient will experience comparatively little pain from the operation. If the puncture is made at too high a point the peritoneum is endangered. After aspiration, the bladder must not be allowed to become distended again for fear of leakage through the puncture into the prevesical space, and consequent infiltration of urine or infection. Care must be taken not to plunge the needle too deeply for fear of wounding the prostate or posterior wall of the bladder. An overdistended bladder must not be emptied too rapidly nor entirely, as the return flow of blood to the wall causes an engorgement favorable to hemorrhage and inflammation.

Fig. 110.—Curved Trocar, with Ensheathing Cannula.

Trocar Puncture. — When the puncture is made with a trocar one of three routes may be selected: the suprapubic, the perineal, or the rectal. The slightly curved trocar, ensheathed in a cannula, possesses the advantages of simplicity, safety, and efficiency. (Fig. 110.) The instrument is in the possession of every practitioner and can readily be sterilized. The objection to its use is that it opens the way for extravasation of urine and the occurrence of infection. It is not safe to leave a short cannula in the bladder, as frequently recommended, because the instrument is liable to slip out of the bladder when the viscus contracts. When the urine is normal I have on some occasions passed several strands of silkworm gut into the cannula and have then withdrawn the instrument, leaving the strands in the bladder as a drain. By this means the urine seeps out gradually by capillarity for as long a time as may be desired. If however, the urine contains pus, tube drainage should be substituted for capillary drainage. This drainage is installed by first inserting a very large cannula and then pushing the tube into the bladder through the cannula; afterward the cannula is withdrawn and the tube is left in place. Through this tube or catheter the septic urine may be siphoned into a vessel placed on the floor, and irrigations may be carried on at will, with the least possible disturbance. As an additional safeguard, one may enlarge the wound and surround the tube with iodoform gauze down to the bladder. Suprapubic drainage, no matter how carried out, is at best a makeshift, and has nothing to recommend it save the simplicity of its technique. A more rational method for drainage is secured through the perineum, but, to establish it and make it work effectively, both skill and surgical knowledge are necessary. In the large majority of cases of retention, a simple median perineal section (Cock's or Wheelhouse's operation), followed by drainage, is the best and safest plan of treatment. Certain conditions may render this procedure impossible; and, when this is the case, a trocar may be thrust into the bladder and a catheter slipped in through the cannula, as described above. Should the patient be affected with some prostatic disorder, a grooved staff placed in the urethra as far down as the obstruction, and a finger introduced into the rectum and pressed against the apex of the prostate, will serve as safe guides when one is about to pass the trocar into the bladder. The objection to using a trocar for making a puncture through the perineum is that hemorrhage into the diseased middle lobe of the prostate may follow,—an occurrence which may prove dangerous,—and also that a channel is thereby opened up for infection. Some years ago, puncture of the bladder through the rectum was practised, but it has, very properly, been abandoned. The rectovesical pouch of peritoneum, in front of the rectum, was frequently injured, and in some instances death followed from peritonitis. Then again, the prostate sometimes received the entire trocar and the bladder escaped altogether; besides which infection is imminent.

Cystotomy.—The bladder in the female may be opened by either the suprapubic or the vaginal route. Suprapubic cystotomy may be performed in one or two stages. The one-séance operation is preferable in clean and urgent cases, while the two-stage operation is indicated only when the urine is septic. In the female, ample room is usually obtained for the removal of stone and tumors *per vaginam*. Vaginal cystotomy for drainage alone is unsurgical, for, with the assistance afforded by our improved cystoscopes, all inflammatory conditions may be locally treated through the urethra.

The indications for suprapubic cystotomy are too numerous to describe in detail; let the following suffice:—

(1) For retrocatheterization, in cases of traumatism to the peritoneum, in which a catheter cannot be passed into the bladder even after median perineal section.

(2) For the removal of foreign bodies which cannot be safely removed through the perineum or by the urethral route.

(3) For the removal of stone, especially in boys.

(4) For drainage in the cystitis of old men whose urine has become foul,

and in whom ascending infection has resulted in grave constitutional symptoms In these cases nothing short of cystotomy affords the prompt relief demanded.

(5) For the removal of prostatic papillomata and other tumors.

(6) For affording direct access to the bladder for the treatment of certain tuberculous conditions, ulcers, etc.

(7) For palliative treatment in certain prostatic and bladder conditions; diverticula, for example, may be diverted into the bladder. In one case the writer dilated the mouth of a diverticulum through the bladder and pulled the club-shaped pouch into the bladder.

In considering the advisability of cpening the bladder, for any purpose, the surgeon will have to choose between the suprapubic route and external urethrotomy. Other things being equal, it is better to choose the lower route.

Minor Cystotomy.—A minor cystotomy for the removal of a foreign body or small stone, or for the purpose of drainage, is quite a simple thing and differs in technique from a major cystotomy where such conditions as a tumor or a prostatic hypertrophy have to be dealt with. The steps of the operation are as follows:—With the bladder properly distended, pass a long, narrow-bladed knife through the prevesical space into the bladder at a point about an inch and a half above the pubes and in the median line. The drainage tube is guided into the bladder by the probe, which is passed along the blade of the knife. The latter instrument is then withdrawn. This completes the operation when drainage alone is required.

When a catheter can be passed into the bladder, vesical irrigation is proper; then, after all the fluid is removed, the bladder should be filled with air before the cystotomy is attempted. Should a foreign body or stone be present, the incision should be made large enough to admit the index finger as the knife is being removed. The beginner had better pass a long hook into the bladder along with the knife; this catches the bladder wall, acts as a guide for the surgeon's finger, and·prevents the bladder from receding before the advancing finger.

Major Cystotomy.—This operation requires an opening in the abdominal wall and bladder large enough for the necessary inspection and manipulations. The writer prefers to distend the bladder with air (Pilcher) and to illuminate the bladder with an electric cystoscope. One has no adequate appreciation of the value of this instrument until he gives it a fair trial. The skin incision commences one inch above the symphysis in the median line and extends upward for four inches. With a fresh knife, an incision is then made through the linea alba, or through one rectus muscle, down to the bladder, care being taken to avoid the peritoneum. When the bladder is filled with air it projects like a balloon into the wound. The incision made into the bladder should be large enough to admit two fingers; a broad, but short, retractor is slipped into the viscus and turned squarely across the wound. This retractor keeps the recti muscles out of the way and protects the peritoneum. With the aid of lateral retractors, the entire interior of the viscus may be inspected. The final steps of the operation will be described under Suprapubic Lithotomy (page 328).

Transverse Skin Incision.—In very fleshy persons. it is an advantage to raise a broad flap by means of a transverse crescentic incision, with the convexity downward. When the thick flap of the skin is raised upward, an exposure of the upper margin of the symphysis pubis and the abdominal muscles immediately above is obtained. A short transverse cut across the inner margins of the recti muscles enables the operator to expose the bladder with ease and accuracy, especially when the bladder is inflated with air. I believe that it is unnecessary to use guy threads or hooks to steady the bladder. The difficulty of suturing the transverse cut in the recti is overcome by Watson, who raises an osteoplastic flap from the pubis and, at the end of the operation, wires the bone back into place. The sheaths of the recti furnish ample material without injuring the bones.

Drainage in Cystotomy.—The simple drainage furnished by the late Hunter McGuire (Fig. 111), by means of a curved silver tube with a stop-cock, is suitable

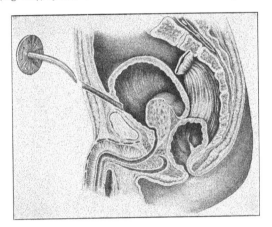

Fig. 111.—Suprapubic Drainage of the Bladder. (After Hunter McGuire.)

in those cases in which drainage alone is necessary. Senn's sigmoid tube (Fig. 112, *a*) was at one time extensively employed. The multiplicity of methods of drainage is limited only by the ingenuity of the surgeon. Some insert a self-retaining rubber catheter into the bladder and fasten it to the anterior wall of the viscus; others extend a straight tube or catheter to the bottom of the bladder. When the bladder is septic, the double drain, as employed by McRae (Fig. 114), is safest and best. All suprapubic methods of drainage are contrary to physical and surgical principles. The author recommends to the reader to select some one of the methods of drainage illustrated in these pages.

Median Lithotomy.—The patient is constitutionally and locally prepared as for any other major operation. The strictest attention is paid to the genito-urinary tract. Efficiency of the kidneys and asepticity of the bladder are secured so far as may be possible.

While the patient is under the influence of a general anæsthetic, the urine is withdrawn by a catheter, the bladder is washed out, and a feeble antiseptic solution (six to eight ounces) is left in the viscus. The catheter is removed without allowing the fluid to escape from the bladder, and a large, grooved staff is introduced in its place. If the meatus is small, it is preferable to enlarge it, rather than to use a staff which is too small. A staff suitable for this purpose is shown in Fig. 116. Search is made for the stone with the staff. When the calculus is located, the patient is placed in the lithotomy position and held there by a crutch or by two assistants,—prefer-

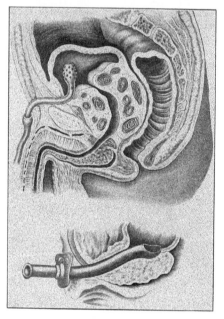

FIG. 112.—Different Patterns of Drainage Tubes. (a) Senn's and Watson's; (b) Sigmoid Drainage Tubes. (After Deaver.)

ably the latter. In old people care must be taken not to sprain the hip-joint or the knee-joint.

The surgeon, sitting directly in front of the perineum, passes a pledget of gauze into the rectum to prevent the escape of liquid feces over the field of operation. The middle finger of the gloved left hand is inserted into the rectum until it rests upon the tip of the prostate. The index and ring fingers rest upon the perineum. The point of a long, narrow knife, with a straight-backed blade (Fig. 113), is inserted into the median rhaphe at a point from one inch and a half to two inches in front of the anus. The knife is pushed upward a distance of from two and one-half to three inches, according to the thickness of the perineum. The knife reaches the staff in the membranous urethra, missing the bulb in front and the rectum behind. If a median lithotomy is intended, the knife splits the perineal body from before backward as it is withdrawn. Great care is taken not to injure the rectum or the sphincter ani muscle. The opening thus made should be large enough to admit the index finger into the wound as the knife is withdrawn. Should there be insufficient room to admit the finger into the prostatic urethra, a blunt-pointed lithotomy knife (Fig. 113) is passed alongside the finger and any obstruction found is severed. During this time the stone is fixed by the grooved staff. (Fig. 128.) The finger now locates the stone. A lithotomy forceps, guided by the finger, is passed into the bladder. The stone is then seized and the instrument is cautiously withdrawn. Should the stone be of large dimensions, it should not be forcibly withdrawn for fear that it may injure the neck of the bladder. The lithotrite should

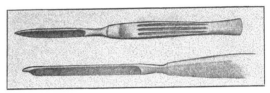

FIG. 113.—Sharp-pointed and Blunt-pointed Knives Used in Operations on the Urinary Bladder.

be applied to the stone and, after careful crushing, the débris may be scooped away with a suitable evacuator or spoon. (Figs. 115, 116.)

The technique to be employed in extracting a stone from the bladder varies according to its shape and size. As little damage as possible should be done to the perineum and prostatic urethra, and especially to the neck of the bladder. We do not hesitate to break up large stones through a small opening in the perineum and wash out, or suck out, the débris with the apparatus devised by Bigelow. (Fig. 115.) In patients over forty years of age the condition of the prostate is ascertained, and, if it is found to obstruct the urinary flow, prostatectomy should then be performed. Some surgeons abandon the curved staff and use one much straighter. Even if the cystoscope has revealed only a single stone, search ought to be made, by means of the finger and with the aid of my prostatic depressor (Fig. 128), for further calculi.

If pyuria, diverticula, or cystitis be present, drainage should be established through the perineum for a few days.

The perineum is closed by a few deep catgut sutures placed above the drainage opening; these sutures approximate the levator ani muscles. The skin wound is closed with horse-hair.

The after-treatment should be as simple as possible. No interference with the drainage or bladder is necessary as long as the patient is comfortable. If no pus is present in the urine then the perineum alone should be drained for a short period. A suitable catheter is inserted into the penis and the urine is carried off in this manner.

The operation just described is, in my opinion, the only perineal operation that should be performed for stone. If any difficulty arises in inserting the finger into the bladder after the primary incision is made, a broad, grooved staff, or a blunt-edged gorget, forced into the bladder, makes a safe and reliable guide for the finger. If there are a large number of stones, of considerable size, in the bladder, perineal section combined with litholapaxy is safer than litholapaxy alone.

Personally, I prefer to split the perineum from behind forward, with the

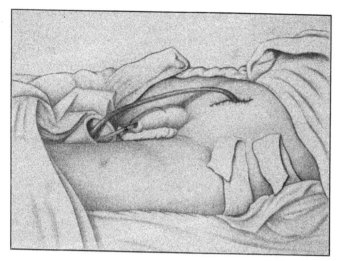

Fig. 114.—Double Drainage of the Bladder. (After Floyd McRae.)

back of the knife toward the rectum. This operation should not be performed upon children unless there are concretions in the prostatic urethra.

Lateral and Bilateral Lithotomy.—Both lateral and bilateral lithotomy, especially the latter variety of operation, were practised with eminent success before the Listerian era by the late Prof. James R. Wood, of New York, and the late Professor Briggs, of Nashville, Tenn., by means of instruments peculiar to themselves. Indeed, the modern surgeon can well afford the time, and perhaps the effort in certain cases, to emulate their success, fortified by suitable implements and modern methods of cleanliness and care.

Suprapubic Lithotomy.—This operation is one which was perfected in America and is indeed the one of choice in this country. Personally, I prefer perineal lithotomy combined with litholapaxy. Indeed, it is not a bad plan to crush the stone through the penis, and then to open the perineum and remove the débris. If the bladder is filled with sterile oil and iodoform, the stone may be crushed with less danger of injury to the bladder. When the perineum is opened the olive oil facilitates the removal of the crushed fragments, and sufficient iodoform is left in the viscus to aid in maintaining it in an aseptic condition.

Litholapaxy.—Litholapaxy was first performed by Bigelow, of Boston, in 1878. The name covers all operations for the removal of stones in the urinary bladder, whether they are crushed before being pumped out or not. The

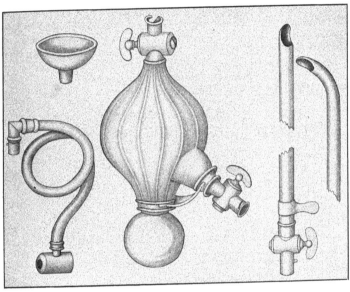

Fig. 115.—Bigelow's Evacuator.

evacuator (Fig. 115) described by Bigelow was the first apparatus invented for this purpose that actually did accomplish the work of evacuation.

Indications:—(a) After an attack of nephritic colic, small stones may often be washed out of the bladder without crushing. (b) All stones of comparatively little hardness may be safely crushed. (c) In young children litholapaxy is preferable; and (d) it is nearly always so in females. (e) In performing prostatectomy, where there is a large stone in the bladder, one may crush the calculus through the perineal wound.

Contra-indications:—(a) Stones having a diameter greater than one inch and a half should not be treated by litholapaxy. (b) The extreme hardness of the "mulberry stones" renders it dangerous to crush them. The writer had occasion to revoke this contra-indication in one case. In removing a prostate, a large mulberry stone was found in the bladder. It was too large to pass through the perineal wound. It was seized by the lithotrite and a hood of gauze was thrown around the end of the instrument containing the stone. It was crushed without damage to the bladder. (c) In severe cystitis it is better to remove the stone perineally, and to drain the bladder.

The technique of litholapaxy is described farther on, under the heading of Combined Litholapaxy and Cystoscopy (page 335).

Cystoscopy.—The method of procedure as devised by Kelly, of Baltimore, is as follows:—(1) Introduce a simple cylindrical speculum into the bladder; (2) produce atmospheric dilatation of the bladder solely by posture; (3) illuminate and inspect the vesical mucosa. A direct view of the interior of the bladder is thus obtained. The method is particularly useful in female cases; it is a more difficult matter to apply it to the male bladder. There are two clear contra-indications, viz., post-operative cystitis and acute gonorrhœal cystitis.

Instruments Required.—The following instruments are required:—(a) A suitable light; (b) a head mirror; (c) a urethral calibrator; (d) a vesical speculum

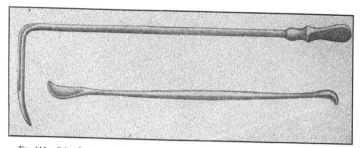

Fig. 116.—Other Instruments Employed in the Operation of Lithotomy.
The upper picture represents Buchanan's lithotomy staff, the lower one Ferguson's double-ended lithotomy scoop.

with obturator; (e) an evacuator for removing urine; (f) a long, slender, mouse-toothed forceps; (g) a ureteral searcher.

The best light is the white electric light; in an emergency, however, an oil lamp or even a candle will be found useful. The light is reflected by a head mirror. Kelly's specula range in size from five to twenty. They are so well known that a description of them is unnecessary. The accompanying figures show, not only one of these specula, of natural size, but also the manner of using it, and the various instruments which are employed in connection with it, in treating the bladder. (Figs. 117, 118, 119.) In this connection he says: "a specialist will also find it convenient to have on hand the following sizes; 6½, 7½, 8½, 9½, 10½, and 11½. The sizes below 12 are used for examination, and those above to secure wide illumination in operating upon the bladder."

The urethral dilator may be dispensed with and the different specula and obturators used instead. While it is best to have the evacuator recommended by Kelly, the urine may be removed by means of a catheter or in any other

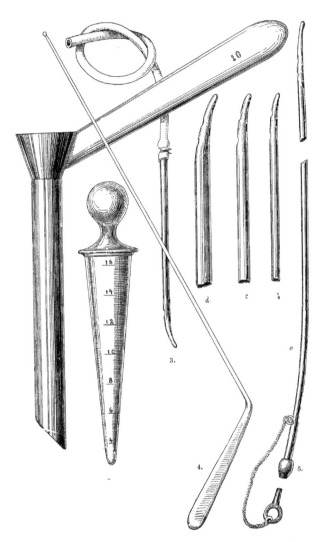

FIG. 117.—Kelly's Cystoscope, with Various Accessory Instruments. (From "Reference Handbook of the Medical Sciences," Wm. Wood & Co., New York.)
1, Bevelled cystoscope; 2, urethral calibrator and dilator; 3, short metal ureteral catheter; 4, searcher for locating ureteral orifice; 5, a, b, c, d, long metal ureteral catheters.

simple way that the surgeon may choose. Applicators and forceps should be employed to carry medicated cotton to various parts of the bladder. The cystoscope is simple, inexpensive, and easy to use. Every physician should master its employment. No harm can follow its use provided the aseptic precautions used in ordinary catheterization are taken. One should be careful not to cause abrasions of the mucosa of the urethra. The liability to infect patients with septic instruments should ever be remembered. Syphilis and gonorrhœa have been passed from one patient to another by instruments that had not been sterilized. The one important preparation which the patient needs

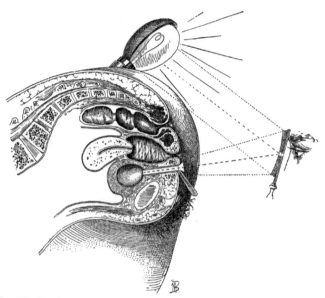

Fig. 118.—Examination of the Urinary Bladder with Kelly's Cystoscope, the Patient being in the Knee-chest Position. (From the "Reference Handbook of the Medical Sciences," Wm. Wood & Co., New York.)

before the operation is that his bowels should be evacuated. It is best for the bladder to be full of urine, for then the capacity of the bladder is learned and a specimen of urine is obtained which may be examined at once.

The Employment of an Anæsthetic.—Local anæsthesia is usually sufficient, but some patients are so nervous, or the genito-urinary tract is so sensitive, that the employment of a general anæsthetic is imperative. When cocaine, or preferably eucaine, is used, the meatus urinarius and the external mucous membrane may be moistened while the catheter is being introduced. I usually anæsthetize the entire urethra, while the catheter is slowly being introduced, by forcing a two-per-cent solution of eucaine through the catheter, a few drops at a time.

After the urine has been allowed to escape and the bladder has been gently washed out by the siphon method until the water returns perfectly clear, the trigonum of the bladder may be anæsthetized with eucaine before the catheter is withdrawn. In chronic cystitis and prostatitis associated with calculi, the parts may be bathed for some time before the cystoscope is introduced. It is wise to give morphia hypodermically half an hour before the examination of the bladder.

Position of the Patient.—While the bladder is being prepared to receive the cystoscope, the patient is in a dorsal position. If a female is being examined, Kelly prefers the high dorsal or knee-chest position before the cystoscope is

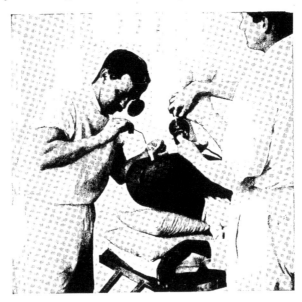

Fig. 119.—Examination of the Urinary Bladder with Kelly's Cystoscope and Reflected Light, the Patient being in the Dorsal Position. (From the "Reference Handbook of the Medical Sciences," Wm. Wood & Co., New York.)

inserted into the bladder. It is true that the Trendelenburg position, with the knees flexed upon the abdomen (Pryor) or the semi-prone one (Sims) may be used, but the knee-chest position ·(Kelly) has many obvious advantages if one wishes to make a perfect examination. (See Fig. 118.) The ascent of the intestines, the relaxation of the abdominal muscles, and the excellent dilatation of the bladder afforded by the knee-chest position, leave no room for argument against its employment when the patient is awake. It is important to dilate the rectum and vagina with air first, and the bladder last, to prevent the orifices of the ureters from being carried upward instead of downward.

The patient kneels, with the knees separated about ten or twelve inches, close to the edge of the table, her buttocks being raised as high as possible; she allows the back to curve forward and rests the side of the face upon the table. If she squats a little, allowing the buttocks to droop toward the feet, she will be more conveniently disposed for the examination. Sometimes it is necessary, in order to get a good expansion, to push the thighs in the opposite direction beyond the vertical. If the patient is under the influence of an anæs-thetic, "the best way to hold her in the knee position is for two assistants, one on either side, to stand close up to the body, to prevent it falling over, each grasping the body with one arm thrown across the back, and holding the leg in the crotch of the knee with the other hand to keep it from slipping up and down." (Kelly, Vol. I.)

Before introducing the speculum, the examiner measures and dilates the urethral orifice when necessary. Care must be taken not to tear the mucous membrane of the meatus; it is better to use a small speculum, especially for a simple examination. The conical dilator used by Kelly, lubricated with glycerin, is passed into the bladder with a boring motion, time being given for the urethra to stretch until a medium-sized lumen is obtained. The dilator is then removed and the speculum, properly lubricated, is slowly inserted. If tearing of the meatus occurs, subgallate of bismuth should be rubbed into the abrasions at once. This checks hemorrhage, is non-irritating, and forms a protecting crust under which repair rapidly takes place. The obturator must be kept in place while the speculum is being introduced. When the speculum enters the bladder the obturator is removed, and the air rushes into the bladder and dilates it, provided the patient is not in a faulty position. If the patient is induced to take a number of long deep breaths, the abdominal type of inspiration being used, more air is aspirated by the bladder.

Examination of the Bladder.—An electric drop light is held close to the end of the sacrum and the examiner reflects the light into the bladder by a head mirror. It requires a little practice before the best illumination is obtained. The examiner may use direct illumination with an electric head light if he has difficulty with the head mirror. If some definite plan of examination of the interior of the bladder is adhered to, the examination takes but a short time, and the whole field is observed. It is probably more satisfactory to push the speculum beyond the ureteral orifices and thus bring into view the posterior pole of the bladder, beyond the trigonum. If to-and-fro, up-and-down, and lateral movements are made, nothing will escape the examiner's eye. The speculum is now slowly withdrawn and its inner end is brought into close contact with the remainder of the mucosa. The beginner must first learn the appearance of the normal bladder.

Appearance of the Normal Bladder.—When the normal bladder is dilated with air, the mucosa presents a dull-white appearance; large and small blood-vessels are seen to branch and anastomose irregularly. The minute vessels are emptied by the pressure of air, and consequently the rosy appearance seen in a contracted bladder is not visible. Kelly calls attention to an acquired red spot which is often seen, and he describes it as follows:—" At a point one or two centimetres above the posterior pole, a rounded, red spot is often seen, which may easily be mistaken for a localized inflammation, but is merely a suction hyperæmia induced at this point by contact with the end of the speculum during the withdrawal of the obturator. The large veins are quite prominent and are seen to fade away as they become smaller. It is not uncommon to see the pulsation of an artery. Shallow, interlaced ridges are observed, situated between the right and left posterior hemispheres; these ridges are formed by irregular muscular bundles. Numerous little glistening points are due to the moisture on slight inequalities of surface which catch and reflect the light." (Kelly.) Through the open speculum the entire surface of the mucosa is examined. By lowering the handle of the cystoscope, the examiner is able to bring the trigonum into view. It is more injected than the rest of the bladder, owing to the close connection between the mucosa and the underlying structures. In order that one may be able to inspect the mucosa in the immediate vicinity of the internal urethral orifice, the speculum must be tilted sharply in every direction. The ureteral orifices should now be looked for. Turn the speculum through fifteen or twenty degrees, to the right and left alternately, and, at a point near the outer and posterior angle of the trigonum, a little pink elevation is noticed; this is the *mons ureteris* and marks the orifice of the ureter. The orifice may look like several things: (*a*) a faint transverse line about 2 mm. long; (*b*) a faint water line on paper; (*c*) a paler area about 1 mm. broad, with a rosy border; (*d*) a blood-vessel may be seen emerging from a small hollow. Watch the spot for about half a minute and a jet of urine is seen coming from it; then one is sure that the ureteral orifice is in full view. The ureteral line or ridge is usually of a deeper color than the bladder behind it. In a normal bladder a beautiful rosy hue appears at each contraction of the organ, and, as dilatation occurs, the color fades away. The bladder will not fully dilate when the patient is pregnant, or ascitic, or has a pelvic tumor. Overdistention of the bladder renders the examination difficult because the ureteral orifices and the trigonum are carried high up. When this occurs, the patient should be placed in the dorsal position, and then the bladder does not overdistend. Before withdrawing the cystoscope, the patient being in the knee-chest position, allow her to resume a side posture; then instruct her to expel the air and instruments by bearing down. This prevents after-pains due to retained air.

The above is the description of a normal female bladder as it appears through the speculum.

Combined Litholapaxy and Cystoscopy.—The idea of crushing a stone while it is being inspected in the bladder, is a sequence to the development of cystoscopy. There are four instruments on the market which combine the lithotrite and the cystoscope—viz., one by Nitze, one by Bierhoff, one by Casper, and one by Walker, of Baltimore. The accompanying cut (Fig. 120) represents Walker's instrument. It is so constructed that the operator looks directly between the jaws. The instrument is sufficiently strong to stand the strain of one-hundred and seventy pounds and will crush any stone in the bladder except one of the hard oxalate type. The following is a brief description of the instrument and of the manner in which it should be used. For a detailed description see *Annals of Surgery*, Sept., 1907.

A (Fig. 120) is an illustration of the complete instrument closed; *C* is a sectional view, as seen when one looks directly between the jaws upon the surface of the cystoscope; *D* shows the jaws open (side view). The principal parts of the instrument are: a female blade carrying a handle; a male blade which is worked by means of a screw; two attachments (*E*)—one for the cystoscope and one for the evacuator; a cystoscope and a steel rod. The handle is composed of two parts, a fixed part and a revolving part. Manipulation of this revolving cap (*B*) closes the jaws. Running along the female blade and handle is an open slot into which a ridge on the under surface of the male blade fits. This male blade consists of a steel tube and is forced along the slot by means of a screw working in conjunction with the revolving cap. The length of the female blade, exclusive of the handle, is 9½ inches; the calibre of the straight portion is No. 25 French, while that of the curved portion is No. 26 French. Thompson's lithotrite is shown in Fig. 121.

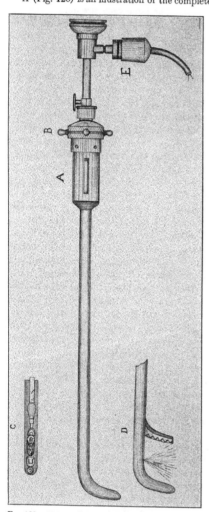

Fig. 120.—Walker's Combined Lithotrite and Cystoscope.

Mode of Using the Instrument. — Walker thus describes the mode of using the instrument:—"The bladder is thoroughly irrigated until the returning fluid is entirely clear, 150 c.c. of clear, sterile water being finally left in. The instrument, adjusted as shown, is then introduced; the jaws are opened by turning the screws from right to left; the cystoscope is adjusted in such a way that the line of vision is between the open blades. The stone is then located, the male blade, which can be seen, is placed squarely in front of it, and the jaws are closed by turning the screw. Before the jaws are entirely closed the cystoscope is turned so that the prism surface will be protected. In some instances it is better to pull the cystoscope well back into the male blade so that it cannot be injured by the stone. After the primary crushing the larger fragments are sought for and broken. If during the crushing some fragments are forced into the tubal portion of the male or female bladder, the cystoscope is removed and the steel rod passed through so as to clear the canal; after which the cystoscope is re-introduced. When the crushing is finished the cystoscope is removed and the evacuator attached. After this, the lithotrite is turned around so that the con-

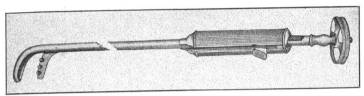

FIG. 121.—Thompson's Lithotrite.

vex surface rests on the floor of the bladder and the beak projects upward into the cavity. The jaws are separated a distance of from three-quarters of an inch to one inch and the fragments are washed out in the usual manner.

"The object of this instrument is not to supplant suprapubic section or the use of the ordinary lithotrite, except in certain cases. It is intended to be used, not for large or hard stones, but for small ones of the soft variety.

The results of lithotomy and lithotrity were never better than they are to-day. Even the statistics of so great a man as Sir Henry Thompson are exceeded—because of our improved technique and increased knowledge—by the fact that other conditions which contributed to his operative mortality, such as enlarged prostate, may now be eliminated.

The treatment of stone alone, without complications, is practically without any mortality. That the worst cases must be treated by cutting operations, and the less serious ones by lithotrity, still holds good. It is true, again, that the field of crushing operations has been extended by Bigelow, litholapaxy superseding lithotrity.

III. ANATOMY AND PATHOLOGY OF THE PROSTATE.

ANATOMICAL CONSIDERATIONS.—The prostate is situated in front of and below the neck of the bladder and surrounds the vesical end of the urethra. It is cone-shaped and in its form resembles very much the ordinary horse-chestnut. The apex is directed downward and forward and the base is in relation to the bladder. It normally measures one inch and a half from base to apex and about one inch in depth. Its weight varies from fifteen to twenty-four grams (four to five drachms). It has been variously described as a bilobed and trilobed structure; all anatomists not being agreed upon this point. At birth it is distinctly a bilobed organ and is situated behind the urethra. That portion which surrounds the urethra and which is situated between the two lateral portions or lobes is frequently designated as the third or median lobe. It is claimed by some that this third lobe is in reality a pathological development; by others, that it is an occasional occurrence. However, it is certain that, when the organ is enlarged, there are three very distinct lobes, one of these being the so-called median lobe. The posterior surface is in relation to the anterior wall of the rectum, to which it is attached by firm connective tissue, while the convex lateral surfaces are covered in part by the levator ani muscles. The apex of the organ impinges on the urogenital triangle.

The first vestige of the prostate appears during the third month of fœtal life as a thickening of the posterior wall of the urethra. The further development is similar to that of acinous glands. The lateral lobes are formed first, and later the median lobe is formed. According to Griffiths, the normal glands on the posterior surface of the urethra, especially on each side of the veru montanum, grow outward, backward, and then forward, so as to enclose the sides of the urethra and finally coalesce on its anterior surface. During their growth, these glands project into and between the muscle bundles of the thickened portion of the urethra, which bundles are continuous with the circular muscular coat of the bladder and are inserted at or near the vesical orifice of the urethra.

With the further development of the gland, the Wolffian ducts finally come to empty into the urethra on, or even with, the margins of the coalesced Muellerian ducts (uterus masculinus), while the orifices of the prostatic gland retain their original situation on each side of the opening of the uterus masculinus. This accounts for the passage of the ejaculatory duct through the prostate.

Piercing the prostate from base to apex, somewhat anteriorly to its central axis, is the urethra, the first part of which, extending from the vesical orifice behind to the deep layer of the triangular ligament in front, is called the prostatic urethra. The ejaculatory ducts empty into the floor of this portion of the urethra on either side of the uterus masculinus, and sometimes into that structure. The upper prominent part of the uterus masculinus is termed the veru montanum or caput gallinaginis. On both sides of the veru montanum are the orifices of the ducts coming from the prostatic acini. The depressed portions of the urethra into which these ducts empty are known as the prostatic sinuses. By compressing the gland, one may see fluid oozing from these orifices, and thus easily be able to locate them. The usual number of these ducts is from fifteen to twenty. When glandular acini are present in the median lobe, their ducts empty into the floor of the prostatic urethra at a point just posterior to the veru montanum.

The prostate is in relation to three layers of fascia that are continuous with the recto-vesical fascia. (Fig. 106.) The superior layer of fascia passes along toward the median line, above the prostatic plexus of veins, and over the upper surface of the prostate, fusing with the external coat of the bladder. The middle layer of the fascia passes below the prostatic plexus of veins, beneath the prostate and bladder, and above the rectum, joining with its fellow of the opposite side. The third layer of this fascia covers the superior or internal surface of the levator ani muscle and becomes continuous with the upper coat of the rectum. The second and third layers form what is known as the aponeurosis of Denonvilliers, which is situated between the prostate and the rectum. This aponeurosis is originally a serous sac derived from the peritoneum. The three layers of the recto-vesical fascia are distinct and separate at the sides and below the prostate; toward the median line above they are indistinguishable as three layers, and form the pubo-prostatic ligaments, intervening between the most anterior fibres of the levator ani muscle and the space of Retzius. They blend at the median line, between these muscle fibres, with the fascia on the other side of these muscles—the deep layer of the triangular ligament, which is a prolongation of the obturator fascia, and which, with the recto-vesical fascia, forms the pelvic fascia.

Beneath this sheath of the prostate and its capsule, various fibrous prolongations pass, surrounding the veins in a mesh and binding the prostate in place. Above the prostate these fibrous prolongations pass to form a more or less fibrous septum, separating the pericapsular space around one lateral lobe from the other, and serving, moreover, as a medium of support. The prostate, therefore, is enveloped, first, by its own capsule; second, by its venous plexus, laterally and anteriorly, and by the bladder above; third, by the sheath of the prostate. (Fig. 107.)

The dorsal vein of the penis divides into two branches, one of which passes to each side of the prostate and, uniting with the veins emerging from the substance of the gland, form the venous plexus of Santorini. In the aged these veins frequently become varicose, and phleboliths may then form.

The arterial brânches supplying the prostate arise from the internal pudic, inferior vesical, and middle hemorrhoidal arteries. These branches are numerous but small, the largest being the vesico-prostatic artery, which is derived from the inferior vesical and passes along the lower part of the sides of the bladder to the prostate. The branches of the pudic and inferior hemorrhoidal arteries are rarely of sufficient size to be noticed.

Histologically, the prostate is a compound tubular gland. The acini of the gland are surrounded by a network of muscular and fibrous tissue, which is a continuation of the capsule of the gland. In these trabeculæ are found the blood- and lymph-vessels. When glandular tissue is present in the isthmus, which binds the two lobes together, there is formed a definite third or median lobe. The acini are lined by a single layer of cubical epithelium, although occasionally this epithelium is stratified, consisting of irregular or transitional cells such as are found in the bladder. The ducts of the gland are lined by transitional epithelium, which gradually changes to columnar and cubical as the acini are reached.

The exact function of the prostate has not been determined, although it is generally believed to participate in the function of the generative organs, rather than in that of the urinary organs. The fluid secreted from the gland, commonly known as the prostatic fluid, is believed to serve as a diluent of the testicular secretion and of the secretion from the seminal vesicles. It has been shown by several observers that the prostatic fluid is necessary for the motility of the spermatozoa. However, the removal of the gland does not seem to interfere with the function in any way. The fact that the prostate in some animals shrinks in winter and increases in size during the warm seasons has

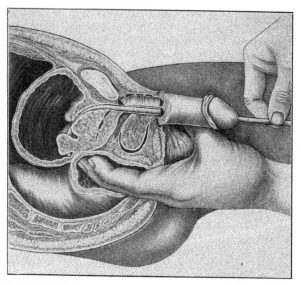

Fig. 122.—Conjoined Examination. with Catheter in the Bladder and Finger in the Rectum. (Original.)

been taken as evidence that there is a correlation between the prostate and the testis.

The prostate may be examined by means.of the finger introduced into the rectum or bimanually, or it may be inspected with the aid of the urethroscope. By rectal examination it is possible to determine the consistency and size of the gland. A fluctuating area may be determined also in this way. If the individual has a thin abdominal wall, bimanual examination will be of assistance. Under certain conditions, the urethral examination is of service if used in conjunction with a rectal examination. (Fig. 122.) With the aid of a large metal catheter in the urethra and a finger in the rectum, much can be learned by skilful manipulation. The evidence of the urethroscope must be regarded as confirmatory of that obtained by the other methods.

Congenital Anomalies.—Congenital anomalies of the prostate are exceedingly rare. The most frequent of these is entire absence, but this condition is found only when there are defects in the development of the rest of the genito-urinary system.

Injuries to the Prostate.—Owing to the situation of the prostate, traumatism occurs very infrequently, even when there is extensive laceration of the perineum. Only a few cases have been observed. When the gland is injured, severe hemorrhage occurs, either through the perineal wound or through the urethra. Although the gland is quite close to the bladder, the latter is rarely involved in the injury, and the blood from the gland seldom flows into the bladder. The blood that is voided with the urine comes through the urethra directly.

Injuries of the prostate are usually followed by infection unless the greatest care is exercised and the wound is carefully cleansed and drained after the injury. Because of the nature of such injuries, foreign bodies are often carried into the deeper structures and must be removed if infection is to be avoided. Simple wounds of the prostate heal very quickly.

The treatment is entirely expectant. Hemorrhage is controlled by pressure. If other structures, such as the prostatic urethra, are injured, the wound must be sutured as is described elsewhere.

Prostatitis. (Albarran.)—There are two varieties of prostatic inflammation—the acute, and the chronic.

Acute Prostatitis.—Owing to the anatomical situation of the prostate, acute inflammations are very infrequent, and depend for their existence mostly upon the presence of diseases in neighboring structures, particularly in the bladder and urethra. Trauma, such as that caused by horseback riding or by blows upon the perineum, may, in exceptional instances, result in inflammation of the prostate. The passing of instruments through the urethra, or the injection of irritating fluids into this channel by one unskilled in the use of such measures, may cause inflammation.

The inflammation may involve all the structures of the gland, or be limited to the parenchyma, or involve only the interacinar tissues. When the inflammation involves the gland in its entirety, it usually terminates in abcess formation. Protracted involvement of the connective tissue of the organ or repeated attacks of inflammation may give rise to chronic prostatitis, with hypertrophy of the gland. The most common cause of chronic prostatitis is gonorrhœa of the posterior urethra. To this infection may also be ascribed the formation of abscess in the prostate. As a rule, however, an acute specific prostatitis will terminate in a short time or become chronic.

Symptoms.—The symptoms of acute prostatitis will vary with the severity of the attack. There is always a feeling of fulness in the perineum, with tenderness on pressure and more or less pain, which is increased in severity during urination and defecation. Rectal examination or the introduction of the catheter into the urethra, is extremely painful, and the latter frequently is a source of hemorrhage. The examining finger in the rectum encounters a hard, firm, tender mass consisting of either one lobe of the prostate or of the entire gland. There may be some elevation of temperature or even chills, although these symptoms are usually indicative of abscess formation.

Differential Diagnosis.—Acute posterior urethritis is the disease which may most readily be mistaken for an acute prostatitis. The features which distinguish these diseases, the one from the other, are given below in tabulated form.

ACUTE POSTERIOR URETHRITIS.	ACUTE PROSTATITIS.
Urination.—Urgent and frequent, with tenesmus.	Not so frequent; tenesmus infrequent.
Pain.—(a) Slight in perineum.	(a) Severe and constant.
(b) Present at end of micturition.	(b) Relief until the bladder contracts on the prostate.
(c) No referred pain.	(c) Referred to rectum, and severe during defecation.
(d) Moderate on catheterization.	(d) Pain from catheter may cause spasm.
Retention.—Absent.	Common.
Blood and Pus.—In urine at end of urination early in disease.	Absent, unless complicated with cystitis or abscess; and then it would be late should it burst into the urethra.
Fever.—Very slight, if any.	Always great.
General Disturbance.—Slight; patient can walk about.	Severe and protracted, as a rule.
Rectal Examination.—	
(a) Slightly tender to touch.	(a) Very painful.
(b) No heat.	(b) Hot sensation.
(c) Prostate of normal size.	(c) May be very large.
(d) Slight œdema of the prostate possible.	(d) Œdematous.
Muscular spasm.—Not present as a rule.	Always present.

The three-glass method of examination is valuable if the specimen shows pus (microscopically) and prostatic elements as well. Acute prostatitis is diagnosed if the urethritis has extended into the prostate.

Treatment.—It is necessary to put the patient at rest and briskly to clear out the alimentary canal with magnesium sulphate. The diet must be restricted and the patient induced to drink large quantities of water. The urine is rendered alkaline by the administration of sufficiently large doses (from twenty to thirty grains) of potassium acetate. Hot or cold rectal lavage through a return rectal tube is carried out during the day and an opium and belladonna suppository is inserted at night. In some cases nothing affords the relief obtainable by a hypodermic injection of morphia. Other diuretics and balsamics may, to advantage, be given internally. Irrigation of the bladder by means of the catheter, or by hydraulic pressure without it, should not be undertaken before the acute symptoms subside, and even then I think that direct applications to the prostate through a proctoscope secure speedier and better results. A microscopic examination of the discharge, made from time to time, aids in determining the progress of the case.

Massage of the prostate is begun as soon as the tenderness on pressure subsides, and is carried out daily until no discharge is obtainable. To secure the best results rest in the horizontal position under strict supervision should be enjoined.

Chronic Prostatitis.—The most constant symptom of chronic inflammation of the prostate is the discharge of glairy fluid from the urethra, the amount varying from a few drops to several ounces in twenty-four hours. The general health of the patient is usually more or less affected, and patients have been known to lose mental as well as bodily power from protracted chronic prostatitis. A rectal examination discloses the presence of an irregular swelling of the gland and may elicit some tenderness. The three-glass test is useful in making a diagnosis. To obtain any secretion from the prostate the base of the gland is massaged through the rectum and the urethra washed out by the urine. The quantity obtained is small and is composed of epithelium, strings of mucus, a few amyloid bodies, and spermatozoa expressed from the seminal vesicles. In chronic prostatitis a much larger amount is obtained by massage and stripping the urethra without allowing the patient to urinate. Under the microscope this fluid contains, in addition to many epithelial cells, large masses of hyaline material, amyloid bodies, lecithin granules, spermatozoa, and Boettcher crystals. It has been shown that these crystals are due to cholin in the seminal fluid (Bocarins) and also to organic extracts. By means of the Florence reaction these crystals may be detected in specimens of semen after twenty years, even when the specimen is putrid. This test for semen is valuable for medico-legal work. To the suspected material add a few drops of a mixture consisting of iodine, 2.54, potassium iodide, 1.65, and aqua destillata, 30; place on a slide and examine with the medium-power lens. If semen is present Boettcher's crystals are detected. These are of a dark-brown color, of various shapes and sizes; some being single, lance-shaped bodies, others having the form of rosettes, still others being double, and finally a few having the form of rhombic crystals.

Tuberculosis and sexual neurasthenia have been known to complicate the chronic form of the disease.

Abscess of the Prostate.—Before an accumulation of pus sufficiently large to be dignified by the term abscess and to demand the consideration of an operation for its evacuation, forms within the capsule of the prostate, an infection of the prostatic tubules by gonorrhœa has usually taken place. Œdema of the entire gland must follow and the tubules and stroma break down, forming one or more pus cavities in each lobe. The more rapid the destruction of the gland substance, the larger the accumulation of pus in one or both lobes of the prostate. While one lobe is usually more involved than the other, still it is only a matter of degree. It is common to find multiple abscesses first.

The infection having extended from the urethra, the abscess empties itself into this passage, thus occasionally effecting a spontaneous cure. In the writer's experience, infection is not so easily overcome, and Nature must be aided with the knife. In the majority of cases many abscesses are found throughout the gland, and these must be treated surgically, because, if they are left untreated, the capsule and surrounding tissues soon become involved. In this manner perineal and ischiorectal abscesses develop. Extraprostatic suppuration may, in acute cases, cause a fatal periprostatic phlegmon, or the pus may escape spontaneously into the bladder, rectum, groin, peritoneal cavity (rare), or externally through the perineum.

It is true that one abscess after another may find its way into the urethra until the entire prostate becomes a suppurating sac. The infection in most cases has extended by this time into the ejaculatory ducts, seminal vesicles, vas deferens, epididymis, testicles, and bladder, causing chronic inflammation of one or all of these connecting structures.

In the course of a gonorrhœal infection, prostatic abscesses may form, in the first infection, in upward of fifty per cent of the cases. Subsequent abscesses form, next in frequency, after relapsing discharges (small abscesses emptying into the urethra); but an abscess may also form in any gonorrhœal infection that occurs at a still later date.

Acute posterior urethritis leads to an acute prostatitis, and this in turn may cause prostatic suppuration (abscess).

The progressive stages should be differentiated one from the other, so that, when the abscess or abscesses form, prompt relief by incision and drainage may be carried out. It is not necessary, for the purposes of this paper, to describe each and every etiological factor that has been delineated in the pathogenesis of prostatic abscess. Suffice it to furnish Segond's table, viz.:—

PROSTATIC INFECTIONS.
    A. *Exciting Causes.*
        I. *Pathogenic Bacteria.*
            (a) Gonococcus.
            (b) Streptococcus.
            (c) Staphylococcus.
            (d) Colon bacillus.
            (e) Pneumococcus.
            (f) Anaërobic organisms.
    B. *Predisposing Causes.*
        (a) Adult age.
        (b) Cold.
        (c) Contusions (falls, riding, cycling).
        (d) Marching.
        (e) Constipation.
        (f) Superpurgation.
        (g) Hemorrhoids.
        (h) Sedentary habits.
        (i) Excessive coitus.
        (j) Masturbation.
        (k) Balsamics.

The avenues of infection, as laid down by Segond, are:

I. Ascending:—Acute posterior urethritis, gonorrhœal sounds, catheterization, etc.

II. Circulatory:—The acute exanthemata, typhoid fever, etc.

III. Lymphatic:—Prostatitis, periprostatitis, hemorrhoids, perirectal inflammation, fistula, pericystitis, etc.

IV. Direct infection:—Traumatism from without and from within, injuries, false passages, etc.

While this table is not complete, it is an excellent guide to the student in ferreting out the many causes of prostatic abscesses. If, in the course of pneumonia, typhoid fever, one of the exanthemata, tuberculosis, or some other constitutional infection, retention of urine occurs simultaneously with an aggravation of the general symptoms of the patient, a prostatic abscess should be suspected. Again, when a man who has been exposed to cold, fatigue, travel, or work, experiences a chill (not explainable by any other known cause) which is followed by fever, thirst, etc., and he cannot pass his urine, search should be made for a prostatic abscess.

In 1891, the writer saw a man, 32 years of age, who had been clearing railroad tracks of snow for three days, and had then, after experiencing a chill, become desperately ill, with retention of urine; within eighteen hours he became delirious, maniacal, and unmanageable. When first seen, about thirty-seven hours after the initial chill, he was being restrained by two powerful men; he was confused, delirious, muttering unintelligible sentences; he was shivering, his teeth were chattering, and he could not be persuaded to lie down; he stood or attempted to walk. His face was blue and congested; the eyes were bloodshot and the extremities were cold. Assisted by Dr. J. C. Todd, of Winnipeg, and the men in attendance I administered chloroform before I deemed it safe to attempt catheterization, and even then I found it impracticable to pass a soft-rubber catheter. A silver catheter was passed with some difficulty, and then only after I had aided my direct efforts by pressure made with the finger in the rectum. The discovery of a well-defined swelling in the region of the prostate left no doubt that this organ was the seat of an abscess. A scalpel was immediately passed into the swelling, a large quantity of grumous pus was evacuated, and the cavity was drained by a rubber tube held in place by a stitch of silkworm gut. The rectal temperature was 107.2° F. The patient broke out into a profuse perspiration, fell asleep, and remained in that state for seven hours. When he awoke he was rational, but prostrated. The body-temperature was by this time subnormal. In two days the drainage tube was removed. At the end of two weeks he was back at work again. No further treatment, beyond the making of the incision and the establishment of drainage, was found necessary.

In this case there was no history of urethral infection, either before or at the time of his illness. The nature of the infection was not determined.

In consultation with the late Dr. Tulloch, I saw another very interesting case of prostatic abscess, which had followed the ligation of hemorrhoids many years previously. An ischiorectal abscess formed first. A couple of days afterward it was evacuated by an incision through the perineum to the right of the median line. When I first saw the patient, he was suffering intensely from acute sepsis. He had had to be catheterized every eight or twelve hours since the operation. Catheterization became more and more painful; he dreaded its repetition. There was a history of an old gleet, probably a chronic urethritis (gonorrhœal). A rectal examination under chloroform revealed the existence of an enlarged, tense prostate. Through the incision that had been made for opening the ischiorectal abscess, I passed a long, slender knife into the prostate, but no pus escaped. I then pushed a closed artery forceps into the mass and opened the abscess by Hilton's method. A tube was inserted and the cavity drained for over a week, pus escaping through the fistula. About two months later another operation was performed for the purpose of getting rid, if possible, of a troublesome fistulous discharge. The perineum was incised in the median line, the membranous and a portion of the prostatic urethra being divided by the knife. The finger was passed into the bladder. The curette was freely applied to the fistulous tract and a considerable amount of granulation and prostatic tissue was scraped away. I was amazed at the time (1886) to find a cavity of such large size and I believed that the case was one of carcinoma of the prostatic tissue. However, the microscope showed the tissue to be simply inflammatory, and the patient made a tedious but complete recovery.

The writer has seen three cases in which a traumatism inflicted upon a hypertrophied prostate was followed by direct infection that caused a suppurative inflammation and the formation of an abscess in that organ. In the first of these cases the abscess was simply drained, the gland itself being removed three weeks later. In the remaining two it was found necessary to perform immediately a median perineal prostatectomy, the result of which, in both instances, was a complete cure.

A calculus in the prostate is often the cause of prostatic abscess. In these cases the removal of the stone is necessary to effect a cure. Prostatic abscess of a tuberculous nature is chronic, and the clinical behavior of the disease shows plainly that the tubercle bacillus is the causative factor. Farther on, I will go into this subject more fully.

While cases of prostatic abscess develop without the clinical picture of suppurative inflammation (Fuller), insidious causes other than gonorrhœal prostatitis being responsible, still it is the rule to find a history of an acute or chronic gonorrhœal infection. When a man suffering from gonorrhœa, acute or chronic, becomes the subject of sexual excitement, of alcoholic excesses, of exposure to cold or to extreme fatigue, or of instrumentation, and soon thereafter manifests inflammatory symptoms and signs, abscess formation should be immediately apprehended. As the pus accumulates, the discomfort in the rectum and perineum increases, and these parts become tender; urination becomes painfully laborious or even impossible; retention of urine, if it occurs, adds another train of agonizing symptoms to those already present; defecation is tardy and painful; enemata are not well borne; and any attempt to pass a catheter produces spasm. It is not unusual for grave constitutional symptoms to arise concomitantly with, or before, the local manifestations begin. They may be ushered in by a chill or rigor. The man has a dry, dusky skin, and his tongue is dry, furred, and red; he is thirsty, excited, prostrated; he does not eat or sleep; his temperature is high (103° to 107° Fahr.); in short, he presents every appearance of being very ill.

An examination of the blood shows a leucocytosis of probably 20,000. A rectal examination reveals the fact that the prostate is enlarged—sometimes to a surprising degree,—œdematous, hot, and tender. In many cases fluctuation is present. Tumefaction and enlargement of the periprostatic structures, especially the vesiculæ seminales, are also likely to be present. In an acutely developed prostatic abscess, the perineal, abdominal, and pelvic muscles are all on guard, and all the local reflexes are increased. A sudden cessation of pain and a rapid diminution of the fever, with the escape of pus from the rectum or urethra, indicate that a prostatic abscess has spontaneously ruptured.

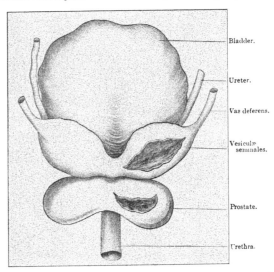

Bladder.

Ureter.

Vas deferens.

Vesiculæ seminales.

Prostate.

Urethra.

Fig. 123.—Tuberculosis of the Bladder and Seminal Vesicles; External View of the Affected Parts. (After Senn.)

The treatment of prostatic abscess is either expectant or operative, and the details of the two methods may be stated as follows:—

I. Expectant treatment.

    (a) Same as for glandular prostatitis.

    (b) Suprapubic puncture for retention of urine.

II. Operative treatment.

    (a) Opening the abscess internally through the urethra. (Velpeau.)

    (b) External urethrotomy and rupture of the abscess by pressure through the urethra with the fingers. (Alexander.)

    (c) Perineal prostatectomy and drainage without opening the urethra.

    (c, d) Perineal prostatectomy and drainage. (Alexander.)

Tuberculosis of the Prostate.—Tuberculosis of the prostate is a very rare affection and is always secondary to tuberculosis in some other part of the body, especially in the testis. In the opinion of Sir Henry Thompson, the prostate is never the seat of a primary tuberculosis, but the affection is secondary to disease of the kidney or testicle. In 18 cases of prostatic tuberculosis collected by him, the kidney in 13, the testicle in 7, and the lungs in 10 were affected before the prostatic invasion. From Czerny's clinic (according to Senn), Marwedel has reported two cases of primary tuberculosis. (Fig. 123.) Socin has also reported two similar cases. The disease here is rarely diagnosed; it remains unrecognized unless the prostate is incidentally examined in the course of an examination of other organs.

The chief symptom is unduly frequent and painful urination. The signs of cystitis are also usually present, and blood is found in the urine from time to

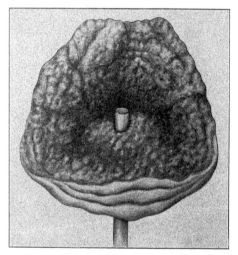

FIG. 124.—Tuberculous Necrosis of the Prostate; view of the organ after it has been laid open. (From Fuller: "Diseases of the Genito-Urinary System," The Macmillan Co., New York.)

time. Emaciation, debility, and hectic fever are constant. Catheterization is painful and causes bleeding. During the early stages there may be spasmodic retention of urine, but later on, when the sphincter vesicæ muscles are involved, incontinence may result. In my own cases, six in number, tubercle bacilli were present in the urine and there were prostatic discharges. The course of the disease when it affects the prostate is the same as that of tuberculosis involving some other part of the body: the tubercles form, coalesce, break down, and form an abscess which requires evacuation. This is readily done through a curved incision in the perineum just anterior to the anus. The bulb of the urethra is separated from the anal sphincter, and the surgeon, with one finger in the rectum to prevent injury to that structure, continues the dissection upward until the abscess is reached. It is opened widely and drained.

The abscess may be reached by making a puncture wound through the rectum, but this method should not be one of choice, because in this way infection may extend into the bowel and produce a fistula, causing considerable trouble to the patient.

In carrying out the treatment it is important to exercise great caution. After the diagnosis has been made through the urethroscope, instrumentation is no longer permissible, and even urethral irrigation should not be practised, because this only aggravates the disease. The injection of a few drops of silver-nitrate solution, or of Lannelongue's solution of zinc chloride, by means of a catheter introduced into the urethra, does good in most cases. Perineal section, to be followed by careful scraping of the diseased area and suitable medicinal applications, is indicated, especially when an abscess forms. Iodoform emulsion may be injected into the diseased gland (Senn), but in two of

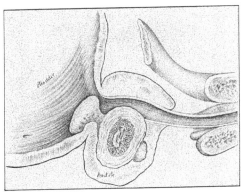

Fig. 125.—Prostato-vesical Calculus. (After Joseph D. Bryant.)

my cases it caused too much suffering to warrant a repetition of the procedure. The employment of bismuth paste, thirty per cent in vaseline, is of decided advantage in some cases. The prostatic urethra may be filled with it, either by way of the urethra or through a perineal opening, once or twice a day; and marked improvement of the symptoms and an apparent arrest of the disease may be expected, in most cases, to result from this procedure. I have had no experience with the x-ray. Prostatectomy and the removal of the vesiculæ seminales should not be recommended. I am sure that, in three of my cases, it hastened a fatal termination, which occurred three months after the operations. It is important to know that the subjects of tuberculosis are liable to have tubercle bacilli in the testis without involvement of the prostate. (Jani.)

English writers have called attention to a tuberculous periprostatitis which is very virulent, as shown by its tendency to produce a general dissemination of tuberculosis. Tuberculous prostatitis may be controlled, and sometimes even cured, by the adoption of suitable measures, but the treatment must not be too vigorous. The local treatment should be supplemented by efforts to increase the patient's resistance, as by a change of climate, a liberal diet, etc.

Tuberculous Necrosis of the Prostate.—Fuller ("Diseases of the Genito-Urinary System," 1900) gives the following description of a case of tuberculous necrosis of the prostate:—"Twelve hours after prostatectomy an autopsy was obtained. The entire prostate was found to have been involved by the necrosis. The inner layer of the prostatic fibrous capsule was lined with granulations,· showing that Nature had detached the dead from the living tissue. The prostatic urethra and neck of the bladder, aside from showing evidences of surface inflammation, were normal. The mucous membrane of the bladder was congested and inflamed. Both seminal vesicles were filled with purulent material, and one of these showed evidences of ulceration in connection with its mucous

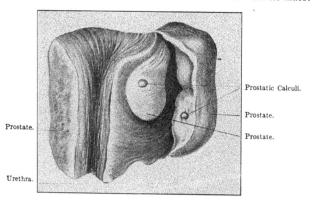

Prostatic Calculi.

Prostate.

Prostate.

Prostate.

Urethra.

Fig. 126.—Prostatic Calculus Embedded in the Substance of the Gland, and Exposed by a Deep Longitudinal Incision. (After Fuller: "Diseases of the Genito-Urinary System," The Macmillan Co., New York.)

membrane. The area of the prostatic necrosis was, however, widely separated from the seminal vesicles." (Fig. 124.)

Syphilis of the Prostate.—Although there seems to be no reason why syphilis should not affect the prostate, it appears that such a condition has never been noted even by the most careful observers.

Calculi in the Prostate Gland.—Prostatic calculi are rare; they may be found in the prostatic urethra, in the ejaculatory ducts, or in the substance of the gland. Some are embedded in the gland only in part, while a portion of the stone projects into the bladder, or the urethra, or both (Fig. 125-127). These calculi, which are lodged in spaces that communicate with the tracts lined by mucous membrane, are usually of urinary origin, while the "true prostatic calculi" develop in the tubules of the prostate and are there found sometimes in great numbers. They originate from the corpora amylacea and are at first only microscopic in size. When they attain the size of the follicles which enclose them, they act as foreign bodies and become encrusted with calcium phosphate and calcium carbonate. These calculi, which are of about the size of millet seeds, are scattered irregularly throughout the lateral lobes, but may be present anywhere within the capsule where there are tubules. The true prostatic calculi may, by causing pressure atrophy, appear exposed on the mucous membrane of the prostatic urethra (Fig. 125), where they may be felt grating upon a metal catheter or sound when the instrument is being introduced.

In the course of my practice I have observed four cases of prostatic calculi. In two of these the calculi were probably of renal origin; one of them was lodged

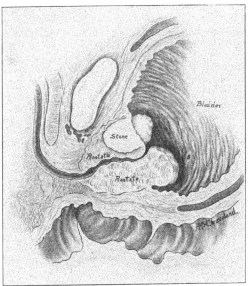

FIG. 127.—Prostatic Calculus. (Original.)

in the prostatic urethra and pressed down into the substance of the gland to the extent of nearly half an inch, while the other protruded into the bladder from the anterior portion of the prostate. (Fig. 127.) In the third case there were many small calculi in the lateral lobes, and two of these protruded through the mucous membrane of the prostatic urethra, in a manner similar to that represented in Fig. 125. In the fourth case the lateral lobes contained numerous (thirty-six) small uric-acid calculi, for the most part smaller than pin-heads.

In the first two cases there was a history of renal lithiasis, cystitis, dysuria, etc. In the third case no such history was given, but the lad, nine years of age, was for three years greatly troubled, night and day, with incontinence of urine and inflammatory attacks about the neck of the bladder, which frequently confined him to bed. So irritable and painful were the urethra and bladder that no examination could be made without the aid of a general anæsthetic. I operated upon this youth three times before I succeeded in removing all the calculi. The relief afforded was complete. This was the first case of this nature (date, 1895) that I had encountered in my own work.

In 1908 the prostatic calculus represented by Fig. 127 was found in a man 67 years of age, in the practice of Dr. N. F. McClinton, of Alma, Mich. This patient also suffered from enlargement of the prostate and had led a catheter-life for seven years. Since I removed his prostate and the stone which was lodged in it through the perineum, he has had complete relief.

The fourth case referred to above was that of a physician, 63 years of age, who had been complaining of dysuria for nine months. During the three months preceding the time when I first saw him he had lost over fifty pounds in weight, and had spent much of his time in urinating, which was painful. After considering the signs and symptoms present and especially the fact that there was no residual urine, I was led to make a probable diagnosis of prostatic calculi. No instruments could be passed through the prostatic urethra without producing excruciating pain. Even under cocaine anæsthesia considerable pain was caused by passing a soft-rubber catheter. On Saturday, August 21st, 1909, I made a median perineal incision, and came in contact with a nest of small calculi. They were well distributed throughout the lateral lobes. Enucleation of the gland was impossible, owing to the dense character of the fibrous tissue which surrounded it. I removed it piecemeal with my prostatic forceps. (Fig. 128, No. 2.) A small pathological middle lobe was encountered and removed. The calculi were small, only two being larger than the head of a pin. There were thirty-six in all, and they consisted principally of uric acid. They had evidently come down from the right kidney at different times during the preceding ten or twelve years. The patient had never had a distinct nephritic colic, but was conscious for a number of years of a tenderness in the region of the right kidney and ureter. He stood the operation well and made a complete recovery.

Prostatitis is nearly always present in these cases of calculi. Occasionally the perineum has been opened for the purpose of removing a vesical calculus, and the presence of a stone in the prostate has then been discovered.

SYMPTOMS AND DIAGNOSIS.—Frequent urination and "wetting the bed" are early symptoms of prostatic phleboliths, especially in boys. Pulling at the penis when asleep and suddenly grasping it has been noticed in many of the cases reported. As the calculi produce more and more local trauma, inflammation and suppuration of the gland are sure to result, and in consequence the patient suffers from sudden spasms at the neck of the bladder, similar to those experienced in cystitis. The dysuria is not unlike that of other disorders of the prostate—e.g., tuberculosis, prostatitis, etc. In some of the cases it will be found that inflammation has extended to the vesicles, vas, and epididymis. It should be remembered that prostatic stones have been mistaken for incrustations in the urethra. Examination per rectum reveals a firm, tender prostate, usually of normal size. When prostatitis and cystitis are present as a complication, it is almost impossible to pass a catheter without causing much suffering and more or less hemorrhage. In old men simple hypertrophy of the prostate must be excluded; it can easily be eliminated by the history of the case, by a cystoscopic examination, by the use of the x-ray, and, in addition, by the ordinary means of diagnosis with the catheter, sound, and finger. Decided pain, or at least discomfort, in the region of the prostate, together with sexual irreg-

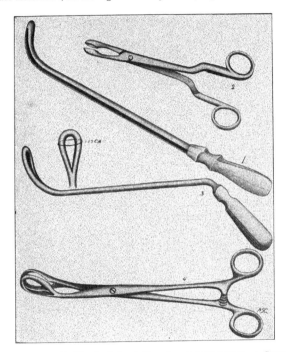

FIG. 128.—Instruments Used by the Author in Operating upon the Prostate. 1. Grooved staff; 2, prostatic cutting forceps; 3, prostatic depressor; 4, large retention forceps.

ularities, is also caused by diseases of the kidney alone, or by these in combination with some disorder of the bladder.

Errors in diagnosis occasionally occur. Thus, it is not long since an advanced case of cancer of the prostate and bladder was sent to me with the diagnosis of vesical calculus. If all the means of diagnosis recently developed are faithfully employed, I am sure that errors in the diagnosis of prostatic calculi will be less frequent.

TREATMENT.—The removal of the calculus by one of the three following routes constitutes the only rational treatment of this diseased condition:—

1. Extraction from the urethra by means of forceps (Brodie, Lister, Fergusson, Morgan, and others) is recommended only when a small concretion is lodged in the prostatic urethra. These small stones usually pass down from the kidney and become obstructed in the urethra.

2. Perineal section (median).—Median perineal section is the preferable procedure for removing prostatic calculi, even when they protrude greatly into the bladder.

3. Suprapubic cystotomy.—When a prostate which also contains a calculus is to be removed, the surgeon who is more familiar with the suprapubic route will no doubt give it the preference. Considerable skill is required to deal with a prostatic condition through the median perineal incision, but I am convinced that it is the safest and best method of operating.

Tumors of the Prostate.—The most common tumors of the prostate gland are carcinoma and sarcoma. Fibromata have been noted occasionally; and, inasmuch as they rarely cause symptoms, it is possible that they are more frequent than is generally supposed.

Fibroma.—Fibromata in the prostate do not differ in any respect from fibromata in other parts of the body. This variety of new-growth does not cause any enlargement of the gland, or at most only a slight enlargement, and is detected solely because of its firmness. It is always encapsulated.

Sarcoma.—Sarcoma of the prostate is not so common as might be inferred from the fact that the prostate normally contains a small amount of connective tissue. Many cases of sarcoma of the prostate have been recorded in the literature, but, unfortunately, a microscopic examination was not made in every instance, and consequently it is impossible in these cases to differentiate correctly between carcinoma and sarcoma. As has been stated elsewhere, hypertrophy of the prostate is quite unusual in very young persons. One of the most striking features of sarcoma is its rapid growth; another is the rapidity with which the surrounding pelvic structures are involved. The sarcomatous prostate varies in size from that of an apple to that of two fists. It has been found that the larger tumors are more likely to occur in young than in old individuals. Sometimes the entire gland, with the exception of one lateral lobe, is involved. The tumor is usually of the round-cell variety, although examples of both the spindle-cell and the large-cell types have been noted. Myxosarcoma, lymphosarcoma, and angiosarcoma have been reported, but they are exceedingly rare. Sarcoma spreads very rapidly, metastases having been found in the ureters, bladder, pelvic connective tissues, and bones. The lymph nodes and the rectum are not often the seat of metastases.

The treatment, which is always of an operative nature, is very unsatisfactory, because the patient sooner or later reaches the stage in which his symptoms, particularly those of pain and pressure, are unbearable, and because catheterization then becomes impossible. Removal of the tumor makes the patient comfortable for a while and prolongs life. In fact, as a rule, the pain never again becomes so severe as before the removal of the tumor. Death, which results from the extension of the disease to other structures, takes place in from three to six months. A few cases have been reported in which a cure was effected by prostatectomy, but in such instances there was either a mistake in diagnosis or the tumor was removed before any extension had taken place.

Carcinoma.—Carcinoma of the prostate usually occurs in older persons, but it has been noted in persons under forty years of age. One observer (Wolff) collected 67 cases, more than half of which occurred between the ages of seventy and eighty. It has been stated that carcinoma frequently appears in patients who have suffered from hypertrophy of the prostate, and that, therefore, the diagnosis of carcinoma is not made as a rule during life. This is also true of other conditions which may be found post mortem.

Gross, of Philadelphia, in 1850, was one of the first to write of cancer of the prostate. Thompson, in 1881, drew further attention to the subject by publishing a report upon twelve cases. Since then, during the last decade, many cases have been reported. Since complete prostatectomy has become a recognized surgical procedure the frequency of cancer has been demonstrated. Carcinoma was formerly considered rare in the prostate, but now it is variously reckoned as being present in from five per cent to twenty-five per cent of all prostatic enlargements. It is claimed (Musée Guyon, by Albarran) that as high as fourteen per cent of the cases of supposed hypertrophy of the prostate are more or less malignant in character. From a clinical viewpoint this relative frequency is too high. In my own cases, cancer appeared to arise independently of prostatic enlargement. In none of the six cases examined microscopically did carcinomatous degeneration have its seat in a hypertrophied middle lobe.

Pathology and Diagnosis.—According to Albarran two forms of prostatic carcinoma are recognized, viz.:—

I. Circumscribed carcinoma (within the capsule).

(*a*) Malignant nodule appearing in benign hypertrophy.

(*b*) Entire gland involved but not enlarged.

(*c*) Malignant nodules protruding from the gland which is itself enlarged and involved.

II. Diffuse carcinoma, extracapsular as well as intracapsular.

The surrounding tissues—rectum, vesiculæ seminales, lymph nodes, etc.— are also involved.—The epithelioma of Albarran, Halte, and others, may have originated in a lobe otherwise benign. Seven years ago the writer removed (intracapsular operation) a prostate which the microscope showed to be a cancer of the epitheliomatous type; and, despite this fact, the man is to-day in excellent health. The diagnosis of cancer of the prostate, in its early development, is a puzzling problem; but, when the disease is advanced, the diagnosis is self-evident, even to the inexperienced. An early diagnosis and an early extirpation may save life. No plan of treatment thus far discovered offers any hope of a cure when the cancer involves the extracapsular structures. When considering the question of diagnosis the surgeon must be on the lookout for stone, tuberculosis, cystitis, chronic prostatitis, spinal disease (locomotor ataxia), kidney stone, and even Bright's disease. Any condition that causes pain in and around the prostate must be carefully excluded before a diagnosis of carcinoma is made. One case of malignant disease (cancer) of the prostate was sent to me with a diagnosis of stricture of the urethra,—an error, which cast discredit upon a well-informed practitioner simply because he made no examination. In two of my cases the patients were previously operated on for hemorrhoids, which represented only secondary manifestations of the cancerous condition; and in both instances the operation was performed at a time when malignancy should have been suspected, if not diagnosed. The fact must not be overlooked that, at the present time, cases of carcinoma of the prostate are sent to the surgeon at such a late stage of the disease that he is not justified in recommending a radical operation—prostatectomy. A diagnosis of prostatic hypertrophy, instead of carcinoma, is the error most frequently made. There is considerable excuse for this error, when we consider that carcinoma is often recognized only by a microscopic examination of a prostate which ran the clinical course of simple hypertrophy. In all the cases of cancer that I have seen, the pain has been out of all proportion to the other manifestations of prostatic disease.

The tumor may be confined to one lobe or it may involve the whole gland. Metastases are found most commonly in the seminal vesicles and bladder, the lymph nodes of the pelvis, the inguinal lymph nodes, and even the remote lymph nodes. They are also found in bony structures, and, when one of the long bones is the seat of such a metastasis, it is very likely to undergo a pathological fracture.

In cases in which the prostate is the seat of a tumor, it is preferable to make the examination while the patient is under the influence of a general anæsthetic, for then the patient will be subjected to a minimum amount of pain and a thorough examination will be possible. Bimanual examination may disclose the fact that a mass is projecting from the posterior surface of the prostate into the rectum, and in very rare instances a similar mass may be felt (through the abdominal wall) projecting into the bladder. Catheterization is usually painful and causes hemorrhage. Cystoscopy is unreliable in the diagnosis of tumors of the prostate.

The following table may be found useful as an aid in diagnosis:—

DIFFERENTIAL DIAGNOSIS BETWEEN CARCINOMA AND SIMPLE HYPERTROPHY OF THE PROSTATE.

	Carcinoma.	Hypertrophy.
Pain.	Constant and referred.	Only during urination.
Urination.	No relief and infrequent.	Gives relief; frequent.
Onset.	Months.	Years.
Obstruction to flow of urine.	Rare.	Very common.
Residual urine.	Rare.	Very common.
Retention.	Rare and late in the disease.	Common off and on, and early in the disease.
Progress.	Steadily worse.	Better and worse; worse and better.
Prostatitis.	Rare:	Common.

	Carcinoma.	*Hypertrophy.*
Cystitis.	Rare.	Common.
Catheterization.	Not often necessary.	Often necessary. (Instrument bent like prostatic curve.)
Cystoscope.	No enlargement; ulcer late sign.	Shows middle or other protrusions.
Age.	About fifty. Rare before or after. Extends laterally and involves seminal vesicles.	More frequent over than under fifty. Extends toward the bladder and more uniformly.
Stricture.	Permanent; affects vesical neck; later, the ureters.	Spasmodic, occurs early, ureters never involved.
Rectal examination.	Stony; indurated, fixed, tender; vesicles and trigonum often thickened. May be nodular.	Firm, elastic, movable, not always tender. Usually smooth.
Sound in urethra.	Usually passed with ease. Beak on trigonum not easily felt *per rectum.* Bladder neck fixed, not sacculated. Marked central prostatic thickening.	Hard to pass. Beak easily felt. Bladder pouches, moderate in periurethral type; no median thickening, as a rule.
Hemorrhoids.	Rapid development, no remission of symptoms and signs.	Slow in developing or relapsing.
Emaciation.	Marked when cancer is usually diagnosed.	Begins after years of suffering.

TREATMENT.—In advanced cases of cancer of the prostate, palliative means only can be employed. A carcinomatous stricture of the vesical neck is best treated by the catheter, as long as this can be done without pain; the object being, of course, to draw off the urine and keep the urethra patent. It is sometimes of advantage to leave the catheter in the bladder for from twenty-four to forty-eight hours at a time, or even longer, after which a respite from the catheter may be enjoyed for a few days. The benefit of this treatment is no doubt due to the fact that the instrument causes a pressure atrophy of the tissues involved, thus enabling the meatus to remain patulous for a variable period of time. This treatment may relieve the patient for several weeks or months; a nurse can best carry out this treatment, not alone on account of her natural gentleness, but because she has more patience and more time at her disposal than the practitioner; and then, besides, she is always at hand to give relief regularly and promptly. Sooner or later, the catheter cannot be passed, and something more efficacious must be done to carry off the urine. After a careful consideration of the results obtained by the Bottini operation and by partial prostatectomy, above and below, I am constrained to recommend neither of them. Judging from my own experience, and from evidence furnished by other surgeons, I am convinced that the sufferer from prostatic cancer will live longer and more comfortably with a suprapubic fistula, after the method practised by Hunter McGuire (Fig. 111) for prostatic obstruction of a benign nature, than after any other surgical procedure. A partial prostatectomy, while it temporarily relieves the obstruction, hastens the final issue by increasing dissemination of the carcinoma. A few cases of apparent cure, following complete prostatectomy, have been reported by Fuller, Young, and others. In early operations the suprapubic route was selected, but the more recent cases have been dealt with through the perineum. The radical operation for cancer of the prostate, indicating, as it does, the removal of part of the bladder, will in future—when performed at all—be executed through the perineum. The mortality is very high. The patients who live thereafter deserve more praise and credit for the value they place upon their lives, than does the intrepid surgeon who seeks glory out of obvious defeat. Prostatectomy must not be undertaken when the bladder is involved, if one would save his patient much suffering and himself surgical disgrace.

Hypertrophy of the Prostate.—Enlargement of the prostate gland, the result of a hyperplasia of its tissues, is by far the most important, although by no means the most serious, condition the surgeon is called upon to treat. This hyperplasia may affect the glandular elements, the non-striated muscle, the interstitial connective tissues, or all three. It may be confined to one lobe, or it may involve both lateral lobes and the central or middle lobe. When only the glandular tissue is involved, the resultant tumor is soft in consistency, more so than when the interstitial or muscular tissue is affected. When only the interstitial tissue is affected in the hyperplasia, the tumor is usually hard and firm in consistency. When only the connective and muscular tissues are involved the enlargement is often confined to the middle lobe, because here few, if any, glandular elements are found. The new product consists chiefly of connective tissue with a moderate amount of muscle fibres.

SYMPTOMS.—The objective symptoms are often very pronounced and the cystoscope reveals a mass projecting into the bladder. As a rule, hypertrophy of the prostate is the result of hyperplasia of the muscular and connective tissues. The tumor varies in size, sometimes being, in extreme cases, as large as two fists. The increase in connective-tissue elements corresponds to what is observed in a fibroma elsewhere; the increase in the muscle alone is termed a myoma—a condition which is exceedingly rare; and an increase in the connective tissue and glandular elements has been termed a fibro-adenoma. Socin describes adenoma of the prostate as consisting of a hyperplasia of the glandular elements in excess of the increase in the muscle and connective-tissue elements.

As might be expected, increase in the size of the prostate gland alters the shape, size, and course of the prostatic urethra. It is increased in length, is more or less curved, and is sometimes bent at a sharp angle. When only the lateral lobes are involved, the prostatic urethra is compressed from side to side; when the middle lobe is enlarged, the urethra is compressed antero-posteriorly and is bent considerably. It is this change in the course and the shape of the urethra, that makes it so difficult to pass a sound or hard metallic instrument. Much of this difficulty, if not all, can be overcome by allowing the weight of the instrument to carry it into the bladder without the use of any manual force whatever. False passages in the urethra are always due to attempts to force the sound through the urethra. It is also necessary that the beak of the instrument should hug the anterior wall of the urethra, because it presents fewer pathological changes than the posterior or lateral walls.

The enlargement of the prostate pushes the opening of the urethra in the bladder forward and upward, and this, in combination with forcible attempts to empty the bladder, produces behind the prostate the familiar pouch in which the urine is retained. The internal sphincter of the bladder soon loses its identity entirely because of the fact that it is involved in the hypertrophy. It appears as an irregular mass of pathologically formed tissue encircling the neck of the bladder and presents considerable obstruction to the passage of sounds or other instruments and to the escape of urine.

The retention of urine stimulates the bladder to increased efforts to empty itself, giving rise to eccentric hypertrophy of the bladder wall. The muscle is thickened and the increase of intravesical pressure leads to the formation of diverticuli. Finally, the muscle becomes weakened as the result of ineffectual attempts to free the retained urine. The residual urine is increased in amount, and this adds greatly to the patient's suffering. Depending on the patient's age and the duration of the disease, the relaxation of the bladder may become so great that this viscus is converted into a functionless sac. In the most pronounced cases, the abdominal wall becomes relaxed, the bladder dropping forward over the symphysis. Inguinal hernia not infrequently develops.

Guyon advances the theory that hypertrophy of the prostate is the result of an arteriosclerosis, while others maintain that it is a typical hyperplasia or a new-growth. Geiger is of the opinion that it is caused by a chronic inflammation following gonorrhœa. While this may be correct in cases in which a gonorrhœal inflammation was present at some previous time, it must be acknowledged that prostatic hypertrophy is frequently met with in individuals in whom gonorrhœa can safely be ruled out. Other forms of inflammatory processes may, however, begin the trouble. Chronic constipation, diabetes, alcoholism, and conditions affecting the prostatic circulation, undoubtedly often cause enlargement.

In the main, the symptoms caused by hypertrophy of the prostate are due to the obstruction to the outflow of urine, although pruritus of the perineum, a sensation of fulness in the perineum, and not infrequently discomfort and even pain, are just as important and prominent subjectively, as is the difficulty in urination. Tenesmus is usually the first symptom of any importance. This is soon followed by difficult urination. The patient first complains of difficulty in starting the stream, although in some cases there is a constant dribbling of urine, especially at night. Next, the urine is discharged with difficulty, until finally it is utterly impossible to empty the bladder. Then the catheter must be resorted to.

Bladder symptoms make their appearance in the final stage of the trouble, the stage of complete obstruction. The bladder is distended and a urethritis and a cystitis, both the result of infection following the use of the catheter, may complicate the clinical picture considerably. There is then a possibility of the infection extending upward and involving the ureters and kidneys, although this occurrence is by no means common.

DIAGNOSIS.—The diagnosis of hypertrophy can usually be made quite readily. The shape and consistency of the gland can be felt by the finger in the rectum, and are characteristic. The organ is irregular, nodular, firm, and movable. Simple hypertrophy must be differentiated from chronic prostatitis, calculus, abscess, and new-growths. The history of the onset of the trouble, the uniform enlargement of one or both lateral lobes, the nodular, rough, firm surface, and the consistency of the mass will readily differentiate the conditions named from hypertrophy, except in the case of sarcoma and carcinoma, when the diagnosis must be made microscopically after enucleation. If the tumor is small, or if a calculus is contained in the gland, a hard mass surrounded by soft prostatic tissue will be revealed. In a case of chronic prostatitis, the urine will at all times be found to contain pus, often gonococci, and tissue shreds.

TREATMENT.—Although in hypertrophy of the prostate, little can be gained by expectant or symptomatic treatment, nevertheless, most patients will prefer to try all other known measures before consenting to operation. If the diagnosis is made early, dietetic treatment, with careful regulation of the patient's mode of life, will afford some relief for a while; but, as a rule, the hypertrophy continues to increase and the patient is forced to consent to an operation or to live a catheter life. Catheter life is not only most unenviable but also undesirable, and always dangerous, because of the possibility of causing infection of the bladder, urethra, ureters, and kidneys. Yet many "prostatics" go on in this way for several years without any complications or even inconvenience, except that resulting from the use of the catheter.

Local treatment, by means of ointments or suppositories, or the injection of iodine or other reactive substances into the gland, gives some temporary relief, but not infrequently it leads to the formation of an abscess in the gland.

When the patient first resorts to the catheter, it is only at rare intervals, following some indiscretion in eating or the excessive ingestion of fluids, particularly alcoholic drinks. Gradually the catheter must be used more often, until finally voluntary urination is practically impossible.

PATHOLOGY.—There are many theories regarding the pathological processes which are active in prostatic hypertrophy. The most recent of these is that "prostatic hypertrophy is almost always the result of chronic inflammatory changes." (Chickanowski.) This view is strongly supported by Greene and Brooks, but it does not meet with the approval of Albarran and Halte, who, from a study of 100 cases, found four varieties of prostatic hypertrophy. Their classification is as follows: (a) Glandular hypertrophy; (b) fibrous hypertrophy; (c) mixed hypertrophy; (d) prostatic epithelioma. The hypertrophy of the prostate has been variously described as: hyperplastic myoma (Virchow); glandular and fibromuscular hypertrophy (Rindfleisch); spheroidal developments in the prostate (Volpius). Sir Henry Thompson describes four changes in the enlarged prostate: (a) development of all the elements of the gland;

(b) stroma more abundant; (c) glandular elements more abundant; (d) spheroidal bodies not unlike uterine fibromata.   In a recent study of 120 cases, by Geraghty and Young, three types were distinguished: (a) glandular in 100; (b) fibromuscular in 14; (c) inflammatory in 6 cases.

The inflammatory theory is gaining ground.   Recently Metz has observed that prostatic hypertrophy nearly always begins in the glands lateral to the urethra, and that those below the urethra and ejaculatory ducts are seldom enlarged.   It is most likely that only one pathological process is at work, and that the various transitional appearances called types of pathological tissue all owe their origin to some form of infection.   Primary infection passes away in some cases, and then another set of germs develop in the prostate.   Thus, mixed infection is the rule in the presence of suppuration.

PATHOLOGICAL ALTERATIONS.—The different gross appearances of the hypertrophied gland are the following:—(1) The gland appears sponge-like, owing to dilatation of the acini.   (2) The specimen shows the gaping orifices of retention cysts.   (3) The secretion of the gland oozes out.   (4) Many spheroidal tumors are seen projecting beneath the capsule; they are encapsulated and are easily enucleated.   Some tumors are distinct.   Under the microscope the lobules and acini appear segregated in area; the acini are dilated, lengthened, and ovoid, with an infolding of their lining quite cylindrical in character; cuboidal cells may form only a single layer.   In the various offshoots or sprout-like processes, where proliferation is seen to be active, many polygonal cells present themselves, with heaps of small epithelial cells here and there.   The stroma separating the epithelial acini is formed of both fibrous and muscular (nonstriated) tissue in varying quantities.   Some of the tubules may have undergone cystic degeneration.   In most instances these are lined with a single layer of flattened epithelium.

SYMPTOMS AND SIGNS.—The symptoms and signs of prostatic hypertrophy are based on the pathological conditions which are present in the gland, and more particularly on those which cause obstruction to urination.   The endeavor should be to learn, by studying the clinical evidence in each case, just where this obstruction is located.

The clinical features of the case may develop slowly or quickly, and may run an intermittent or a continuous, but usually chronic course, with or without complications, until complete retention occurs.   The function of the bladder is interfered with first.   It begins to empty itself more frequently, both day and night, and the act of urination becomes difficult and prolonged.   The stream starts slowly, flows less forcibly, sometimes intermittently, and ceases in an involuntary dribble.   The more the patient hurries to complete the act, the more time it requires to perform it.   The frequent and difficult urination is followed by a general vesical distress, which eventually becomes quite painful.   When cystitis ensues, an additional train of symptoms is added to make up what is designated "prostatism."   These symptoms are present in nearly every case of prostatic obstruction.   Frequent and painful urination may be the most prominent symptom in chronic nephritis, but the difficulty in urination and the dribbling of the urine are absent. It is probably too dogmatic to say that "nocturnal frequent urination is always pathognomonic of hypertrophy of the prostate." In order that the clinical indications for prostatectomy may be of practical value, some classification of the cases is desirable. I select the following:—

(1) *Cases Manifesting Genito-urinary Disturbance.*—Cases with simply functional disturbance may go on for months or even years, and still not give sufficient cause for operation. Besides frequent, difficult, and prolonged urination, such symptoms as sexual irritability, too frequent erections, premature orgasm, and unsatisfactory coitus add much to the discomfort and annoyance of the patient. A feeling of fulness in the bladder and rectum is present during the daytime, and, when the patient awakens after the first sleep, there is pain. With all his hurried calls to urinate, which are slow and imperfect in accomplishment, the man of fifty or sixty years often does not consult a surgeon until he is sorely tried; indeed, not until he finds that rest at home or at one of the hot springs, the taking of the various vaunted cures for bladder and kidney diseases, and restricted diet are of little avail. Exposure, local and general excitement, and alcoholic stimulants increase his difficulty. In such a case no residual urine is found in the bladder when the catheter is introduced, and no positive enlargement of the prostate can be detected by a rectal or bimanual examination, aided by the sound in the bladder; but the bladder is intolerant to the sound and the prostate is tender under manipulation. The urine is normal. The cystoscope may reveal a congestion of the internal vesical meatus and of the surrounding bladder mucosa, with some prominence of the latter. The diagnosis of congestion of the prostate is now made. This is the first stage of prostatic hypertrophy. As long as there is no marked obstruction to the flow of urine, even though the gland can be felt, *per rectum*, to be enlarged, prostatectomy is not indicated. In the absence of other signs of congestion, the fact that urination is prolonged is almost conclusive proof that the prostate is slightly hypertrophied. In this class of cases, the genito-urinary specialist finds a great field for usefulness, and, by proper hygienic and local treatment, he may, in some individuals, be able to obviate the need for prostatectomy.

The percentage of cases that remain rebellious is high. It is self-evident that these patients should be operated on early before residual urine forms or infection occurs.

(2) *Cases with Partial Retention.*—A man whose "bas fond" has formed so insidiously as not to interfere with his work or with his rest at night, aside from a slight interference with urination, is likely to have acute retention of urine on exposure to cold or as an after-dinner surprise. Relief is obtained spontaneously by antispasmodics or by the use of the catheter, but ever afterward, in almost every case, the catheter draws off residual urine after micturition. To avoid a return of his acute suffering from retention, he must promptly obey Nature's call to empty the bladder, and must avoid wine and exposure to wet and cold, as well as indulgence of any kind. A sagging of the bladder behind the prostate will hold residual urine. This change, which develops slowly, is usually mani-

fested by an exaggeration of the symptoms and signs already pointed out as characteristic of cases of this kind. There are two forms of partial retention— acute and chronic.

Acute Retention.—As soon as the existence of prostatic dysuria and partial retention has been determined in any case, the dangers following permanent catheterization should be explained clearly to the patient. The habitual use of the catheter—whether in the hands of the patient, the nurse, or the physician, it matters not—should be disapproved. Even when the comparative comfort of the patient requires catheterization, cystitis is almost sure to develop in spite of all precautions. My rule is to impress on the patient the nature of his malady, to explain to him that only temporary relief can be expected from the use of the catheter, to point out the dangers to life incident to the employment of this instrument, and then to state the beneficial results that are obtainable from prostatectomy. Harrison, Lydston, and others have shown that the expectation of life when the catheter is used is only four or five years.

Repeated hemorrhages into the bladder of a prostatic patient are sometimes profuse and dangerous. Instead of this sign being a contra-indication to prostatectomy, as some operators aver, I have found that the sooner the gland is removed and the bleeding is checked, the safer it is for the patient. In this respect it must be remembered that erosions and ulcers due to catheter traumatisms are not prone to heal when the mucous membrane is chronically congested, as it is in all these cases. When the bladder becomes acutely inflamed, whether the catheter has been used or not, the patient should be ordered to bed, preferably in a hospital, sparingly fed, moderately purged, and his bladder systematically irrigated for a week or more until the acute symptoms have subsided. Then the prostate should be removed before he resumes his work.

The cases that are difficult to treat successfully are those which are complicated with chronic cystitis. If the bladder is once chronically inflamed, it remains so until the prostatic obstruction is removed. The sufferer should know the permanent damage that is sure to be done to the bladder by chronic inflammation—such, for example, as contraction, trabeculation, and the formation of diverticula (Fig. 129) and stone (Fig. 134). He should also be informed that ultimately ascending infection is likely to lead to a fatal involvement of the kidneys.

(3) Cases of Chronic Retention.—In the chronic form of obstruction, the quantity of residual urine gradually increases until eventually the bladder becomes distended to its utmost capacity. Some relief is often obtained when the pressure of the urine forces open the vesical meatus, causing overflow in little streams, or drop by drop (false incontinence).

Cases of this class develop into cases which give histories like the following:

The bladder is full all the time; every five, ten, or fifteen minutes during the day, involuntary urination occurs, while at night a constant dribble is noted; atony or contraction of the bladder is more or less extreme, depending on the length of time retention has been complete or on the duration of the cystitis. The passing of a sound through the penis and the insertion of the finger into the rectum, may reveal prostatic obstruction in the urethra and hypertrophy of the prostate, respectively.   It is in this class of cases that we should recommend prostatectomy.   If, however, advanced age, feebleness, or disease of the kidney or heart forbids the employment of a general anæsthetic, the operation is contra-indicated; but neither the age of the patient nor the prostatic enlargement, *per se*, is a bar to prostatectomy.   If the person is able to survive the operation, experience teaches that the kidneys will be benefited, the atony will subside to a remarkable degree, and the bladder, oftener than not, will be able to contract and empty itself of its contents.   Acute and partial retention

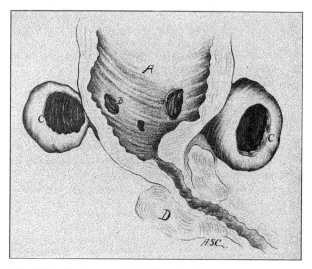

Fig. 129.—Multiple Diverticula from the Bladder.   In this case the prostate was removed perineally.   Cystitis was of long standing and persisted after prostatectomy, because decomposed urine remained in the diverticula.   A radical operation (diverticulectomy) was not granted.   (Original.)
A, Bladder; *B*, mouth of diverticulum; *C*, diverticulum cut open; *D*, site of prostate, which has been removed.

usually repeats itself many times and then becomes chronic; and chronic retention may at any time become acute and complete.

(4) *Cases of Absolute Incontinence and no Residual Urine.*—In all cases of marked prostatic enlargement, associated with urinary disturbances, there are— except in the cases of this class—the following changes: residual urine is present, the prostatic urethra is elongated, enlarged, and often tortuous, and its curve is increased.   These abnormal conditions are detected by the use of the catheter, the sound, and the cystoscope.   In the present class, however, there is no frequent urination nor any dysuria; there is no residual urine; elongation of the prostatic urethra is lacking; and there is no fulness or pain in the bladder or perineum.   When a catheter is passed, the bladder is found to be empty.   It

will usually be found that the patient has been treated for months or years for paralysis (the usual cause of true incontinence). It is in this class of cases that the prostatic enlargement is in front and protrudes into the bladder anteriorly to the vesical orifice. Since the sphincter cannot close the vesical meatus, the urine no sooner enters the bladder than it flows away. If there be an overhanging development of prostatic tissue as is here represented, the vesical meatus may become blocked by it and retention thus caused. The enlargement may be felt above and behind the symphysis pubis. Cystoscopy may show the site, shape, and perhaps also the size of the prostatic hypertrophy.

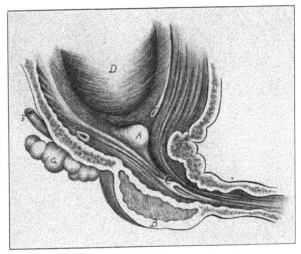

Fig. 130.—Pathological Middle Lobe of the Prostate. (After Maclise.)
A, Middle lobe; B, lateral lobe; C. prostatic urethra; D, bladder; E, E, ureters; F, vas deferens; G, vesiculæ seminales.

In this class of cases there is no posterior, abnormal middle lobe, no bar, and no vesical meatal pouting or stricture. Prostatectomy offers the only relief. Two instances of these pathological conditions have come under my observation, and in both I was able to remove the prostate successfully. The bladder regained perfect control of the urine in both cases.

Prostatectomy is not always called for on account of the large size of the gland, for the latter may be very large and yet offer no obstruction to the flow of urine. Obstruction is the "sine qua non" for the operation. In one case of diffuse prostatitis I found the rectum partially obstructed by the great size of the lateral lobes, and still the man had control of the urine and emptied the bladder completely. There was no abscess in the gland.

The different kinds of prostatic obstruction and the pathological conditions associated therewith may be tabulated as follows:—

I.—Located at the vesical meatus.

(a) A polypus-like growth, acting like a valve, obstructs the meatus from behind. (Fig. 130.)

(b) A bar. (Fig. 131.)

(c) An overhanging anterior growth, as in class 4 (page 365). (Fig. 132.)

(d) Nipple-like projection, or a mass like a cervix uteri, pushing into the bladder. (Fig. 133.)

(e) Various alterations in the shape of the vesical meatus, such as flattened,

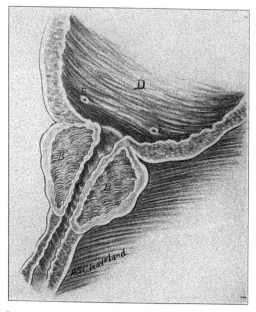

Fig. 131.—Lateral Section of the Prostate.
A, Middle lobe forming a transverse bar; B, lateral lobe; C, prostatic urethra; D, bladder; E, E, ureteral orifices.

straight, crooked and crescentic slits, sometimes oval, star-shaped, or even spiral in cross-section.

II.—Located in the prostatic urethra.

(a) Circumferential pressure.

(b) Bilateral pressure.

(c) Unilateral pressure.

III.—The obstruction is due to chronic inflammation causing cicatrization and then contraction.

Prognosis.—For the prognosis see under Perineal Prostatectomy.

Cysts of the Prostate.—Large cysts of the prostate are very rare; but microscopic cystic degeneration of the gland in cases of hypertrophy are frequently met with. Hugh Cabot, of Boston, presents the following classification of cases of prostatic cyst:—

(a) Echinococcus cysts.

(b) Retention cysts.

(c) Cystic dilatation of the utricle.

(d) Cysts or cystic cavities connected with carcinoma of the prostate.

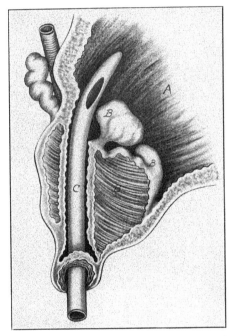

Fig. 132.—Hypertrophy of the Anterior Portion of the Lateral Lobes of the Prostate. (After Maclise.)

A, Bladder; B, anterior portions of the lateral lobes, enlarged, projecting into the bladder, and causing obstruction; C, bougie in the prostatic urethra which is straighter than normal.

Hydatid cysts of the prostate are very rare. Thompson, in 1883, found that only one case had been reported in literature. Belfield says that he can find but three authentic cases.

Retention cysts are caused by obstruction of the orifices of the ducts of the prostatic acini. These are insignificant in size and are of common occurrence in old prostates.

Cystic dilatation of the utricle is met with in children. In seventy-five post-mortem examinations made on the bodies of the new-born, Englisch reports but five instances of this condition.

Cystic cavities that are in some way related to carcinoma of the prostate are no doubt more common than heretofore reported. In 1906 Cabot reported two cases, and others have since been observed. In the first of these cases, which occurred in a man 87 years of age, who was leading a catheter life owing to complete obstruction of prostatic origin, the patient began to experience considerable

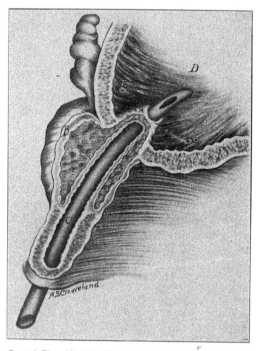

Fig. 133.—Prostatic Ring; Nipple-like Vesical Orifice. (Original.)
A, Vesical orifice contracted, fibrous, and protruding into the bladder; B, lateral lobes enlarged, but not causing obstruction; C, bougie in the prostatic urethra; D, bladder, E, E, ureteral orifices.

pain while the bladder was being emptied with the catheter. He then developed. in a short time, a prostatic swelling which simulated an abscess. Within a month this was opened through the rectum with a trocar. The instrument entered a large cavity which contained about two ounces of a glairy fluid. The cavity was then opened and drained. In seventeen days pyelonephritis caused his death. "The autopsy revealed cancer of the prostate in the early stage. Besides the cavity that had been opened, there was another smaller pocket, which was a pouch made up of smaller cavities that had coalesced. The cavity was filled with thick, opaque, yellowish-white fluid, which contained epithelium, leucocytes, and débris, but no bacteria." It would appear that the irritation caused by the catheter might have been an etiological factor in this case. The second case referred to by Dr. Cabot is one of especial clinical interest.

A man, 46 years of age, with a history of gonorrhœal infection five years previously, followed by a chronic urethritis, began to complain of frequent urina-

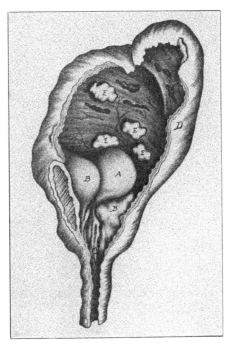

Fig. 134.—Three Lobes of the Prostate Enlarged, Obstructing the Vesical Orifice. Bladder sacculated, contracted, and containing calculi. (After Maclise.)
A, Median lobe; *B*, lateral lobes; *C*, prostatic urethra; *D*, bladder; *E*, calculi in pouches.

tion, with a feeling of distress in the bladder following the act. Annoyed by a constant desire to urinate he presented himself for examination. Upon examination of the prostate, normal massage brought out two drops of a glairy fluid. A catheter (No. 27 F.), was easily passed. In a month's time the quantity of residual urine amounted to as much as ten ounces. After the patient had passed three ounces of urine the cystoscope was introduced. The instrument revealed a projection into the bladder from the prostate, to the left and behind the urethral orifice. After this examination there remained three ounces of residual urine in the bladder. The patient, fearing the loss of sexual function, postponed operation. Some time later there occurred a stoppage of urine which required the use of the catheter. Instrumentation was difficult owing to the spasmodic condition of the deep urethra. Cystoscopy now revealed the existence of a distinct tumor to the left of the internal vesical meatus. This tumor, as remarked by Cabot at the time, resembled a cyst. When the bladder was opened on the following day, a tumor about the size of a cherry was removed. The tumor ruptured during the removal. The wall was cut away with scissors and the lining was burned with the Paquelin

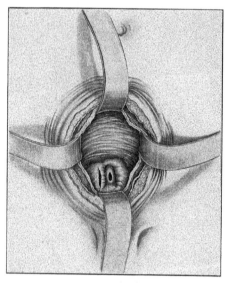

Fig. 135.—Suprapubic Prostatectomy. The bladder has been opened, and, by the use of retractors, the field of operation is exposed sufficiently to show the enlarged prostate and the catheter projecting from the internal vesical orifice. An incision has been made in the bladder mucosa over the right lobe of the prostate down to its capsule. (After Deaver.)

cautery. Subsequently to the operation the patient remained well for at least seven months. Although no pathological report was made, the case is most interesting clinically.

IV. OPERATIONS ON THE PROSTATE.

Prostatectomy.—The two operations in vogue for the removal of the prostate are suprapubic prostatectomy and perineal prostatectomy. The former was begun in America by Belfield, of Chicago, in 1886; was further employed in Great Britain by McGill, of Leeds, in 1889; and finally was perfected by Freyer, of London, who, in 1900, developed the total enucleation operation.

Total Enucleation of the Prostate by the Suprapubic Route.—In order to do justice to the deviser and champion of this operation, I am constrained to publish his exact words as found in "A System of Surgery," by F. F. Burghard, Vol. III., pages 527 to 536 inclusive.

"Operation.—The pubes having been previously shaved and the parts rendered aseptic, the bladder is thoroughly washed out with an antiseptic lotion, as in this disease the urine is almost invariably foul. The catheter employed for this purpose should be made of rather stiff gum elastic, and be of the largest size that the urethra will freely admit.

"Suprapubic cystotomy (Fig. 135) is now performed. After the bladder has been washed out the catheter is left in situ, and the viscus is distended with boric-acid lotion. The nozzle of the large syringe which is employed for this purpose, filled with the lotion, is inserted in the end of the catheter, thus acting as a plug to prevent leakage from the bladder, and the syringe being ready to further distend the bladder with fluid, if necessary, as the operation proceeds. An incision, varying in length from two and one-half to three and one-half inches, according to the stoutness of the patient and the size of the prostate, is made in the median line of the abdomen, its lower end reaching to the level of the pubic arch. This incision is rapidly carried down through or between the recti muscles till the prevesical space is opened. Any bleeding vessels are clamped by catch-forceps, the forefinger is introduced into the lower angle of the wound, and the prevesical fat scraped upward off the bladder by the finger-nail for the whole length of the wound. The peritoneum, which should not be seen, is thus pushed upward out of harm's way, and the bladder appears deeply in the wound, quite tense, glistening, and of a pale, somewhat whitish hue, with large and tortuous veins coursing in its substance. An area devoid of veins having been selected, the point of a scalpel is plunged boldly into the bladder, and an incision about one inch long is made in the vertical direction toward the symphysis. The wound in the bladder can be subsequently enlarged if necessary; and this is best effected—as being attended by the least bleeding—by separating two fingers placed in the wound, and thus tearing the bladder wall to the required extent. On withdrawal of the scalpel the forefinger is introduced into the bladder as the lotion rushes out through the wound, and a general survey of the viscus is made. Should calculi be present they are at once removed by forceps and scoop.

"The forefinger of the other hand is then introduced into the rectum to render the prostate prominent in the bladder, and to keep it steady during the manipulation of the finger in the bladder. (Fig. 136.) The mucous membrane over the most prominent portion of one lateral lobe, or over the so-called 'middle lobe' if there be but one prominence, is scored through by the finger nail, and gradually detached by it from the prominent portion of the prostate in the bladder. This portion of the enlarged prostate is covered merely by mucous membrane, so that, when this is scraped through and detached, the true capsule of the prostate is reached at once.

"The finger's point being kept in close contact with the capsule, the enucleation of the prostate from the enveloping sheath outside of the bladder is proceeded with by insinuating the finger tip first behind, next outside, and then in front of one lateral lobe, thus separating the capsule from the sheath. The finger is then swept in a circular fashion from without inward, in front of, and to the inner side of the lobe, detaching this from the urethra, which is felt covering the catheter, and pushed forward toward the symphysis between the lateral lobes, which will, as a rule, have separated in the course of the manipulations, along their anterior commissure. The other lobe is attacked and treated in the same manner. The finger is then pushed downward behind the prostate and the inferior surface of the gland is peeled off toward the triangular ligament. When the prostate is felt free within its sheath, and separated from the urethra, by means of the finger in the rectum, aided by that in the bladder, it is pushed

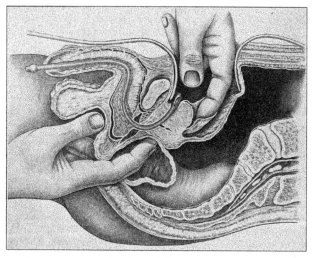

Fig. 136.—Suprapubic Prostatectomy. Median sagittal section of the pelvis showing the finger enucleating the prostate from its sheath; counter-pressure is made by the other hand in the rectum and against perineum. (After Deaver.)

into the bladder through the opening in the mucous membrane, which, during the manipulations, will have considerably enlarged.

" The prostate, which now lies free in the bladder, is withdrawn, by strong forceps, through the suprapubic wound. And here I might remark that it is astonishing through what a comparatively small wound a very large prostate can be delivered, owing to the elasticity and compressibility of the adenomatous growth between the blades of the forceps. Sometimes the lobes become detached along both anterior and posterior commissures and come away separately.

"The question now arises: What becomes of the ejaculatory ducts in the course of this operation? When the lobes come away separately they are probably left behind uninjured. attached to the urethra. When the prostate comes away as a whole, they may be torn across, or pulled out of the gland. But, as will subsequently appear, in the vast majority of my later operations the distorted portion of the urethra behind the verumontanum has been removed with the prostate, the urethra being severed at the position at which the ejaculatory ducts enter it, the ducts as a rule remaining adherent to the portion of the prostatic urethra that is left behind.

"Almost from the commencement I have abandoned the employment of any cutting instrument for incising the mucous membrane, finding the finger-nail alone most convenient and expeditious. Besides, when a scalpel or scissors is employed, there is danger of cutting the capsule, and, the guiding lines being thus lost, the finger flounders about inside, enucleating adenomatous tumors instead of the whole organ in its capsule.

"When I first conceived the possibility of removing the whole prostate, my ideal operation consisted, as already stated, in enucleating the large gland in its capsule out of the enveloping sheath, leaving the urethra behind; and this was the procedure undertaken in my earlier cases.

"I have lately almost abandoned the attempt to preserve the urethra entire in the enucleation of the prostate. The excellent permanent results obtained from partial removal of the urethra with the organ, have convinced me that no advantage is to be gained by leaving the vesical end of the urethra behind. In a large proportion of cases of enlarged prostate the vesical end of the urethra is extremely dilated, being trumpet-shaped, or distorted out of any shape resembling a more or less circular tube in the normal prostatic urethra. Even when it is left behind I have always had my doubts as to its ultimate fate in most instances. The probability is that, through want of support and adequate blood-supply, it sloughed in large part and came away in the washings during the after-treatment.

"Examinations of prostates which, in the course of removal, have opened along the anterior commissure,—to which category the great majority belong,—will show that the dilated portion of the prostatic urethra—viz., that portion lying between the verumontanum and the vesical outlet—has come away with the prostate, the urethra in front of this being left behind. The portion of the urethra behind the point at which the ejaculatory ducts enter it, is much more adherent to the prostate than that in front of it, between this point and the triangular ligament. In fact, in the greatly enlarged prostate this latter portion lies quite loosely attached to the lateral lobes on either side. When a prostate is enucleated in its capsule from the sheath all round, and the lobes are gently separated from the triangular ligament by the point of the finger, the organ can be felt hanging on by the urethra and the ejaculatory ducts, and the finger tip can be easily inserted on either side between the inferior border of the prostatic lobe and the urethra. If now the finger be placed behind the prostate in the median line above the ejaculatory ducts, and the prostate be propelled upward into the bladder by the finger in the rectum, the urethra will be found to snap across at the verumontanum, leaving the ejaculatory ducts, as a rule, adherent to the portion of the prostatic urethra left behind.

"Toilet of the Wounds.—With the delivery of the prostate from the bladder the essential part of the operation may be regarded as completed. The forefinger of one hand is re-introduced into the bladder forthwith, and that of the other hand into the rectum. The opposing surfaces of the cavity from which the prostate has been enucleated, are then pressed together all around the vesical orifice between the tips of the fingers. By thoroughly kneading the opposing surfaces together in this manner, the contraction of the cavity and its diminution in size are facilitated, and hemorrhage is thus arrested, just as a dentist presses the gums together after extraction of a tooth, or the accoucheur does the flaccid womb after parturition, with a similar object in view.

"The bladder is then irrigated with hot boric-acid lotion (temperature above 110° F.) through the catheter still in situ, for the purpose of removing clots and further to control bleeding. This process should not, however, be continued for more than two or three minutes, as I find from experience that these irrigations not infrequently promote bleeding, instead of diminishing it, if the irrigation is continued too long.

" The bladder having been cleared of clots, and whilst the irrigation is still proceeding, a stout India-rubber drainage tube is introduced through the suprapubic wound. The dimensions and management of this tube I regard as matters of the utmost importance in the after-treatment of this operation. I have been gradually increasing the calibre of this tube, till now I invariably employ seven-eighths-inch tubing, with a lumen of five-eighths inch in diameter. Two large perforations or eyes are made as near as possible to the vesical end of this tube, on opposite sides of it. Only about one inch of the tube should project into the bladder, just sufficient for the side openings to lie completely within its cavity. When the bladder is allowed to contract, the tube is gripped by it, so that the whole of the urine escapes through the tube. In this way infection of tissues in the prevesical space is obviated and cellulitis prevented. On no account should the tube be inserted into the prostatic cavity, our object being to facilitate by every means the contraction of this cavity. If more than one inch of the tubing be introduced into the bladder, it will press on its base and give rise to constant straining, and in the end of the penis a pain like that caused by vesical stone.

"The edges of the parietal wound are now brought together round the tube by silkworm-gut sutures, one or two of which should pass through the recti muscles. On no account should buried sutures be employed, as they are certain to be infected by urine. One of the sutures should pass through the drainage tube to keep it in position. No sutures are inserted in the bladder.

"Before the catheter is withdrawn and the dressings applied the bladder is once more irrigated, in order to remove clots and to ascertain that drainage is quite free. Finally, a piece of broad iodoform gauze tape, a couple of inches long, is inserted in one angle of the wound against the side of the tube, and left there for twenty-four hours. This is done for the purpose of preventing the accumulation of fluids in the prevesical space. The wound is now covered with cyanide-of-zinc gauze, and the patient deeply swathed in absorbent dressings,—

in front and on the sides and back. The whole dressing is kept in place by a broad flannel binder or many-tailed bandage, loosely applied. Cotton-wool, wood-wool, tissue, or cellulose may be employed. The last is most absorbent and keeps the patient driest. A thin layer of cotton-wool should be placed between it and the skin; otherwise, the cellulose, when wet, forms a pulp, which adheres to the skin and feels cold and clammy.

"After-Treatment.—The dressings should be changed when saturated with urine, every four or six hours, according to the quantity of fluid secreted. During the first twenty-four hours after operation there will generally be some clots of blood lying in the drainage tube; these should be removed by long, slender, forceps at each dressing.

"The bladder should be irrigated at least once daily, by the surgeon himself, with warm boric-acid lotion or a weak solution of potassium permanganate. For this purpose a long glass nozzle attached to the rubber tubing of an irrigating can is best, the nozzle being introduced through the drainage tube. During the first few days, there should be very little pressure of fluid on the bladder, the irrigating can being held, or placed, upon a table, a little above the level of the patient's abdomen, so that the lotion flows into the bladder and out again through the drainage tube with very little force. It is all-important that, in the early days, the drainage should be absolutely free, and that no pressure should be thrown on the cavity from which the prostate has been removed, either by accumulation of urine in the bladder or by pressure from a high column of lotion, so that the cavity may remain at rest, and that blood-clot adherent to its surfaces may be undisturbed, thus obviating bleeding and facilitating the healing process. This is the main object with which I employ a stout drainage tube— that the urine and clots may escape through it freely, and that, consequently, there may be no straining, which would have the effect of dilating the cavity. Patients who pass no urine *per urethram* for ten or twelve days after operation almost invariably do best.

"The patient should lie on his back for twenty-four hours, after which he should be placed alternately on either side, and on his back. During the first four or five days he should not be allowed to make any exertion, all movements being effected by the nurses. Should there be any oozing of blood after the operation, the foot of the bed should be raised on blocks and hypodermic injections of ergotin given. Shock, when it occurs immediately after the operation, should be treated by warmth from hot-water bottles and extra clothing, by hypodermic injections of strychnine, and by enemata of coffee and brandy. Pain or spasms of the bladder should be relieved by hypodermic injections of morphia. Should there be any bronchial catarrh or other lung affection, the patient's head and shoulders should be well raised by pillows after the first twenty-four hours succeeding the operation. And in any case this position should be encouraged early, so as to obviate hypostatic congestion of the lungs.

"As a rule, I remove the large tube four days after the operation. If the patient be thin the tube may be dispensed with in three days; if he be very stout, it should be left in for five days. By this time a plastic lymph will have been thrown out around the tube, thus shutting off the prevesical space from contact with the urine, and in this way avoiding the occurrence of cellulitis. Before removal of the large tube, a smaller one should be passed through its lumen and left in the fistula for a few days, to facilitate free drainage from the bladder, the wound in which may then be allowed to close as rapidly as nature can accomplish this by granulation.

"The sutures are removed on the seventh or eighth day, by which time the primary union will have taken place in the parietal wound,—save. of course, in the track of the tube.

"Irrigation of the bladder may be continued daily—twice daily, if the urine be at all foul—by inserting the long glass nozzle of the irrigator through the fistula right down into the viscus. The return stream will, in the early days, flow out beside the nozzle; but, as the fistula contracts, the nozzle will fill it, and the irrigation is then accomplished by alternately filling the bladder with the lotion and then withdrawing the nozzle, when the fluid will rush out with more or less force. As the case advances, more and more pressure on the bladder may be employed. The irrigation should be continued until the boric-acid solution returns quite clear, or the permanganate lotion unaltered.

"Nine or ten days after the operation Janet's method may be employed, if possible. This consists of introducing the glass nozzle into the urethra and gradually raising the irrigation can till the pressure exerted by the fluid forces the lotion into the bladder and out through the suprapubic opening. This is, perhaps, the best method of flushing out the bladder; but some patients will not tolerate it, owing to the pain produced. It should never be employed during the first week after operation, for fear of bleeding; and if it cause pain it should not be employed at all. Patients vary much in their tolerance of this method of irrigation.

"After a fortnight or so, after the bladder is distended by the lotion injected through the nozzle placed in the suprapubic opening, the patient will frequently pass the lotion *per urethram* as rapidly as it enters the bladder. When this takes place it is an effectual method of flushing out the bladder.

"It will be observed that I have not hitherto referred to the employment of the catheter for the purpose of washing out the bladder during the after-treatment. In the early days of the introduction of this operation I was in the habit of introducing a large-sized gum-elastic catheter through the urethra daily from the third or fourth day of the operation, and irrigating the bladder through this. The catheter was introduced partly in consequence of my apprehension that, if it were not employed, there might be a contraction of the deep urethra during healing of the prostatic cavity. Experience has taught me, however, that my apprehension in this respect was quite unfounded, for in not a single instance has there been any contraction to interfere with the free flow of urine. I do not now introduce a catheter till the suprapubic fistula has contracted to such narrow dimensions that it will not admit the nozzle, so that irrigation cannot be practised in this way. It is employed only during the few days before the patient begins to pass urine *per urethram* in volume, in order to keep the bladder clean during this transition period. When once natural micturition is established the bladder is, of course, automatically washed out.

"The management of the bowels is of the utmost importance. For three or four days previous to the operation the bowels should be freely moved once daily at least, by means of a laxative pill given at night and a mild saline in the morning. On the morning of the operation the lower bowel should be emptied by means of an enema.

"The bowels then should be left undisturbed for two or three days, when they should be freely moved by castor oil or liquorice powder, or anything that can be depended upon to act with certainty and efficiency. After this the bowels should be moved gently once a day by means of a pill taken at night or a saline in the morning, or both if necessary. Patients of the prostatic age confined to bed are liable, owing to want of tone in the bowel, to have the feces accumulate in the rectum until they form a hard mass. Should the presence of such a mass be suspected a finger should be introduced into the rectum and the mass broken down, when it may be removed by an enema.

"Patients should, as a rule, be confined to their rooms, but not necessarily kept in bed, for three or four days before the operation. Poor, broken-down hospital patients will require to be kept under observation for several days, in order that they may be well fed, and their general health improved before operation.

"I have entered somewhat at length into the details of the after-treatment, because I consider that an intelligent appreciation of, and attention to, them is not less essential to success than the skilful performance of the operation.

"Secondary Hemorrhage.—Secondary hemorrhage has occurred in a few instances. It is a very rare sequela of the operation, and may be serious enough to require proper attention.

"Slight arterial hemorrhage may occur from the suprapubic wound upon removal of the large drainage tube on the fourth or fifth day. This is purely traumatic and due to the fact that the tube is gripped by the bladder. The utmost gentleness should be employed in removing the tube, which should be withdrawn slowly and with a slight rotary motion, if it be gripped very tightly by the wound. The bleeding from this cause is always trifling and ceases automatically in a short time.

"Should there be any obstruction to the free flow of the contents of the bladder through the tube in the early days after operation, the prostatic cavity is liable to be dilated, resulting possibly in venous hemorrhage from its walls. This is controlled by readjusting the tube in such a manner that a free outlet is given to the urine, and by irrigating the bladder through the tube with boric-acid lotion as hot as the patient can bear.

"But the most serious form of hemorrhage takes place, strange to say, in the case of patients in whom healing is most rapid, resulting in the suprapubic wound closing earlier than usual. Urine is passed through the urethra before the prostatic wound is sufficiently healed to bear the resultant pressure on its surface, and hemorrhage may take place owing to spasm of the bladder and consequent undue pressure on the prostatic cavity. Should this occur, a full-sized rubber or gum-elastic catheter should be introduced through the urethra and tied in the bladder, so as to give free exit to its contents.

"But should the hemorrhage persist, giving rise to pain and spasm from the accumulation of clots in the bladder, no time should be lost in re-opening the suprapubic wound, and inserting a large drainage tube for a few days, to relieve the pressure on the walls of the prostatic cavity. Hypodermic injections

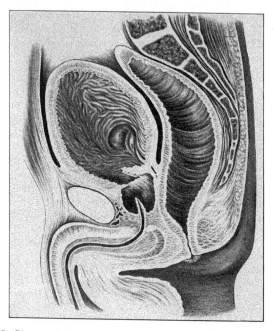

Fig. 137.—Diagrammatic Drawing, showing, above, a flap of mucous membrane left by shelling out a prominent third lobe, and below, a remnant of the urethral mucous membrane extending back into the cavity from which the prostate has been removed—either of which projecting masses would tend to form a valvular closure of the urethra. (After A. T. Cabot.)

of ergotin and the administration of calcium chloride by the mouth should also be employed."

Perineal Prostatectomy.—Different surgeons employ different incisions of the skin and subcutaneous structures for gaining access to the enlarged prostate. The median incision is the one of choice in the vast majority of cases, because through it rapid and efficient work can be executed with excellent results: especially by a man whose hand is not too large and who is dexterous. Some excellent surgeons have such large fingers that they are practically excluded from attempting perineal prostatectomy. While a short slender finger is at a disadvantage compared with a long, slender digit, still, with the aid of instruments which drag the gland down into the perineum, the former can do satisfactory work As one surgeon has aptly said, "a short finger becomes longer by experience"; but I might add that a stout finger acts as a cork.

Several kinds of incisions are employed for making an opening through the perineum. These are: (a) the median; (b) the transverse; (c) the Y-shaped, (d) the T-inverted; (e) the semilunar; (f) some modification of these.

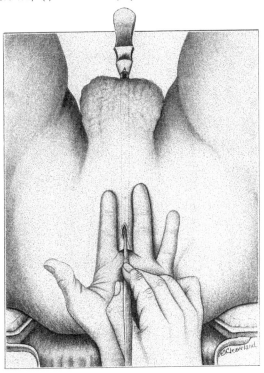

FIG. 138.—Perineal Prostatectomy; Making the Median Incision. (Original.) A, Prostatic grooved staff in the urethra and bladder; middle finger of left hand in the rectum.

From a sufficient number of cases to enable me to have an opinion, I am compelled to say that the median perineal incision is my preference. In a very limited number of cases the entire prostate can be removed without injury to the prostatic or membranous portion of the urethra. (MacEwen and Fergusson.) This can never be done suprapubically. Nearly all the operations by the perineal route require the opening of the membranous and prostatic urethra —the one, for the purpose of introducing instruments which aid in the operation;

the other, to afford ample room for the enucleation of the gland. In the intracapsular method the capsule must be opened to find a cleavage through which
the finger may be introduced for the purpose of separating the gland from its
capsule. While this is true we must admit that some cases are suitably dealt
with by the suprapubic route. In my opinion they are vastly in the minority.
From my experience I would advise that almost all cases should first be explored
through the perineum. If it then be found that certain portions of a hyper-

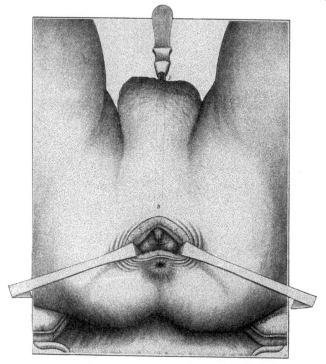

Fig. 139.—Perineal Prostatectomy; Extra-lithotomy Position. (Original.)
  B, Grooved staff; C, median incision retracted; E, enlarged prostate; F, lateral incision in the
capsule; I, median incision in the urethra.

trophied prostate cannot be removed through the perineum, it does not compromise either the surgeon or the patient to make a suprapubic opening and
complete the operation. It seems to me that this is much safer than to undertake a suprapubic prostatectomy alone, or the combination operation reversed.

  More knowledge can be gained of the size, shape, and extent of prostatic
protrusions into the bladder, by the finger in the perineal wound than by cystoscopy before operation.

Steps of the Operation.—The bladder is washed out with an antiseptic solution. A quantity of the fluid amounting to six or eight ounces is then left in the viscus. A plug of gauze is next inserted into the rectum. A grooved staff (Figs. 138 and 139) is passed *per urethram* into the bladder. Then the patient is placed in the extreme lithotomy position and held by assistants.

Now pass the middle finger of the left hand into the rectum. (Fig. 138.) Split the perineum in the median line from behind forward. Open the membranous urethra and prostatic urethra as far back as the sinus pocularis, and pass the index finger of the left hand into the wound as the staff is withdrawn.

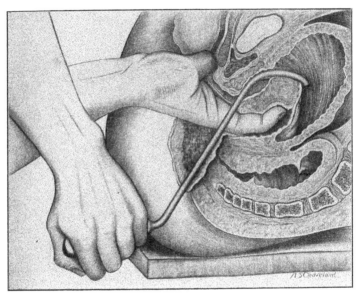

Fig. 140.—Perineal Prostatectomy; Extravesical Enucleation of the Diseased Middle Lobe.
(Original.)

In exposing the membranous urethra by the median incision it is probably better to teach that the skin be cut first and that a careful dissection be made through the other soft structures down to the urethra in order to insure against injury to the bulb. Remove the finger from the rectum and pass the prostate depressor into the bladder as the finger is withdrawn.

Remove the glove from the left hand, reinsert the finger into the wound, and search for a line of cleavage within the capsule of one or both lobes of the gland. Usually the cleavage can be found near the apex of the prostate and to the left, because the knife generally cuts a little to this side as it opens the prostatic urethra. If cleavage is not found, a small transverse incision is made alongside of the finger through the capsule. (Fig. 138.) By means of the prostatic depressor, the gland is pulled down as it is being enucleated by the finger (Fig. 140); this enucleation is sometimes accomplished in less time than it takes to describe the process. It will be found that the separation of the gland is interfered with where it is covered with vesical and prostatic urethral mucosa. Pulling and tearing should be avoided at this stage; large portions of prostatic tissue may be grossly cut away by means of my prostatic cutting forceps. (Fig. 128, No. 2.) Both lobes having been removed, the interior of the bladder may be readily explored by the finger. If there are protrusions or prostatic tissues in the

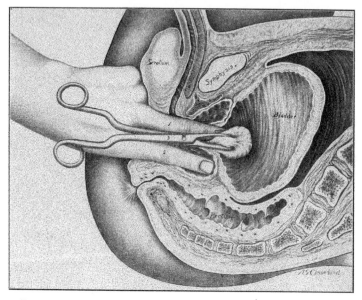

Fig. 141.—Perineal Prostatectomy; Pedunculated Middle Lobe. (Original.) 1. Middle finger in the bladder; 2, index finger in the space from which the prostate has been removed, 3, prostatic forceps grasping the middle lobe of the prostate.

shape of a pathological middle lobe, or prolongations from either or both lateral lobes, the first thing to be determined is whether the growth is sessile or pedunculated. (Fig. 141.) If it is sessile, it is an easy matter to enucleate it with the finger or remove it by morcellement; if it is pedunculated and cannot be safely delivered through the perineal wound without unduly stretching and perhaps tearing the neck of the bladder, then the operation should be completed suprapubically.

Where enucleation is easy and the bladder is not septic, deep sutures (No. 0 chromicized catgut) are employed to close the urethra and bring together the edges of the levator ani muscles. A small cigarette drain is employed to take care of the discharge from the perineum alone, the skin is closed by horse-hair, and a retention catheter is passed into the bladder. (Fig. 142.)

In septic cases and in very old men with marked prostatic deformity, the gland must be removed as rapidly as possible. The safety of the rectum from injury, and the rapidity of the operation may be increased by the use of a double-edged gouget with a beaded point which strikes the groove in the staff, and the knife is passed through the prostatic urethra in a firm, gentle curve. The gouget splits the prostatic urethra laterally; its flat posterior side is toward the rectum and protects it from injury. This is not the operation of choice.

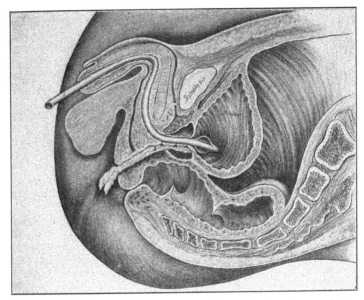

FIG. 142.—Perineal Prostatectomy. (Original.) 1, Drainage tube in place; 2, gauze packing.

Total enucleation of the prostate gland by Freyer has taught us one thing, viz.: that the preservation of the prostatic urethra is not of so great importance as the advocates of perineal prostatectomy believed. With this in mind, we can attack the enlarged prostate through the perineum with less regard to the prostatic urethra and raise it from its bed where all the structures are within reach of the finger. One type of gland, the chronically inflamed prostate, usually atrophied, can be removed only piecemeal. A chronically inflamed prostate cannot be removed suprapubically at all. This is also true of pros-tatic abscess and calculi, and the recent experience of Young demonstrates that a malignant prostate can best be removed through the perineum.

In my opinion it seems unsurgical to attack a contracted bladder from above except possibly in two steps. The plan of making bilateral incisions of the capsule, as devised by Proust and exploited by Young (Fig. 143), in order to save the ejaculatory ducts, does not appeal to decent old men. While the many tractors and depressors devised are often clumsy and inefficient,—though some of them answer the purpose well enough,—I prefer my own.

Mortality.—The worst result that can be obtained in prostatectomy is death. "While old age waits to hear the keel upon the other shore," the old man chances death by operation rather than suffer constantly; and, even though inconvenient post-operative sequelæ arise, life is endurable after the operation.

It is interesting to note that for years the mortality of suprapubic prostatectomy (McGill) has been less when the operation was combined with lithotomy than when no calculus was present. Burckhardt gives 13.8 per cent mortality (four deaths in 29 cases) for the former operation, and 20.8 per cent (16 deaths in 77 cases) for the latter. "This difference can only be explained on the assumption that the presence of the stone necessitated operative interference earlier and while the patients were better able to endure an operation than when no calculus existed. . . . The death-rate from McGill's operation (partial suprapubic prostatectomy) has always been higher and always will be, it seems.*

Belfield collected 111 cases in which McGill's operation had been performed, with 12 deaths—a mortality of 13.6 per cent; Moulin, in 1892, collected 94 cases, with 19 deaths—a mortality of 20.2 per cent. Watson collected from various sources 243 cases of total suprapubic prostatectomy, with 28 deaths—a mortality of 11.5 per cent; while among perineal operations he found 33 deaths—a mortality of 6.2 per cent.

Young thus states his experience:—"I have now had 185 consecutive cases of perineal prostatectomy, with seven deaths—a mortality of 3.7 per cent. This includes all of the early cases, when the operation was in a developmental stage and much less satisfactory; the patient being confined to bed and the drainage not being removed for much longer periods. It certainly does not represent the true mortality. . . . During the past two and one-half years there have been one hundred cases with only two deaths—a mortality of two per cent. But the most convincing evidence of the benignity of the operation is the fact that in the last sixty consecutive cases there has not been a single death or bad result." †

The results obtained by A. T. Cabot are as follows:—"My experience has been that the restoration of function is more complete and lasting after the perineal than after the suprapubic operation. . . . In the past four years I have operated on thirty-five cases of perineal prostatectomy. Two of the patients have died, one three days after operation, the other at the end of a month." ‡

---

* Deaver: "Enlargement of the Prostate," pages 210–212.
† Hugh K. Young: "Study of 145 Cases of Perineal Prostatectomy," John Hopkins Hospital Reports, vol. iv., 1906, page 115.
‡ A. T. Cabot: "Modern Operations for Complete Removal of the Prostate," 1907.

Miles F. Porter * gives the following account of the results of prostatectomy: —"A study of 485 cases of prostatectomy for hypertrophy of the prostate, occurring in the practice of thirteen different operators, wherein the cause of death is given, show in all thirty-three deaths. Of these deaths ten were due to such causes as cancer of the liver, pulmonary tuberculosis, etc., diseases in no way connected with the operation or with the pathological condition for which the operation was undertaken; eight of the deaths were due to exhaustion, pneumonia, pulmonary embolism and sepsis, conditions caused by the operation

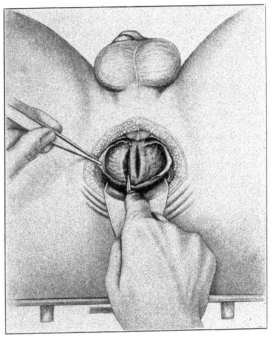

Fig. 143.—Perineal Prostatectomy. Incision in capsule advocated by Albarran.

itself or the anæsthesia. It would be nearer the exact truth, perhaps, to say of the deaths due to sepsis, that most of them were due to conditions existing before the operation was done; but, for the present, at least, we will consider them as deaths due to the operation *per se*. The remaining fifteen deaths were due to pyelitis, pyelonephritis, and other conditions secondary to and caused by the hypertrophy of the prostate, and existing at the time of the operation. The total death rate in this series of cases, then, is less than seven per cent. · · · ·

* Miles F. Porter, in Journal of Amer. Med. Assoc., May 23d, 1908.

"The death rate of the operation is less than two per cent; while the conditions secondary to and caused by the enlarged prostate is three and one-half per cent. In other words, half of all the deaths following prostatectomy are due to conditions set up by the enlarged prostate. The deaths from these conditions outnumber the deaths from the operation *per se*, two to one. This means that the death rate in hypertrophy of the prostate treated without operation is about four per cent, while timely prostatectomy will yield a death rate of two per cent or less. If there is any error in these statistics, it consists in attributing to the operation itself too many deaths, and charging to the pathological conditions secondary to the enlarged prostate, too few."

Fuller, speaking of his personal experience with prostatectomy in over 300 cases, says: "I feel that, if cases complicated with very marked uræmia are excluded, I can operate with an average risk to the patient of not more than, and probably under, five per cent. *Death from the operation itself is practically nil.*"

Goodfellow has done 105 perineal prostatectomies with but two deaths. Watson gives the death rate in enlarged prostate, treated by catheterization, as 7.7 per cent.

C. H. Mayo, including his brother's cases with his, says: "In 291 cases, including 26 for carcinoma, we have had 28 deaths."

Willy Meyer writes as follows: "I have done, outside of some 85 Bottini operations for prostatic enlargements, 41 suprapubic and 8 perineal prostatectomies. . . . Personally, I prefer the suprapubic to the perineal operation."

Crile says: "In my experience in about 25 operations for prostatectomy, the patients themselves were pleased with the result."

Miles F. Porter further says: "My own experience is limited to 25 cases. There were three deaths, all due to septic conditions (pyelonephritis and cystitis) which existed at the time of the operation and because of which the patients finally asked for relief. . . . The fatalities following prostatectomy are largely due to conditions resulting from the hypertrophy and existing at the time of operation. Prostatectomy, in the absence of serious complication, entails a risk to life of *less than two per cent.* The death rate in enlarged prostate treated by catheterization is over five per cent." .

In a more recent communication * Young makes the following statement:— "Including cases of cancer of the prostate in which the typical operation of conservative perineal prostatectomy was employed; 13 recent cases which have not been tabulated; 20 cases in which operation has been performed since my paper appeared some months ago; and a few cases in which the technique was not the typical one and which have not been tabulated, . . . there have been 400 cases of perineal prostatectomy, with 13 deaths—a mortality of 3.25 per cent. . . . During a period of two years and eight months 128 consecutive cases were subjected to the operation of conservative perineal prostatectomy without a single fatal result. Forty-three of these 128 patients were *over seventy years of age* and two were over eighty years of age."

* H. K. Young: "Perineal Prostatectomy," Jour. of Amer. Med. Assoc., March 5th, 1910.

Dr. Stanley Stillman, of San Francisco, refers to the fact that Sir William Macewen was in the habit of performing the suprapubic operation in all cases in which the urine could be rendered fairly healthy; but, when this could not be done, he performed a double lithotomy incision in the perineum for drainage purposes, and then allowed an interval of a week or ten days to elapse. During this time the surfaces of the incisions which he had made became covered with granulations and the capsule of the prostate retracted, causing the cut surface of the gland to protrude from the wound. While it was in this state he reduced its size materially by means of a thorough dissection, and then, ten days later, he shelled out, with his index finger, each lobe of the gland, with no bleeding

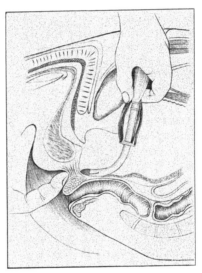

Fig. 144.—Perineal Drainage. (After Ransohoff.)

and little danger of infection, inasmuch as the urine had, in the interval, become fairly healthy. Dr. Stillman says that he has himself followed this plan for two years, with much better results than he ever obtained from other methods of prostatectomy. His preference is distinctly for the suprapubic method of operation in cases in which the urine is healthy, and for Macewen's method in those in which the urine cannot be rendered healthy prior to operation.*

General Remarks.—Re-establishment of spontaneous urination and relief of vesical infection are the rule. The loss of generative power is habitual. The advanced age of the patient is not a contra-indication to operating. The relative integrity of renal activity is necessary. Patients with grave organic diseases, such as diabetes and renal disease, succumb to what is apt to be termed shock.

* Jour. of Amer. Med. Assoc., July, 1909.

It may be said that the two methods of operating, the perineal and the suprapubic, have each their advantages and disadvantages.

According to Ricketts * there were, in Freyer's series of 644 operations of suprapubic enucleation of the prostate to date, 48 octogenarians, and 9 bordering on this period, with 6 deaths. "In connection with these 644 operations there have been 39 deaths varying from six hours to thirty-seven days after operation, or a mortality of 6.05 per cent. The mortality has been gradually diminishing from ten per cent in the first 100 cases, to 4.24 per cent in the last 200."

M. Tuffier † believes that the suprapubic operation is easier to perform and requires less time than the perineal. When the gland is very small and the abdomen very fat, he selects the perineal operation; and he quotes from Proust, Watson, Horwitz, Leque, Hartmann, Pauchet, Rafin, Young, and Albarran, to the effect that, in a series of 2,222 cases, the average mortality was 6.23 per cent;

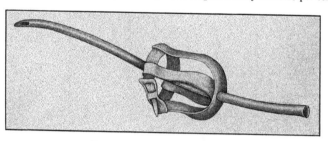

FIG. 145.—Soft-Rubber Catheter Holder.

out of the total number of cases operated upon, the cause of death was about the same in both operations (thirty-five per cent of the number being perineal and thirty-three per cent suprapubic). Shock is given as the cause of death in 17.8 per cent operated on the suprapubic method.

No permanent fistulæ have been observed after operation in those cases in which the bladder was inflamed (purulent secretion), trabeculated, pouched or diverticulated, or contained stones. The natural tendency of the perineum is to close spontaneously, but, so long as pus escapes from the opening, a fistula is likely to persist or to recur. I have had two cases of this character. Injury to the rectum during operation is more of a blunder than an accident, and secondary rectal fistulæ are caused more frequently by rough treatment from the eighth to the twelfth day, when the granulations are exuberant. Secondary fistulæ have occurred in two of my patients in whom the after-treatment was not carried out by myself. Three patients, at the time when I first saw them,

* Journal of the Amer. Med. Association. Jan. 29th, 1910.
† Ann. des Mal. gén.-urin., October, 1902.—The Journal of the Amer. Med. Assoc., Oct. 25th, 1902.—Centrbl. f. Krankh. d. Harn- u. Sex. Org., 1901, p. 571.—Phila. Med. Journal, June 8th, 1901.—"Traitement de l'Hypertrophie de la Prostate," Rapport au Congrès International de Médecine, 1905.

were wearing urinals on account of partial incontinence. They and their relatives found this more acceptable than death. One of these patients—a man aged seventy, accepted the operation only when life became unendurable from pain, etc. In this case considerable sloughing took place at the seat of the operation, from the skin inward. In one case a stricture developed as a result of the operation; it was cured by perineal section. Five patients had epididymitis. One had unilateral intrarenal and extrarenal abcess, which developed three weeks

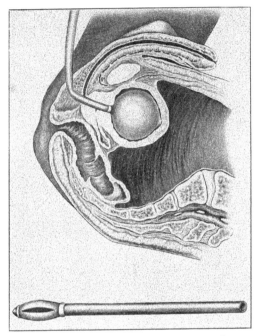

Fig. 146.—Syms' Prostatic Tractor in Use. Details of construction of end of the tractor are shown in the small figure at the lower part of the illustration.

after the operation. A cure was effected by incision and drainage. Stone in the bladder was present in six cases.

Drs. Tenney and Chase, in discussing the question of mortality after prostatectomy, accept as possibly due to the operation every death reported as occurring within six weeks. From their table we find that 2,342 patients were operated on through the perineum and 667 suprapubically. The mortality experienced in this series was a little over 7.9 per cent for the cases which were operated upon by the perineal route, and a little over 13.2 per cent for those operated upon by the suprapubic route. In other words, the mortality of the suprapubic was nearly twice as great as that of the perineal operation.

In my own cases I had no deaths in the first series of 21. Then, afterward, I lost three cases—one from renal insufficiency, in forty-eight hours. This was considered a very unfavorable case for operation. Another patient died in twelve hours from an overdose of morphine; and a third—an unfavorable case because of old age and emaciation—succumbed on the third day. This makes my mortality between three and four per cent in one hundred and three cases, and does not include five deaths following prostatectomy—three from carcinoma and two from acute tuberculosis.

SURGERY OF THE OVARIES AND FALLOPIAN TUBES.

By BENJAMIN R. SCHENCK, M.D., Detroit, Michigan.

EMBRYOLOGY.—While various embryologists differ concerning certain minor details in the development of the reproductive organs, they all agree as to the main facts. The essential points in the formation of the tubes, ovaries, and uterus are given in the following brief account.

The internal generative organs develop from the intermediate cell-mass— a group of mesoblastic cells situated on either side, just external to the paraxial mesoblast. Some of these cells form into a ridge running longitudinally from the head region, posteriorly to the caudal extremity. Mesially this ridge is paralleled by the primitive aorta, cardinal veins, and beginnings of the vertebræ. The outer edge projects into the cœlom or body cavity, which space separates it from the somatopleure, or body wall. This ridge is known as the Wolffian ridge. It is covered by the mesothelium, a portion of which, situated on the inner side of the Wolffian ridge, proliferates and thus forms a second cord, known as the genital ridge. The Wolffian ridge is largely concerned with the development of the urinary system; the genital ridge with the reproductive organs. (Fig. 147.)

In the various parts of the Wolffian ridge three sets of tubules form by ingrowths from the cœlomic or peritoneal mesothelium. These are known, from before backward, as the head-kidney, the mid-kidney, and the hind-kidney. The first of these has but a transitory existence; its duct, however, represents the beginning of the Wolffian duct, presently to be described. The mid-kidney acquires considerable size, acts at first as an embryonic excretory organ, and later takes an important part in the formation of the genital system. It is known as the Wolffian body. The hind-kidney becomes the true or permanent kidney and its further development does not here concern us.

The duct of the head-kidney, or Wolffian duct, extends posteriorly, and, between the third and fourth weeks, in the human embryo, reaches the urogenital sinus into which it opens. At the same time, or a little later, a second duct is being formed in the following manner: When the Wolffian body has become fully developed, the peritoneal epithelium (mesothelium), which covers its outer and anterior portion, becomes thickened and an invagination takes place forming a tube, lined by these same cells which are columnar in shape. The lumen of this tube, known as the Muellerian duct, connects with the peritoneal cavity. This duct runs, for the most part, parallel to the Wolffian duct, and, like the latter, enters the urogenital sinus—a portion of the primitive hind-gut, formed by an ingrowth of a fold from either side. (Fig. 148.)

While these changes have been progressing, certain alterations have been taking place in the mesothelium covering the Wolffian ridge on its inner side. The epithelial cells in this position proliferate and become several layers in thickness, thus forming the genital ridge referred to before. These cells constitute the germinal epithelium of Waldeyer. They grow downward into the mesoblastic stroma in columns, sometimes called the egg-tubules of Pflueger, while the stroma grows upward among the epithelial cells, thus forming something of a network of epithelium and connective tissue. Even before this downgrowth of the epithelial cells takes place, certain of them are distinguishable by their large size, vesicular nuclei, and characteristic chromatin network. These cells are the primordial ova, and each one of the egg-tubes contains one or more of them. By the growth of the connective tissue, the egg-tubes become separated

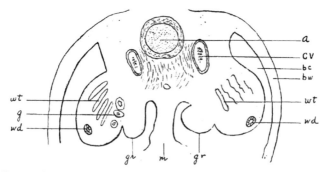

Fig. 147.—Diagrammatic Cross Section of a Rabbit Embryo, 12 millimetres (½ inch) long. The picture shows the Wolffian body and the genital ridge. (After Mihalkovicz.) a, Aorta; cv, cardinal vein; bc, body cavity; bw, body wall; wt, tubules of Wolffian body; wd, Wolffian duct; g, glomerulus of Malpighian corpuscles; gr, genital ridge; m, mesentery.

from their peritoneal attachment, thus forming nests of germinal epithelium, in the centre of each one of which are one or more primordial ova, while the other cells of the nest become the epithelial cells of the Graafian follicle. It has been computed that the ovary at birth contains from 70,000 to 100,000 primordial ova, only a very small proportion of which ever reach maturity.

The first stages in the growth of the Wolffian body, the Wolffian and Muellerian ducts, and the ovary, having thus briefly been described, it remains to trace their further development and ascertain how these primitive structures change into the organs as we see them at birth.

We have seen that the Muellerian duct consists of a tube of epithelial cells, having a lumen which connects at its anterior end with the cœlom or peritoneal cavity. As this duct grows posteriorly it is contained in a fold of connective tissue, known as the genital funiculus, which extends from the body wall out into the peritoneal cavity. This fold, with the contained Muellerian duct, develops mesially until it meets the one of the opposite side, when fusion occurs. Fusion of the ducts also takes place to a similar extent, forming the epithelial lining of the uterus and upper vagina, while the mesoblastic tissue of the genital funiculi forms the musculature and connective-tissue framework of the uterus and broad ligaments. The unfused portion of the Muellerian duct forms the Fallopian tube, its lumen connecting, as we have seen, with the peritoneal cavity.

The Wolffian body remains rudimentary in the female. It is important, however, on account of certain new-growths which develop from its remains. Some twelve or fifteen of the tubules comprising it persist in the broad ligament, between the ovary and the tube, and may be readily demonstrated by stretching this part of the ligament and holding it to the light. These tubules form the epoöphoron (Waldeyer) or parovarium (Kobelt) or organ of Rosenmueller. (See Fig. 150.)

The Wolffian duct also remains rudimentary. Its lower end, where it enters the urogenital sinus, early becomes cut off by the formation of the uterus and disappears. Its upper portion forms a fine tube, running at right angles to the tubules of the parovarium. This is known as the duct of the epoöphoron or Gaertner's duct. Vestiges of it may sometimes be demonstrated in the lateral walls of the uterus.

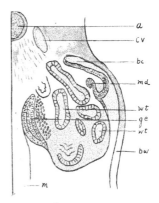

Fig. 148.—Cross Section of Embryo Chick at a Somewhat Later Period than that shown in Fig. 147. The diagram shows the development of the Muellerian duct and the thickening of the germinal epithelium. (After Waldeyer.) *a*, Aorta; *cv*, cardinal vein; *bc*, body cavity; *md*, thickening and invagination of the epithelium to form the abdominal end of the Muellerian duct (Fallopian tube), *wt*, tubules of the Wolffian body cut variously, one of which is the Wolffian duct; *ge*, thickening of the epithelium over the genital ridge, being the earliest stage in the development of the ovary; *bw*, body wall; *m*, mesentery.

The ovary and abdominal end of the tube originally lie in the lumbar region. A band of tissue, corresponding to the gubernaculum Hunteri in the male, extends upward from the internal abdominal ring to the Wolffian body, and, as it passes by the united portion of the Muellerian ducts, it becomes attached, on each side, at this point. With the increase in the growth of the body this band pulls on the ovary and causes it to descend toward the pelvis. The portion of the band extending from the fundus of the uterus outward becomes the round ligament, while the upper third forms the utero-ovarian ligament. During the remainder of embryonic life, and during childhood, the ovary is above the superior strait, and is an abdominal rather than a pelvic organ. It gradually settles lower and lower, probably as a result of the increase in size and weight.

TOPOGRAPHY AND SURGICAL ANATOMY OF THE INTERNAL ORGANS OF REPRODUCTION.—When viewed from above, as through the ordinary laparotomy incision, the internal organs of reproduction are seen to have the following relations to one another. In the centre lies the uterus, markedly anteverted; its anterior surface rests against the bladder and is not visible; the fundus is forward, immediately behind the symphysis; the upper half or third of the posterior surface is visible, while the remainder disappears into the deep fossa lying between the uterus and upper third of thevagina and the rectum. (Fig. 149.)

Extending to the right and left from the uterus is the upper part of the broad ligament, attached to the sides of the pelvis, the outer portion being lost to view beneath coils of the intestine. The upper and anterior edge of the broad ligament presents three ridges, separated by two well-marked grooves. The anterior ridge is the round ligament and is seen to extend in a gentle curve outward, upward, and forward, to become lost in the internal abdominal ring. The middle ridge is the tube. It runs outward and backward, then turns downward and slightly inward, when it ends, free, in a funnel surrounded by a delicate fringe of tissue, thus forming the fimbriated extremity. The posterior

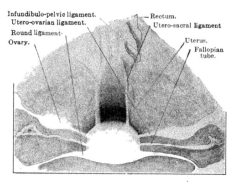

Infundibulo-pelvic ligament.
Utero-ovarian ligament.
Round ligament·
Ovary.
Rectum.
Utero-sacral ligament
Uterus.
Fallopian tube.

FIG. 149.—Diagram Showing the Pelvic Organs as Seen from Above, as if through the Ordinary Laparotomy Incision. Note the relations of the ligament. (From Kuestner.)

ridge, the shortest of the three, is the utero-ovarian ligament. It ends at the inner pole of the ovary.

To the surgeon, the ligaments of the organs are most important structures, for in them are contained the important vessels and nerves. Disease of the organs frequently causes much distortion of these ligaments, and, as an essential part of practically all pelvic operations, at least all operations for the removal of structures, is the recognition of these ligaments, a thorough knowledge of them is necessary.

These ligaments are six in number, namely, the utero-vesical, broad ligament, round ligament, utero-ovarian, utero-sacral, and infundibulo-pelvic.

The so-called utero-vesical ligament is illy defined and consists merely of the duplication of the peritoneum extending from the posterior surface of the bladder to the anterior surface of the uterus. It corresponds to the level of the internal os. and forms the lower boundary of the broad ligament.

The broad ligament extends from the side of the uterus and upper part of the vagina, laterally to the pelvic wall. It consists of a small amount of connective tissue and the two lamellæ of peritoneum which are reflected respectively from the anterior and posterior walls of the uterus. The pouch behind the uterus being relatively deeper than the one in front, the anterior surface of the broad ligament has only about half the extent of that of its posterior surface. In the upright position the broad ligament, corresponding to the anteflexion of the uterus, is nearly, if not quite, a horizontal plane. Its lateral attachment is to the fascia and peritoneal covering of the iliopsoas muscle. The upper and posterior portion extends upward and is attached to the pelvic wall higher up, making a distinct band—the infundibulopelvic ligament.

Between the peritoneal lamellæ of the broad ligament is found the parovarium or organ of Rosenmueller, which consists of from ten to twelve delicate tubules, running more or less parallel to one another and at right angles to the tube. These represent, as we have seen, the remains of the Wolffian body. Parallel to the tube and a short distance below it, may often be seen the vestiges of the Wolffian duct, gradually disappearing as the uterus is approached. In some cases one may also see yellowish or brownish bodies, varying in size from that of a wheat kernel to that of a split pea, located in the broad ligament on the mesial side of the parovarium. These represent other remnants of the Wolffian body, and, from their macroscopic appearance, may readily be mistaken for caseated tubercles or diminutive fatty tumors.

The portion of the broad ligament immediately beneath the tube is known as the mesosalpinx.

The round ligament extends outward, slightly upward, and forward, in a graceful curve, from the cornu of the uterus to the internal abdominal ring. Passing into the ring it carries with it a little pouch of the peritoneum with which it is covered. In embryonic life this pouch extends some distance down the inguinal canal, corresponding to the processus vaginalis of the male, and known as the canal of Nuck. Normally, it becomes obliterated, but occasionally the lumen persists and, if distended by fluid, a so-called hydrocele of the canal of Nuck results. The intra-abdominal portion of the round ligament varies in thickness from 4 to 7 millimetres; the portion within the inguinal canal, which becomes lost in the connective tissue of the labium majus and mons veneris, is somewhat thinner. It consists of white fibrous and elastic tissue, with considerable unstriped muscle fibres, the latter being more abundant at the uterine end. These latter fibres are derived from the uterine musculature. When the round ligament is severed, it often bleeds freely, owing to the fact that it contains an artery of considerable size. It also contains lymphatic vessels which drain into the inguinal lymph nodes.

The utero-ovarian ligament is contained in the posterior sheath of the broad ligament and connects the uterus and the ovary, being attached to the former, behind and a little below the insertion of the tube. It runs outward and slightly backward, for a distance of 2 or 3 centimetres, and becomes lost at the median pole of the ovary.   It consists of connective tissue with a few strands of unstriped muscle fibres.

The utero-sacral ligament, one on each side, is found deep in the pelvis, on each side of Douglas' cul-de-sac—the deep peritoneal pocket found between the upper part of the vagina and the rectum.   The ligament runs backward from the cervix uteri, encircles the rectum, and is attached to the sacrum at the level of the third vertebra.   It contains considerable muscle tissue and has been called the retractor uterine muscle.

The infundibulo-pelvic, or suspensory, ligament of the ovary is the thickened free margin of the broad ligament extending from the outer pole of the ovary outward, upward, and backward to the side of the pelvis, where it is attached to the fascia and peritoneum covering the ilio-psoas muscle.   It is along this path that the ovary descends during fœtal life.

The parametrium is the name applied to all that portion of connective tissue which is located in the floor of the pelvis, between the levator ani muscle below and the peritoneum above.   It forms a horizontal layer, which, on account of the various depressions between the organs, is very irregular and variable in thickness.   It is thickest between the lateral border of the cervix and the side of the pelvis, where it forms the base of the broad ligament,—being sometimes called the cardinal ligament of the uterus,—and supports the ureter, the uterine artery, and a complex network of veins.   In front, it extends upward anteriorly to the bladder, its loose strands filling up the space of Retzius, and becomes lost on the anterior abdominal wall, as the retroperitoneal connective tissue.   The septum between the bladder and the fundus uteri forms a loose connection between the two organs.   Posteriorly, the parametrium separates the vagina from the rectum and merges with the retroperitoneal connective tissue and with that beneath the gluteal muscles through the sciatic foramen.   Laterally, there is a considerable mass continuous with that covering the iliac bone.

The parametrium is soft and normally not palpable.   It readily becomes infected, and exudates may burrow in the various directions indicated.

The ovary, located behind and below the tube, varies in size and appearance according to age.   In the child it is long and narrow, later becoming of an ovoid shape.   In the adult the average measurements are 3 to 5 centimetres in length, 1.5 to 3 centimetres in width, and 1 to 1.5 centimetres in thickness.   It generally lies somewhat obliquely, with its long axis parallel to the external iliac vessels.   Frequently, it lies in a shallow depression on the obturator muscle, termed the fossa ovarica.   The ovary is attached, along its straight border, to the broad ligament, by the mesovarium, upon which for a variable distance the peritoneal covering of the broad ligament extends.   One of the fimbriæ of the tube is frequently attached to the ovary, forming the fimbria ovarica.   (Fig. 150.)

The tube and ovary receive an abundant blood-supply from two sources—the ovarian and the uterine arteries.

The ovarian artery, after taking its origin from the aorta, immediately below the renal artery, or sometimes from the latter, runs downward behind the peritoneum covering the psoas muscle, crosses the ureter at an acute angle near the brim of the pelvis, and enters the infundibulo-pelvic ligament. Small branches are given off to the outer end of the tube, and others enter the hilum of the ovary. It then anastomoses with the ovarian branch of the uterine artery.

The uterine artery arises from the internal iliac and passes in the base of the broad ligament to the side of the cervix uteri, where it sends a large vaginal branch downward. It then pursues a markedly tortuous course upward along the side of the uterus, to which it sends numerous branches, and finally anastomoses by its ovarian branch with the ovarian artery. From this anastomosis many branches are given off to the tube, and one enters the round ligament, in which it runs to the internal abdominal ring.

The veins of the pelvic organs form extensive plexuses. In the broad ligament is the ovarian or pampiniform plexus, and around the uterus is located the uterine plexus. These freely anastomose and empty into the ovarian vein

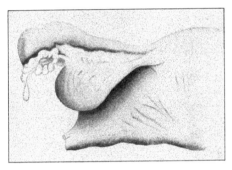

Fig. 150.—Left Tube and Ovary seen from Behind. The drawing shows the utero-ovarian ligament, the severed infundibulo-pelvic ligament, a hydatid of Morgagni, and a few of the tubules of the parovarium. (Original.)

and into the internal iliac through the uterine vein. These veins are without valves.

The lymphatics from the tube, ovary, and fundus uteri empty into the lumbar nodes, a group of about twenty large nodes forming the lumbar plexus, situated along the common iliac vessels, just below the bifurcation of the aorta.

The nerves of the tube and ovary are derived from the sympathetic system through a plexus surrounding the ovarian vessels.

Congenital Anomalies of the Tube and Ovary.—The anatomical anomalies of the tube and ovary are comparatively rare, of little practical importance, and, in the majority of instances, are associated with defects in the development of the uterus.

Absence of both tube and ovary may occur on both sides in cases of absence of the uterus, but more commonly the defect occurs in the Muellerian ducts alone, the tubes and uterus failing to develop, while the ovary is formed, but remains rudimentary. Failure of development of the Muellerian duct—

and hence the tube—may occur on one side alone, as in uterus unicornis. In such a case the ovary may or may not be present. In other instances the tube may be represented by a solid cord, a persistence of the fœtal condition.

Complete reduplication of the tube has not been described.

Occasionally accessory tubes are seen as little outgrowths on the side of the

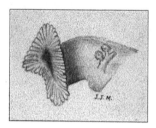

main tube, either ending blindly or having a poorly defined fimbriated extremity. They are of no importance except as a possible starting-point for a tubal pregnancy. Accessory ostia are now and then encountered. (Figs. 151 and 152.)

. In cases of infantile uterus, the ovaries usually retain their fœtal characteristics, and may or may not contain functionating Graafian follicles. Amenorrhœa or severe dysmenorrhœa usually results.

FIG. 151.—Accessory Fallopian Tube.
(From Kuestner.)

Superfluous ovaries occasionally occur. Winckel divides them into two classes: (1) supernumerary, or those which are independent of the normal pair; and (2) accessory, those which become separated from the normal by disturbances of the fœtal blood-supply, or by inflammatory adhesions during post-fœtal life. Most cases belong to the latter class and probably explain the continuation of menstruation after double oöphorectomy, a phenomenon now and then observed.

Displacements.—Alteration in the position of the tube and ovary is frequently the result of inflammation with adhesions, or it may owe its origin to a complication of tumors in the neighboring organs. Certain abnormal positions, however, are primary and of considerable importance.

In very rare instances the ovary fails to descend and is retained in the lumbar region, near the attachment of the infundibulo-pelvic ligament. I have observed one such case, the ovary being buried beneath the sigmoid. Such a condition is usually but a part of other errors in development.

Descensus of the Ovary.—Malposi-

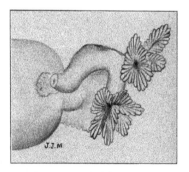

FIG. 152.—Accessory Tubal Ostia.
(From Kuestner.)

tion of the ovary frequently accompanies retroposition or descensus of the uterus and then constitutes an important factor in the general pelvic condition. Aside from such secondary descensus, cases occur in which the uterus is in good position, but one ovary, or both, are found out of the normal location.

Saenger divides these cases of primary descensus into two groups: (1)

descensus lateralis, or the falling of the ovary to the outer side of the utero-sacral ligament, and (2) descensus posticus, or the displacement of the ovary into Douglas' cul-de-sac, often termed prolapse of the ovary. Cases of the first class are relatively common, but no sharp distinction can be made between the two groups. The left ovary is more frequently affected.

The causes operating to induce descensus are those which produce an increased weight of the ovary (such as œdema, hyperæmia, hemorrhage, or cyst-formation) and those which cause a relaxation of the ligaments (such as malnutrition or general lack of tone, sometimes seen in the nullipara, or a relaxation of the infundibulo-pelvic ligament, seen after the birth of twins, hydramnios, or in poor involution generally). Occasionally a sudden jar or fall may cause the prolapse. I observed one case, with marked symptoms, in which it resulted from sliding down a "down-and-out tower," a popular summer-resort diversion.

The results of ovarian prolapse may be chronic passive congestion, especially if the pedicle becomes twisted, leading to connective-tissue hyperplasia and the formation of multiple cystic follicles. Inflammation and adhesions may later take place.

Symptoms may be wanting or complaint may be made of backache; dull dragging pain, when the patient is long on her feet, may be present; painful defecation and dyspareunia are common. There may also be painful menstruation and more or less disturbance of the nervous system.

The diagnosis, by bimanual palpation, is usually easy, although in many cases it is somewhat difficult to determine whether or not inflammatory changes have taken place.

Bimanual reposition of the organ is not easy, but may sometimes be accomplished after a few treatments with glycerin tampons, hot douches, and other measures directed toward increasing involution. The tampons should be inserted in the knee-chest posture and the patient directed to assume this position several times during the day. The symptoms may be sufficiently severe to justify operation. Resection of the ovary with a shortening of the infundibulo-pelvic ligament is the operation most frequently done, but it is open to the objection of a possible disturbance of the circulation through interference with the ovarian vessels. If the uterus has a tendency to fall backward, Webster's operation of bringing the round ligaments through the broad ligaments beneath the ovary, and suturing them together and to the posterior surface of the uterus, gives excellent results, as I can testify from the experience of a number of cases.

The steps of the operation are thus described by Webster:—"After performing curettage, which is ordinarily indicated, the abdomen is opened while the patient is in the Trendelenburg position. The fundus uteri is then raised toward the abdominal incision and is held toward the pubes by a tenaculum forceps. An ordinary long forceps is then placed against the broad ligament on one side close to the uterus, immediately under the utero-ovarian ligament, emerging just above the round ligament. The latter is grasped and pulled back, through the broad ligament, so as to lie doubled on the back of the uterus. The surface of the latter is scratched with the point of a knife adjacent to the attachment of the utero-ovarian ligament. The round ligament is then spread over this area and attached to it with a collodion-linen suture, the smooth peritoneal surface of the flattened ligament remaining superficial. One or two sutures may also be used to attach the round ligament to the edge of the perforation in the broad ligament. The other round ligament is then similarly dealt with. As a result of this procedure, the uterine body is practically slung between the round ligaments, shortened by their partial transplantation to the back of the organ."

A few gynæcologists have advocated making an incision in the broad ligament between the tube and the round ligament, bringing the ovary through the slit, and suturing it to the anterior surface of the broad ligament. The technique of this operation, as advocated by Burrows,* is simple. The tube is caught up between the thumb and finger, thus putting the mesosalpinx on the stretch and allowing the operator to avoid the branches of the pampiniform plexus of veins that run from the tube. The proper distance from the uterus having been selected, a pair of blunt scissors is thrust through the ligament and withdrawn with the blades open. The ovary is then passed through the slit without exerting any tension on the mesovarium, which in these cases is very lax. The slit should be wide enough to prevent any constriction of the pedicle of the ovary, and the latter is held in place by catgut sutures, one placed on each side. If deemed necessary, a fold may be made in the broad ligament and the utero-ovarian ligament as well.

Hernia of Tube and Ovary.—The tube, the ovary, or both may be found in the sac of any variety of hernia. In Andrews' exhaustive study † of the literature of the subject of hernia of both tube and ovary, there are recorded eighty-eight instances of inguinal, five of femoral, four of obturator, and two of ischiatic herniæ. They may be bilateral, in which case they are frequently congenital, or unilateral, either congenital or acquired. The congenital cases are often associated with defects of development of the genital organs, such as infantile uterus or absence of the uterus, uterus unicornis, or pseudo-hermaphroditism. An interesting complication is pregnancy in a herniated tube, noted five times in Andrews' compilation. An ovary present in a hernia sac is frequently enlarged and contains dilated follicles or hemorrhagic cysts, or it may be the seat of a neoplasm.

The symptoms and signs are fairly characteristic. There is often a history of the presence, throughout childhood, of a small, painless tumor, which with the onset of puberty becomes larger, tender, and the cause of a dull, sickening pain. Palpation shows a firm, rounded, often movable mass, somewhat resembling an enlarged lymph node. Reduction is usually impossible. On bimanual palpation, absence of the ovary on the affected side is noted. When the tube is present in the sac, it is usually located deeper than, and to the median side of, the ovary.

---

* For a discussion of this whole subject see Ward, in Journal of the American Medical Association, Nov. 2d, 1907, vol. xlix., p. 1507.

† Andrews, in Journal of the American Medical Association, Nov. 24th, 1906, vol. xlvii., p. 1707.

A truss cannot be worn. The treatment is always operative and is the same as that for the more common types of hernia.

A point to be kept in mind in advising operation is the great liability of a misplaced ovary to undergo malignant degeneration.

Circulatory Disturbances.—Congestion of the ovary occurs physiologically during coitus, menstruation, and pregnancy. Active hyperæmia occurs also during the first stage of inflammation, and passive hyperæmia in connection with many pelvic affections, such as tumors, chronic infections, and misplacements.

Hæmatoma occurs less commonly, but is, nevertheless, fairly often found at autopsy, or during operation. The distinction between the bleeding which normally takes place whenever a follicle ruptures, and the pathological form is rather difficult to make. The latter may be diffuse and extra-follicular, or it may be circumscribed, within either a follicle or a corpus luteum. At times it may appear as if several follicles or corpora had fused, thus forming a hæmatoma of considerable size. On account of the pressure, the surrounding follicles are either flattened or atrophied, while, in the larger hæmatomata, the ovarian tissue may be practically all destroyed and functionless.

The clinical manifestations of ovarian hemorrhage are not clear. Frequently no symptoms are present; sometimes there may be a dull, aching pain in the ovarian region accompanied by dysmenorrhœa, menorrhagia, or metrorrhagia.

In most cases the hemorrhage ends in the resorption of the blood, only pigmented areas remaining in the stroma. The prognosis is therefore good, and treatment, when necessary, should usually be rest in bed, with the application of ice to the lower abdomen. When encountered accidentally the hæmatoma should be excised, the remaining portion of the healthy ovarian tissue being brought together by sutures of catgut. If all the functionating tissue is destroyed, the ovary should be removed.

Dilatation of the veins in the broad ligament and hilum of the ovary—the so-called ovarian varicocele—should be considered in this connection. Its clinical significance is not well established, but it is said to be the cause, in some cases, of a dull, dragging pain experienced in the ovarian region. Both ligation and excision of the veins have been done, but neither operation is on a firm footing.

Œdema of the ovary, in slight degree, accompanies inflammatory conditions and misplacements, as well as various tumors, both of the ovary and of neighboring organs. It has been described as the result of torsion of the ligaments, and has been found bilaterally present in cases of syphilis.

Atrophy and Hypertrophy of the Ovary.—*Atrophy.*—Atrophy of the ovary occurs physiologically at the climacteric. Pathologically, it may result from the presence of various pelvic tumors, or from adhesions caused by infection. It may follow severe systemic infections, grave anæmia, chronic nephritis, myxœdema, akromegaly, morphinism, and tabes dorsalis. It is occasionally associated with obesity, and may follow repeated exposure to the Roentgen ray.

An atrophied ovary is smaller and firmer than the normal organ and, on microscopic examination, is found to be either devoid of follicles or to possess them in greatly reduced numbers.

Clinically, there is either amenorrhœa or very slight menstruation, with accompanying sterility. The patient is often markedly neurotic.

The treatment is directed toward amelioration of the nervous symptoms, by means of hydrotherapy, etc. The results of the administration of the ovarian extract have not in the past fulfilled the expectations at one time entertained, but more recent work, particularly that of Morley,* has again awakened the hope that an extract made, not from the whole gland, but from corpora lutea alone, may be of great therapeutic value. At present, the question is *sub judice*.

Hypertrophy.—Considerable variations in the size of the ovary are normal. As the result of pre-existing inflammation there may be enlargement, due to the increase in the connective-tissue stroma; in many cases of uterine myoma, the ovaries are enlarged and firmer than normal. Clinically, the condition is unimportant, unless the increased weight is sufficient to cause misplacement, with consequent dragging on the ligaments.

Retention Cysts of the Ovary.—The various retention cysts are often classi- fied among the neoplasms of the ovary, but, inasmuch as they are formed by distention and dilatation of normal ovarian structures, they should not be con- sidered as new-growths. Such retention cysts may be divided into: (1) Multiple Cystic Follicles; (2) Graafian Follicle Cysts; and (3) Corpus Luteum Cysts.

(1) *Multiple Cystic Follicles.*—Much has been written concerning sclerotic, cystic ovaries, a condition frequently encountered, but of doubtful clinical importance. Synonyms are: microcystic ovarian follicles, and follicular ovaritis.

The ovary is usually enlarged and its surface is studded with cysts having thin, translucent walls, and varying in size from that of a millet seed to that of a cherry. On section, the ovary is found to be studded with cysts of various sizes, which are filled with a clear limpid fluid, and the walls of which are firm. Pfannenstiel believes that the fluid contained in these cysts is a transudate from the vessels within the tunica interna.

Microscopically, the cyst wall is seen to be made up of ovarian stroma and to be lined by a single layer of cuboidal cells, representing the membrana gran- ulosa of the normal follicle.

Cystic ovaries of this description are frequently associated with interstitial fibroids, inflammatory conditions of the tubes, and displacements of the uterus. Chronic inflammation, resulting in an increase in the amount and the density of the ovarian stroma, is the probable cause of the condition.

There is still much difference of opinion as to whether or not cystic ovaries, *per se*, produce symptoms. Ovarian pain, tenderness, backache, and disorders of menstruation have been attributed to their presence, but that such is the case would appear doubtful. My own belief is that the congestion, increased weight, and malposition which sometimes accompany the severer cases, are the cause of the symptoms.

* Morley. in Detroit Medical Journal, August, 1909. Preliminary report.

Rarely will the removal of such an ovary be required.   If the condition is encountered during the course of an operation for some other lesion, the cysts should be opened, either with the point of the knife or with the thermocautery. The results of resection of a portion of the ovary have, in the experience of most operators, been disappointing.

(2) *Graafian Follicle Cysts.*—To be distinguished from the small multiple cystic follicles before described, are the cases of single (or rarely multiple) Graafian follicle cysts, which reach the size of a hen's egg or a small orange. Such cysts are usually single, are attached to the ovary over a comparatively large area, and have smooth, thin, translucent walls, especially at the most prominent part.   The wall is made up of connective tissue with an inner lining of cuboidal cells, often much flattened and sometimes demonstrable with difficulty.   The fluid is clear, or, when hemorrhage has occurred, chocolate-colored.

Pain of a dragging character, increased at the menstrual period, is the usual symptom.

The diagnosis is generally easy and is made on finding a smooth, readily movable, non-sensitive, rounded body on one or the other side of the uterus and attached to it by a pedicle.   When this body is adherent, however, it must be distinguished from tubal pregnancy, an enlarged tube, and ovarian abscess. The history, carefully taken, will materially aid in the differential diagnosis.

Such cysts may be deliberately ruptured by bimanual pressure; they may be removed through the vagina, or through an abdominal incision.   Vaginal cœliotomy is the operation of choice.

(3) *Corpus Luteum Cysts.*—It sometimes happens that a corpus luteum fails to undergo the usual retrogressive changes and, either remaining stationary in size or becoming larger, forms a cyst.   As a rule, such cysts are smaller than those developing from the Graafian follicle, but they may exceptionally reach the size of a fœtal head.   They are comparatively soft in consistency, have a smooth exterior, and vary in color from a light-yellow to a dark-brown.   The walls are friable and are readily injured, allowing the contents, usually consisting of thick, tarry fluid, to escape.   The lining membrane is velvety in texture and dark in color.

Histologically, the wall is seen to be made up of ovarian stroma with a vascular inner layer.   The lining cells are large, cuboidal in shape, and possess a vesicular nucleus and yellowish pigment granules.

There are no characteristic symptoms.   In the past, many normal corpora lutea have been removed, under the impression that they were tumors.   If the size of the normal corpus (2.0 to 3.5 cm. in diameter) is kept in mind, this error will not occur.   When unmistakably pathological, the cysts should be excised, the rent in the ovary being sutured with fine catgut.

Pelvic Infection.—The term pelvic infection is a broad one, but may properly be used to cover a number of allied conditions which produce similar symptoms, but which have more or less distinct pathological characteristics.   A similar term, equally broad in its application, is "pelvic inflammatory disease."   This term, however, is open to the objection that, according to the views now held, inflammation is not a disease, but rather a reparative and curative process, a remonstrance on the part of the tissues to the invasion of the infection.

Infections of the internal pelvic organs form a most important group of gynæcological affections. The lesions produced are among the most frequent encountered by the gynæcologist and the results are more serious than in any other class of cases, for the impairment of health is extreme and the consequences of improper treatment are frequently grave. Moreover, the operative measures employed for the relief of infections are among the most dangerous undertaken in pelvic surgery. In no group of cases is better judgment required in the treatment, and in none will the careful handling of the individual case produce more satisfactory results. Therefore, an intimate knowledge of the etiology and pathology is essential in order that the surgeon may know when to be radical and when to be conservative. An unnecessarily radical operation is often more to be deplored than a timid conservatism, whereas an unwarranted mortality may follow the failure to resort to an operation when plainly indicated.

The subject of pelvic infection is frequently discussed under numerous headings, such as Salpingitis, Pyosalpinx, Ovaritis, Ovarian abscess, Pelvic abscess, and Pelvic peritonitis. This is done in the attempt to emphasize the predominant feature of the infection, but it should be kept in mind that, although one structure may be the principal focus of the infection, rare indeed is the case in which the neighboring parts escape. Occasionally, it is true, one may find a pyosalpinx lying free in the pelvic cavity, but in the vast majority of instances the tube is adherent to the peritoneum and the ovary to both, as a result of the inflammation set up in the adjacent peritoneum in the attempt to wall in and thus ward off the infection.

Clinically, no sharp distinction can be drawn between an infection in the pelvis from which a pus tube has resulted, and one which has caused a thickening of the broad ligaments with adherent tube and ovary. The history of the case, however, will often differentiate certain probable conditions, for, as we shall see, gonorrhœal infection most frequently travels by continuity of tissue, thus producing a pus tube, while an infection acquired during labor or from an abortion generally extends through the lymphatics, producing lymphangitis, often incorrectly termed cellulitis. Patients, however, seen in the subacute or chronic stage of both of these forms of disease, present much the same symptoms. Because of this difficulty in sharply distinguishing between the pathological conditions, due to their frequent association, and because of the similarity of symptoms produced, it seems logical to consider pelvic infection as a pathological unity.

This does not mean that it is impossible to differentiate, both from the history and by the examination, the various forms of infection, for frequently this can be done with a remarkable degree of accuracy. The aim should be to obtain a broad knowledge of infections in general, differentiating and refining the diagnosis and treatment whenever possible.

CLASSIFICATION.—The most scientific classification of pelvic infections is that based upon the etiology—i.e., upon the variety of micro-organism producing the infection. The determination of the bacteria involved, however, is often difficult, for the reason that, in many of the subacute and chronic cases, the micro-organisms have either disappeared or are so few in number that cultural tests are negative. Moreover, some infections are caused by several species of micro-organisms and others by anaërobic varieties, which are difficult to grow or about which we know little.

For practical purposes—that is, for purposes of treatment—it is convenient to divide pelvic infections into three general groups, namely, (1) The Non-Puerperal, (2) The Puerperal, and (3) The Tuberculous. In the discussion of the general subject, however, it will be better to ignore these distinctions.

ETIOLOGY.—In reviewing the causes of disease, one naturally considers both predisposing and exciting factors. In many cases of pelvic infection it is difficult to discover predisposing causes which seem of importance. However, it is fair to assume that the following have a certain bearing toward favoring infection of the internal organs:—

Predisposing Causes.—(1) Menstruation. The congestion which takes place at every menstrual period produces a swelling of the mucous membrane of the uterus and an accompanying activity of the lymphatics. Moreover, the blood which is present in the uterine cavity is an excellent culture medium for bacteria. The importance of menstruation in this connection is evidenced by the great frequency of cases in which the patients date their illness from a certain menstrual period.

(2) The presence of tumors of the uterus or ovaries is an important factor and frequently the exciting cause of the extension of infection from the uterine cavity, from the vermiform appendix, or from the intestine.

(3) Tubal pregnancy, with death of the fœtus or with tubal abortion, furnishes a focus of excellent culture media which may readily become infected.

(4) General ill-health, because of lowered vitality and increased susceptibility, may predispose to the extension internally of an existing external infection.

(5) Chronic constipation, especially if caused by an adherent and extra long sigmoid, may be a factor in favoring infection.

Direct Causes.—The internal genital organs are normally free from bacteria. Infection results from the invasion of micro-organisms either from the exterior or from the blood stream. Various bacteria occur, their relative frequency differs according to different authorities. Thus, Menge found micro-organisms in 47 of 122 cases of salpingitis. Of these 47 cases, there were 44 pure cultures and 3 mixed. In 28 instances the gonococcus was found alone and in nine the tubercle bacillus alone. In Andrews' exhaustive report,* the cases of tuberculosis are not included. Of 684 cases collected from various sources his findings were as follows:—

Sterile	55.0 per cent
Saprophytes alone	6.0 " "
Gonococcus	22.5 " "
Staphylococcus and Streptococcus	12.0 "
Pneumococcus	2.0 "
Colon bacillus	2.5 " "

* Andrews, in American Journal of Obstetrics, vol. xlix., No. 2.

Inasmuch as a relatively large proportion of the sterile cases were unquestionably gonorrhœal in origin, and as fifty per cent of the cases which gave cultures were due to the gonococcus, it is evident that this organism plays the most important rôle in the causation of pelvic infection. Next in importance is the tubercle bacillus. Especial emphasis should be laid upon this point, for I believe that the general practitioner seldom has this in mind when dealing with his cases of pelvic infection.

The important practical points to be considered as regards the etiology are these:—

(1) Of whatever importance exposure to cold, chills, wet feet, excessive coitus, surf bathing during menstruation, etc., may be as predisposing causes, they are never sufficient in themselves to produce even the mildest salpingitis.

(2) Bacteria are always present at the onset of a pelvic infection.

(3) A careful history as to the onset will, in a large majority of cases, strongly point to the variety of the infection. First, infection following confinement or abortion is in most cases easily excluded. If the infection is non-puerperal in origin, what are the probabilities of gonorrhœa? Here caution is required, but there are usually suspicious circumstances which may be elicited, circumstances pointing to the probability of infection with the gonococcus. If both puerperal and gonorrhœal infections are excluded, the case is either one of tuberculosis or one of the rare instances of infection with the colon bacillus or the staphylococcus, or with some variety of saprophytes.

So much has been written on the subject of pelvic infections and so many text-books give such a confused idea of the conditions, that it would seem practical to formulate the etiology in this simple way, for rare indeed are the cases which will not be cleared up by the application of these simple rules.

PATHOLOGY.—As before stated, in pelvic infections we do not deal with any one organ, but rather with a condition which involves all the organs to a greater or less extent. Moreover, the same case may at different periods present different pathological features. For example, the gonococcus may extend from the uterus and produce, at first, a salpingitis, with which is associated a certain amount of pelvic peritonitis. The amount of pus produced within the tubal lumen may be minimal, and the "residue" may be adhesions between the tube and the neighboring peritoneum, the ovary being involved in the process. Or pus formation may continue until large pus tubes are produced, and, if the abdominal ostium is early sealed, the pus may be confined to the tube, the reaction on the part of the neighboring organs being slight. This pus may become sterile, gradually liquefy, and a hydrosalpinx result. On account, therefore, of the association of several conditions and because of the often rapid change in the picture, we must remember that a diagnosis of salpingitis or of pyosalpinx does not mean that the designated condition covers the whole· field, but rather that it represents the predominant feature of the case. If we keep in mind, then, that sharp distinctions cannot usually be drawn, it will be profitable to consider briefly the pathological characteristics of these predominant features.

Salpingitis.—In salpingitis the mucosa of the tube is primarily affected. This membrane becomes congested, the cells are swollen, and an effusion of serum, in small amounts, is poured out into the lumen. Round-cell infiltration takes place, the muscularis and serosa become affected, and the tube becomes thickened and stiff. The ovary is involved in adhesions because of the inflammation set up to ward off the infection. The mucosa of the tube may desquamate and adhesions of the walls to one another may occur, thus producing a loculated condition. All stages of acute, subacute, and chronic inflammation may be found, according to the time when the tube is examined. In general, the earlier the infection, the more conspicuous are the evidences of congestion and serous effusion; the later the infection, the more round-cell infiltration, the greater the thickening and rigidity, and the oftener adhesions are encountered. Various micro-organisms produce much the same changes. These differences, however, are to be noted, viz., that, in general, infection with the gonococcus is confined more strictly, and for a longer period of time, to the mucosa, while the streptococcus and the staphylococcus very early invade the muscularis and serosa, producing a more widespread inflammation.

Hydrosalpinx.—The theories as to the formation of hydrosalpinx differ according to different authorities. Some believe that the condition is a primary one, and others that it results from a previous pyosalpinx, the contents being transformed. From the histories of several of my own cases, I am inclined to believe that this is a probable, although not the only explanation. That it may be primary is shown by the cases (now and then seen) of hydrosalpinx in young girls, cases in which no evidence is obtained—and no suspicion arises —of a pre-existing pus tube.

In hydrosalpinx the tube becomes an elongated, pear-shaped cyst, having thin, translucent walls, often smooth and lightly adherent, especially at the abdominal end. The fimbriated extremity is closed, probably as a result of inflammation, possibly as the result of imperfect development, as pointed out by White. As the distention increases, the muscular coat atrophies and the plicæ of mucous membrane become simply thin ridges on the inner surface. The compartments containing the fluid may be single or multiple, and may involve the whole tube or only a portion of the outer extremity.

An interesting form is the intermittent hydrosalpinx, or hydrops tubæ profluens, as it has been called. In this form, constriction at the uterine end is intermittently relieved, allowing the escape of the fluid through the uterus and vagina, with an accompanying relief of the pressure symptoms. Some observers, among them Bland Sutton, do not believe that it is possible for fluid to be emptied from the tube into the uterus, but the cases of intermittent hydrosalpinx reported by Meier,[*] Kelly,[†] Findley,[‡] and others are difficult to explain on any other hypothesis.

[*] American Medicine, December 27th, 1902, p. 1005.
[†] "Operative Gynæcology," 1906, vol. ii., p. 199.
[‡] American Journal of Obstetrics, February, 1906.

Pyosalpinx.—In pyosalpinx the tube is distended with pus, the amount of the distention varying with the extent of the invasion of the tubal wall. If the latter is but little affected, it may become atrophied, allowing of extreme distention. Especially is this true in the outer third of the tube. On the contrary, when the wall becomes early inflamed and thickened, great distention is impossible. It is for this reason that the streptococcus practically never produces large pus tubes, while the gonococcus is usually found to be the causative agent in cases of marked pyosalpinx. (Fig. 153.)

The distention may be uniform, producing a club-shaped tumor, but more often there are twists and constrictions, causing multiple swellings. Acute pus tubes are reddened and "angry-looking" and are covered with thin adhesions; while the more chronic tubes are yellowish-blue and densely adherent to the ovary, bladder, intestine, and pelvic peritoneum.

The mucosa in acute cases is hypertrophied and infiltrated with leucocytes, especially of the eosinophile variety. In the long-standing cases, it is atrophic

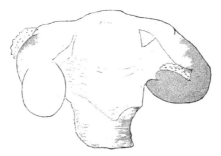

FIG. 153.—Diagram Illustrating a Double Pyosalpinx, as Seen from Behind. Slight adhesions bind the distended tubes to the uterus. (Original.)

and infiltrated with small round cells. The muscularis shows a variable amount of either acute or chronic inflammation.

The pus is usually thick, of a deep-yellow color, and odorless. If perforation has taken place or if the colon bacillus has entered from the intestine, the odor, peculiar to this organism, may be strong.

A pus tube may rupture into the intestine (more frequently on the left side), into the bladder or vagina, or, rarely, through the abdominal wall. Rupture into the pelvic cavity is the most frequent. A general peritonitis may result or, more commonly, when adhesions have formed, a pelvic abscess occurs.

Pelvic Abscess.—The term pelvic abscess is somewhat loosely used to designate any collection of pus in the pelvis, whether it be confined to the tube, to the tube and ovary, or to the cellular tissue beneath the peritoneum. It is properly used in cases where the pus is localized in the pelvis, but not confined to any organ,—as, for example, a purulent collection in the cul-de-sac. Such an abscess may contain the tube and ovary of one side or it may contain both pairs. The walls are formed by the peritoneum and its adhesions, there being no mucous membrane in the lining, as in pyosalpinx.

Tubo-ovarian Cysts and Abscesses.—Not infrequently one encounters a pelvic mass which, on removal and examination, is found to consist of a cyst the walls of which are made up in part of tubal and in part of ovarian tissue. The lumen of the tubal part communicates directly with that of the ovarian portion. The cavity may be filled with a turbid or clear, thin fluid or with thick pus.

The origin of such cysts or abscesses has given rise to much discussion, there being not less than seven different theories to account for the condition. Rosthorn's views, as given by Watkins, seem to cover the ground. They are:—

(1) A pyosalpinx may become adherent to an ovary by perisalpingitis and perioöphoritis and cause infection of the ovary, producing an ovarian abscess; perforation of the septum between the two abscesses forms a tubo-ovarian abscess.

(2) The infection may take place primarily in the ovary or in an ovarian cyst and may produce an ovarian abscess; then it may extend to the tube and cause occlusion of the abdominal ostium. The formation of a pyosalpinx and the perforation of the dividing septum complete the formation of a tubo-ovarian abscess.

(3) A tubo-ovarian cyst may occur from the union of a papillomatous cystoma of the ovary with a sactosalpinx and from the perforation of the septum by papillary excrescences.

(4) Hydrops tubæ may come in communication with a hydrops folliculi and form a tubo-ovarian cyst.

SYMPTOMS OF PELVIC INFECTIONS.—In the acute stage of a pelvic infection there is usually intense pain, due to the involvement of the peritoneum. The symptoms are those of localized peritonitis, including the extreme tenderness, the pinched expression of the face, and, frequently, marked gastro-intestinal disturbance. The body-temperature is variable, depending upon the resistance. Often there is considerable fever with a full, bounding pulse; again, there may be but slight rise of the temperature, with a small pulse, which, except in the severest cases, is not rapid.

In the gonorrhœal form the symptoms may be directly preceded by an acute inflammation of the urethra, bladder, vulva, and Bartholin glands. Sometimes, however, a distinct interval of fairly good health intervenes between the vulval inflammation and the onset of the pelvic symptoms. The latter develop gradually. Pain, of a sharp or burning character, is complained of; it is located in one or the other ovarian region, and is often dated from a menstrual period. This pain may be continuous or may be felt only when the patient is on her feet. There is usually marked tenderness, compelling the wearing of loose clothing. The appetite gradually fails, constipation becomes marked, micturition may be frequent and painful, and the patient passes on into a semi-invalid condition.

The degree of fever and the presence of rigors depend upon the amount of the toxins, and this again depends upon how completely the pus is walled in.

It is not uncommon to find women with comparatively large pelvic abscesses, going about in seemingly fair health. Pain, tenderness, and backache, however, are rarely absent, and dysmenorrhœa is the usual accompaniment.

While gonorrhœal infection, following confinement or an abortion, is not rare, it is practically always an auto-infection,—that is to say, it is the spreading of an infection previously localized in the glands of the cervix or in those of the urethra or vulva. Except in its mode of onset, such infection does not differ from the non-puerperal form. By puerperal infection, we usually understand an infection by the streptococcus, which extends by means of the blood- and lymph-vessels, rather than, as in gonorrhœa, by continuity of tissue. It, therefore, involves the connective tissue of the broad ligaments, the walls of the tube, the ovary, and the adjacent structures. Such an infection generally results from a badly managed accouchement or from criminal abortion.

The acute symptoms are more alarming than those of the non-puerperal form. The onset is rapid; rigors are frequent; the body-temperature is intermittent and may reach a high point; the pulse is rapid and thready, and the prostration is grave. The pain, however, is usually less severe than in gonorrhœal infection, for the reason that the tension of the peritoneum is generally less.

The symptoms of a chronic puerperal infection do not differ from those of the non-puerperal. The objective signs are, as we shall see, fairly characteristic.

The attacks of pain and pelvic peritonitis tend to recur at intervals.

DIAGNOSIS.—The importance of obtaining a careful history as to the onset of the symptoms has already been noted. In some cases there will be a distinct history of infection of the urethra and cervical glands, followed within a certain time by evidences of inflammation higher up, within the pelvis. An onset dating from a menstrual period immediately after marriage is most significant. In other cases, the date of the beginning of the trouble will be within a short time after a confinement, an abortion, a minor operation, such as a curettage, or after some form of intra-uterine treatment.

Having obtained a careful history, the surgeon should make a general physical examination, including the chest and abdomen. The latter should be carefully palpated, areas of tenderness and resistance being sought, particularly in the iliac regions. Especial attention should be given to McBurney's point and to the two points referred to by Morris—the two points, namely, which are situated, one on each side, about an inch and a half, in an outward and downward direction, from the umbilicus, beneath which the lumbar lymph nodes are located. I have found these sensitive in about sixty per cent of the cases of infection which I have examined during the past eighteen months.

Bimanual examination should not be made until the external genitalia have been inspected. If done with artificial light, beneath a carefully draped sheet, this does not offend the patient and is an important step in the examination. The presence or absence of a discharge should be noted, and, if a discharge be found, a smear should be made on a glass slide, before the parts are touched. Bartholin's glands should be carefully palpated for evidences of infection, the ducts being inspected for discharge and induration sought. The urethra should be "stripped," the organ being pressed against the symphysis with the forefinger. In this way any secretion which may be present in Skene's ducts is forced out and may be utilized for a smear examination. A bivalve speculum is next introduced into the vagina and the cervix uteri is inspected, note being made of any discharge and of any enlargement of the cervical glands. Many examiners dispense with the speculum, believing that the information secured by its use is not of sufficient importance to warrant the discomfort to which the patient is thereby subjected.

The condition of the vaginal walls is first observed, then the size, position, consistency, and general condition of the cervix are noted. With the abdominal hand pressing downward and inward just above the symphysis, and the vaginal finger placed behind the cervix, the two hands are brought together until the fundus uteri is located. Its size, position, mobility, and sensitiveness are noted. The condition of the tubes is next ascertained. Except in the rarest instances, normal tubes cannot be felt, nor is any tenderness elicited by bringing the vaginal finger and the abdominal hand together between the uterus and the ovary. Induration and tenderness in this location are evidences of inflammation.

The ovaries are next palpated, the same points being kept in mind.

In salpingitis all of the organs will be sensitive, especially when the uterus is rocked to and fro between the examining hands. The tube may or may not be felt, but the attempt to feel it will cause pain. Mobility will be limited and the ovary, when palpated, will be found fixed in one position, or its normal mobility will at least be somewhat lessened. On account of the tenderness, it will often not be practicable to push the examination any further; and, under these circumstances, one will have to be content with the discovery that general induration and tenderness exist.

In hydrosalpinx, the lateral fornices will be filled with a soft, non-sensitive mass, in which fluctuation can sometimes be made out. The differentiation between a coil of intestine and a hydrosalpinx is often difficult to make. The attachment of the mass to the cornu of the uterus is an important differential point.

In pyosalpinx one can usually feel the thickened uterine extremity of the tube, which, if traced outward, ends in a boggy, fixed mass. Often the two tubes, together with the ovaries, lie posteriorly to the uterus. It may be impossible to distinguish the demarcation between the mass and the fundus, all that can be made out being the fact that the pelvis is more or less filled by a fixed, sensitive mass, in parts of which fluctuation may be elicited. A marked hardness of the vaginal vault is an important sign.

In some cases a tubo-ovarian abscess may be quite movable and difficult to distinguish from a small ovarian cyst. Usually, however, the latter is more movable and much less tender.

In streptococcus infection the result of the examination without an anæsthetic may be quite unsatisfactory. One must be content with finding a hard and immovable vaginal vault, a stony hardness in the broad ligaments, and a fixed and tender uterus.

The following table from Kelly is useful in making the differential diagnosis between gonorrhœal infection and streptococcus infection:—

KELLY'S DIFFERENTIAL DIAGNOSIS BETWEEN GONORRHŒAL INFECTION AND STREPTOCOCCUS INFECTION.

Gonorrhœal Infection.	Streptococcus Infection.
1. Slow in its onset; often preceded by inflammation of the external genitals and urethra.	1. Onset abrupt, following miscarriage, normal labor, or topical applications.
2. Pain localized in one or both ovarian regions.	2. Pain more general and severe in the lower abdomen.
3. No signs of general peritonitis.	3. Usually signs of peritonitis.
4. Suffering more or less constant, but there may be no fever.	4. Suffering constant, with usually a septic fever.
5. Temperature 98.5° to 102° F.	5. Temperature 101° to 105° F.
6. Pulse accelerated, but of good quality.	6. Pulse never feeble and more rapid.
7. Attack lasts for from five to fifteen days.	7. Attack seldom lasts less than a month, and may continue three months or more.
8. Patient often presents the appearance of good health.	8. Patient anæmic and weak.
9. Gonococci usually found on coverslip preparation from the cervical, urethral, or vulvovaginal glandular secretions.	9. Gonococci not found in the secretions; streptococci occasionally.
10. History of marital gonorrhœa.	10. Husband sound.

Blood Examination.—In every acute case of suspected infection a blood examination should be made, and careful attention should be given to the number of leucocytes and the relative proportion of the several varieties. In general, it may be said that a white-blood count of 15,000 always indicates the presence of infection, and that every count above 11,000 is strong presumption of it.

The present views as to the significance of the differential count may be briefly summarized as follows:—

Decided leucocytosis, with a slight relative increase in polymorphonuclears, indicates a mild infection with active resistance.

Decided leucocytosis, with a marked relative increase in polymorphonuclears, indicates severe infection with active resistance.

Decrease in the number of leucocytes and decrease of the polymorphonuclears indicate a good prognosis.

Decrease in the number of leucocytes, with relatively increased polymorphonuclears, indicates a grave prognosis.

In chronic infections, such as gonorrhœal pyosalpinx, the value of the blood count is less, but a moderate leucocytosis is to be expected in all cases where pus is present.

PROGNOSIS.—The course and termination of pelvic infection depend upon a number of conditions, mainly upon the variety and virulence of the causal micro-organisms. Gonorrhœal pyosalpinx may undergo a change into a hydro-salpinx, or the pus may become inspissated and the thickened, stiffened tube remain unaltered for years. Usually, there are symptoms resulting from the adhesions, such as backache, abdominal tenderness, flatulency, and dysmenorrhœa. Streptococcus infection is often fatal, but a certain percentage of cases clear up, leaving but a small residual focus of disease. A patient having an inflammation in the pelvis is never free from the possibility of general peritonitis or septicæmia.

TREATMENT.—*Treatment of Non-Puerperal Infections.*—The treatment of non-puerperal sepsis naturally divides itself into three sections, namely, the prophylactic, the non-operative, and the operative.

(1) Prophylactic Treatment.—Inasmuch as a very large proportion of the instances of infection of the internal organs of generation come from the direct extension of infection of the external organs, every case of the latter should be treated at the earliest possible moment. Even when this is done in the most careful and vigilant manner, a certain proportion of cases will not be aborted and extension will take place.

In view of the fact that the three most common situations of an acute gonorrhœa are Skene's ducts in the urethra, Bartholin's glands, and the glands of the cervix, vigorous local treatment should be instituted. There should be daily applications of one of the silver salts, either the nitrate, argyrol, or protargol, care being taken to empty the glands, in so far as is possible. Rest in bed, copious and frequent douching with a one-per-cent lysol solution, and applications of glycerin and ichthyol to the cervix by means of a tampon, meet the local indications. The following combination should be applied to the tampon each evening, and the latter should be kept in place until morning, when it is to be removed and the douching carried out through the day:—

> Ichthyol ,
> Ext. belladonnæ fl..āā ℥ ss.
> Glycerini..℥ iv.
> M.

At the same time a diuretic mixture should be given. In some instances I have found the gonococcus vaccine to be of value, but its use has not yet become established.

A serious error which is often committed in the treatment of acute gonorrhœa is the performing of curettage. The scraping-away of the endometrium accomplishes nothing of importance, while it does harm by leaving a raw surface covered with coagulated blood and detritus, an excellent medium for the growth of the organisms present. Intra-uterine applications are open to the same objection and are used but rarely at the present time.

The social and economic aspects of gonorrhœal infection are most important, but a discussion of them cannot here be entered upon.

(2) Non-Operative Treatment.—When extension has taken place and there are signs of active inflammation in and about the tubes, what should be the method

of procedure? It is not so many years ago that operations were done at this stage, but, with a careful study of the results obtained by many surgeons, came the conviction that the treatment of acute pelvic infections is essentially non-operative. Such treatment frequently does not cure the patient, for there is often left a residuum of disease consisting of thickened, misplaced, adherent organs. It has for its object the prevention of the spreading of the infection from the pelvic to the abdominal peritoneum, the elimination of the toxins produced, and the sustaining of the strength of the patient until the acute stage is passed.

Absolute quiet and rest in bed must be insisted upon. In the severer cases the illness is sufficiently grave to make this easy, but it should be enjoined even in the mildest forms. An ice bag or a cold-water coil should be kept constantly over the area of greatest pain. Often no other analgesic will be required, but, if something additional be found necessary, reliance should be placed upon codeia, little, if any, morphine being given. A light diet, with a daily evacuation of the bowels, either by means of a saline or by enemata, is indicated. Copious vaginal douches of saline, at a comfortable temperature, should be given twice daily. It is my custom to order urotropin in every case of pelvic infection, for I believe that a certain number of troublesome bladder infections are thus prevented.

Careful watching is the keynote of success in the treatment of acute cases. The number which, on this régime, will go on to a symptomatic cure is considerable, yet a constant look-out must be kept for the development of an abscess outside the tube, and to this end frequent examinations should be made.

In case an abscess develops in such a position that it can be reached through the vagina no time should be lost in providing a vent for the pus.

Technique of Vaginal Puncture.—In the great majority of cases a pelvic abscess can be reached through the vagina, and this is always the route to be chosen, if possible. (Fig. 154.) The patient is placed in the lithotomy position and the vagina is carefully disinfected. General anæsthesia may be advisable, but in grave cases it is sometimes better to proceed with cocaine infiltration. Nitrous oxide gas is the anæsthetic of choice. After carefully mapping out the uterus and abscess, a posterior speculum is introduced, and the posterior lip of the cervix seized with bullet forceps. Traction is made on this until the posterior fornix is tense, when a transverse incision is made through the vaginal wall. This is stretched with the fingers, and, with the vaginal finger inserted in the incision, the abscess is again carefully examined. If there is any doubt as to the presenting mass, it is well to insert an aspirating needle. The abscess having been recognized, its wall is punctured with an artery forceps, and, as the pus pours out, the opening is enlarged by spreading the blades of the artery clamp, or by means of a Goodell dilator. Many advocate the washing-out of the cavity, but, as there is a certain danger in this, it is better to be content with a single evacuation of the contents. A pack made of a sterile roller bandage is next introduced, or, if the cavity is large, a T-shaped rubber drainage tube, surrounded by gauze, may be introduced. The gauze should remain in place for three days, when it is to be removed and a smaller one inserted. The opening usually tends to close rapidly. A second operation is sometimes necessary.

In doing this operation particular attention should be given to the bladder, in order to make sure that it is empty. A partially filled bladder may be mistaken for the fundus, and a retroverted fundus, especially if pregnant, may be mistaken for an abscess.

Drainage through the rectum, formerly much employed, is to be reserved for those cases in which a small opening already exists. In such a case it is permissible to enlarge the opening.

Abdominal drainage is to be reserved for those rare cases in which an abscess points above Poupart's ligament.

A certain number of cases are symptomatically cured by vaginal puncture;

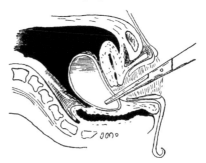

Fig. 154.—Diagram Showing the Puncturing of a Pelvic Abscess Through the Vagina.

in others, the adhesions give trouble, and a second, more radical, operation must be done.

The non-operative treatment of chronic pelvic infection, or of the condition which results from infection (*i.e.*, the inflammation), is now being employed in many cases where formerly a radical operation would have been done. Not a few of these cases occur in comparatively young women, and no pains should be spared to preserve, if there is any possibility of doing so, the function of the tubes and ovaries. Operation should be reserved as a last resort.

Rest in bed, general tonic treatment, hot sitz baths, hot vaginal douches, glycerin and ichthyol tampons, and the application of hot fomentations over the hypogastrium, are all to be employed.

The weight-posture method of Pincus often gives excellent results. It should be carried out as follows:—With the patient in the knee-chest position, the cervix is cleansed and about one ounce of the glycerin-ichthyol solution is poured into the fornices. They are then tightly packed with sterilized gauze, introduced under the guidance of the eye, care being taken to lay the folds in smoothly and to surround the cervix and fill the upper vagina tightly. The patient then assumes the lithotomy position and a bag of shot weighing about two pounds is placed above the symphysis. The position is maintained for at least thirty minutes, the patient in the mean time breathing deeply with the abdominal muscles. The packing remains in until the following morning, when it is removed and a hot vaginal douche given. The treatments should be given three times a week. The plan should not be adopted if pus is present or if the body temperature is above normal.

This method of Pincus accomplishes the same results as pelvic massage. The latter has been strongly advocated by some authorities, but it has many objections, not the least of which is its indelicacy. Electricity is used by few men of authority.

The object of the hot sitz baths, the hot douches, and the hot applications is to produce hyperæmia of the surface of the body. For the same purpose the suction apparatus of Bier has been employed, but the reports available at this time are not especially encouraging and the method is of doubtful value.

(3) Operative Treatment.—If general measures and local treatment, such as have been outlined, do not relieve the symptoms after a fair trial, the question of operation must be considered. It having been advised and accepted, the surgeon should have a clear idea of what the conditions are which are to be met, and he should explain clearly to the patient the nature of the operation which he is about to perform—i.e., whether it is a radical or a so-called conservative procedure. Conservatism has many brilliant successes to its credit, but it must also be blamed for many dismal failures. Whether or not it is to be the keynote of the operation should be discussed with the patient and the decision should be left with her, the surgeon frankly telling her that there are about four chances out of ten, that nothing short of a radical operation will relieve all the symptoms. In general, this is about the proportion of successes of conservative surgery on the tubes and ovaries; but, of course, each case must be judged for itself alone, as one case may promise excellent, and the next hopeless, results. It may be said that the present-day tendency is rather against the ultra-conservatism of a few years ago, but the reaction has not set back as far as the reckless sacrifices which were so common in the early days of abdominal surgery.

Conservative Operations.—If, when the abdomen is opened, both tubes are found diseased, one possibly being normal except at its abdominal extremity, the former may be removed and the latter resected. If one tube is healthy, it is better surgery to remove the diseased side, rather than attempt a resection.

Technique of Resection.—The diseased outer end of the tube is removed by an oblique incision. If the opening is small, it is enlarged by a longitudinal incision on the dorsum of the tube, the mucosa and the peritoneum being united by a row of very fine, interrupted catgut sutures.

Technique of Salpingectomy.—When a tube alone is to be removed the adhesions are first carefully separated and the field of operation walled off with gauze pads. The uterine end of the tube is seized with artery forceps and a V-shaped incision made into the uterine muscle, at the root of the tube. The mesosalpinx is then divided just beneath the tube, for a distance of about 2 centimetres. This will free the attachments of the uterine end of the tube sufficiently to allow the operator to close the V-shaped incision in the uterus with interrupted catgut sutures. The remaining portion of the tube is then cut away from the mesosalpinx, any bleeding points being caught up and tied as they are encountered. One small artery, a branch of the utero-ovarian anastomosis, will usually be divided about 2 centimetres from the uterus. This should be carefully secured. The upper edge of the broad ligament, from which the tube has been severed, should then be stitched, over and over, with a running suture of fine catgut.

In case there is pus in the tube, it should be aspirated before the attempt is made to break up the adhesions. In most chronic cases the pus is sterile, so that no harm results from soiling the wound with it. Nevertheless, it should be the aim to remove the pus tube intact, if possible.

In some cases of pyosalpinx the ovaries are in a fairly normal condition. When such is the case the tubes alone are removed, and, while there is no possibility of a pregnancy taking place later, the menstrual function is preserved and the patient spared the discomforts of the artificial menopause. In other instances it may be possible to preserve one ovary; in which case a salpingectomy is done on one side and a salpingo-oöphorectomy on the opposite.

Technique of Salpingo-Oöphorectomy.—After the adhesions have been dealt with in the manner described under the Technique of Hysterectomy (p. 418), the field of operation is isolated with gauze pads. The enucleation is begun by placing two artery forceps on the infundibulo-pelvic ligament and cutting between them. The uterine end of the tube is then severed as in simple salpingectomy, the utero-ovarian ligament is tied and severed, and the tube and ovary are cut away from the broad ligament, as much of the latter being preserved as may be found possible. The round ligament is also kept intact, if possible. A No. 3 catgut ligature is then placed on the infundibulo-pelvic ligament, in the stump of which the ovarian artery is recognized and separately tied with a No. 2 catgut ligature. The endeavor should be made to cover all raw areas with peritoneum.

If there is reason to believe that infection is still present, particularly if, from the history of the case, one is suspicious that the original infection was streptococcic, it is safer to puncture the posterior wall of the vagina, behind the cervix, and push through the opening the end of a small gauze drain, the remainder being loosely arranged in the cul-de-sac. Gauze provides but poor drainage, but its presence opens up a tract for the escape of any infected fluids which may accumulate.

The advantages of the abdominal route for the removal of the tube and ovary are these: more careful work can be done, and complications and unexpected conditions are more easily recognized. Some who are especially experienced in vaginal work prefer the vaginal route, and open the abdomen through an incision anterior or posterior to the uterus. That such an operation is safer for the patient seems illogical.

There is no indication for the removal of the ovaries without the tubes, for, when the former are extirpated, the latter become useless.

When the ovaries are both involved in the disease process, being either converted into abscesses or densely adherent to the tubes and surrounding peritoneum, and it is evident that to obtain a good result both of these structures must be removed, a hysterectomy should be done. This is the operation of choice for the following reasons:—The uterus, so far as we know, becomes useless after removal of both ovaries. If left in place it is very apt to become adherent to the raw areas left after removal of the appendages. The endometrium is diseased and is liable to cause a chronic leucorrhœa. It is often easier and safer to remove the organs *en masse* than to dissect out both sides separately. It is often impossible to avoid doing much injury to the uterus, and hence it is dangerous to leave in place a damaged and mutilated organ. Better drainage is secured by its removal.

Technique of Hysterectomy and Double Salpingo-Oöphorectomy.—In preparing the patient the bladder should be emptied and the vagina, as well as the abdomen, thoroughly cleansed. The incision should be large enough to secure ample exposure; indeed, a proper exposure of the field is one of the most important points in the operation. The Trendelenburg position should be employed and large abdominal retractors used.

After the abdomen is opened the whole field should be carefully inspected and palpated. If the uterus can be recognized, a traction forceps is applied to the fundus and it is lifted as high into the incision as possible. The tube and ovary on the less adherent side are then freed and the enucleation begun by tying off and severing the infundibulo-pelvic ligament of that side. It will now be possible partially to wall off the field of operation with gauze. The round ligament is tied and cut and the broad ligament severed as close to the tube as possible. The reflexion of the peritoneum between the bladder and the uterus is next severed and the former pushed down by blunt dissection. The separation is often readily made by "wiping" with a gauze sponge. One then feels for the pulsation of the uterine artery at the side of the uterus, near the internal os, and, having located it, passes a provisional ligature through the uterine musculature and around the artery. The uterus is then amputated above this ligature, care being taken to cut upward as the opposite side is reached. In this way the uterine artery is exposed and may be readily clamped. The remaining tube and ovary can usually be readily enucleated from below upward, the round and infundibulo-pelvic ligaments being clamped. Catgut ligatures are now substituted for the clamps. The cervical stump is "cupped out," only a shell being left. In this way the mucous membrane is destroyed and leucorrhœa from the cervical glands avoided. The anterior and posterior lips of the cervical stump are united with three or four interrupted catgut ligatures. The stumps of the infundibulo-pelvic and round ligaments are united to the edge of the cervical stump on each side, thus drawing up the cervical stump and providing a support for the bladder. The severed peritoneum is next united over the raw area thus left. It is usually easy to bring the anterior portion of the peritoneum over the stumps and unite it to the posterior layer. In this way the pelvis is left smooth and resembles the pelvis of the male.

If it is found impracticable to cover all of the raw area or if active infection is suspected, it is safer to open the posterior fornix and insert a small drain through the vaginal vault. (Consult also the article on "Surgery of the Uterus.")

In some cases the operation just described cannot be performed because of the dense adhesions which cover in the pelvic organs. No plane of cleavage can be discovered from above, and any attempt to separate uterus, tubes, and ovaries from the intestine involves a serious risk of opening the latter. For these cases Kelly has devised hysterectomy by bisection—an operation which I have done a number of times with the most gratifying results. The technique is thus described by Kelly:—

"If the uterus is buried from view, the bladder is first separated from the rectum and the fundus found; then, if there are any large abscesses, adherent cysts, or hæmatomata, they are evacuated by aspiration or by puncture; the rest of the abdominal cavity is then well packed off from the pelvis.

"The right and left cornua uteri are each seized by a pair of stout museau forceps and lifted up; the uterus is now incised in the median line in an antero-posterior direction, and, as the uterus is bisected, its cornua are pulled up and drawn apart. With a third pair of forceps the uterus is grasped on one side on its cut surface, as far down in the angle as possible, including both anterior and posterior walls. The museau forceps of the same side are then released and used for grasping the corresponding point on the opposite cut surface, when the remaining forceps are removed. In this way two forceps are in constant use at the lowest point. I commonly apply them three or four times in all. As the uterus is pulled up and the halves become everted, it is bisected further down into the cervix. If the operator prefers to do a panhysterectomy, the bisection is carried all the way down into the vagina. The uterine canal must be followed in the bisection, if necessary, a grooved director being used to keep it in view. The museau forceps are now made to grasp the uterus well down in the cervical portion, if it is to be a supravaginal amputation, and the cervix is bisected on one side. As soon as it is divided and the uterine and vaginal ends begin to pull apart, the under surface of the uterine end is caught with a pair of forceps and pulled up, and the uterine vessels, which can now be plainly seen, are clamped or tied. As the uterus is pulled still further up, the round ligament is exposed and clamped; then, finally, a clamp is applied between the cornu of the bisected uterus and the tubo-ovarian mass, and one half of the uterus is removed. The opposite half of the uterus is also taken away in the same manner.

"The pelvis now contains nothing but rectum and bladder, with right and left tubo-ovarian masses plastered to the sides of the pelvis and the broad ligaments, affording abundant room for investigation of their attachments, as well as for deliberate and skilful dissection; the wide exposure of the cellular area over the inferior median and anterior surfaces of the masses offers the best possible avenue for beginning their detachment and enucleation.

"The operator will sometimes find, on completing the bisection of the uterus, that he can just as well take out each tube and ovary together with its corresponding half of the uterus, reserving for the still more difficult cases, or for the more difficult side, the separate enucleation of the tube and ovary after removal of the uterus.

"The operation which I have just described is not recommended to a beginner in surgery; the surgeon who undertakes it must be calm and deliberate, and must bear in mind at each step the anatomical relations of the structures."

The great advantage of this method of hysterectomy is that the adhesions are dealt with from below upward. Working in this direction it is often an easy matter to find the point of cleavage and to separate the diseased organs from the neighboring structures safely and rapidly. Whenever adhesions are encountered they should be separated under direct observation; blind tearing should never be done. They may be separated with the fingers, by means of a blunt dissector, or by "wiping" with gauze. When dense, they are divided with scissors, and, if necessary, a small bit of the tube or ovary may be left on the intestinal wall, rather than run the risk of breaking through the latter.

Treatment of Puerperal Infections.—Both the non-operative and the operative treatment of puerperal or streptococcic infection is similar to that of the non-puerperal form. One must bear in mind, however, that the puerperal form often leaves behind less severe lesions than those resulting from gonorrhœa. Another point not to be lost sight of is, that the danger of general infection as a result of operation is much greater in the puerperal cases. No abdominal work should be done, if it is possible to avoid it, when there are still signs of active infection. At. times, interference cannot be avoided; then ample drainage should be provided.

Tuberculosis of the Tube and Ovary.—Tuberculosis of the tube is comparatively common. It is the cause of about ten per cent of all cases of salpingitis and pyosalpinx. Thus, Menge found 7 cases among 70, and Williams 7 cases among 91 cases of salpingitis. In a very large proportion of all cases of peritoneal tuberculosis in women, the apparent focus, so far at least as the abdominal cavity is concerned, is in the tubes. It is bilateral. The internal surface of the ovary is usually involved, but the infection in most cases is secondary to that of the tube.

The tubal infection is generally secondary to tuberculosis elsewhere in the body and is brought to the tubes through the blood- and lymph-streams. While direct infection from without would appear to be probable, thus far no case has been proven to have been thus caused. Patients are frequently enough seen in whom no lesions can be found other than in the tubes and peritoneum; but autopsy records show that there is practically always an extraperitoneal primary focus, usually a healed or partially healed lesion in the lungs. Tubal tuberculosis occurs in childhood, and the reports of Schmorl and Friedman would indicate that it may be congenital. (Fig. 155.)

PATHOLOGY.—In considering the pathology of the disease, it may be said that some cases, at the operating table, cannot be distinguished from cases of gonorrhœal salpingitis or pyosalpinx. In a study of a series of 80 cases of infected tubes which were removed at Kelly's clinic at Johns Hopkins University, it was found, on microscopic examination, that 9 were tuberculous. Five of these macroscopically were typical, two were suspicious, and in two tuberculosis was not suspected from the gross specimen. On the other hand, three cases in which tuberculosis was diagnosticated at the time of the operation, were microscopically non-tuberculous. Unless sections are made, therefore, of all removed tubes, there is a large percentage of error in diagnosis. Williams has brought out this point very clearly.

The typical case of tuberculous tube is one in which this structure is thick, stiff, and nodular. The interior is filled with cheesy material, on the removal of which tubercles may be seen on the partially denuded mucosa. The peritoneal covering often shows numerous discrete and conglomerate miliary tubercles. The bladder, pelvic peritoneum, and neighboring coils of intestine are also frequently studded with tubercles. The ovaries usually are adherent. As pointed out, however, the picture may vary considerably. Large pus tubes, containing thin, serous pus, are not infrequent.

SYMPTOMS.—There are no characteristic symptoms, but in every case of pelvic inflammation where gonorrhœa and puerperal infection can be reasonably excluded, tuberculosis should be suspected.

Watkins has given a good table of the differential points between tuberculous and non-tuberculous salpingitis. We shall take the liberty of reproducing it here:—

WATKINS' DIFFERENTIAL DIAGNOSIS BETWEEN TUBERCULOUS AND NON-TUBERCULOUS
SALPINGITIS.

Tuberculous Salpingitis.	*Non-Tuberculous Salpingitis.*
1. May be no history of infection.	1. Usually history of infection.
2. Often no history or signs of vulvitis, vaginitis, or endometritis.	2. Usually history and signs of vulvitis, vaginitis, and endometritis.
3. Hereditary history of tuberculosis may be present. (Of little value.)	3. Usually no history of hereditary tuberculosis.
4. Often history and signs of an old tuberculous disease.	4. Seldom history or signs of tuberculosis.
Fever: usually continuous and remittent.	Fever during the acute, but usually not during the chronic stage.
Pain: more or less continuous, but (usually) not severe.	Severe during acute stage.
Tenderness moderate.	Marked during acute stage.
Ascites common; coils of intestine visible.	Ascites uncommon; abdominal distention usually absent except during the acute stage.
Physical signs: swelling m re nodular in character and there is more exudate; boundary is usually not so well-defined as in non-tuberculous salpingitis. Usually more emaciation than in non-tuberculous salpingitis.	
There may be diarrhœa.	Usually constipation.
Disease may occur before puberty.	Disease seldom occurs before puberty.

TREATMENT.—Unless the disease is very far advanced, operation is indicated. There is a difference of opinion as to whether or not tuberculous tubes should be removed, but, from my own experience, I am convinced that they should be excised, even in the presence of extensive peritoneal involvement. I have operated thus upon four patients who were apparently desperately ill, and all are now either in good or in fair health. In one case where the whole peritoneum was covered with tubercles, from the pelvis to the diaphragm, an abdominal section four years later, for hernia, failed to reveal a single tubercle. In every case of tuberculous peritonitis in women the tubes should be carefully inspected and if diseased, even though there are no pelvic symptoms, they should be removed.

Ovarian Neoplasms.—When one considers the wonderful physiological activity of the ovary and the continual changes which its cellular structure undergoes, he is not surprised at the frequency with which neoplasms occur in the organ. Not only are new-growths here common, but they occur in great variety; indeed, no other organ of the body presents a greater number or a greater diversity of tumors than does the ovary. Gurlt's figures show that

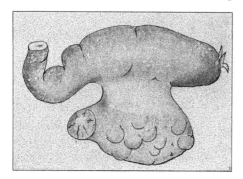

Fig. 155.—Tuberculosis of the Tube and Ovary. (Original.)

8.5 per cent of all tumors of the female are ovarian, and these tumors contribute from five to nine per cent of gynæcological affections. In contrast to myoma and carcinoma of the uterus, neoplasms of the ovary are found from birth to old age, while the former occur only at certain periods of life.

CLASSIFICATION.—There is no better classification, either from a practical or from a scientific standpoint, than that of Pfannenstiel. In a somewhat simplified form it will be here followed. Accordingly, neoplasms of the ovary are divided into:—

I. Tumors developing from the parenchyma. The parenchyma consists of germ epithelium, follicular epithelium, and ovum.

    (1) Epithelial Tumors.

        (a) Simple serous cysts.

        (b) Cystadenoma.

            (α) Pseudomucinous cysts.

            (β) Papillary cysts.

        (c) Carcinoma.

(2) Tumors developing from the Ovum.
(a) Dermoids   }
(b) Teratomata } Embryomata.
II. Tumors developing from the Stroma.
(a) Fibroma.
(b) Sarcoma.
(c) Perithelioma and endothelioma.
(d) Rare tumors, such as myoma, angioma, chondroma, etc.
Combinations of these tumors may occur in the same ovary.

I. Tumors Developing From the Parenchyma.

Closely related clinically to ovarian tumors are the cysts which develop from the parovarium. Simple retention cysts of the Graafian follicle and corpus luteum have been described elsewhere (page 402 *et seq.*) and tubo-ovarian cysts considered under the inflammations of the ovary. (Page 409.)

Before describing the characteristics of these different tumors, I believe I may advantageously consider their relative frequency. The cystadenoma (pseudomucinous) is by far the most frequent, comprising 62 per cent of the cases included in the table given by Leopold, 59 per cent of Martin's, and 52 per cent of Schauta's cases. Of Kelly's 556 cases, 322 were cystadenomata, and of these 54, or 9.7 per cent of the total number, were papillomata. Carcinomata and sarcomata (in other words, the malignant tumors) make up about 20 per cent of the whole number, and three-fifths of these are carcinomata. Dermoids comprise about 12 per cent. If, then, we take a large series of cases, we shall find that the relative frequency is about as follows:— Cystadenoma (pseudomucinous) 54 per cent; carcinoma and dermoids, each 12 per cent; papilloma, 9 per cent; and sarcoma, 8 per cent; which leaves 5 per cent for the rarer forms.

(1) *Epithelial Tumors.*—The epithelial tumors consist of the simple serous cysts, the two forms of cystadenomata, and the carcinomata.

(a) Simple Serous Cysts.—Simple serous cysts resemble the Graafian follicle retention-cysts, except that they are lined with epithelium and that their walls display active proliferation. The cyst wall is of fibrous tissue, and the lining is composed of a single layer of cuboidal epithelial cells. There are no proliferating gland-like spaces in the walls, such as occur in the cystadenoma. The contained fluid is a thin, yellowish serum, containing albumin, but no pseudomucin.

Such cysts are usually monolocular and never contain more than two or three loculi. They are unilateral, grow slowly, and are commonly of moderate size, although very large specimens have been described. I have removed one weighing, with the contained fluid, eighty-eight pounds, from a patient aged seventy-seven years.

(b) Cystadenoma.—Pseudomucinous cystadenoma, as we have seen, is the most frequent of the ovarian tumors. It is the classical cyst of the ovariotomist and is a well-defined pathological entity. It is occasionally found in early and also in advanced life, but is usually seen between thirty and fifty years of age. We no longer see the large cysts of this description, formerly so common. They may, however, attain an immense size, the early gynæcological literature containing many descriptions of tumors weighing more than the patient after operation. They are always multilocular, although usually there are one or more large cyst-cavities. While these tumors are, in general, of a spherical form, the development of daughter cysts often produces bosses on the exterior, making the contour irregular. The differences in tension of the contained fluid may cause a great variation in the firmness of these bosses, some fluctuating and others feeling as hard as a fibroid of the uterus. They are practically always unilateral. (Fig. 156.) Externally, they are smooth and glistening, but the color varies greatly. Not infrequently they are uniformly of a bluish or gray tint; again, the color of the various loculi may vary, producing a mottled appear-

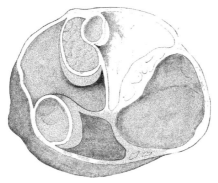

Fig. 156.—Diagrammatic Cross Section of a Multilocular Pseudomucinous Cystadenoma. (Author's case.)

ance. Areas in which the blood-supply to the wall is poor are often of a pearly white. Dark areas, almost black in color, may be produced by blood extravasated into the cyst walls. Again, the whole of a loculus may be of a chocolate color, due to degenerated blood, admixed with the normal contents of the loculus. Running over the surface are arteries and veins of various sizes, often exquisitely outlined. The larger cavities are frequently formed by the rupture of the partition walls, and a tendency is generally manifested for the tumor to rotate, so that the large loculi are directed forward, occupying the concavity of the distended abdominal wall.

On cross section, a pseudomucinous cyst is found to be made up of cavities of various sizes and shapes separated by septa and trabeculæ, some of which are ruptured and project free into the cyst spaces. The external walls and the trabeculæ here and there contain small cystic spaces, appearing like the cross sections of glands. Some specimens contain no large loculi, a cross section appearing like cut honeycomb.

On microscopic examination, the outer wall and the trabeculæ will be found to be made up of fibrous tissue, containing blood-vessels in varying numbers. The cells are of the usual type, and have long, rod-shaped nuclei. If the specimen is stained with hæmatoxylin, deep purple areas will generally be seen, especially in those parts where the blood-vessels are less abundant. There are deposits of calcareous matter. Spots of degenerated blood are also frequent. The lining of the cell spaces is best studied in one of the smaller cysts, where the cells have been less influenced by pressure. The lining cells are in one layer and are of the high cylindrical variety, having a small basal nucleus. The protoplasm of the cells takes the eosin stain poorly, the pseudo-mucin which they contain having an affinity for the hæmatoxylin, and appearing bluish in color. Droplets of the pseudo-mucin are visible. These cells may or may not be ciliated.

In former years cysts were much more frequently tapped than at present and the examination of cyst fluid was an important laboratory procedure. Hence distinctions were made which are now of little practical importance. This form of cystadenoma typically contains a thick, mucoid substance, pale-blue in color, but many of the loculi may be filled with a thin, serous fluid, varying in color according as to whether or not there has been hemorrhage into the loculus. The specific gravity of the fluid varies from 1010 to 1040, and chemically it contains a substance first carefully studied by Pfannenstiel and known as pseudo-mucin. Microscopically, the fluid is found to contain degenerated red and white blood-corpuscles, degenerated lining cells, and sometimes crystals of cholesterin.

Papilloma.—The second variety of cystadenoma is the papilloma. While papillary growths may either occur on the surface or project from the inner wall into the interior of the other varieties of cysts, the true papilloma differs from the simple serous cysts in the character of the lining cells and from the pseudo-mucinous variety in the character of the contents. It receives its name from papillary masses which grow either on the outer surface or on the inner surface of the cyst. These papillæ may be small and sessile or of considerable size and pedunculated. In the latter instance they consist of a main stem connected with the cyst-wall, and they give off numerous branches. Although, as a rule, they are rich in blood-vessels, there is frequently degeneration, sometimes of the myxomatous type, the ends of the papillæ being transformed into blebs. Often, too, these papillomata are of the calcareous type, hard, gritty areas being formed in the wall. (Fig. 157.)

Papillomata are usually moderate in size, seldom being larger than an adult head. In about half of the cases they are bilateral. They are multilocular, but the loculi are fewer in number than in pseudo-mucinous cysts.

The cyst wall is made up of fibrous tissue, and the lining is composed of high cylindrical epithelium which is generally in one layer, but may be in several layers. The cells are frequently ciliated. These same cells cover the papillary outgrowths. The contained fluid is thin and serous, resembling that of the simple serous cysts.

Such tumors have a tendency to develop in the broad ligament. While not malignant, in the sense that metastases are formed in distant organs or within the structure of adjacent organs, the papillary growths may be reproduced on the peritoneum of uterus, bladder, parietes, and intestine. Ascites then results. The rapidity of growth varies. As long as the papillary masses are inside the cyst the growth may be slow; when they appear on the surface they usually spread rapidly, and quickly produce ascites. While occurring at any age they are most frequent during the fourth and fifth decades.

Carcinoma.—Carcinoma is found in about one out of eight ovarian grówths. The cases may be divided into three groups: (1) the tumors which have devel-

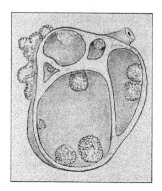

FIG. 157.—Diagrammatic Section of a Papilloma of the Ovary. (After Findley.)

oped from the epithelial structures of the ovary—the idiopathic form; (2) the tumors which develop from carcinomatous degeneration of one of the other forms of neoplasm—the secondary form; and (3) tumors which result from a primary growth in some other part of the body—the metastatic form.

The idiopathic or primary cancer is the most frequent. It may form either a cyst or a solid tumor, but most frequently it is a semi-solid, soft, irregular mass containing cysts of various sizes. In color these tumors vary from pearly-white to dark-red, the difference being due to the degree of vascularity. The surface is often furrowed, the tumor presenting distinct lobes; knobs and bosses may produce bizarre shapes.

On cross section the appearance of the tumor is somewhat like that of brain substance, but on close inspection there may be seen small nests of cells separated by delicate trabeculæ. Areas of degeneration are frequent. Histologically, the structure is seen to be of the adeno-carcinoma type, i.e., there are masses of cells which originally were of the cylindrical form, but many of them are atypical. They grow in a more or less tubular fashion, producing spaces not unlike those seen in glands. Evidences of cell division are frequently very plain. Delicate trabeculæ, often œdematous and carrying the blood-vessels, separate the cell nests. In certain specimens the connective-tissue framework is almost entirely lacking, the tumor being very soft and friable.

Carcinomata are bilateral in about half of the cases. They grow rapidly and quickly produce ascites, which is often blood-stained. They occur at all ages.

Carcinomatous degeneration of other ovarian neoplasms is fairly frequent. A simple cyst, a pseudo-mucinous cyst, or a dermoid may contain areas of carcinoma which, owing to their homogeneous, opaque, granular appearance, may be recognized by the naked eye. Smaller areas of epithelial cells, of a typical growth, may be discovered in the laboratory during the course of a systematic examination.

Metastatic carcinoma may follow cancer of the uterus, stomach, or intestine. Recently numerous authors have called attention to the frequency of metastatic cancer of the ovary. Bland Sutton [*] states that this form is the most frequent, but that its secondary character is overlooked. In every case, a careful search should be made, both before and at the time of the operation, for carcinoma elsewhere.

(2) *The Ovigenous Tumors.*—The ovigenous tumors are divided into dermoids and teratomata. The former are comparatively common, the latter rare.

(a) Dermoids.—As their name indicates, dermoid tumors contain certain tissues commonly found in connection with the skin. They may be found at any period of life, are of slow growth, and usually are of small size. They have been found in infants and in a few instances in the fœtus. Usually they do not produce symptoms before puberty. Very large specimens have been described. They are unilateral, generally monolocular, and produce no characteristic symptoms. In some specimens no trace of the normal ovary can be found; in others, practically normal ovarian tissue will be seen at some point on the tumor.

Dermoids are usually oval or spherical in shape and have, when free from adhesions, a smooth exterior. The consistency varies according to the contents.

Microscopically, the cyst wall resembles the skin. Externally, there are, first, a layer of fibrous tissue, then a layer resembling the subcutaneous tissue of the skin. The lining is composed of several or many layers of flat epithelial cells; and sebaceous and sweat glands, hair follicles, muscle fibres, and fat cells are found in the walls. Cartilage, bone, teeth, horns, and finger-like processes tipped by nails are frequent. Hair in varying amounts nearly always occurs. It may be short or long and the color differs greatly, often being entirely different from that on the head of the patient.

At the body temperature the contents resemble melted lard, but on cooling they usually become granular and of the consistency of putty.

Dermoids frequently become infected and the clinical picture is then one of pelvic infection. Adhesions result and not infrequently fistulæ, through which hairs or teeth may be discharged.

(b) Teratomata.—The teratoma is a modification of the dermoid and bears somewhat the same relationship to the latter as carcinoma does to cystadenoma. In the dermoid the secretory products predominate, while in teratoma the solid elements prevail. There are comparatively few cases on record, and each one is more or less in a class by itself. Teratomata occur in young women and may reach an enormous size, growing very rapidly. They are made up of tissue derived from any or all of the blastodermic layers, bits of skin, bone, muscle, and cartilage being all mixed together in a confused mass.

* Sutton, in British Medical Journal, January 4th, 1908.

II. Tumors Developing from the Stroma.

The tumors developing from the stroma of the ovary are for the most part solid.

(a) *Fibroma.*—Fibroid tumors of the ovary comprise, according to Pfannenstiel, from two to three per cent of all ovarian neoplasms. They are homogeneous in structure, and are to be differentiated from so-called fibrosis of the ovary, a condition in which there is an overgrowth of the stroma with retention of the Graafian follicles. Fibroids vary in size from a mere excrescence on the surface of the ovary to a large pedunculated tumor weighing twenty or thirty pounds. They are very dense and hard, grayish in color, and irregular in shape. They may appear at any age, usually somewhat earlier than fibroids of the uterus,

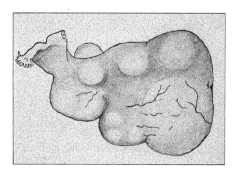

Fig. 158.—Fibroma of the Ovary.   Actual measurements: 13 cm. x 11 cm. x 10 cm.
(Dr. Peterson's case.)

and grow slowly. Saenger reports an instance which was under observation for thirty-seven years. Not infrequently ovarian fibromata are bilateral. (Fig. 158.)

On cross section, fibromata may display a texture that is quite homogeneous, although it is usual to find interlacing bands of connective tissue, sometimes arranged in whorls. Degenerations are frequent. Deposits of calcareous matter and cystic spaces caused by fatty degenerations are common.

Ascites was present in forty per cent of the 84 cases collected from the literature by Peterson.*

(b) *Sarcoma.*—Sarcomata are somewhat more frequent than fibromata. The statistics as to their frequency vary between six and fourteen per cent of all ovarian neoplasms. Their general appearance is much like that of fibromata, although they are usually smoother, more glistening, and softer. When a large amount of fibrous tissue is present—as in a fibrosarcoma—it may be impossible to make the differential diagnosis without microscopic sections. When the fibrous tissue and sarcoma cells are diffused throughout the whole

* Peterson, in American Gynæcology, July, 1902.

specimen, one may assume that the tumor has been sarcomatous from the beginning, and that the condition is not sarcomatous degeneration of a fibroid.

Sarcoma is found at all ages and is the most frequent ovarian growth encountered in childhood, forty per cent occurring under twenty-five years and six per cent under ten.

There are two varieties: the spindle-cell sarcoma and the round-cell sarcoma. The spindle-cell variety is the more frequent, and, on microscopic examination, is found to be made up of long cells with long, thin nuclei, the cells being arranged in bundles and sheaths. The round-cell variety is softer, more vascular, and more malignant. It tends to invade surrounding organs and is frequently densely adherent. On histological examination, a varying amount of connective-tissue framework is found, there being very little in the softer and more rapidly growing tumors.

Both forms are often bilateral and grow rapidly. Chrobak reports an instance of the round-cell variety in which the tumor grew from the umbilicus to the costal margin in twenty-three days.

Hyaline and fatty degeneration is frequent. Cystic spaces often occur.

(c) *Perithelioma and Endothelioma.*—Perithelioma and endothelioma are related to sarcoma clinically, but, on account of their pathology, they belong in a class by themselves. They develop from the mesoblast of blood- and lymph-vessels. They are rare, occur at all ages, may be of any size, and are malignant. Barrett * has collected the cases up to 1907.

(d) *Myoma, Angioma, Chondroma, etc.*—Other connective-tissue tumors are occasionally observed in the ovaries, but they are so rare as to be pathological curiosities.

Parovarian Cysts.—As we have seen, the parovarium is a collection of tubules, the remains of the Wolffian body, situated in the broad ligament between the tube and the hilum of the ovary. One of these tubules may be the starting-point of a cyst, which develops between the layers of the ligament and may attain a large size.

A parovarian cyst is monolocular and filled with a thin, serous fluid. It may be recognized by a double layer of vessels on its outer surface—one belonging to the cyst-wall proper, and one to the peritoneal leaf of the broad ligament. The tube runs over the surface and may be very long. The ovary is independent of the growth.

On microscopic examination, the thin wall is found to be covered by peritoneum externally, and to be lined by a single layer of ciliated, low, cylindrical epithelium.

HISTOGENESIS OF OVARIAN GROWTHS.—The histogenesis of ovarian growths, from a scientific standpoint, is one of the most interesting questions in gynæcological pathology. It has no important practical bearings, however, and cannot here be discussed in more than the merest outline.

The simple serous cysts and the pseudomucinous cystadenomata are believed to be derived from a proliferation of the cells of the follicular epithelium, which

* Barrett, in Surgery, Gynæcology, and Obstetrics, May, 1907.

in turn are generally believed to arise by down-growths of the germinal epithe lium. If we accept the views of Foulis and others,—viz., that the cells of the membrana granulosa are derived from the connective tissue of the ovary,—this origin would be impossible; and these tumors must therefore be regarded as developing from the germinal epithelium. Pfannenstiel holds that they develop from the membrana granulosa, while others maintain that they arise from the corresponding cells of unripe follicles.

It has long been held that the papillomata develop from remains of the Wolffian body in the hilum of the ovary, particularly the so-called *Markstraenge*. Williams and Pfannenstiel believe that they arise from altered germinal epithe lium. Marchand claims that they are derived from misplaced tubal epithelium and are therefore of Muellerian-duct origin.

To account for the ovigenous tumors, dermoids and teratomata, many in genious theories have been brought forward, the principal of which are thus given by Hirst:—(1) that the ovum undergoes a parthenogenetic development; (2) that a polar body becomes impregnated at the same time as the ovum and undergoes a certain development in the ovary; and (3) that there is a separation and inclu sion of one or more blastomeres in the course of embryonal development.

MALIGNANCY OF OVARIAN GROWTHS.—The term malignancy, as applied to ovarian growths, is a relative one, for we have at one end of the line tumors which are absolutely benign, i.e., the proliferation of the tumor cells is absolutely confined to the tumor itself, and no tendency to invade surrounding tissues is manifested; the cellular elements are not transported to distant parts of the body to form metastases; and there is no return of the growth after removal. At the other end we have the extremely malignant growths, which invade all the surrounding organs, and the cells of which are transported to distant parts, become embedded there, and reproduce a tumor similar to the original. Such growths practically always return after a seemingly complete removal. The best examples of the absolutely benign growths are the simple serous cysts, the fibromata, and the dermoids. The malignant growths are carcinoma, sarcoma, teratomata, and some of the endotheliomata. Midway between these extremes, often leaning toward malignancy and then again having only a slight tendency in this direction, are the following varieties: the papillomata, which do not form metastases, but generally produce implantation growths; a certain, very small number of the apparently benign pseudo-myxomatous cystadenomata, which, after removal, recur as papillary tumors in the scar or produce the con dition known as pseudomyxoma peritonei; and certain of the fibrosarcomata, a complete removal of which is not followed by recurrence.

Pseudomyxoma peritonei is the term applied to the implantation growths found in certain cases of cystadenoma. The epithelium from the tumor becomes attached to the peritoneum in various places, proliferates, and produces pseudo mucin. Olshausen reports having removed a mass of pseudomucin which had formed in this manner and which weighed eighty pounds.

SYMPTOMS OF OVARIAN GROWTHS.—In many cases of uncomplicated ovarian neoplasms the first symptom noticed by the patient is the enlargement of the abdomen. In other cases, where the tumor becomes wedged in the pelvis or develops within the folds of the broad ligament, there are indefinite pains in the pelvis, vesical tenesmus, and constipation. As the tumor releases itself from the pelvis and becomes an abdominal parasite, these symptoms may disappear and the patient have little or no complaint other than the swelling of the abdomen. Dyspeptic troubles are frequently associated with the development of an ovarian tumor; the patient gradually loses weight and manifests symptoms of nervous disorder; and there is a more or less characteristic expression of the face long known as the *facies ovariana*. There may be swelling of the breasts and the development of colostrum within them. Backache is a frequent complaint. The very large ovarian cysts may embarrass the lungs and the heart. Menstruation is usually little affected. In the case of double tumors there may be amenorrhœa, or the circulation of the pelvis may be interfered with and menorrhagia develop. Sterility is the rule, but there are many

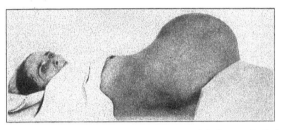

Fig. 159.—Large Multilocular Pseudomucinous Cystadenoma of the Ovary. (Author's case.)

exceptions, pregnancy not infrequently developing. Even in the case of bilateral neoplasms the patient may, in rare instances, become pregnant.

The symptoms produced by complications will be discussed later.

DIAGNOSIS OF OVARIAN GROWTHS.—There being no well-marked nor pathognomonic symptoms of ovarian tumor, the examination is, as in other gynæcological affections, the most important step in making the diagnosis. There is such a great diversity of size, shape, mobility, and consistency among these growths that it is difficult to determine what are the usual clinical findings. The most important points in making a diagnosis as to the seat of the tumor are the palpation of the pedicle and the demonstration that it is attached to the side of the uterus. Pedicles differ in length and breadth according to the manner of growth of the tumor. If the growth develops from the free margin of the ovary the pedicle is usually long and narrow, while one starting near the hilum generally has a short, broad attachment. Intraligamentary tumors may or may not have a pedicle. (Figs. 159 and 160.)

One should form the habit of never approaching the examining table without having in mind two physiological tumors, namely, a full urinary bladder and pregnancy. If the possibility of finding either of these conditions is never forgotten, many embarrassing mistakes will be prevented.

The clinical picture differs so greatly according to the size of the growth that it is convenient to describe the physical signs under three headings corresponding to the small, medium-sized, and large tumors.

The Clinical Picture in Tumors of Small Size.—By a small-sized tumor is meant one which is contained wholly within the pelvis. The various steps usual in making a pelvic examination should be carefully and systematically carried out. The cervix uteri is first sought, its size, direction, and consistency being noted. Next, the fundus is located. In the presence of a pelvic ovarian tumor the uterus will be found pushed to one or the other side, while the opposite fornix is filled by a globular, firm mass, smooth in outline, and of variable mobility. Sometimes this globular mass will be found situated directly posterior to the uterus, in which case the fundus is high, the cervix drawn well up under the symphysis, and the posterior vaginal wall pushed forward by the tumor. If possible, two fingers should now be introduced and an attempt made to lift up the tumor. By pushing downward with the abdominal hand, the growth may

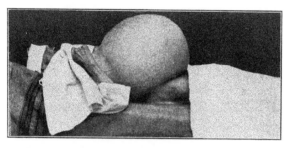

Fig. 160.—Simple Serous Cyst of the Ovary, Practically Unilocular, Successfully Removed from a Patient Seventy-seven Years of Age. Weight of tumor eighty-eight pounds. (Author's case.)

readily be outlined and an attempt made to elicit fluctuation. Such tumors, when cystic, are usually so tense that this is not practicable. Often one fails to palpate the pedicle, either because, at this stage, it is too short or because it is impossible to stretch it, there not being room enough to separate the growth from the uterus. The line of demarcation between tumor and fundus uteri should be carefully made; it is very distinct in cases of intraligamentous growth.

The diagnosis rests upon finding such a mass separate from, but apparently connected with, the uterus, no ovary being discoverable upon the affected side, and a normal ovary being found upon the opposite side.

Bilateral growths, when of any size, choke the pelvis and are separated from the uterus with difficulty.

Differential Diagnosis.—It is important to distinguish an ovarian tumor from the following pathological conditions:—Myoma uteri, a tumor of the broad ligament, hydrosalpinx, pyosalpinx, a pelvic hæmatocele, a pelvic abscess, and an incarcerated pregnancy.

Even the best diagnosticians are often unable to make a diagnosis between ovarian tumor and fibroid of the uterus. A fibroid develops more slowly, is firmer, has a thicker pedicle, and is more intimately connected with the uterus. Other small fibroids, if present, as well as an elongated uterine cavity, point to the probability of the tumor in question being a myoma. If attached at some other point than at the cornu of the uterus, and if both ovaries can be palpated, the tumor is a fibroid.

The greatest difficulty is experienced in differentiating a tumor in the broad ligament from an ovarian tumor. Here the consistency is practically the only guide; for, although a cyst is more frequently spherical and is smoother than a fibroid, there are no distinguishing features that are to be depended upon.

A hydrosalpinx is softer and less movable than an ovarian tumor, and, as a rule, it is distinctly club-shaped.

The history, the signs of infection in the external organs, and the fact that both sides are affected point to pyosalpinx rather than to an ovarian tumor. Moreover, inflammatory masses are tender, fixed, and irregular in outline. An infected cyst, especially a dermoid, cannot always be differentiated from an inflammatory mass, especially if it be of a tuberculous nature.

In the case of a pelvic hæmatocele or a pelvic abscess, the history is of some assistance in making a differential diagnosis. Both of these pathological conditions are usually less distinct than an ovarian tumor, especially as regards their upper limits. Rectal examination may reveal the "tissue paper" sensation conveyed by blood clots, or the induration of the surrounding tissues.

A normal pregnancy of the third or fourth month can hardly be mistaken for an ovarian tumor. When, however, the fundus is in retroposition and wedged in the hollow of the sacrum, and when at the same time the bladder is hypertrophied, as is often the case, the latter organ may be taken for the fundus and the mass in the cul-de-sac for an ovarian growth. If one is in doubt, a sound should be introduced into the bladder. The relation of the cervix to the mass gives the clew to the condition.

The Clinical Picture in Tumors of Medium Size.—These tumors fill the pelvis and project into the lower abdomen. The presence of a swelling in the hypogastrium is evident on inspection, and the so-called "breathing line" is visible, caused by the tumor splinting the abdominal wall and by the latter moving only above the tumor. On palpation, the swelling may be regular or irregular; it is sharply defined and fluctuation may be elicited. Unless adhesions are present or the lower part of the tumor is wedged in the pelvis, there is considerable mobility. Palpation is painless. On percussion the mass is dull and more or less surrounded by an area of resonance. (Fig. 161.)

The pelvic relations are next made out by vaginal or rectal palpation. The pedicle should be sought in the following manner:—After the vagina has been cleansed, a bullet forceps is attached to the cervix and the uterus is pulled down, the forceps being held by an assistant. The examiner or assistant then pushes the tumor upward by pressing and pushing upward above the symphysis. In this way the tumor and fundus are separated, and by palpating, through the rectum, first one and then the other cornu of the fundus, the band may usually be made out. If no insurmountable obstacles exist, a certain diagnosis of the ovarian origin of the tumor is made and the side from which it springs demonstrated. An attempt should be made to locate the other ovary.

Differential Diagnosis.—It is of great importance to differentiate an ovarian tumor from pregnancy. The history may readily be confusing, especially in cases of hydramnios and dead fœtus; moreover, the patient may try to conceal the true condition and give an inaccurate history. Abdominal palpation may be of little aid. Fœtal heart sounds, if heard, will of course immediately estab-

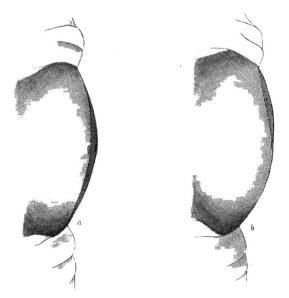

FIG. 161.—Diagram Showing the Respiratory Movement of the Abdomen; (a) when no tumor is present, and (b) when there is an intra-abdominal tumor which extends up as high as the umbilicus. (From Giles: "Gynæcological Diagnosis," William Wood & Co., 1906.)

lish the diagnosis, but they are rarely heard earlier than the eighteenth week, and often not until the twentieth. The consistency of the cervix and the color of the mucous membranes will afford aid, but will not answer the question either way. In case of doubt, great care should be exercised in pulling down the cervix, and in no case should a uterine sound be passed. When unable to decide, the examiner should insist on making an examination a month or six weeks later. In fleshy patients, a rapidly growing hydatidiform mole may be most confusing.

When the diagnosis lies between an ovarian tumor and a myoma uteri, it should be remembered that an intramural fibroid of medium size is not infrequently cystic and may closely resemble an ovarian cyst. The diagnosis is cleared up by investigating the relations of the tumor to the cervix and by attempting to discover, by palpation, the existence of a pedicle.

Phantom tumors are generally easy to differentiate from ovarian tumors, but now and then there occurs a case which requires an examination under an anæsthetic before the diagnosis can be made. Such phantom tumors are produced by contraction of the abdominal muscles, by deposits of fat in the abdominal walls, the omentum, or the mesentery, and by distention of the intestines with gas.

Hepatic and splenic tumors are sometimes found in the pelvis. They are differentiated from ovarian growths by the facts that no connection with the uterus or with an ovary can be demonstrated, that both ovaries may be palpated, and by pushing the tumor up into the region from which it originated.

The Clinical Picture in Tumors of Large Size.—A large tumor fills the whole abdomen and extends upward under the ribs, often causing the costal cartilages to bend forward. The solid tumors practically never grow to be so large; indeed, rarely do any ovarian growths other than the cystadenomata attain these dimensions. The skin over such a cyst is generally thin, and shows prominent blood-vessels and marked lineæ atrophicæ. On palpation the tension may be found to be uniform, or distinct bosses may be here and there made out, some hard and others softer. When there is one large cyst, as is usually the case, distinct fluctuation can be made out. On percussion there is dulness over the whole tumor, with tympany in the flanks.

The vaginal examination reveals little. Often the uterus is crowded down and there may be marked œdema of the vulva. The pedicle generally cannot be felt.

The differential diagnosis most frequently to be made is that between a large ovarian cyst and ascites. The points may be tabulated as follows:—

OVARIAN CYST.	ASCITES.
Dome-shaped.	Plateau on top.
Umbilicus prominent.	Umbilicus depressed.
Slight bulging in flanks.	Sagging in flanks.
Fluctuation less distinct.	Fluctuation very distinct.
Wave sluggishly transmitted.	Wave quickly transmitted.
Flatness in umbilical region.	Tympany in umbilical region.
Tympany in flanks.	Flatness in flanks.
Very slight, if any, movable dulness.	Marked movable dulness.
Liver, heart, and kidneys normal (?).	Signs of disease in these organs.

The diagnosis of the variety of the tumor is of scientific interest and one should always attempt it. From a practical standpoint, however, it is not of great importance, because all ovarian tumors should be removed as soon as possible after they are discovered. Some points to be considered will be given, but no attempt will be made to discuss the question exhaustively.

Most large cysts are either parovarian cysts or pseudomyxomatous cyst-adenomata. When thin-walled and apparently monolocular, as evidenced by the fluctuation wave, the cyst is probably parovarian. When bosses and irregularities are felt, it is probably a cystadenoma. The papillary masses on the surface of a papilloma can sometimes be felt *per rectum*. A dermoid is usually hard and very frequently adherent, and sometimes it is felt in front of the uterus. Ascites accompanies the malignant tumors, fibromata, and papillomata. Its presence is not an absolute sign of malignancy, as is sometimes taught.

The diagnosis of malignancy is important. There is usually, in the case of a malignant tumor, marked rapidity of growth, associated with failing strength and falling weight. Often the distention of the abdomen from ascites is the first symptom noted. There is more often pain, especially that radiating from the pelvis down the leg, than in benign growths. The tumor is often found fixed in the pelvis. Signs of metastases may be found elsewhere in the body. One must keep in mind the fact that the ovarian growth may itself be metastatic.

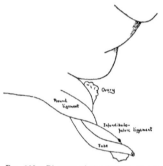

Fig. 162.—Diagram of the Pedicle of an Ovarian Tumor which had Undergone Torsion. (From Kelly.)

COMPLICATIONS.—Of the complications of ovarian tumors, torsion of the pedicle resulting in hemorrhage or gangrene, rupture of the cyst wall, and infection are sufficiently common to deserve brief mention in this place. The association of ascites and pregnancy will also be here considered.

Torsion of the Pedicle.—This accident most frequently happens to the smaller and moderate-sized tumors. According to Schauta, it takes place, to a greater or less extent, in one-fifth of all tumors. That the twist is sufficiently marked to cause symptoms in so large a percentage, is doubtful. It was present 37 times in 257 cases at the Jena Clinic (14.4 per cent). Storer* has collected 248 instances from the literature. The following are thought to be the causes: the tendency of the largest loculi to rotate anteriorly, the peristaltic action of the intestine, and possibly the alternate distention and emptying of the bladder. (Fig. 162.)

The result of torsion of the pedicle is the shutting off of the return flow of blood through the thin-walled vein, the artery remaining open. The continuous pumping of blood into the tumor causes it to enlarge. Weeping may take place from the surface, or a vein may rupture and alarming hemorrhages follow. If the twist becomes sufficiently pronounced to shut off the artery, gangrene may result.

The usual symptoms are severe abdominal pain, pallor, and an increase in the size of the tumor. The cause of the pain is not clear, but the pain itself is

* Storer, in Boston Medical and Surgical Journal, November 5th, 1896.

probably analogous to that caused by the dragging on the intestinal mesentery. Not infrequently there are symptoms of intestinal obstruction, without any mechanical cause being found.

When a twist takes place in an unsuspected tumor on the right side, the attack may resemble very closely one of acute appendicitis. Careful vaginal examination will usually make the diagnosis clear.

Rupture of the Cyst Wall.—It is probable that the rupture of a cyst takes place quite frequently without producing any symptoms. In most cases the cyst-fluid is sterile and is absorbed. The origin of implantation growths from carcinoma and papilloma may be explained by a rent in the wall and the discharge of the cellular elements through the hole. Hemorrhage may be caused by a rupture.

Infection.—The contents of a cyst may become infected through the blood-stream or through adhesions formed with the intestines. Colon-bacillus infections are the most frequent; typhoid infections are not extremely rare.

When a tumor co-exists with infection of the tubes, dense adhesions may result, sometimes completely covering the tumor and producing the pseudo-ligamentary type. Adhesions to the anterior abdominal wall and omentum are often extensive; in rare instances, new blood-vessels may form in these adhesions and the nutrition of the tumor be mainly carried on in this way. "Parasitic tumors" of this kind have been described.

Dermoid tumors are especially prone to become adherent.

Ascites.—The throwing out of free fluid in small amounts occurs in many cases. In appreciable amounts it is commonly found in cases of papilloma, carcinoma, and fibroma. Numerous ingenious theories have been brought forward to account for the ascites. Among them may be mentioned the following:—that the solid tumors rest upon and compress the superior vena cava; that the peritoneum is irritated and the lymphatics blocked; and that early metastases in the liver press upon the portal vein. Emphasis should again be laid upon the fact that the presence of ascites does not always mean malignancy.

Ovarian tumors are not infrequently complicated by pregnancy, even when both ovaries are the seats of new-growths. The effect of pregnancy on the rapidity of growth of a benign tumor is not marked, but numerous authors have stated the belief that malignant changes in such tumors are more frequent when pregnancy becomes associated with the condition. Torsion of the pedicle is common under these circumstances; Williams stating that it is three times more frequent when a pregnant uterus is present than when this organ is empty. This accident happens more frequently among multiparæ than among primiparæ, in the early than in the late months, and in small than in large tumors. It may also occur during the puerperium. Rupture of the cyst is also more frequent when pregnancy co-exists.

Abortion sometimes results; more frequently, however, the patient goes on to term, when there may be a normal labor, or delivery may be impossible.

TREATMENT OF OVARIAN TUMORS.—When the diagnosis is made previous to the eighth month, radical operation should be done. In the ordinary case this does not interrupt the pregnancy. When the diagnosis is not made until near term, radical operation and Cæsarean section are the operations of choice. An ovarian tumor is a constant menace, not only to the health of the patient, but to her life as well. Infection, torsion of the pedicle, rupture of the cyst, or pregnancy—each one of which is a grave condition—may occur at any time. Furthermore, malignant changes in every form of tumor are sufficiently common to be the sole indication for operative intervention at an early date.

The Operation of Tapping.—In former times the tapping of an ovarian cyst was an operation that was frequently done. It is a dangerous procedure and, besides, is useless, so far as a permanent cure is concerned. If, for any reason, radical operation is refused and it is necessary to relieve the tension by letting out the fluid, it is better to do so through a small incision, made, under infiltration anæsthesia, in the abdominal wall, the cyst wall being penetrated with trocar and cannula. By thus making a small opening the relations of a tumor can be made out and much valuable information obtained. Moreover, there is less danger of introducing infection into the cyst than by puncturing skin, muscle, and fascia.

The Radical Operation.—An operation having been determined upon, a choice of two possible routes—depending upon the size, variety, and position of the ovarian growth—is open to the surgeon. Small cysts, which are freely movable or lie low in the pelvis, as well as small non-adherent solid growths, may be removed through the vagina. The vaginal operation has the advantage of being quickly performed and of leaving no abdominal scar; moreover, the convalescence is somewhat more rapid. This manner of operating, however, is applicable only to certain selected cases, while the abdominal operation, preferred by most surgeons, has the very great advantage of allowing the operator to deal more easily with unforeseen complications and to inspect all of the abdominal organs.

The Vaginal Operation.—In the preparation of the patient, the abdomen should be shaved and thoroughly cleansed, and so also should the perineum and vagina. This precaution is obligatory, because one never knows when complications which cannot be dealt with except by laparotomy, may arise during the course of a vaginal operation. As the first step in the operation, a posterior vaginal retractor is introduced, and the cervix is caught with traction forceps and pulled down to the vaginal outlet. An incision is then made through the vaginal mucous membrane, close to the posterior surface of the cervix, and by blunt dissection the peritoneal cavity is opened. One or two fingers are next introduced and the pelvic organs examined, care being taken to sweep them around the tumor and thus make sure that no adhesions exist. By hooking the finger over the pedicle, a small tumor may be delivered. In the case of a cyst, a trocar is introduced and the contents of the cyst evacuated, after which the sac may be delivered and the pedicle exposed. The latter is then clamped and severed; if small, it may be doubly ligated. The clamp is then removed and the raw cut surface is covered by a cuff of peritoneum. If the pedicle is thick, it is better to release the clamp sufficiently to allow of recognition of the separate arteries, each one of which is separately secured. After the pelvic cavity has again been explored the edges of the peritoneum are brought together, and the vaginal incision is closed without drainage.

The Abdominal Operation.—The removal of ovarian cysts was one of the first abdominal operations undertaken, and has been practised since 1809, when McDowell did his first operation. Sporadic cases were reported during the next sixty years. With the advent of Listerism, the operation became more frequent, but, in the two decades following, the mortality was very great. To-day, except in complicated cases, the mortality is practically nil. The operation is usually spoken of as an "ovariotomy"—a word, however, which is' etymologically incorrect and is rapidly passing into disuse. Oöphorectomy or oöphoro-cystectomy should be substituted.

The preparation of the patient and the making of the abdominal incision are the same as in other abdominal operations. (See the article on "Abdominal Section" in Vol. VII.) In the case of cysts the incision should be large enough to admit the whole hand; but, before the hand is introduced, the edges of the wound should be retracted and a careful inspection made of as much as can be seen of the tumor, the bladder, the uterus, the opposite ovary, the parietal peritoneum, and the omentum and intestines. Areas of hemorrhage and necrosis in the tumor, implantation growths on the peritoneum or adjacent organs, and adhesions are the lesions which should be specially looked for. The whole hand is next introduced and swept around the tumor, slowly and carefully, thus separating the very light adhesions which sometimes exist, or revealing the presence of denser adhesions. The uterus is palpated and the location of the pedicle of the tumor ascertained.

If the tumor is a solid one, or if the slightest suspicion of malignancy exists, the incision should be enlarged and the growth delivered intact. There are surgeons who insist that all tumors should thus be removed unopened; but, when the case is clearly one of a simple cyst containing a serous fluid, or of a tumor of the pseudo-myxoma-cystadenomatous type, the characteristics of both of which are usually recognized without any difficulty, this course would seem to be unnecessary.

It having been determined to evacuate a cyst, gauze pads are carefully inserted around the wound between the tumor and the cyst wall, and the assistant is directed to make pressure upward and inward by pushing upon the flanks. A trocar, one that has a lumen of at least half an inch and to which a rubber tube is attached, is thrust through the cyst wall, care being taken to avoid any blood-vessels which may be seen coursing over the surface of the cyst. The contents are allowed to drain into a basin. As the cyst walls gradually collapse, they are picked up with forceps and delivered, fold after fold, upon the surface of the abdomen. Several loculi may require separate evacuation. In this way the pedicle is in due time exposed to view and the opportunity is afforded for studying its relations. The remaining pelvic organs are closely examined, and, if they are found to be normal, the pedicle of the cyst is clamped off and severed. A portion of the pedicle—not less than half an inch in length—should, if possible, be allowed to remain.

If it be found, however, that the pedicle consists of the broad ligament, the tube, the utero-ovarian ligament, and the infundibulo-pelvic ligament, the course to be pursued will be somewhat different. If the pedicle is long and narrow, all the structures which have just been enumerated may be included in a single clamp; if they are short and thick, it is better to clamp the infundibulo-pelvic ligament, which contains the ovarian artery, separately. Catgut ligatures are next substituted for the clamps, care being taken to isolate and then separately to tie the ovarian and utero-ovarian arteries. The latter vessel is normally located in the pedicle, at a point from 1 to 2 centimetres distant from the uterine cornu, but the relations may be greatly altered. After all bleeding points have been carefully secured, the stump of the ovarian artery is sutured to the stump of the tube, and the whole is neatly closed over with peritoneum.

In case of solid growths or of cysts which it is proposed to remove unopened, the treatment of the pedicle is, of course, essentially the same as that described.

An operation like that which we have just been considering may be done with absolutely no shock to the patient, provided care be taken to prevent loss of moisture and heat from the intestinal and parietal peritoneum. This is a most important detail, and yet one which is often neglected. Next to infection a disregard of this precaution is the most frequent cause of post-operative trouble. As fast as the tumor is removed the intestines and the incision should be covered with large gauze pads wrung out of hot salt solution; and, if the operation is in any way prolonged, these gauze pads should be covered by sterile towels, also wrung out of the solution and frequently changed. This duty of keeping the intestines warm and moist should be thoroughly drilled into the assistant; by-standers should never see the bowel at any stage of the operation. The gauze pads furnished at most hospitals are entirely inadequate as regards both size and thickness. In no other operation is there greater danger of leaving pads and instruments behind in the abdominal cavity, and this is especially true in those cases in which the incision is of unusual length and the operation prolonged by complications. Especial care in this regard should be enjoined upon the one in charge of these objects. Tapes and clamps should always be attached to every pad and a careful count should be kept as well.

Before the abdomen is closed, all organs should be inspected, any fluid which has accumulated in the cavity should be wiped away, and the omentum should be carefully spread out over the intestines. The fluid which has been evacuated should be measured and its specific gravity ascertained, by which means the weight of the tumor may be estimated.

Complications of the Operation.—The most frequent complication—aside, of course, from pathological changes in other organs—is the presence of adhesions. The light attachments, resembling spider webs, which are so frequently found between the wall of the tumor and the abdominal wall may be separated by the fingers with impunity. Sometimes, however, they are so dense as to require painstaking dissection. If they can be separated only with great difficulty, it may be found impossible to avoid leaving bits of the tumor wall attached here and there to the parietes. When this happens, the lining of the wall should be removed. A Pacquelin cautery is here useful to check bleeding.

In some cases it will be found that the tumor has contracted attachments to the bowel. If, in the endeavor made to separate the two, the bowel is injured, the rent should be repaired at once, lest, in the further course of the operation, the intestinal contents escape and soil the field of operation. If the omentum is adherent it is best to tie it off at two points about 2 or 3 centimetres from the tumor, the division with the knife being made below the ties and tags of omentum that are left attached to the tumor. For the repair of the rent in the bowel interlocking sutures should be employed.

If the growth is adherent at the base of the pelvis, great care should be exercised in effecting a separation, especially in the region over the iliac vessels and

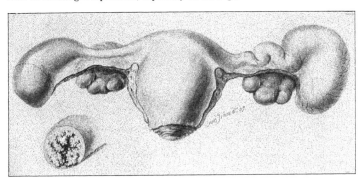

Fig. 163.—Carcinoma of the Fallopian Tube. The small figure to the left shows the appearance of a cross-section of the papillary cancer. (Case of Dr. C. C. Norris, of Philadelphia.)

ureter. If the plane of cleavage cannot be demonstrated, it may be necessary to leave behind a portion of the cyst wall. The lining of the cyst should then be removed, and, if the oozing cannot be checked by the application of very hot gauze, a tampon should be left in position, the end being carried into the vagina through an incision in the posterior fornix.

When it is found that the tumor has developed within the folds of the broad ligament, the foregoing description of the operative technique is not applicable. The removal of a tumor having a distinct pedicle and lying free in the abdominal cavity is often one of the simplest of operations. This is not true, however, when the new-growth has developed between the lamellæ of the lateral ligament. Here no pedicle exists and it is usually found that the tumor wall and the fold of peritoneum which forms the ligament are tightly adherent. Occasionally one finds, after slitting the peritoneal covering, that cleavage of the ligament may be effected and the tumor rapidly shelled out of its bed, this procedure being accompanied by almost no bleeding. This separation is usually accomplished most easily along the line where the ligament is attached to the uterus, and it is at this point that the dissection should begin, the work being continued in a downward direction. When its lower part has been freed the tumor may be readily rolled out and the more densely adherent places dealt with from below. If the uterus is spread out over the tumor, as sometimes happens, supravaginal amputation of the organ (with the tumor included) should be

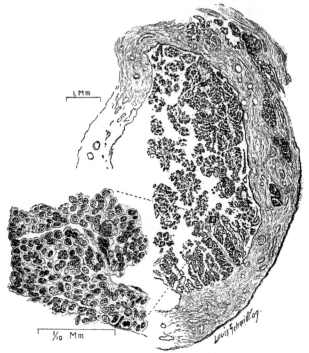

FIG. 164.—Transverse Section of the New-Growth shown in Fig. 163. Above and to the right the parts are so little magnified that one may obtain a good idea of the relations of the cellular elements to the walls of the tube and to the connective-tissue framework which supports them. Below and to the left a higher degree of magnification is shown. (From specimen removed by Dr. C. C. Norris.)

carried out. Such an amputation, which should be begun on the side opposite to that on which the tumor is placed, will enable the operator to get below the tumor and roll it out from its bed. After the removal of the growth, the folds of the broad ligament should be brought together, care being taken to obliterate the "dead space" which has been left.

If the tumor prove to be a carcinoma or a sarcoma, the opposite ovary should also be removed. In this case and in cases where both ovaries are the seats of a malignant growth, hysterectomy should be done by one of the methods described in the next article.

The principles governing the treatment of ovarian new-growths during pregnancy may be summed up by the statement that the tumor should be removed as soon after it is discovered as circumstances will permit. The operative technique does not differ from that required in uncomplicated cases except in one respect: great care should be exercised to handle the uterus as little as possible.

The Results of Oöphorectomy.—In uncomplicated cases, the primary mortality of the operation in the hands of competent men is very small; the deaths being due to such accidents as may follow any operation—*e.g.*, pneumonia, embolism, etc. The ultimate results are among the most satisfactory in surgical practice. The convalescence is usually rapid and the restoration of the patient's health complete. In the cases of primary or secondary malignancy, where there are no metastases and no implantation growths, the results are better than in cases of sarcoma or cancer of almost any other organ.

Neoplasms of the Fallopian Tube.—New-growths of the Fallopian tube are not frequent. Isolated cases of various neoplasms have been described, but, with the exception of carcinoma, they are so rare that they will not be here considered.

Primary carcinoma of the tube, while the most common of the growths found in the organ, is not often encountered, for there are less than one hundred well-described cases on record. Norris * has recently gone over the literature and he admits eighty-six cases to the list of undoubted carcinoma. Of these instances seventeen were bilateral. Cancer secondary to disease in the uterus is more frequent. It may also arise as a degeneration of a benign papilloma. Inflammatory changes, due to infection, are probably predisposing factors. In the one case which I have reported,† there was no history pointing to the existence of infection. (Figs. 163 and 164.)

The symptoms and signs are not pathognomonic, and Norris is authority for the statement that no case has been diagnosed previous to operation. The symptoms usually observed are leucorrhœa, often blood-stained, irregularities in the amount of the menstrual flow, and a variable amount of pain. The latter may be entirely absent.

Radical operation, with removal of all the pelvic organs, should be done. The ultimate results are not encouraging.

* Norris, in Surgery, Gynæcology, and Obstetrics, March, 1909.
† Schenck, in Detroit Medical Journal, May, 1905.

SURGERY OF THE UTERUS AND ITS LIGAMENTS.

By JOHN B. MURPHY, M.D., and FRANK W. LYNCH, M.D., Chicago, Ill.

I. MALFORMATIONS OF THE UTERUS.

MALFORMATIONS of the uterus are fairly common, and frequently have an important bearing upon the phenomena of reproductive life. They result from failure, or arrest of growth, of one or more parts necessary for perfect development of the organ, and the great majority occur in the early months of antenatal life. The resultant condition therefore presents a relative disproportion of the organ. In order clearly to understand the production of the uterine malformations, it will be necessary to refer briefly to the embryogenesis.

EMBRYOGENESIS.—The uterus is formed by the junction and fusion of the Muellerian ducts, which is accomplished in large part before the twelfth week of embryonal life. During the first four weeks of this period these structures are but solid cords lying in the neighborhood of the Wolffian ducts. (Fig. 165.) Occasionally they are canalized in the parts which later appear as the fimbriated extremities of the Fallopian tubes. In the second and third months they become hollow, and blend in their lower parts to form the utero-vaginal canal, the upper parts remaining distinct as the Fallopian tubes. Until the twentieth week there remain evident traces of the fusion of the two ducts, as the uterus extends laterally toward the Fallopian tubes, on each side, in the form of two cornua, and the uterus at this period is in consequence distinctly bicornuate. During the remainder of the fœtal life the change in the uterus is one of gradual development and enlargement. The two cornua gradually become merged into the body of the organ, with the result that the anterior-posterior sides of the fundus are first concave, then flattened, and finally become convex with the development of the organ. After birth, and up to the tenth year, the infantile uterus is characterized by a greater development of the cervix than the body. Thereafter, and up to the sixteenth year, a gradual increase in the relative size of the body of the uterus is noted, until finally the entire organ presents the characteristics of the adult virgin organ.

Malformations of the Uterus.—Malformations of the uterus vary in appearance in accordance with the pathological process which causes them and the period of life at which they are paramount. The great majority result from disturbances during the first four months of intra-uterine development,—*i.e.*, the embryonal period,—but they may occur later in fœtal life, or even after birth before the complete development of the organ has been attained. In general, there are three types of pathological processes which cause them, and commonly more than one have operated in any given case. These are: De-

SURGERY OF THE UTERUS AND ITS LIGAMENTS.   445

struction, or agenesis, of the Muellerian ducts on one or both sides; hypoplasia of all or part of them; imperfect fusion.

Destruction, or agenesis, of the Muellerian ducts on one or both sides gives rise to unilateral or bilateral aplastic defects of various degrees of gravidity. Hypoplasia of the ducts or of portions of them leads to rudimentary conditions of the genital tract or of some of its parts. Either of these pathological processes may occur before or after the fusion of the ducts. Imperfect fusion of the Muellerian ducts may cause a series of anomalies of development whose common feature is the duplicature of the genital tract in its uterine, or its vaginal, por-

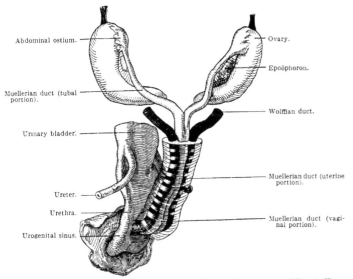

Fig. 165.—Drawing from a Fœtus 29 mm. in Length, Showing Development of Female Urogenital Tract. (From Kollmann's Handatlas, etc. Jena, 1907.)

tions, or both. The majority of the known uterine malformations are due to imperfect fusion of the ducts, associated largely or only partially with hypoplasia of limited portions of them. Two classes of malformations due to imperfect fusion of the Muellerian ducts may be distinguished. In the first class there is no trace of external division, although internally the organ is divided more or less completely by a longitudinal septum. If this division is complete the organ is termed *uterus bilocularis* or *uterus septus duplex*. (Fig. 168.) An incomplete division limited to the cervix and the external os, or to the fundus, constitutes *uterus subseptus*. (Fig. 169.) The second group of cases presents a division of the canals distinguishable externally. This division is usually situated at the uterine fundus, which presents cornua (*uterus bicornis*), or resembles the shape of an anvil (*uterus incudiformis*). (Figs. 170 and 171.) Cases may occur, however, in which the division merely gives rise to a slight incurving at the middle of the fundus (*uterus arcuatus*). When a septum extends in the uterine cavity from the fundus of a bicornuate uterus to the external os, the condition is termed *uterus bicornis duplex* (Figs. 172 and 173), and if the septum is incomplete the organ is designated as *uterus bicornis semiduplex.* In rare instances the external duplication may be complete and there may exist two ununited uteri (*uterus didelphys* [Fig. 175], and *uterus bicornis duplex separatus*). The division may or may not extend into the vagina.

We are as yet unacquainted with the exciting cause of these pathological processes. Some investigators have taken the ground that they result from the action of germs and toxins upon the tissues in the course of evolution, but of this there is no actual proof.

In a work of this character it will be unnecessary to detail all the varieties of uterine malformations, and it will be sufficient if the leading types are described in outline.

Absence or Rudimentary State of the Uterus.—Complete absence of the uterus is a very rare condition, which has thus far been described only in monstrosities.

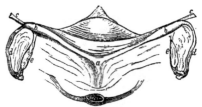

Fig. 166.—Rudimentary Uterus. (From Veit, after P. Mueller.) *a*, Solid remnant of uterus; *b*, rudimentary horns; *c*, round ligament; *d*, Fallopian tube; *e*, ovary.

It has been frequently noted in sympodial fœtuses and acardiac twins, and it is doubtful whether it ever exists in the adult woman. The condition of absence can be recognized only at autopsy or operation, as the uterus may be present at least in part, although it may not be recognizable by clinical means. When the uterus is absent, the bladder and rectum come into apposition. The vagina is either absent or but partially developed. The tubes may be absent, rudimentary, or represented only by solid cords. The ovaries also may be absent, rudimentary, or of normal size, as they develop independently of the Muellerian ducts.

On the other hand, it is not uncommon to meet with adult patients in whom the uterus is present in a rudimentary state. (Fig. 166.) The condition presents various findings, but the organ is frequently bipartite or bicornuate, or appears as a mere cord connecting the two Fallopian tubes. It is rare for the cornua to be absent while a middle portion of the uterus corresponding to the body and the cervix persists. Occasionally the undeveloped organ may contain a rudimentary cavity. The tubes and the vagina may be absent, or present: if present, they are usually in an undeveloped condition. It is not unusual to find a well-formed vulva and even a short vestibular vagina which has been enlarged by attempts at coitus associated with this anomaly.

Symptoms.—The symptoms vary with the presence or absence (or at least physiological absence) of the ovaries, and are first noted at puberty and only in those cases in which the ovaries functionate. Menstrual molimina are met with and there may be a great deal of pelvic pain. There is of course no menstruation, although vicarious hemorrhages are not infrequent. The secondary sexual characteristics are generally present, although the vulvar hair may be defective.

Diagnosis.—The diagnosis may be extremely difficult, and cases in which either of these conditions is suspected should be examined under anæsthesia. The method of procedure is as follows: A sound having been passed into the bladder, the tissues which lie between the sound and the rectum are carefully palpated through the bowel. A rectal-abdominal examination is then made, in order to palpate the pelvic cavity above the level of the bladder, as the sound in the bladder reaches only to a limited height in the pelvis. By this means, we can usually determine at least one fact, viz., that the uterus is

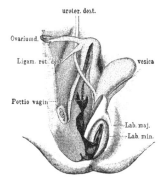

Fig. 167.—Uterus Unicornis in a Child.
(From Nothnagel, after von Winckel.)

seriously defective. In the marked cases no thickness of tissue can be felt between the rectum and bladder, but, when two bodies can be felt laterally without a distinct mass between, it may be impossible to say whether these are rudimentary horns or ovaries.

Treatment.—The treatment is directed only to the symptoms, as the condition per se does not demand treatment and in fact will not respond to it. When the pain at the menstrual periods is so severe as to be a menace to health, the removal of the functionating ovaries is indicated and in the great mass of cases affords relief.

Uterus Unicornis.—This condition is the result of arrest of development of one of the Muellerian ducts, with the subsequent formation of a uterus from the other duct. (Fig. 167.) The one-horned uterus has no fundus proper, as it inclines to one side and tapers to a point which is continuous with the Fallopian tube. The other horn may be absent or present in a rudimentary condition, and its Fallopian tube is usually absent. Occasionally the rudimentary horn is present and hollow for a short distance, or indeed for its whole length, but often appears only as a solid band. In examining specimens it is often difficult to determine where the horn (rudimentary or developed) ends and the Fallopian tube begins. This is best effected by ascertaining the site of insertion of the round ligament. All below this point is uterine horn, and all above it is Fallopian tube. Other failures of development are frequently noted in association with this condition. The vagina may be absent, small, or septate. The ovary of the imperfectly developed side may be rudimentary or absent; sometimes it may lie in the lumbar region. The kidney and ureter have been absent occasionally on the same side as the rudimentary horn, as the development of the kidney is closely associated with that of the generative system. Maldevelopment of the bladder also has been reported. The well-developed horn may perform all the functions of a normal uterus, as menstruation is not necessarily affected in unicorn uteri, and pregnancy may develop and pass to a normal termination. The condition will not cause symptoms if the genital tract is patent through its entire extent.

Symptoms.—Symptoms may arise only in those cases which present two tubes, one of which is in a rudimentary condition, and when the tract is occluded by reason of the retention of menstrual fluid, or because a pregnancy

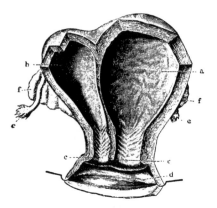

Fig. 168.—Uterus Septus, Puerperal. (From Cruveilhier.)

exists in the imperfectly developed horn. If there is no communication between the rudimentary and the developed horn, menstrual fluid may collect in the cavity of the former with the consequent production of a distended sac and pain. Pregnancy may occur in the rudimentary horn, generally from external migration of the ovum and spermatozoa, and give rise to a very serious condition. As the fœtus lies in a blind sac and cannot be extruded into the vagina, the horn commonly ruptures early, as does a tubal pregnancy. Rarely does pregnancy progress to term. If the fœtus dies in utero, the condition rarely may simulate a fibroid tumor. The continuance of irregular hemorrhages from the developed horn, and the absence of the fœtal heart may obscure the condition of pregnancy if the fœtal parts cannot be distinguished. There have been reported several such cases in which the diagnosis was made only at abdominal section. The presence of a unicorn uterus is not often diagnosed unless it is discovered accidentally during a laparotomy. When an accumulation of blood occurs in a rudimentary horn, abdominal section should be performed, and the mass removed. Pregnancy in the same location should be so treated if diagnosed.

Uterus Septus.—This is the common type of double uterus which presents no external signs of division, although internally there is a more or less complete septum which divides it into two cavities. (Fig. 168.) Externally the uterus is more globular than usual, and sometimes presents a slight grooving which corresponds to the site of the internal septum. The two cavities of the uterus are usually situated side by side, and the septum may or may not extend as far down as the cervix—uterus septus, and subseptus (Fig. 169) respectively. There may or may not be indications of duplicature in the cervix or vagina.

Symptoms.—The condition usually does not cause symptoms if both halves of the divided uterus open into the cervical canal, although dysmenorrhœa and amenorrhœa may be present, or there may be hemorrhages which recur

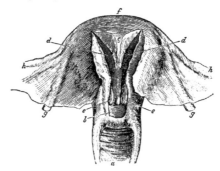

Fig. 169.—Uterus Subseptus. (From Veit, after Kussmaul.)   *a*, Vagina; *b*, single cervical opening; *c*, septum; *d*, right and left uterine cavity.

twice monthly and which have been interpreted as menstruation of a nonsynchronous type from the two uterine cavities. Unless the two cavities open into the cervix, hæmatometra unicornis will occur at puberty. This condition may be perplexing, as the statement that the patient menstruates regularly confuses the practitioner, who should always insist upon a careful examination, bearing in mind that the menstrual fluid may escape from one cavity but accumulate in the other. It is most likely that the majority of patients who menstruate during pregnancy have double uteri, and flow from the empty uterine cavity. Pregnancy may progress normally, although some believe that it is more apt to result in abortion. Malpresentations of the fœtus are common, especially breech presentations. Retention of the placenta after labor is also very frequent in this condition. During curettage the curette has been known to pass from one cavity of a septate uterus into the other, giving the sensation of perforation of the uterus.

Diagnosis.—The diagnosis of a septate uterus is usually made accidentally, although it may be suggested by the presence of a vaginal septum, or cervix with a duplicate os and a rather large, rounded uterus. A sound may easily pass into either cavity, or constantly into the same one, and thus be of no aid in effecting a diagnosis.

Uterus Bicornis.—In this condition the upper portion of the uterus is divided externally, and the cavity is in consequence Y-shaped, as the lower uterus and cervix usually contain but a single cavity. (Fig. 170.) The common cavity

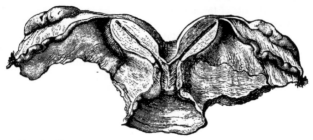

FIG. 170.—Uterus Bicornis Unicollis. (From Chrobak and von Rosthorn.)

of the uterine body is rarely further divided by an internal septum. The bicornuate uterus may have one os or two external ora, and the resulting deformity is termed uterus bicornis unicollis or bicollis, respectively. (Fig. 171.) This condition is regarded as an intermediate form between the uterus septus and the uterus duplex. Many varieties are noted, from a uterus which presents merely a slight external notching between the two cornua, to one showing a well-formed external division extending nearly to the cervix. One of the horns is commonly larger than the other, and one may be solid or partially perforate, and in the

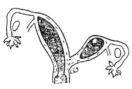

FIG. 171.—Uterus Bicornis Unicollis with Rudimentary Horn. (After J. W. Williams, Appleton & Co., 1908.)

latter case may be the seat of a pregnancy or retention of menstrual fluid (hæmatometra), just as is the unicorn uterus with a rudimentary horn. In seventy-eight per cent of the eighty-four cases collected from the literature by Kehrer in 1900, the proximal end of the rudimentary horn did not communicate with the uterine cavity.

Symptoms.—Symptoms do not result unless one cavity is obstructed and causes interference with menstruation or pregnancy. When both horns are patent, menstruation may occur simultaneously from both, or independently from each. Both horns may contain impregnated ova of different stages of development, and many cases of so-called superfœtation are thus explained, as are the curious cases in which an ovum has been expelled during the course of a pregnancy which progresses to full term. (Fig. 172.) The same complications of labor are noted as in septate uteri. Pregnancy in the rudimentary horn generally results in rupture within the first four months. Rupture of the more developed uterus is threatened when extraction of the fœtus is attempted before complete dilatation of the cervix, because the axis of the impregnated horn generally does not correspond to that of the pelvis, and the force exerted in extractive efforts is thus directed against the lower uterine segment.

Diagnosis.—The diagnosis is made accidentally, as a rule. A bicornuate uterus with one horn closed and distended may be confused with a normal uterus associated with a fibroid, ectopic pregnancy, or some other pelvic swelling. Occasionally the findings are most confusing, especially when this condition exists in a bicornuate uterus with a double cervix, as the gradual accumulation of the menstrual fluid may have forced a comparatively thin and elastic membrane downward, whence it protrudes into the vagina in the form of a cyst. In these cases a mere incision of the cyst wall suffices for treatment.

Uterus Duplex.—This condition is also termed uterus didelphys, or separatus,

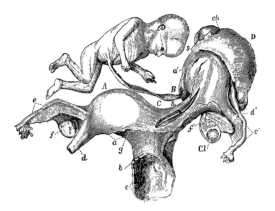

Fig. 172.—Pregnancy in a Rudimentary Horn of a Bicornuate Uterus, Resulting in a Rupture. (From Veit, after P. Mueller.)
The canal of the rudimentary horn (K) did not communicate with that of the developed uterus.

and is the most complete form of double uterus. (Figs. 173 and 174.) It is much more rare than the bicornuate uterus, and it is impossible to distinguish the two by clinical means. The anomaly results from failure of the Muellerian ducts to unite in the portions which form the body and cervix of the organ. The vagina is also septate in consequence. The two uteri are seldom of the same size and both are usually undersized. One vaginal canal may not open into the vulva, and may be the seat of retention of menstrual fluid.

Here, as in the other two double uteri described previously, the condition causes symptoms only when there is obstruction to menstruation or to the expulsion of the products of conception, due to an atresic band in one cavity. Pregnancy may develop and progress normally in case both uterine cavities open into the vagina. Giles has collected eight cases of pregnancy in one half of a uterus duplex, and two cases of simultaneous occurrence in both halves.

If there is retention of blood in the atresic half, an opening may be made by way of the cervix. When the corresponding tube is much distended, abdominal section is preferable.

Fœtal and Infantile or Pubescent Uterus.—In these conditions an undeveloped type of uterus persists, presenting a large conical cervix together with a small corpus. (Fig. 175.) In the fœtal type the cervix is usually much larger than

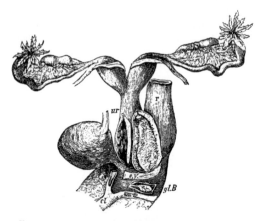

Fig. 173.—Uterus Duplex Bicornis cum Vagina Septa. (From Veit, after P. Mueller.)

the corpus, while in the pubescent form the two are nearly equal in size. The os is frequently smaller than normal. Associated with either of these conditions may be deficient development of the tubes, ovaries, and vagina. The breasts are small and the pubic hair scanty. Menstruation is usually retarded and may be most irregular; dysmenorrhœa is common, and vicarious hemorrhages may occur. Systemic disorders, as chlorosis, and stomach disorders, cardiac palpitation, and headaches, are frequent. These patients are usually neurotic. and show a marked tendency to obesity. Sterility is the rule, although pregnancy may be possible.

Diagnosis.—The diagnosis can be made by the bimanual method of examination, aided in selected cases by the use of the sound. The various types may be separated by the relative size of the cervix and corpus.

Treatment.—Treatment should be directed toward establishing the growth of the uterus. The smaller the uterus, the less is the chance of forcing development. Iron, arsenic, and nourishing foods may be useful, and in case of obesity gymnastics are indicated to bring the bodily condition to a normal standard. Various methods of local treatment have been recommended, chief of which are massage, the periodic passing of the sound, and uterine faradization. Frequently a stem pessary inserted into the uterine canal, after dilatation of the cervix, stimulates the organ to growth. It must be confessed, however, that the results as a rule are most disappointing, and the prognosis must be guarded, although it may be borne in mind that in certain instances the uterus has suddenly developed after having remained more or less rudimentary for years. These cases of delayed development, however, are unusual.

Minor Malformations.—In addition to the marked deformities already described, the uterus may be the site of lesser anomalies. The most important

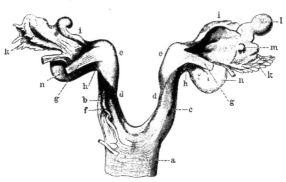

Fig. 174.—Uterus Didelphys Solidus; Front View, Half Natural Size. (From Heppner.)   *a,* Solid vagina; *b,* right, *c,* left uterus; *d,* cervical portion; *e,* body of the uterus; *f,* ovary.

of these, from a clinical view-point, are those which alter the lumen of the cervical canal. Thus, complete occlusion of the cervical canal, or atresia, may result in the retention of menstrual fluid. Fortunately, it is rarely observed in a uterus which otherwise appears normal.

Stenosis, or narrowing of the canal, may also be encountered, the constriction being either at the internal os or at the external os, although sometimes it extends throughout the entire length of the cavity.

Abnormal folds in the cervix, forming a sort of second internal os, may be found in the cavity. This condition may be mistaken for a polyp, and sometimes gives rise to hemorrhage; consequently it should be removed when recognized. This condition is normally present in the sheep.

The vaginal portions of the cervix may be rudimentary and small, but may also be elongated and conical. Uterus biforis is the condition in which a median partition divides the external os into two parts. Uterus accessorius, or trifid uterus, is very rare, and to explain its origin we must assume that one of the Muellerian ducts was originally double, and that from it developed two uterine bodies.

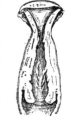

Fig. 175.—Infantile U t e r u s. (From Hart and Barbour, Keener & Co., publishers, Chicago, 1905.)

Premature Development of the Uterus.—The uterus rarely may develop into the adult type in early life. In such a condition the associated changes are not uniform in all cases, as the rest of the generative tract does not always develop *pari passu.* Usually the patient exhibits some of the general changes which are normally encountered at puberty, together with the development of some secondary sexual characteristics.

II. DISPLACEMENTS OF THE UTERUS.

The uterus forms part of the elastic pelvic floor and consequently moves up and down with it in all actions which alter intra-abdominal pressure. As the fundus lies more anterior in the pelvis than the cervix, there is a slight anterior or posterior swing of the corpus combined with descent, as the floor gives or retracts under the influence of variations of intra-abdominal pressure. Wide

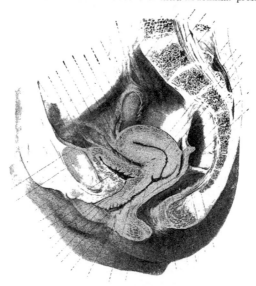

Fig. 176.—Median Frozen Section of Female Pelvis, showing Normal Anteflexed and Anteverted Uterus. (From Spalteholz, Leipzig, 1903.)

variations from a limited range are resisted by the ligaments which are inserted into the lower portion of the uterus and reinforce its lower attachments. The normal uterus therefore is anteverted and slightly anteflexed, and, in mobile equilibrium, moving with each inspiration in walking, singing, deep breathing, etc. (Fig. 176.) To a certain extent its position is altered by the distention of the bladder or rectum. Wide departures from the above have been considered pathological and described as displacements.

These displacements may be divided into three groups, as the organ is displaced anteriorly, laterally, or posteriorly. Upward displacements are theoretically possible, yet are not included in this discussion as they are almost invariably due to tumors. Formerly much attention was paid to these conditions, yet during the past few years the subject of displacements has been under revision, with the result that, at the present time, more attention is paid to the presence of associated complications than to the position which the uterus maintains.

Anteflexion and Anteversion of the Uterus.—These exist normally, and we must be extremely cautious therefore in stating that anteversion and anteflexion really constitute pathological conditions. Theoretically, the whole organ may be displaced forward, anteposition; it may be inclined forward as a whole with-out flexion on its own axis, anteversion; or it may be sharply bent forward on itself, anteflexion. These may occur together or independently.

Anteposition.—In this condition the vaginal portion of the cervix may be felt at its normal level, but displaced forward immediately behind the symphysis.

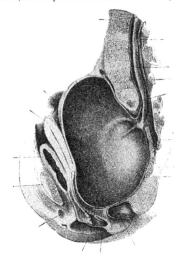

Fig. 177.—Median Section through Pelvis, Showing Anteposition of the Uterus due to Sacral Meningocele. (From Hegar, 1905.)

The fundus, in such cases, is close to the anterior abdominal wall, and, in consequence of the preceding, the vaginal vault is also displaced forward so that the vagina runs upward behind the symphysis. Not infrequently some part of the uterus may be crowded against the floor of the bladder, or the urethra, with the result that the evacuation of the bladder is interfered with, and that organ therefore becomes much distended. The common cause of the uterine displacement is generally some mass posterior to the uterus and in the pouch of Douglas, which pushes the organ forward as it develops. Among these we may mention pedunculated uterine fibroids incarcerated in the pouch of Douglas, ovarian tumors, pus tubes, pelvic exudates, etc. (Fig. 177.) The greatest displacement occurs with retro-uterine hæmatoma, or serous or purulent pelvic exudates. More rarely, the displacement is due to the retraction of adhesions between the uterus and anterior abdominal wall.

Anteversion.—Symptoms were formerly attributed to this condition, and were thought to be due to the more or less straightened uterine axis. This view is no longer held, as it is well known that the normal uterus may have but little flexion. Were this condition able to cause symptoms, we should have found them resulting from vagino-fixations, in which the uterus was firmly anchored intentionally in anteversion beneath the bladder wall. This operation formerly enjoyed great vogue in the treatment of the posterior dislocations, and its popularity was restricted only by the dystocia which uniformly resulted if pregnancy ensued; yet rarely, if ever, did the woman thus operated upon complain of symptoms which in any way could be referred to the anteversion. Anteversion cannot be considered as a special disease, but merely as one of the results of chronic metritis, which causes a thickening of the walls of the uterus. The treatment of anteversion, therefore, is merely that of the accompanying changes which are causing symptoms.

Anteflexion.—This term is used to describe an exaggeration of the normal flexion of the uterus. Yet, nearly all degrees may be found in conditions of perfect health and reproductive activity. It is impossible, therefore, to say that symptoms may result from this condition *per se*, if the organ remains movable. Formerly many symptoms were ascribed to anteflexion, but this teaching has been overthrown largely by the efforts of Schultze. We are indebted to him for advancing the view which limits the application of the term of pathological anteflexions to those cases which present lessened mobility of the organ. The condition may be congenital or acquired. Congenital anteflexion is frequently found in nulliparous women of unstable nerve control. In such cases the genitals are frequently of the infantile type. Schultze advanced the view that the congenital form depends upon the shortness of the anterior vaginal wall and a puerile development of the cervix, yet all cases do not present these findings. Acquired anteflexion commonly results from pelvic inflammation, usually cellulitis rather than peritonitis. The seat of the inflammation is usually the utero-sacral ligaments, although it may be chiefly in the parametrium. As a result of the induration and contraction of the previously inflamed bands, the cervix is drawn backward so that the broad fundus of the uterus settles lower in the pelvis and down upon the bladder, owing to the force of gravity and the greater surface of the organ which is exposed to the downward force of intra-abdominal pressure. Increased flexion, therefore, commonly results at the level of the internal os, at which point Rokitansky has shown that the connective-tissue framework is thinnest. It may, however, occur higher up.

Symptoms.—The symptoms usually complained of are dysmenorrhœa and sterility, which, it will at once be observed, are the symptoms of pelvic and uterine inflammation, and are therefore not pathognomonic of anteflexion. Many patients, moreover, who present extreme flexions do not complain of symptoms. Therefore the treatment is of the associated pelvic inflammation, and few at the present time believe that uncomplicated anteflexion should be the subject of operative procedures, as Schultze and others have shown that the symptoms of acquired anteflexion improve as the inflammatory products are absorbed, even though the flexion of the uterus remains of the same degree.

Treatment.—The treatment of dysmenorrhœa and sterility is considered in its appropriate section. For many years intra-uterine stem pessaries have been used for the purpose of straightening the uterus. Their employment cannot be justified by our present conception of pelvic pathology. Moreover, they must be regarded as dangerous because of the injury they cause to the endometrium, giving rise to irritation or abrasions of the surfaces and thus affording a portal for the entrance of infection. When stenosis of the cervix is an accom-

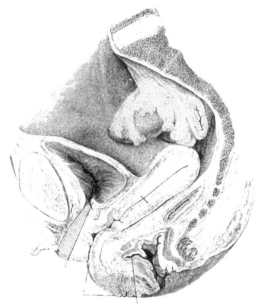

FIG. 178.—Retroverted Uterus with Descent. (From Halban and Tandler, Wien, 1907.)

panying complication, the cervix should be thoroughly dilated with or without incision of the internal os. Various operative procedures have been advocated by Dudley, Thirian, and others, which, however, we do not believe to be of value, save possibly in the treatment of sterility, as they are not concerned with the treatment of the pelvic inflammation, which is regarded as the only thing producing symptoms.

Lateral Flexions and Versions.—Lateral flexions and versions are more frequently associated with tumors or exudate. Their treatment, therefore, is also that of the associated condition.

Retroversion and Retroflexion.—In marked contrast to the so-called patho-logical positions previously described, retroversions and retroflexions are most commonly observed in multiparæ. Retroversion is a condition in which the unflexed long axis of the uterus is directed posteriorly, so that the fundus lies in the hollow of the sacrum. Retroflexion implies that the organ is bent on its own axis posteriorly. Save in a few rare conditions, retroflexions occur only in cases in which the uterus is also retroverted, and consequently the two conditions must be considered together. Descent of the uterus is generally observed in cases of posterior displacement, and is so frequent that many writers consider this section under the caption "Retroflexio-versio-descensus." (Fig. 178.) Descent results from the prolonged action of intra-abdominal pressure upon a uterus which has been so displaced that its long axis more or less coincides with that of the vagina. With this are usually combined changes which lessen the normal rigidity of the pelvic floor.

Retroflexion alone is probably less frequent than retroversion, and E. Schroeder has found it in the relative proportion of one to three, although Fraenkel found the reverse in his earlier experience. Together, however, they are noted in nearly one-fifth of gynæcological cases, constituting 17.75 per cent of the combined material of Winckel, Loehlein, and Saenger, and 18 per cent of Fraenkel's cases.

Etiology.—The causes of retro-displacements of the uterus are various, but may be congenital or acquired. We frequently and often erroneously assume it to be congenital when we find, on examination of a virgin, a retro-posed uterus, and either no symptoms, or those dating back to puberty. The organ may be enlarged and tender, or of normal or subnormal size. That it is not a rare condition is shown by the fact that Kuestner found it in 21 per cent of private and 13 per cent of clinic cases, and Hewitt in 23 per cent of his private cases. The most common of the acquired causes is undoubtedly the changes resulting after childbirth. Winter examined 300 women from two to ten months following delivery and found posterior displacements in 12 per cent. The frequent occurrence in the puerperium is undoubtedly due to the increased weight of the uterus, combined with the laxity of the uterine supports, the pelvic floor, and the abdominal wall. The condition doubtless is favored when the patient lies during the puerperium more or less continuously in the dorsal position; also by the distention of the bladder which here, owing to the laxity of the ligamental supports, is able to exert more definite pressure upon the fundus, although some—as, for example, Kuestner—deny this and adduce experiments to substantiate their view. Ordinarily, this condition is but temporary, unless metritis develops or the patient rises to go to work before normal involution has resulted, or she subjects herself to tight lacing, etc.

Next in frequency, we believe, are those cases which are due to sudden increase in intra-abdominal pressure, brought about by active exertion, as lifting, or by a sudden fall. Possibly the condition may be favored by tight lacing, especially in cases with relaxation of the pelvic floor. It is necessary to assume that, when retro-displacement results in these cases, the fundus has already been displaced to the posterior limit of its normal mobility. It may also be produced and rendered permanent by adhesions behind the uterus resulting from peritonitis; by contracting cicatrices in the anterior vaginal wall following vesico-vaginal fistula; by fibroids which have developed in the upper part of the fundus and pull the uterus backward on account of their weight; by tumors situated in the anterior uterine wall which displace the organ backward as they develop; etc.

It has been customary to describe three degrees of retroversion, yet, save for purposes of description, there is no justification either clinically or pathologically for this distinction. Once the anterior wall of the uterus is made to resist the intra-abdominal pressure, the uterine body will fall from the effect of gravity and be pushed as far backward and downward as the vagina and Douglas' pouch will permit, unless the uterus is maintained in a fixed position by peritoneal adhesions and the strength of its ligaments.

Symptoms.—The symptoms of retroversion depend not only on the displacement of the uterus, but also upon the complications in the individual case. There is no doubt that the symptoms of uncomplicated retrodisplacement are less marked than those presenting complications. In fact, the view has constantly gained ground within the last few years, that uncomplicated retrodisplacements cause no symptoms. Winter reports that, in 36 cases which were noted from two to ten months after labor, 11 had no symptoms, and only 4 of the remaining 25 had symptoms which could be referred to the displacement. Of 90 other cases under treatment for retroversion, 84 presented complications (as metritis, etc.), which were considered as the actual cause of their complaint. With a view of determining the relation that existed between displacement and symptoms, he examined 710 apparently normal women. Of these, 154 (22 per cent) had posterior displacements, yet 60 per cent of them complained of no symptoms referable to pelvic disorders. In 1900, E. Schroeder investigated this subject in Winter's clinic in Koenigsberg. His material comprised 411 cases, 82 of which were from the gynæcological polyclinic, 184 from the obstetrical, and 145 from the medical clinics. Posterior displacements were found in 118 (or 28.7 per cent) of these; 303 of his total cases presented no symptoms referable to the pelvis, yet 79 cases (or 26 per cent) had posterior displacements; 108 cases complained of symptoms in the lower segment of the abdomen, and posterior displacements were found in 39 cases, or 36 per cent. He concludes, therefore, that about 25 per cent of women who complain of no symptoms referable to their pelvic organs have posterior displacements. Theilhaber and others have adduced similar views.

Yet the fact remains that very frequently one or more of the following symptoms are given by a woman in whom the only demonstrable departure from the average normal condition is the backward displacement of the uterus: a bearing-down feeling, weakness or pain in the back and groins, menorrhagia, metrorrhagia, dysmenorrhœa, leucorrhœa, tendency to abortion, sterility, weakness or pain in the lower limbs. Neurotic phenomena—headache, neuralgias, dyspepsia, etc.,—are often found. In those cases in which considerable blood

has been lost anæmia is present. *When careful physical examination has eliminated all other etiological possibilities, we are justified in treating the displacement.*

Diagnosis.—The diagnosis should be made by the bimanual examination. Through the vagina the cervix is felt low down in the pelvis. It may point in the axis of the vagina, or forward, depending upon the presence or absence of flexions. By the bimanual examination the fundus cannot be felt forward between the fingers of the two hands, but will be found posteriorly in the pelvis. If retroflexion is marked, the fundus frequently can be palpated through the vagina or rectum, lying backward in the cul-de-sac of Douglas. Care must be taken to exclude the following conditions: fibroid of the posterior uterine wall; prolapsed and enlarged ovary; ovarian tumors; a dilated and pro-lapsed tube; exudates in the pouch of Douglas; utero-sacral or perirectal cellulitis; and especially fæces in the rectum. The sound should not be used except in rare cases and only after antiseptic preparation and exclusion of pregnancy. These possibilities having been excluded, an attempt should be made to ascertain whether the uterus is fixed or movable, *i.e.*, whether it can be replaced or not. For this purpose the rectal examination is most important, especially if done in the knee-chest posture, and while the cervix is pulled down by a tenaculum. The presence of adhesions may be suspected if there is much pain in the lateral fornices and the uterus is but slightly movable, but it must be remembered that there is frequently restricted movement without adhesions, when the uterus has fallen so far backward as to be wedged between the thickened utero-sacral ligaments, or when there are adhesions of one or both appendages, or thickening and cicatrization in the broad ligaments. More-over, long and extensive adhesions may be present without interfering with the mobility. Not infrequently are we surprised on opening the abdomen to find unsuspected adhesions between the posterior surface of the uterus and neighboring parts. Considerable variation may exist in size and consistency of the organ. Frequently it is large and boggy, although not uncommonly, and especially in the cases which present no adhesions, the uterus is of normal size and consistency.

Treatment.—The cases logically divide themselves into several groups, and may be classified from the standpoint of accompanying inflammatory changes, associated with or not characterized by loss of support of the pelvic wall. The only drawback to this classification as a basis for treatment is that, as we have before stated, the presence or absence of adhesions cannot always be determined clinically in a given case. Although there are many of the more recent investiga-tors who believe that there are no symptoms from simple retrodisplacements, we believe it is good practice to correct the deformity, when there exist symp-toms which cannot be attributed to other findings, or which do not disappear after systemic treatment.

The treatment may be medical or surgical, depending not only upon the ana-tomical findings in the individual case, but also upon the patient's condition of life. As a rule, medical treatment should be given a trial. The therapeutic test of determining whether the symptoms are relieved by local treatment and

uterus is an extremely rare condition. Indeed, spontaneous reduction is not out of the question, even when, adhesions exist, since they often become softened and stretched and occasionally disappear without any treatment. Spontaneous reduction is rendered possible by an eccentric hypertrophy of the uterus, owing to which the anterior wall grows more rapidly than the posterior, and, emerging above the pelvic brim, eventually draws with it the rest of the organ. (Fig. 180.) There is no doubt, however, that this favorable outcome results less frequently in true retroversions than in the cases which also present retroflexion, as, when the fundus is prevented from rising into the abdominal cavity by contact with the sacral promontory, the cervix becomes displaced forward and upward with the advance of pregnancy, even above the symphysis pubis, and serious symptoms supervene. (Fig. 181.) The common cause of abortions in this complication during the third month of pregnancy is incident to pathological changes in the decidua, resulting from endometritic alterations induced by the circulatory disturbances which may accompany posterior displacements. If, therefore, we subject all cases to manipulative procedures in order to avert the risk of such a rare complication as incarceration, we shall undoubtedly cause many abortions needlessly, as it is only fair to assume that the great majority of the displaced uteri contain decidual tissue which presents some deviation from the normal as a result of the pre-existing circulatory dis-

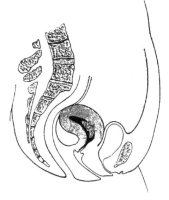

FIG. 182.—Retroflexed Puerperal Uterus, Showing Placental Remnants on the Anterior Uterine Wall. (From Martin und Jung, 1907.)

turbances,—a deviation, however, which may not be sufficient to cause abortion, unless aggravated by the trauma of manipulative procedures.

The treatment of retrodisplacements of pregnant uteri of less than three months affords a field for the use of careful judgment, and cases should be cautiously selected for various procedures. The knee-chest position and careful attention to the bladder and rectum suffice, as a rule, to aid Nature in producing a spontaneous reposition. The knee-chest posture should be persisted in faithfully, night and morning, for gradually increasing periods, until finally the patient is able to maintain it for twenty minutes; it should always be followed by the Sims posture. During this course of treatment all heavy work should be interdicted. If incarceration is threatened, persistent efforts should be made to secure reposition by the methods above advocated (Fig. 183); indeed, the inducement of abortion may rarely be necessary. Laparotomy may be indicated in severe incarcerations when reduction cannot otherwise be secured. (Fig. 183.)

5. *Retroversion of the Movable Uterus when Pelvic Inflammatory Symptoms are Present, but when the Ovaries are not Especially Painful nor Prolapsed.*— Such cases should be treated with ichthyol and glycerin tampons, and after the symptoms of inflammation subside the uterus should be restored to ante-position and a pessary introduced; later, operative measures may be adopted.

6. *Retroversion of a Movable Uterus when Pelvic Symptoms are Present, and Where one or both Ovaries are Prolapsed and Tender.*—These are generally very troublesome cases to deal with. Pessaries should not be employed until a

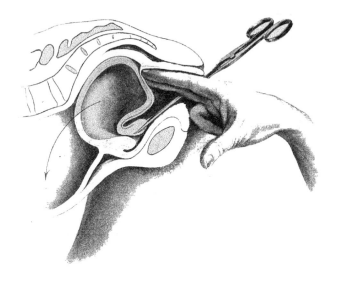

Fig. 183.—The Drawing Shows Manner of Reducing an Impacted Pregnant Uterus in the Knee-Chest Position. (From E. Bumm "Grundriss zum Studium der Geburtshuelfe," 1903.)

thorough course of glycerin tampons and vaginal douches has been tried sufficiently long to reduce all inflammation. Even after this is accomplished and the uterus replaced, it is often difficult to select a suitable pessary. If the prolapse of the ovaries is marked, the majority of pessaries will exert pressure upon them so that the patients complain of pain when walking and are not able to endure them. If the Hodge, the Albert Smith, or the Thomas pessary made with a thick-rubber end cannot be borne without pain, a soft rubber ring should be tried. Failing in this, one should resort to operative procedures, if the symptoms continue.

B. Treatment of Cases in Which Retroversion is Complicated
by Adhesions and Fixation of the Uterus.

It is readily seen that in this class of cases the treatment should be directed
rather to the pelvic inflammatory condition than to the malposition of the uterus,
which in the majority of cases is a secondary and conservative condition brought
about by Nature's effort to wall off the inflammation in the pelvic cavity and
prevent extension of the original infection into the peritoneal cavity. When
the inflammation has been reduced the correction of the displacement may
be considered. Two plans of treatment are given: palliative and operative.

Palliative Treatment.—Tampons should be inserted every other day into
the posterior vault of the vagina. These are best given, medicated with from
ten to fifteen per cent of ichthyol in glycerin. The patient should be instructed

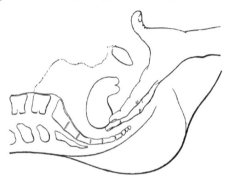

Fig. 184.—First Step in Bimanual Reduction of a Retroflexed and Retroverted Uterus. (From
Veit's "Handbuch der Gynaekol.," 1897.)

to remove the tampon, by means of the string attached to it, at the end of
from eighteen to twenty-four hours and to take a vaginal douche of one gallon
of water medicated with lysol, formalin, or boracic acid. The douche should be
taken twice daily, while the patient is lying on her back, and as hot as can be
borne. Sometimes a douche is of great value when given by means of an enema
syringe, by which a stream can be thrown intermittently into the vagina, as
originally advocated by Emmett, although usually it is best given from a metal
irrigating can. If, after a six-weeks' or three-months' trial of the tampon and
douche treatment, the uterus cannot be restored to its normal position, operation
should be strongly advised.

Method of Replacing the Displaced Uterus.—A most convenient method
of replacing a retroverted uterus is by the bimanual manœuvre of Schultze.
After the rectum and bladder have been emptied, the patient's clothing is
loosened and she is placed in the dorsal position, with the thighs well flexed on
the abdomen, the legs on the thighs, the pelvis slightly elevated, and the trunk
flexed just above the pelvis. Two fingers of one hand are inserted into the vagina

and are then used in elevating the retroverted uterus as high as possible by pressure through the posterior vaginal wall. (Fig. 184.) The fingers of the other hand then depress the abdominal wall until their tips are hooked behind the fundus, which is pulled forward while the internal fingers are quickly shifted from the posterior to the anterior vaginal vault, pressing the cervix and lower uterine segment back as the fundus is pulled forward. (Fig. 185.) To assure himself that the position is good, the physician then grasps the fundus and body between the internal fingers and those on the abdominal wall. (Fig. 186.) Sometimes it is necessary to make the fundus describe a semicircle from the sacrum to the symphysis as it is brought forward, this result being effected by rotating the uterus upon an anterior-posterior axis instead of the transverse. This manœuvre can be more easily effected if a tenaculum is first applied to

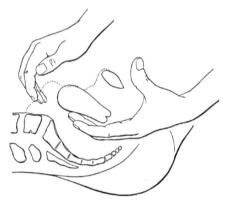

Fig. 185.—Second Step in Bimanual Reduction of Retroflexed and Retroverted Uterus. (From Veit's "Handb. der Gynaek.," 1897.)

the anterior cervix and traction exerted, which brings the uterus lower in the pelvic axis and at the same time straightens out the angle of flexion and brings the fundus into easier reach. (Fig. 187.) The fingers are then introduced into the rectum, and the fundus is pushed forward so as to cause anteflexion, when it can be easily reached with the fingers of the abdominal hand. This manœuvre is best effected in a woman with a thin, lax abdominal wall and capacious vagina. The employment of an anæsthetic may be necessary in those patients who are fat or who cannot relax completely.

A more satisfactory method, which is applicable to a larger percentage of cases, is the employment of manipulation in the knee-chest posture. After preparation, as in the first method, the vagina is distended to allow the entrance of air. Frequently this distention of the vagina will cause the fundus to fall forward, especially if the cervix is tilted toward the sacrum by a finger pressed into the vagina, or while traction is made upon a tenaculum inserted into the anterior lip of the cervix. In some cases it is necessary to use recto-vaginal manipulation to displace the fundus from the sacrum. (Fig. 188.) Great force should not be attempted with either of these manœuvres. There are on record many cases in which the rectum has been perforated by the finger during such procedures.

No attempts at replacement of the uterus should be made if adhesions or inflammatory or other swellings are present in the pelvis. The recommendations of Schultze and others that adhesions should be broken by bimanual manipulation under anæsthesia should be strongly condemned on account of the blind trauma which may excite hemorrhage or infection, the extent of which cannot be ascertained until symptoms develop.

Fitting of the Pessary.—The patient should lie in the lithotomy position.

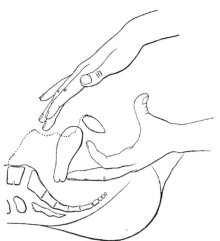

Fig. 186.—Reduction of Retroflexed and Retroverted Uterus. (From Veit's "Handbuch der Gynaekol.," 1897.)

The finger is then introduced into the vagina as far as the posterior vaginal vault and the distance between this point and one 2 cm. from the external urinary meatus is measured while at the same time the width of the vagina is estimated, so that a pessary may be selected which roughly conforms to the length and breadth of the vagina. (Fig. 189.) Frequently the instrument first selected will not be found suitable. The pessary is most easily introduced with the wide posterior bar more or less parallel to the long axis of the vulva. Prior to the insertion, the perineum is strongly retracted downward by a finger of the left hand, so that the pessary may be introduced without impinging on the sensitive areas about the urethra. The instrument is now held by the anterior bar and inserted until the posterior bar comes in contact with the cervix, when the instrument is rotated transversely, so that the posterior side curve comes to point upward. (Fig. 190.) Two fingers are now introduced into the vagina, and, while one elevates the cervix, the other pushes upon the posterior bar and carries it into place in the posterior vaginal fornix.

A pessary acts by stretching the posterior vaginal walls, and, by slightly

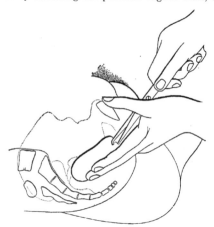

FIG. 187.—Reduction of Retroverted Uterus with the Aid of a Tenaculum. (From Veit's " Hand-buch der Gynaekologie," 1897.

elevating the fornix, compensates in a measure for the relaxed utero-sacral ligaments. It does not correct a displacement, but merely holds the uterus in the faulty position which it occupies. Diligent care must be exercised to have the uterus well forward when the pessary is introduced. The pessary should

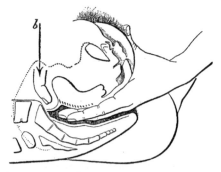

FIG. 188.—Reduction of Retroverted Uterus by Recto-Abdominal Manipulation. (From Veit's "Handb. der Gynaek.," 1897.)

not forcibly distend any part of the vagina, or abrasions and resulting inflamma-tion will follow. Frequently the instrument first selected will prove unsuitable, and others may then be tried. It should give no symptoms of its presence, nor interfere with coitus. Immediately after a pessary is inserted, the patient should walk about for some short distance in order to see whether there are any unpleasant symptoms resulting from the presence of the instrument. The next day the patient should be examined again to see whether the position of the instrument is good, and six weeks or two months later it should be taken out, cleansed, and replaced. This should be done at the same intervals as long as the instrument is worn. Frequent douches for cleansing purposes should be advised.

It is needless to say that pessary treatment is indicated only in cases in which the vaginal outlet is strong enough to retain a pessary. Many cases with so-called relaxed vaginal outlet are unable to retain any save a ring pessary, and the treatment of these cases eventually narrows down to operative procedures. It must be remembered, however, that this latter type of cases are most apt to have symptoms, and many emphasize the fact that the symptoms in association with retroposition of the uterus without inflammatory changes, may be due to the tugging upon the broad ligament of a uterus working its way down into the outlet. Sometimes an operation which restores the relaxed outlet relieves both the discomforts and the tendency to prolapse, although the flexion persists. Yet, we believe that it is better practice, if an operation is necessary, to do both at one sitting.

OPERATIVE MEASURES.

Operations for Retrodisplacements.

Symptoms associated with retroversio-flexio and descensus uteri are generally met with during the child-bearing period. Consequently, if the woman is capable of becoming pregnant the operation must leave the fundus not only anteverted, but so movable that it may rise in the abdominal cavity without great difficulty in case pregnancy supervene. In no field of surgery has there been so much controversy as to the choice of operation. Nearly one hundred and twenty-five have thus far been described and many procedures are interdicted only because of the dystocia which has arisen in pregnancies that have followed. Generally speaking, there are three chief methods of retaining a displaced uterus in the normal position: (1) by shortening the round ligaments; (2) by suspending the uterus from the abdominal wall; or (3) by fixing it to the vagina.

(1) **Operations for Shortening the Round Ligaments.**—*Alexander-Adams Operation.*—This is the oldest of the operations which enjoy vogue at the present time, and was first described in 1840 by Alquie, of Montpellier, France, who performed it only upon animals and in the dissecting room and never upon the living woman. It was not early accepted, as the commission from the Académie de Médecine, composed of Baudelocque, Bérard, and Villeneuve, which was appointed to consider it, condemned it *in toto*. The first to attempt the operation upon a living woman was De Neffe, in 1864, but it was a complete failure, as neither ligament could be found. Adams had practised and taught the operation on the cadaver to his classes previous to February, 1862, when he

first performed it unsuccessfully on a living woman. To Alexander belongs the credit of first performing it successfully in November, 1881. The operation, therefore, is frequently called the Alquie-Alexander-Adams operation, and its design is to pull the uterus forward by traction exerted on the round ligaments, applied near their insertion outside of or in the inguinal canal. This operation has obtained immense popularity, largely on account of its low mortality in the early days of antiseptic surgery, when the opening of the peritoneal cavity was rare and was quite apt to be followed by septic infection. It has not caused serious dystocia in resulting pregnancies. Its employment has been attended

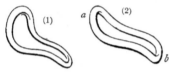

with a large proportion of failures, and many believe that its use should be restricted, for both theoretical and practical reasons. It is at once apparent that the application of this operation is confined to such cases as present a movable uterus, without adhesions. We have indicated that there are many who adduce evidence to show that simple uterine displacements without adhesions do not cause symptoms, and it appears

FIG. 189.—Two different Types of Pessaries. (1) Smith's pessary; (2) Hodge's pessary. The end a lies against the posterior wall of the vagina, with the concavity resting against the portio vaginalis of the cervix uteri; b lies in the introitus vaginalis, with the concavity directed backward. (From Veit's "Handbuch der Gynaekologie," 1897.)

that the propriety of surgical interference in this group of cases is at least debatable. We have already alluded to the difficulty of determining the exact condition of the pelvic contents even by examination under ether. The most expert frequently find, upon opening the abdomen, conditions which they failed to recognize in the previous physical examination; this is particularly true in regard to adhesions. Tubal accumulations of fluid are also frequently overlooked, especially when the quantity is not sufficient to cause tenseness of the sac wall. There is always the chance, therefore, if we use this operation to correct "simple" displacements which should not cause symptoms, that we have overlooked the true cause of the trouble through errors in diagnosis. The usual operation is not applicable to such cases as present prolapse of large and tender ovaries which also demand suspension.

The operation is contra-indicated in the larger group of cases in which the displacement is complicated by inflammatory changes, as it does not permit of their treatment; it is designed only to correct the least important of the possible pathological findings. Alexander himself states that the most suitable cases are those in which displacement is not complicated by other lesions; but his opinion that the operation may be also performed when complications exist, in the hope that improvement may follow, is not shared by the majority of trained workers in the field. This leaves but a restricted field for its employment, and, unfortunately, there are other factors which limit it still further. The patient must not be obese, or there may be much difficulty in finding the ligaments, nor should the operation be elected in those cases in which the uterus is large and heavy, as the round ligament is not always of strength sufficient to bear the strain imposed upon it, and quite frequently appears as an atrophied cord. Moreover, the method is not applicable to cases with marked uterine descent combined with an inherent weakness in the pelvic floor. Therefore this operation should never be performed unless the peritoneal cavity has been opened and the condition of the pelvic contents ascertained.

Technique.—As the operation is performed at the present time, the various stages are as follows:—The patient, when anæsthetized, is placed in the lithotomy position in order that the displaced uterus may be corrected by bimanual manipulation; the vagina is then firmly packed with one long strand of dry gauze to hold the uterus elevated. The patient is then placed in a dorsal position and an incision is made from the pubic spine outward in the direction of Poupart's ligament, one inch above and parallel to it, just as in a modern hernia operation. The incision is continued through the skin, subcutaneous fat, and superficial fascia, down to the fibres of the aponeurosis of the external oblique. All bleeding points are carefully compressed or ligated with catgut. This

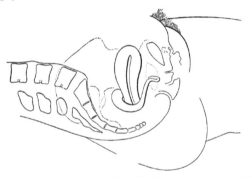

Fig. 190.—Pessary in Situ. (From Veit, "Handbuch der Gynaekologie, 1897.)

is most essential, and upon it the success of the operation may depend, as, if the wound is not kept dry, it may be very difficult to distinguish the round ligament even when it is exposed. When the glistening fibres of the external oblique aponeurosis are seen, the fat should be detached from it throughout the length of the incision and laterally for 1 or 2 centimetres. The external ring is now located just above the spine of the pubes, and its pillars are caught up with hæmostat forceps, preparatory to their section. Incision should be made through the intercolumnar fibres, and the parallel fibres of the external oblique muscle should be retracted so as to expose the canal for one inch. The round ligament, with its distinct corrugated vessels, is thus brought into view, turning obliquely with the nerve and vessels over the lower pillar. If it is not seen, the outer border of the internal oblique muscle should be rolled upward and in toward the median line, as the round ligament normally lies on Poupart's ligament, just within and beneath the outer border of this muscle; it is recognized by its glistening sheath. Should there be much difficulty in finding it, the internal ring is located and the ligament sought for there, as sometimes the ligaments do not run throughout the inguinal canal, but turn upward and outward toward the anterior superior spine of the ilium.   The guide to the internal ring is the epigastric artery, which curves around its inner border. Usually the ligament can be located by pulling upon the tissues in the bottom of the canal, or by tracing the ilio-inguinal nerve upward toward the internal ring.   When the ligament is found, the nerve is drawn to one side, and the ligament pulled down until the reflexion of the peritoneum comes to view. The peritoneum is then detached from the ligament by means of a gauze sponge, and the ligament is drawn out until it is sufficiently shortened.   The peritoneum is then opened sufficiently to admit the index finger, the position of the uterus

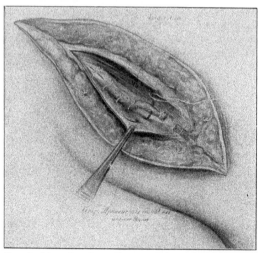

Fig. 191.—Alexander-Adams Operation.   Exposure of the canal and fixation of the round ligament.   (From Doederlein und Kroenig, "Operat. Gynaekol.," Leipzig, 1905.)

is ascertained, the pelvic floor and organs are carefully palpated, and the opening is closed with fine catgut.   The ligament is usually drawn out 8 or 10 centimetres. As tension increases, the color changes from a paler to a pink hue.   When both ligaments have been drawn out sufficiently they are sutured through half their substance to Poupart's ligament by four or five stitches of catgut; or the operation may be completed by performing the Andrews operation for hernia—closing the inner layers by imbrication, and passing the sutures which attach the internal oblique to Poupart's ligament through the round ligament to fix it firmly and to obliterate the canal.   (Fig. 191.)   The nerves should not be included in these sutures.   It may be convenient to pass a single silkworm-gut suture through the skin of one side, next into the pillar of the ring of the same side, thence through the centre of the ligament at its point of emergence, and finally into the pillar of the ring and into the skin of the side of the wound opposite to that in which the needle was introduced. The loose end of the ligament is cut off or folded upon itself, or passed across through the fat anterior to the recti, and the end secured with the suture on the opposite side. The wound is then closed in layers.

The operation may not be without difficulties. Frequently the cord cannot be drawn out because of adhesions in the inguinal canal or in the peritoneal cavity. Occasionally the cord is poorly developed or atrophied, when it may be broken by careless manipulation, especially if it is held up with forceps. If it should be broken, the ring should be opened in order to discover the upper end of the ligament. Absence of the cord has been reported in a few cases, yet it is doubtful whether these reports are entirely correct, as a thin cord may so

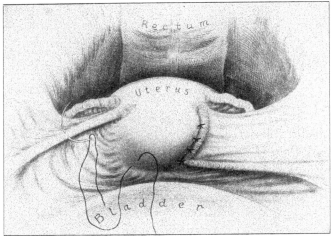

Fig. 192.—First Step in Coffey's Round- and Broad-Ligament Plication.   (From *Surgery, Gynæcology, and Obstetrics*, Oct., 1908.)

easily be frayed by careless dissection as to be unrecognizable; these difficulties are practically all produced by careless work. In a small percentage of cases the canal of Nuck is patent from the interior ring to the pubes, and the round ligament is so firmly embedded in the wall of the passage that it cannot be easily separated and shortened. Sometimes the problem is complicated by the presence of an inguinal hernia, in which event the ligament will be found on the hernial sac. It is a popular belief that wounds in the groin, whether for the Alexander operation or for hernia, are more apt to suppurate than wounds elsewhere; in the procedure described above, the incision is well above the fold in the groin. Suppuration should not result if the wound is prepared by sterilization with tincture of iodine and sealed with celloidin, or if the dressings are broad and are fixed not only laterally but above and below.

Silkworm-gut sutures should be removed at the end of two weeks.   If the stem pessary has been used it should be removed just before the patient leaves her bed.   The vaginal pessary, if used, should not be removed for two months, when it should be taken out and cleansed and reinserted, and should be worn thereafter for a period of a few months, with occasional removal for cleansing. Its presence is a guard against recurrence.   Hernia following the operation has been rarely observed.   The final results vary.   Noble reported one failure to secure anatomic results in two hundred cases.   Other authorities have reported results less satisfactory, some with even more than ten per cent of failures.   Pregnancy following the Alexander operation has, as a rule, given rise to no serious dystocia.   As a rule, the only complication noted during

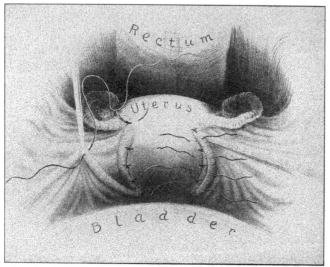

Fig. 193.—Second Step in Coffey's Round- and Broad-Ligament Plication.   (From *Surgery, Gynæcology, and Obstetrics*, Oct., 1908.)

pregnancy has been a certain tugging sensation in the groins, caused by the traction of the growing uterus upon the shortened ligaments.   This symptom has been quite annoying in some cases, and, while as yet there is no record of a large series of pregnancies following this operation, the result of those thus far recorded has been satisfactory.

Intraperitoneal Shortening of the Round Ligaments.—Because of the fact that the typical Alexander operation or its modification involving the opening of the inguinal canal is applicable only to women with normal appendages and a non-adherent uterus, various intraperitoneal operations have been devised. Mann has advocated folding each ligament upon itself in front of the uterus, so that there shall extend, from the parietes of the uterus, three folds of the ligament, carefully stitched together with non-absorbable sutures. This method has been attended with many failures. Palmer Dudley folded the ligaments anteriorly and sutured the end of the loop to the anterior surface of the uterus. Byford folds the ligaments anteriorly and stitches the loop to the abdominal parietes opposite or below, and a little above, the inguinal ring. The procedure advocated by Goffe is somewhat similar to that of Mann, save that he recommends the vaginal route.

Coffey Plication Operation.—Coffey, in 1904, described an operation which consists in the plication of the peritoneum of the round and broad ligaments upon the anterior aspect. Its various stages are well shown by the accompanying illustrations. (Figs. 192, 193, and 194.)

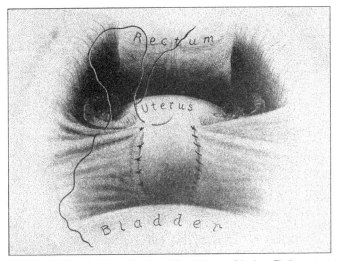

Fig. 194.—Third Step in Coffey's Round- and Broad-Ligament Plication. The ligament, on the observer's right, shows the position which it should occupy after the operation is completed. (From *Surgery, Gynæcology, and Obstetrics*, Oct., 1908.)

Technique.—The technique is described as follows:—The abdomen is opened in the midline in the usual manner. Before the operation proper is begun all adhesions are broken up and other pathological conditions are corrected. The uterus is lifted up and a gauze sponge is packed back of it. The round ligament is then seized about an inch and a half from the uterus and stitched with No. 2 chromicized catgut sutures to the antero-lateral border of the uterus, at the beginning of the vesico-uterine fold. Three or four similar sutures are placed between this point and the uterine end of the ligament, thus bringing a double fold over to the side of the uterus. The free ligament is now seized an inch and a half farther on and brought to a point just above and internal to the uterine end of the round ligament and fastened with a chromicized-catgut suture.

Three or four similar sutures are placed between this and the first suture at the vesico-uterine fold, thus bringing two more broad-ligament layers over to the side and front of the uterus. A fold of peritoneum is now brought from the side of the plication and is sutured to the uterus with fine chromicized sutures, placed by a running stitch. This continuous suture should include only enough peritoneum to render it taut, and the bladder should be carefully avoided. Care should be taken not to include the entire thickness of the round ligament in any of the rows of sutures.

Ferguson-Gilliam Operation.—Ferguson divides the round ligaments about 6 centimetres from the uterus, and sutures the proximal or uterine end to the anterior abdominal wall, perforating the aponeurotic sheath, the rectus muscle, and the peritoneum on each side of the median line, after which each end of the

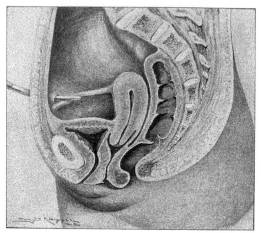

Fɪɢ. 195.—The Ferguson-Gilliam Operation; First Step—Seizing the Round Ligament.

round ligament is drawn through the abdominal wall and sutured to the aponeurosis of the external oblique. This operation has been modified by Gilliam and is now much employed under the name of the Ferguson-Gilliam operation, which is advocated by many surgeons of wide experience. The technique in this case is as follows:—The abdomen is opened and, after the other necessary procedures have been followed out in the pelvis, a long-blade hæmostat is shoved through the outer edge of the rectus muscle, as close to the inguinal ring as practicable, to emerge in the peritoneal cavity, 2 or 3 centimetres from the outer side of the median line. The round ligament is then seized and pulled out through the rectus muscle. (Fig. 195.) The peritoneum covering the lower part of the abdominal incision is now closed, and the loop of the round ligament is joined to its fellow of the opposite side and is further secured by inclusion in the running stitch which joins the edges of the divided fascia and closes the abdominal incision. Various modifications of this operation have been proposed. Thus, the round ligaments have been tied together over the muscle in a loose double knot instead of being sutured, or they may be brought through the fascia instead of under it, as proposed by Gilliam. The ligaments, instead of being pulled through the muscle, may be anchored immediately under it, as proposed by Doleris and Richelot. This operation has the merit of simplicity, and, from theoretical consideration, would appear as if it should cause no complications in pregnancy provided the uterus does not become fixed in the peritoneal wound; and yet the operation, up to the present time, has not been sufficiently tested from this view-point. Theoretical objection has been made on the ground that it divides the pelvic cavity into three segments,—one external to each round ligament and one between them,—

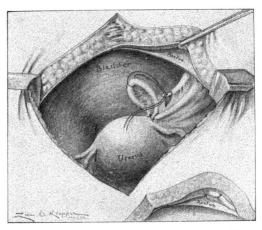

Fig. 196.—Simpson's Operation for Retrodisplacement of the Uterus.

in any one of which the bowel may become incarcerated. This has led others to devise retroperitoneal shortening of the round ligament.

Simpson's Operation.—Simpson's operation (Fig. 196) is in effect a modification of the Ferguson-Gilliam operation. It is designed to avoid the creation of new ligaments in the abdomen, by passing the doubled-up round ligament under the peritoneal covering of the broad ligament, up and through the internal ring, instead of directly upward to the superimposed abdominal wall. The abdomen is opened in the usual midline incision, and the sheath of the recti muscles is separated on each side well down toward the pubes. Whatever abdominal complications, other than the uterine displacement, are present, are then corrected. The first step of the operation is the creation of a double loop of round ligament, which may act as the suspensory band. The entire round ligament, from the uterine cornua to the internal inguinal ring, is roughly divided by the eye into three equal divisions, and the part where the inner and middle thirds join is elevated with tissue forceps and a provisional chromicized-gut suture tied around it, the ends being left uncut. The point of junction of the middle and outer thirds of the ligament is now sutured to the uterine cornua, thus leaving a doubled-up loop of round ligament, 5 or 6 centimetres long, attached to the uterus. At the end of this loop is the provisional ligature with uncut ends. The abdominal wall is next elevated rather than retracted, and the rectus fascia is freed from the muscle down to the region of the internal inguinal ring, when an aneurysm needle is passed between the rectus and its fascia, through the outer edge of the muscle, through the ring, and back under the peritoneum of the anterior broad ligament to a point at its crest near the uterine cornu. The peritoneum at this point is opened to admit the passage of the doubled-up ligament, the needle is threaded with the provisional suture,

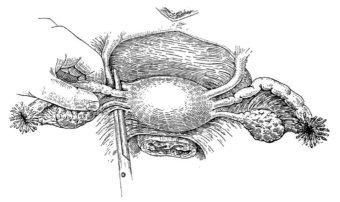

Fig. 197.—Webster's Operation. The picture is intended to illustrate the method of drawing the round ligament through the broad ligament.

and the round ligament is thus led back into the abdominal incision. (Fig. 196.) It may be necessary to strip the peritoneum from the doubled-up loop to permit its retraction. The peritoneal punctures are then closed, the round ligament is sutured to the rectus fascia and muscle, and the incision is closed in the usual manner. This operation has much to commend it, but has not been tested from the view-point of pregnancy.

Barrett makes a median incision, draws each round ligament through the opening into the peritoneum at the interior ring, and stitches it to the inner surface of the aponeurosis in front of the rectus muscle. C. H. Mayo's operation is very similar.

Webster's Operation.—Webster, in 1901, described his method of shortening the round ligaments by stitching them to the posterior wall of the uterus. He operates through the abdominal incision and first corrects any pathological conditions which are present. The uterine fundus is then raised and held toward the pubes by the tenaculum. A long forceps is now pressed against the broad ligament on one side, close to the uterus, immediately under the utero-ovarian ligament, and is pushed forward and through it, emerging just above the broad ligament and thus causing the round ligament to lie doubled on the back of the uterus. (Fig. 197.) The surface of the latter organ is scratched with the point of a knife at a spot adjacent to the attachment of the utero-ovarian ligaments, and the round ligament is then spread over this area and attached to it with a *linen* suture. The smooth peritoneal surface of the flattened ligament remains superficial. The other round ligament is then similarly dealt with, so that the two loops come in contact in the median line. The opening of the broad ligament is now carefully closed, and care is taken to cover the raw surfaces with the peritoneal mesentery of the flattened ligaments. (Fig. 198.) As a result of this procedure the uterus is slung between the round ligaments, shortened by their partial transplantation to the back of the organ. The ovaries are well elevated.

When the operation is accompanied by the removal of the tube and ovary

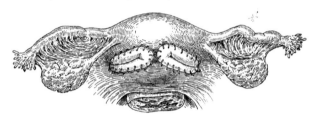

FIG. 198.—Webster's Operation Completed.

on one side, the broad ligament should be divided somewhat vertically, and the round ligament doubled back over the former, so that it may be stitched to the posterior surface of the uterus, as already indicated. If bilateral removal of the appendages is carried out this method is employed on both sides and perforation of the broad ligaments is, therefore, unnecessary. Great care should be given to the covering of all raw surfaces formed in the removal of diseased parts.

Webster does not recommend this operation in cases where the outer portions of the round ligaments are noticeably thin. In 1903 Baldy proposed to modify this method by cutting the round ligaments, drawing them through the broad ligament, and then stitching them to the back of the uterus. This plan differs from the Webster method only in one respect, viz., that Baldy cuts the ligaments and does not double them through. This method can be performed readily through the vaginal incision, although we question the advisability. Webster's operation has not yet caused serious difficulties in pregnancy, although the series of reported pregnancies is not great. It is the operation of choice when the ovaries are prolapsed.

For more than a decade one of us has recognized and taught that in retroversion the attachment of the round ligament gradually slides toward the cervix so that the dome of the fundus extends an inch or more above the level of the ligamental attachments, thus diminishing the leverage power of the ligament in holding the uterine fundus up. Any operation which simply shortens the ligaments does not restore the normal leverage power. We operate by picking up the round ligament one inch and a half from the cornu, folding it over the highest point of the fundus dome, and suturing it with catgut to the dome half an inch behind the intertubal line. The other ligament is treated similarly; it holds the uterus forward for ten years at least.

(2) **Operations for Suspending the Uterus from the Abdominal Wall.**— Olshausen in Berlin and Kelly in Baltimore, in 1886, independently reported operations for the establishment of fibrous bands between the uterine fundus

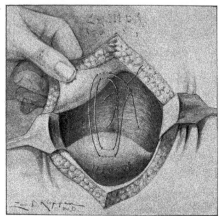

Fig. 199.—The Technique of Ventral Suspension.

and the anterior abdominal wall. Kelly's first operation was performed April 25th, 1885, and at once became most popular, owing to the ease with which it is performed. The abdomen is opened in the midline and the various pathological conditions in the pelvis are corrected before suspension is attempted, and the vaginal outlet is repaired, if necessary, in a preceding step of the operation. The uterine fundus is then brought forward and two silk sutures are introduced through the posterior fundus, each suture starting from the outer surface of the peritoneum and emerging from it to pass through the fundus, when it is continued into the peritoneum on the opposite side, so that the knot will be tied between the parietal peritoneum and the uterus. This suture should be placed at the lower angle of the wound and but a short distance above the symphysis. (Fig. 199.) The incision is then closed. It is not intended that the uterus be fixed to the abdominal wall, but merely suspended from it by the peritoneum. Consequently, as the uterus sinks down into the abdomen under the forces of gravity and intra-abdominal pressure, there is created, in the course of a few months, a suspensory ligament. On this account many claim that the operation is defective, as the ligament may stretch and allow the organ to return to its former position. Yet it must be remembered that gravity and intra-abdominal pressure will maintain the uterus in a forward position, if the accessory ligaments are sufficiently tense to prevent it falling backward past the upright position, and if the pelvic floor is of normal strength. There is no doubt that many failures have occurred because pessaries have not been used temporarily to augment the effect of the operation. These should be worn for six months after the operation, and failure to do so has caused many bad results. The operation is not advisable in case there is considerable tendency to prolapse, as the ligament will elongate beyond a point of usefulness. In such cases, if the woman is capable of bearing children, one of the intra-abdominal round-ligament operations offers more hope of cure.

In general, the results have been good, although there are about five per cent of recorded failures or recurrences. Yet, in presenting the objections to this operation, it is only fair to say that it has been more thoroughly tested than any other method for the correction of retrodisplacements, possibly more than all others combined. All of the objections to it are known, while we have much to learn of the remote effects of the intra-abdominal round-ligament operations, which appeal more strongly to us. These have not been thoroughly tested, as they have not been performed in anything like the same number of cases as the ventral suspensions. The opponents of ventral suspension rightly claim that the uterus is elevated from the pelvis and thus becomes what it was not intended for in the adult resting stage—an abdominal organ. Yet we have already indicated that if the operation is correctly performed the uterus will not remain fixed to the abdominal wall. Theoretically, there is more to fear from the creation of new ligaments in the abdominal cavity; the uterus is fastened to the abdominal peritoneum by two sutures, and consequently, as the organ sinks back, there may result two ligamentous bands, between which a loop of intestine may be caught, with the consequent complication of late intestinal obstruction. Thus Lynch, in 1903, collected ten such cases at a time when the operation had been performed doubtless many thousand times. Ventral suspension has received its greatest setback on account of serious complications which have resulted in subsequent pregnancies. The difficulty has been in limiting the amount of adhesions. The mere passage of the needle through a large boggy uterus may produce hemorrhage sufficient to cause fixation rather than suspension. The majority of cases which are operated upon for retroversion or flexion present other pathological conditions and necessitate other operations which are performed at the same time, frequently with the production of raw areas which may make it impossible to determine at the time the amount of fixation which will result. If fixation ensues and is followed by pregnancy, the uterus may be prevented from rising into the upper abdominal cavity, and serious complications may result. These approximate five per cent of all cases, with two per cent maternal mortality for cases of pregnancy thus far collected. Moreover, the results in the complicated cases have been extremely bad, as has been shown by Lynch, who, in 1903, collected from the literature twenty-one cases in which Cæsarean section was done, with a mortality of thirty-eight per cent for the mother and forty-five per cent for the child, even though several of the primary operations had been only intended for suspensions. Other observers recently have nearly doubled this list. The claim of Holden that no serious dystocia has resulted from any case operated upon in Kelly's clinic in Baltimore is somewhat vitiated by the fact that one of us had observed such a case which was operated upon in Kelly's clinic, previous to the time of his report. For

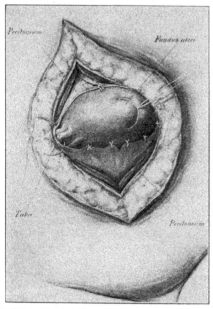

Fig. 200.—Ventrofixation, Applicable to Cases with Marked Uterine Descent, after the Patient has been Sterilized. (From Doederlein und Kroenig, "Operat. Gynaekol.," Leipzig, 1905.)

these reasons many believe that the field for ventral suspension is far more limited than is generally supposed, and some claim that it should not be performed if pregnancy can occur. Franklin Martin performs ventral suspension by attaching to the uterus a strip of peritoneum one centimetre wide, which is turned down from the abdominal wall.

Ventro-fixation may be performed if the woman is rendered or is incapable of becoming pregnant. In this operation the silk or chromicized catgut sutures may include the recti muscles in which the knot is buried, although a better technique is obtained by suturing the peritoneum to a wide area of the previously scarred fundus, which is then included in the closure of the abdominal muscles. (Fig. 200.)

(3) **Operations for Fixing the Uterus to the Vaginal Wall.**—Various methods of fixing the uterus through the vaginal incision have been introduced, but they have been followed with such grave results, in case of ensuing pregnancy, that they are no longer attempted in women capable of becoming pregnant. Formerly the operation enjoyed wide usage in cases of retroversion, but now it is performed only in certain cases of prolapse. It is sufficient, therefore, to describe the following method:—The patient is placed in the lithotomy position, the cervix is drawn down, and the anterior vaginal wall is divided mesially in its upper three-fourths. The base of the bladder is separated both from the

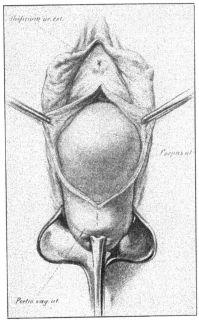

Fig. 201.—Vaginal Fixation. The uterus has been inverted underneath the bladder wall. The closure of the anterior vaginal wall is the next and final step of the operation. (From Doederlein und Kroenig, "Operat. Gynaekol.," Leipzig, 1905.)

vaginal wall and from the cervix. The peritoneal fold from the bladder to the cervix is then pushed up as high as possible and the cervix is pulled down with a tenaculum. The cervix is now pushed well back and large catgut sutures are passed through the edge of the vaginal incision, through the cellular tissue between the cervix and the bladder, and through the surface of the uterus below the peritoneum. (Fig. 201.) The remaining ununited edges of the wound are then closed with continuous catgut.

(4) **Shortening of the Utero-Sacral Ligaments.**—This procedure has been attempted for many years and is extremely helpful as an adjunct to other

operative methods in the treatment of marked retrodisplacements, yet recent results indicate that it is not of great value when performed alone. In 1893 Froemmel proposed a shortening of the utero-sacral ligaments by the abdominal route, and in 1888 Byford reported two cases in which the ligaments were shortened through the vagina. Since then it has been adopted by very many surgeons. It has been extensively employed at the same sitting with ventral suspension, when it is of great value.

The operation may be done either after abdominal or after vaginal section. If the operation is carried out by the vaginal route the patient should be in the lithotomy position. Bovée described it as follows:—An anterior-posterior incision is made through all the structures of the posterior vaginal fornix, except the peritoneum. Careful section of the peritoneum exposes the ligaments.

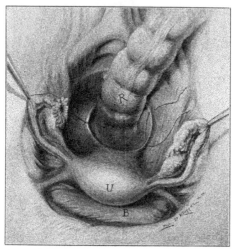

FIG. 202.—Intra-Abdominal Shortening of the Utero-Sacral Ligaments.   (Original.)

These are grasped one at a time with a forceps, midway between the extreme points to be united, and by lessening the traction on the cervix the folds of the ligament are brought into the vagina. A kangaroo-tendon suture is then passed through one ligament, and down and through the posterior portion of the cervix below the insertion of the ligament. The other ligament is treated in a similar manner, and the sutures are then tied. The incision in the vaginal fornix is closed in the transverse manner, just as if it had not been run anterior-posteriorly.

When the operation is to be carried out by the abdominal route the patient should be in the exaggerated Trendelenburg posture. The uterus is held forward and upward, thus putting traction upon the utero-sacral ligaments and bringing them more prominently into view. (Fig. 202.) A non-absorbable suture is passed from without inward through one ligament, about 2 centimetres from the uterus, and then at the same distance from the rectum from within outward. This suture, when tied, will give the necessary amount of shortening in the average case, but this must be arranged to suit the particular case. Other sutures must be employed to give neat approximation. The operation has not had extensive trial as an entity, and is best employed in connection with other abdominal operations.

III. PROLAPSUS UTERI (PROCIDENTIA).

When the uterus is displaced downward to such a degree that the cervix descends to or beyond the vulva, and the descent is accompanied by some degree of inversion of the vagina, the condition is termed prolapsus uteri, or "falling of the womb." Various grades of downward displacement, varying from simple descent to the extreme form of prolapse in which the uterus and vagina, together with a considerable portion of the bladder, lie without the vulva (procidentia), have been grouped under this heading. Properly speaking the term "prolapse" is incorrectly used, as, contrary to the older view, *the condition is, in reality, a hernia of the displaceable portion of the pelvic floor.* This is most clearly seen in the marked forms of the deformity; and anatomical studies have shown that the same fundamental principles govern the production of the various types and degrees of displacement. On account of variations in the plan of treatment, we distinguish between partial and complete prolapse.

FREQUENCY.—Prolapsus uteri is almost invariably an acquired condition and rarely has been noted as a congenital defect. It is extremely rare in women who have never been pregnant. It is rare in multiparous women who are in good circumstances and lead lives of comparative freedom from hard work. It is more common toward the fourth and fifth decades of life, possibly on account of the normal atrophy of the tissues of the genital canal and the rearrangement of the fat. The accompanying charts from Doederlein and Kroenig show the percentages of prolapsus in Doederlein's material in Tuebingen, arranged according to age and parity. (Figs. 203 and 204.) Prolapsus cases formed twelve per cent of the total material of the clinic.

ETIOLOGY.—In order properly to understand the production of prolapse, it is necessary to refer to certain features of the pelvic floor. The pelvic floor in its simplest form may be regarded as a fascial and muscular framework in which are suspended the bladder, vagina, uterus, and rectum. The structure is elastic and movable and varies in its nature, thickness, and shape, inasmuch as it closes the irregularly shaped outlet of the bony pelvis. For the most part there is everywhere a well-developed muscular layer, save immediately behind the pubes and between the two pubo-coccygeal muscles. Here the supports are practically tendinous and only slightly elastic. The area is termed the urogenital trigonum. Upon it lies the bladder, and through it run the urethra and vagina. (Fig. 205.)

The inherent weakness of the pelvic floor is due to the fact that it must permit of the complete distention of the vaginal canal in childbirth. The vagina pierces the pelvic floor at a very obtuse angle, so that the force of intra-abdominal pressure normally falls upon it at right angles and tends to close the lumen. The structure is supported by fascial and muscular attachments, the most important of which are lateral. Its fixation is assisted by its relation to

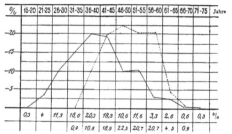

Fig. 203.—Chart Showing Age Curve in Prolapsus Uteri. Complete prolapse is indicated by dotted line. (From Doederlein und Kroenig, "Operat. Gynaekol.," Leipzig, 1905.)

the urethra, bladder, and rectum. At its upper end it is attached to the uterus, from the broad support of whose utero-sacral ligament it gains strength. The orifice is held forward by fascial and muscular fibres that spring from the posterior aspect of the pubic bones. The contraction of these muscles pulls the orifice forward and tends to close it, thus rendering the direction of the canal more nearly horizontal. The central portion of the pelvic floor is the perineal body. Here meet several important structures of which the fascial are most important. They are: the anterior and the posterior layers of the posterior portion of the triangular ligament, the rectovaginal layers of the visceral fascia, the anal

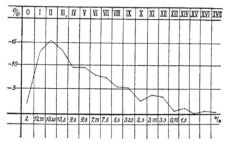

Fig. 204.—Chart Showing Prolapse Cases Arranged according to the Number of Labors. (From Doederlein und Kroenig, "Operat. Gynaekol.," Leipzig, 1905.)

fascia, the deep superficial fascia, the transverse perinei profundus muscles, small offshoots from the levator ani muscles, the sphincter vaginæ and the sphincter ani muscles.

The uterus forms part of the pelvic floor. It is suspended by the vaginal and bladder attachments, and by the broad and utero-sacral ligaments, which tend to fix the cervix and offer resistance to the force of intra-abdominal pressure. These connections are more elastic and less firmly fixed to the rest of the floor and to the bony wall of the pelvis, than the supports of the vagina, bladder, or rectum. This defect, however, is normally compensated for by the position of the uterus. The long axis of the normally anteflexed and anteverted uterus is at right angles to that of the vagina. The fundus lies close to the partially empty bladder. Increase of intra-abdominal pressure tends, therefore, to drive the fundus down upon the bladder and vagina and increase the anteversion, and thus preserves the angle between the long axis of the uterus

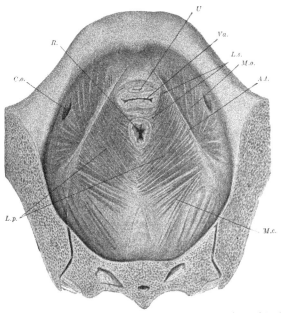

Fig. 205.—Musculature of Pelvic Floor as Seen from Above. (From Halban und Tandler, "Anatomie und Aetiologie der Genital-Prolapse beim Weibe," Wien, 1907.) *A.t.*, Arcus tendineus; *C.o.*, canalis obturatorius; *L.p.*, levator muscles; *L.s.*, margin of pubococcygeus; *M.c.*, coccygeal muscles; *M.o.*, obturator internus muscles; *R*, rectum; *U*, urethra; *Va.*, vagina.

and vagina. (Fig. 206.) On the contrary, the long axes of the uterus and vagina tend to coincide when the uterus is retroverted, so that increase of intra-abdominal pressure is apt to drive the uterus down through the vaginal canal with inversion of the upper portion of the latter. (Fig. 207.) The problem of prolapse is, therefore, more or less intimately concerned with the strength of the supports of the urogenital trigonum.

The causes of prolapse are predisposing and exciting. The exciting factor is the increase of intra-abdominal pressure. This is due to various causes, yet it is most commonly due to the strain of muscular work, involving lifting, carrying, etc. Chronic coughing may cause it, as can constriction of the abdominal wall by tight clothing. It may be due to that form of pelvic deformity which is associated with diminution of the normal angle of the pelvic inlet, which thus allows intra-abdominal pressure to act more directly on the floor.

The chief predisposing factor in prolapse is the rupture of important parts of the fascial and muscular framework of the pelvic floor. Pregnancy and labor are usually responsible. Under the influence of pregnancy, the floor softens and is displaced somewhat downward by the increased intra-abdominal pressure. Actual rupture almost invariably occurs during labor. The rupture may be at various parts of the floor, and is of varying importance. Of great importance, however, is the injury to the fasciæ and muscles which surround the lower vagina and hold its outlet forward toward the pubic bones, thus partially

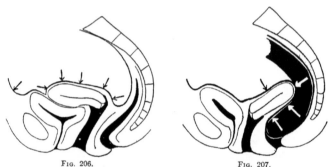

FIG. 206.   FIG. 207.

FIG. 206.—Diagram to Show the Effect of Increased Intra-abdominal Pressure when the Uterus is Anteverted. (From Halban und Tandler, "Anatomie und Aetiologie der Genital-Prolapse beim Weibe," Wien, 1907.)

FIG. 207.—Diagram Showing Effect of Increased Intra-abdominal Force when the Uterus is Retroverted, the Bladder empty. (From Halban und Tandler, "Anatomie und Aetiologie der Genital-Prolapse beim Weibe," Wien, 1907.)

supporting the urogenital trigonum. These structures in birth are invariably distended to what appears as their bursting-point, so that later they may undergo incomplete involution. (Fig. 208.) Frequently, they rupture, thus weakening the anterior segment of the pelvic floor. Rupture may occur subcutaneously and without external sign, yet it more commonly follows extensive injury of the perineum. Rupture of one portion of the floor is apt to weaken others and disturb the fixation of some of the bodies suspended by it. A pelvic floor thus weakened is commonly followed by prolapse when it is subjected to a more or less constant strain of increased intra-abdominal pressure, and especially when the uterus is retroverted. The outlet of the pelvis is no longer closed; the perineum and rectum drop downward and backward; the vaginal canal no longer runs at right angles to the direction of the intra-abdominal pressure. The long axes of the vagina and uterus tend to coincide when the uterus is retroverted. Therefore, the weakened anterior segment of the floor drops down under straining efforts and eventually the one or the other of the vaginal walls rolls out with resultant prolapse of the pelvic· contents.

Owing to the variations in the mode of life of different patients, the rupture of the supporting structures of the pelvic floor is not always followed by prolapse. In women who undergo little physical exertion, such defects may exist for a long while without prolapse, especially if the uterus is normally anteverted and involuted. Given conditions of hard work, and prolapse will result, as the floor is not sufficiently strong to resist the strain of increased intra-abdominal pressure. Prolapse, therefore, is more common among the poor.

Congenital defects of the pelvic floor may supply the predisposing factors

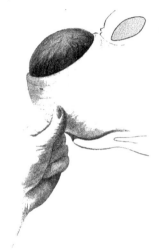

Fig. 208.—The Drawing Shows Distention of Pelvic Floor during Labor.· (From E. Bumm, "Grundriss zum Studium der Geburtshuelfe," Wiesbaden, 1903.)

for prolapse. Prochownik reports a most interesting case in which congenital defect had been present for twenty years without symptoms. Prolapse, however, followed a few months of hard physical labor.

Increased weight of the uterus from the presence of a tumor occasionally is followed by prolapse. There is frequently, in these cases, increased pelvic circulation, which in a measure causes some softening and relaxation of the supports of the pelvic floor. Subinvolution of the uterus and utero-sacral and broad ligaments is apt to cause descent. Prolapse, however, does not result unless there are structural defects of the pelvic floor.

` VARIETIES OF PROLAPSE.—The pelvic floor is rarely displaced downward, as a whole, and the more frequent condition described as prolapse is in reality a hernia of the urogenital space. All cases of this type do not present the same findings. Hernias of the urogenital space differ among themselves in several respects, and may be classified accordingly as the apex of the exciting force (intra-abdominal pressure) was chiefly applied anteriorly or posteriorly to the uterus. When the brunt of the downward pressure has been chiefly directed against the vesico-uterine space, the resulting picture varies with the extent of the prolapse. (Fig. 209.) Cases of this type are always associated with cystocele. The uterus, in incomplete prolapse, is retroverted and elongated, and the elongation may be cervical or both cervical and uterine. When the uterus is completely prolapsed it may assume either the anteverted or the retroverted position. Cystocele, however, may exist without prolapse. When the apex of the dis-

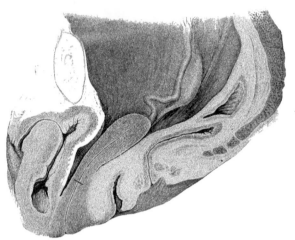

Fig. 209.—Total Prolapse of Anterior, Incomplete Prolapse of Posterior Wall of Vagina. Partial prolapse of the uterus with elongation of the corpus and cervix uteri. Total prolapse of the bladder, with cystocele. (From Halban und Tandler, "Anatomie und Aetiologie der Genital-Prolapse beim Weibe," Wien, 1907.)

placing force has been directed chiefly toward the recto-uterine fossa, the uterus is always anteverted and anteposed. No cases of complete prolapse of this type have yet been described. The uterus is elongated as a whole, or in the cervix alone, and is invariably associated with prolapse of the posterior vaginal wall. (Fig. 210.) The more extensive forms also present cystocele, yet need not necessarily do so.

Mechanism.—In the common type of prolapse, in which the apex of intra-abdominal pressure has been directed chiefly against the vesico-uterine space, we note the following points of interest in the mechanism of the condition. If we may replace the prolapsed parts, beginning first with the posterior vaginal wall, then with the uterus and the posterior vaginal wall, the parts will come down in the following order, as the patient strains:—First, appears the anterior wall and, as if dragged down with it, the uterus and posterior vaginal wall also come into view, the cervix following the axis of the pelvic curve. The uterus now becomes more and more displaced backward until, at the vaginal orifice, it lies in the axis of the vagina. The posterior vaginal wall forms a pouch, with a depth of one-half of its own length behind the uterus. Finally, the uterus becomes displaced outside the cervix, points upward and forward, and the posterior vaginal wall now becomes completely inverted. On vertical section, the following conditions would be found: First, almost complete extrusion of the anterior part of the floor, the upper and anterior part of the bladder still remaining behind the symphysis; second, complete extrusion of the uterus, which some-

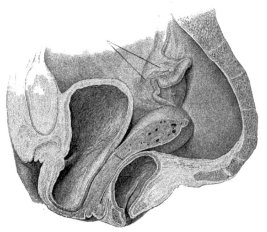

Fig. 210.—Slight Inversion of the Anterior Vaginal Wall. Total prolapse at the posterior vaginal wall. Partial prolapse of an anteverted uterus with elongated cervix. Hernia of Douglas' cul-de-sac. Beginning rectocele. No cystocele. (From Halban und Tandler, "Anatomie und Aetiologie der Genital-Prolapse beim Weibe," Wien, 1907.)

times lies with the fundus below the level of the anus; third, the rectum in position, although the posterior vaginal wall has peeled downward from its attachment to the rectum, as far as that portion which is attached immediately above the sphincter ani muscles. In the great majority of cases, the explanation of this mechanism is the following: the displacement is caused by the force of intra-abdominal pressure pushing down that portion of the pelvic floor which has lost its supports. This part consists of the entire displaceable portion of the pelvic floor, together with the uterus and appendages. Thus, if intra-abdominal pressure is excessive, the following sequence of protrusion at the vaginal orifice is apparent: first, anterior vaginal wall from below up; second, the cervix uteri; and, third, the posterior vaginal wall from above downward. The cervix, as it is forced down, follows the pelvic curve, but constantly changes its own long axis. This is frequently described by saying that the uterus becomes more and more retroverted in its downward course. The real fact is that, as the anterior portion of the pelvic floor is forced downward, the cervix is subjected to tension, with the effect of throwing the fundus back and making it rest on the adjacent structures. As these, in a general manner, coincide with the pelvic curve, the uterus thus constantly alters its axis as it descends. As a result of tension the cervix elongates.

The enlargement of the uterus is not purely cerv.cal, but may affect the whole organ. Probably this is a consequence of the prolapse and not a factor in

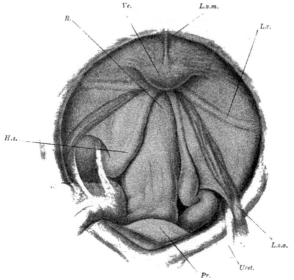

FIG. 211.—The Picture Shows the Relation of the Different Organs and Structures to one another as seen when one looks down into the Pelvic Cavity in a Case of Prolapse. The uterus is not visible. (From Halban und Tandler, "Anatomie und Aetiologie der Genital-Prolapse beim Weibe," Wien, 1907.)

Pr., Promontory; *L.r.*, round ligament; *L.s.o.*, infundibulo-pelvic ligament; *H.s.*, hydrosalpinx; *R*, rectum; *Uret.*, ureter; *Vc.*, urinary bladder.

its production. If we view a completely prolapsed uterus from above, looking through the pubic brim, it can be seen that it lies at the bottom of a depression the sides of which are formed by the broad ligaments. (Fig. 211.) The various parts of the uterus do not lie in the same horizontal plane, although the cervix lies lowest. It is thus probable that the venous supply of the uterus is interfered with, as a result of which there is venous stasis, which quite possibly accounts for the increased size of the uterus in prolapse.

SYMPTOMS OF PROLAPSE.—As might be expected, the symptoms may vary greatly. Common y, the discomfort caused by the protrusion and excoriation of the parts is predominant. The patient usually complains of something coming down in front, and there may be a feeling of dragging and of weight in the limbs and pelvis or back. Usually there is frequency of micturition on account of inability completely to empty the bladder, and occasionally there is incontinence on account of the traction on the urethral sphincter and pressure on the bladder. Symptoms of cystitis and stone may be present. Diarrhœa, or difficulty in defecating, may exist. Menorrhagia is often present, as a result of associated metritis and endometritis and venous stasis. Leucorrhœa may arise from the same cause, from endocervicitis, or from the inflammation or ulceration of the vaginal walls. As a rule, there is sterility, but conception may occur and be followed by much discomfort in the early months of pregnancy.

COMPLICATIONS ASSOCIATED WITH PROLAPSE.—We have noted, above, the increased size of the uterus; and possibly, as its result, there may be endometritis or endocervicitis. The prolapsed vaginal wall loses its rugæ, thickens. and

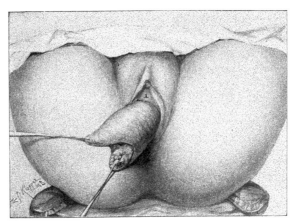

FIG. 212.—Procidentia Uteri, with Hypertrophy of the Cervix and Cervical Ulceration. (Original.)

becomes skin-like. (Fig. 212.) Frequently the cervix is infected or ulcerated. Cystitis is also not an uncommon accompaniment, because part of the bladder is prolapsed below the level of the urethra and is rarely emptied completely. It is traumatized between the symphysis pubis and the uterus and usually becomes infected. There may be calculus formations. The rectum rarely presents complications. Rectocele is rare and prolapse of the rectum is very uncommon. The uterine appendages are usually displaced downward. Plastic peritonitis may develop and form adhesions in the hernial sac and among the viscera, rendering it dangerous to reduce the hernia. Thus, Simpson has reported such a case which ended fatally.

Physical Signs in Prolapse.—It is evident that many different conditions may be found, varying in accordance with the degree of prolapse. If the condition be partial there may be nothing more than the descent, sometimes termed the first stage of prolapse. When the uterus is retroverted, which is the rule, or retroflexed, it usually occupies a lower plane than normal. The lower part of the anterior vaginal wall bulges downward when the patient is in the erect position, when she coughs or strains. The cervix lies lower than normal and may cause the posterior fornix to appear unusually deep. The uterus is enlarged and lies with its long axis in line with the vagina.

The true hernial nature of the affection is readily understood in cases of complete prolapse. The hernial sac is the peritoneum. Its boundaries are the pubes, the anterior rectal wall, the obturator internus, and the levator ani muscles. Its coverings are the bladder and the anterior and posterior vaginal walls, and its floor is the uterus. In the sac are the intestines. After replacement, prolapse recurs when the patient rises, coughs, or bears down. The uterus may be considerably enlarged, and the vaginal walls hypertrophied, ulcerated, or excoriated. The position of the bladder may be distinguished by passing into it a catheter. A rectocele may be palpated through the rectum.

DIFFERENTIAL DIAGNOSIS.—Usually there is little difficulty in making the diagnosis unless there is marked erosion of the uterus as well as some confusion of landmarks. Then the condition may be confounded with inversion of the uterus, or with a uterine tumor projecting from the cervical cavity. The incomplete varieties must be differentiated from hypertrophy of the cervix, cystocele, and rectocele.

PROGNOSIS.—When once a prolapse is established there is no more tendency to spontaneous recovery than that noted in inguinal hernia in men. The prolapse, however, may be markedly modified by pregnancy. During the first three months the uterus tends to sink lower and lower, and abortion may occur. If the position of the prolapsed parts, however, has been restored and held in place by a pessary, the uterus, as it increases in size, ascends above the pelvic brim, and then, during the rest of the pregnancy, it shows no more tendency to prolapse. After delivery, however, the prolapse is usually found to be greater than it was before the pregnancy. The menopause also exerts certain modifications upon the condition. The parts generally undergo a degree of atrophy, although the enlarged size of the cervix remains in the majority of cases. There may be some relief in symptoms. Often, however, the prolapse becomes more marked.

TREATMENT.—Prophylaxis is most important. Labor should be carefully conducted, and lacerations of the vaginal mucosa and deep muscular separations of the perineum should be repaired as early as possible. After labor the patient should not be allowed to rise from bed until normal involution is quite advanced. Tight abdominal binders should not be employed. The woman should not go up and down stairs, nor adopt a mode of life which will cause a sudden increase in intra-abdominal tension, until at least five weeks post partum have elapsed. The actual treatment of the condition, however, resolves itself into, first, treatment by pessaries or tampons and, second, operation.

Treatment by Pessaries.—When the prolapse is slight and the anterior vaginal wall protrudes only a little, an Albert Smith or a Hodge pessary (Fig. 189) may be useful, with or without the transverse bar. If there has been an extensive rupture of the deep fascia of the vagina, these instruments will not be retained and a ring pessary should be tried. This is best of hard India rubber, bent in the shape of a doughnut, with a small core and large thick sides. It is apparent at once that this method depends for success upon the distention of the upper vaginal wall to such a further extent that its inversion cannot take place. Ro_ tation of the ring often allows it to escape; this can be avoided by fixing a hard rubber tripod to its lower margin; it then becomes the best type of support. (Fig. 213.) Other types of pessaries have been recommended, usually of the ring, ball, or Zwanck type.

In some cases of procidentia there may be so much congestion and œdema of the parts that it is necessary to put the patient at rest for a few days and take measures to restore the venous circulation. Infrequently a tumor or some

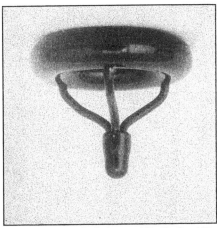

Fig. 213.—Tripod Ring Stem Pessary, for Prolapsus and Procidentia.   (After Martin, Berlin.)

other intrapelvic condition may prevent replacement. Alum injections (one drachm to the pint) and applications of boracic acid and zinc oxide to the raw surfaces are indicated for the relief of congestion and excoriation. In cases of marked prolapse of old standing, no pessary, except the tripod ring (Fig. 213), will stay in the vagina unless it is held in place by supporting bands. Operation alone will cure these cases. When operation is refused, a cup pessary attached to an abdominal or T-binder should be tried, if there is no excoriation of the cervical tissue which would contra-indicate the employment of this method. If the patient has passed the menopause, periodic packing of the vagina with gauze or oakum should be tried; and this, if thoroughly done, may hold it up for several days.

Operative Treatment.—In recent times the employment of pessaries in the treatment of advanced prolapse has been superseded by operative measures, for the reason that the condition does not permit of spontaneous recovery, but tends to become aggravated with advancing years. Moreover, treatment by mechanical means, as by pessaries or tampons, is in no sense curative; it depends upon putting the vaginal tissue upon the stretch and thus supporting the uterus. It is safe, therefore, to assume that, after a number of years of such treatment, many cases will outlive the usefulness of the method. Surgical interference, on the contrary, is curative and is attended with comparatively little risk in the hands of skilled men, even though the patient be well advanced in years. Trained men frequently operate without anæsthesia, or under local anæsthesia, thus avoiding the risk of a general anæsthetic.

Operative treatment is divided into two classes, conservative and radical,

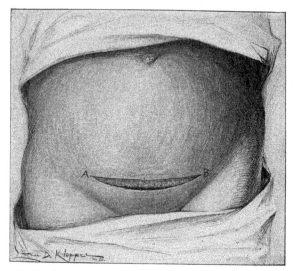

Fig. 214.—The Murphy Operation; First Step. The drawing shows the line of the semilunar incision, six inches in length and about one inch above the symphysis pubis. (Original.)

according as the uterus is allowed to remain or is removed. Conservative operations are applicable generally in cases of incomplete prolapse, while the radical procedures are usually reserved for complete procidentias, unless there is some indication for extirpation, such as is afforded by ulceration, etc. Both operations are supplemented by procedures which restore the pelvic floor and narrow the lumen of the vagina.

Conservative Operations.—The operative treatment which up to recent times has enjoyed the greatest vogue consists in fixing the uterus to the abdominal wall after a preliminary curettage, amputation of the cervix, and resection of the anterior and posterior vaginal walls. (Fig. 200.) As we have already indicated, fixation of the uterus should not be done upon a woman capable of becoming pregnant. Therefore, as a preliminary step in the operation on women who have not passed the menopause, the tubes should either be resected or a wedge-shaped portion should be removed. If this is not done and if sutures are tied about the tubes, the lumen of the tubes may later be restored and pregnancy result. Zweifel, a number of years ago, reported a most interesting case in this connection.

A woman presenting pelvic indications for Cæsarean section was operated on by the Saenger method. After the removal of the child, the tubes were tied off with silk ligatures, thus completing, as was supposed at the time, the process of sterilization. Much to Zweifel's surprise, a year or two later, she presented

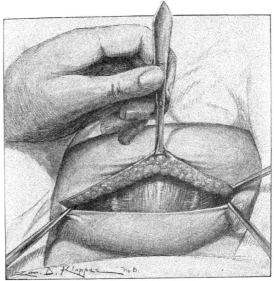

Fig. 215.—The Murphy Operation; Second Step. The drawing shows the skin and fat divided down to the aponeurosis of the recti. (Original.)

herself in early pregnancy. When she arrived at term, Cæsarean section was again performed and the tubes were removed. Microscopic examination showed that the sutures could not be located in the scar and that the lumen of the tubes had become patent. Following this case a series of experimental researches upon the integrity of the tubes following their ligation was carried out upon rabbits and other laboratory animals, and it was found in each instance that the ligature became absorbed and that the integrity of the lumen was restored by nature.

Therefore, if the tubes are to remain, a wedge-shaped area should be removed from the cornua and the gap should be closed over by plastic sutures; the ligated end of the tube should be buried in the broad ligament.

The study of chronic cases has shown that the method of fixing the uterus, as performed in this country up to ten years ago, does not lead to good results. The fixation, as a rule, is not firm and there is formed a suspensory ligament which later elongates. It is better, if this method is decided upon, to make upon the fundus a raw area several centimetres in diameter, and, around the edge of this denuded area, to fix the peritoneum with a continuous suture of catgut. Then, in closing the recti muscles, seize the scarified top of the uterus in the intermuscular suture, so that the fundus shall be firmly attached to the recti muscle. (Fig. 200.) It must be admitted, however, that the remote results of this method in unselected cases are not so satisfactory as to make it the opera-

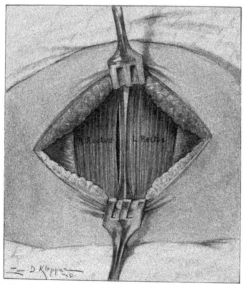

Fig. 216.—The Murphy Operation; Third Step. The drawing shows the line of incision in the rectus muscle and peritoneum. (Original.)

tion of choice for cases of complete prolapse. Not infrequently the operator finds, some years after operation, that, although the uterus is well held up, the bladder is again prolapsed.

The anterior extra-abdominal fixation of the uterus suggested and practised by Murphy is a simple and secure means of curing procidentia in those who have passed the child-bearing period. It does not necessitate a vaginal operation as an accessory. It holds the uterus, vagina, bladder, and rectum permanently up. It is performed as follows:—

The patient is placed in the Trendelenburg position. A transverse semilunar incision is made one inch above the symphysis and measuring six inches from A to B (Fig. 214). The tissues should be divided down to the aponeurosis of the recti; the latter should be freed from fat over an area one inch wide for the full length of the incision and the edges retracted, as shown in Fig. 215. The right rectus is then incised for two inches close to the median line and parallel to its long axis. This incision is extended through the peritoneum. (Fig. 216.)   The uterine fundus is then grasped with a vulsella forceps and brought out through the opening until the cervico-corporal portion is clearly in view.   The round and broad ligaments are then clamped with heavy hæmostats on either side and cut free from the uterus down to the tip of the forceps. The stumps are ligated, and the tips sewed over and displaced back into the

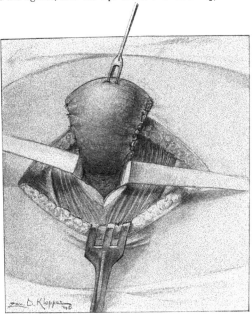

Fig. 217.—The Murphy Operation; Fourth Step. The drawing shows the uterus divested of the broad ligament on both sides down to its junction with the cervix. (Original.)

abdominal cavity, thus leaving the body of the uterus bare and free, standing above the level of the divided rectus.   (Fig. 217.)   The peritoneum is next sutured accurately around and to the circumference of the cervico-corporal portion of the uterus, thus closing the peritoneal cavity.   The uterus is then split through the middle from before backward down to the cervix.   It is opened out laterally, thus forming two wings. The mucosa is next cut off clear out through the divided cornua down to the cervix, and removed.   The two lateral flanges of uterine muscularis are then sewed firmly to the aponeurosis of the rectus all the way around, making a bat-like flange over the recti. (Fig. 218.)   Finally, the incision in the rectus is tightly closed down to the cervix.   The skin and fatty tissue are united, a small drain being left at the lower angle of the wound. The uterus can never again get back into the abdomen. The traction on the anterior vaginal wall holds the bladder in position and the posterior vaginal wall supports the rectum. The only intra-abdominal work is the detachment of the broad ligaments. The stumps of these are covered by suturing, so that no abraded surface is left within the peritoneum at the completion of the operation. If the operation is performed before the menopause, great care should be exercised in removing all the uterine mucosa, as otherwise periodic hæmatomata will form

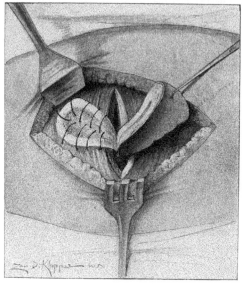

Fig. 218.—The Murphy Operation; Fifth Step. The drawing shows the right half of the divided uterus sutured on the anterior surface of the right rectus; the left half being ready for suturing. (Original.)

at the menstrual periods. The operation can be done in twenty minutes by trained hands.

The conservative operations first advanced by Fritsch and elaborated by Freund, Watkins, Wertheim, and Landau have given fair results. Freund's operation (Fig. 219) consisted in effect in closing the vaginal orifice with the inverted uterus. After separating the bladder from the cervix, the peritoneum is opened and the uterus is inverted into the vagina. It is then firmly sewn to the posterior wall of the bladder. The tubes are either removed, or a wedge-shaped area is removed from each of the cornua. The fundus is then incised to secure an opening through which the contents of the uterus may be discharged. Later, Wertheim proposed a method of vesical fixation, which, however, was advocated in this country by Watkins at least one year before Wertheim's report was published in Germany. The technique of this operation is here given in the author's own words :—

"After the usual preparations, including dilatation and curettage of the uterus if indicated, the anterior lip of the cervix is grasped with a vulsella forceps and drawn downward, and a transverse incision is made across the vagina at the junction of the anterior wall and cervix. The edges of this incision are caught with artery forceps and held taut (as shown in Fig. 220), and sharp-pointed six-inch scissors, closed, are pushed up between the anterior vaginal

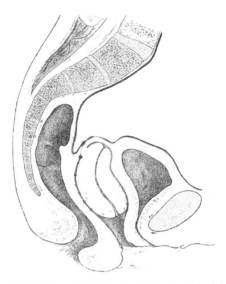

Fig. 219.—Schematic Illustration of the Freund Operation. (From Doederlein und Kroenig, "Operat. Gynaekol.," Leipzig, 1905.)

wall and the bladder about as far as to the urethral body. The handles of the scissors are now separated and the instrument is withdrawn. This generally causes enough separation of the anterior vaginal wall from the bladder. The amount of separation which this produces will vary in different cases, depending upon the size of the cystocele and the resistance of the tissues. Care is used, in inserting the scissors, to keep the points in contact with the vaginal wall in order to guard against injury of the bladder, and, in the separation of the handles of the scissors, not to use much force, for fear of tearing the bladder wall. The amount of force required in opening the handles to secure enough separation is generally very little.

"The anterior vaginal wall is incised along the median line and the edges of the flap are caught with forceps, as shown in Fig. 221. With gauze over the finger further separation of the vaginal wall from the bladder may be easily accomplished, if desired. Personally, I prefer not to make complete separation of the vaginal wall from the bladder, as such an amount of separation endangers the ureters, increases the bleeding, favors the accumulation of bloody serum in the wound, and thus increases the dangers of slight infection, which sometimes necessitates extensive plastic vaginal operations. The extensive separation of the bladder also increases the danger of exfoliation of the bladder epithelium which may follow much traumatism of the bladder wall. I have gradually been making the amount of separation of the anterior vaginal wall less, and I now generally free just enough of the vaginal wall to cover the uterine body,—except in cases of very extensive cystocele.

"With the cervix held downward the bladder is separated from the uterus

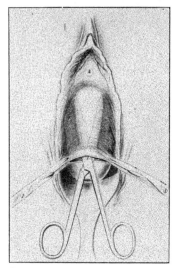

Fig. 220.—Watkins' Operation; First Step. (From *Surgery, Gynæcology, and Obstetrics*, May, 1909.)

by blunt dissection with the scissors. (Fig. 222.) The points of the scissors are kept pressed against the cervix so as to avoid injury of the bladder. They are pushed upward one-quarter to one-half inch and then opened, then a little higher and again opened, and so on until the peritoneum is reached. The peritoneum is detected as a thin membrane which moves freely underneath the finger over the anterior wall of the uterus. As long as any of the bladder wall remains attached, the tissues under the finger feel thick and fixed. I have never known the points of the scissors to puncture the peritoneum. Further separation of the bladder from the uterus is made by inserting two fingers into the wound and separating them. The amount of separation should be enough to allow the delivery of the body of the uterus. The use of blunt dissection with scissors has, in my experience, shortened the time of operation and simplified the technique. One oftener strikes the 'planes of the fascia' with scissors than with blunt dissection with the aid of gauze. Less bleeding also results.

"The peritoneum is now opened, which is not always such an easy task as descriptions would indicate. If one tries to puncture it with the finger it will at times separate readily from the bladder and broad ligaments, push on in front of the finger, and be punctured with much difficulty. At other times the finger can be readily pushed through the peritoneum. At still other times it is very easy to grasp a fold of the utero-vesical peritoneum between two fingers, pull it down, and incise with scissors. I sometimes push a blunt-pointed dressing forceps through the peritoneum and make a sufficient opening by separation of the handles.

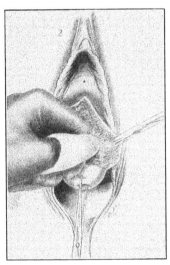

Fig. 221.—Watkins' Operation; Second Step. (From *Surgery, Gynæcology, and Obstetrics,* May, 1909.)

"The anterior uterine wall is next grasped with a single vulsella forceps inserted under the guidance and protection of the left index finger. As this is pulled downward and forward the cervix is pushed upward and backward. The anterior uterine wall is now exposed by elevating the bladder wall with an eight-inch forceps or a 'ribbon retractor,' and a second vulsella forceps catches the uterine wall near the fundus. This is repeated, if necessary, in order securely to grasp the fundus. The fundus can, in most cases, be easily delivered into the vaginal canal. One should use care not to attempt delivery of the anterior surface of the uterus, as the diameters of this are much greater than are the diameters of the fundus.

"A catgut suture is placed as shown in Fig. 223 and tied. Care should be exercised not to fix the uterus in such a manner that it will press upon the urethra, as that may interfere with urination. The vaginal opening is closed with a continuous catgut suture. The suture occasionally catches up a small bit of uterine tissue. The transverse vaginal incision is often closed in the same line of suture so as to lengthen the anterior vaginal wall and to displace the cervix further backward and upward. In cases of very large cystocele some of the vaginal mucosa is excised. If the cervix is eroded or much hypertrophied a part of it is excised before the above suture is completed, and the wound in the cervix is closed with the same suture. Occasionally one or two interrupted sutures are used in the cervix. Amputation of the anterior lip of the cervix is often sufficient for the relief of an erosion or hypertrophy. If there is any

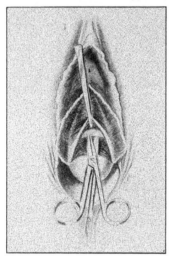

Fig. 222.—Watkins' Operation; Third Step. (From *Surgery, Gynæcology, and Obstetrics,* May, 1909.)

bleeding about the cervix this is easily controlled by catching the tissues deeply, to either side of the cervix, so as to include the vaginal branches of the uterine arteries."

In 1905 Landau proposed a new procedure for the treatment of prolapse,—one which, in effect, constituted simply an improvement of the Watkins-Wertheim method. He stated that, although the results of the various vaginal fixation methods were, in the majority of instances, satisfactory, nevertheless, in certain cases the patients complained later that the dragging sensations, which constituted the chief symptoms before operation, had returned. He noted this especially in cases where the uterus was large and heavy. He therefore proposed a method the essential feature of which is the creation of a new pelvic floor by utilizing a portion of the uterine musculature and by obliterating the cul-de-sac of Douglas, both of which results are accomplished by stitching the utero-sacral ligaments to the upper portion of the anterior vaginal wall. So far as the technique is concerned the operation is not difficult; it is performed as follows:—

After disinfection, the anterior vaginal wall is made tense, and is incised from a point immediately below the urethral orifice to one within 2 or 3 centimetres of the external os. The incision is then carried around the external lip of the cervix, the vaginal wall is detached, and the bladder is stripped back.

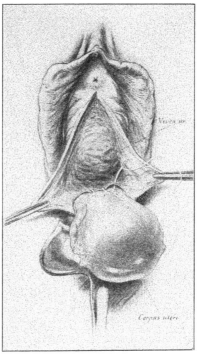

Fig. 223.—Wertheim Operation; Third Step. (From Doederlein und Kroenig, "Operat. Gynaekol.," Leipzig, 1905.)

The plica vesico-uterina is now opened and the fundus drawn forward so as to bring the peritoneum of the latero-posterior walls of the cul-de-sac within easy reach. This latter is then caught with one or two silk or linen sutures, the track of the needle also including the uterine muscles, and is fixed to the upper angle of the vaginal incision. By sharply anteflexing the uterus, the organ is brought outside the peritoneal cavity. The adnexa are next removed and the greater portion of the uterus, together with the upper portion of the vaginal wall, is resected, the cutting being done from before backward. The anterior vaginal incision is now closed, the sutures including the remains of the uterus, which thus remains firmly fixed between the bladder and the anterior vaginal wall. A high colporrhaphy finally completes the operation.

Radical Operations.—The operations which depend upon the removal of the uterus differ only in the method of attaching the remains of the vaginal fornices to the stumps of the broad ligaments. They all are supplemented by extensive vaginal resection. That which is employed at the present time is

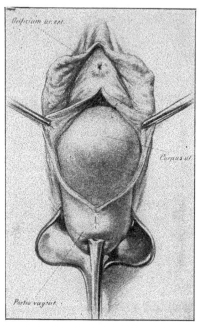

Fig. 224.—Vaginal Fixation. The uterus has been inverted underneath the bladder wall. The closure of the anterior vaginal wall is the next and final step of the operation. (From Doederlein und Kroenig, "Operat. Gynaekol.," Leipzig, 1905.)

generally done by the vaginal method, the description of which can be seen under its proper heading (page 647). After the removal of the uterus the stumps of the broad ligaments are brought down into the angle of the wound and joined together so that they are considerably overlapped, care being taken that no raw areas are allowed to remain. The vaginal incision is now closed, the sutures passing through the base of this stump. This method, as a rule, has been attended with good results, but not infrequently an inversion of the vagina has taken place, and the patient is then in worse condition than before the hysterectomy, possibly because the stumps of the broad ligaments later retracted, owing to the fact that the lumen of the vaginal wall had not been sufficiently resected.

A method which will give better results is advocated by Webster. After the extirpation of the uterus has been completed, a vertical strip of the upper part of the vaginal mucosa is removed on each end of the vaginal stump. The broad ligaments are then drawn down and firmly stitched into the raw surface of the lateral fornix. (Fig. 225.)

The opening in the peritoneum is then closed and the sutures which unite the cut edges of the vaginal wall are made to include the mar-

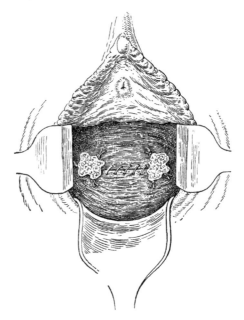

FIG. 225.—The Drawing Shows the Appearance of the Vagina after the Broad-Ligament Stumps have been Stitched into the Vaginal Vault after Hysterectomy. (After Webster.)

gins of the stumps of the broad ligaments. This operation gives excellent results. The broad ligaments by their new insertion into the vagina, act as a support of the pelvic floor. Following this procedure, the vagina is extensively resected on both the anterior and posterior walls. The after-treatment is important, inasmuch as the raw areas which are exposed in the vaginal canal are somewhat liable to infection and subsequent sloughing through the action of saprophytic bacteria. Consequently, two copious hot formalin douches should be given daily, and the woman kept at rest for ten days.

IV. INVERSION OF THE UTERUS.

Inversion of the uterus is a condition in which the uterus is more or less completely turned inside out, the inverting portion extending downward and outward toward or through the cervix. As a rule, the cervix is not involved, but remains as a collar around the isthmus of the inverted corpus. Complete inversion is a very rare condition, and many experienced gynæcologists have never seen a case. Thus, Braun and Spaeth report that not a complete inversion of the uterus has occurred during the supervision of 250,000 labors in their clinics, and it has been observed but once in 191,000 deliveries in the Rotunda in Dublin.

The process may be acute or chronic, and most often develops during the puerperium, usually shortly following labor, but it may take place in a uterus

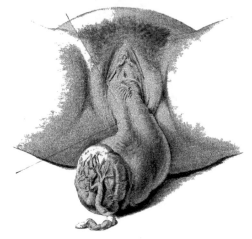

Fig. 226.—Complete Inversion of the Puerperal Uterus with Placenta still Attached to the Fundus. (From E. Bumm, 1903.)

which has a tumor attached to the fundus and enclosed in its cavity. Various degrees of inversion are described in the puerperium cases. Sometimes the deformity is merely a cup-shaped depression in the fundus, which may be pushed down into the cervix or may extend for a short distance into the vagina. It is generally believed that, in such partial cases, the predisposing factor of the deformity is a paralysis of the placental site, and that the inverted area is the portion of the uterus to which the placenta formerly was attached. In the more marked cases the fundus will be turned completely inside out and protrude through the cervix and into the vagina, or even hang outside the vulva. (Fig. 226.) Such inversion cannot result unless contraction and retraction of the uterine musculature has been held in abeyance. This may occur momentarily as a normal condition immediately after the fœtus has been expelled and while the uterus is being readjusted to the new condition. If it exist longer we must assume that there has been some factor predisposing to uterine inertia—such, for example, as too frequent pregnancies, prolonged labor, or a condition in which the uterus has been markedly distended, as in hydramnion, multiple pregnancy, etc. The exciting factor is usually due to unskilful management of the third stage, although it would appear that spontaneous inversion may in rare cases result from any of the many factors which greatly increase intra-abdominal pressure, such as straining in vomiting, coughing, etc., during or after the third stage. As a rule, however, the condition arises from traction on the cord of an adherent placenta, or from exaggerated pressure upon the

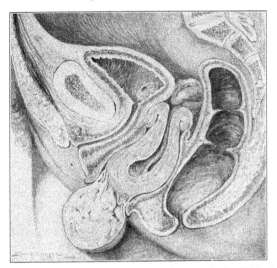

Fig. 227.—Inversion of Uterus Caused by a Submucous Fibroid. (Original.)

fundus during or following the separation of the placenta and while there is associated failure of the normal contractile forces. In 1881, Murphy operated upon a case of complete inversion, seven months after it occurred. The patient, 20 years of age, unmarried, was hurriedly delivered of an eight-months fœtus by a midwife. Great traction was made on the cord and the uterus was completely inverted and protruded from the vagina, and the hemorrhage was profuse. The midwife, not recognizing the true nature of the tumor, pushed it back into the vagina after several ineffectual efforts to pull it off. I believe that the firm fixation of the placenta to the uterus at eight months was a materially contributing factor in the production of the inversion. (J. B. M.)

It is possible to conceive of inversion occurring spontaneously if delivery occurs while the woman is standing, especially if the cord is short, although usually the cord breaks from the weight of the child and the shock of the fall. Whenever the placenta remains attached to the fundus and partial inversion occurs, we may expect that the weight of the placenta and the pressure of the intestines sinking into the inverted area will augment the descent.

In non-puerperal cases this condition generally is due to the efforts of the uterus to expel a tumor attached to the region of the fundus. In these cases the weight of the tumor produces a depression of the fundus, which, from the infiltration of the muscular tissue by the tumor growth, is no longer able to contract. (Fig. 227.) As Trent has shown, the lessened contractile ability of this portion of the uterine wall, coupled with the force of intra-abdominal pressure and the tugging of the tumor, may bring about the beginning of a partial inversion. The mass consisting of the prolapsed portion of the uterine wall and the tumor acts as a foreign body and the normal portion of the uterus is stimulated to contractions which, however, merely augment the extent of the paralysis, as this phenomenon is apt to result from contractions. The paralyzed site thus increases in area and inversion results. It is necessary, however, that the incurved circle be absolutely paralyzed to permit inversion.

In the majority of puerperal cases the inversion, whether complete or partial, is rapidly produced. Inversion due to the presence of a tumor progresses slowly. Occasionally the condition, in a puerperal case, may require several days for its development, although almost always there are symptoms during the period of development.

SYMPTOMS.—The characteristic symptom in both puerperal and non-puerperal inversions is hemorrhage, immediate and secondary. This is usually sufficient to cause marked anæmia. Aside from the hemorrhage, the other symptoms depend on the extent of the inversion. There may be no symptoms whatsoever save a slight hemorrhage in the incomplete inversions. When the inverted fundus reaches the cervix, the patient may complain of distress in the lower abdomen and back, and dragging and bearing-down pains in the pelvis, although sometimes there are no symptoms In cases of complete inversion, there may be a sensation as if something had given way, accompanied by severe pain, hemorrhage, and collapse. The patient may complain of the sensation of a mass in the vagina and of a marked desire to urinate; sometimes retention of urine occurs. Very rarely is complete inversion produced without any signs or symptoms. If the case is later complicated by infection, the signs and symptoms of sepsis develop. Chronic inversions present symptoms such as menorrhagia, metrorrhagia, leucorrhœa, backache, inability to stand for a considerable period or to make exertion while in the upright posture, bearing-down pains, and other pelvic complaints. The patient always becomes weak and anæmic. Reflex and neurotic symptoms may develop.

DIAGNOSIS.—The diagnosis is usually determined by palpation aided by inspection. If the inversion has not passed through the cervix, the finger introduced into the vagina may be passed into the cavity of the uterus up to the point where it meets the depressed area. When both hands are employed, the one placed upon the abdomen feels the cup-shaped depression at the site of the fundus. A sound cannot be passed into the uterine cavity to the normal distance. Advanced cases generally present a tumor mass either in, or projecting from, the vagina. As a rule, the rim of the cervix may be outlined, and occasionally the finger may explore the circumference of the inverted uterus, although this is unusual. The condition is easily recognized if a red and bleeding, rounded tumor protrude through the cervix as through a collar, and fill the vagina, while at the same time a depression, corresponding to the site of the fundus, can be felt by the hand placed on the abdomen. When there is a placenta resting upon the tumor mass the diagnosis is positive. When the abdominal wall is so thick that the bimanual examination is unsuccessful the pelvis should be palpated through the rectum. If a sound which has been placed in the bladder can be palpated above the tumor mass by the finger introduced into the rectum, we may conclude that inversion exists. The appearance presented by the inverted uterus varies according to the stage at which this condition is noted. Thus, in a recent case, if the tumor is covered by the placenta, it will present a smooth and glistening appearance, while if the latter has been removed the surface will be red, soft, raw, and bleeding. Clots may be seen at the mouths of the large sinuses, and sometimes the openings of the Fallopian tubes are visible. Later, when the vessels have been constricted by the cervical cuff, the inverted area becomes dark and swollen from engorged vessels and œdema. If the condition becomes chronic, the inverted mass may present the appearance of being covered with vaginal epithelium; it may lose its glands and become firm and hard, inasmuch as the uterus may undergo puerperal involution even in the inverted position. Ordinarily, however, the surface appears as if the exposed mucous membrane was œdematous and hypertrophied. When the inversion has resulted from a tumor attached to the fundus, traction upon the tumor often pulls down the point of attachment to the fundus and exposes the inverted fundus. The appearance presented by the tumor and the sensation which it conveys to the palpating finger are in sharp contrast to the conditions noted in the adjacent uterus, especially if there are sloughs on the surface of the tumor from the impaired circulation of the prolapsed uterus.

Differential Diagnosis.—Inversion may be confused with uterine polyps which extend down into the vagina, but is differentiated by a digital examination of the normal fundus. If the polyp is associated with inversion of the uterus, the character of the growth may be suggested by the polypoid shape observed when the growth is pedunculated. In case it is sessile the differentiation may be more difficult, and an examination with the aid· of an anæsthetic should be made in order to determine the depth of the depression in the fundus. Rarely is inversion confounded with prolapsus uteri.

PROGNOSIS.—The prognosis, if inversion of the uterus is left to nature, is very unfavorable. Instances of spontaneous replacement are on record, but are extremely rare. Death from hemorrhage or sepsis must be anticipated if replacement is not effected. Croisie has collected 400 cases with a mortality of 35 per cent. Of 109 fatalities, 72 died within a few hours and the majority within half an hour. Eight died in from one to seven days, and six in from one to four weeks. Crampton, from 120 collected cases, obtained a mortality of 32. There were, however, only 7 deaths in 104 chronic inversions. Statistics show that if the inversion is not reduced, the danger, after the first month, is slight, but increases again with the resumption of menstruation, which is often hemorrhagic.

TREATMENT.—The treatment naturally differs accordingly as the case is recent or chronic. In recent cases the uterus as a rule can be easily replaced. If the placenta is still attached to the uterus it is generally advisable to defer its separation until reposition has been effected, because the contractile function of the inverted uterus is in abeyance, and there is great risk of profuse hemorrhage if the placenta be removed at this stage.

Reduction by Taxis.—In carrying out taxis, the patient should be anæsthetized, after the bladder and rectum have been emptied. One hand is then placed on the abdomen, for the purpose of steadying the cervix, while the other grasps the inverted uterus and pushes it up, reducing the inversion in the inverse order of its occurrence, and following the axis of the pelvis. Many recommend that better results may be had by first starting to shove up the uterine wall at a point near the cervix, while the hand, through the abdominal wall, attempts to enlarge the cervical ring. Should these attempts fail, the patient should be kept in bed on a low diet for several hours, hot antiseptic fomentations being applied to the uterus; then manipulation, under strict antiseptic precautions, should again be attempted. If these efforts fail, on account of the tightness of the constricting cervix,—which is usually the case when they fail,—division of the cervix should be accomplished in the median line, in order to facilitate reduction. Division may be made anteriorly or posteriorly, or indeed in both of these places. The uterine wall must be handled gently in all manipulations, lest it be torn, perforated, or injured. It is always well after reposition to tampon the cavity for forty-eight hours and give ergot.

In chronic cases, before any attempt at replacement is made, the patient should be kept at rest in bed for a few days, with the hips elevated. If the inverted uterus does not extend beyond the vulva, a sterilized Braun's bag should be distended in the vagina each day. In rare cases this may be sufficient to cause reduction. If it fails, an attempt to secure the desired result may be made by taxis, under anæsthesia. When the hand becomes tired from pressing the fundus, pressure may be exerted by means of a cup and stem attached to a spiral, which is supported against the operator's chest. Bynne, White, Aveling, and others have devised such instruments. If partial reposition only can be obtained at one sitting, the patient should be put to bed and a colpeurynter again placed in the vagina to prevent the partial reduction already gained from being lost. Emmet proposed, in such cases, to close the cervix with wire sutures over the partially reduced uterus. When manual manipulation fails to replace the uterus, continuous slight pressure may be applied through a cup and curved stem attached by means of elastic bands to an abdominal belt. A pad soaked in an antiseptic ointment is first placed in the cup to prevent injury to the inverted fundus. Success has been achieved with these various appliances, but the result is always problematic, and the method, even though it is unattended by marked danger, should never be attempted in complete inversion. The chronic inversions are best treated by operation.

Reduction by Operative Measures.—Various operative procedures, varying from simple division of the cervix to abdominal section and vaginal hysterectomy, have been advocated. Of these, division of the cervix is the least formidable and should often succeed. The cervix is split in the median line, posteriorly, and the incision is carried higher on the internal than on the external surface, thus almost completely severing the contracted ring without opening the peritoneal cavity. Hirst, who recommended this operation, succeeded, after thus splitting the cervix, in reinverting the uterus by exerting comparatively little pressure on the lower segment, just below the uterine angle of the wound. When reduction cannot be accomplished by this means, a free incision may be made into Douglas' pouch and the peritoneal cavity packed off with gauze. The median incision in the cervix is then continued upward sufficiently far to permit the reinversion of the uterus. The cervical incision is now closed. If it extends too high up to permit closure *in situ*, the fundus of the uterus is brought down sufficiently far into the posterior colpotomy wound to permit of careful closure. The peritoneum is then closed off and the vagina sutured. It is probably better to drain the cul-de-sac with a small gauze pack.

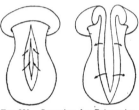

Fig. 228.—Operation for Reinversion of the Uterus. (From Kuestner.)

Kuestner's method of operation is as follows:—A wide transverse incision is made into the cul-de-sac, and any adhesions present are separated with the finger. The posterior uterine wall is then opened in the midline, beginning 2 centimetres below the inverted fundus and extending to within the same distance of the external os. (Fig. 228.) The uterus is reinverted by fixing the cervix with the finger in Douglas' pouch and pressing the fundus in and upward by the thumb of the same hand. The uterine incision is closed with deep and superficial sutures applied from the peritoneal surface, as in the preceding operation (Hirst's), and the vaginal incision is closed in the same manner. Excellent results may be obtained by either of these methods. For a résumé of the literature of the subject the reader is referred to the paper of Oui, in the *Annales de Gynécologie*, 1901.

V. FIBROIDS OF THE UTERUS; UTERINE FIBROMYOMATA.

A uterine fibromyoma is a benign, circumscribed tumor which develops in the wall of the uterus. It is composed of muscular and fibrous tissue in varying proportions and contains blood-vessels, lymphatics, and probably nerves. Fibromyomata are rarely single, and may be found in large numbers. These tumors are also known as fibroids (fibroma, myoma, leiomyoma, hysteroma lævecellulare, etc.). The terms fibromyomata, fibroids, and myomata are often used interchangeably, and will be so used in this article.

FREQUENCY.—Fibromyomata are generally regarded as the most common neoplasms in the human body, yet it is difficult to estimate their frequency, because many of them present no symptoms. Varying percentages have been given by different authors. Thus, Bayle states that they occur in twenty per cent of all women over thirty-five years, and Klob that they are present in forty per cent of all women over fifty. The proportion which causes symptoms is much less. In the records of 1860 autopsies made at St. Bartholomew's Hospital, Champney found them present in eight per cent. Haultain found fibromyomata in eight per cent of 2,230 gynæcological patients in the Edinburgh Royal Infirmary. Herman reports that 7.5 of his female patients over thirty-five were afflicted with them.

AGE.—Fibroids may develop at any period of life, but rarely are observed before the twenty-fifth year. Pick, Anspach, and others have described them in newborn children. Sasaki has noted one case of large multiple growth in a girl of nine. Gusserow has described one at ten, one at fourteen, one at sixteen, three at eighteen, and eight at nineteen years. Tillaux reports a case of fibroid of the cervix, in a girl of nineteen, which had caused symptoms for six years. Roger Williams has analyzed 100 cases and found that the average age at which symptoms develop is thirty-seven and one-quarter years. Schroeder states that, of 196 cases, 104 were between forty and fifty, and 62 were between thirty and forty years.

ETIOLOGY.—We have little definite knowledge concerning the etiology of this form of tumor, although the majority of investigators believe that they are congenital. Yet it is difficult to determine what part heredity plays in their production. There are frequent instances of fibroids occurring in members of the same family, but these must be looked upon more as coincidences than as examples of cause and effect, for, as may readily be seen, a growth which constitutes eight per cent of all gynæcological cases, or which exists in from twenty to forty per cent of women past middle life, will be described very frequently in large families in which the family life history is well known.

There is, furthermore, a dispute as to the site of origin and the factors which predispose to the growth and development of the tumor. The site of origin has been ascribed chiefly to two sources, viz., the blood-vessel walls and the uterine muscle. There is, however, almost unanimity of opinion among the more recent investigators in ascribing the origin to the blood-vessel walls. Virchow's opinion that they develop from the uterine muscle stands almost alone. It would appear that Roesger first directed the attention of investigators to the possibility of the origin from the blood-vessel wall. Because of the absence of the adventitia in the smaller arteries of the small fibroids, he came to believe that the tumors originate in the longitudinal or cross muscle-bands of the arterial wall. Gottschalk regarded the starting-point as the very tortuous part of certain arteries of the uterine wall. He found the lumen of some vessels considerably narrowed at certain points or else entirely obliterated, and concluded that such a corkscrew-like section of an artery constituted the nucleus of a fibroid, about which the growth developed. Kleinwächter, in studying small nodules, thought he could recognize in the band connecting a fibroid with the normal uterine tissue, an obliterated capillary, and stated that the origin of muscle-cell formation could be recognized surrounding the vessel. Pilliet states that the adventitia gives rise to a zone of embryonic cells which develop into the concentric rows of muscle fibres. The outermost of these are transformed into fibrous tissue from lack of proper nourishment. Bishop says that, although some tumors may arise from embryonic remains (adenomyoma), the majority are derived from blood-vessels, and in favor of this view he adduces the fact that, in the ordinary hard fibroids, there is usually only one connective-tissue pedicle through which blood-vessels enter the tumor. He, moreover, calls attention to the fact that when calcification occurs it always begins almost at that part of the periphery which is farthest away from the blood supply; also that, if the vessel supplying any nodule becomes thrombosed, the entire nodule softens and liquefies, leading to the formation of a cavity into which surrounding nodules tend to project. Furthermore, he states that the whorled appearance is strongly suggestive of a vascular development, inasmuch as the majority of uterine vessels are markedly convoluted.

There is considerable discussion as to the factors which predispose to the growth of the tumor. Sexual irritation is about the only cause which has been admitted, although even this has been denied by many. The advocates of this theory attempt to prove that fibroids are more common in women who have not borne children, and they advance the view that the uterine muscle which has been denied the opportunity of physiological hypertrophy in this manner, is prone to the pathological development of musculo-fibrous tissue as a result of sexual stimulation. Yet the subject of the relation of sterility and fibromyoma must be approached carefully, and statistics must be cautiously considered. From the evidence before us at the present time and from extensive experience with women belonging to the religious orders, in whom uterine fibroids are very common, it is our conviction that sterility is a great predisposing cause of fibroids, and that fibroids are not so common a cause of sterility as is generally believed. The theory just advanced leaves unexplained the occurrence of fibromyoma in young women and women who conceive early and frequently.

GROWTH OF UTERINE FIBROIDS.—As a rule, uterine fibromyomata grow slowly and steadily, and the greater the relative proportion of fibrous tissue, the slower the growth. Variations, however, are noted. Schorler concluded, from the observation of eighteen cases in Schroeder's clinic, that a fibroid tumor will not attain a size sufficient to be recognizable on examination in less than three months, and may not be much larger at the end of a year. It will reach the size of a man's fist at the end of five years, while at the end of thirteen it may be as large as an adult head. Yet Kleinwächter, from the observation of forty cases, concluded that Schorler was dealing with tumors of unusually slow growth, and that commonly they develop more rapidly. Uterine fibroids increase rapidly in size during pregnancy and often decrease during the involution of the uterus in the puerperium. The majority also diminish in size following the menopause, although they often grow rapidly in the years immediately preceding this change. Thus, Bland Sutton, in 1903, found that, in ten per cent of the cases requiring operation, the women were in or near the menopause. It was formerly believed that many growths atrophied and disappeared following the climacteric, yet this belief is now questioned, as many grow rapidly immediately after this period. Spontaneous atrophy of a fibromyoma is extremely rare, either in the involution of the puerperium or at the time of the menopause. Cases supposed to be of this nature have been reported, yet there is always the possibility that there was a mistake in the diagnosis, or that the growth was submucous and was expelled from the uterus.

Sudden increase of size is not rare and is usually due to œdema from some disturbance of the local circulation. Even in pregnancy, œdema is largely accountable for the apparent growth. The advent of certain degenerations also causes increase in size. The size of the tumor may vary during menstruation, and this is especially true of adenomyomata, which are swollen and congested at this period. Rest in bed frequently will cause diminution in the size of a tumor which is swollen from some circulatory disturbance.

The tumors are usually small, but may occasionally attain enormous size. Rarely, however, do they weigh more than forty pounds. There have been recorded a number of cases in which the weight was between eighty and ninety pounds. McIntyre has reported one in which the tumor weighed 104 pounds. The largest tumors on record are the following: one reported by Stockard, who observed, in the case of a negress, a tumor that weighed 135 pounds; and one recorded by Hunter which weighed 140 pounds when separated from a body which, after the removal of the tumor, weighed but 95 pounds. The larger tumors are almost invariably cystic.

CLASSIFICATION.—Fibromyomata may be classified from several standpoints. Histologically, we may group them according to the predominant tissue of their composition. Thus, those tumors in which the smooth-muscle elements predominate are termed myomata, in contrast with the fibromata, or those in which the fibrous tissue is in excess. When the component tissues are both well represented the growth may be termed a fibromyoma. Practically, however, this classification is not observed by the clinician, who uses the terms myoma, fibroid, and fibromyoma interchangeably. The growths containing glandular tissue are termed adenomyomata. Fibroids are also classified according to their situation either in the body of the uterus or in the cervix, and both the latter classes may be subdivided according to their location in the wall of the uterus or their relation with the peritoneum or mucosa. All of these tumors, in the beginning, are situated in the body of the uterine wall. As they increase in size they expand in the substance of the wall and remain there, or else spread toward one of the two surfaces (peritoneal or endometrial) and become subperitoneal or submucous. Hence, we have three chief varieties—interstitial or intramural, subperitoneal or subserous, and submucous. (Fig. 229.) This classification is an artificial one, as we must remember that practically all fibroids are inter-stitial in their beginning, and it may be difficult to say just at what point a growth becomes either subperitoneal or submucous. Thus, some—as, for example, Gusserow—would limit the term subperitoneal to those growths which are invested in peritoneum and hang in the abdominal or pelvic cavities upon a definite pedicle. This suggestion, however, has not obtained adoption. Growths, in their development, may extend to and through the outer periphery of the uterus, and still not become covered with peritoneum if they develop on the lateral uterine wall and between the folds of the broad ligament. This type of tumor is termed intraligamentous. Subperitoneal, intraligamentous, and

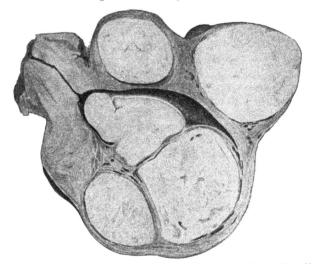

Fig. 229.—Multiple Intramural Subserous and Submucous Fibroids of the Uterus. (From Martin und Jung, Berlin, 1907.)

submucous tumors may also be classed accordingly as they are sessile or pedun-culated, although the latter may represent the later stage of development.

The cervical tumors may be classed like those of the uterine body, although the terminology of tumors which develop on the periphery of the cervix varies according to the structures with which the growth comes in contact. Thus, in addition to the subperitoneal and intraligamentous forms, we may recognize subvesical tumors—i.e., tumors which develop under the bladder, and fibro-myomata of the vaginal cervix—i.e., tumors which grow downward into the vagina. Finally, we may classify the tumors according to the degenerative and pathological changes which they have undergone. These degenerations will be considered in a later section.

For the sake of convenience we will describe, first, the tumors which arise in the body of the uterus, and will consider separately the comparatively rare forms which are cervical in origin. Adenomyomata also will be considered separately.

Fibromyomata Arising in the Body of the Uterus.

Subperitoneal Fibromyomata of the Body of the Uterus.—These tumors originate in the uterine wall and grow outward toward the peritoneum. At first they are sessile, and attached to the uterus by a broad base. Later, if the outward growth continues, they become pedunculated and are attached to the uterus by a stump of uterine tissue in which run the nutrient vessels of the tumor. The subperitoneal pedunculated fibroids vary in form, but are usually roughly spherical or ovoid. The form is dependent in a manner upon pressure from contiguous structures. The tumors are usually multiple, and of small size, yet occasionally they attain considerable dimensions. Thus, Spencer Wells described one that weighed thirty-four pounds. The outer surface of the growth is covered with peritoneum which has extended over from the uterus in the growth of the tumor. As a rule, the peritoneum is rather firmly attached to the fibromyoma. The vascular supply is generally scanty and varies according to the size and component structure of the tumor and the character of the degenerations which may be present. The length of the pedicle varies considerably, as does its thickness. The range of movement of the tumor depends largely upon the length and thickness of the pedicle. Subperitoneal tumors vary considerably in the location and direction of their growth. Quite commonly they develop from the fundus, and, if the pedicle is stout and thick, they grow upward. They may, however, grow from other parts of the wall and extend in any direction. Subperitoneal tumors may grow laterally into the broad ligament. They may lie in the pelvis, having developed there primarily, or may fall into the cavity on account of the comparative weakness of the pedicle; this is especially true of fundal growths which first develop upward. Various changes may take place in the uterus as a result of the growth of pedunculated subperitoneal tumors. The uterus may become elevated and elongated, and finally, in the large tumors, present itself only as the continuation of the pedicle.

Various complications arise from injury to the pedicle. Torsion or twisting of the pedicle may occur in tumors with long pedicles, although much less frequently than in ovarian tumors. The resulting changes vary according to the number of turns the tumor makes, the tightness of the twist, and the suddenness with which the torsion is accomplished. In the milder forms there are congestion and œdema due to disturbance of the venous circulation, and the tumor may even be distended with blood. The arteries are less liable to compression on account of the thickness of their walls; yet the blood-vessels of the pedicle usually become thrombosed in the later stages of this complication. Very rarely, the tumor becomes separated from the pedicle and lies free in the abdominal cavity. More commonly, however, it will be found that, as a result of the congestion and œdema, adhesions have formed between the tumor and some of the neighboring organs, prior to the division of the pedicle. Blood-vessels may develop in these adhesions, especially if the latter extend, as they usually do, to the omentum, and the tumor then becomes parasitic. Parasitic tumors of large size have been reported. Sometimes the uterus itself is the seat of torsion, especially if that organ has been so thinned by the traction incident to the upward growth of the tumor, that it really has become the pedicle of the tumor. Torsion of 120 degrees or more has been frequently observed, and Lennander has described a case in which the corpus was thus finally seprated from the cervix. Adhesions to the intestines have frequently occasioned symptoms of intestinal obstruction. Subperitoneal pedunculated growths often are the seat of pathogenic degenerations. They may also, especially if de-

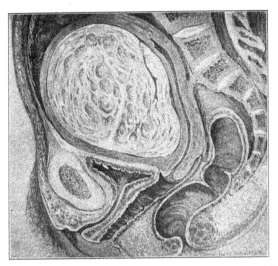

Fig. 230.—Large Interstitial Fibroid of the Uterus Simulating Pregnancy. (Original.)

generated, become infected through the blood or from the intestines, and thus cause peritonitis.

Interstitial Fibromyomata of the Body of the Uterus.—These forms of fibromyomata remain in the substance of the uterine wall and do not become pedunculated. As they grow, the musculature expands rather evenly around them. (Fig. 230.) The intramural fibroids are separated from the normal muscle by a thin layer of loose connective tissue, from which, as a rule, they can be easily shelled out when the incision is carried down to the tumor; even the spontaneous retraction of the normal muscle when cut through may force them entirely out of their bed. The only apparent connection between the tumor and its matrix consists of minute blood-vessels which supply the tumor with its nourishment. As a rule, these growths are multiple, yet one tumor often develops while the others remain of small size. As a result of the growth of the tumor, if only one is present, the uterus may be uniformly enlarged, yet frequently it assumes an irregular outline. The shape of the tumor may depend upon the pressure exerted upon it. The uterus may be displaced in various directions, largely owing to the direction of the tumor's growth. Thus, it may grow downward into the pouch of Douglas, into the vesico-rectal septum beneath the peritoneum, or into the cervix and vagina, or it may gradually fill up the pelvis, while in other cases it may grow laterally into the broad ligament.

Submucous Fibromyomata of the Body of the Uterus.—From the clinical standpoint fibromyomata of the body of the uterus are of the greatest importance. They are most frequently seen at or near the fundus, from which they tend to project into the cavity of the uterus. Frequently they are pedunculated, when they are known as fibrous polyps; yet occasionally they are attached over a broad base. Their shape, owing to the pressure of the uterus, is usually rounded. When a submucous growth projects into the uterine cavity, it acts as a foreign body and produces uterine contractions. This leads, as a rule, to an elongation of the pedicle, and even to its extrusion from the uterine cavity. As a result of the tumor's growth the uterine wall is increased in area, yet is usually thinned at the site of the pedicle. Occasionally inversion of the uterus occurs, this result being due to the paralysis of the thinned muscular wall from which springs the tumor. (Fig. 227.) As a rule, there is but one submucous polypoid growth in the uterine cavity. Such growths are round or ovoid in shape and softer and more vascular than the forms previously described. Consequently they are less prone to atrophy. Their blood supply is generally better than that of the subserous type, and therefore the growth is fairly rapid. During menstruation the tumor becomes congested and enlarged, and stimulates the uterine musculature to marked contractions. The capsule covering the tumor on the side of the uterine cavity is frequently thin. Occasionally it ruptures or ulcerates, so that spontaneous enucleation and expulsion of the tumor may occur. Sometimes the contractions of the musculature may constrict the pedicle, and gangrene or suppuration may then ensue.

FIBROMYOMATA OF THE CERVIX UTERI.

Fibromyomata of the cervix are rare. Courty, in a series of 131 cases, found but 16 per cent; Schroeder found them in 8.1 per cent, and Lee in 5.4 per cent. They may arise from either wall, but Roger Williams states that they are more common in the upper and posterior parts. Like the fibromyomata of the uterine body they may remain interstitial, or extend into the cervical cavity, or grow outward beneath the peritoneum. On account of the distortion of the resultant growth, the diagnosis may be difficult. Tumors extending toward the periphery may grow anteriorly between the bladder and the uterus, laterally into the broad ligament, or posteriorly into the pouch of Douglas. On account of the situation of these tumors the uterus is not greatly enlarged. Menorrhagia is consequently not common, but symptoms from the bladder and rectum are frequent. Especially are the intraligamentous forms a source of great danger on account of the proximity of structures of great importance. The submucous growths may produce elongation of one cervical lip and form a polypoid tumor in the vagina. Such cases may easily be mistaken for inversion or prolapsus. The tumors are especially dangerous in pregnancy and labor. Cervical myomata are said to develop more rapidly than those of the uterine body on account of their proximity to the larger blood-vessels.

STRUCTURE OF UTERINE FIBROMYOMATA.—The ordinary fibroids are composed of the same elements as the normal uterine wall. The proportion of the fibrous and muscular elements varies, however, in the different cases. The smaller tumors are composed of an irregular interlacing mass of fibrous tissue and smooth muscle, which in the larger growths is grouped in definite bands or whorls. Surrounding the whole mass is a zone of connective tissue, constituting the capsule of the tumor and connecting it with the uterine wall. The blood-vessels are comparatively few, but in rare forms large dilated blood-sinuses are found in all parts of the tumor (telangiectatic myoma). Apparently the minute blood-vessels, many of which end in the centre of the whorls, constitute the only connection between the tumor and its matrix. The larger the tumor the more attenuated is the uterine musculature which covers it, and, in the growths which extend from the surface of the uterus, it may be so thin as scarcely to be recognizable.

On section the tumor cuts with difficulty. The cut surface shows a glistening, white, coarsely fibrillated structure, arranged in distinct whorls. The longitudinal and cross sections of muscle bundles are clearly recognizable. Surrounding the tumor is the darker capsule in which blood-vessels may be seen.

Under the microscope the muscle cells are fusiform in shape, with elongated, rod-shaped nuclei. Their length varies from 0.25 mm. to 0.45 mm. The ends of the muscle cells are frequently branching. There is a more or less abundant fibrous tissue, poor in cellular elements, which forms a fine network between the muscle bundles and the individual muscle cells. There is considerable difference in the cell activity of the fibroid tumors, some appearing dense and fibrous while others are very cellular, with the nuclei as a predominating portion of the individual cell. The muscle cells are arranged in bundles which run in various directions. These bundles or whorls are surrounded by connective tissue. Nerves may be traced into the muscular fibres. Lymphatics and blood-vessels lie in the connective-tissue framework.

PATHOLOGICAL CHANGES IN UTERINE FIBROIDS.—Fibromyomatous tissue frequently undergoes degenerative changes, which, as a rule, result from disturbance of the circulation of the tumor. Practically all types have been described, many of which are merely various stages of the same general pathological process. The frequency of degenerations has been emphasized by many recent authors, all of whom call attention to the fact that they are more common than has been supposed. Including malignancy, Webster found 52 degenerations in 210 cases; Noble found 47 in 258 cases; Scharlieb found 26 in 100 tumors; and Cullingworth described 52 in 100 cases. Noble, who has done much to call attention to these degenerations, has described the following in 2,247 collected cases:—

Form of Degeneration.	No. of Cases.	Per Cent.
Hyaline degeneration	72	3.1
Hyaline degeneration with calcareous infiltration	8	0.3
Calcareous degeneration...................................	39	1.7
Myxomatous degeneration	89	3.4
Cystic degeneration......................................	58	2.5
Hemorrhagic degeneration	13	0.57
Necrosis of tumor	119	4.7
Fatty degeneration........	7	0.25
Œdema	17	0.74
Sarcoma......... .. .., ...	34	1.4
Carcinoma corporis....	42	1.8
Carcinoma cervicis.....	16	0.7

The chief types are outlined below.

Atrophy and Sclerosis.—When the nourishment of the tumor is diminished as a result of physiological involution of the genital organs, the tumor frequently undergoes atrophy and decreases in size. This change is commonly noted after the menopause, whether artificial or normal, yet may occur following the puerperium. As its result the muscle cells are reduced in size and number, which gives the tumor a hard and indurated character. This change is most common in the pedunculated subperitoneal growths, yet does not always result after the menopause. Schroeder held that it followed a fatty degeneration of the muscular tissue comprising the growth itself; yet the majority believe that the primary step is the constriction of the smaller nutrient blood-vessels from endarteritis.

The extent and situation of the new-formed fibrous tissue vary. In some areas the increase of the connective tissue is seen chiefly between and around the muscle bundles, while in other parts the muscle is split up and compressed by intranodular bands. The cases of so-called absorption of fibroids following the menopause are due to this process. Unfortunately, it does not always result after the menopause, and indeed is rarely noted.

Associated with sclerosis we commonly find hyaline degeneration.

Hyaline Degeneration.—The most common pathological change noted in fibroids is undoubtedly hyaline degeneration. It occurs in varying amounts in practically all growths, irrespective of their size. In the early stages the change may not be visible to the naked eye, but later it is distinctly recognizable as yellowish-white areas of homogeneous appearance. With extension of the process, necrosis of the centre of the areas frequently supervenes, and finally there results a cyst with irregular softened walls. Under the microscope the connective tissue is recognizable as the preponderant tissue of the tumor. The cells are more dense and contain fewer nuclei than normal. The muscle is fairly scanty. Extending between the muscular bundles, and replacing to a large extent the connective tissue, may be seen the characteristic homogeneous hyaline areas. These may be generally distributed, or may be chiefly localized. The muscle cells and bundles, interstitial connective tissue, and the blood-vessels themselves may all be converted into the degeneration areas. The process is attributed to arterio-sclerosis and the resulting impairment of circulation.

Calcification.—Calcareous deposits are frequently found in fibroids which have been the site of atrophic and sclerotic changes. As in the preceding degeneration, pedunculated subperitoneal growths with narrow pedicles, and detached tumors, are more commonly affected, although interstitial forms are not immune. Most rarely, however, does it occur in the submucous polypoid growths. Like simple atrophy it is most common in women of advanced years. This form of degeneration has been known, from the time of Hippocrates, as "womb stones." The deposit consists of phosphates and carbonates of lime. The calcareous infiltration may begin at any part of the tumor which has become degenerated—in the periphery, or in the centre, or at various points throughout the substance. There is, first, a deposit of lime salts which infiltrates the degenerated fibrous tissue of the tumor. From constant additions this deposit grows in size, forming concentric plaques, until finally the whole tumor becomes infiltrated with a granular, calcareous material. In case the calcareous infiltration begins in the periphery, there may result a complete calcareous shell about the mass, with coincident irregular areas of calcification scattered throughout the centre of the growth. As in the case of central calcification, the degenerated areas spread until they finally coalesce into a large single mass. Very seldom, however, does the tumor become completely calcified. A profound disturbance of circulation of the tumor results almost invariably from the calcification in the periphery, and necrobiosis commonly supervenes. Under the microscope, the concentric placques present a characteristic appearance. As is usual with this form of degeneration, the tissue takes an intense nuclear stain in the earlier stages. Fine calcareous granules are noted in the degenerating muscle and connective-tissue cells. This is best seen in areas which have been deprived of the blood-supply, as calcareous degeneration here, as elsewhere, supervenes only in degenerated tissue.

Œdema and Cystic Degeneration.—Œdema and cystic degeneration usually affect subserous tumors, generally those of considerable size. It is rare in the submucous and very rare in the interstitial forms. Piquand claims that it is more common in single fibroids of the uterus. The œdema is generally regarded as a result of interference with the return circulation in the tumor, leading to a passive congestion. The tumor presents a smooth and rounded appearance, with the surface reddish and traversed by many large, branching blood-vessels. The veins are dilated and engorged. The consistency of the tumor is soft and sometimes fluctuant. The œdema may be limited, or may extend throughout the whole tumor. In the early stages the tissue appears to be slightly soft, and serous fluid may exude from the interstitial tissue on section. In more advanced types there are extensive translucent, homogeneous, soft areas in which cavities ultimately develop. As a final result, the tumor may be converted into a thin-walled cyst, the interior of which is traversed by thin fibrous bands that represent the remains of obliterated blood-vessels. The microscopical findings are fairly constant. In the earlier stages, the blood-vessels are dilated, and the tissue cells are swollen. The cells stain less clearly than normal, and the protoplasm appears granular. In the late stages the cells are indistinct and granular, and the nuclei are diminished in size and stain poorly. As the final process, the cells become completely disassociated, the nuclei disappear, and the few cellular fibres which remain are separated by the serous exudate. The last stages of this process have been frequently termed myxomatous; yet, Meslay and Hyenne have shown that this is inaccurate. A true myxomatous degeneration has been pointed out by Virchow. It has been regarded as very rare.

Necrobiosis.—Necrobiosis is thought to result from some disturbance of the circulation, with consequent cell-death without subsequent infection. The tumor, however, softens and becomes red-colored from the dissemination of pigment of the broken-down blood cells, and finally undergoes liquefaction. Necrobiosis is usually seen in interstitial growths and begins in the centre of the tumor. Rarely is it found in subperitoneal or submucous tumors, as these are more prone to secondary bacterial invasion following profound disturbances of circulation. Fairbairn, in 1903, concluded that the vascular changes do not explain this form of degeneration. The tumors were not engorged with blood, nor were there vascular changes of importance in any of his nineteen cases.

The process occurs most frequently in the child-bearing era, and pregnancy is called a predisposing factor. There is no doubt but that this condition is frequently described as "soft fibroids." The old classification of myoma according to the consistency of the tumor should be abandoned. Save in adenomyoma, softening indicates a degeneration.

Infection and Suppuration.—Infection and suppuration result from bacterial infection and are common occurrences in tumors of low vitality which have been subjected to some disturbance of their local circulation. They occur most frequently in the puerperium. Submucous tumors are more prone to infection, while the interstitial and subperitoneal types are rarely affected. The source of infection varies and may arise from the genital tract of the blood stream, or from extension from pre-existing infection of the neighboring viscera. Thus, a pyosalpinx, or an adherent and inflamed appendix, or a firmly agglutinated intestine may furnish the exciting factor, yet the common source of infection is through the genital canal. Usually this follows abortion or labor. All fibroids are prone to infection during childbirth. The pressure from the uterine contractions, and the disturbance of the local circulation are undoubted predisposing factors. Moreover, the low vitality of a fibromyomatous uterus increases the susceptibility to infection. Infection may follow the use of sounds and minor operations such as curettage. It has been claimed that the continued use of ergot increases the susceptibility to infection. Electrical treatment is also regarded as a predisposing cause.

The resulting infection may remain local or become general. Sometimes the local infection is limited to the interior of the capsule of the tumor, and may extend about it so that, as a final result, the tumor may be liberated from its site and extruded from the uterus. Suppurating tumors have been expelled through the uterine cavity, or into the bladder, bowel, or peritoneal cavity, Gangrene may result from the invasion of the degenerative area by pathogenic germs.

Fatty Degeneration; Lipomyomata.—Fatty degeneration of a uterine fibromyoma has occasionally been described, but appears to be a rare condition. It is seen most often in cases which present large areas of hyaline degeneration. These become liquefied in the centre, and, in the broken-down material, fat globules and cholesterin crystals may be found. There are also a few cases which have been described as lipomyomata and in which the tumor was composed of fibromuscular and adipose tissue. In Knox's case the large globular tumor was composed of typical adipose tissue, divided into small areas of varying size by bands of smooth muscle and connective tissue. The tumor sprang from the uterine wall. R. Peterson describes a submucous lipomyoma which was accidentally discovered in a case operated upon for procidentia.

Telangiectasis and Lymphangiectasis.—Virchow described as myoma telangiectodes that variety of fibroid which contains numerous vessel spaces. On section these tumors resemble cavernous angiomata. They are most commonly of a soft consistency, as would be expected. Occasionally they may pulsate. They vary in size from time to time, according to the amount of blood contained in their vessels. Occasionally the lymphatics are increased in number and size, and are then, according to Fehling and Leopold, classified as belonging to the lymphangiectatic variety.

Hemorrhage.—A fibromyoma may be the seat of an actual hemorrhage, especially when torsion of the pedicle occurs in tumors of the cystic variety. The size of the growth may thus be rapidly increased. More commonly there are observed dark-colored infarcted areas, with extravasation of blood into the surrounding softened tissue.

Fibroids and Malignancy.—Within the last few years there has been a revulsion from the old impression that fibroids were not wont to undergo degenerative changes of a malignant nature. Careful laboratory work and the routine examination of all tumors have given us a more complete understanding of these malignant degenerations. As a result of such study our knowledge, although far from complete, will now allow more or less definite statements.

Relations of Uterine Fibromyomata to Sarcoma.—Fibroids may undergo sarcomatous degeneration or be the seat of a primary sarcomatous growth. The frequency of this complication is variously given, the variation being due in large measure to the fact that, in the past, fibroids were rarely subjected to routine examination. The routine examination of all tissue removed at operation is giving us a knowledge of pelvic pathology. This fact is well illustrated by the statistics of Winter. This author, in 1907, found sarcoma in 3.2 per cent of 500 cases in which only grossly suspicious areas of the tumor were subjected to examination, while complete routine examination of 253 cases disclosed sarcoma in 4.3 per cent of cases. As a result of his work he states his belief that, if sections were made from various portions of all fibroids as a routine procedure, sarcoma would be found in 4 per cent of cases. The percentage of sarcoma in fibroids is usually given at a lower figure, doubtless because all parts of the tumors have not been examined microscopically. Thus, Noble, in 2,274 collected cases, states that sarcoma was found in 2 per cent. Fehling found it in 2.3 per cent of 409 fibroids, and Noble in but 2 per cent of his own 337 cases. Webster also noted only two instances of sarcoma in 210 cases. Yet the number of reports of instances of sarcomatous degeneration is constantly growing. Williams believes that the form of sarcoma commonly found in myomata is the myosarcoma in which round and spindle-shaped cells predominate. He found it more frequently in the encapsulated subperitoneal and submucous polypoid growths, yet the interstitial forms were not immune. Evelt believes that the growth begins in the muscle rather than in the connective tissue. He reports 120 collected cases, one of which was melanotic. The disease is not confined to the young, and Schauta describes a sarcomatous growth in a fibroid that developed eleven years after removal of the ovaries.

Sarcomatous degeneration is often associated with the non-malignant pathological degenerations of fibromyomata, especially the myxomatous and cystic forms. We should suspect its presence when the tumor presents areas of hemorrhagic degeneration, with the formation of small cysts. Seminecrotic hemorrhagic areas without fibrillar arrangement are also highly suggestive.

Relations of Uterine Fibromyomata to Carcinoma.—Carcinoma is not one of the forms of degeneration of fibroids, as it must arise from epithelium. It may, however, begin in the epithelium of adenomyoma, or in the epithelium of the cervix or body of the uterus that is the seat of a fibromyoma. Piquand, among others, thinks that the presence of a fibroid favors the development of cancer of the cervix, yet other authorities combat the statement. Fibroids may be invaded by cancer of the cervix or uterine body, just as may the normal uterus. Noble has recently emphasized the greater relative frequency of cancer of the fundus in fibromatous uteri. Cancer was present in 2.8 per cent of 4,880 cases of fibroids collected by him. Cervical cancer occurred in 1.29 per cent, and cancer of the corpus in 1.54 per cent. In 337 of his own cases, cancer of the cervix existed in 1.4 per cent and cancer of the corpus in 2.6 per cent. Noble believes that this altered proportion of cervical and corporal cancers is highly suggestive, and indicates that fibromatous growths favor the production of adenocarcinoma of the endometrium. In his series corporal cancers were more frequent than cervical, whereas the reverse should be expected, as epitheliomata of the cervix are from five to ten times more common than adenocarcinomata of the fundus. (For statistics as to the relative frequency of cervical and corporal cancers of the uterus see page 582.)

The Effect of Uterine Fibromyomata upon Neighboring or Distant Organs.—Effect upon the Uterus and Adnexa.—Under the influence of fibromyomatous growth the uterus hypertrophies as in pregnancy. This condition is more marked with the submucous and interstitial types than with the subperitoneal. Kelly reports an interesting example in which the uterus weighed 645 grams after the removal of a fibroid of moderate size—an increase of uterine growth fifteen times the normal weight. The uterus changes in outline according to the variety of the tumor which it harbors. As a rule, the enlargement is asymmetrical, yet, in the case of interstitial and submucous growths, the normal outline is often retained. Fibromyomatous uteri are frequently mistaken for pregnancies. The uterine cavity is usually much lengthened in interstitial and submucous tumors and may be much distorted in shape and direction. Occasionally it may be entirely obliterated. Microscopically, we observe hypertrophy of the individual muscular fibres and the intermuscular cellular tissue. This change may not be marked in the myometrium lying between small and numerous interstitial fibroids, because the side pressure exerted by the presence of a number of tumors may inhibit the hypertrophy. Carl Ruge has described a rhomboid arrangement of the muscles in an interstitial growth. The hypertrophy of the muscle cells is most marked when the tumor is large and of the submucous variety, and Bertelsmann regards it as an example of "work hypertrophy." This enlargement is due possibly to the frequent contractions

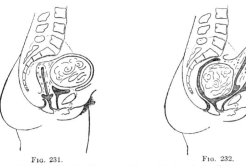

FIG. 231.   FIG. 232.

FIG. 231.—Subserous Fibroid Displacing Uterus Backward in Retroversion. (From Veit, "Handbuch der Gynaekol.," 1897.)

FIG. 232.—Myoma of Posterior Cervical Wall Displacing the Uterus Upward and Forward. (From Veit, "Handbuch der Gynaekol.," 1897.)

made by the uterus in its efforts to expel the tumor. Individual muscle cells have attained a length of 166μ and a breadth of 13.5μ.

Displacements of the uterus by the tumor may occur in any direction (Figs. 231 and 232), although the uterus, through its attachments to the vagina and bases of the broad ligaments, is more or less limited in its capacity for upward displacements. The uterus may become twisted on its long axis (torsion), and in rare cases the body of the organ may be partly or entirely separated from the cervix. Inversion is not infrequently caused by submucous polypoid fibroids. Rarely there may be obstruction of the cavity of the uterus, causing a retention of the fluids and giving rise to hydrometra, pyometra, or hæmatometra.

The changes in the uterine mucosa vary. In the majority of cases there will be found hyperplasia, which is often incorrectly described as of inflammatory origin. All the elements of the mucosa may be increased and many variations from the normal are seen, ranging from simple œdema to gland hypertrophy, or polypoid thickening of the endometrium, associated with dilatation of the glands and vascular changes. Not infrequently there are localized projections which are described as mucous polypoids. Hyperplasia is generally found in the mucosa of the uterus when a submucous myoma is present. It rarely occurs with the subperitoneal forms. Even though the uterus is elongated, the mucosa rarely undergoes hypertrophy in this class of tumors; more frequently the reverse is noted, the mucosa being atrophied. True endometritis resulting from infection may be observed, yet it results, not from the presence of the tumor, but from secondary infection. The mucosa covering a submucous fibroid is usually thinned upon the prominent portions of the growth. Indeed, it is sometimes absent, having ulcerated away after the great stretching to which it has been subjected and from the trauma of the pressure. About the neck of the growth, on the contrary, the mucosa is thickened and may form a thick ridge or collar which is usually very vascular and bleeds easily. Counter-pressure against the uterine mucosa causes atrophy of the endometrium at the point of contact. Landau has described a case in which serial transverse sections of the whole uterus failed to show a uterine cavity under the microscope.

Effect upon the Tubes and Ovaries.—The tubes are frequently elongated and the ovaries commonly diseased. Tait found appendage disease in fifty-four per cent of cases. Fabricius found that the tubes are commonly diseased in the case of the larger growths and that both tubes are apt to be affected. The lesions are generally those of endosalpingitis and interstitial salpingitis, with resulting thickening of the walls and a partial destruction of the mucosa. Under the microscope one finds that the epithelial cells have been thrown off from the mucosa or are the seat of mucinous retentions. The connective tissue is œdematous and distended by an exudate or by extravasations of blood. "Mast cells" are common, as are groups of round cells. The muscle is first œdematous, and later may be the seat of much round-cell infiltration.

For the most part, the ovaries are longer than usual and, according to Bulius, thicker. This may be due in part to the retention of growing follicles, yet is aided by a chronic inflammation. Sometimes the ovaries are peculiarly flattened and sclerotic, or they may be greatly stretched out and elongated. The stroma is infiltrated with round cells, and the blood-vessels are contracted and commonly the seat of hyaline degeneration. The corpora fibrosa are generally thickened. The frequency of tubal and ovarian complications is shown by the following: In McDonald's series of 280 cases they were found in 137; Webster found them in 99 out of 210 cases; Meredith reports tubal disease in 56 per cent and chronic ovaritis in 46 per cent of Lawson Tait's series. Coincidently with the presence of the fibromyomata there is commonly tubal disease, while the changes in the ovaries may be the direct result of these growths.

With the growth of the fibroids, the blood-vessels of the broad ligament and uterus tend to enlarge and sometimes are found of great size; the veins especially may form varicose masses. Œdematous areas are commonly seen in the broad ligament, and by some are considered as distended lymph spaces filled with serum.

Effects upon the Contents of the Pelvis.—As the tumor grows it is apt to compress the structures which normally lie in the pelvis. As a rule, pressure effects develop gradually, but sometimes the reverse is noted. They are most commonly observed in the case of large tumors which have remained within the pelvis, although serious complications often arise with the growth of intraligamentous tumors. Even small fibroids of this type may give rise to serious complications. Pedunculated subserous growths may also cause difficulty, especially when they fall into the pouch of Douglas and finally become incarcerated in the pelvic cavity. The bladder, ureters, and rectum are most exposed to compression. The bladder symptoms may vary with the different types of growth. Frequently the viscus is prevented from filling in a normal manner. A fibroid of the anterior uterine wall may compress or elevate it. Pressure may lift it out of the pelvis, so that it occupies a position between the summit of the growth and the anterior abdominal wall; sometimes it lies as high as the umbilicus. Obstruction of the urethra may further the displacement through retention of urine. Occasionally bladder symptoms are the first complaint made by the patient who has a uterine fibromyoma. The round ligaments may be hypertrophied, but more often they are thinned. If the growth is fundal, the ligaments elongate. Frequently they are so thinned by being stretched over the tumor that they are scarcely recognizable.

The vagina may also be displaced. Sometimes it is drawn up and elevated, yet may be pushed down by the weight of a large tumor in the pelvis or partially inverted in the case of certain submucous growths. Lateral displacements are not uncommon, and the vagina may be distended by a submucous polypoid growth.

The ureters are frequently involved. Their lower insertions may be displaced by growths which exert pressure upon the base of the bladder. Intraligamentous tumors may displace them outward, upward, or downward. Sometimes the ureter will be found overriding the growth. Pressure on the ureter may cause hydro-ureter, hydronephrosis, or even destruction of the kidney, and it would appear that these complications are more common than has been taught in the past. Knox has shown that some obstruction was present in a large proportion of his series of cases.

The rectum may be compressed, although complete obstruction probably never occurs from fibroids except when there are secondary complications. Yet the bowels may be compressed to an extent that favors the advent of conditions causing symptoms. Auto-intoxication and anæmia have been ascribed to partial obstruction by impacted fibroids, and chronic constipation and difficult defecation are quite common. Hemorrhoids are frequently observed.

The pelvic circulation may be impeded, with resulting œdema and varicosities in the lower extremities, rectum, vagina, or vulva. Phlebitis is occasionally noted, especially after infection of the myomatous growth.

Effect upon Remote Organs.—Cardio-Vascular Degenerations.—Cardio-vascular changes are frequently found in relation with fibromyoma, and in recent years they have been the subject of much investigation. Yet, at the present time, they are not thoroughly understood.

For a long time it has been well known that the mortality following the removal of fibroids has been greater than should be expected from the mere removal of the tumor. As early as 1835 Hofmeier stated that cardiac disease is frequently observed in cases of abdominal tumor, and especially in fibroids of large size. Many pathological findings have been described by the pathologist and clinician. Brown atrophy and fatty degeneration of the heart, arterial sclerosis of the blood-vessels, myocarditis, and endocarditis are commonly observed. Clinically, one finds many cardiac murmurs, presumptively of hæmic origin.

There is little doubt but that such pathological changes in the heart are very frequent. Strassman and Lehman found definite cardiac lesions in 48.8 per cent of 71 cases in Gusserow's clinic. Fleck obtained similar percentages in a series of 325 cases. Boldt, in a study of 79 cases, found some circulatory disturbance in 47 per cent. Wilson reports that in 72 cases, which were treated surgically, there were cardiac disturbances in 46 per cent. They were also noted in 25 per cent of Webster's 210 cases. Roger Williams thus reports the cardiac findings in 32 autopsies of women with fibromyomatous uteri: Valvular disease, mostly chronic, 6 cases; fatty degeneration, 5 cases; hypertrophy and dilatation, 3 cases; atheroma of aorta, 3 cases; small heart, 3 cases; normal, 12 cases.

Pallanda, as a result of his study in 1905, concluded that, in the natural evolution of fibroids, thrombosis of the pelvic venous sinuses, pulmonary embolism, cardiac lesions, and sudden syncope followed in 11 per cent of cases. Wilson believes that myocardial degeneration was responsible for death in 4 of the fatal cases of his series. Three of the 5 cases of Boldt's series that succumbed after operation, died from cardio-vascular degeneration. Fenwick, in 1888, reported 22 cases of large cystic abdominal tumors, in which fatty degeneration of the heart was found at autopsy. Yet all do not agree as to the frequency of these complications. Winter reports his clinical results in a series of 266 fibromyoma cases, in which the diagnosis was made by an internalist. The heart was normal clinically in 60 per cent of cases, while 30 per cent presented murmurs of presumptive hæmic origin. Cardiac dilatation and hypertrophy were noted in 6 per cent of cases, and were mostly attributed to anæmia. True valvular disease was determined in only one per cent of the series.

There is much controversy as to the cause of these lesions. Are these primary changes in the heart and blood-vessels due to the same cause which produces the tumor, or are they merely secondary results and symptoms of the tumor? At the present time the majority believe that the changes are secondary to the anæmia which results from hemorrhage or from disturbance of digestion from pressure of the tumors. Fleck suggests that they may result from a disordered ovarian secretion.

Large tumors may lead to cardiac changes through pressure on various organs. The expansion of the lungs may be curtailed, and large vessels may be compressed. The alimentary functions may be impaired, and toxic matter absorbed from the bowel. Other organs, as the kidneys, ureters, and bladder, may be compressed. Pressure on the sympathetic ganglia may cause reflex irritation of the heart. The different authorities, however, do not agree. In Fleck's series, for example, cardiac changes were demonstrated clinically in 34.6 per cent of cases in which there had been no hemorrhage. Nor was there a history of bleeding in six of eleven cases in which cardiac lesions were demonstrated at autopsy. Cardiac lesions, moreover, have been demonstrated in cases in which the tumor was of small size. More work is necessary before definite conclusions can be adopted; yet many, as Noble, believe that cardio-vascular degenerations do not play a large part in producing fatal results, save in neglected and late cases.

Renal Disturbances.—Renal disturbances are more common in fibroids than is generally believed. Webster found albumin, casts, diminished urea, or diminution of the amount of urine, in thirty per cent of his cases in which symptoms of pre-existing renal disease had been eliminated, as far as could be done, by careful histories. Nor did treatment, prior to operation, produce marked improvement. He concludes that the facts producing these lesions are identical with those causing the cardio-vascular disturbances. They are chiefly operative in large growths which fill the pelvis and abdomen.

SYMPTOMS OF UTERINE FIBROMYOMA.—The symptoms of fibromyoma are extremely variable, and depend upon the site and character of the growth, its size, and the presence of degenerations. Not uncommonly there are no symptoms, especially in subperitoneal tumors, which, even when of large size, may occasionally produce merely discomfort from the abdominal distention.

The range of symptoms includes the following: menorrhagia and metrorrhagia, anæmia, dysmenorrhœa, pain, leucorrhœa, and various pressure symptoms.

Hemorrhage.—The most common symptom is hemorrhage from the uterus, which Winter says is present in two-thirds of all cases presenting symptoms. Usually it begins as increased and prolonged menstruation, and never as the sudden flooding which is seen in carcinoma. The interval between the periods gradually shortens until finally there results a continuous dribbling of blood with exacerbations at the times corresponding to the menstrual periods. The rule is, however, that there is no bleeding between the monthly periods. The greatest variations may occur, and rarely are the cases typical. The law of the bleeding in single tumors is, roughly speaking, as follows: In interstitial growths the menorrhagia increases in accordance with the size of the tumor. It decreases as the growth approaches the peritoneal uterine covering, and may be lacking when the fibroid is subperitoneal and pedunculated. When the tumor approaches the mucosa and becomes submucous, there is a disproportionate increase of bleeding. Typical cases are rarely seen, as frequently all three forms of the growth exist in the same uterus. A single submucous tumor of very small size may occasion more serious hemorrhage than great subperitoneal or many interstitial forms. The hemorrhage is therefore increased in direct ratio to the proximity of the tumor to the uterine mucosa.

The hemorrhage results from the congestion of the endometrium due to the disturbance of the circulation caused by the presence of the tumor. The thin-walled veins are more easily compressed than the thicker-walled arteries, and the return flow is consequently impeded. The bleeding comes from the hyper-trophied endometrium of the increased uterine cavity. Disturbance in the local circulation of the tumor may cause serious hemorrhage, especially in en-gorgement due to twisting of the pedicle. Under the latter circumstances the bleeding may be sudden and considerable.

In uterine fibroids the duration of the menstrual period and the quantity of flow are increased as the patient approximates the normal age for the meno-pause. There is no intermission in the regularity; one flow may continue into another, but, when that period ceases, the flow does not begin anew until the regular term for menstruation arrives. The menopause is greatly postponed, and, where patients are menstruating regularly and without interruption past the age of forty-eight years, there is a rapidly increasing percentage of fibroids as the cause of the postponement of the menopause with the increasing age. So uniform is this that ninety-four per cent of the patients menstruating regu-larly and without interruption at fifty-four years of age have fibroids. In car-cinoma of the uterus, the interruption of normal menstruation takes place under the climacteric age. These patients may have sudden and severe hem-orrhage months or years after the cessation of menstruation. This never occurs in fibroids and rarely in uterine fibrosis, so that postponement of the menopause is of itself an evidence of fibroid.

Anæmia.—Death from acute hemorrhage is very rare, and usually there results more or less profound anæmia. Pallanda, in 1905, states that death resulted directly or indirectly from hemorrhage in 6.4 per cent of 171 fatal cases which had not been operated upon. The resulting anæmia may constitute a serious feature, and generally is sufficiently marked to add considerably to the risk of operation. Often it is amenable to treatment, yet it may resist the effects even of curettage. Noble reports two cases in which the hæmoglobin was reduced to ten and fifteen per cent respectively.

Dysmenorrhœa.—Dysmenorrhœa is common in adenomyomata, as the blind sacs in the glandular areas become engorged with blood at the time of menstrua-tion. It is also marked in submucous polyps which also swell from engorge-ment of blood, and stimulate painful uterine contractions as the organ tries to expel the growth. These pains may resemble those of labor. Yet pain may result in the presence of subserous and interstitial growths, from causes which we cannot always explain. As a rule, it is ascribed to engorgement of the tumors with blood; yet fibrous growths have few blood-vessels, although they may occasion pain. Dysmenorrhœa may often result from an associated tubal or ovarian inflammation.

Intermenstrual Pain.—Intermenstrual pain is a variable symptom. It may be present or absent. Especially is it noted in connection with degenerative changes. Thus, Cullingworth noted pain as a marked symptom in two-thirds of his necrobiotic cases, in three-fifths of the cystic fibroids, and in one-third of the cases classified as œdematous. In the majority of the degenerated growths the mass is tender to pressure, even though no actual inflammation exists. The advent of complications is often associated with pain, especially in peritoneal complications. Torsion of the pedicle may, if produced suddenly, occasion great distress. The incarceration of the tumor in the pelvis may cause intense pain, largely due to pressure.

Leucorrhœa.—Leucorrhœa is a symptom of little actual diagnostic value. It is more common when the endometrium is the seat of glandular changes. Then it represents the glandular secretion, yet may occur from old cervical infections. Sometimes it is the transudate from the distended capillaries of a submucous growth. The discharge is foul-smelling when ulceration or gangrene occurs. Like leucorrhœa in general it is most noticeable just before and after menstruation.

Pressure Symptoms.—Pressure symptoms are common and depend upon the extent and location of the growth. A small intraligamentous tumor may occasion far more symptoms than a large pedunculated subperitoneal growth that is not incarcerated in the pelvis. Sometimes the symptoms are slight, such as a sense of fulness in the pelvis or a dragging sensation in the loins or back. Pressure on the bladder may lead to frequency of micturition and even vesical tenesmus. Sometimes retention may occur, especially when pressure is exerted upon the urethra. These symptoms are often aggravated at the menstrual period, and may be due to large growths or to the small subvesical forms which compress the neck of the bladder. Intraligamentous tumors may compress the ureters, yet as a rule the ureters are pushed aside. More or less obstruction may result, however, with secondary changes in the upper urinary tract, as hydro-ureter, hydronephrosis, and even destruction of the kidney. We have already called attention to the frequency of such complications in Knox's series. Infection of the urinary tract is apt to follow. Deaths from uræmia have been reported. Pressure on the rectum is not common, although incarcerated fibroids have occasioned obstruction. Growths from the posterior uterine wall may cause irritation of the rectum and constipation, and mucous proctitis has been ascribed to it. Hemorrhoids often occur. Pressure on the nerves and veins may cause painful symptoms of the lower extremities. Œdema and varicose veins are commonly noted in incarcerated pelvic growths. Phlebitis and thrombosis are seen even in cases before operation. Intra-abdominal growths may attain a size sufficient to give symptoms of pressure on the organs in the upper abdominal and thoracic cavities.

DIAGNOSIS OF UTERINE FIBROMYOMATA.—The diagnosis of uterine fibromyomata is usually easy, although occasionally it is extremely difficult, especially in the small submucous and large interstitial forms, when nearly all methods of examination may be exhausted before the diagnosis is final. A careful history is often of great value, yet the pelvic condition must be determined by a bimanual examination. The symptoms are subjective and objective. As subjective, we commonly obtain the history of hemorrhage, dysmenorrhœa, or other pelvic symptoms which have extended over a considerable space of time in a woman usually of middle age. Commonly there is a history of sterility or of frequent spontaneous abortion. The patient may or may not have symptoms of pressure, or be conscious of a growing tumor. Usually she has gained weight. Emaciation rarely occurs save in the later stages of growths of enormous size. Objectively we may find symptoms of anæmia when the bleeding has persisted for a considerable space of time. The color of the skin differs from that of cachexia following malignancy, which is seen only in the later stages of this disease, and is attended with loss of weight and strength. The skin is pale-yellow and white in the anæmia following fibroids, rather than the yellowish-brown of the true cachexia of cancer.

On bimanual examination we commonly find an enlarged uterus of firm consistency and frequently of irregular outline. As the growths are usually multiple we often find the bosses or knobs of subperitoneal tumors plainly appreciable; yet all fibroid uteri are not hard, nor of irregular outline. Frequently they are soft and rounded, when they may be confused with various conditions and cause much difficulty in the diagnosis. Sometimes the diagnosis cannot be made until the cervix is dilated and a polypoid growth felt within it.

As regards the appearance of fibromyomatous growths the range is so extensive and the physical aspects so variable that, in their relation to the diagnosis, we may best review the question according to the size and situation of the tumor. Thus, we may classify these growths as (a) small myomata, and (b) the larger myomata which extend as distinct tumors into the abdomen.

(a) *Diagnosis in the Case of a Small Uterine Fibromyoma.*—Small submucous, pedunculated fibroids above the level of the surface are often recognizable only when the uterine canal is sufficiently dilated to admit a palpating finger. The whole uterus is usually more or less symmetrically enlarged, and, although softer than normal, is harder than a pregnant uterus. There is no Hegar's sign of pregnancy, nor are there intermittent contractions. The enlargement is occasionally mistaken for a metritic uterus.

When a tumor projects through the cervix, the condition can be confused with inversion of the uterus, a pedunculated sarcoma, a uterine polyp, or the placental remains of an abortion. The appearance varies accordingly as the tumor is covered or not covered with mucosa. Tumors covered with a mucosa are red and sensitive to pain, while those which are not so covered are pale and not sensitive. An inverted uterus is readily recognizable in the majority of cases. On sweeping the finger around the base, in the case of a polypus, the cervical canal is felt, unless the tumor has become adherent at its neck and has thus obliterated the canal, when the condition may be mistaken for an inverted uterus. The recto-abdominal examination, in inversion of the uterus, will show the absence of the fundus above the cervix, and sometimes we can recognize the tubal ostia in the inverted mass. An ulcerated or gangrenous tumor may be confused with a malignant growth. When the diagnosis is in doubt, the patient should be examined under anæsthesia, and the cavity of the uterus should be explored with the finger or the sound. Such exploration should never be undertaken without aseptic precautions, nor unless pregnancy has been absolutely excluded.

Small submucous, non-pedunculated tumors may be very difficult of diagnosis. The uterus is increased in size and more rounded than normal, and often the condition is recognizable only when the cervix has been dilated and the uterine cavity explored with the finger. Small interstitial tumors may escape recognition. The higher they lie in the uterus, the more difficult is the diagnosis. When situated low down they may bulge into the cervix and simulate inversion. Quite frequently they cause bulging of one lip of the cervix, displacing the os to the other side and changing its appearance to a slit, which easily escapes recognition. Such cases must be examined most carefully and under anæsthesia. The os must be found, when the sound will show the position of the uterine cavity. By this means the thickness of the uterine wall can be determined and areas of local hardness located.

Small subperitoneal tumors produce a slight bulging on the surface of the uterus or are felt as pedunculated projections. The latter are more or less movable, but their form and consistency depend upon the condition of the growth. Usually they are hard and unyielding, but when cystic they may have an elastic consistence. When the growths are confined to one side of the uterus, or to the fundus, the womb may be clearly outlined as a distinct body to which the tumors are attached. Sometimes pedunculated growths may simulate ovarian swellings. The diagnosis is easy when both ovaries can be palpated, yet frequently this is impossible. The consistency and irregular outline of the pedunculated growth may furnish sufficient evidence of its nature and the mass will follow the uterus when it is pushed from side to side. Enlarged Fallopian tubes may simulate this condition, yet there are generally the history and symptoms of tubal disease. The sound is of the greatest help in determining the diagnosis, but this instrument must be most cautiously used.

Intraligamentous fibroids are readily diagnosed. They usually are situated low down in the pelvis and consequently are within easy reach of the examining finger. Sometimes they even project into the vagina. On account of their location and attachments they are but slightly movable.

(b) *Diagnosis in the Case of a Large Uterine Fibromyoma.*—A large uterine fibromyoma may be regular or irregular in outline and can usually be distinctly defined. The greatest confusion results in the case of tumors of regular outline, which may be confounded with pregnancy or with ovarian cysts. When the growth is subperitoneal we can generally recognize its connection with the uterus, although sometimes this may be impossible. The tumors vary in their range of movements according to their size, the length of their pedicle, and the extent and character of the adhesions when present. An abdominal examination is frequently of the greatest aid in the diagnosis, and often we are able to recognize the connection of the tumor with the uterus when an assistant makes traction upon it through the abdominal wall and upward toward the diaphragm. The pedicle is thus made tense and appreciable under bimanual examination which should proceed according to the usual methods of medical diagnosis (inspection, palpation, etc.).

Inspection.—The contour of the abdomen frequently gives diagnostic aid. A fibroid tumor large enough to distend the abdomen, but not completely to fill it, is commonly located to one side of the median line. This is partially due to the projection of the promontory of the spinal column into the abdominal cavity, which throws the fibroid to one side, as it does the pregnant uterus, and partially on account of the more irregular shape of the tumor growth. The contour of the abdomen also may be suggestive. Thus, the abdominal wall drops suddenly to its normal level above the upper confines of the tumor, while in ovarian cysts and pregnancy the descent is more gradual. This is best recognized under anæsthesia. A linea nigra may be present, although it is rarely as well marked as in pregnancy.

Palpation.—The outline may be regular or irregular. The irregular shapes are the easier to diagnose. On pushing the tumor from side to side, one may find, on examining through the vagina, that the cervix moves coincidentally. Small nodules upon the tumor mass, especially when pedunculated, are strongly presumptive of fibroids. We must bear in mind also that large subserous, pedunculated growths may be detached from their connection with the uterus and become parasitic; in which event the diagnosis will be more confusing. A sign of great diagnostic value is the absence of intermittent contractions,—the characteristic of pregnancy. Yet some, as Hart and Barbour, have observed this phenomenon in soft fibroids. The breasts occasionally are enlarged and may contain colostrum.

Percussion.—The percussion note is flat, unless the growth is covered with distended intestines. Tympanitic resonance is present in the flanks, unless the abdomen contains free fluid. When the examiner is in doubt, he should turn the patient upon her side and then make percussion. Movable dulness is apparent in ascites and in subperitoneal tumors which are mobile.

Auscultation.—A uterine souffle is heard most distinctly at the side, although sometimes it is present over the surface of the tumor. This is not of diagnostic value, as it is present in all conditions presenting enlarged veins of the broad ligament. The presence of a fœtal heart should be looked for.

Vaginal Examination.—The vaginal mucosa is often discolored and softened as in pregnancy. In rare cases it presents the characteristic purplish hue. The cervix may be variously displaced, according to the position of the tumor. Usually it has a firm consistence, although it may be softened. The lower uterine segment is rarely symmetrical as in pregnancy, although occasionally it may present such symmetry. On the bimanual examination, the uterus is found to be enlarged and, in the case of pedunculated subserous growths, is frequently distinct from the tumor. Sometimes, however, we simply feel a large mass continuous with the cervix.

The Use of the Sound.—The sound should not be used unless the possibility of pregnancy has been excluded. In doubtful cases, unless there is urgency for operation, it may be well to wait until the positive signs of pregnancy have had time to develop. Frequently the canal is so displaced that a metal sound cannot be passed. A bougie, therefore, may be useful. The length of the cavity is always increased in submucous and interstitial growths of large size. The direction in which the uterine canal runs may also be strongly suggestive, as not uncommonly, in fibroids, the canal is markedly displaced to one side.

DIFFERENTIAL DIAGNOSIS.—We have already discussed certain essential points in the differential diagnosis between fibromyoma, ovarian cysts, and normal pregnancy. There are certain other conditions, however, which may cause confusion in the differential diagnosis.

Ectopic gestation may be mistaken for myoma, or *vice versa.* The difficulty is greater if pregnancy is in an undeveloped horn, in which condition it may not be possible to reach a diagnosis until abdominal section has been made. As a rule, the hardness of the myoma, its slow growth, and the absence of the signs and symptoms of pregnancy may suffice to establish its nature. In soft tumors, however, the condition is more confusing.

When the uterus is greatly enlarged by the tumor the condition may resemble that of an advanced ectopic pregnancy, in which there are death of the foetus and the absorption of the liquor amnii. Many such cases have been reported. If, after a careful routine examination, some doubt still exists, the case should be subjected to the x-ray.

Pelvic inflammatory masses are, as a rule, easily differentiated. Occasionally, however, it may be difficult or even impossible to make such a differentiation, especially when there has been peritonitis with an extensive exudate which is undergoing absorption. In most cases the history aids the differentiation. The diagnosis is most difficult in cases in which it is thought that adhesions exist about the tumor.

A displaced kidney or spleen may lie in close relationship to the pelvis and may be mistaken for a fibroid. If the organs are easily palpated the diagnosis is clear. The notch on the spleen is usually palpable in enlargement of that organ. In the presence of adhesions, however, the case may be confusing, as either condition may be attended with torsion of the pedicle and attacks of severe abdominal pain.

Cancer of the ovary may be difficult of differentiation from fibroids complicated with pelvic suppuration and extensive parametritis. The true condition may not be recognized until the abdomen has been opened.

Sarcoma associated with fibroids may also be confusing, unless the disease has extended to the endometrium. Tissue removed by the curette and subjected to microscopical examination will reveal the true condition. Frequently, however, the malignant areas are not reached by the spoon, and the diagnosis is not made until the advent of metastases which give symptoms.

PROGNOSIS, WITHOUT OPERATION.—The prognosis varies according to different factors. We must take into account: (a) the site, the prognosis being unfavorable when the tumor is of the submucous or the intraligamentary variety; (b) the size and rapidity of growth; (c) the size and position in the pelvis—whether impacted in the pelvis, or situated low down and likely to become wedged within it; (d) the symptoms already present, of which hemorrhage is the most important; and (e) the presence of degenerations in the tumor or in the cardiovascular organs.

The prognosis of fibroids without removal is still a matter of contention. Thus, Roger Williams, in 1901, concluded that only one of 3,000 cases of fibroids proved fatal without operation. This report was based upon the Registrar-General's statistics for Great Britain, in which 339 deaths were attributed to uterine fibromyoma, in a population of 17,000,000 women. In the calculation the frequency of the growth was taken as 20 per cent of women over 35 years of age. There are objections to these figures, interesting though they are, as unfortunately death statistics are usually incomplete. That deaths without operation are not uncommon is shown by Pallanda's study of 171 such fatal cases. Winter states that death resulted from the effect of the tumor, after a longer or shorter period, in 10 per cent of cases. Noble estimated that 12 per cent of 2,274 of his collected cases would have died without operation from degenerations or complications which existed in the tumor or the uterus at the time the operation was performed; and that 11 per cent would have died without operation as a result of complications which were found present in the uterine appendages or in the abdomen. He states that there existed numerous other complications which caused invalidism, in addition to those classified as fatal, and concludes that approximately 30 per cent of all women having fibroid tumors, as seen in the operating room, would die without operation in the natural course of the disease, or from the complications.

Many have claimed, on the other hand, that the latter author has exaggerated the influence of these tumors. Yet, it would appear that the widely held view of the harmlessness of fibroids must be greatly modified. We may say conservatively that, although these growths possibly cause death directly in only very rare instances, their influence may be so harmful as to render the system less able to withstand the effect of other diseases. The frequency of degenerative changes in the heart and arteries, as well as in the liver and kidney, must be borne in mind; nor can we lose sight of the frequency of malignant degeneration, to which cause must be assigned a mortality percentage nearly equal to that of operative interference. The loss of blood, the resulting anæmia, and the pressure effects frequently cause most serious conditions. Moreover, the presence of a fibromyoma undoubtedly increases the dangers of pregnancy, labor, and the puerperium to a considerable degree.

TREATMENT.—The treatment of fibroids may be expectant, palliative, or radical. Many of the small growths produce no symptoms and their recognition is purely accidental. Probably the great majority of these require no treatment whatsoever.

Expectant Treatment.—When a small growth is accidentally discovered, the case should be kept under observation, even if there are no symptoms. If the woman has no discomfort, or if the symptoms are slight and there is no evidence of pathological degeneration, radical treatment is not justified, and even palliative treatment is uncalled for. The patient should be seen at intervals of five or six months, and careful notes should be kept showing the size of the tumor and the advent of new symptoms. A certain proportion of these growths may decrease in size after the menopause. Yet there is no certainty that this will occur, and moreover the patient and the physician must often be reconciled to the postponement of the menopause.

Palliative Treatment.—The main object of this treatment is control of the hemorrhage, as the other symptoms are not apt to respond to treatment. Occasionally the bulk of the tumor may be reduced, but such a result is not to be expected. Pressure symptoms may sometimes be relieved by the elevation of a tumor which has become incarcerated in the pelvis, although this is frequently impossible save at operation. Palliative treatment may be instituted with the use of drugs and hygienic measures and the application of electricity; and, later, one may resort to curettage, intra-uterine applications, operations which diminish the blood supply of the uterus and tumor, or to the removal of the ovaries and tubes.

Systemic Medication.—At the present time medicines play a very small rôle in the treatment of myoma of the uterus. In the past certain medicines enjoyed a wide vogue in the treatment of symptoms, the most important of which was hemorrhage. For many years ergot was a drug of universal adoption. It was first advocated by Hildebrandt, in 1872, when it was thought that it controlled menorrhagia and checked the nutrition of the tumor by diminishing its blood supply. It was also believed that the drug favored the pedunculation and expulsion of submucous growths. Yet at the present time this view no longer obtains, and the employment of ergot is restricted to treatment of the hemorrhage during or between the menstrual periods. Undoubtedly the drug may cause contraction of the small arteries of the uterus, and consequently exert a valuable hæmostatic action in many cases of bleeding, yet the results from the administration of ergot are most uncertain. The variations are mainly due to the condition of the uterine mucosa, but also to the nature of the preparation of ergot. In case the capillaries of the endometrium are so dilated as to form small sinuses, or when there is marked enlargement of the veins of the uterus and broad ligament, the drug will be followed with few if any results. Ergot at the present time is the most uncertain of drugs. Many preparations are absolutely inert, while others contain the active principles in proportions which are not useful for the control of bleeding. Marckwald and Helme have shown that the variations in the action of ergot depend upon the relative proportion of the chief constituents, ergotinin and sclerotinic acid. The former is not hæmostatic but increases the rapidity of the blood flow, while the latter contracts the arteries and thus diminishes the flow. Sclerotinic acid has not been much used alone. Some advise the use of ergot preparations in submucous tumors, with the view that the powerful uterine contraction which the drug is supposed to incite may push the tumor out farther into the uterine cavity than would result if the case were left to nature, and thus render it amenable to removal through the cervical canal. Various pills are recommended, and a combination of ergotin (gr. i.), stypticin (gr. i.), and hydrastinin (gr. ss.), is often useful. It should be given, in the form of a pill, four times a day during the week preceding the expected flow, and should be continued until the flow ceases. The protracted use of ergot is apt to cause disturbed digestion, irregular heart action. and some general impairment of the health.

Hydrastis canadensis was formerly praised by many clinicians; yet the experimental work of laboratory pharmacologists has demonstrated that this drug is useless in controlling hemorrhage. A long list of other drugs has been advocated by various authors, yet the very length of the list shows that none acts as a specific. In the last few years various glandular extracts have been employed, yet they have failed to bring about absorption of tumors. Adrenalin has been used with advantage in these cases to control the bleeding, yet the effects are very temporary. But all the medicinal treatment of hemorrhage is uncertain and is attended with an extremely large per cent of failures.

Hygienic and Dietetic Treatment.—Hygienic and dietetic treatment should be attempted, and every effort should be made to build up the blood. A simple, non-stimulating diet should be advised and the greatest attention paid to the details which will promote comfort and prevent fatigue. Special attention should be given to secure proper elimination, and everything that causes pelvic congestion should be avoided. The patient should be kept in bed during the menstrual period and at other times when there is bleeding. The assumption of the knee-chest position for five minutes night and morning should be encouraged in all cases in which there is a possibility of impaction of the tumor in the pelvis. Various baths have been advised, but they are productive of good results only through the improvement of the general health. Pressure symptoms occasionally may be relieved by the wearing of a pessary, provided the tumor is of small size. An abdominal bandage should be recommended when a large abdominal growth becomes pendulous, in case operation is declined.

Electrical Treatment.—At the present time it is generally believed that electricity is of use only in the control of the bleeding. Formerly it was commended as a means of reducing the size of the tumor, was introduced for that purpose by Tripier of Paris, and was soon adopted generally. Apostoli, however, brought it prominently before the profession, and it soon obtained almost universal vogue. Yet at the present time the claims of the earlier advocates are largely discounted and the reports of commissions of societies appointed to investigate the subject are discouraging, save for the occasional use of this agent in the control of hemorrhage.

The galvanic current, applied through the positive pole to the uterine cavity, is, in selected cases, a valuable means of controlling the bleeding. It acts as a cauterant and destroys the superficial tissue with which it comes in contact, leaving in its stead an eschar. Yet it is unfortunately not of the greatest use in those cases in which the bleeding is caused by submucous tumors, which constitute the largest per cent of the cases in which hemorrhage is the prominent symptom. The method is contra-indicated in any degenerative process, or in tumors complicated by inflammatory disease of the appendages. A rheostat and galvanometer are necessary to govern and to indicate the strength of the current. A special sound is required—one provided with a platinum point, a movable insulating sheath to limit the area of application, and an insulated handle. The positive pole is connected with the sound by a wire; the negative pole is attached to a large pad which is wet with salt water and placed over the abdomen. The treatment must be given under aseptic precautions. The vulva, vagina, and cervix are carefully cleansed and disinfected and the instruments are boiled. The technical details are as follows:—

The cervix is exposed with a speculum, seized with a tenaculum, and brought down into view. The sound is next introduced into the uterine cavity as far as it will go without force, and the movable insulating sheath is pushed upward on the sound as far as the cervix to protect the vagina. The speculum is withdrawn and the current is turned on until the galvanometer registers 20 or 30 milliampères, and is maintained there for five minutes during the first treatment. After the sound is withdrawn, a vaginal douche of bichloride solution (1 in 1,000) is given and the patient is placed in bed until the following day. In subsequent treatments the current should be gradually increased to 50 or 60 milliampères, and maintained for five or ten minutes, although Apostoli recommended 250 milliampères. Treatments should be given three times a week, and twenty-five or thirty are usually necessary.

Curettage.—Like the preceding, this method may be of value in checking hemorrhage, but it cannot be relied upon in those cases in which bleeding is a prominent symptom,—as, e.g., in submucous polyps,—and is often attended with failure. It is most useful in cases in which the uterine cavity is simply elongated and not distorted. In many cases curettage is rendered impossible by the tortuous course and the inequalities of the canal, or even by a greatly enlarged cavity. There is always the risk of inflicting injury upon a submucous tumor, which may then undergo necrosis and secondary infection. The procedure has been known to cause profuse bleeding which was alarming, and controllable only by firm packing.

Other Measures.—Intra-uterine applications have been recommended by Veit, as a means of controlling hemorrhage from tumors of moderate size in women near the menopause. The uterus is dilated with laminaria tents, and the uterine cavity is first explored with the finger. If the tumor is of the submucous variety, removal is effected; if not, a considerable quantity of iodine in tincture, or of chloride of iron, is injected into the wound. Veit states that the iron is more efficient, but causes severe uterine colic.

Atmokausis has been tried for the same purpose, and has been followed with varying results. At the present time the value of the treatment is under dispute.

Non-Radical Operative Treatment.—Salpingo-Oöphorectomy. — Salpingo-oöphorectomy was first described by Tait, in 1872, and practised by him for the purpose of checking the hemorrhage from bleeding fibroids. Four years later, Trenholme of Montreal and Hegar of Freiburg adopted it, and did much to secure its employment. For a long period it enjoyed wide vogue, but lately it has been almost entirely supplanted by hysterectomy, save in rare and selected cases. The operation, unfortunately, is attended with variable results even in the cases in which it is possible. It is applicable in interstitial growths in which there are no marked degenerations, and in those cases in which the patient has not passed the menopause. It is applicable, however, to cases which promise to withstand a longer operation badly, provided the pelvic conditions are found suitable for its employment after the abdomen is opened.

The beneficial result of the operation is believed by many to be due to the establishment of an artificial menopause through the removal of the ovaries, and we have elsewhere alluded to the fact that the natural climacteric is frequently followed by cessation of bleeding and atrophy of the tumor. Others hold that the most important factor is the ligation of the ovarian arteries, with the consequent diminution of the blood supply. The influence of the latter factor has been demonstrated in cases in which one or both ovarian arteries were ligated, and the ovaries not removed, as will be described below.

The technique of removing the appendages is the same as in abdominal salpingo-oöphorectomy for other causes. Various authors state that it will check the hemorrhage or cause a reduction in the size of the tumor in from seventy-five to ninety per cent of suitable selected cases. As a rule, the beneficial results are noted soon after operation, but they may be delayed for months and sometimes for one or two years. Occasionally, they are only temporary, and the bleeding ceases for a while but returns later; in other cases the tumor does not shrink in size, but may even continue to grow. The operation is by no means either as safe or as easy as an ordinary salpingo-oöphorectomy. The tubes and ovaries are frequently so embedded in adhesions as to be neither visible nor palpable without manipulation, which may cause large abraded areas. The large blood-vessels in the broad ligament are easily injured, and serious hemorrhage may result from their puncture with the pedicle needle. Infection is more likely to occur than in the ordinary broad-ligament operation. All ovarian tissue must be removed in order to make the operation a success, and this sometimes is nearly impossible.

Ligation of the Blood-Vessels of the Uterus.—Schroeder and Antal early attempted the ligation of the ovarian vessels, and in 1889 Rydygier ligated the ovarian, uterine, and round-ligament arteries, although the operation was not ultimately successful. In 1893, Franklin Martin proposed the ligation of the uterine vessels, and this operation has been subsequently advocated by Goubaroff, Goelet, Gottschalk, Hartmann, and others. It is recommended for interstitial tumors of small size which are not the site of extensive degenerations. Gottschalk emphasizes the size of the tumor as an indication, and would restrict the procedure to growths no larger than an orange.

This operation is also followed by variable results. In some cases menstruation is suppressed and there is permanent benefit. Occasionally, the pains are diminished, but sometimes they continue with even greater severity. The procedure, however, has been attended with unfavorable results. Necrosis of the tumor has resulted, with profuse uterine discharge as well as general toxic symptoms, and several cases have succumbed from secondary infection of the necrotic tumor.   For these reasons the operation has been largely abandoned.

This procedure may be carried out by either the vaginal or the abdominal route.   The former of these is the method of choice, and the latter should be attempted only when the cervix is markedly elevated, as the operation then occasionally may be wellnigh impossible through the vaginal incision.

(A) Ligation by the Vaginal Route.

The patient is in the lithotomy position.   The cervix is pulled down and steadied by a tenaculum, and the uterine cavity thoroughly curetted.   A circular incision is made through the mucosa covering the upper part of the vaginal portion of the cervix, and it is extended for about half an inch on each side into the lateral fornices.   The muscular wall of the cervix is thus exposed.   The bladder is now stripped back from the cervix as far as the level of the internal os, where the uterine arteries can be felt pulsating.   The vessels are then exposed and the main trunk is isolated and ligated with catgut.   When this is impossible, or not deemed wise, a mass ligature has been injudiciously advised, but it should never be used.   Closure is then made by the method elsewhere described (p. 565).

(B) Ligation by the Abdominal Route.

The patient is in the Trendelenburg position.   The abdomen is opened by a medial incision.   The round ligament is pulled forward and an incision is made through the anterior peritoneal layer of the broad ligament, close to the side of and parallel to the uterus.   A blunt dissection is then made deeply until the uterine artery is found; it should then be ligated.   Care must be taken not to include the ureter in the ligature.

RADICAL TREATMENT.

There are differences of opinion as to how often radical surgical treatment is justified.   Some hold that all fibroids should be removed unless there are contra-indications to surgical interference, while others would restrict operations to such cases as present symptoms which constitute a distinct menace to life or health.   The advocates for operation in all cases call attention to the fact that the removal of small tumors is attended with practically no mortality, while in the case of the larger growths it is out of proportion to the size of the tumor.   Yet the opponents of this teaching insist that the mortality from non-operative treatment is less than that following operation, and conservatively believe that the indications should be restricted to the removal of all large or rapidly growing tumors, as well as to the smaller ones which give rise to troublesome or serious symptoms.   There is no doubt that, in recent years, the frequency of degenerative changes in the tumor, as well as those in the heart and kidneys, has convinced many that surgical treatment should be resorted to earlier and be employed more extensively; yet there are many who believe that the frequency of the more important degenerations has been overemphasized. Webster, in 1905, stated that, among 1,228 myomata, there were degenerations or pelvic complications in 562, but many of them were not dangerous. In 1,068 cases there were 62 with malignant disease, although 42 were probably but accidental associations. Hirst states that conditions actually dangerous to life or inevitably fatal were present in but 7 or 8 per cent of 203 cases operated upon in his series. Yet, in the very recent past, surgical technique has made such strides and has been productive of such a greatly reduced mortality that we believe, with the majority, that surgical procedures should be extended beyond those cases which are threatened with invalidism or death, and that all fibroids in the pre-menopause period should be removed unless there is some positive contra-indication to operation.

The more important degenerations are positive indications for operation, but, according to Olshausen, they do not occur in more than five per cent of cases. Hemorrhage that cannot be controlled by palliative measures, certainly demands operation before the woman's chance is impaired by severe anæmia; and operation is also demanded when there are pressure symptoms of high grade. Moreover, secondary complications in the adnexa, as well as the presence of a growing tumor, offer indications which are scarcely disputable. The various factors of age, social state, and other similar matters must be carefully considered in deciding in favor of an operation which is not actually demanded by conditions that threaten life or promise invalidism. Thus, single women with nobody dependent upon them may take risks which a mother of a large family is not warranted in taking; and, in like manner, one who must toil for a living should be given the opportunity of doing it with as few symptoms disturbing to health as possible. In the case of a young woman one may suggest an operation which, in one approaching the menopause, would not be advisable until the chance of a spontaneous shrinkage of the tumor had been afforded. It should be borne in mind that the menopause is greatly postponed, even to the age of fifty-three or fifty-five, in those who are suffering from interstitial and submucous fibroids, and that it rarely ever takes place as early as forty-six or forty-seven in this class of cases. The surgeon of ordinary ability should remember that the mortality attending the removal of myomata is greater in his hands than in the hands of an expert; and it is certainly sufficiently great in the latter's hands. The primary operation is not practised by most conservative men in more than fifty per cent of cases which come under investigation.

The contra-indications to operating are those of any serious surgical procedure. Before an operation is instituted the condition of the heart, lungs, and kidneys should be thoroughly investigated. Anæmia may afford a contra-indication, yet one should remember that there is the possibility that bleeding cannot be checked and the blood brought up to normal unless the tumor is removed.

The surgical procedures employed at the present time are myomectomy and hysterectomy, and the relative advantages of these have been the subject of much dispute. There is no doubt that, from the standpoint of pure theory, myomectomy has many advantages of a conservative nature. For example, it leaves the woman able to bear children and avoids the induction of an artificial menopause which frequently entails many distressing nervous complications. Myomectomy, therefore, is applicable especially to women under thirty-five years, whereas, in a person of forty or somewhat older, who is affected with a uterine fibroid, it should not be considered. Nor is the operation advisable in multiple growths or those of large size on account of the strong possibility that the uterus would not stand the strain of the pregnancy which would be likely to follow. Tubal or ovarian disease also contra-indicates the procedure, as does any other condition which is a barrier to pregnancy. Extensive cystic or other advanced degenerations of the tumor are also contra-indications on account of the great chance of secondary malignant changes. One must always bear in mind, in case of multiple tumors, that the removal of the larger tumors in no way restricts the growth of the smaller ones which are left behind. On the contrary, as long as the blood supply remains good, these may grow to such an extent as to demand a later secondary operation. Moreover, the pressure of the numerous sutures necessary for closing the uterine wound makes abdominal adhesions an almost certain sequel.

Recent investigation has shown that myomectomy is attended with greater primary mortality than hysterectomy. Hunner, in 1903, showed that the operation could not be considered benign, as it was followed, in Kelly's clinic in Baltimore, by 5 deaths in 100 cases. Winter, in 1904, reported 451 collected cases of Hofmeier, von Rosthorn, Martin, Olshausen, Schauta, Zweifel, and others, in which there was a mortality of 9.8 per cent as contrasted with one of 4.5 per cent for the cases in which supravaginal hysterectomy was performed by the same men. Kelly, in 1907, gives a mortality of 4.5 per cent for 306 myomectomies and one of 3.1 per cent for 691 hysterectomies. Kelly and Cullen, in 1909, give a mortality of 5.4 per cent for 296 abdominal myomectomies in their hands. Fifty per cent of these deaths resulted from intestinal obstruction, peritonitis, or both. Subsequent operation was necessary in 18 of the 280 patients who survived the primary operation. The same authors had a mortality of 6 per cent in a series of 84 vaginal myomectomies; 48 of the surviving cases were followed. Subsequent hysterectomy was necessary in two of these cases and carcinoma developed in one other. The primary mortality for their series of 901 abdominal hysterectomies was 5.5 per cent, with no deaths in a series of 24 cases treated by vaginal hysterectomy. The cases operated upon during the last two and one-half years gave a mortality of less than one per cent of all cases.

Winter, in 1904, carefully investigated the question of the relative values of myomectomy and hysterectomy, and drew certain conclusions from the subsequent histories of 296 cases. Two hundred of these patients had been subjected to the operation of hysterectomy and 96 to that of myomectomy, and 73 per cent of the myomectomies were cured symptomatically, while

97.3 per cent were cured by the more radical operation. His conclusions are as follows:—

(1) Myomectomy preserves menstruation.

(2) Subsequent pregnancy is possible in women under forty years of age. Pregnancy is more often noted after the removal of subserous and submucous growths of comparatively small size; it is unlikely to occur after the removal of interstitial growths larger than a child's head. The operation *per se* should not cause disturbances that are likely to interrupt subsequent pregnancy.

(3) Myomectomy prevents the unpleasant symptoms that attend the artificial menopause which occurs in twelve per cent of cases after the radical operation.

(4) There is no guard against recurrence, even if every visible and palpable tumor is removed. If a second radical operation is required, the conservative operation must be looked upon as a failure.

(5) There is no certainty that myomectomy will relieve the suffering of the patient.

(6) The immediate results of myomectomy are worse than those of the radical operation. This applies to cases operated upon by the vaginal route as well as to those operated upon by the abdominal route.

MYOMECTOMY.

Myomectomy may be performed through an abdominal or a vaginal incision. Generally speaking, the abdominal incision is preferable, and there are special indications for the vaginal operation.

Abdominal Myomectomy.—The technique of abdominal myomectomy depends upon whether the tumor is pedunculated or sessile. Preliminary to the following procedures the uterus should be curetted and its interior irrigated as part of the disinfection of the operative field. The vagina should be packed with gauze as a routine procedure, as there are many cases in which it will be deemed more wise to do a hysterectomy after the abdomen is opened, and in that event drainage may be necessary. The abdominal cavity is opened in the midline and the intestines are pushed back into the abdomen and retained by large gauze pads, so that the field of operation is isolated from the abdominal cavity. The myomatous uterus is then delivered and brought up through the wound. It is well to place gauze on the edge of the skin incision to prevent the uterus from coming in contact with the skin.

(a) Technique in the Case of Subperitoneal Pedunculated Fibroids.—The tumor is firmly held by a tenaculum and an incision is made through the peritoneal covering about the margin of the pedicle. The peritoneum is then stripped backward as a cuff, the exposed base of the pedicle is secured with one or two catgut ligatures, and the tumor cut away externally to the ligatures. The flaps of the wound are then approximated by a row of continuous catgut sutures. When the pedicle is broad, the incision should be planned so that, when the tumor is removed, there results a crater-like cavity. This raw excavation is then completely closed by a continuously running catgut suture placed deeply, and the peritoneal cuff is inverted so as to leave exposed only serous surfaces.

(b) Technique in the Case of Subperitoneal Sessile and Interstitial Fibroids. —The technique is more complicated in these cases. If there are a number of tumors to be removed, the incisions should be planned so that there shall be

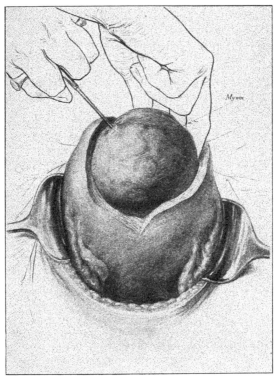

Fig. 233.—Abdominal Myomectomy. (From Doederlein und Kroenig, "Operat. Gynaekol.," Leipzig, 1905.)

as few as possible and that they shall run in the same direction. The incision is then made through the capsule until the tumor is exposed. The growth is now seized with a tenaculum and the opening in the capsule is enlarged sufficiently to allow the removal of the tumor. (Fig. 233.) The growth is separated from its bed by blunt dissection, although occasionally it may be necessary to cut it with scissors. The uterine cavity should not be opened, if it is possible to avoid it. In case there is much hemorrhage from the wound, an assistant should grasp the supravaginal cervix and maintain pressure on the uterine arteries. The ovarian vessels may also be controlled by direct pressure if necessary, although the hemorrhage is rarely considerable save in large growths. After the tumor is removed the bleeding vessels are tied off with ligatures passed through the muscle; after which the raw bed of the fibroid is closed with continuous catgut sutures and the peritoneal edge of the incision is inverted. In rare cases oozing cannot be checked in this manner and ligation of the uterine arteries is necessary.

This operation may be employed in cases in which several fibroids in the uterus are removed, yet multiple myomectomy is not advisable if the patient is anæmic and if a long period of anæsthesia is necessary. Large fibroids, even when single, should not be removed by myomectomy, because a considerable opening is apt to be made in the uterine cavity and good closure cannot always be obtained. A considerable amount of blood is usually lost during the procedure, and the uterus is not likely to be a satisfactory organ if pregnancy should subsequently result. Myomectomy should never be performed if there is any doubt as to the sterility of the uterine cavity. The mortality of this method is quite as large as that of supravaginal amputation, or complete removal, which are the methods of choice for the large growths.

Occasionally it will be found more advantageous, in performing myomectomy, to split the uterus in half at the very beginning, cutting down directly through the tumor. The edges of the wound are now widely separated, and the divided growth freed from its bed. This method is preferable to the former in difficult cases, and especially in those in which the uterus is impacted in the pelvis. Yet the majority of operators advocate the supravaginal hysterectomy in cases requiring so large a wound in the uterine muscle. Round needles are preferable to those with a cutting edge in controlling the oozing, and care should always be taken that the eye of the needle is of the same size as the suture material.

(c) Technique in the Case of Intraligamentous Fibroids.—Myomectomy is suitable only for the smaller of these growths which present definite pedicles. The tumor can easily be removed when it has been dissected from the surrounding tissue, after which the incision should be covered by the loose peritoneum which has been elevated by the growth of the tumor. Large intraligamentous growths should not be removed in this manner unless the pedicle is small. When these tumors present complicated relationships with the surrounding structures, as is usually the case, the uterus together with the tumor should be removed. There is apt to be less bleeding after hysterectomy than after myomectomy, and the important neighboring structures are not so likely to suffer injury.

Vaginal Myomectomy.—Vaginal myomectomy is indicated for the removal of:

(A) Infected submucous myomata which are contained in the cavity of the uterus or are undergoing expulsion into the vagina. These growths may be removed by the vaginal route more safely than through the abdomen. Removal should not be attempted, however, until the field of operation has been disinfected in a satisfactory manner by irrigations and local applications continued over a considerable period of time.

(B) Myomatous polyps contained in the cavity of the uterus or projecting through the cervical canal down into the vagina.

(C) Submucous tumors, when single and not of great size. Veit claims that any tumor which can be pressed into the pelvic canal from above may be removed in this manner. Medical literature shows that tumors weighing as much as six or eight pounds have been removed by vaginal myomectomy. The usual limitation of size. is that of the fœtal head, or, roughly speaking, 10 or 12 centimetres in diameter. Important factors in deciding in favor of vaginal myomectomy, in the case of a relatively large tumor, are the age of the patient and her desire to have children, as well as the situation of the growth.

(D) Cervical myomata of moderate size, which usually can be reached by means of hysterotomy and can be enucleated with comparative ease and safety.

(E) Subperitoneal myomata of moderate size, which are situated on either the anterior or the posterior wall.

(F) Single intramural myomata of moderate size, and especially those which are situated on the anterior wall.

The chief contra-indication is the size of the tumor. Although large tumors have been safely removed through the vagina by various men, the results which they have secured merely demonstrate the possibilities of the operation and not its relative desirability. Since the operative technique of the abdominal operation has been so improved, the removal of large tumors through the abdomen is more safe than the removal through the vaginal orifice. A small vagina has been given as a relative contra-indication to vaginal myomectomy, yet here, as in cervical cancers, room may be secured through the Schuchardt incision.

Details of the Operation.

(a) *In the Case of a Pedunculated Submucous Myoma.*—The growth may be removed through the dilated cervix or through a cervix which has been split by means of hysterotomy.

When the polyp does not project through the external os, the cervix may be dilated if it is thought that sufficient room can be obtained in this manner for securing the pedicle and for removing the growth. Laminaria tents should not be used to dilate the cervix, for the rapid dilatation by means of dilators has all the points of advantage. When the cervix has been sufficiently dilated, the tumor is seized with a polypus forceps and twisted off by rotation, or else its pedicle snipped with scissors. This should not be attempted until the condition of the growth and of its pedicle has been ascertained by palpation with the finger or by the use of the sound. The cavity of the uterus is then carefully curetted, mopped with formalin and perchloride of iron, and then packed with gauze.

When the cervix is already dilated and the tumor protrudes wholly or partly, a similar method may be adopted, although in cases of doubt it is wise to secure extra room by splitting the uterus. If the tumor is small it can be pulled down easily along with the cervix, and its pedicle divided after torsion inside the uterus, as previously described.

If the tumor is large, its size had best be reduced before one attempts the ligation of the pedicle. The growth is seized with a tenaculum and its connections to the uterus are explored with the finger or a sound. This had best be done while traction is exerted upon the tumor. Then the capsule of the growth should be incised in a circular manner, successive portions of the growth being cut away and as much of the tumor as possible then shelled out. Bleeding can be controlled with the forceps. When the pedicle is reached it may be ligated and divided with scissors or a snare. Torsion is frequently helpful in controlling the bleeding. The cavity of the uterus should then be carefully curetted and irrigated and firmly packed with gauze to control any oozing.

When the growth does not project through the external os and the cervix cannot be dilated sufficiently for securing the pedicle, the tumor may be removed after a hysterotomy. As a rule, the anterior hysterotomy is preferable, although the posterior incision may be indicated in certain cases. The cervix is seized with a tenaculum and the anterior vaginal wall is divided transversely at its junction with the cervix. Sometimes a circular incision around the cervix is necessary, so that the entire vaginal fornix can be elevated. The bladder is next separated from the cervical wall as high as the level of the internal os, care being taken, in dissecting, to direct the cutting edge of the knife against the cervix, thus avoiding the danger of opening the bladder. The anterior lip of the cervix is now divided in the midline. As a rule, the incised uterine tissue bleeds but little, and the oozing can be readily controlled by traction upon tenacula applied to each side and at the margin of the uterine incision. When the tumor is exposed it should be removed in the same manner as previously described. Traction, torsion, enucleation, and morcellation are the principal methods employed in accomplishing this. The pedicle should not be divided too close to the uterine wall. Some operators advise transfixion of the pedicle and ligation. If sufficient room has not been secured by the cervical incision previously described, the peritoneal reflection may be opened behind the bladder, and the uterine incision continued upward until the parts are sufficiently exposed to view. After the removal of the tumor the incision should be closed with catgut, care being taken to leave exposed, in the abdomen, only serous surfaces. The vagina is reattached to the cervix after oozing has been checked. If the hæmostasis is not complete, a gauze tent should be placed in the wound for drainage. As in the previous operation the uterus should be curetted after the removal of the tumor and mopped with formalin; packing is not indicated except in cases of hemorrhage.

(b) *In the Case of a Non-Pedunculated Submucous Myoma.*—Non-pedunculated submucous myomata are more difficult of removal than the pedunculated ones previously described. In the case of very large tumors laparotomy is preferable to the vaginal operation. The smaller tumors can be removed after a hysterotomy. When sufficient exposure has been obtained by splitting the anterior wall of the uterus, the prominent portion of the growth is seized with a tenaculum and an incision as long as possible is made through the mucosa and the capsule of the fibroid. The tumor is then shelled out from the capsule with the fingers or an enucleator, and is gradually drawn down with the forceps as it is liberated. If the growth is too large to be pulled down *en masse*, it may first be divided.

It is better to remove the large tumors by morcellation. After the growth has been exposed, either by hysterotomy or by a transverse slit across the body of the cervix, the capsule is incised over its prominent portion. The incision had best be made at right angles to its longest axis. One edge of the tumor beneath the incision is now grasped by forceps, pulled down, and cut away with the scissors, a portion of the tumor being seized immediately above before this is done, so that the tissue may not retract and bleed. This procedure should be continued until complete removal has been effected. (Fig. 234.) The greatest care should be observed that the removal of the tissue shall be confined to the centre of the tumor, in order to avoid accidental injury of the uterus beyond the growth. Sometimes, when the lower part of the tumor has been removed, the remainder of the growth may be separated by torsion. When the mass has been removed, all bleeding parts should be controlled with forceps. The cavity should be cleansed and a gauze tampon tightly packed about and around the forceps. Occasionally the peritoneal cavity is accidentally opened; and when this happens the opening should promptly be closed. The operation should not be attempted in growths of large size or even in those of moderate size, except when the tumor is undergoing degeneration and is septic; even then it is a more difficult and dangerous procedure than a cautiously conducted transperitoneal removal. When a large tumor, which has caused a very extensive destruction of the uterus, has been removed, it is good treatment to remove that organ at once, if possible, by vaginal hysterectomy.

After-Treatment.—Ergot should be administered and the forceps and gauze should be removed at the end of from thirty-six to forty-eight hours, after which daily douches of boracic acid or sterile salt solution should be given.

(*c*) *In the Case of an Interstitial Myoma.*—The methods described in a previous section are applicable to the removal of tumors of this nature. One may either split the cervix as far as the edge of the capsule, and thus remove the tumor, or may perform a vaginal cœliotomy, pull the growth down between the margins of the incision, and then remove it *en masse* or piecemeal, after morcellation. The removal of fibroid tumors by morcellation is an obsolete procedure, though we still retain its description in the text books. (Fig. 234.) As stated in the preceding section, it may be necessary, when the tumor is of large size, first to ligate the uterine arteries. After closure of the myomectomy wound, in those cases in which the growth was removed through the peritoneal surface of the anterior uterine wall, it may be safer to suture the vesical peritoneum to the anterior wall of the uterus above the former location of the tumor. Then, if secondary oozing occurs, it will be extraperitoneal, and will drain into the vagina.

(*d*) *In the Case of a Subperitoneal Fibroid.*—Subperitoneal fibroids may be removed either from the anterior or from the posterior uterine wall. Whenever possible, the anterior vaginal cœliotomy (Fig. 235) is preferable, after which, if it be found practicable, the uterus is inverted through the incision into the vagina and the growth is removed as described under Abdominal Myomectomy in this class of tumors. Occasionally, the smaller subperitoneal growths on the posterior wall of the uterus may also be removed in this fashion, yet frequently an incision into the posterior cul-de-sac is preferable. This is performed as follows: A transverse incision is made in the upper posterior vaginal fornix

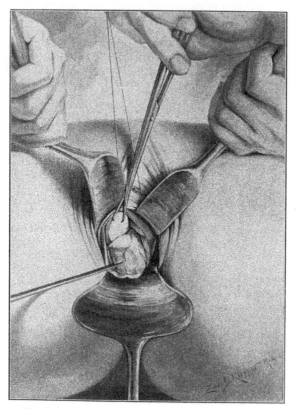

Fig. 234.—Morcellation of a Non-Pedunculated Submucous Fibroid of the Uterus. (Original.)

close to the uterus, and the incision is continued upward until the peritoneum is encountered. This is then seized, opened in the midline, and incised laterally, after the condition of the cul-de-sac has been explored with the index finger. As a rule, there is some hemorrhage from two small veins which are severed in this step. These had best be controlled by suturing the posterior flap of the peritoneum to that of the vagina. The uterus is brought through the incision in the vagina until the growth is well exposed. When this is not practicable the growth should be seized with a tenaculum, brought down into the wound, and removed in a manner similar to that for the removal of submucous growths after dilatation of the cervix. When the mass has been severed as far as the pedicle, the uterus may be inverted through the incision and the pedicle removed in the manner described in the section relating to Abdominal Myomectomy for this class of cases. The danger of myomectomy after vaginal cœliotomy consists in secondary oozing and peritonitis. For the control of the oozing from

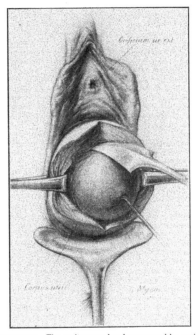

Fig. 235.—Vaginal Myomectomy. The peritoneum has been opened by vaginal cœliotomy, and the fundus drawn down and incised. (From Doederlein und Kroenig, "Operat. Gyn.," Leipzig, 1905.)

the anterior uterine wall one may cover the bleeding area with the bladder, as has been mentioned above in the description of the removal of an intramural myoma. If the tumor removed was situated upon the posterior wall, or upon the fundus, a drain should be left in the pouch of Douglas.

(e) *In the Case of a Cervical Myoma.*—Cervical myomata may be removed in a manner similar to that described above, especially if they are pedunculated. The interstitial ones tend to grow into the broad ligament and may be palpated through the vagina as distinct masses projecting laterally from the cervix. The first step of the operation, therefore, should be either a hysterotomy or a direct transverse incision into the cervix, the knife being carried through that portion which gives readiest access to the growth. The capsule is then incised and the mass removed by enucleation. The greatest care should be taken to avoid the bladder and ureters. The cavity is then closed with continuous catgut or tightly

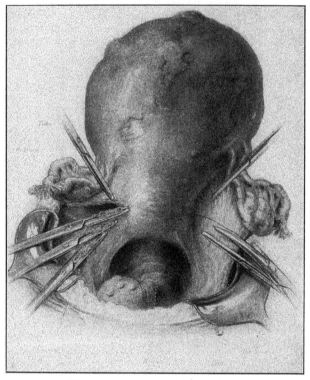

Fig. 236.—Supravaginal Hysterectomy. (From Doederlein und Kroenig, "Oper. Gynaekol.," Leipzig, 1905.)

packed with gauze. In case there is persistent oozing it may be necessary to ligate the uterine vessels.

ABDOMINAL HYSTERECTOMY.

Two methods of abdominal hysterectomy are open for adoption in the varying classes of cases. One carries with it the removal of the tumor and that part of the uterus which lies above the cervix; the other removes the tumor with the entire uterus. Successive improvements in the technique of this operation have made abdominal hysterectomy the most satisfactory of all operations for fibroid tumors. It is adapted to tumors of any shape, size, or position, but involves a mutilation of the patient which should be avoided in women in the child-bearing era, in whom it is possible to leave the uterus in good condition. Hence, the operation is usually restricted to large interstitial growths, to submucous tumors too large to be removed by the pelvic route, to subperitoneal tumors with too large a pedicle for safe ligation, to intraligamentous growths which cannot be removed separately, and to tumors which have undergone some form of degeneration. We have already indicated that myomectomy in the larger tumors carries with it a mortality greater than that of hysterectomy. The two methods shortly to be described also show differences in the primary mortality, and are indicated by different conditions. The complete removal of the uterus carries with it a higher mortality and a more difficult technique, in the hands of most men, than the supravaginal hysterectomy.

The abdominal hysterectomy for fibroids has been developed as a result of the successful removal of ovarian tumors. The abdomen was first opened in 1825, by Lizars, for a fibroid that had been mistaken for an ovarian tumor, but at this time the removal of a fibroid of the uterus was not thought of, and the operation was abandoned. In 1837 Granville successfully removed a pedunculated subserous tumor, and in 1855 the first deliberate hysterectomy for an interstitial myoma was performed by Kimball. Within the last fifteen or twenty years there have been remarkable advances in the operative technique, and the complications of sloughing and degeneration of the stump, and of protracted healing, are now avoided by our modern methods. As in ovariotomy, the pedicle was first treated extraperitoneally, because the size of the uterine stump and the difficulty of controlling the hemorrhage from it made operators hesitate to drop it back into the abdomen. Consequently it was held outside the abdominal wound by a clamp, which was tightened from time to time as the pedicle sloughed. Subsequently, elastic ligatures and the *serre-nœud* of Cintrat replaced the clamp. There resulted from this procedure a sloughing mass which exposed the patient to the risk of sepsis, and carried with it a high mortality. Schroeder first advocated covering the cut surface of the pedicle with peritoneum and then replacing the stump in the abdominal cavity. But even then bad results followed because the cervix was tied *en masse*. Subsequently improvements in the technique were made. These consisted largely in the ligation of isolated blood-vessels and the subsequent covering of the cervical stump with flaps of peritoneum. At the present time supravaginal hysterectomy carries with it a smaller mortality than the more complete removal, yet recent study has shown that it is not always the operation of choice. In case of pre-existing cervical infection, the troublesome leucorrhœal discharge may continue if the cervix has been left in place. Moreover, the association of malignant disease with myoma is so frequent (4 per cent in all cases, and 12 per cent in those over 50 years of age, according to Sutton) that its possibility must be borne in mind; for the condition commonly is not suspected nor discovered until the specimen has been examined after its removal. Therefore, if the operator does not practise total extirpation as a routine procedure, he should at least curette the uterus thoroughly as a preliminary measure and carefully examine the scrapings and the tumor itself for signs of malignancy.

Supravaginal Hysterectomy in Uncomplicated Cases.—The technique of this operation varies slightly accordingly as the ovaries are removed or allowed to remain.

Preliminary Preparations.—After the usual routine preparation, the vagina is thoroughly disinfected and as much of the uterine cavity as can be reached is carefully curetted and finally mopped with a formalin solution. The curetting is indicated, not only to reduce the opportunity of infection through the cervical canal after the removal of the corpus, but also to diminish the chance that the malignant degeneration of the endometrium may be overlooked. As the final stage of the vaginal preparation, the vagina is packed with a long strip of gauze, on account of the chance that conditions found after the abdomen is opened may demand a complete extirpation of the uterus and vaginal drainage.

The Preparation of the Abdomen.—On the day preceding the operation, the abdominal wall is thoroughly cleansed with tincture of green soap, shaved well over the symphysis, and washed first with hot water and afterward with ether and alcohol. A dry dressing is placed on the abdomen and allowed to remain in position until the patient is anæsthetized, when it is removed and the abdomen is mopped over with tincture of iodine. This dries in a minute and a half or two minutes, and renders the field sterile and ready for incision. The abdomen should *never be wet on the day of the operation* if the iodine sterilization is to be used.

Opening the Abdomen.—An incision large enough to permit the delivery of the tumor is made in the midline, or in the rectus close to the midline. In the majority of cases a cut from the symphysis to the umbilicus will suffice. The incision should be carried well down toward the symphysis, inasmuch as the last inch in the lower angle of the wound permits a better exposure of the pelvis than if the wound were extended a much greater distance at its upper end. When the fascia is exposed, the incision should be extended in the linea alba, and each rectus muscle should be partially isolated from its sheath. This allows good exposure during the operation and secures flaps which permit of the direct union of fascia with fascia, at the subsequent closure of the wound. The operating table is now raised for the purpose of elevating the pelvis and allowing the intestines to gravitate back into the abdominal cavity, after which the peritoneal cavity is opened. This is best done by seizing the pre-peritoneal fat and peritoneum with thumb forceps and elevating it, while a nick is made in the peritoneum in an oblique or shelving manner, and never between the two thumb forceps. This reduces the chances of the bowel or bladder being injured, as the latter viscus sometimes extends several inches above its normal site. Indeed, this occurs so frequently in the case of the larger tumors that the exact position of the fundus of the bladder should be ascertained as a routine procedure. This can usually be done by passing a sound immediately after catheterizing during the preliminary preparation. As soon as the peritoneal cavity is opened, the air rushes in and separates the peritoneum from the abdominal viscera. The peritoneal incision is now extended in both directions, the angles of the wound being raised upon two fingers and the cutting being done between them with the scissors, under the guidance of sight. The hand is then introduced within the abdomen, and the surface of the tumor is explored, with a view of determining its size and shape, the possible presence of adhesions, and the probable difficulty of the operation. Retractors are next inserted under the sides of the wound and the field of operation is isolated.

Isolation of the Field of Operation.—In the simpler cases, the isolation of the field of operation consists merely in replacing the intestines in the abdominal cavity. When adhesions of the omentum to the abdominal wall, the tumor, or the bladder exist, these must first be separated and the raw surfaces covered with peritoneum. The intestines may be replaced with advantage if one starts at the right side and works upward and to the left, as this method permits of an early inspection of the appendix, which, if diseased, may be bound down by adhesions or attached to the tubes or tumor. The intestines are displaced upward with large gauze packs wrung out of hot saline solution, or, with dry rolls of gauze, from one to two yards long, five inches wide, and folded so as to make six layers; they are retained in position by the same means. To one end of each of these packs is attached a tape with an artery forceps fastened at its end, so that the latter may hang without the wound and prevent the pack from subsequently being lost among the intestines. If the packs are well placed, the intestines will not come into view during the remainder of the operation. The table is now further elevated in the Trendelenburg position, and the tumor is delivered.

Delivery of the Tumor.—The delivery of the tumor can readily be effected with the hand, although a myoma forceps is frequently an aid during this procedure. Tumors limited to the body of the uterus can be lifted out readily through the wound, as the unaffected lower portion of the uterus forms a natural pedicle for the tumor. When there are multiple growths a succession of deliveries may be necessary before the entire mass is outside the wound. Too great traction must not be made upon a pedunculated tumor for fear of inflicting injury upon the pedicle and thus causing hemorrhage. If the tumor is too large to be delivered through the wound, the incision may be elongated by cutting the upper angle of the wound after the abdominal wall has been raised upon two fingers. Occasionally it is necessary to ligate and divide the upper part of the broad ligament before the tumor can be delivered. Adhesions may complicate the delivery. They are relatively uncommon, and are usually due to infection of the uterine appendages. Occasionally they are so numerous that the operation cannot be performed in the typical manner. When the adhesions are slight and non-vascular, or are not attached to the bowel or other structures that may be easily injured, they can be broken up with the fingers. Otherwise they must be treated as their special characters demand.

Supravaginal Hysterectomy when it is Found that the Ovaries are Diseased.—The tumor is drawn strongly to one side with tenacula. This exposes the ovarian vessels, which should then be ligated with catgut. To accomplish this, the outer extremity of the broad ligament should be seized between the thumb and forefinger, and a pedicle needle should be passed through the thin clear space in the ligaments immediately below the vessels. The vessels themselves should not be ligated close to the pelvic wall, as they retract after division and thus impart added tension upon the ligature. It is always well to pass two ligatures around them and to tie each of these three times. A second ligature or clamps are now placed one inch to the uterine side of the first ligature, and the vessels are cut through. The round ligament is next ligated close to the uterus, so that the major portion of this structure and the adjacent peritoneum may be left as a flap with which to cover the raw area incident to the subsequent removal of the tumor. The uterine end is clamped, and the ligament is cut through, thus opening the top of the broad ligament. These procedures are repeated on the opposite side.

Separation of the Bladder and Ligation of the Uterine Vessels.—The uterus is drawn upward and backward, and an incision connecting the incisions of the round ligaments is made about half an inch above the utero-vesical reflection of the peritoneum. The bladder is pushed away from the uterus by blunt dissection or by pressure with a sponge, until the cervix is bared nearly as far as the vaginal juncture. The tumor is pulled to the opposite side and the uterine vessels are exposed by pushing away the broad ligament from the tumor or uterus with a sponge. The large uterine veins on the side of the uterus are clearly recognizable and the pulsations of the smaller artery can be felt plainly. These vessels are now ligated in their course along the uterine wall, the ligature being passed close to the cervix or even through a part of its tissue, so as to avoid the ureters. If the broad ligament is pushed away from the uterus or tumor, and the suture is placed close to the cervix, there is little risk, in the uncomplicated cases, of injuring the ureter. The undivided portions of the broad ligament are then cut from the uterus down to the level of the uterine vessels, which are divided. The process is repeated on the opposite side.

Section of the Cervix and Closure of the Stump.—The tumor and the uterus are held up, and the level at which the amputation is to be made is determined. One should always be certain that the bladder is well below this level. A pair of bullet or small vulsella forceps should be attached to the cervix to prevent its prolapse in the wound immediately after the amputation. The cervix is then divided well below the level of the internal os, so that there will remain a crater-like cavity which facilitates the subsequent closure. While the cervix is elevated with tenacula the cavity is touched lightly with the actual cautery, or with ninety-five per cent of carbolic acid, to secure asepsis. The wound should now be carefully examined for bleeding points, particularly after the stump is returned to its normal level, as tension upon the smaller vessels frequently checks the bleeding while the stump is elevated. All bleeding points should be ligated with fine catgut and the cervical stump should be closed with interrupted or continuous catgut sutures, thus uniting the anterior and posterior walls and accurately producing hæmostasis. The sutures should not include the mucous membrane of the canal.

Murphy has simplified the technique of this procedure. After the uterus has been elevated into the abdominal incision, a heavy uterine clamp is placed on the broad ligament, either inside or outside the ovary, according as that organ is or is not to be removed. The clamp should extend down to the cervico-corporal junction of the uterus, and, if possible, it should not include the uterine artery. A similar clamp is likewise placed on the opposite side, care being taken that neither includes the wall of the bladder in front. The broad ligament is then divided down to the tip of the clamp, thus permitting the uterus to be lifted clear out of the abdomen and the cervix to be brought up to the level of the abdominal incision. The peritoneum on the posterior surface of the uterus is next incised from the tip of one clamp to the tip of the other and half an inch above the point of amputation. This peritoneal edge is grasped with two hæmostats. The cervix is then divided from behind forward (see Fig. 237) until the cervical canal comes into view; then the incision is extended gradually to the margin of the cervix, when the uterine artery may be seen and grasped, or, better still, first cut and then grasped, as one would manage a radial in amputation of the forearm. The incision should not be extended farther to the side, as the ureter is just outside the uterine artery. The opposite side of the cervix is divided in the same manner and the other uterine artery is secured. The cervix, including the canal, is then grasped with a vulsella forceps and lifted upward, while the incision is continued forward through the muscular tissue of the cervix until the sub-vesico-areolar tissue is reached, when it peels easily off the bladder. One should then inspect the anterior surface of the uterus and decide where the peritoneum may best be divided to protect the bladder and allow a sufficient fold of perito-neum to cap the cervical stump. The uterine arteries are next ligated with catgut, each one separately and with no other tissue included in the ligature. Occasionally, just anterior to the uterine artery, there is a small vessel which may need separate ligation. Not more than two ligatures at the side are needed. The funnel-shaped cervical tissue is then closed with a continuous or interrupted catgut suture, as described above. The edges of the broad ligament are then grasped with two hæmostats to steady it and the clamp is removed. There will be bleeding from two small points only; these are secured individually with catgut ligatures. There is no mass ligation of the broad ligament. An overstitch is then made with catgut; it covers the cut edge down to and across the cervix, the anterior and posterior folds of peritoneum being utilized for accurately covering the stump. (See Fig. 238.) The other broad ligament is freed from the clamp, its vessels are tied and the cut surface is embedded in a similar manner.

The advantage which this procedure has over the primary anterior or pre-vesical division of the peritoneum and localization of the uterine arteries for ligation, is to be found in the fact that, in dividing the cervix from behind, one comes upon the uterine arteries without searching for them, and they in turn signal the location of the ureters before the latter are reached, as they always lie to one side and in front of the artery and never behind it. By this method there is the least excavation or pocket formation in the cellular tissue of the broad ligament. Mass ligatures in the neighborhood of the uterine artery or in the broad ligament should always be avoided. They are unscientific and dangerous.

Covering Over of the Abraded Areas.—Each round ligament is brought down and stitched to the top of the stump, while the latter is completely covered by the vesical flap of peritoneum which is drawn over and stitched to the posterior flap of cervical peritoneum by continuous sutures. The stumps of ovarian vessels are next turned in and covered with peritoneal flaps from the broad ligament. The raw edge of the broad ligament is then closed by the union of the anterior and posterior flaps by a continuous suture. Care should be taken, during these

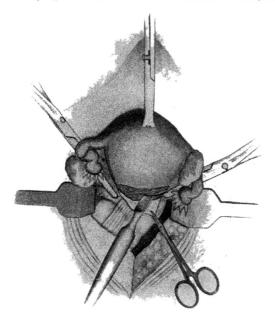

Fig. 237.—The Drawing Shows the Cervix Uteri being Divided from Behind Forward, according to Murphy's Method.   Patient is in the Trendelenburg position. (Drawn by Alfred de Roulet.)

steps, to avoid the production of dead spaces. As the result of this procedure the pelvic floor is entirely covered with peritoneum and there are no exposed raw surfaces. All free blood and clots are now removed from the pelvis and preparation is made for the closure of the abdomen. No solution whatever should be used in the abdominal cavity. Previous to the actual closure of this cavity the gauze packs are removed and counted by an assistant, who should make sure that the number removed agrees with that of the supply on hand before the operation and thus prevent the possibility of any having been overlooked in the abdominal cavity.

Closure of the Abdominal Incision.—The abdomen is closed in layers. After the small intestines are drawn down into the lower part of the abdomen, and the omentum has been spread out between them and the abdominal wall, the peritoneum is elevated with tenacula placed at each end of the wound, and the opening is closed with a running suture of fine catgut, the cut edges being everted so that no raw surfaces may be left in the cavity. The anterior aponeurosis of the rectus should be closed with a continuous catgut suture, No. 2; the muscles should not be included in the suture. A series of figure-of-8 silkworm-gut sutures are next passed. The lower loop of the 8 should include the anterior

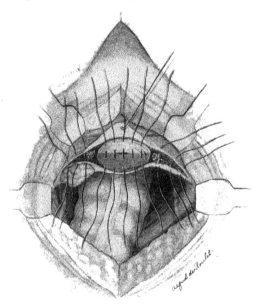

Fig. 238.—The Drawing Shows the Appearance of the Cervical Stump and Broad Ligament after Completion of the Amputation, with Sutures Inserted for Closure of Both.

aponeurosis of the rectus or linea alba, the upper loop of the figure of 8 all of the fat and skin. The edges of the skin should then be accurately approximated with horsehair sutures, and over this should be spread a fold of gauze as thick as the index finger and covered with the subiodide of bismuth powder. The silkworm-gut sutures are tied over this gauze. The latter prevents the transverse cutting of the silkworm-gut, makes an excellent splint for the immobilization of the edges, and obliterates the dead space between the rectus fascia and the skin.

Various methods are applicable to the dressing of the wound. In the majority of cases a dry dressing of sterile gauze suffices, if the edges of the pad are sealed with sterile collodion. Silver foil makes an excellent dressing for the immediate wound, as numerous experiments have demonstrated that this substance possesses bactericidal properties without being detrimental to the body tissues. Various dusting powders are also commended, all of which are covered by the gauze pad just described. This in turn is covered by loose dry sterile gauze which is held down by a gauze or cotton pad and secured by strips of adhesive plaster. A broad cotton pad is now superimposed over all and held in place by a scultetus bandage.

Supravaginal Hysterectomy When it is Found that the Ovaries are Healthy. —When it is not desired to remove the ovaries, the first suture applied to the upper part of the broad ligament is placed near the horn of the uterus and below the tubes, so as to secure the utero-ovarian ligament. Each tube is then removed, after which the operation continues as described in the previous section. After the closure of the peritoneal cuffs, subsequently to the removal of the tumor, each ovary should lie free, a short distance external to the stump.

Complete Removal of the Uterus and Tumor.—The complete removal of the uterus and tumor may be indicated where there has been rupture of pus sacs during the operation, or where, for some other reason, vaginal drainage is deemed necessary. It is also indicated in all cases in which there is a suspicion of malignant degeneration.

The first stages of the operation are identical with the corresponding stages of the supravaginal hysterectomy, i.e., up to the point where the cervix is divided. After the uterine vessels are ligated and the broad ligaments are freed from the uterus as far down as the upper part of the cervix, the bladder is carefully separated from the cervix until the upper end of the vagina is exposed. This level is easily determined by palpation of the cervix and by the recognition of the vaginal pack placed there previously to the operation. Ligatures are now placed by the side of the cervix and for some little distance on the sides of the vagina, to secure the supravaginal vessels, after which the uterus with the tumor is drawn backward and upward, and the vagina is opened by a transverse incision into the anterior fornix. Occasionally the conditions present may make an incision into the posterior fornix more desirable, yet as a rule this is more difficult, as it lies deeper in the wound. The incision is next continued around the cervix, the knife or the scissors being kept close to that structure, and the cut ends of the vagina being held up with tenacula. Sometimes it is advantageous to seize the vaginal cervix with a tenaculum as soon as the vaginal cavity is opened, and draw it toward the abdominal wound as the incision is carried about it. The uterus is thus completely severed from all attachments and is removed. Bleeding vessels are now secured with forceps and tied off with catgut ligatures. Figure-of-8 sutures may be found advantageous in controlling large oozing areas in the depths of the wound. If there are no conditions present which demand drainage, the cut edges of the vagina are secured with interrupted or running catgut sutures passed antero-posteriorly and in such a manner as not to pierce the vaginal mucosa. The vagina is now depressed to its normal level, in order to relax the tension upon the blood-vessels and to ascertain if hæmostasis is complete. All instruments which have come in contact with the vagina are now discarded, and preparation is made for the peritoneal covering of the pelvic floor. The edge of peritoneum attached to the bladder is stitched to the anterior vaginal wall and the round ligaments of each side are drawn down and sutured to the sides of the vagina to prevent subsequent prolapse; after which the posterior flap of peritoneum is joined to the posterior vaginal wall and to the peritoneum attached to the bladder. The raw surfaces in the broad ligament are then closed in such a manner as to leave a pelvic floor everywhere covered with smooth peritoneum. When drainage through the vagina is indicated, the sides of the vagina are closed, a loose coil of gauze is attached to the vaginal pack, and the knot is placed in the vagina, while the free ends of the drain are lightly placed in the field of operation in the parametrial space. The peritoneal flaps are then closed above the pack in order to isolate the vagina from the abdominal and pelvic cavities. When the peritoneal flaps are not sufficient for this purpose, the sigmoid may be utilized by stitching its free edge to the peritoneum attached to the bladder, and to the right broad ligament.

Doyen, in 1892, published a method of abdominal panhysterectomy for uncomplicated cases, in which operation the structures are cut through in the order of removal through a vaginal incision. (Fig. 239.) In this operation the myomatous uterus is pulled through the abdominal incision and swung forward and over the pubes. The posterior vaginal fornix is then opened through the pouch of Douglas. The cervix is seized with a stout tenaculum and drawn forcibly backward into the pelvis while the vagina is cut away close to the cervix. The uterus is then freed from below upward, care being observed to keep the incision tightly hugging the uterus and the vessels being ligated as they are encountered. No attention is paid to the adnexa during this incision, which passes through the tubes and round ligament at the uterine cornua. After the removal of the uterus the adnexa are dealt with as required, and the operation is completed by the usual closure.

Operations in Atypical Cases.—The typical classical operation described above suffices for the great majority of cases. Not infrequently, however, complications are met with which confuse relationships and render this procedure either very difficult or impracticable of accomplishment. In general, these complications may be grouped as due to adhesions or inflammatory conditions, or to the size, site, or degenerations of the tumor. Generally, they exist in combination.

When the tumor is complicated by inflammatory disease of the adnexa, an effort should be made to break up the adhesions about the tubes and ovaries before attempting the removal of the tumor, provided this can be done without inflicting a serious trauma upon the intestines or the ureter, but the adnexa must be completely freed before any attempt is made to remove the uterus. When the adhesions can be reached without great difficulty, an adherent tube or ovary, or a hydrosalpinx, or even a pyosalpinx can be freed by gently working the fingers down, in the lines of cleavage, between the inflamed structures and the posterior pelvic wall until their under surface is reached. Then the mass is carefully freed from the adhesions to the pelvis or the uterus and brought up and out of the pelvic cavity. Such a procedure is facilitated by strongly elevating the uterus, provided it is not impacted or can be released from the pelvis. Occasionally it may be necessary to open the tops of the broad ligaments before the tumor mass can be elevated. Adhesions to the sigmoid or rectum are not uncommon. Occasionally the sigmoid covers the diseased

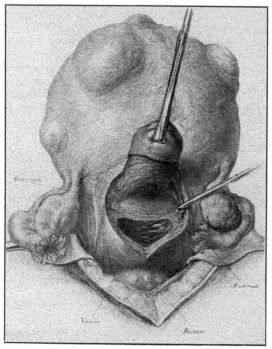

Fig. 239.—Doyen's Panhysterectomy. (From Doederlein und Kroenig, "Operat. Gynaek.," Leipzig, 1905.)

adnexa of one side, or indeed a considerable part of the tumor. If these adhesions cannot be released by working from above without the chance of inflicting serious injury upon the intestines, it is better to ligate the ovarian vessel of that side and open up the broad ligament so that they may be reached from in front or below; or else the capsule of the tumor may be split and displaced with the intestine, and the tumor extirpated, the capsule being left to support the intestinal wall. The method of Kelly, which has been described as suitable for intraligamentous growths, may be found advantageous in dealing with these cases.

Cases complicated with abscesses in the cul-de-sac should not be subjected to radical operation until after vaginal incision and drainage have been tried some months previously. The risk of infection from the dissemination of pus or infectious material, in a radical removal of a myomatous uterus, is extremely great, on account of the wide area of cellular tissue opened in the removal of the tumor mass.

Adhesions of the omentum and intestines to the tumor may occasion serious complications. Generally, they can be freed by cutting under slight tension and with the guidance of the eye before one attempts the removal of the tumor, although not infrequently this step may better be performed later. The greatest care should be taken to avoid the production, on the surface of the bowel, of raw areas which may later lead to ileus or serious adhesions. When the intestines are matted down by broad and dense adhesions, it may be wiser not to cut them in the usual way but to dissect them from the tumor in such a manner as to leave wide flaps of the latter's serous coat, which may later be turned back to form a smooth peritoneal coating about the bowel. Occasionally the omentum is attenuated, and presents itself only as a thin sheet composed of strands of blood-vessels. Open spaces in this structure must be closed if practicable, and, if this cannot be done, the omentum must be amputated above the level of the spaces and the raw edges covered.

Ovarian cysts of moderate size may usually be removed with the tumor. If they are of large size they should be reduced by tapping. The general rule is that the first efforts of the surgeon, in cases which present unusual complications that obscure the landmarks, should be directed to the removal of the tumor mass and appendages. After the enucleation the complications can be managed with greater facility.

The appendix may be the seat of an old inflammatory process which has resulted in the formation of dense adhesions between it and the structures composing one side of the tumor. Occasionally these adhesions may be so dense that they can be treated better after the removal of the tumor by Kelly's plan of attacking it from below, as will be described later.

Sometimes, through the development of multiple growths, the tumor presents itself as a large irregular mass that fills a large part of the pelvis. Occasionally the removal is simplified if some of the individual tumors are first removed, as advocated by Pean.

The most difficult cases are usually those in which the uterus and tumor are fixed in the pelvis by a mass of adhesions, the presence of which obscures the landmarks and the more important vessels. The incarceration of the tumor in the pelvis may force the bladder up into a position in the abdomen which further obscures the relationships. The danger from trauma in blindly attempting to break up adhesions is very great, as the tearing of important structures may excite uncontrollable hemorrhage or may scatter infection throughout the entire wound. While it is true that such masses can be removed according to the classic method for uncomplicated cases after the adhesions are separated, nevertheless much valuable time will be lost in the ligation of single vessels and in the blunt dissection that will be necessary to expose the cardinal vessels. When the ovarian vessels can be exposed they should be ligated together with the round ligaments, and the top of the broad ligament should be opened. By pushing the cellular tissue to one side the tumor may be partially freed so that it can be brought out of the pelvis, although Kelly's method of bisection of the mass may greatly simplify the procedure. In cases with obscure land-marks the position of the round ligaments may afford valuable aid.

The bladder is sometimes displaced upward upon the tumor, and, when this is the case, its separation may be attended with considerable difficulty. For example, it may be displaced upward by a growth developing below it; it may also be displaced upward by a growth which fills the pelvis and forces it to expand in this direction; or it may be dragged upward by adhesions. The line of reflection of the vesical peritoneum is often raised so high that, in making the usual incision, the bladder may be opened. One cannot always rely upon the sound to show the height of this viscus, as the progress of this instrument may be arrested by the tumor. Frequently the vessels of the bladder are enlarged, sinuous, and congested. These may assist in locating the line of the vesical reflection, and the incision must always be made above them, as, when they are cut, great vascular sinuses are opened, which can be controlled with difficulty even by numerous clamps. In case of doubt the incision to free the bladder should always be made well above the possible location of the viscus. The great chance that the ureters are elevated together with the bladder must always be borne in mind. As a rule, they will be displaced downward in the separation of the bladder.

Serious complications have been so difficult to meet that various operative methods have been proposed, most of which have many points of advantage over the attempt to reduce the complicated to a simple state before proceeding to the removal of the tumor. These methods involve the principle of attacking the adherent masses last and from below, after the important landmarks have been recognized and dealt with.

When there is a large intraligamentous growth of one side the methods of Pryor and Kelly will be found advantageous. They are practically the same in principle, but the Kelly method is one of supravaginal hysterectomy, while that of Pryor is essentially a panhysterectomy.

Kelly's Method of Operating.—Kelly's method (Fig. 240) was advocated by him for all cases, even the uncomplicated ones, but is especially valuable in the removal of one-sided intraligamentous growths. It consists in a continuous posterior incision down through one broad ligament, across the cervix and up through the other broad ligament; the procedure being in contrast with the classic method of supravaginal hysterectomy, in which an incision is made from above downward on each side of the broad ligament before the cervix is amputated. By the employment of this method there is a great saving of time (Kelly states from sixty to eighty per cent), but there is also greater ease in the removal of intraligamentous tumors and of tumors complicated by the presence of inflam-matory masses behind the broad ligament, without involving much risk of injuring the uterus. The inflammatory masses back of the cervix are also readily attacked from below after the division of the cervix and the recognition of the hitherto obscured landmarks. The details of the procedure are as follows: —*The start should be made on the side which is more free from complications.* The broad ligament is ligated as in the more usual operation, and the bladder is separated and pushed down to expose the supravaginal cervix. The uterine artery is exposed and ligated as in the classic operation. It is not always necessary to ligate the uterine veins. The cervix is next cut across, while the uterus is elevated and pulled over to the fixed side. As the last fibres of the cervix are severed, the other uterine artery is exposed and is caught with artery forceps about one inch above the level of the cervical incision and consequently above the point at which the artery crosses the ureter. The intraligamentous nodule is now peeled from between the layers of the broad ligament without risk of in-

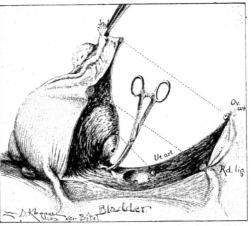

Fig. 240.—Kelly Technique for Hysterectomy, from Left to Right.

juring the ureter; after which, by rolling the uterine body still further out, the round ligament and then the ovarian vessels are clamped and cut. Sutures are now applied and the incisions are closed in the manner already described.

When the fibroid develops mainly within the pelvis, whether intraligamentous or not, it may disturb the relationships to such a degree that the ovarian or uterine vessels, or both, cannot be found easily or tied. In such cases Kelly has proposed a sagittal bisection of the uterus and tumor. The bladder is freed from the cervix in the usual manner and the uterus and tumor are then bisected as far down as the level of the cervix. In order to avoid any risk of injuring the vessels through losing landmarks, a probe is inserted into the uterine cavity through which the bisection is carried. When the cervix is reached it is amputated in successive halves, and each half is removed according to the method employed in the preceding procedure. This plan is also advocated when the adnexa are diseased and held down by firm adhesions below and behind the myomatous mass, which is also firmly held to the pelvic wall by dense adhesions. By this means the enucleation is simplified and the large cardinal vessels are easily reached. There is, however, the danger of exposing accumulations of pus or necrotic material in the bisection of the organ through the uterine cavity, as has not infrequently happened, thus adding greatly to the risk of operation and frequently necessitating the entire removal of the uterus and cervix and subsequent drainage.

Occasionally a large myoma is encountered, the upper pole of which is firmly adherent to the bowel. Kelly reports such a case in which the growth reached to the umbilicus, and was firmly attached at its upper pole to the transverse colon, upon which pus was discharging from the body of the tumor. This was operated upon as follows:—The cervix was located behind the symphysis at the vesical reflection. After the bladder had been stripped back the cervix was divided transversely by plunging a knife through its centre and continuing the incision to either side. As soon as the cervical division was completed, the uterine arteries were ligated, and then, by forcibly pulling the cervix upward, the broad ligaments, the round ligaments, and the ovarian vessels were clamped from below and behind, thus permitting the detachment of the colon and the closure of the bowel without embarrassment from the presence of the tumor and with lessened risk of infection.

Pryor's Method of Operating.—Pryor's method of panhysterectomy for intraligamentous tumors of one side is as follows:—The ovarian vessels and the round ligament are ligated on both sides, after which the bladder is separated in the usual manner and pushed downward until the vaginal cervix can be palpated through the anterior wall of the vagina. The broad ligament on the free side is next pushed back until the uterine vessels are exposed and ligated. The vagina is then opened in front, and the incision is carried around to the side on which the vessels are ligated. While the uterus is forcibly pulled toward the side on which is located the intraligamentous nodule, the cervix is seized with tenacula and forcibly drawn through the vaginal incision, thus putting the intact portion of the vagina on the stretch. The cervix is then cut free, thus exposing the uterine artery, which is ligated and cut close to the cervix under direct sight. The intraligamentous growth can now be shelled from its attachments without fear of injuring the ureters. The incision is then carried upward and the tumor is removed. Although the six cardinal vessels are ligated, other smaller vessels may require separate ligation, particularly at the base of the broad ligament, in the posterior vaginal wall, and in the utero-sacral ligaments. After hæmostasis is complete, the raw areas and the incision are closed as previously described.

When intraligamentous growths are present on both sides, Pryor advocated a method which first removed the nodules, and allowed the ureters to return to their normal positions before the removal of the uterus. The ovarian vessels and round ligament are ligated and the bladder is detached from the cervix. The anterior wall of the uterus is then split from the fundus down through the cervix into the vagina. An incision is made through the endometrium laterally, through the uterus to the base of the tumor, which is fixed with a corkscrew and enucleated. The posterior wall of the uterus is then divided and the half of the uterus first cut laterally is removed. The procedure is then repeated on the other side.

Fibroids Originating from the Posterior Cervico-Corporal Junction.—These fibroids extend downward from the point of origin, burrowing in between the rectum and the uterus, carrying the latter up against and above the symphysis, and elevating the Douglas fold of peritoneum. They are very difficult of removal without inflicting an injury upon the rectum, as there is no peritoneum between the tumor and the rectum. The safest method of procedure is, first, to detach the upper portion of the tumor—its point of origin—from the uterus; next, to remove the uterus by a supravaginal amputation; and then to grasp the upper portion of the fibroid, split its connective-tissue capsule, and enucleate it, leaving the capsule to support the anterior wall of the bowel behind, the uterus on the side, and the posterior wall of the vagina in front. The tumor can be removed without the hysterectomy. The most dependent portion of the pocket should be drained into the vagina by a tube extending up to the peritoneum.

RELATIONS BETWEEN A UTERINE FIBROMYOMA AND STERILITY.

The question of the relationship between fibroids and sterility is of the greatest interest and has long been a matter of contention. For many years it has been a common teaching that fibroids predispose to sterility, yet the more recent investigations indicate that there are so many exceptions to the rule that we must consider the subject as still open to debate. There is no doubt that the older teaching is supported by statistics. Thus, Olshausen, in compiling the tables of nine other investigators, found that sterility was noted in 520 of 1,731 patients affected with uterine fibroids, and in like manner Charpentier found it in 476 of 1,554 other cases. Other students of this question have cast considerable doubt on the true value of these statistics, which, they claim, are largely vitiated by the error of omitting controlling data, and, with Hofmeier, show that pregnancy is most frequent in the third decade of life, while fibroids are usually met with at a far later period, when there may be many other reasons to account for even relative sterility.

The exact relationship between this disease and conception is unknown, since pregnancy or sterility may be found with all varieties of uterine fibromyomata. Thus, if we recall the frequency of symptoms in uterine fibroids, it will be seen that there are many factors which bring about more or less important changes in the uterine endometrium and consequently may produce sterility—such, for example, as menorrhagia, metrorrhagia, leucorrhœa, etc. Generally speaking, pregnancy is less likely to occur in a uterus that is the seat of a submucous or a large interstitial growth, which is rapidly developing toward the uterine cavity. It is not uncommon in women in whom the growth is subperitoneal and pedunculated, and in others in whom the tumors are situated near the fundus of the uterus and are not growing rapidly. Exceptions to all of these, however, are encountered.

If we include the smaller tumors, we find that fibroids are very commonly encountered during pregnancy. The older observers considered only the larger growths and found the complication but infrequently. Thus, Pinard observed but 84 in 13,814 consecutive cases of labor in the Baudelocque clinic—a proportion of six-tenths of one per cent.

The effect of pregnancy upon the fibroids varies within wide limits. Rapid increase in size, however, is frequently observed. As would be expected from a purely theoretical consideration, the changes resulting in the tumor depend primarily upon the increased vascularity in the pelvic cavity, and vary accordingly with the site of the tumor and its structure. Rapid increase in size is usually due more to œdema than to actual hypertrophy, although both factors must be considered. The large tumors are usually softer in consistency than they are in the non-pregnant condition and frequently present alterations in form due to the compression exerted by the growing ovum. Central necrosis occasionally is found in the large soft growths. Tarnier and Budin have observed, in soft fibroids, rhythmic contractions resembling the intermittent contractions of a pregnant uterus. Yet it is still uncertain whether this phenomenon is actually due to the contractions of the tumor tissue or to those of the uterine musculature.

The influence of the fibroid upon the pregnancy is also variable and depends upon many modifying conditions. It is generally stated that abortion, or premature labor, commonly results, yet some, as Hofmeier, state that this is an exaggeration, as it ensued in but 6.9 per cent of 796 cases collected by him. Nauss, however, describes it in 47 of 241 cases. It may be anticipated in growths which have caused profound alterations of the endometrium. Retroversion of the uterus may occur in the early months of pregnancy, and is then due to the weight of a fibroid in the fundus of the uterus. Several cases of prolapse have also been recorded. In advanced pregnancy pressure symptoms may result from the presence of large or multiple tumors.

At the time of labor the effect produced by a fibromyoma depends entirely upon the size and situation of the growth. Generally speaking, the subserous pedunculated growths of the fundus do not seriously complicate birth unless they have prolapsed into the pelvis. On the other hand, large cervical growths, or interstitial forms which have developed in the pelvic cavity, may constitute a serious obstruction to normal labor. (Fig. 241.) Occasionally the uterine contractions may cause the partial extrusion of a submucous tumor into the vagina, where, if the new-growth be of large size, it may prevent the descent of the fœtal head. The uterine contractions are also frequently weak, irregular, and ineffectual.

Even when the tumor, for reasons already given, does not interfere with the progress of labor, it frequently causes abnormal presentations. Olshausen, in tabulating the reports of four observers, found 24 per cent of breech and

19 per cent of transverse presentations in 304 cases of labor occurring in women affected with uterine fibroids. Pujol records 27.18 per cent of breech and 19 per cent of transverse presentations in 100 similar cases. Placenta prævia is also more common in this condition than when the uterus is normal. Fibroids predispose to post-partum hemorrhage, partly because the nodules interfere with the normal contraction and retraction of the uterus, and partly because they offer mechanical obstacles to the separation and expulsion of the placenta.

During the involution of the uterine musculature in the puerperium, fibroids frequently undergo degenerative changes and may give rise to serious symptoms. Gangrene may result if the labor is continued for a sufficient length of time or

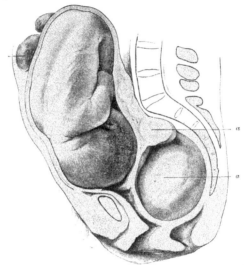

Fig. 241.—Obstruction to Labor due to the Presence of an Impacted Subserous Fibroid (a, a).
(After E. Bumm, "Grundriss zum Studium der Geburtshuelfe," 1903.)

if the growths are subjected to much pressure. The importance of these degenerative processes is unfortunately not universally recognized.

The recognition of the association of fibroids and pregnancy is not always easy, and is usually not made in the early months. Hemorrhage may occur at intervals from the elongated uterine cavity and may be mistaken by the patient herself for the menstrual flow; and the recognition of the true cause of the bleeding may not take place until the advent of characteristic symptoms. A sudden increase in the size of a fibroid which has been under observation should always arouse the suspicion of pregnancy. Subperitoneal fibroids are frequently mistaken for fœtal parts, or are overlooked if they are situated on the posterior uterine wall, although—as shown by Olshausen—pedunculated bosses are usually flattened out with the advance of pregnancy, unless the fibroid mass is of large size. Frequently a simple fibroid, in an early pregnancy, is mistaken for an enlarged metritic uterus, but not uncommonly the tumor simulates a portion of the uterus and may lead to the diagnosis of ectopic pregnancy. Occasionally a fibroid nodule in the lateral fundus may simulate a bicornuate uterus, with pregnancy in one horn. In the later months fibroids in the pregnant uterus may be confused with multiple pregnancy.

The treatment, in the presence of an association of the two conditions, varies with the individual case. In the great majority of instances no special symptoms are caused nor is there any dystocia, and consequently no special treatment is required. When impaction of the growth is threatened, the knee-chest position should be ordered and an attempt made to raise the tumor above the pelvic brim by careful manipulation. Even after failure of these procedures, the tumor may rise spontaneously out of the pelvis with the subsequent development of the uterus. If the symptoms are not threatening, active treatment may be deferred until there is hope of saving the child. Operation should then be postponed until the time of expected labor, as the uterus frequently changes its size and position and renders operative measures unnecessary from the obstetrical point of view. When, on the contrary, threatening symptoms supervene so early in pregnancy as to preclude all reasonable chance of saving the child, the case should be treated from the surgical standpoint. Frequently it is better treatment to evacuate the uterus and wait for involution before removing the growth, than to open the abdomen as a primary measure. Occasionally myomectomy is possible during the pregnancy. Stavely, in 1894, reported 33 cases of myomectomy performed during pregnancy (between 1885 and 1894). The maternal mortality was 24.25 per cent. Of these 8 deaths, 2 were due to hemorrhage, 1 to peritonitis, 3 probably to infection after abortion, and 1 to "long-standing aortic disease," and in one case the cause was not given. In 3 cases in which the mother died, no mention is made as to whether abortion took place, or not. Abortion was mentioned in ten cases. Duncan Emmett has recorded 44 cases, which occurred between 1890 and 1900, with a maternal mortality of 9 per cent. Thumin's series includes 62 myomectomies between the years 1885 and 1901, with a mortality of 10 per cent.

Better results are reported from the employment of supravaginal hysterectomy, especially when the operation is performed early in pregnancy.

Myomectomy must have a limited sphere of usefulness during pregnancy for two reasons: first, because there is no indication for the removal of the smaller growths; and, second, because in the larger forms operative removal is contraindicated on account of the danger of rupturing the scar in the strain of subsequent labor. Practically, there are few cases in which the procedure is justified, as better results will be obtained after the termination of pregnancy. Unless there are pressure symptoms or disease of the heart or kidneys, the case should be closely observed until the viability of the child is assured, when a Porro-Cæsarean operation should be considered upon the advent of symptoms of dystocia.

ADENOMYOMA OF THE UTERUS AND ACCESSORY ORGANS.

Adenomyomata, as the name implies, consist of glandular elements and myomatous tissue. They form a distinct class of myomata, and are easily recognizable under the microscope, and very often macroscopically in the gross specimen. Indeed, within the last few years, owing to the better understanding of this class of tumors, the condition is often diagnosed, prior to operation, from the symptoms and findings upon examination. It would appear that, with the recognition of this type of tumor, many of the old classifications of cystic myoma will disappear, for recent advance has shown that the cystic tumors which present a lining of epithelium in the cyst spaces are usually adenomyomata. The growths are found in any part of the uterus, the tubes, or the round ligament. (Fig. 242.)

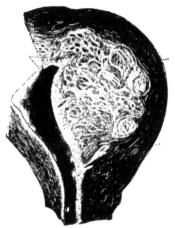

FIG. 242.—Diffuse Adenomyoma of the Posterior Uterine Wall. (From Cullen, "Adeno-Myome des Uterus," Berlin, 1903.)

The occasional presence of glandular tissue in uterine myomata has long been recognized, and up to 1884 Schroeder, Herr, and Grosskopf were able to collect one hundred such cases. Yet these growths were not recognized universally as distinctive tumors until von Recklinghausen directed the attention of the medical world to them in 1896, since which time they have been the subject of considerable investigation.

ETIOLOGY.—The causative factor is unknown, but is usually ascribed to congenital causes. The origin of the epithelial elements is also still under dispute. Some claim that the tumor is composed essentially of epithelium, and therefore is a true adenoma with a secondary development of smooth muscle; while others take the view that it differs from the ordinary myoma only in the secondary extension of glandular tissue from the endometrium. According to von Recklinghausen there are two types. In one the epithelial elements are derived from portions of the original Wolffian bodies which had become pinched off in some way and had then, after long remaining dormant, finally developed into glandular areas. In the other type the glandular elements arise from the uterine mucosa. Von Recklinghausen's report was based upon the examination of thirty tumors, of which twenty-three were from the uterus and yet a connection between the uterine mucosa and the glandular spaces of the tumor could be demonstrated in but a single instance. The majority of the larger growths presented a characteristic arrangement of the glandular tissue. There was one main canal, into one side of which ran many subsidiary tubules, radiating out like the fingers of a fan. The tubules were closely approximated like those of a kidney, and the resemblance was further increased by numerous cystic dilatations in the secondary channels, which dilatations appeared to mark off a medullary and a cortical zone. The whole picture strongly suggested the possibility that the epithelial elements originated from the Wolffian bodies. This suggestion was strengthened by the site of the tumors. While the growths whose glandular tissue was connected with the endometrium lay deep in either the anterior

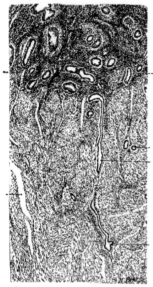

or the posterior wall, the larger tumors were found near the tube and on the posterior surface of the uterine wall. This theory of the origin from the Wolffian epithelium was presently supported by Pick and others, although reports of the origin from the glandular tissue of the endometrium followed—for example, by Cullen, Baldy, Loncope, and others. (Fig. 243.) Cullen, in 1903, reported a series of twenty-two cases. In nearly all of the specimens the glands of the tumor were found to be directly continuous with those of the uterus. The epithelium of the tumor also resembled that of the uterine glands, and the presence of blood in the glands of the tumor further suggested that these detached islets of uterine mucosa maintained the menstrual function. Cullen, therefore, took the stand that the glandular elements of the tumor represented aberrant endometrium, which in some way had extended through the crevices or chinks in the

FIG. 243.—Extension of a Uterine Gland into a Diffuse Adenomyoma. (From Cullen, 1903.)

myomatous tissue. This dislocated endometrium either retained its connection with the parent glands, or else became atrophied in part of the connecting gland, possibly through compression of the muscular bands, detached areas of glandular tissue being thus left in the depth of the tumor. This hypothesis is strengthened by the case reported by Whitridge Williams, in which the uterus of a woman dying shortly after labor proved to be the seat of a diffuse adenomyoma, in which the stroma of the glandular areas was found to be converted into decidua. Cullen also has reported a similar finding in an adenomyoma complicated by a tubal pregnancy. Since the appearance of Cullen's book, his theory has rapidly gained ground, and is now held to account for the great majority of cases, although possibly a smaller number can best be explained by von Recklinghausen's hypothesis. In Cullen's able work, published in 1908, the drawings of the sections plainly show the method of extension. In fifty-five of fifty-six cases of diffuse adenomyoma of the uterus the endometrial epithelial origin could be demonstrated.

FREQUENCY.—We have comparatively few data bearing upon the frequency of the tumors, most of which have been accidentally discovered in the routine examination of the laboratory. Cullen, in 1908, reported that 5.7 per cent of the 1,283 specimens of fibroids which came under his observation were actually demonstrated to be adenomyomata, yet he called attention to the fact that this percentage is probably lower than the actual one, as there is the possibility that some adenomatous patches were overlooked in the routine examination of the fibroids in his series. It will be seen at a glance that, in order positively to exclude adenomyomata, all tumors should be carefully cut into thin cross sections, and all suspicious areas subjected to careful microscopic examination. Largely on account of the enormous labor entailed by such methods, only the more suspicious cases were so treated.

PATHOLOGICAL ANATOMY.—The great majority of adenomyomata are diffuse growths, which infiltrate the normal uterine walls and presently replace them. They are not included in a capsule as are the ordinary fibroids. This form of new-growth may occur in any portion of the uterus. When it arises in the cervix, the glandular areas may resemble the cervical glands. The appearance of the tumor varies according to its location in the uterus. Von Recklinghausen distinguished four varieties:—(1) Hard tumors in which the myomatous tissue preponderates; (2) cystic tumors with dilated glands; (3) soft tumors in which the glandular structures predominate; (4) tumors of the angiomatous type, in which the mass as a whole is very soft and contains dilated vessels.

Cullen, in 1908, thus divided these tumors from the clinical standpoint:— (1) Adenomyomata in a uterus of relatively normal contour; (2) subperitoneal and intraligamentous forms; (3) submucous forms. We will consider them here according to Cullen's classification.

Adenomyomata in a Uterus of Relatively Normal Contour.—In these cases the uterus is rarely enlarged beyond three times its normal size, and is often covered with adhesions. Indeed, the growth may be so firmly embedded that the removal of the uterus in which it is seated is attended with much difficulty. Occasionally growths have been recorded which, in their advance, have lifted up the peritoneum of the cul-de-sac of Douglas, and have become adherent to the rectum. The extent of the myomatous transformation varies, and the thickening may occasionally extend from the mucosa as far as the peritoneal covering. Either wall of the uterus may be involved. If the growth has developed almost entirely in one wall, that side of the organ is unusually thick. On section of the uterus the diagnosis can be made macroscopically. The rounded outline of the enlarged organ and the uniform increase in density, with no evidence of a circumscribed tumor, are characteristic features. The difference between the glandular tissues and the normal muscle is clearly marked. The endometrium is generally seen to be normal or slightly thickened, although occasionally it may appear to be attenuated. Rarely are there polypoid projections, and the adenomatous growth extends to, but not into, the endometrium. The outer muscular coats are also generally normal, and between the endometrium and the external layer of muscular tissue lies the tumor. This is of variable thickness and appears as a mass of coarsely fibrillated fibres arranged in whorls, with occasional areas of homogeneous translucent substance resembling mucous membrane. In these areas small cystic spaces are occasionally found, but in this form of tumor rarely are there cysts of any considerable size. The glandular areas frequently present a brownish discoloration which, in the cystic zones, is due to the presence of a chocolate-colored fluid.

Histologically, the growth is composed of myomatous tissue and glandular structures. The former differs from the type found in the ordinary fibroids only in that there is no definite encapsulation, the tissue merging gradually into the surrounding muscular wall. The glandular tissue occurs in the form of irregular masses of variable size and shape, which may be scattered throughout the tumor, but usually are more abundant near the uterine cavity. The glands present the characteristics observed in the normal endometrium, save that their outline is more irregular, which difference, however, is readily explained by the conditions accompanying their development. The glands are embedded in cellular tissue, as in the normal endometrium. They are of tubular form, and frequently several of these open into one chief canal which later may become a cyst of some size. The arrangement of these tubules is not uniform, and occasionally they may enter the terminal canal on one side, in the manner in which the ducts of the glomeruli of the mesonephron communicate with the main canal. It was from this characteristic that von Recklinghausen concluded that the origin of the adenomatous structures was in the Wolffian body. The microscopical picture varies, of course, according to the plane in which the section is made. Thus, when the growth is cut in its long diameter, the field will present a number of cross sections, while in other specimens, in which the cut has been made in a different plane, the glands will appear as long and narrow tubules. Very often ingrowths of glandular structure are seen advancing inward from the endometrium. The greater part of the epithelial structure lies near the endometrium in the periphery of the whorls of the connective tissue. The glandular elements are lined with a single layer of ciliated columnar epithelium (like that of the normal endometrium), with oval vesicular nuclei in the base of the cells. The stroma also resembles that of the lining membrane of the cavity of the uterus, and contains thin-walled vessels. The cyst spaces of the central duct contain old blood and pigmented cells which probably result from menstrual changes. As a rule, the glandular areas of the tumor may be traced directly to the endometrium of the uterine cavity.

Subperitoneal and Intraligamentous Adenomyomata.—The process by which these tumors extend is practically the same as that which characterizes the extension of an ordinary fibroid; both grow toward the outer surface of the uterus. If the tumor is situated above the middle of the uterus, the resulting form is subperitoneal, whereas if it is located below this point and on the lateral side of the uterus, the growth is likely to spread out between the folds of the broad ligament.

The subperitoneal adenomyomata may be of various sizes and shapes. The site of attachment is usually broad, although occasionally it is so narrow as to suggest a pedicle. The type of growth differs from the diffuse type previously described, in that cystic formation is almost the rule, especially in the large tumors. The cysts vary in size from a mere pin-point to practically that of the whole mass, and they usually contain chocolate-colored fluid. (Fig. 244.) They are commonly multiple. Occasionally the cystic growths can be seen shining through the peritoneal covering of the uterus. Usually they are dark-colored, but various pictures are presented according to the amount of myomatous tissue which separates the cystic centres from the peritoneal covering. There is no

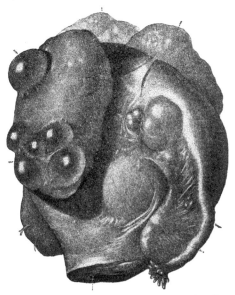

Fig. 244.—Cystic Subperitoneal Adenomyoma. .(From Cullen, "Adeno-Myome, des Uterus," Berlin, 1903.)

doubt but that these cases of adenomyoma form a considerable percentage of those which formerly were described as peritoneal inclusions.

The cyst walls are composed of myomatous tissue and are lined with a well-defined membrane, the inner zone of which consists of a single layer of cylindrical epithelium that is commonly ciliated. The rest of the tumor is similar to that of an ordinary myoma.

The intraligamentous forms of adenomyoma are similar in character to those of the subperitoneal variety. Sometimes the cysts are of extremely large size. Breus has described an adenomyoma that contained several cysts from which seven litres of fluid were evacuated at operation prior to the removal of the tumor. Both the subperitoneal and the intraligamentous forms have one characteristic in common, viz., that all the larger growths are cystic.

Submucous Adenomyomata.—Submucous adenomyomata are the rarest forms of uterine adenomyoma. They differ from the types previously described only in the fact that they are forced into the uterine cavity in their development, and finally make their appearance in the form of polyps. It is quite probable that this type starts as a diffuse growth, and becomes polypoid when the contractions of the uterus tend to force it from its bed, in precisely the same manner as the ordinary myomata are extruded from the uterus. There is commonly but little cyst-formation, as the growth is constantly subjected to pressure from all sides of the uterus. The condition of the mucosa covering the polyp varies just as it does in the ordinary myomatous polyps. The structure of the tumor is identical with that of the other diffuse forms.

Cervical Adenomyomata.—Cases have been described in which the glandular elements are derived from the cervical epithelium, although sometimes the growth extends downward from the uterine endometrium above the internal os. Various forms may result, depending upon the direction of the tumor's growth. Landau and Pick have reported a case in which the cervical canal was entirely obliterated by a tumor which completely shut off the uterine cavity from the vagina.

The histological picture is similar to that of the preceding forms, save that the glandular areas may resemble the normal cervical glands.

Other Forms of Adenomyomata.—Adenomyomata of the uterine horn and of the round ligament have also been described. In their essential features they do not differ from any of the preceding types.

DEGENERATIONS OF UTERINE FIBROMYOMATA.—Degenerations, aside from that of cyst formation, are infrequently encountered in this class of tumors. This is undoubtedly due to the close relation which exists between the uterus and the tumor, and to the consequent good circulation and nourishment. As already noted, the cysts are due to the deposits of menstrual fluid in the blind pockets of the growth. Their ultimate size is dependent upon the resistance offered by the uterine wall and the *vis a tergo* of the menstrual secretion. The subject has been fully considered above.

Carcinoma has been encountered rather infrequently in adenomyoma. It may originate primarily in the epithelial elements of the tumor or may extend into the mass as a secondary invasion from a carcinoma of the uterus proper. An adenomyoma may be observed in a carcinomatous uterus in which the cancer has not yet invaded the benign tumor. Primary carcinomatous degenerations have been recorded by Rolly, Kaufmann, Babescu, and Schwab, while von Recklinghausen, Cullen, Meyer, and Babes have reported instances of secondary cancerous invasion of an adenomyoma. Cullen, Gruenbaum, and von Recklinghausen have observed adenomyomatous uteri that contained carcinoma which had not involved the adenomyoma by extension.

Only very infrequently has sarcoma been observed to invade an adenomyoma. Kaufmann, Iwanoff, and Bauereisen have reported cases.

According to Clark, tuberculosis of an adenomyoma has been observed but five times, up to 1908.   The cases were recorded by von Recklinghausen, Hoesli, Archambauld and Pearce, and Gruenbaum.

CONDITION OF THE TUBES AND OVARIES IN ADENOMYOMA.—Cullen carefully examined the tubes and ovaries in forty-five cases.   Fifteen were normal and thirty presented numerous adhesions, which, in his belief, had developed as a result of a mild degree of pelvic peritonitis caused by the diffuse myomatous growth.   As a result of his study he concludes that adenomyoma does not materially increase the incidence of pathological changes in the tubes and ovaries.

Adhesions were found on the uterus in twenty-four of forty-nine cases.   As a rule, they involved the posterior aspect of the organ and rarely implicated the anterior face.

SYMPTOMS OF UTERINE ADENOMYOMA.—The symptoms of uterine adenomyoma vary according to the size and location of the growth, and also according to whether the uterus does or does not contain, in addition, the ordinary fibroids. Usually the latter are also present.

Hemorrhage is common and is usually present at first as a lengthened menstrual period.   In association with the hemorrhage there is generally a certain amount of pain, sometimes limited to the uterus, but more often referred to the back and legs.   The pain may be a dull ache, or it may be grinding in character. With the development of the tumor, the menorrhagia may be replaced by more or less constant bleeding, the amount of which sometimes causes alarm.   The hemorrhage is readily explained when we take into consideration the greatly increased area of uterine mucosa, both that of the uterine cavity proper and the patches scattered throughout the tumor.   It is thought that the pain results from Nature's effort to expel the tumor as a foreign body, at a time when it is engorged with blood.

Leucorrhœa is not a usual finding, unless there are old foci of infection in the cervix.   Rarely is there any intermenstrual discharge.

PHYSICAL FINDINGS.—When the growth is contained in the uterus, the bimanual method of exploration will reveal a normal cervix and an enlarged uterus. In the early cases the uterus is freely movable, but later the organ is more or less firmly held by adhesions.   Frequently it also contains ordinary fibroids, some of which can be palpated as hard bosses.   In the later stages, and when the tumor has attained considerable size, differentiation from an ordinary myoma, or, for that matter, from an ovarian cyst and myomata, may be impossible. The intraligamentous forms are more firmly fixed in the pelvis than are the ordinary myomata, although on palpation they may simulate a large pelvic abscess. The history, however, may aid materially in making the differentiation.   On curetting the cavity of the uterus we obtain, as a rule, a thick but normal mucosa.

DIAGNOSIS.—Generally speaking the findings are those of an ordinary fibroid, and the diagnosis is not made until after a specimen of the tumor has been examined in the laboratory.   Frequently, however, the case presents certain features which at least are strongly suspicious of this condition.   Cullen believes that, when a physical examination has disclosed an enlarged adherent uterus, the following clinical facts point strongly to adenomyoma:—(1) The bleeding is usually confined to the menstrual period; (2) there is commonly much pain, which, at that period, is referred to the uterus; (3) there is usually no inter-menstrual discharge of any kind; and (4) the uterine mucosa is perfectly normal and is rather thick, although this finding can be determined only after curettage.

After a similar review of cases, Freund came to the conclusion that patients affected with uterine adenoma usually presented a history of (a) a sickly childhood, (b) a tardy establishment of menstruation, (c) a profuse and painful menstruation, and (d) a general health below par, rendering ordinary activities more or less impossible.

The view that the diagnosis is possible in a considerable number of cases is combated by others, among whom may be mentioned Pick, Landau, Kudoh and Polano, Gruenbaum, and Ernst, all of whom dispute the points submitted by Freund. These state that all of the so-called characteristic symptoms mentioned by Freund were absent in many typical instances of adenomyoma of the uterus and were present in several cases of simple fibromyoma. They practically agree that the most striking features noted in the adenomyoma cases observed by them were the frequent occurrence of adhesions and adnexal inflammations, and the absence of degenerative processes in the tumor. Gruenbaum observes that eleven of his twenty cases complained of menorrhagia or irregular bleeding, which was not controlled by either curettage or cauterization.

TREATMENT.—The treatment is operative, as the history of cases thus far recorded shows that the symptoms do not respond to palliative measures. Hysterectomy is indicated on account of the lack of a definite capsule from which the tumor could be enucleated and the frequent association of adhesions and adnexal disease.

VI. CARCINOMA OF THE UTERUS.

GENERAL CONSIDERATIONS.—Carcinoma of the uterus occurs most frequently as a primary affection, and has been observed very rarely as a result of involvement from other cancers, either through direct extension or from metastases.

Primary carcinoma may develop in the cervix or in the body of the uterus, and arises from the squamous epithelium of the vaginal cervix, from the columnar epithelium of the uterine canal, or from the glands.

Cervical carcinomata are much more common than those of the uterine body, although the statistics furnished by the different observers regarding this point do not agree. Thus, Roger Williams found the proportion, in Great Britain, as 98 to 2; in Germany, Hofmeier observed but 3.4 per cent of cancers of the fundus in 812 uterine cancers, Krukenberg 6.7 per cent in 848 cases, Freund, Sr., 7.9 per cent in 227 cases, Kuestner 9.4 per cent in 234 cases, and Winter 29 per cent in 210 cases; while Cullen, in Baltimore, found 25 per cent in a series of 176 cases.

There are several reasons which may be advanced to explain these differences of percentage. There is no doubt, for example, that cancer is more frequent in some localities than in others. Yet the relative percentage observed in some clinics cannot be accepted as the true ratio, because the cases may be drawn from an extremely wide area of country, and not constitute a large percentage of all the cases that exist in those localities. Again, there is reason to believe that cancer is more common at present than previously, as is shown by the statistics adduced by Roger Williams, who found that, in Great Britain, in 1840, 1 in 129 of the total mortality was due to cancer, while in 1894 it has risen to 1 in 23,— *i.e.*, an increase of more than fivefold. As a result of his study he concluded, at the time when he wrote (1896), that 1 in 35 of all women over 35 years of age dies of uterine carcinoma in England and Wales.

It must be said, in passing, that many believe that this increase is more apparent than real, and may be due in large part to the greater frequency of correct diagnoses at the present time. Moreover, it would appear that, with the greatly reduced mortality attending those infectious diseases which formerly amounted to plagues, a greater number of women now live to the age at which they are liable to cancerous growths. Nevertheless, even with these qualifications, cancer appears to be on the increase.

There is also the same difference of opinion as to the relative frequency of cancer of the stomach, breast, and uterus. Roger Williams states that cancer of the breast is more commonly observed in women than uterine carcinoma; yet, there are many other authors who believe that uterine carcinoma is more frequent. Welch found, in 31,482 collected cases of primary cancer, that 29.5 per cent were uterine cancers, and 21.4 per cent were of the stomach. This series, however, includes both men and women, and the percentages obtained cannot be adduced as the correct proportion of these diseases in women, because, while cancer of the stomach may occur in both sexes, cancer of the uterus can occur in but one. Spencer quotes the sixty-eighth annual report of the Registrar-general of England and Wales to show that cancer of the uterus is more frequent than cancer elsewhere in the female body. During the years 1901–1905, 19,645 women died of cancer of the uterus, as opposed to 14,308 of cancer of the breast, and 12,048 of cancer of the stomach.

ETIOLOGY.—We are still in the dark concerning the cause or origin of cancer of the uterus, as we are of cancer in general. An attempt has been made to explain it by Cohnheim's theory of the embryonic inclusion of epithelial elements, as well as by Ribbert's theory that embryological cells become separated from the organic continuity and develop in an atypical growth after a long latent period. Cullen and many others have been unable to reconcile the histological findings with either of these theories. Nor is there satisfactory evidence that the disease is of parasitic origin.

Even after much experimental and statistical study our positive knowledge concerning this most important disease is limited to comparatively few facts. Chief of these is the fact that the great majority of cases of carcinoma of the uterus occur about the time of the menopause. In 100 cases collected by Roger Williams the disease was first noted:

```
Before the menopause in ............................50 cases
About the time of the menopause in.....................21   "
After the menopause in ..............................29   "
```

Gusserow has analyzed 3,471 cases according to age with the following result: —The disease occurred at:

17 years	in 1 case	40–50 years	in 1,196 cases
19 "	" 1 "	50–60 "	" 856 "
20–30 years	" 114 cases	60–70 "	" 340 "
30–40 "	" 770 "	Above 70 years	' 193 "

Roger Williams has analyzed 500 cases, and shows the percentage in groups of five years:—

20–25 years	0.2 per cent	50–55 years	13.0 per cent
25–30 "	7.0 "	55–60 "	9.0 "
30–35 "	11.0 "	60–65 "	5.0 "
35–40 "	20.0 "	65–70 "	1.0 "
40–45 '	17.0 "	Above 70 years	0.8 "
45–50 '	16.0 "		

Kroemer has analyzed 776 cases according to age and has illustrated his results by a chart that shows at a glance the great proportion of cases that occur at the time of the menopause. (Fig. 245.)

A few cases of carcinoma have been reported in women less than seventeen years of age, although in many of them there is the possibility that the disease was really sarcoma. One case reported by Ganghofner was described as papillomatous, and there is the possibility that it was not malignant. Cancer develops later, on the average, in the corpus of the uterus than in the cervix, the majority of cases occurring between fifty and sixty years. Roger Williams gives the following table:—

20–30 years	8.3 per cent	50–60 years	51.2 per cent
30–40 "	3.6 "	60–70 "	16.7 "
40–50 "	19.0 "	Over 70 years	1.2 "

There is as yet no unanimity of opinion as to other etiological factors. The influence of heredity was deemed paramount by earlier authors, but some recent compilers lay much less stress upon it. Cullen has recorded three cases that were observed in sisters whose father died from cancer of the face. Gusserow was able to prove this factor in only 7.6 per cent of 1,028 cases investigated; Schroeder, in an examination of the combined statistics of Barker and Sibley, found it in 8.2 per cent; Picot found it in 13 per cent and Williams in 19.7 per cent of 142 cases investigated by him; while Cullen records it in 19 per cent of his series of 176 cases. It is important, however, to remember that the majority of these hospital statistics are based upon the statements of a class of people who, as a rule, know but little of the history of their families, and that these figures may err on the side of conservatism.

Williams states that primary tuberculosis has been more common in families which show a tendency to cancer, and he finds that a large proportion of cancerous patients are the surviving members of tuberculous families; also that apoplexy, joint diseases, and insanity are more commonly observed in these families. Yet it appears that there is a very large percentage of longevity in the parents of cancerous patients.

There is a prevalent idea that cancer is more frequent among the poor and ill-nourished classes than among the wealthy. Schroeder has supported this theory by statistics showing the relative frequency of myoma and carcinoma. In his polyclinic, which is limited to the poorer classes, carcinoma and myoma

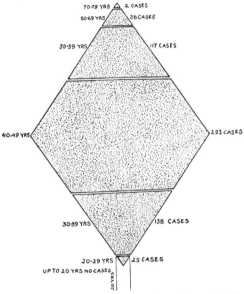

Fig. 245.—Analytical Diagram Based on a Total of 776 Cases of Cancer of the Cervix Uteri and Showing the Proportion of Cases at Various Ages. (After Kroemer.)

were noted in the proportion of 100 to 61. In the wealthier cases, comprising his private practice, the proportion was 100 to 332. In the analysis of any one man's statistics the reputation of the man must be taken into account, as it influences his source of material. These figures have been adduced to prove that whatever tends to diminish resistance and impair the vital forces favors the occurrence of the disease. Yet it may be said in passing that the power of resistance may be diminished as frequently in the rich as in the poor, and that statistics may be fallacious unless they are prepared to prove a single point. Nor is there unanimity of opinion concerning the view that cancer is more common among the poor. Roger Williams, among others, denies it, and adduces statistics to show that it is more frequent among the rich.

It has also been stated that the disease is more frequent among those who eat meat than among those who limit their diet to vegetables; yet we must remember that the great majority of people are meat eaters. Williams states that cancer is more common in brunettes than in blondes, and Chisholm and others have called attention to their statistics which show that it is seen more than twice as frequently in the whites as in the blacks. There are, however, comparatively few large clinics which contain a large proportion of colored people, and which at the same time have furnished careful statistics as to the frequency of carcinoma. Statistics from the Johns Hopkins Hospital show that cancer is observed in the negroes at least as frequently as in the whites, if indeed not more frequently. It is also said that the disease is more common in temperate climates than in the tropics, and among the civilized races than among the uncivilized, although the paper of Dudley, in 1908, gives but little support to this belief. This author states that the disease is quite commonly observed in the Philippine Islands, and that carcinoma of the cervix is more common than the other cancers. He voices the belief that the impression that cancer is either very rare or absent in the tropics and subtropics, is not borne out by the facts. Thus it will be seen that one may readily find ample justification for objecting to the value of many of the statistics of this disease.

There is also much diversity of opinion concerning what are generally described as local predisposing causes, which have been emphasized because we are as yet unacquainted with the true etiological factors of carcinoma. Multiparity, cervical lacerations and erosions, and chronic inflammatory conditions of the uterus are mentioned among these, yet they may be grouped under the general headings of trauma, and of stimulation of the genital organs, either in consequence of pregnancy or as a result of inflammation.

The great majority of cases are noted in married women, yet the disease does occur in the virgin, although rarely in those who have not undergone some gynæcological operation requiring dilatation of the os. Sampson shows that, in 412 cases, only 3 per cent had not been pregnant. In 96 per cent of 334 cases collected by Williams the women had been married, and the greater proportion of them had borne children, although the percentage was in no way proportionate to the degree of multiparity. The great majority of cases presented no sign of the disease until several years after cessation of child-bearing. Gusserow finds an average of 5.1 per cent children to every case of carcinoma of the uterus. Cullen reports that, in 49 of a series of 50 cases of squamous-cell cervical cancer, the women were married and had borne children, as had 12 of 14 cases of adenocarcinoma of the cervix. Two of the latter group were single. In Cullen's 19 patients affected with adenocarcinoma of the body of the uterus, 10, or 52 per cent, had not had children, and 6 of the 17 married ones had never been pregnant.

Admitting that repeated parturition is a factor in the causation of the uterine cancers, we are unable to say whether it is due to the greater functional activity of the uterus, or to the production of fissures with their resulting chronic inflammatory changes.

Unfortunately, we have no large available statistics bearing upon the relation between cervical lacerations and erosions and the development of carcinoma, although this possible factor has been mentioned by Ruge and Veit, Breisky, and hosts of others. Williams states that he never found the disease starting from the epithelium covering an old tear in any of his cases, and he thinks that there is no evidence that lacerations play any part in its causation; yet Boldt, among others, has found such a positive case, and we are inclined to the belief that many others have not been described simply because cases are rarely seen early enough to determine the exact point of origin. Indeed, it appears to us that, if all women who have had children were to have their cervices removed before the age of forty, cancer of the cervix would be a comparative rarity; yet, for manifest reasons, this procedure cannot be recommended.

There is little actual knowledge concerning the part that previous inflammation plays in the etiology. With this point in view, Cullen studied the endometria of his sixteen patients affected with cancer of the corpus, but found no endometritis in any of the specimens. Yet there is strong belief that the constant irritation of the leucorrhœal discharge predisposes to the development of malignant growths.

Secondary cancer of the uterus is rare, this fact being in harmony with the usual rule that those organs which are liable to primary cancerous degenerations rarely are the site of secondary growths. It may result from extension, from the involvement of contiguous structures, or from metastases from distant growths. Williams states that metastases are generally multiple, and are commonly found under the peritoneum of the corpus uteri.

CLASSIFICATION OF UTERINE CANCERS.—At the present time we are still ignorant of many of the fundamental laws governing the growth of uterine cancers, and it would appear that we can hope ultimately to possess knowledge sufficient to prognosticate concerning individual cancers only by a careful study of the methods of growth of similar forms. To this end a detailed classification is most essential. The chief objection to detailed classification has thus far been that many late cancers will not permit of more than conjecture as to their site of origin, and must in consequence remain unclassified. Yet for the present our chief object of interest is the early growths which alone offer hope of cure. These permit of extensive subdivision. Various classifications have been proposed and cancers may be grouped from different standpoints, thus: (1) According to the site of the original growth; (2) according to the histological features of the growth; (3) according to the morphology represented in the special growth.

1. *Classification According to Topography.*—All uterine cancers may be grouped according to their origin in the corpus or the cervix, and in like manner we may classify cervical cancers according to their origin, either in the vaginal portion of the cervix or in the cervical canal.

2. *Classification According to Histological Features.*—The vaginal portion of the cervix is normally covered with stratified epithelium, which undergoes transition in the neighborhood of the external os into the high columnar cervical epithelium which is continued into the uterine cavity. The site of this transition is not constant, and in exceptional cases the change may take

place some distance above or below the external os. According to this classification, cancer arising from the stratified epithelium is known as epithelioma or squamous-cell carcinoma. Likewise, cancer arising from the cylindrical epithelium, no matter from what anatomical origin, is known as cylindrical-cell carcinoma or adenocarcinoma.

3. *Classification According to the Morphology.*—Cancer of the cervix may also be divided according to the morphology of the growth, irrespective of its situation or its histological structure. In one type of cases the tumor everts as it grows, giving rise to a papillary or cauliflower-like mass. In another group of cases, which are of the same histological type, the tumor inverts as it develops and forms a nodular mass of cancerous tissue in the cervix, the external surface of which presents but little evidence of the disease. The malignant process may be circumscribed in one instance, while in another it may be scattered diffusely throughout the cervical and neighboring tissues; and yet, both cases present the same histology. This division is not always clearly defined, and intermediate forms occur; indeed, both processes may be present in the same specimen. Sometimes, in the progress of the disease, the growth may undergo a transition from one morphological type to another. In the great majority of cases, however, we may divide these cancers into the following morphological divisions: (*a*) everting, or vegetating; and (*b*) inverting, contracting, or infiltrating. Various synonyms have been given for these different types, and the former are also described as cauliflower, papillary, and proliferating growths, while the latter are termed nodular, ulcerating, and parenchymatous. They may further be subdivided according to the nature of the predominating cell. Thus, in cases in which the cancer cells predominate and the stroma constitutes but a small proportion of the tumor, the mass is soft and may easily become necrotic with the resultant formation of a slough. This type has been termed medullary in contradistinction to the so-called scirrhous cancer, in which type the stroma predominates.

Combining the above classifications, we will consider this subject under the following heads: squamous-cell cancer, and adenocarcinoma.

The squamous-cell carcinoma may arise from the vaginal portion of the cervix, or from the lining of the cervical canal, or, very rarely, from that of the uterine cavity. Each subdivision may be again divided, according to the morphology, into everting and inverting types. The cylindrical-cell cancer or adenocarcinoma may also be divided, in a similar fashion, into growths which arise in the cervix from the epithelium of the cervical canal or glands, and growths which arise from the epithelium of the uterine canal or glands. These also may appear as of the inverting or everting type.

In addition to these forms of cancer, malignant adenoma, endothelioma, and chorio-epithelioma have also been described.

Squamous-Cell Carcinoma of the Uterus.—The squamous-cell carcinoma generally develops on the vaginal portion of the cervix, although it may arise in the cervical canal or even in the cavity of the uterus. It is the most common type of uterine cancer. Cullen, in 141 cases of cervical cancer, found that 123 were of the squamous-cell type, a proportion the correctness of which is confirmed in the majority of the larger clinics of this country, although it does not exactly coincide with some statistics from abroad.   Thus, Hofmeier, out of 422 cervical cases, described 236 as developing in the portio vaginalis and 186 in other portions of the cervix.   Baecker reports 682 cases, of which 379 were cervical, and 282 of these developed from the portio vaginalis.   The following types of squamous-cell carcinoma are recognized:—

A. Squamous-Cell Carcinoma of the Cervix.

Everting Type of the Portio Vaginalis.—These cancerous growths usually originate externally to the external os, and begin as a proliferation of the epithe-

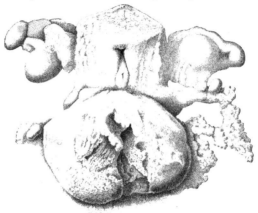

Fig. 246.—Everting Carcinoma of the Vaginal Cervix. (From Doederlein und Kroenig, "Operat. Gynaekol.," Leipzig, 1905.)

lium of the vaginal portion of the cervix.   Associated with this proliferation are a reaction and proliferation of the cervical connective tissue, the development of which gives rise to a papillary outgrowth in the vagina.   (Fig. 246.)   The early stage is rarely seen, because at this period the disease does not cause symptoms or signs which attract the attention of the patient.   The nodules consist of a number of small papillæ, which on section present a yellowish-white and somewhat translucent appearance.   As the disease develops the tumor increases in size, and the surface becomes irregular and lobulated, so that, as a final result, it suggests a cauliflower.   The growth may be pedunculated or sessile, and may extend over the surface of the vaginal portion of the cervix or down the vaginal walls, or into the cervical canal, until finally it fills the vagina either partially or completely.   Sometimes isolated nodules may be found in the vaginal wall some distance from the main growth, and at the same time there may be extensions into the substance of the cervix and the parametrium.   As a result, therefore, the cervix becomes markedly altered, and its normal outlines are destroyed. Erosions soon appear, and, as a result of sloughing, the cervix may be represented only by a cavity covered with necrotic tissue and pus, and bounded only by an irregular nodulated wall.

Microscopic Appearances.—In the earliest stage there is a proliferation of the deepest cells of the surface epithelium, which forms irregular columns and extends inward. (Fig. 247.) The columns are round, oval, or irregular on transverse section, and presently they not only invade the underlying tissue but give rise to papillary or polypoid outgrowths on the surface of the portio vaginalis.

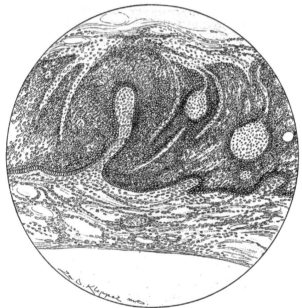

Fig. 247.—Transition of Normal into Carcinomatous Epithelium in Squamous-Cell Carcinoma of the Cervix.

These little epithelial projections are soon provided with a delicate stem of vascularized stroma that extends up into the epithelial mass. Variations in the size of the cells and in the appearance of their nuclei are noted. Sometimes the epithelial cells conform rather closely to the normal type of the parent cell, while at other times they show marked variations, even in early growths. The cells are closely packed together, and contain, as a rule, relatively small amounts of protoplasm. Giant cells containing several nuclei are occasionally found, and the connective-tissue stroma between the columns is infiltrated with round cells. Epithelial pearls may be found, but they are not nearly so frequent as in the epitheliomata which develop in the skin, on account of the scanty development of the stratum corneum in the cervical mucosa. The normal stratified epithelium of the vaginal portion is often well preserved, even as far as the very edge of the neoplasm, and, apart from a round-celled infiltration, which becomes denser as the tumor is approached, is practically unaltered. At the margin of the growth there is a lengthening of the interpapillary processes which invade the underlying tissue in all directions, sometimes as long; slender, anastomosing cords. The epithelium at this point is markedly altered, and the change is noticeable, even to the naked eye, on microscopic sections. This is due to the increased number of cells which take a nuclear stain, in part owing to the increase in size and the staining properties of the individual nuclei, and in part to the increased mass of epithelial cells. Surrounding the epithelial downgrowths there is a more or less dense zone of infiltrated round cells, mixed with eosinophiles in certain cases. Degenerations are noticed in the older portions of the growth,

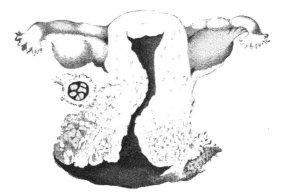

Fig. 248.—Inverting Carcinoma of the Vaginal Cervix. (From Doederlein und Kroenig, "Operat. Gynaekol.," Leipzig, 1905.)

particularly in tumors in which the blood supply is scanty. Cell inclusions of leucocytes, hyaline droplets, and even other epithelial cells are common. The principal degenerations are coagulation necrosis, hyaline and fatty changes, vacuolization, and nuclear fragmentation. Sampson has made interesting observations concerning the method of growth of these cases. His material consisted of twenty-seven cases of cancer of the uterine cervix, which had been removed by wide excision of the primary growth at operation, and with few exceptions without preliminary curettage. The uterus and parametrium were cut in sagittal and cross sections and the growth was reconstructed and studied. Sections from the entire uterus and parametrium were cut in one piece and stained for microscopical study, from which the relations of the disease to the cervix and the method of extension through the tissue can well be seen from the illustrations in his article. (Johns Hopkins Hospital Report, Jan., 1907.)

Inverting or Infiltrating Type of Squamous-cell Carcinoma of the Portio Vaginalis.—This type of carcinoma also begins as a proliferation of the epithelium of the vaginal portion of the cervix, although the papillary formation here is absent or plays but a minor part. In the early stages there is usually some hypertrophy of the cervix, together with a diffuse induration of the invaded portion. (Fig. 248.) The surface is livid and glazed, and feels infiltrated to the touch. The growth appears to invert itself into the tissue of the cervix, although all cases do not furnish the same picture. Sometimes, as the disease progresses, there is necrosis of the central portion, with the consequent production of a deep ulcer bounded by ragged and infiltrated margins. This

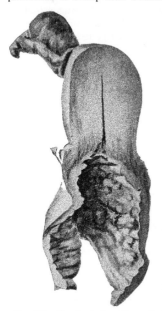

gradually extends until there finally results a large crater-like cavity in the vaginal vault and at the site of the sloughing cervix, with a cicatricial contracting base of connective tissue. (Fig. 249.) The clinical manifestations of this type of carcinoma, consisting, as they largely do, of the discharge of blood and necrotic tissue, depend upon the extent of necrosis and ulceration. Therefore, a cancer which undergoes necrosis at an early period gives symptoms sooner than one in which this process takes place later. In other instances the cervix is shrunken, hard, and surrounded by densely indurated tissue, the product of the excessive connective-tissue production excited by the epithelial invasion. As the disease progresses it invades the deeper tissues of the cervix, extending directly inward and avoiding the cervical canal. As a result of the advance of the new-growth, therefore, the cervical canal may be entirely surrounded by cancer and yet remain intact until late in the disease, —until finally the central core including the canal sloughs away. Unfortunately, this type of cancer occurs at least as frequently as the preceding, is more malig-

FIG. 249.—The Cervix has Ulcerated and Sloughed, and in its Place is seen an Infiltrating, Crater-shaped Ulcer. (From Martin und Jung, "Path., etc.," 1907.)

nant, and is more difficult to diagnose. Such cases may present, on the surface, only a small nodule, and yet the growth may have already deeply invaded the cervical and adjacent tissues. Then again, the new-growth may manifest itself in the form of a large nodular mass, which is frequently described as nodular cancer. More often, however, the process of invasion, necrosis, and ulceration go on together. This type of cancer is often described as ulcerative cancer.

The microscopical sections present, as a rule, the same picture as that seen in the former type. Solid cell-cords and cell-nests are common and there is a marked reaction of the connective tissue at the margins where the new-growth is invading the normal tissue.

Combined Everting and Inverting Squamous-Cell Carcinoma of the Portio Vaginalis.—As the growth develops, transition forms are frequently seen; in fact, both types may be found in the late stages of one specimen. Thus, the disease may begin as a growth which inverts into the cervical tissue, but later breaks through its outer shell and assumes the everting type. In similar manner papillary outgrowths may spring from the floor of an ulcer resulting from the necrosis of an inverting growth. Yet these variations do not impair the classification. In combined forms the cancer must be classed according to the prevailing type of growth.

B. Squamous-Cell Carcinoma of the Cervical Canal.

Squamous-cell carcinomata of the cervical canal also may be divided into the everting and the inverting forms.

The everting form, as it develops, may fill the canal or may even protrude through the external os well into the vagina. As a result of the growth of the tumor there is occlusion of the cervical canal, and pyometra generally supervenes.

The same changes occur in the inverting type which arises in the cervical canal, as in that which we have already described as involving the vaginal portion of the cervix. There is this important difference, however: the growths which arise from the vaginal portion of the cervix nearly always extend outward by invasion of the deeper tissue of the cervix, rather than by direct extension downward over the mucous membrane, or upward into the cervical canal. As a result of the growth of the tumor, therefore, the cervical canal may be entirely surrounded by cancer and yet remain intact until late in the disease, when finally the central core, including the canal, may slough away. On the other hand, cancer which arises from within the canal first attacks the surrounding mucosa, and from this locality spreads on all sides into the cervical tissue. Changes caused by infiltration and ulceration result, and finally the cervix is converted into a thin shell lined with cancerous tissue which cannot be distinguished macroscopically from the later stages of the inverting type of epithelioma of the portio vaginalis. In notable exceptions, however, the cervical tissue may not be deeply invaded in cases in which the disease has arisen within the canal, and the picture presented may be merely that of retraction and puckering of one or other of the cervical lips within the external os.

The diagnosis of this type presents all the difficulties which are encountered in the inverting cancers of the portio vaginalis, with the additional feature that it is more difficult on account of the origin of the tumor within the cervical canal. Only rarely, and in the late stages of the growth, does the disease appear on the vaginal surface of the cervix. Yet induration, retraction, and puckering of the vaginal mucosa is almost constantly observed. Sometimes there are distinct

folds of mucosa adjoining a retracted area, suggesting the retraction of the nipple
or skin in certain of the mammary cancers.

C. Squamous-Cell Carcinoma of the Uterine Corpus.

In rare instances the normal uterine mucosa may be replaced by a lining of
squamous epithelium, which either in part or completely covers the cavity of
the corpus. Such a condition has been reported by Zeller, von Rosthorn, and
others, but its rarity was shown by Ries, who found, in the routine examination
of two hundred uterine scrapings, but one specimen which even slightly suggested
this change. The majority of observers believe that pre-existing endometritis
is in some way connected with the etiology.

If cancer develops in the mucosa of a uterus which presents such departures
from the normal, the resulting neoplasm will be an epithelioma. Gebhard,
Kaufmann, von Flaischen, and a few others have reported cases which appeared
to be instances of primary squamous-cell carcinoma of the uterine mucosa, while
others have reported cases which were regarded by the reviewers rather as secondary extensions than as the primary growths which the observers took them to be.

D. Adeno-Carcinoma of the Cervix.

(a) The New-Growth arises from the Surface Epithelium of the Cervix or
from the Cervical Glands.—Cancer may develop from the cylindrical epithelium
of the surface of the cervix, in cases in which the transition from squamous
to cylindrical epithelium occurs at a point outside the external os. Or it may
develop from the cylindrical epithelium of the cervical glands. The growth
may be everting or inverting. (Fig. 250.)

Carcinoma of the everting type macroscopically resembles the squamous-
cell carcinoma of the portio vaginalis. Small papillary outgrowths are seen in
the early everting forms, and the cervix looks "worm-eaten." In the later
stages the growth assumes the cauliflower type. The large cauliflower masses
which spring from the cervix are made up of branching papillæ, composed of a
core of fairly dense connective tissue, surmounted by several layers of epithelium.
They break less easily and bleed less freely than the similar projections in the
squamous-cell carcinoma. The surface epithelium is continuous with that which
lines the glands in the depths of the tissue. The appearance of the individual
cells varies according to conditions. Sometimes the epithelium is present in only
a single layer, and in that case the individual cells are cylindrical and contain
oval vesicular nuclei. When there are several layers the cell outlines become
polygonal, but both the cells and the nuclei may be of almost any shape and
form. Cells containing two or three nuclei are commonly encountered, and
nuclear figures are frequently seen. Karyorrhexis occurs frequently in degenerating cells. Sometimes the nuclei stain faintly, yet they nearly always stain
deeply along the advancing margin of the growth.

More frequently the growth is inverting, and arises either from the cylindrical
epithelium of the surface or, more commonly, from that of the glands lying in the
cervical lips. In the latter event the surface of the portio vaginalis is quite

smooth or thinned out over a deep-seated nodular tumor. These growths early invade the neighboring structures. Frequently there is no ulcer-formation until late in the disease, and on inspection the cervical lips merely appear glazed, thickened, and infiltrated. On palpation, there can be detected hard nodular masses which do not project from the surface nor tend to bleed. Very rarely do these inverting growths attain a size sufficient to fill the upper part of the vagina. The diagnosis is usually made from scrapings. Sometimes a growth which has

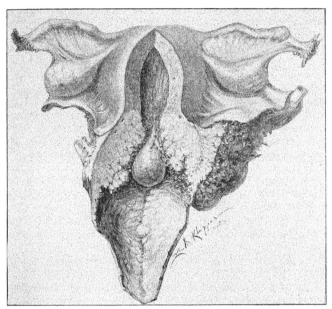

Fig. 250.—Adenocarcinoma of the Cervix Uteri, presenting everting and inverting growths.

originated in the cervical glands breaks through into the vagina and assumes the everting type.

When the growth has developed from the glandular epithelium histological preparations show an atypical reproduction of glands which run rampant and invade the tissue in all directions. The first stage of this development appears to be a proliferation of epithelial cells, which presently form small teats or club-shaped growths which project into the lumen of the gland. These excrescences give off side-growths which gradually coalesce with their neighbors and form small cancerous glands, so that at one end of a normally-sized gland there may be a mass of cancerous tissue which appears to consist of ten or more newly formed cancerous glands, with but little or no connective tissue bounding their lumen. The continuation of this growth completely fills the original gland.

In more advanced specimens the cervical tissue has been invaded in all directions by glands which present various outlines on microscopical section. Serial sections show that what appear to be small round glands are in reality but the cross sections of branches from larger glands, and it is at once seen that these new-formed cancerous glands have sent off shoots in all directions. Sometimes the lumen may be filled with cancerous cells, and their cross sections may at first glance be taken for nests of the squamous-cell carcinoma. The true condition is easily determined in the younger growths, in which a glandular arrangement can be recognized.

Sometimes the growth can be traced, from a normal gland which is lined by only a single layer of epithelium, into the cancerous portion where the cells constitute a layer five or six cells deep. The individual cells of this new-formation vary in appearance. As a rule, they do not stain intensely and have oval vesicular nuclei. Karyokinetic figures are not uncommon, and the cells may vary considerably in size. In general, it may be said that the epithelial cells in adenocarcinoma of the cervix differ greatly from those of the normal cervical epithelium, and cannot be recognized morphologically as their derivatives.

The surrounding stroma is usually infiltrated by small round cells which are most frequent along the advancing margin of the growth. The extent of this infiltration appears to be in inverse proportion to the rapidity of the growth. Degenerations are commonly seen both in the stroma and in the epithelium. The former frequently present areas resembling mucoid tissue; while, in the latter, degeneration may progress to necrosis which extends to a considerable depth in the underlying tissue.

(b) The New-Growth Develops in the Cervical Canal.—These tumors, together with those belonging to the type just described, are the most malignant of uterine cancers, and the diagnosis unfortunately is more difficult than in those which develop on the vaginal portion, because the tumor is so situated within the cervix that it cannot be recognized on visual examination. When the growth begins in the upper part of the cervix, marked lateral extensions occur before the disease extends as far downward as the external os. Frequently, even with the uterus in one's hand after operation, no pathological changes can be detected before the specimen is opened, for the cervix may appear intact and the uterus of normal size. The growth begins as a small nodule which is of waxy appearance and of firm consistency. It tends to invade laterally before there is downward extension or necrosis. With the progress of the disease upward and outward there is a coincident downward extension, and carcinomatous nodules presently are seen about the general os.

When the disease develops in the lower part of the cervix, the cervical lips are soon involved and appear thickened, glazed, and infiltrated, and the picture in general is that described under Adenocarcinoma developing from Cervical Glands in the Cervical Lips.

(c) The New-Growth Develops in the Body of the Uterus.—This type of uterine cancer will be considered separately under the heading of Adenocarcinoma of the Corpus Uteri. (Vide page 663.)

Method of Extension of Cervical Cancer.

The disease does not remain localized for long, but at an early stage spreads to the surrounding tissues, by lateral extension, or by means of detached cells which are carried by the lymph or blood stream to more distant structures, where they develop. Microscopical study shows that the disease may extend in thick masses, or by thin threads of cancerous tissue, and that in not more than forty per cent of "operable" cases is the disease limited to the uterus.

In the early growths extension is most marked in a lateral direction, and consequently the bases of the broad ligaments are early involved. They may be invaded by direct extension alone, or partly in this way and partly by way of the lymphatics. The disease may also progress through the lymphatics of nerve sheaths. The majority of text-books lay much stress upon induration of the broad ligaments as a sign of cancerous involvement, yet thickenings of the parametrium in connection with cervical carcinoma may be non-malignant in character. Late in the disease the parametrium is infiltrated and brawny, yet it has been shown that invasion may occur without macroscopical change, and microscopical study is necessary to prove the presence or absence of involvement. Thus, Wertheim, in his series of cases, found the parametria involved in sixty per cent, and in another fourteen per cent, although there was considerable infiltration, no cancer cells could be determined by microscopical study. On the other hand, the microscope showed that the parametria were involved in twenty-two and one-half per cent of cases, in which these parts were found, clinically, to be soft and distensible and apparently normal. Unfortunately, there may be no relation between the size of the primary growth and the involvement of the neighboring tissues. A small tumor may invade at a very early period, while a large growth may remain localized for a long time.

Carcinoma of the cervix rarely invades the body of the uterus, and in the great majority of cases the upper limit of the disease is below the internal os. When extension does occur above this level, it is generally into the musculature, although rare cases are seen in which the whole inner surface of the corpus has been involved in secondary extension.

The vagina is early invaded, generally by direct extension, either over the surface or through the deeper structures; yet, in many cases, the secondary growths appear to have resulted from retrograde lymphatic metastases. As the disease advances, the bladder, urethra, ureter, rectum, peritoneum, intestines, liver, and other structures may become involved. The ovaries and tubes are rarely affected. The bladder and urethra may be involved by direct extension from the cervical growth, as well as by metastases. Secondary necrosis of this cancerous extension may lead to the formation of a vesico-vaginal fistula. The ureters are early surrounded by the extension of the growth into the parametrium, and soon become involved; compression of the lumen is common, although complete obstruction is rare; and dilatation of the ureter and pelvis of the kidney, together with degenerative changes in the latter, is not an unusual result. (Fig. 251.) The rectum is less commonly invaded than the bladder, as it is more or less effectually protected by the peritoneum of the cul-de-sac of Douglas. It is more apt to be involved when the uterus is retroposed, yet may result from involvement of the parametrium through the posterior vaginal wall. Secondary necrosis may cause a recto-vaginal fistula. The pelvic bones are rarely affected, as the disease generally results fatally before the advent of this complication.

Involvement of the Lymph Nodes.

The Pelvic Lymphatics. The regional lymph nodes of the uterus which may be invaded by the cancerous process are: (1) parametrial; (2) iliac; (3) hypogastric; (4) sacral; (5) lumbar; and (6) inguinal; each group consisting of from three to five individual nodes.

The following lymph nodes may be found in the parametrium: (1) a relatively large node is frequently found near where the uterine artery crosses the ureter;

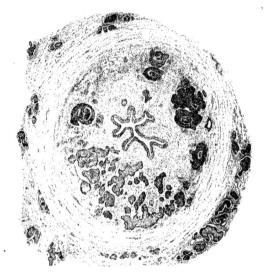

FIG. 251.—Carcinomatous Infiltration of the Ureter. (From Doederlein und Kroenig, "Operat. Gynaekol.," Leipzig, 1905.)

(2) small nodes are scattered throughout the parametrium; (3) there are new-formed atypical nodes, which develop apparently in the walls of the main lymphatic channels and protrude like a sponge into their lumen.

According to Baisch there are from five to eight lymph channels which run from the portio vaginalis and cervix laterally along the uterine artery, and which may be divided into three sets on account of the fact that they empty into lymph nodes in three different areas. The first set empties into the iliac nodes upon the anterior surface and inner border of the external iliac artery, between this and the hypogastric (anterior branch of the internal iliac) artery. The lowest of these nodes are also known as the obturator lymph nodes. The second set runs more posteriorly and empties into the hypogastric lymph nodes on the inner border of the hypogastric artery. The third division of the lymphatics springs more from the dorsal side of the cervix, runs over the posterior vaginal fornix, through the utero-sacral ligaments to the posterior pelvic wall, and empties into the nodes lying by the side of the sacral ganglia, or higher up and more in the median line beneath the promontory.

The lymph channels of the corpus uteri leave the uterus in four or five branches. They pass through the broad ligament beneath the tube, but above the ovary, alongside of the ovarian vessels, and thence upward, ending in the lumbar lymph nodes just above the bifurcation of the aorta. In addition to these main branches from the corpus, there are some lymphatics which arise near the middle of the uterus. Their origin is partly with the cervical radicles, but they finally pass along the round ligaments and empty into the superficial and deep inguinal lymph nodes. From the consideration of the anatomical distribution of the lymphatics, it would appear that the parametrial, iliac, hypogastric, and sacral nodes would be the most likely seats of metastases in cancer of the cervix. These groups are frequently termed the lower or first group, in contradistinction to the lumbar and inguinal nodes, which are designated as the upper or remote group. The latter would appear to be more directly concerned in cancer of the corpus uteri. Laboratory study of clinical cases supports this belief. Yet at the present time we have little actual knowledge as to the exact stage of the disease at which the pelvic lymph nodes become involved, as we are not yet in possession of the laws which govern metastases. Thus, small growths are frequently seen which have early given rise to metastases, while other larger tumors may remain definitely localized for a comparatively long period. On this subject we have no positive information either clinical or experimental. In general, we believe that the regional lymph nodes are involved only fairly late in the disease, although there are many known exceptions. It appears that in the so-called operable cases the pelvic lymph nodes are involved in from thirty to fifty per cent of cases, as is shown by the following table. It is possible that these figures are too low, for they were obtained from the study of lymph nodes removed at operation, and it is more than probable that many nodes which perhaps were cancerous were overlooked. The cases are not limited to cervical cancers, but also include cancer of the corpus.

Authority.	Per cent.	Number of cases.
Doederlein	22.8	115 cases.
Do.	33.	for cervical cancers.
Wertheim	28.	
Kleinhans	28.	32 cases.
Pankow	28.2	70 cases (67 cervical).
Zweifel (Glockner)	30.	59 cases.
Sampson	33.	27 cases.
Bumm	33.3	32 cases (cervical).
Freund	35.8	
von Rosthorn	42.4	28 cases (cervical).
Brunet.	51.	47 cases.

Recent study has shown that the determination of the cancerous involvement of lymph nodes can be effected only by the microscopical examination of serial sections of the entire node. Cancer is found in lymph nodes with such varying frequency that, unless this is done, the disease may easily be overlooked. Cancer cells may be carried from the primary lesion and become lodged in the afferent vessels outside of the tissue of the node proper; or they may be found penetrating the connective tissue of the hilum of the node. Invasion of one or more follicles or medullary cords may be noticed, while in the more advanced stages the whole node may be replaced by carcinomatous tissue. It does not follow that all enlarged lymph nodes are cancerous, as all recent observers have shown that the size of the node does not serve as a criterion to the presence of cancer. A large node may not be cancerous, while a small one may be, notwithstanding the absence of any change in either its size or its consistence. In thirty per cent of Wertheim's cases there were enlarged lymph nodes which were proven, by the study of serial sections, to be the site of hyperplasia and infiltration without cancerous involvement.

The regional lymph nodes may be affected without involvement of the parametrium, although it appears that they are more apt to be diseased if the latter is involved. Kundrat found that in ten per cent of Wertheim's cases the nodes were cancerous, although the parametria were not. Sampson also observed cancerous involvement in three of ten cases in which the parametria were free. On the other hand, the lymph nodes are not involved in all cases in which the parametria are affected. Kundrat showed that the nodes were not involved in. 27.5 per cent of cases in which cancer was demonstrated in the parametria. Indeed, it would seem as if involvement of the parametria had checked, at least temporarily, the extension through the lymphatics in certain cases. Cancer tissue, which has gained access to a lymph channel, may grow there for a time in contiguity with the primary growth, or be set free, and not become arrested until it reaches a lymph node. The newly formed lymph nodes which develop in the wall and project into the lumen of the lymph channels of the parametria early become the seat of metastases. Kundrat observed this condition in fifteen of his eighty cases. Sampson found these nodes in four of his twenty-seven cases, and in three of them metastases were present. On the other hand, cancerous cells may pass through the lymphatics of the parametrium without involving them, and not become lodged until they are obstructed by the pelvic lymph nodes.

In the past many investigators have claimed that there is no definite order of involvement of the pelvic lymph nodes. Yet it would appear from the result of more recent studies that these findings were largely vitiated by the grouping together of all uterine cancers, as well as by the mixture of autopsy cases with those considered operable. Baisch and others who have recently investigated this question find that metastases to the lymph nodes in cervical carcinoma follow the physiological and anatomical distribution, that there is no break in the chain, and that the second or remote group of nodes is not involved save in very rare exceptions, when the first or lower group is free. Oehlecker, Vinay, and others, however, have shown that the second group of nodes are frequently the seat of simple hyperplasia, when the first or lower set are involved by cancer. With the extension of the disease they also may become carcinomatous.

General Metastases.

The likelihood of general dissemination of cancer is not great in the early stages, and indeed many of these patients die before there is a general dissemination. We are not in possession of statistics embracing large series of cases considered from the standpoint of cancer of the portio vaginalis, cervical canal, and fundus. Roger Williams found general metastases in 20 per cent of fatal cases, as contrasted with 73 per cent in cancer of the breast, and he reports the sites of metastases in 79 autopsies. The value of these figures is impaired, however, by the fact that all types of cancer of the uterus are grouped together.

Sites of Metastases in 79 Autopsy Cases of Uterine Cancer (Williams).

```
In the lung .................................................. 7 cases.
In the liver ................................................. 7   "
In the peritoneum and omentum............................. 4   "
In the pleura................................................ 2   '
In the skin of breast and abdomen .........................  . . ... .... 1   '
In the tibia and innominate bone ...................  ... .. . .... .. 1
In the heart ...............................................  1
In the kidney ............................................... 1   ··
```

Blau, Dybowski, and Wagner, in 255 cases of all forms of uterine cancer, found metastases in the following parts of the body: In the liver, 24 cases; in the lung, 18 cases; in the kidney, 9 cases; in the stomach, 4 cases; in the intestine, 4 cases; in the thyroid, 5 cases. In addition, there were single cases of metastases to the brain, adrenal, skin, gall-bladder, heart, breast, muscle, and bone. As a result of the study of these cases it would appear that metastases to the liver occur in 9 per cent, to the lung in 7 per cent, and to the kidneys in 3½ per cent. Offergold, in 1908, reports 20 cases of metastasis to the brain which he collected from the literature, as well as 5 metastatic tumors of the dura. From a review of this material he concluded that metastasis to the brain may occur relatively often, even in the so-called "operative" cases, although they are generally associated with other metastases, as in the lung and the liver. The metastases to the dura were found in inoperable cases. There are no records of metastases to the cord, although many cases of secondary cancer of the cauda equina have been described.

Symptoms of Carcinoma of the Uterus.—Unfortunately, the disease develops in an insidious manner. Proof that the symptoms of the early growth are slight is shown by the large proportion of cases which are found to be inoperable when the patient first consults a physician. Although the percentage of cases operated upon in various clinics depends much upon the individual operator and upon the character of the surgical procedure which he favors, not more than from twenty to twenty-five per cent of cases in this country, at the present time, are considered operable. Many of our leading surgeons do not operate upon as many as ten per cent of the cases applying for treatment with the hope of cure. Wertheim emphasizes the truth of this in Germany, and states that, a few years ago in Vienna, only fifteen per cent of cases were considered operable. The classical symptoms are hemorrhage, leucorrhœa, and pain.

Hemorrhage is usually the first symptom noted and may appear when the woman is apparently in perfect health. It may be a mere trace following coitus or defecation, or some other form of trauma. In these cases the blood comes from the bursting of capillaries in the remains of the mucosa covering the growth, or from the laceration of the cancerous papillæ. Sometimes it comes from an actual ulceration. Frequently the first indication is altered menstruation, which is commonly rather profuse and may proceed to metrorrhagia. Waldstein has compiled statistics from 219 cases, in 120 of which there was atypical uterine bleeding, either in the form of a slight flow between periods; or in that of an increase in the amount of regular menstruation. Sampson stated that bleeding, or a blood-stained discharge, was present in 93 per cent of 412 cervical cancers in Kelly's clinic, and in 60 per cent of these there was a history of neglected bleeding for more than six months. In 21 of 78 cases collected by Craig, hemorrhage was the first symptom.

Leucorrhœa was present in 75 of Waldstein's cases, and constituted the first symptom in 45 of 78 cases analyzed by Craig. It may present the ordinary character found in connection with endometritis, yet in the early squamous-cell carcinomata there is frequently an early and profuse watery discharge. When ulceration has occurred, and there is a slough of the necrosed tissue, a characteristic discharge with fetid odor develops. This is variously colored, being yellowish-white, brown, green, or bloody, according to the character of the secondary bacterial invasion. The discharge is composed of serum and shreds of necrotic mucosa, together with more or less blood and pus.

Pain is a variable symptom, and depends upon the character of the tissues involved in the extension of the disease. Rarely is it an early symptom, as it does not occur until infiltration of the uterine wall and parametrium has taken place. In some cases it is scarcely noticeable until the last stages. In Waldstein's 219 cases pain was noted in but 7 instances, occurring as backache in all of them, although it was the first symptom in 12 of Craig's 78 cases. Pain is intense when the growth, in its extension, has involved branches of the sacral plexus; it is commonly experienced in the pelvis or the legs, and is variable in character. Compression of the ureter, with resultant kidney changes, will cause pain in the lumbar regions.

CLINICAL PICTURE OF THE DISEASE.—Clinically, we may divide the course of the disease into three stages. In the first of these stages the patient presents no sign of ill health. Save for a bloody discharge there is nothing to arouse her suspicion. In a large proportion of cases the patient ascribes this most important symptom to an irregularity of menstruation, or, if the menopause has occurred, to a return of the flow. The findings, on examination, will vary according to the site and character of the growth. A few finger-like projections which bleed on touch may be found in cancer of the portio vaginalis, while if the growth is within the cervix, induration and puckering may be the only features disclosed. Negative findings are the rule in the earliest stages.

In the second stage hemorrhages are more and more frequent. They may come on without warning, or may follow coitus or some form of trauma. In the interval between the hemorrhages a vaginal discharge is now noted. At first, it is thin and watery, but generally has a penetrating, offensive odor, and causes itching or scalding of the external genitals. Rarely is the discharge without color and non-irritating, as it is due to disintegration of carcinomatous tissue. Yet, even in this stage, some patients look the picture of health. Others, however, show signs of anæmia and loss of weight. Yet, even when the disease is fairly advanced, many patients complain of no discomfort, and others have only a dull, gnawing pain in the lower abdomen or back, or pain on defecation. Vaginal examination often discloses areas of ulceration.

In the third stage the patient's strength begins to fail. The skin often, but by no means always, has the whitish-yellow or cachectic appearance which is so characteristic of malignant disease, and which, according to Klemperer, is due to the fact that more nitrogen is excreted than is received. The bowels, if not already costive, become so, and there is painful defecation as the loaded intestine presses upon the growth. Hemorrhages are now likely to be more frequent and abundant, and the carcinomatous surface is now greatest in extent. The discharge is profuse and exceedingly offensive, having a smell that is so characteristic that it scarcely can be mistaken for anything else. Accompanying the extension of the growth there is frequently much pain, knife-like and darting, or cramp-like, in the lower abdomen and uterus; often there is complaint of a dragging or radiating pain in the back and of a dull aching in the rectum. When the growth has extended far laterally, there may be pressure on the cervix, giving rise to pain in the hips, thighs, and calves of leg. The involvement of the bladder is often heralded by blood in the urine. Cystoscopic examinations will reveal the presence of carcinomatous nodules, and presently a dribbling of urine into the vagina calls attention to the formation of a fistula. It must be remembered, however, that a carcinomatous ureter may break down and allow the urine to escape into the vagina through a uretero-vaginal fistula. Occasionally, on exploring the vaginal vault, the examining finger will break through the carcinomatous tissue and enter a cavity from which pus and gas may escape. Later in the disease, defecation becomes more and more painful and, in a small percentage of cases, a recto-vaginal fistula develops, allowing the feces to pass into the vagina. By the time the process has advanced to such a point, the patient's strength has been greatly reduced; food is retained with difficulty and there is considerable tendency toward nausea and vomiting; knife-like pains are more frequent in the lower abdomen, and the patient sleeps but little. Inflammation of the colon sometimes occurs, and the patient passes large quantities of mucus. Brown patches may appear on the face and neck, and various symptoms associated with disturbances of the sympathetic nervous system may be present, especially alternating congestion and pallor of the skin, chiefly noted on the face and hands. The skin becomes more yellow, and is harsh and dry. Bed-sores may develop. In some cases periodic attacks of subacute uræmia may be noticed. As the disease advances they tend to become chronic, and the patient gradually becomes dulled in intellect and sensibility, so that toward the end a semi-comatose condition ensues, during which there is no pain. Œdema of the extremities occasionally follows as the result of pressure on the veins. The patient continues to lose ground, and not infrequently has a slight elevation of temperature, due to absorption of septic matter from the sloughing and necrotic surface of the growths. Death is generally due to some intercurrent affection, usually to pneumonia or extensive renal disease. Quite often it may be due to septicæmia, or sometimes to hemorrhage, and it may result from venous thrombosis. Shortly before the end the pain may become so severe that it cannot be controlled by morphine.

DIAGNOSIS.—It is evident from the foregoing that the physician must be constantly upon the alert to detect this disease in its earliest stages. He should remember that recent statistics have shown that, in Britain and Wales, it is the cause of death in 1 of 35 women over thirty-five years of age, and he should consider all suspicious cases as cancer until the fact is disproven.

The early diagnosis of this condition is of the utmost importance, and, in the majority of early cases, can be made only with the microscope. Even though the operative treatment of this disease has been extended in recent years to the limit of surgical interference, the fact remains that hope of cure can be strongly entertained only in the early cases. As may be seen from the symptomatology, there are no pathognomonic signs or symptoms in the earliest and, therefore, most favorable cases. Consequently, all suggestive signs should be exhaustively investigated in every case that comes under observation. Among such signs are the following—:

1. Intermenstrual bleeding, or any deviation from the normal menstrual period.

2. The return of bleeding after the establishment of the menopause.

3. Bleeding after slight exertion, coitus, or defecation.

4. Any leucorrhœal discharge in a woman who never had it before.

5. An exacerbation in amount or change in character of the discharge, in one who has had leucorrhœa. Especially is a free watery, acrid, or blood-stained discharge suspicious.

6. Pelvic pain (although this rarely is an early symptom of cancer).

We should constantly strive to diagnose cancer in the earliest stages. Although cancer of the uterus is essentially a climacteric disease, one must remember that it may appear at any time from twenty to seventy-five years of age. Any irregularities upon the surface of the uterus which bleed during a routine examination should be subjected to microscopical examination, as the early cases can be recognized only by the aid of this instrument. It is of small benefit to the patient to diagnose the condition when it is so clearly outlined that it can be recognized by an examination with the speculum.

When the presence of a cancer in the uterine cavity is suspected, careful curetting should be employed, and care should be taken that the entire superficies of the inner wall of the uterus has been covered with the curette. All the scrapings should be preserved and mounted upon blocks, which are then cut, and every third section stained and studied.   If cancer is suspected in the cervix, tissue should be removed in such a manner that the line of excision will pass entirely through the suspected area and remove the growth at its advancing edge.   The tissue removed should then be subjected to immediate careful microscopical examination.   There should be no delay in the preparation of the microscopical slides, as the tissue can be fixed, mounted, and stained within two days without using the freezing method.   We insist upon the necessity of this careful routine in all suspicious cases, because of the fact that hope of cure is offered only by early diagnosis.   The reason why cancer is so seldom seen in the early stages is due to two reasons: First, the patients disregard unusual discharges, feeling secure in the belief that they are subject only to a deviation of normal menstruation, which, unfortunately, is often sustained by professional opinions; secondly, the majority of practitioners are not well acquainted with the early stages of this disease, and prefer to take the view that the symptoms represent an approach of the menopause, and generally do not insist upon microscopical examination.   The cases which are recognized most easily are those in which the disease begins at a point external to the os externum, and in which there is a localized induration that projects above the surrounding surface.   Rarely are everting forms seen at a time when the growth consists of the delicate, finger-like processes just described.   An early sign is bleeding on touch, yet it must be remembered that this is rare in cases in which the disease develops in the body of the cervix and merely manifests itself on the portio vaginalis in the form of a nodular area.   When the disease begins at a point internal to the external os, the primary nodule is rarely seen or felt unless the os is patulous.   In more extensive growths the vaginal fornix may be the seat of a well-defined ulceration or cauliflower growth.   We should constantly remember that the everting type is earlier recognized than the inverting form, which, unfortunately, is the more malignant of the two.   Nor should we forget that there may also be extensive growths in cases which present a small ulcerated area by the side of the external os.   In these, the disease may have progressed so far that the deeper tissues of the cervix are invaded in a line parallel to the cervical canal, and extension may have occurred to the parametrium before sloughing exposes the limits of the growth.   Very rarely, indeed, will the appearance of the os give knowledge as to the extent of the invasion of the inverting forms.   All nodules, all irregular and retracted areas, should be viewed with the gravest suspicion.

   After the diagnosis of cancer has been definitely established, an attempt should be made to determine the extent of the invasion.   The vagina should be carefully examined to determine the presence of regional growths.   These are recognized without difficulty when they are raised, yet frequently they exist as indurated plaques which may easily be overlooked.   Much emphasis is placed by many authors on the palpable changes in the broad ligament, yet all recent observers have shown that a soft parametrium may be the seat of carcinomatous invasion, and that induration may be due only to an inflammatory exudate.

Therefore, the latter cannot be taken as an infallible sign of parametrial involvement, although it should occasion the very strongest suspicion.

The utero-sacral ligaments should be carefully palpated, which is best effected by examination through the rectum. They should be traced to their cervical attachments throughout their entire extent, and the presence of enlarged lymph nodes upon the sacrum should be carefully sought for. Bead-like irregularities upon the utero-sacral ligaments suggest cancerous invasion, yet there may be induration from other causes, especially if it is uniform and in close proximity to the cervix. The latter findings are frequently associated with chronic inflammation following cervical lacerations.

When the disease has extended over the surface of the bladder, or down upon the rectum, either with or without the formation of a fistula, the disease is beyond hope of cure. Many have sought to ascertain the extent of bladder involvement by the use of cystoscopy. Fromme, in 1908, reports his results in this connection. He examined one hundred and ten cases of cancer of the cervix by cystoscopy, and in sixty-five cases he was unable to detect any essential modification of the interior surface of the bladder. In all of these cases the detachment of the bladder was easily effected at the time of operation, and the ureters were not dilated. He does not believe that the projection or distortion of the trigonum, by itself, is important as a sign of extension of the cancerous growth to the bladder. Vesical œdema, however, is very important, as in all fifteen of his cases in which it was noted, the detachment of the bladder at the time of operation was most difficult. When there is œdema of the ureteral orifices, he believes that the detachment of the ureters will be found difficult, and sometimes impossible. Such was the case in eleven instances in which this condition was observed.

Differential Diagnosis.—The following conditions must be distinguished from carcinoma of the cervix: congenital ectropion; eversion of the cervical mucosa; erosion of the cervix; simple ulceration of the cervix associated with prolapse; apparent in-growths of squamous epithelium due to a fold in the mucosa; simple hypertrophy of the cervix; lacerations of the cervix; cervical polypi; submucous fibroid polyps; tuberculosis of the cervix; syphilis; condylomata of the cervix; diphtheritic patches; sarcoma; retained portions of placenta; endothelioma.

Congenital Ectropion.—In multiparæ it is not unusual to find, surrounding the external os, a red, sharply-defined zone which varies from 2 mm. to 1 cm. or more in breadth, and appears to be a continuation of the cervical mucosa upon the vaginal surface of the cervix. Palpation reveals a granular surface, but no induration nor any tendency to bleed. The red color stands out in bold relief from the bluish-white color of the vaginal portion of the cervix. A section of tissue taken from such a suspicious area shows that the surface is covered by one layer of high, cylindrical epithelium characteristic of the cervix.

Eversion of the Cervical Mucosa.—This condition is erroneously termed erosion, and is commonly seen in multiparæ with lacerations of the cervix. The mucosa is bright-red in color and presents an arborescent appearance. There is no induration, nor is there bleeding upon touch. The line of demarcation between the mucòsa of the cervical and that of the vaginal portion is irregular, yet sharply defined. The microscopical examination shows that the surface epithelium is practically normal. In many of these cases the condition is confused with ulceration, and it is treated locally, and, as a result of applications, there is a distinct proliferation of the cylindrical epithelium, which is normally but one layer in thickness. As a result of this proliferation there is an increase in the number of epithelial layers, and the tissue assumes the bluish or pinkish color which is normally present on the outer or vaginal portion. Shortly after the treatment is discontinued, the newly formed epithelium becomes exfoliated, and the physician naturally concludes that the ulceration has returned. In reality there has been no loss of substance whatsoever, and no local applications were indicated.

Erosion of the Cervix.—This term has been used most indiscriminately, being applied to nearly all reddened cervices. Properly speaking, it signifies a loss of substance, and the use of the term should be restricted to cases in which this condition is present. All erosions should be considered cancer till disproven by microscopical examination. It is greatly to the discredit of the medical profession that the term "ulcer of the womb" still survives. Emmet, years ago, pointed out that there are very few, if any, benign ulcers or erosions of a lacerated cervix.

Simple Ulceration of the Cervix Associated with Prolapse.—Simple ulceration occasionally results from the external influence to which the prolapsed uterus is subjected. The cervix is usually hypertrophied, and the squamous epithelium tends to become horny on account of friction produced by the clothing, from the evaporation of the normal secretions, and by exposure in the air. The loss of substance may be limited to one area, or there may be several ulcers. These present a punched-out appearance, irregular in contour, and commonly with crenated margins. The edges are not elevated, and the surrounding tissue shows but little inflammatory reaction. The ulcers are usually soft and not indurated. The floor is pink and shows the typical structure of a granulating surface. They are readily dissected out and are very shallow, but may be the seat of carcinomatous changes.

Apparent In-Growths of Squamous Epithelium Due to a Fold in the Mucosa.— These are seen only in microscopical sections taken from cases in which the mucosa of the vaginal portion of the cervix does not present a smooth surface, but is gathered up into little humps and hollows, which cause it to present a wrinkled or puckered appearance. When the section is made the microtome may cut the squamous epithelium at right angles or obliquely, and show cell-nests surrounded by fibrous tissue. On careful examination, however, one will see that the epithelium is of normal type, and with the aid of other sections the true condition will be recognized.

A somewhat analogous appearance may be due to the distortion of the squamous epithelium produced by the curette. Cullen refers to such a case in which a scraping from the body of the uterus included some of the flat epithelium of the vaginal portion of the cervix which became folded into the scraping of the endometrium. Careful study of such a picture will show that the epithelial cells are normal in size and arrangement, and manifest uniform properties.

Simple Hypertrophy of the Cervix.—Occasionally the cervical mucosa is thickened and presents papillæ which are elongated and branching. There are, however, no down-growths of epithelial cells and the individual cells preserve their normal character. When the cervix is studded with Nabothian cysts and is the seat of a chronic inflammation, the condition at first sight may suggest cancer, especially if the cysts are in the depths of an enlarged and indurated cervix. All cases of doubt should be subjected to microscopical examination.

Lacerations of the Cervix.—A gaping, lacerated cervix, with a canal the mucosa of which is exposed, may simulate carcinoma. Yet there will be no bleeding following examination. If a portion of the mucosa is examined under the microscope, the typical structure of the cervical endometrium will be seen. Stellate lacerations of the cervix in early pregnancy, in which the cervical tissue is smooth and soft and gives the appearance of being friable, may also cause some confusion.

Cervical Polypi.—Mucous polypoids growing from the cervical cavity may cause uterine hemorrhages. When they project from the cervix they may bleed upon manipulation. A careful examination shows that they usually spring from a point a short distance within the external os, and that the lips of the cervix are intact. The polypus itself is firm and presents no finger-like projections, nor does it contain friable tissue, as does carcinoma. In cases of doubt the microscope will decide.

Submucous Fibroid Polyps.—A fibroid polyp lying within the cervical canal may be mistaken for carcinoma, especially if it is closely embraced by the cervical ring. These cases present such symptoms as hemorrhage, tissue necrosis, and foul discharge. Careful examination reveals the polypoid character of the mass surrounded by the cervical walls as a ring, and discloses its true nature.

Tuberculosis of the Cervix.—The symptoms of tuberculosis of the cervix may closely resemble carcinoma of the same region, although hemorrhage is a less marked feature. The ulcers are generally well-defined, with undermined edges and a base studded with nodules and covered with pus or caseous matter. There is not usually induration. Microscopically, giant cells and tubercles are found.

Syphilis of the Cervix.—Syphilitic disease may here, according to Winter and Ruge, assume three forms:—

1. The ulceration and initial lesion is usually single and characterized by the density of its base. The ulcer has a convoluted margin and is covered by an adherent, dirty greenish-yellow deposit. It does not bleed easily and forms little discharge. These primary chancres are rare.

2. Secondary syphilides generally occur here in the form of broken-down papules. The ulcers are slightly elevated above the level of the cervix, are usually multiple, and are covered with whitish or yellow necrotic tissue. Non-elevated papules may be found in the vagina, and especially at the vulva.

3. Tertiary gummata are very rare. The ulcers resulting from them are elliptical, sharply defined, and usually covered with necrotic deposits. If this material has been cast off there often develop vascular and sponge-like granulations. They may simulate cancer, especially when there is much breaking-down of tissue. The microscope will decide, although anti-syphilitic treatment will aid the diagnosis.

Condylomata of the Cervix.—Condylomata of the cervix are very rare, but may be mistaken for squamous-cell carcinoma. They occur most frequently in pregnancy. The growth resembles a cockscomb and is whitish or reddish in color. It is narrow and usually consists of a long base with flat epithelial outgrowths springing from it. The tissue at the bottom shows no thickening. On histological examination the stroma shows that it is composed of spindle-shaped cells covered by several layers of squamous epithelium. The condylomata are distinct outgrowths from the cervix, and the epithelium covering them is of normal type.

Diphtheritic Patches.—A cervical diphtheritic infection may produce an appearance simulating a sloughing malignant area. In most cases it disappears rapidly under the use of the antidiphtheritic serum, and the elevation of temperature and other systemic disturbances usually suffice to establish the nature of the trouble. The Klebs-Loeffler bacilli can be isolated. It is a rare affection.

Sarcoma of the Cervix.—Sarcoma of the cervix is very rare. It presents polypoid, grape-like masses which are easily detached from the rapidly growing surface of the tumor. Their nature is soon established by the microscope; even should the case present doubt, the fact remains that no trabeculæ can be seen dividing the growths into small areas. The circumscribed or diffuse varieties which grow slowly gradually produce enlargement, hardening, and fixation of the uterus; these tumors usually require microscopical study before their nature is positively established.

Retained Portions of Placenta.—Retained portions of placenta, or membranes which lie in the cervical canal and are associated with hemorrhage, necrosis, or infection, may simulate cancer. The history of recent pregnancy and the elevation of temperature should suggest the true condition, which will be confirmed by the microscope.

Endothelioma of the Cervix.—Up to the present time our knowledge of this exceedingly rare condition is based upon about a dozen reported cases. The differential diagnosis between this affection and squamous-cell carcinoma may be impossible clinically, and may present difficulties even on histological examination.

PROGNOSIS.—In this section we will consider only the period of time which elapses before a fatal issue, as the disease always terminates in death unless it is completely removed by some surgical procedure. There are no recorded cases of spontaneous cure in which the diagnosis has been confirmed by the microscope. Gaylord and Clowes have collected fourteen cases of cancer which they regard as authentic cases of spontaneous cure, yet in this collection not a single case of squamous-cell or adenocarcinoma of the uterus is included.

The average duration of the disease from the onset of first symptoms is from fifteen to twenty months; this period varies on account of many factors. There is a marked difference between the malignancy of the various types and groups of cancer; and great differences are also observed in respect of the individual resistance of the patient. The squamous-cell carcinoma is moie frequent but of less malignancy than the adenocarcinoma of the cervix. The duration of the disease is longest as a rule in carcinoma of the corpus. Generally speaking, the inverting type of growth is more malignant than the everting form, but there are great variations in the individual cancers of the same general classification. Thus, there are a very malignant type of everting squamous-cell carcinoma of the portio vaginalis and a slow-growing inverting form of adenocarcinoma of the cervix. The malignancy is influenced by the histological structure. The scirrhous forms generally develop more slowly than those possessing less connective tissue. The medullary growths which early present degenerative changes are very malignant. Cancers composed of cells of irregular size and shape, with many karyokinetic figures, grow most rapidly, as a rule. The form of the cell columns also may be indicative of malignancy. Then, again, the local conditions also modify the disease, a local hypervascular condition appearing to favor the growth. Cancer is most malignant in the young and the pregnant, and shortly after the puerperium. It is of longer average duration when it develops after the menopause.

There are several recorded cases in which the disease was of extremely short duration. Thus, Kiwisch records one of five weeks, Martin one of nine weeks, and Henry Morris one of four months. The number of cases in which the disease lasted more than three years is not great; they represent only sixteen per cent of the cases collected by Roger Williams. There are several instances, however, in which the disease lasted five years or more, and Barker has reported one in which the duration was eleven years. Some of these chronic cases may show partial healing due to the development of cicatricial bands. Martin relates a case of carcinoma of the portio vaginalis in which the entire vault of the vagina and cervix were transformed into a crater. Although the patient refused an operation she was alive at the time of the report twenty-two years later. The diagnosis, in this case, had been confirmed by the microscope, but the microscopic interpretation can be and occasionally is erroneous.

VII. OPERATIONS FOR UTERINE CANCER.

HISTORICAL SKETCH AND GENERAL CONSIDERATIONS.

Until comparatively recent times uterine cancer was regarded as practically hopeless, and palliative measures were the only lines of treatment adopted. These did not differ markedly from those of the present, and consisted largely in the curettage of ulcers and their subsequent treatment by some method of cauterization. Occasionally effort was made to remove the growth by more strictly

surgical measures. As early as 1560, Andreas A. Cruce, of Granada, performed
a hysterectomy for carcinoma and described his method, and in 1600 von Schenk
collected and reported twenty-six cases of partial or complete extirpation of
the uterus. Subsequently many other scattered cases were reported, these being,
for the most part, instances of the removal of a prolapsed uterus which had undergone carcinomatous degeneration.   The first widespread interest in surgical
measures followed Osiander's teaching, in 1801, that amputation of the cervix
should be attempted as a curative measure.   The treatment recommended,
however, did not enjoy wide vogue until after its adoption by Schroeder,
in 1878.   In 1813 Langenbeck, the elder, performed a vaginal hysterectomy
by a process of enucleation, removing a carcinomatous prolapsed uterus.
He tied all vessels with ligatures, and the patient recovered and lived for
thirty years.   Sauter, in 1821, performed a vaginal hysterectomy for carcinoma, dividing the base of the broad ligament and ligating the uterine
artery; and, subsequently to this period, many other surgeons practised this
method, especially after the advent of antiseptics and the employment of
anæsthetics.

The first real advance in the principles of treatment beyond this point was
instigated by W. A. Freund, who, after much preliminary investigation, called
attention to the fact that the upper limits of the disease can best be appreciated
by direct exposure obtained by laparotomy, with the pelvis greatly elevated.
On January 30th, 1878, he removed a carcinomatous uterus through an opening
obtained by abdominal section, and six months later he reported five similar
cases, with three recoveries.   Twenty-six years later he presented one of these
cases at a gynæcological congress in Breslau, and demonstrated the specimen
which had been diagnosed by Cohnheim.   There had been no recurrence up to
that time.   Yet the immediate mortality attending this operation, in the hands
of others, discouraged its wide adoption at that time.   Ahlfeld, in 1880, found
that the mortality of all recorded cases was 72 per cent, and Gusserow later
collected 148 cases with a mortality of 71.6 per cent.   The greatest blow, however, followed the publication of Rokitansky, who, in 1882, collected 95 cases
that had been treated in this manner, with 65 immediate mortalities.   Of the
remaining 30 not one escaped without recurrence.   Many, therefore, turned to
the vaginal hysterectomy, as developed by Czerny, in Heidelberg, after Sauter's
method.   Czerny's first case was operated upon successfully August 12th, 1878.
Yet it soon developed that the primary mortality attending this procedure was
also tremendous; and, although it slowly fell, as evinced by the following table,
yet even at the present time it exceeds 5 per cent.   We should remark, in
passing, that the mortality attending vaginal hysterectomy for cancer probably will never be as low as that for non-malignant conditions, such as
chronic metritis, prolapse, etc., for the reason that cervical cancer rarely
permits of a typical operation, and always offers the greatest opportunity
for infection.

The following table shows the primary results from vaginal hysterectomy
during the years 1880 to 1897 inclusive.

Heidler,	1880	52 cases with 36.5 per cent mortality
Olshausen,	1881	41 " " 29 " "
Hahn,	1882	48 " " 29.1 " "
Czerny,	1882	81 " " 32 " "
Saenger,	1883	133 " " 28.6 " "
Engstroem,	1883	157 " " 29 " "
Kaltenbach,	1885	257 " " 23 " "
Gusserow,	1885	253 " " 23.3 " "
Sarah Post,	1887	722 " " 24 " "
Schauta,	1891	724 " " 11.6 " "
Hofmeier,	1892	749 " " 9.2 " "
Hirschmann,	1895	1241 " " 8.8 " "
Wisselinck,	1897	1740 " " 8 " "

For a long period the remote results attending cancer operations were not properly appreciated. Many surgeons from different countries presented their series and claimed a large proportion of cures, while others, who had closely followed their cases, were filled with pessimism. The reason for this variation is easily seen. Ultraconservative men operated only upon the most favorable cases, and consequently upon only a small proportion of all their cancer cases. It is fair to assume that everting growths of the portio vaginalis and cancer of the fundus formed a large proportion of these operative cases, because these types of growths early present characteristic signs or symptoms. Moreover, as we have already indicated, they are of less malignancy than the inverting growths of the portio vaginalis and the cancers of the cervical canal. The remote results of the more conservative operators, therefore, should be far better than those of more radical men who aimed to operate upon the largest possible proportion of uterine cancers, and who treated in consequence many hopeless cases. It became evident, therefore, that a common basis for comparing results must be agreed upon.

This development matured slowly. For a long time surgeons concerned themselves only with the primary mortality and the end-results of the cases operated upon. The discussion hinged largely upon the comparative mortality of the abdominal and the vaginal operations, which was 20 to 25 per cent for the former as contrasted with 8 or 10 per cent for the latter. Yet careful statistical study of the end-results showed that cancer of the uterus was an almost hopeless disease under the existing plan of treatment, and that a common basis for the comparison of results cou'd be found only in the percentage of cures expressed in terms of the operability of cases. Then it was shown that, if a surgeon operated upon only 15 per cent of the cases applying for treatment, with ultimate cures in 30 per cent of the cases thus operated upon, he was in reality curing, not 30 per cent, but less than 5 per cent of such cases. In other words, it was clear that, with the older methods of treatment, more than 90 per cent of this class of patients succumbed to the disease whether they were operated upon or not. Moreover, even though cases were selected for operation with much care it was found that approximately 70 per cent presented recurrences within the first year.

A critical consideration of these and other similar facts directed the attention of many investigators in various countries to the improvement of the situation. The task was approached from two standpoints: one looking to the development of operations having for their object the complete removal of all traces of the disease; the other having for its purpose the instigation of a popular crusade which should make widely known among physicians methods of early diagnosis, in order that patients affected with uterine cancer might thus be brought early to operation. The radical operations have been developed along two lines: the earlier, seeking to remove the parametrium, uterus, and regional lymph nodes *en masse*, and the other paying special attention to the removal of the tissues which surround the primary site of the growth, especially those of

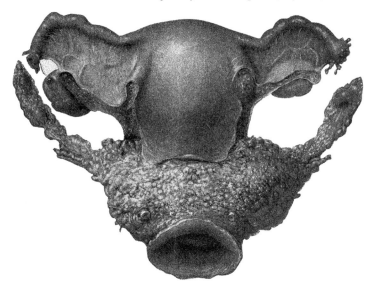

Fig. 252.—Specimen of Cancer of the Cervix Uteri Removed by Sampson's Radical Operation. Note the extensiveness of the removal. The ureters have been cut and later transplanted into the wall of the bladder. The stumps of the ureter are well shown in the parametrial mass. (From Johns Hopkins Hospital Bulletin, Vol. 13, 1902.)

about the vagina. Credit for the development of modern operative measures belongs to Ries. This investigator, having demonstrated to his satisfaction that lymph-node metastases were more common than is generally believed, and were possibly the cause of many recurrences, extended to cancer of the uterus the surgical principles which had been emphasized by Halsted in the treatment of mammary cancers a short period before. He advocated, in 1895, an operation which he had developed upon the cadaver, and which consisted in the removal of the pelvic lymph nodes together with the parametria and uterus. (Fig. 252.) About the same time similar operations were proposed and carried out independently by Clark and Rumpf. Following their lead, others, as Sampson, have developed operations which are still more radical,—operations which demand the extirpation of all cancerous tissue even though it requires the resection of the ureters or bladder. The majority of these operators claim that such extensive procedures can be best effected through the abdominal incision. Schuchardt and Schauta, on the other hand, have developed a vaginal operation of such a character that extensive removal of the parametria may be performed by the aid of paravaginal incisions. These extensive operations have been adopted slowly and have been popularized largely through the efforts of Wertheim. The development of the radical operation has advanced in consequence of a painstaking study of the method of growth of uterine cancers, as well as from a careful consideration of the results following ordinary hysterectomy. Not only are the latter results so bad that nearly all agree that other measures should be attempted, but it has been shown that the simple hysterectomy affords

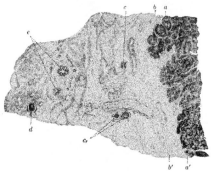

Fig. 253.—Section of Parametrium; twice magnified. (From Sampson. in Johns Hopkins. Hospital Bulletin, Vol. 13, 1902.) *a, a'*, Outer border of the growth; *b, b'*, outer border of the cervix; *e*, cross-section of a double ureter; *c* and *d*, small lymph nodes, which were involved in the specimen.

hope of cure in only a small percentage of cases. Laboratory workers have shown the uncertainty of clinical determinations; they found, for example, that a soft parametrium may be cancerous, and that carcinomatous lymph nodes may be of normal size. It has been shown that the growth has extended beyond the uterus in 60 per cent of cases deemed operable, and that the actual condition of affairs cannot be determined by clinical methods. Thus, Wertheim, in 1907, states that, in 22.5 per cent of his cases, the parametria were soft and distensible, yet were found on microscopical examination to be the seat of cancerous deposits, while carcinoma could not be demonstrated in 14 per cent of parametria which were thickened and infiltrated. (Fig. 253.) The parametria and lymph nodes were both involved in 20 per cent of his cases. Kundrat, in 1903, found that the parametria were free, but that the lymph nodes were involved in 10 per cent of his 80 cases. Cancer existed in the parametria without lymph-node involvement in 27.5 per cent of cases. Kermauner and Lameris found that the parametria were carcinomatous in 72 per cent of von Rosthorn's 33 cases. Schauta, in 96 cases, found one or both parametria invaded in 66.7 per cent of the cases. Cullen states that, in nearly every case of adenocarcinoma in Kelly's clinic, the disease had invaded the broad ligament. Kroemer proved the existence of carcinomatous infiltration of the parametria in all of his cases. This indicates the futility of operations limited to the removal of the uterus. All agree that all possible tissue in the neighborhood of the tumor should be removed. *The necessity of excising the upper vagina is demonstrated by the fact that four-fifths of the recurrences following ordinary hysterectomy have been observed in the vaginal scar.* Brunet found metastases to the upper vagina in 42.6 per cent of 47 of Mackenrodt's cases. The parametria are so commonly involved that all unite in the belief that an operation cannot be termed radical unless the uterus, parametria, and upper vagina are removed. The discussion has become narrowed to the question of the removal of the lymph nodes.

THE QUESTION OF THE REMOVAL OF THE PELVIC LYMPH NODES.

Theoretically the operation should include the systematic resection of the entire cancerous area in one piece from above down. Lymph nodes which are cancerous are as dangerous as the original tumor; the nodes are involved in from thirty to fifty per cent of early cases; and there is no clinical method of determining when they are involved. The results of the modern radical operation indicate, however, that late cancers cannot be cured, no matter what type of operation is performed. It is natural therefore that there should be much discussion as to the value of the removal of the lymph nodes.

The general impression prevails that the disease is hopeless when the lymph nodes are found, at the time of the operation, to be involved; and, although this is true for the great mass of cases, yet there are undoubted instances in which the patient has survived the five-year period after removal of carcinomatous lymph nodes. As has already been indicated, no cases can be admitted as evidence unless the lymph nodes have been examined microscopically in complete serial sections. The enormous labor which this work entails has confined the investigations of cancer of the uterus to a comparatively few of the larger clinics. Many investigators—for example, Olshausen, Hofmeier, Staude, Ott, Richelot, and others—claim that it is impossible to remove all the lymph nodes at the operation, and that the result of post-mortem records in general have shown that, whenever carcinomatous lymph nodes were removed during operation, others were overlooked. Staude states that the lymphatics can be removed from the cadaver by the method advised by Peiser, but that it is not available for living subjects. Staude, moreover, claims that the findings in four post-mortem cases following operation showed that resection of a portion of the radix mesenterii would have been necessary to remove one carcinomatous lymph node. It is also claimed that, just behind the hypogastric artery, there is a small node which is always found post mortem, but cannot be detected at operation on account of its position.

Schauta's investigations have been quoted by many who are opposed to the removal of the lymph nodes. This observer collected the nodes from 60 post-mortem cases. They numbered 1,182, and they were cut into 160,000 sections. Schauta divided this material, for purposes of study, into two groups—those which were accessible at the operation and those which were not. The iliac and sacral lymph nodes were considered accessible, while the lumbar, cœliac, and superficial and deep inguinal lymph nodes were classed as inaccessible. Both divisions were found involved in 35 per cent of cases. In another 8.3 per cent there was involvement of the inaccessible lymph nodes without involvement of the accessible group, so that removal of the accessible nodes would have been valueless in 43.3 per cent of the cases, because the other set was also involved. In another 43.3 per cent of cases both sets were free, and in 13.3 per cent the accessible nodes were involved without affection of the inaccessible group. Schauta concludes, therefore, that only in the 13.3 per cent would removal of the nodes have been indicated, because in 43.5 per cent it would have been unnecessary, and in another 43.5 per cent useless.

Yet there were many defects in Schauta's deductions, as both Baisch and Wertheim have shown. First, as regards the 60 cases, 50 of the number were inoperable and subsequently died from the carcinoma. These should be ruled out of the discussion, because, in the consideration of the value of operations, operable cases alone should be studied. There remain, therefore, ten operable cases for consideration. Of these, eight had no involvement of the lymph nodes, while, in the other two, both sets of nodes (the accessible and the inaccessible) were involved. Two cases, says Baisch, are entirely too few to serve as the basis of the serious conclusion that, when the lower lymph nodes are involved, the upper set must also be affected. Nor does it agree with the findings of others. Baisch, in 52 cases of cervical carcinoma investigated by him, was not able to find a single instance of involvement of both the lower and the upper set of lymph nodes; nor did Winter in 45 cases, nor Oehlecker in 7, save in cancers of the corpus. This leads Baisch to conclude that Schauta's series included carcinoma of the corpus, which cannot be considered with cancers of the cervix. Schauta, in his report, does not mention the site of the tumors. Objection is taken, moreover, to the classification of accessible and inaccessible lymph nodes, according to which classification the latter include the lumbar, cœliac, and inguinal lymph nodes. The lumbar nodes were found involved in 9 per cent of von Rosthorn's cases, and were removed by that surgeon as well as by Jonnesco. The lumbar and inguinal nodes are removed by the methods of Mackenrodt, Sampson, Amann, Strauch, Kroenig, and Doederlein. It appears, therefore, that Schauta's investigations do not support the conclusion that it is useless to remove the nodes, but they are of great interest only in showing that 43.5 per cent of his cases were without involvement of either set of nodes.

It has been claimed that the lymph channels should be removed with the nodes, or else the infected lymph vessels will give rise to recurrences. This does not admit of debate on theoretical grounds. It is undoubtedly true that, if the lymphatics are filled with cancer cells, any operation is valueless; yet it would appear that this condition rarely exists in cases which are deemed operable.

There is every indication for the belief that when cancer first invades the lymphatics, the growth extends in these channels as solid columns only for a short distance; and that the nodes become involved by the arrest, in them, of small groups of cancerous cells, which have been detached from the carcinomatous columns, and have been carried along the lymphatic current until they have been arrested by the constricted lumen in the nodes.   This is strongly suggested by the work of Sampson, who in his carefully studied cases found cancer cells in the lymph channels in but a single instance, and these he interpreted as a backing up from an adjacent lymph node which was the seat of cancerous infiltration.   Cancer cells in lymph tracts have also been found by Kermauner, Lameris and Veit, Schauta, and others.   The routine removal of the nodes is a most formidable part of the operation, as is evinced by the fact that two of Reis' cases collapsed on the table before the dissection had proceeded as far as the uterus.   A large part of the difficulty is due to the fact that the nodes may be so adherent to the vessels on which they normally lie that a vein may be torn through in. the efforts to remove them.   There are several reported cases in which this accident has occurred, and in one of these it was apparently the cause of the fatality.   Kuestner reports that the adhesions were so firm in some of his cases that extirpation could not be accomplished, or, when attempted, was done but imperfectly.

Within the last few years many of the former advocates of the removal of the lymph nodes as a routine procedure have abandoned this feature, and now perform only an extensive local operation even in early cases.   It need not be said that, if the extensive operation were unattended with danger, all would advocate the advanced radical operation with the removal of the entire lymph tract.   Yet it appears that the dangers are in direct proportion to the extent of the operation and the dexterity and celerity with which it is performed. Those who have abandoned the routine removal of the lymphatics claim that, in the great majority of cases, the disease is local and spreads by extension rather than by metastasis; that, on the average, only one-third of operable cases present lymph-node involvement, most of which cannot be benefited by any form of operation.   Thus, Clark states that as yet no operation has saved 50 per cent of the cases; that, of Wertheim's operable cases, 59 per cent showed no lymph-node metastases; and that, even in the far advanced cases of Schauta, 43 per cent were free from lymphatic involvement, while of the remainder which were involved only 13 per cent could have had their chance of a cure enhanced by this more radical procedure, which would have been more than offset by the greater immediate mortality.   Others, as Gellhorn, claim that to remove the lymph nodes as a routine will benefit but few and will subject the remaining two-thirds to an unnecessary operation which carries a high mortality and an enormous morbidity.   At the same time we are obliged to consider the other side, for, unfortunately, the case is not so simple as claimed by the opponents of this step of the operation.   The advocates of the removal of the lymph nodes call attention to the known fact that cancer always kills unless removed, and that, the more the disease is followed along its irregular course, the greater is the chance of cure. They show that from 30 to 50 per cent of cases present lymph-node involvement, but that as yet we have no clinical method of determining which cases are so affected, as from 10 to 20 per cent of the collected early cases show that the nodes are involved while the parametria are yet free, and that 50 per cent of cases with involved parametria also have involved lymph nodes. There is also reason to believe that, with the acquirement of more perfect technique, the immediate mortality of the operation can be reduced somewhat. It is worth while, says Ries, to risk a serious operation when the alternative is a lingering, painful, and disgusting disease, the best feature of which is the semi-idiocy of the morphine-benumbed bearer of the disease. Ries' results bear out this statement, as four of his six cases which presented involved lymph nodes, survived for a greater period than five years, as have three of the four cases operated upon by Wertheim when he performed ablation.

The value of the routine removal of the lymph nodes cannot be decided at the present time. The radical operation is yet new, and has enjoyed vogue only since 1903. The character of the operation, moreover, has been constantly changing and we are not yet in possession of results necessary for the determination of the value of this procedure. The results obtained up to the present time contain variations which must be interpreted cautiously, as the individual character of the surgeon strongly influences his statistics. Some make a selection of cases, while others seek to operate upon all. All surgeons are not of equal dexterity and ability, nor do they follow their cases with equal precision. Moreover, the character of the material is constantly changing. Thanks to the methodical agitation of the cancer problem in Germany, many clinics are receiving large numbers of early cases, which in this country are almost unheard-of rarities. For these reasons larger completed series, grouped according to recent classification, are necessary before this weighty question can be decided. Large series from a few men will be vastly more helpful in throwing light upon this subject than smaller series from many observers. Yet even at the present time the results following radical operations are indicating that late recurrences after extensive operation will be in the lymph nodes. At present the majority of patients affected with cancer of the uterus die from local recurrence before the involvement of the lymph nodes has become paramount. With extensive local removal of the diseased areas we shall have the opportunity of studying the habits of growth in the lymph nodes, of which facts we are at present in ignorance. There are cases in the recent literature which suggest that we may be forced to revise our former conceptions of the manner in which uterine cancers grow, as these reports indicate that carcinoma may remain latent in the lymph nodes for several years;—witness the case of Ries, in which the inguinal lymph nodes became involved nine years after his radical operation, and the observations of Mackenrodt to the effect that recurrences, more than three years after his operation of igni-extirpation, took place almost invariably in the lymph-nodes.

OPERATIONS FOR CERVICAL CANCER.

As we have already indicated, the limit of practical surgical interference has been attained in the most radical of the abdominal operations, and *it is universally believed that the hope of ultimate cure lies only in the employment of extensive operations in early growths.*   Von Rosthorn voices the general view that radical operations should be attempted only in favorable cases.   It is most unfortunate that the terms "parametrial infiltration," "lymph-node involvement," and "cancerous cachexia" are still included under the headings of symptoms of carcinoma.   These are but terminal symptoms in the great mass of cases, and indicate that the chance of radical removal has been lost. The fundamental principle of the surgical treatment of cancer of the cervix, like that of the breast, is block excision of the entire cancer field, in one piece, including the area of lymphatic distribution and drainage.   The knife must never touch the cancerous tissue in an operation that is designed as radical. The exceptions in which an apparent cure has followed an incomplete operation must be disregarded.   The only discussion that exists in regard to the surgical treatment of operative cases of cervical cancer relates to the question whether the routine removal of the lymph nodes should be attempted in all cases, and this discussion continues only on account of the high mortality that attends its accomplishment.   All agree that the parametria, uterus, and upper vagina should be removed in one piece.   Yet there are certain cautions which should be insisted upon in any work of this character, and chief of these is the teaching that these extensive operations should be relegated only to men well and thoroughly trained in abdominal surgery.   Even in the hands of those who have developed their technique upon the cadaver as well as from many living cases, the extensive operations are as difficult as any that exist in surgery, and may require, on the average, upward of two hours for their accomplishment.

Aids to Good Results.—Although the value of all the different points in treatment has not been definitely settled, there are many concerning which there can be no doubt.   First of all, care should be taken in the general preparation of the patient.   Whenever possible, the general condition should be improved, and tonics, mild stimulants, and nourishing food are of undoubted value.   Nor should the patient's strength be exhausted by violent purging immediately before the operation.

The limitation of the quantity of the general anæsthetic administered is most important, and all preliminary preparations should be performed without its aid.   Whiffs of nitrous oxide should be employed during the preliminary curettage, although several continental observers advocate spinal anæsthesia obtained by the injection of stovaine.   Indeed, some have performed the entire operation under such anæsthesia—among others, Veit, who used chloroform as an adjuvant in only five of nineteen cases.   Still others have advocated the use of scopolamine-morphine, or have operated with nitrous oxide and oxygen.

There is little doubt but that infection has caused the majority of deaths following radical operations.   Cervical cancers are often ulcerated, and are, it would appear, commonly the habitat of pyogenic organisms. Preliminary disinfection, therefore, is most important. Mackenrodt's method has been followed by good results. Following the curettage, which is done without a general anæsthetic, the crater and the upper portion of the vagina are packed with tampons wrung out of ten-per-cent commercial formalin. Vaseline is smeared thickly over the vulva and the perineum and the inner surface of the thighs to prevent the irritation which would result unless these surfaces were protected. The tampon is allowed to remain for from twelve to fifteen hours and is removed directly before the operation. Mackenrodt states that only for a few hours is there pain from this procedure, and that the vagina and carcinomatous cavity are rendered of leathery consistency, while an œdematous condition results in the pelvic connective tissue. He states that this is of value from three standpoints: disinfection, a lessened chance of tearing through into the crater, and greater ease in separating the connective tissues of the pelvis. The tampons should not, however, be left in for more than fifteen hours, as otherwise a hardening of the pelvic connective tissue ensues, which alteration constitutes a serious hindrance to the operation. Necrosis of the bladder, the ureters, and the rectum may also subsequently result. Consequently, the tampons should never be applied until the exact time of the operation is positively determined. Immediately before the operation Mackenrodt irrigates the vagina and then packs with bichloride gauze. Seeligman also recommends preparatory treatment by curettage, followed by a formalin (five per cent) tamponade of the vagina and the cancerous crater. Immediately before the operation, the tampon is withdrawn and the vagina and cavity are thoroughly cleansed with a solution of sublimate. At a meeting of the Berlin Gynæcological Society, on the 13th of November, 1908, Mackenrodt announced that he had abandoned his preliminary treatment with formalin on account of the uncertainty of the method, in that the extent of shrinkage of the tissues could not be controlled and that the procedure led quite often to necrosis. His views were shared by the others who participated in the discussion. Mackenrodt now employs tampons of sublimate after the curettage. These he uses for several days, and on the day before the operation he inserts a tampon wrung from tincture of iodine and applied under the guidance of the eye to the affected area. This use of iodine is endorsed by several authorities, among others by Broese and Strassmann. Veit elsewhere recommends washing out with alcohol.

Zweifel has been so impressed with the frequency of fatal infectious processes following radical operations that he has described, for the radical extirpation of the carcinomatous uterus, a technique which is designed to restrict the chance of peritonitis. This was reported to the Gynæcological Society of Leipsic on June 21st, 1909, and published on August 7th, of the same year. This operation, however, with the exception of a few details in the technique, is identical, at least in its salient features, with the operation described by Werder eleven years earlier (March, 1898). Zweifel was led to the adoption of this technique by a study of his cases, which showed that 19 of the 47 deaths in his clinic ascribed to the radical operation were caused by peritonitis. In 21 cases of radical operation with the Mackenrodt-Amann incision there were 5 deaths, 3 of which were due to peritonitis.

Many observers have used antistreptococcus serum as a preventive measure, on the assumption that old cancerous processes are commonly infected with streptococci. The limitations of this measure are apparent to most readers, and the treatment is not commended unless the serum is prepared with cultures of streptococci taken from the cancer to be operated. Hannes and others have followed the lead of Hofbauer and have used nuclein for the purpose of exciting hyperleucocytosis, and thus raise the resistance of the individual before operation. It must be remarked, however, that it is a debatable question whether the resistance can be increased by the production of an artificial leucocytosis. Others, as Veit, have planned their technique so that the vagina is incised at the very last part of the operation.

During the operation the greatest care should be taken to prevent collapse, and not only should the administration of the anæsthetic be curtailed as much as possible, but bodily heat should be conserved by means of warm-water bags, or, better, by the electrically-heated operating table. Crile's operating suit, designed to maintain the blood-pressure, is of undoubted value. No more blood should be lost than is absolutely necessary, and, wherever possible, the vessels should be doubly ligated and cut between. Especially are methods advocated which, like Bumm's, expose the vascular areas before attempt is made at removal.

Many of the sequelæ of the operation have resulted from injury to the ureters, and the question naturally arises what should be done with ureters that are embedded in cancerous parametria. Many workers have shown that the ureters are nearly always involved in such cases, contrary to the older view that these structures long resist invasion. Sampson formerly advocated resection of the ureters at a safe limit from the cancerous mass, and an immediate transplantation into the bladder. (Fig. 251.) The ureters were stripped from their bed with, as he subsequently showed, the resultant impairment of their circulation through injury to the peri-ureteral plexus. Necrosis, therefore, commonly ensued, and, in the cases which escaped this complication, there resulted an upward extension of a secondary cystitis. He therefore concludes that the integrity of the circulation of the ureters should be preserved, and that these structures should be handled as little as possible. Nor are the results shown by Sellheim and others, who subsequently investigated this subject, more gratifying. Return of the growth is common, with resultant stenosis in many of the cases which survive the immediate operation and sequelæ, and we must regard the prognosis of cases presenting involvement of the ureters, as very grave. In general, the resection and transplantation of the ureters has not been widely adopted, and it is agreed that it is advisable to make a vesico-vaginal fistula in the cases which have been so treated in order to control the cystitis which almost invariably supervenes. Better results have been obtained in those cases in which a diseased area has been resected in the bladder wall, and many, as Koblanc, believe that this should always be done, even though the carcinoma cannot be entirely removed from other parts. These men state that the bladder is frequently affected in comparison with the ureters, and that the latter should never be resected until it appears that all of the carcinomatous tissue can be removed. A review of the literature of the present time indicates that practically all agree that, when the disease has extended so far as to require such procedure in order to remove evident carcinoma, there is little, if any, likelihood of an eventual cure.

RADICAL ABDOMINAL OPERATIONS.

At the present time the radical operations show two tendencies, one for the restriction of surgical measures to the removal of the uterus, adnexa, parametrium, and upper vagina, and the other for the extension of such measures to a complete removal of all tissue in the pelvis which may be involved in the growth of the disease. Wertheim's operation is the standard of the former type, while the latter may be represented by the operations of Mackenrodt and Bumm.

The Wertheim Radical Operation.—The Wertheim operation (Fig. 254) is essentially that previously described by Werder, and is modified from the older methods of Ries, Strumpf, and Clark, but differs from them in that the systematic removal of the lymph nodes in one piece is not attempted. The so-called Wertheim operation enjoys wide usage and is the method commonly advocated. The method is as follows:—

As a primary step the uterus is curetted and the cancerous tissue is burned with a Pacquelin cautery. This had best be done on the day previous to the operation and under nitrous-oxide anæsthesia. The abdomen is now carefully prepared and the patient placed in a moderately high Trendelenburg position. As surgical shock is a common sequel, the preservation of the body temperature is important. The patient should rest on an electrically-heated pad, or at least should be surrounded by warm-water bottles which should be kept warm throughout the operation. The abdominal cavity is opened in the median line, by an incision extending between the symphysis and the umbilicus. Much care should be taken in opening the peritoneum in such a manner that injury cannot result to the intestines or the bladder. The best possible exposure of the pelvis is necessary, and the abdominal incision should be carried down close to the pubic bones, as the last half-inch in the lower angle of the wound gives better exposure than does a much greater distance at the upper angle. The intestines are now moved back from the pelvis and held in position in the abdomen by pads wrung from hot saline solution, while a careful examination is made of the pelvic viscera. Each broad ligament should be grasped between the thumb and finger and traced out to the pelvic wall to determine whether there are infiltration and induration of tissue, as well as the state of the lymph nodes. Frequently there may appear wedge-shaped processes extending from the cervix into the broad ligament. These processes may not be cancerous, although they generally are, and the operator should plan to give them the widest possible berth. The lymph nodes at the bifurcation of the common iliac vessels are now palpated. If these are of normal size they can be palpated only with difficulty. The utero-sacral ligaments are next traced to their attachment in the wings of the sacrum. Sometimes the lymph nodes on the sacrum are enlarged, while those of the broad ligament are not; yet one must constantly keep in mind that microscopical examination shows that all enlarged lymph nodes are not cancerous, while nodes of normal size may be. If it appears, however, that the disease has spread to such an extent that there is no likelihood of complete removal, the operation should be abandoned, or limited to an ordinary hysterectomy.

The fundus of the uterus is now grasped by a heavy tenaculum and is drawn

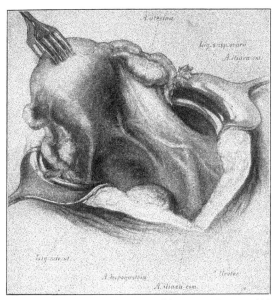

Fig. 254.—Wertheim Radical Operation. The ureter and the great vessels are seen shining through the broad ligament. (From Doederlein und Kroenig, "Operat. Gynaekol.," Leipzig, 1905.)

forcibly upward and to the side opposite that on which the operation is to begin. (Fig. 254.) Wertheim suggests that the peritoneum be opened at a point corresponding to the bifurcation of the common iliac artery and that the incision be continued down into the pelvis to the point where the ureters pass into the broad ligament. (Fig. 255.) By making the peritoneum tense one may see the ureters beneath it, and the incision should be carried down so as to expose them. On account of the danger of necrosis, which may, as shown by Fickel and Sampson, supervene from the destruction of their vascular network, these structures should not be isolated. The infundibulo-pelvic vessels are now doubly ligated and cut between the ligatures. Some recommend cutting between clamps, but, in the event of subsequent hemorrhage in the pelvis, the multiplicity of clamps may impede the work, and be the source of serious embarrassment.

The round ligaments are next doubly ligated and cut an inch and a half from the uterine cornua, and the peritoneal incision is continued in front of the uterus, through the utero-vesical reflection as far as the opposite side. The bladder is then separated from the uterus well down on the cervix by pressure with a gauze sponge, thus opening the broad ligament. Wertheim recommends this

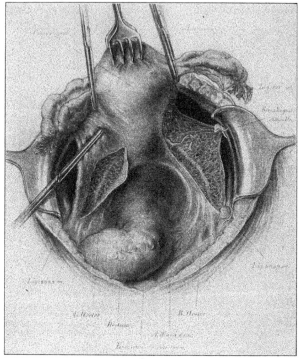

Fig. 255.—Wertheim Radical Operation. The figure shows the preparation of the ureter. (From Doederlein und Kroenig. "Operat. Gynaekol.," Leipzig, 1905.)

procedure as the second step in the operation, yet it appears that there are many points of advantage if it is done in the manner described. The uterus is now pulled well up in the abdomen, the detachment of the bladder from the cervix is completed, and the dissection is carried well down into the paravaginal tissue. In this way the vagina is separated from its fixed points and appears as an isolated sheath. The uterine vessels should be ligated and divided at some distance from the uterus. They can easily be exposed by pushing an index finger of one hand through from the superior surface of the broad ligament down along the ureter and toward the bladder. When the finger is raised these vessels will be brought to view, so that they may be divided without fear of injuring the ureters. The bleeding from the uterine ends of the vessels can be controlled by sutures.

The step just described is now duplicated on the opposite side, and by it the chief source of danger from hemorrhage is overcome. There may result,

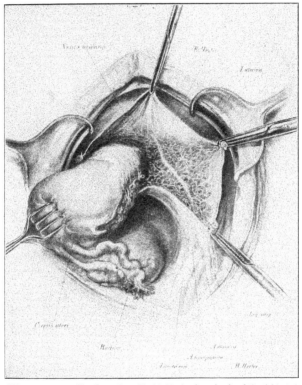

FIG. 256.—Wertheim Radical Operation. The bladder has been freed and the right uterine artery ligated. The right ureter is seen running through the parametrium into the elevated portion of the bladder. (From Doederlein und Kroenig, "Operat. Gynaekol.," Leipzig, 1905.)

however, considerable venous hemorrhage in the lowest angles of the wound. As soon as the vessels are divided the vesical portion of each ureter becomes easily accessible, and in this is the great advantage of the abdominal route, as in this way the ureters can be freed under the guidance of the eye, even in cases in which they are embedded in infiltrated tissue. (Fig. 256.) In the simpler cases they may be separated without difficulty, with gauze on the finger or by blunt dissection; and the bladder is also separated from its deepest attachments to the cervix and vagina.

The rectum is now separated from the vagina by blunt dissection and the parametrium is divided as closely as possible to the pelvic wall,—a step which may be effected without loss of blood if four or five curved forceps are applied to the tissue before the incision. (Fig. 257.) The uterus is now sufficiently

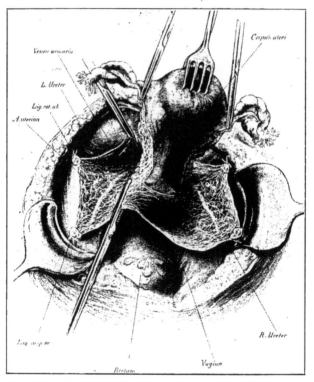

Fig. 257.—Wertheim Radical Operation. The uterus hangs suspended only by the vagina. (From Doederlein und Kroenig, "Operat. Gynaekol.," Leipzig, 1905.)

isolated for removal. The forceps may be replaced later by ligatures. The whole area of the wound is now sponged dry with sterile gauze, and all bleeding points are examined and controlled. The uterus is again pulled upward and forward against the symphysis, and the upper vagina is clamped off by the large forceps, bent at right angles, which Wertheim devised for this purpose. While these are being applied the uterus is pulled as high as possible in the abdomen, thus bringing a considerable portion of the vagina into view. (Fig.

258.) The clamps are applied, one at each side, so that they overlap, and the vagina is quickly burned through with the actual cautery. The edges of the vagina are sutured below the clamps with either running or interrupted catgut, there being left in the centre a small opening through which gauze will be passed. Bleeding from the paravaginal tissue is also controlled by suturing the angles of the vaginal stump. If the patient is in good condition, the removal of the regional lymph nodes may now be attempted, and for this purpose the first

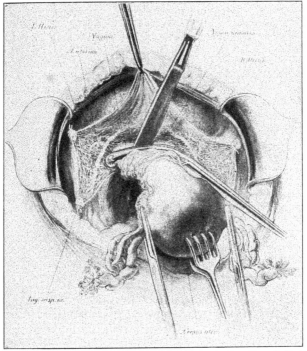

Fig. 258.—Removal of the Carcinomatous Uterus after the Vagina has been Clamped off. (From Doederlein und Kroenig, "Operat. Gynaekol.," Leipzig, 1905.)

incision is extended upward. The great iliac vessels are, as a rule, already bare. If they are not, a blunt dissection of the cellular tissue with the finger suffices to give exposure. All lymph nodes between the bifurcation of the aorta and the obturator foramen should be removed, and all bleeding points controlled. The removal of a few isolated lymph nodes does not render the operation more efficient. The wound is now treated. The cavity created by the removal of the tumor is loosely filled with gauze, which is attached to that previously inserted into the vagina. The peritoneal flaps are then approximated in a careful manner, so that no free raw edges shall be left to promote adhesions.

In case the peritoneal flaps will not come together, the sigmoid flexure may be incorporated between, to make a floor of serous tissue. The abdominal wound is then closed in layers, or, in case the patient is in bad condition as a result of the operation, the more rapid closure with interrupted silkworm-gut sutures may be employed, after the edges of the peritoneum have been united by means of a continuous catgut suture. If the patient is in bad condition submammary normal saline transfusion should be employed. Post-operative nausea may be limited by giving inhalations of pure oxygen before the patient has returned to consciousness; these should be continued for at least twenty minutes.

After-treatment.—The after-treatment differs from that of any other serious abdominal operation in but a few details, chief of which is the care of the bladder. Fluid by mouth should be restricted until the nausea has ceased, and liquid should be given first in the form of small lumps of ice. Murphy proctoclysis should be resorted to immediately on the return of the patient to her bed and it should be continued for from forty-eight to seventy-two hours. During the first twenty-four hours the patient may be turned upon her side, and it is no longer considered necessary absolutely to restrict her movements. The diet should be limited to water for the first day, after which the white of an egg, or a small quantity of milk diluted with lime water, may be given frequently. After the bowels have been opened the amount of nourishment should be increased to a light diet on the fifth or sixth day. Stimulation should not be employed as a routine procedure, but should be resorted to only when specially indicated. At the end of the first twenty-four hours a small quantity of the gauze should be removed from the vagina, and each day thereafter as much as 10 or 12 centimetres should be withdrawn, so that all will be removed at the end of five or six days.

The chief complications come from shock and urinary disturbances. Of the latter, cystitis is so frequent as almost to be the rule; and therefore Sampson and others have suggested the establishment of a vesico-vaginal fistula as a routine procedure after every radical operation. Others still merely advise the insertion of a retention catheter through which the bladder is irrigated with boric solutions at least four times each day. Urotropin in ten-grain doses should be given four times daily, if the stomach permits. If there is any suggestion of the presence of pus, the bladder should be irrigated with a five-per-cent solution of argyrol twice daily. In case this does not control the cystitis, which on the contrary appears to be spreading upward, a vesico-vaginal fistula should be made without further delay. Vesical fistulæ frequently arise from some local injury, but as a rule they heal spontaneously. More serious are the ureteral fistulæ, which were formerly believed to heal spontaneously only in rare cases. It is, however, good treatment to give these latter a chance to heal spontaneously before one resorts to operation. Weibel, in 1908, emphasizes this point and advocates touching them systematically with a caustic. Failing to secure closure, the majority of operators in this country make an attempt to insert the ureter into the bladder. Wertheim and many other continental surgeons formerly favored nephrectomy unless the other kidney had been found diseased. Before resorting to this operation a cystoscopic examination should be made to determine the condition of the bladder and ureter.

Weibel, in 1908, reviewed Wertheim's series of 400 cases of radical operation for cancer of the uterus, with a view of ascertaining the facts in regard to the resulting ureteral injuries. He found that injury of the ureters at the time of the operation was comparatively infrequent, and that it occurred in eleven cases—eight in the first two hundred cases, and three in the second two hundred. It nearly always resulted from insufficient exposure of the ureter. This tube was completely severed in eight cases, cut into in three, and ligated in one instance. Immediate implantation into the bladder was done, as the injury was always recognized at the time, and healing took place in all instances. Ureteral fistula developed in twenty-four cases, or six per cent of the total. It was bilateral in three instances. The appearance of the fistula was fairly well limited between the seventh and eighteenth days following the operation. In the great majority of instances—viz., seventy-five per cent—the fistula made its appearance during the second week. As a rule, they were observed only in difficult cases, although four occurred in cases in which the parametrium was soft and not infiltrated. In eleven other cases this sequela developed as a result of the separation of the ureters from densely infiltrated parametria, although the separation of these tubes from their bed extended only a short distance. The nine remaining cases were some in which the ureters had been isolated from their bed throughout an unusually long distance. Only one-third of the fistulæ were thought by Weibel to have resulted from the isolation of the ureters, and the great majority are credited to cancerous infiltration. The ultimate fate of the fistulæ resulting from necrosis is considered in two divisions—one comprising the cases before 1903, and the other those after that year. Before this period there were eight cases, of which two healed spontaneously and six were treated by nephrectomy with favorable results. The first case treated by nephrectomy was one in which the fistula developed four weeks after the operation, while in the latest case the lesion developed twelve weeks after the operation; pyelonephritis was present in the majority of cases. Since April, 1903, only a single case has been treated by nephrectomy, and that because a severe pyelitis had ensued. Eleven cases were followed by spontaneous healing. One case was treated by the implantation of the ureters into the bladder. This was a case which presented a fistula on both sides immediately following the cancer operation, and at the operation for implantation, three months later, one of the fistulæ was found to be closed. This woman died of a recurrence six months after the radical operation. One other patient died of a recurrence before the fistula closed, and still another died from a pyelonephritis. A nephrectomy was not performed in the latter case because it was thought to be contra-indicated by a bad aortic insufficiency. Of the total thirteen cases in which the fistula healed spontaneously there were six in which the patient succumbed to a recurrence of the cancer. The other cases have been examined to ascertain the subsequent condition of the patients, and it has been shown that one of them is alive and has had no recurrence (*i.e.*, for five years after the operation); that in two of the cases the patient remained free from a recurrence for over two years; and that in one case this freedom lasted for a period of one year. In no case in which the fistula closed, was there a stricture of the ureter. The beginning of spontaneous healing was apparent in one case as early as two weeks after the operation. In three other cases the healing began during the first month, in five within the second month, and in two within the third and fourth months. In several instances an apparent closure of the fistula was followed by a return, although some of the urine did actually reach the bladder. Eventually, however, the fistula closed.

The Mackenrodt Operation.—After the usual vaginal and abdominal preparation (vide Aids to Good Results, page 619) the patient is placed in a moderately high Trendelenburg position, and an incision long enough to' secure the maximum exposure is made into the abdominal cavity. Mackenrodt utilizes a horseshoe-shaped incision, made as follows:—The skin is put upon the stretch transversely, and cut through down to the fascia of the recti, the incision beginning two fingers'· breadths above the symphysis and continuing upward and outward, in a direction more or less parallel to the anterior wall of the pelvis, up to a point opposite the anterior superior spines. Two small cutaneous vessels will be severed, but they bleed slightly and will not require sutures. After the fascia of the rectus has been divided along a line corresponding to the skin incision, the muscles are separated in the mid-line and the index finger is passed through this incision in such a manner as to push the preperitoneal fat and peritoneum to one side and downward, thus isolating the lower portions of the recti muscles. These muscles are now divided transversely with the scissors upon the fingers. They should be severed 3 or 4 centimeters above their insertions, so that there may remain a firm stump for subsequent closure. The peritoneum with the epigastric vessels is then pressed downward and out of the way, and—with the scissors still upon the fingers—the fascia connecting the recti and oblique muscles, as well as the inner edges of the latter muscles, is divided throughout the course of the skin incision. The peritoneum is next divided above the bladder, along the line of the skin incision, out to, but not through, the epigastric vessels. During this step great care must be taken not to injure the bladder, which may be loosened from behind the symphysis during the previous manipulations. If the upper edge of the organ is not visible it can be palpated between two fingers. The tongue-shaped flap with its peritoneal lining is now pressed backward and clamped to the peritoneum of the upper portion of the posterior pelvic wall, thus closing the abdomen from the pelvis. All skin surfaces are carefully covered with sterile towels.

The peritoneal area which it is proposed to extirpate is now outlined in successive stages. When completed the line will pass from between the bladder and uterus, outward over the round and infundibulo-pelvic· ligaments, along the outer border of the posterior layer of the broad ligament at the pelvic wall, and inward across the rectum at the level at which the peritoneum of Douglas' pouch becomes firmly fixed to the rectal wall. The incision first extends to the right. The uterus is seized with a tenaculum and retracted to the left, and the peritoneum between the bladder and uterus is incised from left to right. Clamps are then applied to the right round ligament and to the ovarian vessels just external to the tube and ovary, partially as retractors but also to prevent reflux of blood from the uterus. The uterus having been pulled to the left and posteriorly, the peritoneal incision is carried backward over the round and infundibulo-pelvic ligaments, isolating the ovarian vessels, which, after being securely ligated and cut, are allowed to retract under the peritoneum. The left round ligament is also ligated and severed, thereby rendering the separation of the peritoneum between the bladder and uterus more easy of accomplishment. The peritoneal incision is next continued posteriorly, and that portion of the membrane which is to cover the posterior flap of the broad ligament is picked up and incised, and its outer margin is freed by blunt dissection with the scissors or by the aid of small gauze tampons. When the peritoneal incision nears the rectum great care must be taken not to injure the ureter. The uterus is drawn forward by an assistant, while the operator lifts up the rectum with the left hand and incises the posterior portion of Douglas' pouch just below the point at which it is firmly fixed to the rectum. Mackenrodt believes that the majority of ureteral injuries occur during this step, and that this occurrence is due to the fact that the ureter here is intimately connected with the peritoneum.

When the right side of the peritoneal incision has been completely outlined, and the peritoneum external to the cut has been freed from the underlying broad ligament, the fat and connective tissue of the latter are separated from the pelvic wall. This cellular tissue is not firmly fixed to the pelvic wall, but is held in contact very largely by the peritoneal investment. It is bloodlessly separated by blunt dissection with the scissors, or by stripping it down with gauze as far as the levator fascia and the origin of the uterine artery. This step is facilitated by the use of clamps as retractors, some being attached to the distal stump of the round ligament, while others have a firm hold on the proximal portion of the broad ligament. When the retractors are separated the large bare blood-vessels will be seen on the side of the pelvic wall, and the entire contents of the lateral pelvic cavity will be visible between the common iliac vessels and the bladder. The adjacent lymph nodes are also exposed by this procedure. (Fig. 259.)

No attempt is made toward the isolation of the ureters until the opposite broad ligament has been freed in like manner. Consequently the above steps are repeated on the left side, after which the uterus and parametria will hang suspended only by the bladder, vagina, and bases of the broad ligaments. Up to this point in the operation neither uterine vessel has been ligatured.

The uterine arteries arise from the hypogastrics, or with them from the anterior trunk of the internal iliacs; they measure from 6 to 8 centimetres in length from their origin to the point at which they are lost in the uterine wall.

Their outer half is more firmly embedded in the parametrium than is the inner, which is only loosely attached. The uterus having been pulled to the opposite side, the uterine vessels are freed by blunt dissection near their point of origin, doubly ligated, and then severed between the ligatures in order to prevent reflex bleeding.

The ureters also are rather loosely embedded in the parametrium, although they are firmly attached to the peritoneum of the sides of the pelvic wall. From the point at which they cross the iliac vessels until they penetrate the parametrium, they are connected with the upper lateral wall by a delicate connective-tissue membrane which is practically devoid of anastomosing blood-vessels.

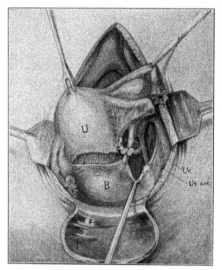

Fig. 259.—The Drawing Shows Exposure of the Vascular Areas and Ureter in the Mackenrodt Operation. (Original.)

Below the point at which they are crossed by the uterine arteries, the connective tissue is fairly dense. By separating the fibres of the parametrium, the ureter is found and easily removed from its sheath as far forward as the anterior part of the parametrium and beyond the crossing point of the artery. This step is now duplicated on the opposite side. Between the ureter and the artery there may be found small lymph nodes which are frequently the seat of carcinomatous involvement. If amputation of the ureter is necessary, on account of extension of the growth to the sheath, it should be made just above this point. The bladder must be freed from its supports before the ureter can be separated from its intimate connection with the paracolpium in this anterior portion of its bed. When the tissues are not infiltrated with the carcinomatous or inflammatory products, this will be a fairly easy thing to accomplish in the midline as far down as the point at which the ureters enter the bladder wall. At this point the connection between the bladder and the vagina is very close and firm. The base of the bladder must be separated most carefully from its bed or injury will result to either the superior or the inferior vesical arteries, or their anastomosing branches. It will be necessary to cut several small veins which spring from the vesico-vaginal plexus and the obturator veins, but the greatest care should be taken to avoid unnecessary ligatures. Bleeding should be controlled by temporary packing or clamping and twisting, whenever possible, as ligatures at this point constitute a menace to the integrity of the bladder. With the completion of this step, the preliminary portions of the operation are accomplished.

Now follows the chief feature of the operation—the separation of the roots of the parametrium and paracolpium from the fascia of the internal obturator and levator ani muscles and the iliac fascia. The paracolpium is the direct continuation of the uterine parametrium and lies to the sides of the vagina; developmentally, as well as anatomically, the parametrium and paracolpium form a single structure. Mackenrodt lays great stress upon the importance of making a clean blunt dissection of the parametrium and paracolpium from the sides and floor of the pelvis. This course is far superior to ligation and division, as, in his opinion, the stumps remaining after the latter procedure are generally the site of recurrences. The lower and external parts of the pelvic parametrium or broad ligament consist of numerous diverging strands of fibres which pass in all directions to, and merge with, the sacral pelvic fascia, the obturator fascia, the rectum, and the peritoneum of Douglas' pouch. These strands correspond in part to the distribution of the lymph- and blood-vessels of this region, and especially to the veins which empty into the hypogastric vein. The fascial sheath of the hypogastric vein is indeed the most prominent point of convergence of the parametrial roots.

Mackenrodt calls attention to certain anatomical points in the pelvis, a thorough knowledge of which is necessary for the successful performance of this operation. There are three groups of veins which pierce the pelvic parametrium and are of great importance from the surgical view-point, inasmuch as the prompt control of these prevents unnecessary loss of blood and enables one to complete the separation of the parametrium in a few minutes. If these veins are not controlled there may result serious loss of blood, sufficient to prolong greatly the operation or even to threaten the life of the patient. The anterior division of these veins empties into the obturator vein, and anastomoses with the vesico-vaginal venous plexus; the middle division drains into the hypogastric; and the posterior communicates with the sacral and hemorrhoidal veins, as well as with those of the rectum. The obturator nerve runs between the hypogastric roots and the pelvic parametrium, and about it are a number of lymph nodes which are generally considered part of the hypogastric group of lymph nodes. Some of the thicker roots of the parametrium pass backward between the folds of Douglas' pouch, and then, surrounding the rectum, take an upward direction toward the promontory; some of these are inserted into the upper part of the sacrum beneath the rectum. This tissue contains the small venous branches above described, as well as numerous anastomosing lymph channels. Lymphatics follow the course of the anterior division of veins to the internal inguinal lymph nodes; around the middle group are radicles which empty into the hypogastric lymph nodes; and with the posterior upper division are tracts which extend to the sacral and prevertebral lymph nodes of the lumbar vertebræ. The larger radicles accompany the uterine vessels and for the most part empty into the iliac lymph nodes. The channels from the ureteral lymph nodes follow this course; less often they empty into the nodes which are located at the bifurcation of the aorta; the iliac nodes also receive radicles accompanying the anterior group of veins from the inguinal region.

The vaginal tampon is now removed, and the uterus is drawn upward so as to put the vagina on the stretch. The anterior vaginal wall is then completely divided from side to side near the level at which the ureters enter the bladder. Clamps are placed at the ends of the incision and used as retractors to support the vagina. The posterior vagina is now made tense and the incision is extended to it; but, before this incision is completed, the rectum is pushed downward and backward by means of gauze tampons. In this manner one-half of the vagina may be removed with the uterus. The upper and lower margins of the wound left by the vaginal amputation are now closed with clamps. These clamps constitute a good means of traction in the further separation of the paracolpium from the rectum and pelvic wall. The rectum can be freed without difficulty, and the connective-tissue bands of the paracolpium, which extend from the rectum to the sacrum, also can be separated from the bone by pressure with gauze. The connective-tissue bands which extend to the side of the pelvis will require more careful attention, as they contain veins which anastomose with the vesico-vaginal plexus and the obturator veins, and which, if injured by strong traction, may give rise to considerable venous hemorrhage. Consequently they must be exposed and carefully ligated without injury to the obturator artery, after which the connective tissue may be freed by pressure with gauze upon a clamp. There are also in this middle root one or two veins which empty into the hypogastric; their early ligation will facilitate the dissection of the anterior roots of the paracolpium. When the sides of the anterior connective-tissue bands of the paracolpium are freed, the whole mass of paracolpium and vagina will be held only by fascial insertions on the anterior sides of the pelvic cavity, and these may readily be severed with the scissors. There are some small veins on the sacrum and about the rectum which may bleed slightly, but they can be controlled by temporary packing.

In the upper connective-tissue band is a small branch of the hypogastric vein which must be ligated. Afterward the connective tissue can be separated from the sides of the pelvic wall; it comes away, under traction, in long strands that extend under the peritoneum and about the rectum, and with it will be found the lymph nodes of the rectal and sacral connective tissue. The parts thus removed, consisting of vagina, uterus, adnexa, and the shaggy connective tissue of the parametrium and paracolpium, form quite a bulky mass.

When all hemorrhage has been controlled, the operation is concluded with the removal of any lymph nodes that may remain. Those of the rectal, sacral, and parametrial areas have already been removed with the mass about the uterus. There remain, therefore, the obturator, inguinal, and iliac nodes, all of which are rendered more accessible after the removal of the parametrium.

Mackenrodt generally discontinues the removal of the lymphatic tracts at the lower third of the common iliac artery, although the dissection may proceed much higher. When the connective tissue has not been thoroughly removed, many lymph nodes will be overlooked, as they lie in masses close about the vessels.

A pack of iodoform gauze is now placed in the vagina and over the raw area of the pelvic region. *The greatest care must be taken to prevent actual pressure*

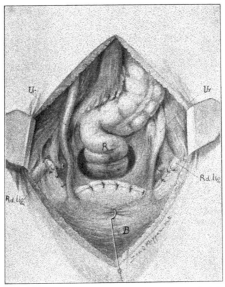

Fig. 260.—View from Above Looking down into the Pelvis after Removal of the Cancerous Area in Mackenrodt's Operation. (Original.)

in the pelvis, and to prevent the gauze from coming in contact with the ureters. The peritoneal surfaces are now closed above the pack, the rectum being united with the vesical flap and covering the entire raw area. (Fig. 260.) Mackenrodt then closes the abdominal wound in layers, using wire to unite the opposite margins of muscle and fascia. A permanent catheter is inserted in the bladder.

Complications.—Mackenrodt's fatalities have come chiefly from albuminuria and nephritis. These were observed twenty times in seventy cases, and eight times with fatal results. Necrosis of the bladder occurred in twenty-two cases.

This, he believes, was due to the involvement of the bladder wall, either by inflammatory processes about the cervix or by carcinoma itself. In fifteen instances the bladder was so fixed to the uterus under the vesico-uterine plica that its separation was possible only with violence and some injury to its wall. Carcinoma was found in the bladder wall in ten cases, while it was observed in the connective tissue between the bladder and uterus in four cases. Nearly all fistulæ heal spontaneously with the use of a permanent catheter and frequent irrigation. Mackenrodt has enucleated the ureter from an infiltrated broad ligament in forty-eight instances. There was necrosis in three cases; in one of these the fistula closed spontaneously, while in the other two the ureter was implanted into the bladder at a secondary operation. The ureters were excised in three cases because they were so firmly bound down by dense adhesions that they could not be separated without serious injury. The freshly incised upper end was immediately transplanted into the bladder, the operation resulting in death in one case, in the formation of a fistula leading into the rectum in a second case, and in complete success in a third. The ureters were accidentally incised during two operations. In both instances they lay in the fold of Douglas and were cut through when this was divided. Transplantation was immediately performed in both instances, with resulting death in one case and recovery in the other.

The after-treatment is practically the same as that outlined for the Wertheim operation.

Bumm's Operation.—Bumm calls attention to the fact that almost any radical operation suffices for an easy case, but that in difficult ones there is much to be desired. The chief difficulty which he has encountered in the Wertheim operation has been serious venous hemorrhage in the depths of the wound resulting from injury to venous plexuses. He therefore believes that the key to the successful operation is the exposure of the so-called vascular areas, and he has evolved an operation which permits a rapid removal of the cancerous field with little loss of blood.

Bumm uses a median incision which is augmented, in stout women, by dividing the inner fibres of the recti muscles just above the symphysis. The fascia is severed only in the median line, and when the peritoneal cavity has been opened and explored the intestines are packed off with gauze. The ovarian vessels on both sides are now doubly ligated and the infundibulo-pelvic ligaments are cut between the ligatures. These incisions are then carried through the peritoneum to the insertion of the meso-sigmoid on the left and the meso-cæceum on the right side, and from these points downward over the round ligament to the attachment of the bladder to the cervix. The round ligaments are then ligated and cut. Upon separating the margins of the incision the iliac vessels and the ureters are easily brought into view. In the outer and upper part of this exposed area lies the common iliac at its point of division. When the posterior layer of the broad ligament, to which the ureter is fastened, is drawn toward the median line, the origin of the uterine artery is exposed. As a rule, this vessel arises, in common with the superior vesical artery, from a short branch of the hypogastric. At the same time the lymph nodes of the vascular triangle and the hypogastric, common, and external iliac arteries are exposed. The ureter and the vessels are next brought into view by dissection, and the lymph nodes which are seen when the vascular triangle is exposed are loosened at the same time. All small vascular branches must be ligated or they will be torn. When the lymph nodes with their contiguous fatty and connective tissue are freed, the division points of the common iliac, the external iliac, and the hypogastric arteries, with their accompanying veins, lie exposed as if by dissection. The uterine artery is now doubly ligated and divided, either in common with the superior vesical artery or separately from it. The accompanying small veins are also tied. The entire vascular cord, with the surrounding fatty tissue, the lymph vessels, and the lymph nodes, may now be drawn toward the median line. The ureter which, as yet, has been exposed only above the point where it is crossed by the uterine artery, is now freed by blunt dissection as far down as the bladder. This separation must be complete, as the underlying tissue must later be extirpated and the largest uterine veins ligated. The uterine vein, as a rule, leaves the uterus in two branches. The smaller of these runs above the ureter and along the artery; the larger one may be as big as the quill of a goose's feather and runs beneath the ureter, but the two unite just before the common stem empties into the hypogastric vein. The larger branch can be exposed and ligated, after which the ureter is fully separated and pushed toward the median line.

The remaining steps of the operation include the removal not only of the cervix and the upper part of the vagina, but also of the paracervical and paravaginal tissues. In Bumm's opinion this is much more important than the removal of the lymph nodes. The excision should be carried out as close to the pelvic wall as possible and down to the pelvic diaphragm. The vaginal walls are divided according to the position of the greatest extension of the growth. This varies in nearly all instances. For example, if the anterior vaginal wall is most affected, the vagina is incised from behind through Douglas' pouch, the paravaginal tissue in this situation having been previously separated from the rectum. Gauze is placed over the cervix, and the entire circumference of the vagina is divided. The uterine mass is pulled upward and the anterior vaginal wall and surrounding cellular tissue are separated from below, the parts being kept in a state of tension and the worst areas being separated last. When the direction of greatest extension of the disease is from before backward or to one side, the procedure must be modified to meet the case. The easy side should always be taken first. After the mass has been removed, all bleeding points should be controlled, the vaginal stump hemmed around, and the free edges of the peritoneum brought together with running catgut sutures, the serous coat of the rectum being united with the serosa of the bladder. After the abdominal incision is closed, Bumm places a gauze tampon in the vagina and removes it after twenty-four hours. Its only object is lightly to press the wounded pelvic surfaces together. He does not use any special drainage for the pelvic cellular tissues, because the secretion easily escapes without it, and drains may cause pressure necrosis of the ureters or lead to prolonged suppuration.

Amann's Method of Covering the Ureters and Draining the Pelvis after a Radical Abdominal Operation.—Amann, in 1908, calls attention to the fact that at the conclusion of any abdominal operation that removes the upper vagina, uterus, parametrium, paracolpium, and lymph nodes, there will necessarily be created deep pits at the side of the vagina and in the lower part of the pelvis,—pits which cannot be drained easily and in which blood-clots accumulate, thus establishing conditions favorable to sepsis. The ureters also, after such an operation, lack their usual supports, and are quite likely to be injured by the gauze that is commonly inserted as a drain, and that quite frequently exerts sufficient pressure to induce necrosis. Amann has, in the past, placed the ureters alongside of the rectum and sutured the bladder to the rectum throughout for as great a distance as appeared expedient. At the conclusion of the operation the depths of the pelvis were drained by paravaginal incisions. Amann now proposes an improved method of closure by which he attempts to lift the ureters out of the way so that the gauze shall not come in contact with them and produce necrosis, and so that at the same time the depths of the pelvis shall be adequately drained.

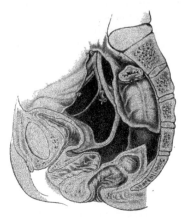

Fig. 261.—The Drawing Shows one Aspect of Amann's Method of Covering Ureters and Draining the Pelvis after a Radical Removal of the Carcinomatous Uterus. (From *Zeitschrift fuer Geburtshuelfe*, No. 61.)

To this end, at the conclusion of the removal of the uterus, he sutures the vesical peritoneum to the anterior vaginal wall, so placing the running catgut sutures that the lower extremities of the ureters are somewhat elevated and in close approximation to the vesical peritoneum. The upper portions of the ureters now sag down in the depths of the pelvis, and, in order to elevate them and displace them to the sides of the pelvic wall, he makes a sort of sling by uniting the lateral borders of the peritoneum with the stumps of the uterine artery. This gently displaces the ureters to the sides of the pelvis and interposes a peritoneal wall between them and the pelvic cavity. The greatest care should be taken during the operation not to injure the superior vesical artery, at the side of which rests the displaced ureter. (Figs. 261, 262, and 263.) The posterior vaginal wall is now seized with two clamps and separated from the rectum for a considerable distance. It is split between the two clamps in a longitudinal manner with the thermocautery, as far down as the level of the denuded pits at the sides of the vagina. The latter cavity is then loosely packed with gauze from above, and the raw areas in the lower portions of the lower pelvis are covered with the same strips. The pelvis is next closed off from the peritoneal cavity; this being effected by uniting first the peritoneal margins of the posterior pelvic wall and the peritoneum in contact with the stumps of the uterine artery, and secondly by bringing the sigmoid flexure down into the depths of the pelvis and uniting it with the vesical peritoneum. (Fig. 264.) In case the sigmoid does not reach, the cæcum can also be used to make a good peritoneal covering for the denuded areas.

The Paravaginal Operation.—We have already indicated the necessity for removing the parametrium in order to prevent local recurrence, and, as this is impossible in the simple vaginal hysterectomy, the latter can no longer be considered a radical operation, save in a small percentage of cases. Methods have been devised, however, which permit the removal of the uterus and wide areas of the parametrium through the vagina. The chief feature of these methods consists in making a lateral incision in the vagina of such a depth that it will give a wide exposure of the cervix and parametrium. Before the description of this incision by Schuchardt, in 1893, more or less deep incisions had been made by Mackenrodt, Fritsch, Duehrssen, Purcell, and Pfannenstiel, but they differed considerably in their extent and in the resultant degree of exposure. The earlier advocates of the paravaginal incision commended

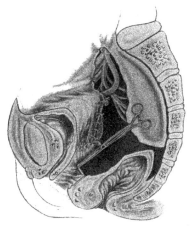

Fig. 262.—The Drawing Shows another Aspect of Amann's Method of Covering Ureters and Draining the Pelvis after a Radical Removal of the Carcinomatous Uterus. (From *Zeitschrift fuer Geburtshuelfe*, No. 61.)

it as a primary step, but Schauta, in 1908, after discussing the possibilities of implantation of cancerous material into the wound, recommends that it be made as a late step in the operation.

The operation is performed in the following manner:—After the patient has been shaved and the parts carefully prepared, she is placed on the edge of the table in the lithotomy position. A speculum is introduced, the cervix steadied, and all possible cancerous tissue is removed with a curette, after which the ulcer is burned with a Paquelin cautery. The vulva and vagina are now again disinfected, and a circular incision is made in the upper vagina below the growth, the tissue being stretched with tenacula and the cutting being done above them. In the early cases this incision is best placed about the junction of the middle and upper thirds of the vagina, but in the later growths it should be located as low as the middle of the canal. The actual cautery may be used instead of the knife. The vaginal cuff thus outlined below the cervix is dissected up as deeply as possible and sutured over the cancerous cervix, so that the infectious material may not escape from the uterus during the operation and contaminate the wound. The ends of the sutures applied to the cervix are left long so that they may be used as tractors. The hemorrhage which results during this step may be controlled by imbrication sutures. This wide dissection is necessitated by the frequent presence of vaginal metastases which are not visible to the naked eye. Schauta advises that the bladder be separated from its attachments before the perineum is incised, as the latter step is useless if subsequently it be found necessary to abandon the operation. The dissection is completed in the midline and carried partially to the sides, and is accomplished in large

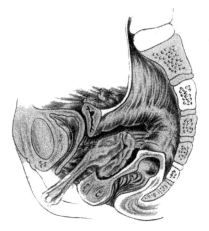

Fig. 263.—The Drawing Shows a Third Stage of Amann's Method of Covering Ureters and Draining the Pelvis after a Radical Removal of the Carcinomatous Uterus. (From *Zeitschrift fuer Geburtshuelfe*, No. 61.)

part by blunt dissection, although actual cutting with the scissors may be necessary. The ureters lie under the lateral supports of the bladder, which are spread out over the parametria and are not exposed until the next step has been accomplished. As much available room is offered by the perineal incision, the bladder is freed sufficiently far out on the sides to permit of palpation of the parametria If the growth can be demonstrated as spreading through the cervix and so far into the parametria that it will be necessary to resect either the ureters or the bladder, or both, it is useless to continue the operation. The best course will be to abandon it at this point, before the peritoneum has been incised behind the bladder.

The paravaginal incision is, in effect, only a wide episiotomy. An incision on one side usually suffices and had best be made on the side of the greatest parametrial induration. Both sides may be cut if necessary, a step which Staude recommends as a routine procedure. Other things being equal, the left-sided incision is more convenient for a right-handed operator. It is made in the following manner:—With the forefinger and thumb of the left hand the operator seizes the posterior portion of the left labium, while an assistant seizes the parts in the midline and puts them on the stretch. An incision is now made, between the two sets of fingers, through the vaginal wall from the circular incision previously made downward and laterally, through the posterior portion of the labium minus to the middle of the coccygeal region. This incision splits the whole vaginal tube and, according to Schuchardt, passes through the left labium minus, the paravaginal and pararectal tissues, the levator ani and coccygeal muscles, the cellular tissue of the ischiorectal fossa and the skin of the perineum, and the left anal region, down to the sacrum. The incision in the pararectal

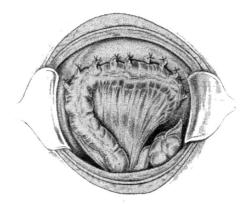

Fig. 264.—The Drawing Shows a still Later Stage of Amann's Method of Covering Ureters and Draining the Pelvis after a Radical Removal of the Carcinomatous Uterus. (From *Zeitschrift fuer Geburtshuelfe*, No. 61.)

tissue is carried to the left only so far that the rectum and sphincter ani may not be injured. It should extend about a finger's breadth from the midline. The copious hemorrhage that results should be controlled, and gauze should be packed into the wound; a weighted hanging speculum being placed over it to control effectually any oozing which may persist, and also to afford sufficient exposure of the parts. The effect of the incision is quite remarkable. Instead of a vaginal tube, there appears a shallow excavation, not more than one inch in depth, at the bottom of which lie the parametria at full extent and within easy reach. (Fig. 265.)

Now follows the preparation of the ureters, which Schauta describes as the most important feature of the operation. This can be safely performed without preliminary catheterization. In fact, some men object to this latter procedure; they claim that ureteritis is more apt to result, and furthermore that the procedure is not necessary, inasmuch as the ureters are constantly kept in sight during the next steps of the operation. The dissection of the bladder is now completed laterally and at the level of the internal os, and immediately under the lateral attachments of the bladder is seen the ureter winding around the uterine artery. In thickened parametria it will be necessary to dissect farther out on the sides in order to expose the ureters. Unless the infiltration is quite marked the ureter can readily be freed from its bed with the finger, which is used to push the parametria away. Sometimes it is better to dissect it loose with the scissors, especially if there is any chance that the infiltration has extended to the ureteral walls, when this tissue becomes extremely brittle and is prone to injury. It is, of course, possible to amputate above the level of involvement and then to do an immediate transplantation into the bladder, but the ulti-

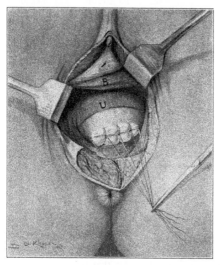

Fig. 265.—Paravaginal Operation. The paravaginal incision has been completed, the cervical area outlined by incision, and the cervical cuff closed with sutures. (Original.)

mate results are not good, and many deem it wiser to abandon the operation if this complication is present. The uterine vessels should now be ligated as far away from the uterus as possible. The pouch of Douglas is opened with the scissors and the incision extended well out on the sides. This procedure will be complicated if the disease has extended out to the rectum, or if the case is complicated by disease of the adnexa and by prolapse of these structures into the cul-de-sac. The index finger of the left hand is next introduced into the incision made in the pouch of Douglas, and the parametrium is separated from the rectum. During this step a branch of the middle hemorrhoidal artery is generally encountered and must at once be ligated. The parametrium can then be hooked down over the finger and cut free with the scissors, care being taken to have the ureter constantly in view so that it may not be injured. This step will be greatly facilitated by pulling the cervix strongly down and to the opposite side, as in this way most excellent exposure is afforded. (Fig. 267.) A clamp placed over the mesial portion of the parametrium is of great use in bringing the lateral margins of these structures into view. Schauta states that, if the uterine vessels have been secured high up, and if the branch of the middle hemorrhoidal has been ligated as a preliminary step, there will result, during this dissection, only venous hemorrhage, which can be well controlled with gauze tampons. Others, however, recommend that the tissue be first ligated and then cut between the sutures. When the dissection has proceeded as high up as the ureter,

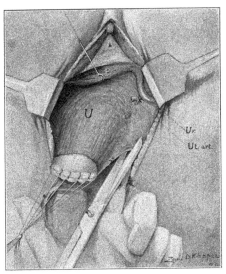

FIG. 266.—In the Drawing the Bladder is Elevated and the Ureter is Plainly Seen after its Dissection from the Parametrium. The incision is passing through the lateral edge of the parametrium. (Original.)

this structure is pushed out of the way and the enucleation is continued. The advocates of this operation unite in stating that it is astonishing how easily an infiltrated parametrium can be removed even as far out as the pelvic wall. If the anterior peritoneal cavity has not been opened, an incision is next made and extended laterally so that the uterus will hang suspended only by the broad ligaments and tubes. The bladder and ureters are lifted well out of the incision and the anterior wall of the uterus is seized with a tenaculum and pulled down beneath the bladder, while at the same time the cervix is pushed up and backward into the vagina, so that the fundus is brought down into the wound. Two large clamps are placed over the upper broad ligament, the round ligament, and the tube of one side, and the tissue is cut between them. The ovarian artery of the other side is now secured by two large ligatures, the broad ligament of that side is ligated with three or four ligatures, and the uterus, parametria, and upper broad ligament of one side, together with one tube and ovary, are removed. The ends of these sutures are left long. The ovarian artery of the other side is then secured in a similar manner, and the ovary and tube are removed in the same fashion. Schauta does not remove the tube and ovaries (Fig. 268); he claims that they are practically never the seat of cancerous extension from cervical carcinoma, but nearly all other advocates of this route remove them as above described.

The stumps of the ligaments are then brought down into the wound, the

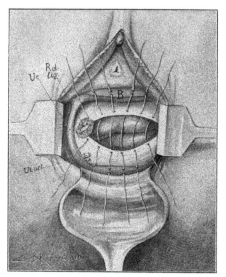

Fig. 267.—Method of Closing Peritoneum and Vagina after Paravaginal Operation. (Original.)

peritoneum covering the bladder is united to that behind the cul-de-sac, and the ligamentous stumps are transfixed in the angles of the peritoneal closure. (Fig. 267.) Great care should be taken that all raw margins are treated extraperitoneally, so that the minimum possibility of adhesions is obtained. The treatment of the upper vagina varies in different hands, yet all agree that, if packs are used, they should be inserted so lightly that they will not exert pressure against the ureters and thus favor necrosis. Gellhorn and Schauta place three small gauze strips in the supravaginal space and do not close the upper vagina, while Schuchardt and several others close the incision, or leave but a very small opening in which a slender gauze drain is inserted. The paravaginal incision is now closed with catgut augmented with non-absorbable sutures on the skin surfaces. It is needless to state that the cut ends of the muscles should be united before the wound is closed. A small gauze strip may be left in the vagina and removed on the following day.

The *after-care* does not differ from that of any serious laparotomy. The same care should be taken to guard against shock, and most careful attention of the bladder is required. In case packing has been inserted in the supravaginal space, its removal should begin two or three days after the operation, small portions 8 or 10 centimetres in length being taken away at a time, so that all shall be removed at the end of a week. By the time the perineal sutures are re-

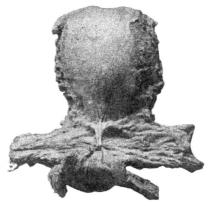

Fig. 268.—Uterus with Parametrium, Removed by Paravaginal Operation. (From Schauta, "Die erweiterte vaginale Totalexstirpation des Uterus bei Kollumkarzinom," Wien und Leipzig. 1908.)

moved, the opening in the upper vagina will have closed, save for a small opening in the granulating area.

The method is not free from accidental injuries, nor can it be hoped that any extensive operation in this region will escape them altogether. In Schauta's series of 258 cases the convalescence was uninterrupted in 150 instances, and complicated in the other 108 cases. Post-operative cystitis developed in 67 cases, and the bladder and ureter were injured in each one of 11 cases, and the intestine in 4 instances. The paravaginal incision broke down in 5 cases, and twice it would appear that the carcinomatous tissue was grafted into the wound.

VIII. OTHER OPERATIONS FOR CANCER OF THE UTERUS.

Removal of the Uterus and the Parametrium by Cautery.—The remarkable results which were claimed by Byrne, in America, following 1872, in the treatment of uterine cancer, have directed the attention of many to the extirpation of the uterus by the cautery. Byrne, by a simple operation, which consisted for the most part in the amputation of the cervix by means of the cautery and the burning out of the interior of the uterus by special cautery instruments, claimed to have operated upon three hundred and sixty-seven cases of uterine carcinoma without a single primary death, and with an operative percentage of cures, at the end of five years, of nineteen per cent. Even though these results have been much questioned, and some doubt cast upon the diagnosis of a considerable number of his cases, Byrne's writings have recently awakened much interest and have led many to employ the cautery treatment of carcinoma. Rawlick, Moore Madden, and others have also obtained relative immunity from local recurrence by the use of the cautery, and they believe that its influence extends beyond the actual field of operation and thus permits a more radical operation than can be accomplished by the more usual methods. Bumm, however, denies this, and believes that the effect of the cautery does not extend more than 1 centimetre into the tissue.

Among the prominent converts to the cautery treatment of uterine carcinoma is Werder, who is well known for the description of the radical operation which was subsequently proposed by Wertheim, and which generally bears the latter's name. Werder has now abandoned his operation and has devoted himself to the perfection of a technique for the performance of hysterectomy by the cautery. At first, he performed the entire operation through the vagina, either with or without the Schuchardt incision, but more recently he has employed a combined operation beginning in the vagina and completed through an abdominal exposure. This change in technique was necessitated on account of the difficulty of protecting the ureters from injury during the application of the heated clamps to the broad ligaments through the vaginal route.

Werder's Cautery Hysterectomy.—After the usual antiseptic preparation and curettage, the patient is brought to the edge of the table and the parts are exposed by a hanging speculum, and the cervix steadied by a tenaculum. An incision is then made around the cervix, as far as possible from the affected area, by means of the cautery knife kept at a dull heat to prevent oozing and keep the wound dry. The requisite heat is obtained by turning on the current only after the knife has been placed against the tissues to be burned. While traction is being made upon the cervix, the dissection is carried up between the bladder and the uterus until the peritoneum is reached, the assistant meanwhile carefully keeping the bladder from the neighborhood of the hot knife. The peritoneum is first opened posteriorly by scissors and the opening is widened by the fingers, after which the lateral vaginal attachments are burned through. The vaginal wound is then carefully inspected and any surfaces that are not black and well charred are thoroughly cauterized. The vagina is now lightly packed with gauze and the abdomen prepared for laparotomy.

An incision is made in the midline and completed in the usual manner. The intestines are replaced in the abdominal cavity and held back by gauze that has been saturated with sterile salt solution. The peritoneum of the bladder is now incised from side to side, thus opening into the cavity previously made by the separation of the bladder from the uterus through the vagina. The broad Downe's electrothermic clamp is then applied to the right infundibulo-pelvic ligament and round ligament, and the tissues included are burned until a thin white ribbon results. Great care should be taken that the surrounding parts are carefully protected by the shield and additional intestinal packs. The clamp is now removed and the ribbon cut through near its inner edge, and, if no bleeding occurs, it is dropped. The other side is then treated in the same manner. The least affected side of the parametrium is now clamped, after the bladder and ureters have been carefully protected. The current is again turned on and the tissue burned through, after which a deeper portion of the broad ligament is treated in the same manner, thus freeing one side of the uterus from attachment. The opposite parametrium is then treated in the same way and the uterus is removed. If the technique has been good, it is claimed that no blood is lost after the primary curettage, and that the cut surfaces remain perfectly dry. The operator is cautioned to observe any vessel for a period of one minute before dropping the stump, after which hæmostasis is as secure as if ligatures had been used.

The stump of the vagina is now exposed, its cauterized edges are turned downward, and the raw surfaces are approximated with a continuous catgut suture. The bladder is brought over the stump of the vagina, its peritoneum is stitched to the rectum, and the broad ligament stumps are carefully covered on both sides, the field of operation being thus completely covered with peritoneum. The abdomen is then closed without drainage. Werder calls attention to the fact that the abdominal operation differs from the ordinary panhysterectomy only in that the tissues are clamped and burned through instead of being cut after ligation.

Up to this time Werder has not made preliminary dissection of the ureters, but has depended upon firm traction on the uterus and side of the bladder with the clamps in position, for the exposure of the parametrium and protection of the ureters. It will be seen that very little parametrium is actually removed, but the advocates of this method claim that the destructive action from the cauterization extends for some distance beyond the actual site of the clamps. Werder's cases are still too few and too recent to justify conclusions as to the permanent value of this method.

Vaginal Hysterectomy.—At the present time vaginal hysterectomy is not considered radical, save in a very small proportion of cases. As a preliminary step it is necessary to curette and remove as much of the cancerous tissue as possible, at least twenty-four hours before the operation, in order to limit the chance of infection from the offensive discharge which is so common in these cases. (Vide Preliminary Measures, page 619.)

The patient is placed on the edge of the table in the lithotomy position with thighs well flexed and the buttocks resting on the perineal pad. The external genitals have been shaved, and, together with the vagina, washed with antiseptic solutions. A large, self-retaining vaginal retractor is introduced so that the vaginal walls and cervix are exposed to view. If the vagina is so narrow that it hinders a view of the cervix, it may be dilated with the hands, or, if the rigidity cannot be overcome in this manner, one or two deep lateral incisions in the midline will give the necessary enlargement. Some surgeons, however, advocate dilating the vagina with a rubber bag two or three days before the operation, in order to avoid the possibility of transplantation of the growth into the vaginal scars; this, however, is not a good practice.

The anterior lip of the cervix is now caught with a tenaculum forceps and drawn down, and the anterior and posterior lips are stitched together, so that

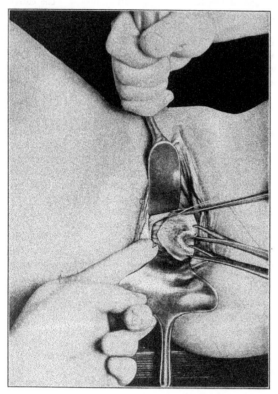

Fig. 269.—Vaginal Hysterectomy. Incision in first step of the operation. (From Wertheim und Micholitsch, " Die Technik der vaginalen Bauchhoehlen-Operationen," Leipzig, 1906.)

the cervical canal will be completely closed and consequently will prevent the escape of cancerous tissue during the operation. In some cases it is advisable to catheterize the ureters before the operation, in order that they may be easily recognized. This is especially desirable when the extent of the carcinoma is not definitely known.

The cervix is next seized with a tenaculum and pulled down, and a circular incision is made around it; this incision passing through the entire thickness of the vaginal wall and extending at least one inch beyond the margin of the disease. (Fig. 269.) With the handle of a knife or dissector, the cellular tissue in front of and behind the cervix and the fornix is pushed back and freed. This is usually accomplished without difficulty and with but little hemorrhage, as the important blood-vessels lie higher up in the broad ligament. Care must

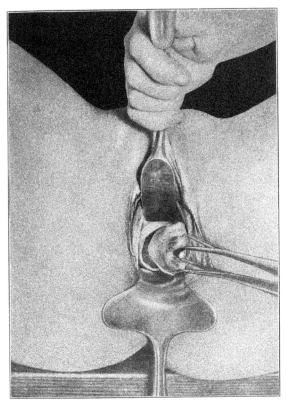

Fig. 270.—Vaginal Hysterectomy. The bladder is strongly elevated while the uterine blood-vessels are being ligated. (From Wertheim und Micholitsch, "Die Technik der vaginalen Bauch-hoehlen-Operationen," Leipzig, 1906.)

be taken during this step to avoid perforation of the bladder or injury to the ureters, especially in the cases in which the carcinoma has extended well into the anterior wall of the cervix. (Fig. 270.) Such cases always are difficult, owing to the operator's desire to keep away from the diseased area. The bladder should be pushed up until the reflection of the peritoneum over the uterus is seen; then, by inserting two fingers, one may stretch the tissues until sufficient space is gained for a rapid exploration of the pelvis. The edge oɪ the peritoneum covering the bladder is pulled down and stitched to the mucosa of the anterior vaginal fornix by two catgut sutures, and the cervix is drawn upward and forward in order to give a good exposure of the posterior fornix. The posterior vaginal wall above the circular incision is separated as far as

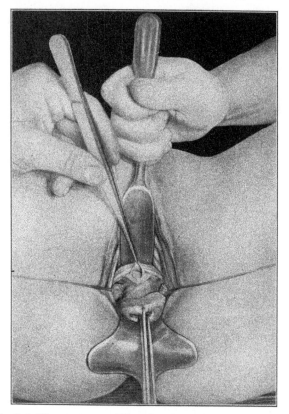

FIG. 271.—Vaginal Hysterectomy. The incision has been made into the peritoneal cavity. (From Wertheim und Micholitsch, "Die Technik," etc., Leipzig, 1906.)

the lower part of the pouch of Douglas, which can be recognized by the fluctuation of a little fluid which may be present, or by the smooth anterior and posterior surfaces gliding over each other. The peritoneal cavity is opened with the scalpel, and its interior palpated with a finger before the opening is stretched to such a degree that it will extend well out to the bases of the broad ligaments. (Fig. 271.) In case the growth chiefly affects the anterior cervix, it may be well to make the primary incision into the peritoneal cavity through the posterior vault. There is usually considerable bleeding from the edges between the posterior wall and the peritoneum, and this bleeding will prove troublesome if the vessels are not secured. It is best, therefore, before proceeding further, to approximate the edges of the peritoneum and the mucosa of the posterior vaginal wall by several interrupted catgut sutures. One or two large gauze pads are now introduced into the pelvic cavity to prevent the intestines from prolapsing into the wound, as well as to prevent the escape of débris from the field of the operation into the peritoneal cavity. A pair of artery forceps should be attached to each of the gauze pads by tapes, in order that they may not be overlooked at the close of the operation. The cervix is then pulled directly downward, and wide lateral retractors are inserted into the wound.

The cervix is drawn strongly to the left and the right broad ligament is pierced by a strong aneurysmal needle, threaded with heavy catgut and passed from before backward on the tip of the finger. The bight should include a mass of tissue about 1 centimetre in diameter, and the needle should enter the broad ligament at a distance of about 1 centimetre from the cervix. The ligature is now tied as tightly as possible, its ends are drawn aside but not cut, and the broad ligament is divided between the ligature and the uterus, but nearer to the latter. All cutting should be done with scissors, and the tissues of the broad ligament should be carefully snipped as they are drawn forward on the index finger. A little oozing of blood following a cut tells us that the blood supply of the last divided tissue is uncontrolled, and another ligature should then be inserted in a similar manner. (Fig. 272.)

Care must now be taken to avoid the ureters. A retractor is carefully inserted between the bladder and the cervix, and the former is held well out of the angle so that the ureters may be elevated as much as possible. If they have been catheterized before operation their exact position can be determined by palpation during the enucleation. An extensive infiltration of the cervix and parametrium complicates this step, and, unless the greatest care is observed, the ureters will be included in a ligature. As soon as the peritoneum is opened the uterine artery can be felt pulsating by the side of the cervix near the internal os. The exact position of the vessel once fixed serves as a guide to determine the amount of tissue to be included in each ligature; the artery will thus be included in the second or the third. When laid bare the vessel is easily distinguishable as a large tortuous trunk, with a lumen of 2 or 3 mm. and pulsating strongly on its proximal side. As soon as the uterine vessels on one side are secured and cut, the other side of the broad ligament is treated in a similar fashion, the cervix being pulled away from that side in order to give good exposure. When the broad ligament has been divided as high as the level of the internal os, and well above the uterine arteries, the bladder should be well elevated by an anterior retractor, and the anterior wall of the uterus grasped with a tenaculum and pulled down, while the cervix is pushed upward and backward into the vagina. In this way the fundus is brought down into the vagina. A finger is now introduced into the pelvis in order to free the tubes and ovaries from adhesions, if any are present. Another gauze pad may be introduced through the upper angle of the wound, well into the pelvis, to prevent the prolapse of the omentum and intestines, and to absorb any blood which may escape. The broad ligament on one side is clamped

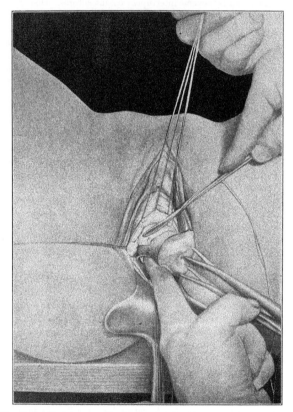

Fig. 272.—Vaginal Hysterectomy. The ligation of the broad ligaments. (From Wertheim und Micholitsch, "Die Technik," etc., Leipzig, 1906.)

with strong forceps from above downward, and is divided between the forceps and the uterus, so as to free the latter entirely on that side. The uterus is then pulled down as far as possible so that the broad ligament of the other side may be ligated and divided. Two ligatures are placed about the ovarian vessels above the tubes and ovaries. Other sutures are now placed in the broad ligament as far down as the ligature previously applied to the uterine vessels, and their ends are kept long.   The uterine tubes and ovaries are then removed.   (Figs. 273 and 274.)

Traction is now made on the forceps applied to the other broad ligament, and it is drawn downward in order that ligatures may be placed around the ovarian vessels of this side.   Following the completion of this step the lower

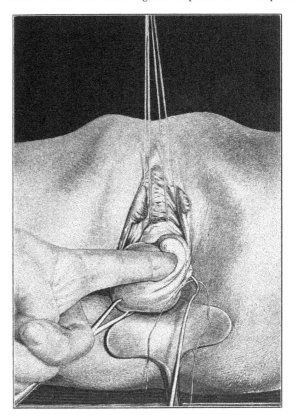

Fig. 273.   Vaginal Hysterectomy.   The finger is reaching for the infundibulo-pelvic ligament. (From Wertheim und Micholitsch, "Die Technik," etc., Leipzig, 1906.)

part of this broad ligament is tied off, and the tube and ovary and upper broad ligament are removed.   The ends of all the ligatures on each side are then grouped together, the condition of each knot investigated, and the broad ligament carefully examined for bleeding points.   Any ligature which seems loose should be at once replaced.   The stump of each broad ligament is drawn down into each lateral margin of the vaginal fornix, so that their raw surfaces will lie outside of the peritoneal cavity and will project into the vaginal cavity, thus lessening the possibility of adhesions. Sutures are applied to maintain the stumps of the broad ligaments in the vagina, a strong catgut suture being passed through the edge of the vaginal wall in such a manner as to include the peritoneum of each broad ligament just above the stump, and then continued

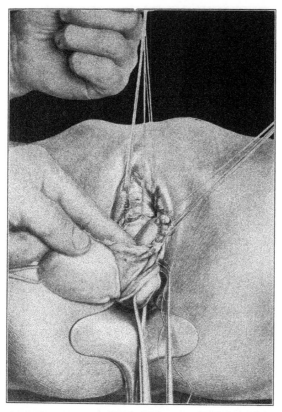

FIG. 274.—Vaginal Hysterectomy. Completion of the separation of the broad ligament of the first side. (From Wertheim und Micholitsch, "Die Technik," etc., Leipzig, 1906.)

through the edge of the upper vaginal wall. This suture is in effect a fixation suture, and before it is tied one similar to it may be inserted in the outer edge of the vaginal wound. Corresponding sutures are now introduced on the opposite side, and these, when tied, compress each broad ligament in a lateral angle of the vaginal incision. The gauze pads are now withdrawn from the pelvis and the latter is sponged out with pads wrung in hot saline solution.

The vaginal openings between the stumps are then closed with a running catgut suture, care being taken to approximate the peritoneal surfaces. The ends of the ligatures are cut short, and the vagina is packed with gauze. The bladder is catheterized, and, if the urine is found to be clear, the operator may feel sure that the organ has received no serious injury. The presence of blood in the urine may indicate injury either to the bladder or to the ureter.

Variations in Technique.—Variations in technique may be necessary. We have already referred to the fact that it may be more convenient to open the posterior peritoneum before attempting to open the anterior. In other cases the fundus cannot be pulled down on account of adhesions, enlargement of the uterus, or the smallness of the vagina, and it may be necessary to ligate the greater part of the broad ligament before the fundus can be pulled down. Occasionally it is more convenient to pull the fundus down behind than in front before securing the infundibulo-pelvic ligaments. If the case is further complicated by salpingitis, or if other infected areas are exposed, it is advisable not to close the vaginal incision at the conclusion of the operation, but to pack with gauze, so that drainage may be maintained for several days.

Many operators advocate the splitting of the uterus before an attempt is made to ligate the vessels; yet this procedure is contra-indicated in carcinoma, not only on account of the risk of transplanting part of the growth, but because of the likelihood of exposing infected areas in the uterus, such as a pyometra above the margin of the cancer.

Complications of the Operation.—The bladder may be torn, cut, or perforated, and the injury may not be discovered during the operation, especially if the patient was catheterized immediately before the operation, as should always be done. This complication is more apt to occur when the disease has spread through the cervix into the bladder. If the injury is recognized, the opening should be closed with two rows of fine catgut. Often, however, it remains unrecognized until the following day, when dribbling of urine is noticed. In the latter event it should be let alone, and, after convalescence is established, if the fistula has not closed, the attempt should be made to accomplish this result by a secondary operation. Similarly, although very rarely, the rectum or an adherent piece of intestine may be injured and a fecal fistula or a peritonitis may result, according to the situation of the injured spot and its relation to the bowel. The ureter may be tied, torn, or cut. This, unfortunately, is not generally recognized at the time of the operation. If the ureter alone is injured, a ureteral-vaginal fistula will develop while the patient is yet in bed. If one ureter is included in a ligature a fistula may also develop. If both ureters are tied,—which, fortunately, is a rare occurrence,—death is most apt to supervene. Fortunately these complications can be avoided ordinarily if the ureters are previously catheterized. Yet the method, even with this precaution, is not without some danger, as shown by a case of Cullen's. Both ureters had been catheterized without difficulty, and throughout the operation their course had been palpated with but little difficulty. At the conclusion of the operation one catheter was easily removed, but the left one had been broken, probably by the bite of a pair of artery forceps. A portion was removed, but a piece 17.5 cm. long still remained in the ureter. The condition of the patient did not warrant the necessary abdominal section for its recovery, and death occurred on the seventh day.

In case the ureters are cut through at the time of operation and recognized, a ureteral anastomosis should immediately be performed. Van Hook's method is satisfactory and simple. In case the incision is close to the bladder, transplantation into that viscus should be immediately effected. (Fig. 275.)

Hemorrhage may be troublesome, especially in the cases associated with indurated parametria, as the ligatures may cut through the tissue and not secure the vessels. One is then in an awkward predicament, and can control the bleed-

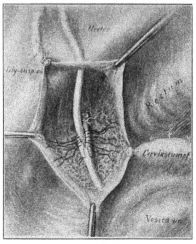

Fig. 275.—Ureteral Anastomosis. (From Doederlein und Kroenig, "Operat. Gynaekol.," Leipzig, 1905.)

ing only by applying forceps to the ligament and leaving them in position for seventy-two hours. This may best be done with the forceps of Pryor, which have detachable handles, or the ordinary long clamps may be used. Each blade of the forceps should be wrapped with gauze. Or the patient may at once be placed in the dorsal position, and abdominal section performed, thus making it possible to control the vessels from above. In the majority of cases, however, this will be unnecessary, as the hemorrhage can be controlled by clamps in the vagina. This complication should rarely occur, as vaginal extirpation of the uterus should not be performed if the parametrium is known to be involved.

The After-Treatment.—When the effects of the anæsthetic have worn away, the patient may be greatly relieved from time to time by turning her gently from one side to the other. After a few days she may be placed on her face and allowed to urinate in that posture. The catheter should be used every eight hours at first, if necessary, and the bowels should be opened on the third day. Just before this time the vaginal pack should be removed and large hot douches of formalin solution (1 in 2,000) should be given twice daily. Morphine should be administered sparingly. As a rule, heroin in small doses, or codeine with trional, will control the pain.

Causes of Death Following Vaginal Hysterectomy.—Rarely does a patient die of shock, because this operation can be performed in from twenty to thirty minutes, and can even be done under local anæsthesia. A general anæsthetic should be given only for as short time as possible.

Infection causes a large proportion of the fatalities, although the facilities for drainage are infinitely better after the vaginal operation than after the abdominal hysterectomy. The mortality, however, resulting from vaginal hysterectomy should be small, because the cases should be selected, and infection should cause an extremely small proportion of deaths if careful preliminary preparation has been observed. Ligation of the ureters may be a most dangerous complication. Sometimes it causes death, but there is always the chance that a uretero-vaginal fistula may develop and fatality thus be avoided. Zweifel states that injuries of the ureters, bladder, or rectum occurred in 4.8 per cent of his cases. Reipen reported them in 8.91 per cent of Kaltenbach and Fehling's cases. In ,69 operations by Baecker they occurred in 9 instances. Sampson reports that, in 157 hysterectomies for cancer of the uterus in Kelly's clinic, the ureters were found to be involved in the disease in 91 cases, so that there was constant opportunity for these structures to receive injuries.

IX. PALLIATIVE TREATMENT OF UTERINE CANCER; TREATMENT OF RECURRENCES FOLLOWING OPERATION; GENERAL MEASURES TO BE EMPLOYED IN CASES OF UTERINE CANCER.

Palliative Treatment.—Every surgeon should familiarize himself with the palliative treatment of uterine cancer; because at the present time, in this country, the great majority of cases are inoperable when they first apply for medical advice. There is little doubt that, in the past, too little has been done for the relief of the unfortunate victims of inoperable cancer. Far too often has the treatment been limited to morphine and douches. The present literature is emphasizing the fact that much can be done to limit the pain and the offensive odor of the disease by comparatively simple measures. Indeed, Lomer, Mond, Roessling, and others have even reported cases in which cauterization has caused the subsidence of the infiltration which proved merely inflammatory and not malignant, and permitted the removal of growths which had been considered inoperable. Yet it would appear that there should be a limit to the extent of the treatment advised, although some, as Freund, have recently advocated the removal of the uterus in cases definitely known to be inoperable, claiming that·hopeless cases demanded heroic treatment. Some basis for such treatment is afforded by the records of isolated cases in the literature, in which it would appear that even the simpler methods of palliative treat¬ment had caused at least an arrest of the growth, as in the well-known case of Lomer's, while, at the same time, the records also show that several have escaped a recurrence of the disease for varying periods after incomplete operations. Thus, Fleischmann, in 1908, reported three cases in which the limit of the growth at one side defied removal at operation, and yet these patients had no recurrence for periods of three, eight, and eleven years respectively. Cases like these do not permit of comparison with those in which attempt is made to remove a uterus from a mass of cancerous parametrium. In Freund's cases two of the seven operated upon shortly afterward presented ureteral necrosis. Moreover, there are not reported in the literature myriads of cases in which death followed as a result of cutting both ureters, or from infection, or from unsuccessful efforts to check the bleeding from the infiltrated parametrium; and the smallness of the number of those cases in which death followed an incomplete removal of the uterus must be considered most marked exceptions to the general rule. These facts make one hesitate to subject the unfortunate individual to the anguish of an operation which offers practically no prospect of relief.

The local palliative treatment consists largely of curettage and cauterization, repeated at intervals of every few weeks. Lomer and many others insist that the treatment should be repeated at least every four weeks. As a rule, it is necessary to employ a general anæsthetic, and then it will be found that nitrous oxide usually suffices. Some surgeons, however, advocate local anæsthesia.

After the usual preliminary preparation for vaginal operations, the patient is placed in the dorsal posture on the operating table, and the limits of the cancerous growth are carefully palpated. Gas is now given, and the friable carcinomatous material is scraped away with a large curette, after which the field is gone over again with a smaller curette, in order to remove the smaller pockets of the ramifications of the disease. Considerable hemorrhage may result before the firm underlying tissue is reached. The greatest care should be exercised to avoid perforation of the uterine wall. That this caution is necessary may be seen from the published statements of Zacharias, who, in 1908, reported seven fatalities following the palliative scraping of inoperable cases, in several of which death was due to peritonitis following perforation.

Up to this point practically all methods are the same, the points of variation consisting largely in the character of the cauterizing agent. For a considerable period of time the thermocautery has enjoyed the greatest popularity, and it certainly is the most helpful agent whenever a portion of the cervix is to be removed. Lomer, in 1903, collected two hundred and thirteen cases in which the results were fairly favorable, yet of course this is undoubtedly a very small percentage of the cases which have been so treated. When the cautery is used, care must be taken to control the bleeding which commonly ensues, and ligatures are often necessary. The bleeding frequently cannot be controlled in this manner, and then artery forceps, left in place for forty-eight hours, will be most helpful.

In 1884 A. Reeves Jackson advocated curettage and zinc-chloride tamponage of the cavity. This treatment has been revived by Czerny. He employs curettage and follows it by a firm tamponade of gauze saturated with a solution of zinc chloride of the strength of from thirty to fifty per cent. This gauze tampon is left in place for three days, after which it is withdrawn and douches are given. This method has been attended occasionally with astonishingly good results. Yet Buttersack, in 1909, who has reviewed this question, calls attention to the fact that the extent of the action of any chemical upon the tissues is quite beyond the control of the administrator; and he concludes that this method has lost most of its popularity. One of us (Murphy), however, does not agree with him.

In 1906 Chrobak reported a series of cases which were cauterized with crude fuming nitric acid—an agent which, in his opinion, is superior to the actual cautery. His series includes four hundred and eight cases, in which life continued for from three to eleven years. One patient who first presented herself for treatment in 1884, was alive at the time of the report, and another who had been under observation since 1886 had as yet shown no evidence of recurrence.

The method which he advocates is the following:—After careful preliminary curetting, the acid is directly applied to the excavated ulcer, care being taken to blow away the fumes of the acid from time to time. The cavity is then packed with gauze for a few hours, after which insufflations of equal parts of iodoform and tannic acid, or iodoform and charcoal, are given instead of douches. Two or three weeks after this treatment a slough is thrown off, and there is left a granulated surface which should be treated with silver nitrate or iodine. This curetting and cauterization should be frequently repeated.

Webster uses the curette and actual cautery followed with tampons wrung from pure formalin; these tampons being allowed to remain in place for three days before removal. As in the nitric-acid method, the greatest care must be employed to prevent the cauterizing fluid from extending below the site of the affected areas, upon the vaginal wall and perineum. For this reason, therefore, the adjacent parts should be smeared with vaseline and a piece of thin gutta-percha tissue should be placed immediately beneath the raw surfaces. Thereafter, and twice daily, formalin douches should be given in the strength of 1 in 2,000. Many others who also employ formalin for cauterization, use it in diluted form for douching.

Gellhorn, in 1907, reported a number of cases which he had treated with acetone. His method is as follows:—The patient being under the influence of a general anæsthetic, the ulcerated area is carefully curetted so as to remove all sloughing tissue, and the crater is gently dried with cotton pledgets; after which the lower third of the vagina and the vulva are thickly smeared with vaseline. The anæsthesia is then interrupted, and the patient is placed in the Trendelenburg posture, when from one-half to one ounce of acetone is poured through a tubular speculum into the cancerous crater. After the acetone has been in contact with the wound for some twenty or thirty minutes, the table is lowered and the excess of fluid is allowed to run through the speculum out of the vagina. All traces of acetone are now washed from the healthy vagina and vulva with sterile water, and a gauze strip wrung from acetone is packed into the crater and held in place by a dry cotton tampon which is firmly packed into the vagina.

Subsequent treatments are made two or three times weekly, beginning four or five days after the first one. These may be conducted at home or in the physician's office, as no anæsthetic is required, nor is curetting indicated. The hips are again elevated and the speculum is filled with acetone, which is again kept in contact with the wound for twenty or thirty minutes. Gell-horn states that the patients themselves may hold the speculum in place. When the table is depressed, care must be taken to prevent the acetone from coming in contact with the healthy tissues, and to this end vaseline should be smeared thickly over the labia, healthy vagina, and speculum. The cavity is next dried, and a cotton tampon covered with vaseline is introduced into the vagina and kept there for a few hours.

Acetone has intense hygroscopic qualities and causes tissue to shrink so rapidly that sections left in it for more than a few hours are too hard for the microtome. All slight oozing is quickly checked by the treatment, and bleeding surfaces are converted into whitish films. Considerable contraction of the cancerous crater soon results, and consequently smaller specula are required for subsequent treatments. More than one curetting is unnecessary, as the walls of the cancerous cavity become smooth and firm and do not present poly-poid excrescences nor friable necrotic tissue. There is no pain attending the treatment unless the acetone has come in contact with the vulva. This passes away rapidly, especially if the parts are washed with cool water immediately after the accident occurs.

Various other local non-operative palliative measures have been attempted. Among these may be mentioned the x-ray, which has been applied to the cancerous tissues through a vaginal tube. The results vary somewhat, yet probably this treatment never modifies the progress of the disease in the deeper tissues, although it would appear that occasionally it has exerted some restriction upon the superficial parts of the growth. Indeed, it is the consensus of opinion that the x-ray should never be advised as a primary measure, if there is any chance of curing the disease by extirpation. Many advise its use after radical operations have been performed.

A still newer form of treatment is the so-called lightning treatment, or fulguration, a method which was devised and modestly exploited by Keating-Hart in Marseilles, although the name "fulguration" was applied by Czerny. The method requires the use of a general anæsthetic and consists in the application of a powerful electric spark to the tissues. The spark is passed at a distance of from 2 to 4 centimetres from the diseased area, and the procedure is kept up for from five to forty minutes, during which time the position of the spark is frequently changed. Following this procedure, the cancerous mass is removed with a knife or sharp curette, and the fulguration is again continued for ten or fifteen minutes. The necessary apparatus can be attached to the ordinary x-ray apparatus. Recent reports indicate that this method, at least in uterine cancers, has no special value over other types of cauterization.

At the present time one of the most talked-of methods is the so-called trypsin treatment. Unfortunately for the success of the method it has been the subject of sensational newspaper articles, both in the lay and the medical press. The editor of the *Journal of the American Medical Association* has shown that a patient with carcinoma who had been treated with trypsin and was reported as cured in a popular magazine, died within four months after the alleged cure, and that an autopsy showed that the body was fairly riddled with the malignant disease. At the present time opinion is divided as to the merits of this remedy, although possibly it is still too early to form a safe judgment as to its merits or demerits. The advocates of the method claim that it causes (1) an arrest or shrinkage of the growth; (2) improvement of the general health; (3) diminution of, or cure of, the pain; (4) diminution of the discharge and a decrease in the fœtor, except in the cases in which much sloughing has occurred. The great interest which has been aroused by the exploiting of this form of treatment necessitates more descriptive space in a work of this character than the recorded results would warrant.

The results of this treatment are not thus far encouraging. Graves, in 1908, reports five cases of recurrent cancer of the breast, and one recurrent squamous-cell carcinoma of the cervix uteri in which this treatment was instituted without favorable results. In all these cases everything that could be done by surgical procedures had been carried out, and the diagnosis had been confirmed by the microscope, before the treatment was instituted. Weinstein, in 1908, administered it in ten cases of cancer of the digestive organs with entirely negative results. The immediate relief of pain, which the supporters of the method claim for it, was never experienced. Pinkuss reported to the Obstetrical Society of Berlin, July 12th, 1907, four cases of inoperable cancer, two of them uterine, which were treated by this method. Although no conclusions were given, the discussion emphasized the toxic effects which may follow the treatment, and the difficulty of determining the dosage, due to the variations in the strength of the ferments, some being nearly inactive while others are the reverse.

However, it does appear to be a fact that trypsin probably has a destructive action on cancer, although an effective method of applying the remedy has not yet been determined. Injections into localized cancerous nodules beneath the skin have been followed by atrophy of the cancer cells without destruction of the normal connective tissue, although it is apparent to all that this type of growth can be removed successfully, and obvious that, if it is a local recurrence or metastasis, any known treatment is not apt to be successful.

The literature of the present time is fairly teeming with the descriptions and reports of other methods of non-operative treatment. Injections of methylene blue, of liver extract, of thymus, of bacterial toxins, of various cancer serums, for the most part taken from the blood of lower animals suffering from the disease, all have their advocates, but, for the most part, they are not yet ready for description in a work of this character. Nearly all agree, however, that the future treatment of inoperable cancer, and possibly all cancer, will be found along the lines of chemical and biological research.

Treatment of Recurrences Following Operation.—In continental Europe, where the percentage of uterine cancers considered operable is high, many have advocated the operative treatment of a recurrence under certain conditions. von Rosthorn, in particular, was an advocate of this procedure under favorable conditions. In order that this method may be carried on under the most favorable circumstances, all operated cases should be examined at intervals of a few weeks, for the purpose of discovering the presence of a recurrence at the earliest possible moment. In this country comparatively few patients are subjected to an operation at an early period, as the diagnosis is generally made late. This question is not of paramount importance here at the present time, as the majority of cases operated upon are really inoperable, and present recurrences so soon that the treatment following operation largely resolves itself into palliative measures.

General Measures.—All emphasize the fact that patients should be kept in ignorance of their true condition in order to spare them much unnecessary anguish. The next of kin, however, should be fully acquainted with the situation. Every attention should be paid to the hygienic surroundings, and the patients should be kept in the open air as much as possible. They should be encouraged to sleep out of doors, and the diet should not only be nourishing but suited to the individual taste. The digestion should be carefully watched and the bowels kept open. The patient should sleep alone in bed. Sexual intercourse should be abandoned, although it is remarkable how few cases of implantation in the male partner have been recorded. In the later stages of the disease much attention must be given to diminishing the foul odor of the discharge. To this end some operative treatment of the palliative type is frequently indicated, which treatment is supplemented by douches, although the effects of the latter are unfortunately extremely transient. The douches may be prepared with diluted formalin, potassium permanganate, iodide of mercury, aluminum acetate, kerosene, or one of many other preparations. After the douche, a mixture of equal parts of sterile glycerin and olive oil should be injected into the vagina and the vulva should be anointed with the same solution. The skin about the vulva may be protected from the irritating discharge by vaseline or by a mixture of oil and lime water. A piece of thin waterproof sheeting tied around the body frequently helps to diminish the bad odor. During the day it may be worn as a petticoat. Late in the disease the pain is the most marked symptom, as a rule. Frequent sedatives are demanded and should be given. Morphine should be saved for the very last resort, and enormous doses are necessary when the habit is formed. A judicious use of codeine, together with trional, or small does of heroin and trional, will frequently give as much relief as morphine. The complications resulting from the extension of the disease to the bowel or urinary tract must be met as demanded by the individual circumstances.

X. FURTHER DETAILS REGARDING UTERINE NEW-GROWTHS.

Adenocarcinoma of the Body of the Uterus.—This is the most favorable form of carcinoma which affects the reproductive organs, largely because it gives symptoms early, does not tend to invade the tissues adjacent to its site, and does not give rise to metastases until late in its course, owing to the fact that, in comparison with the cervix, which is rich in lymphatics, the fundus

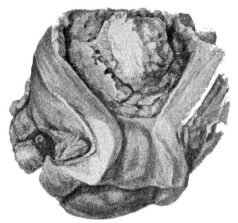

Fig. 276.—Everting Adenocarcinoma of the Fundus Uteri.   From Martin und Jung, "Path. u. Ther. der Frauenkr.," 1907.)

uteri possesses a meagre supply of these vessels. The tumor which, in comparison with some other forms, grows rather slowly, may be everting or inverting in type. (Fig. 276.)

In direct contrast to many of the cancers previously described, adenocarcinoma of the fundus rarely extends to the external os, so that the diagnosis cannot be made from simple inspection. We are entirely dependent upon the symptoms and the microscopical examinations of curettings for the recognition of this form of tumor.

In the earliest stages of the disease the uterus is practically unaltered in size, shape, and consistency; but, as the disease advances, this organ becomes large and firm, although frequently it is boggy. If extension to the peritoneal surface has taken place, irregular and flattened nodules may give the organ a more or less nodular shape. In other cases the uterus may be small or irregular, but appears densely infiltrated. When the organ is cut open, an early growth appears as a circumscribed nodule springing from the surface of the mucosa, and consisting of many delicate finger-like processes, which give it a somewhat shaggy appearance. The tumor gradually becomes thicker as it grows, and presently appears as a branching growth consisting of several main stems with numerous offshoots and delicate terminal branches, suggesting the arrangement of placental villi. The growth is soft to the touch and its cut surface presents the appearance of a pale, waxy, or finely granular area, which is easily distinguished from the delicate, pinkish tint of the normal mucosa. There is usually considerable injection of the surrounding tissue.

As a rule, this type of cancer begins in a localized area, although probably never at a single definite point, and not infrequently it appears as if the entire

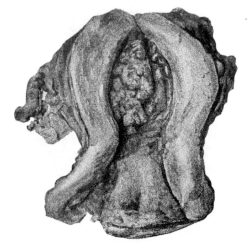

Fig. 277.—Adenocarcinoma of Corpus Uteri. Kaiserling preparation. (From Martin und Jung. 1907.)

mucosa had become simultaneously involved. Early growths may be so limited that they affect only the superficial portions of the endometrium. But if, owing to the development of suspicious symptoms, an examination is made, one is likely to find the entire cavity of the uterus transformed into cancerous tissue, presenting itself as abundant dome-shaped masses, and showing but little trace of the delicate finger-like processes just described. (Fig. 277.) Coincidently with the ingrowth into the uterine cavity, there is a corresponding, though usually more tardy, penetration of the growth into the uterine walls. In sections of the uterus this appears as a whitish-yellow mass, which is slightly granular but soft, and stands out in bold contrast with the surrounding muscle. The extension takes place usually in an irregular fashion, yet ultimately the growth reaches the peritoneal layer, forming rows of small, smooth, waxy elevations upon the surface. Coincidently with this extension there may be degeneration of the primary tumor, which becomes transformed into a necrotic caseous or sloughing mass.

HISTOLOGY.—Cancer developing in the endometrium may begin either in the superficial portions or in the depths of the glandular epithelium, and it usually presents a definite adenomatous appearance. In the everting type the earliest changes appear to be a proliferation of the epithelium in the form of little mounds, although many have described a change in the character of the individual cells. As the epithelial proliferation advances, the mound-like outgrowths are supplied with stroma from the underlying tissue. These little mounds project from the surface of the mucosa into the cavity of the uterus or into the lumina of the tubular glands. The epithelial cells may be uniform in size, but, as a rule, they are very irregular, some being over three or four times as large as their neighbors. The outgrowths may resemble delicate fingers, presenting a rounded outline, although frequently their contour is crenated, showing depressions along the sides or at the ends. The main outgrowth and the various branches are covered with one or more layers of epithelium, the nuclei of which are irregular in size, shape, and staining qualities. As a result of growth there finally ensues an excessive formation of new glands composed of cancerous cells.

With the advance of the disease there is a breaking-down of the older portions of the growth. The surface becomes necrotic and is invaded by polymorphonuclear leucocytes, while the glands themselves serve as foci of coagulation necrosis. Scattered throughout the deeper portions of the tissue, especially in the centre of a necrosed area, are irregular, laminated, calcareous plates which select the nuclear stain. As the progress of degeneration advances still further, the necrosis extends to the uterine muscle and both the muscle and the glands are overwhelmed with polymorphonuclear leucocytes. Just outside this border may be seen an infiltration of round cells.

This type of tumor extends by direct invasion, as well as by extension through the blood- and lymph-streams. As a rule, however, these processes develop much more slowly than they do in cancers of the cervix.

SYMPTOMS.—Fortunately for the patient, symptoms manifest themselves much sooner than they do in the cervical growths. Hemorrhage is most common at a fairly early period of the cancerous involvement. As we have seen, involvement of the lymph nodes occurs comparatively late, so that the majority of cases presenting symptoms of several months' duration are truly operable; for at that time the growth is still frequently limited to the uterus, in marked contrast to what is observed in the cervical types.

TREATMENT.—The hope of a cure is much greater than it is in the cervical type, and a genuine cure frequently results after a simple vaginal hysterectomy. Indeed, many—as, for example, Doederlein and others—find that the percentage of cures is from eighty to ninety per cent of the patients who are so treated and who do not succumb to the primary effects of the operation. Such results, however, are not seen in this country on account of the rarity of the cases in which the presence of the new-growth is discovered at an early period. The recommendation of the more extensive operations, therefore, becomes a necessity.

Sarcoma of the Uterus.—Sarcoma of the uterus is generally primary, but may result from the degeneration of a fibroid uterus, or secondarily from an extension of sarcomatous disease in some neighboring structure, more particularly one of the ovaries. The tumor, as in the case of a carcinoma, may consist of a fungoid everting, or an inverting and infiltrating, mass, and generally presents a uniform, homogeneous structure in contrast to the alveolar or gland-like formation of a carcinoma.

FREQUENCY.—Sarcoma of the uterus is regarded as a very rare condition, and is described by many authors as the most infrequent of all uterine tumors. Yet it is more than possible that if a careful microscopical examination were carried out as a routine measure in the case of every tumor removed from the uterus, it would be found that the percentages obtained in the past are too low to represent the true frequency of this disease. Thus Winter, in 1907, found sarcomatous degeneration in 3.2 per cent of 500 fibroid cases in which only grossly suspicious areas of the fibroid tumor were subjected to microscopical examination, while a complete routine examination of 253 cases disclosed the existence of sarcoma in 4.3 per cent. It is certain, however, that cases of uterine sarcoma have been very infrequently reported in the past. In 1894, for example, J. Whitridge Williams was able to collect but 144 cases from the medical literature. Roger Williams found but 2 instances of primary sarcoma in 2,649 consecutive cases of uterine neoplasms, while Gurlt observed but 8 in 1,933 cases. Various American authors place its frequency at from 2 to 4 per cent of all uterine tumors.

The frequency of sarcoma as compared with that of carcinoma is variously given, but Gessner places it as one to forty. In marked contrast to carcinoma, sarcoma is more commonly observed in the body of the uterus than in the cervix. Thus, Poschmann, in Halle, found that sarcoma was observed in but 16 of 403 malignant uterine tumors, the other 387 being cases of carcinoma. Of these 16 instances of sarcoma, 11 involved the fundus and 5 the cervix, while, of the 387 instances of carcinoma, 10 were of the fundus and 377 of the cervix.

ETIOLOGY.—The causation of sarcoma is unknown. The disease may develop in the uterus at any time from early infancy to old age, although a larger number of cases occur in youth. Gusserow collected 73 cases, 4 of which occurred under twenty-nine years of age; 15 between thirty and forty; 28 between forty and fifty; 18 between fifty and sixty, and 3 in women over sixty. There is on record a case in which a sarcoma of the uterus was observed in a woman of over seventy. Hollander has reported a case in an infant of seven months. Up to the present time no evident causal relationship has been established between uterine sarcoma on the one hand, and trauma, inflammation, or child-bearing, on the other.

Many theories have been advanced to explain the pathogenesis of sarcoma of the uterus, but they may be grouped under the following three heads:—(1)

Sarcoma cells develop by proliferation of cells of the vessel walls; (2) they develop by proliferation of the cells of the intermuscular fibrous tissue; or (3) they develop by the transformation of smooth-muscle fibres.

It would appear possible that each of these theories may correctly explain the origin of certain cases, yet it is also evident that all cases cannot be explained by one theory. Virchow's theory of the development of the malignant process by multiplication of cells of the interstitial connective tissue has been supported by the facts observed in a number of cases. The vascular origin was claimed for the cases reported by Kleinschmidt and Pilliet and others, and Williams and Piquand offer evidence in favor of the transformation of the muscle fibres themselves in the malignant growth. Certain authors—as, for example, Ribbert—limit the term sarcoma to the proliferation of ordinary connective-tissue tumors, and describe those growths which develop by the proliferation of muscle fibres as a distinct variety of tumor, which they designate "*leiomyoma malin.*" Ribbert takes the view that the latter tumor is not due to a degeneration of muscle cells caused by the sarcoma, but is the result of proliferation of muscle fibres. In a case described by Pavoit and Bérard, not only the primary tumor itself but the metastatic nodules as well were composed of proliferating muscle.

CLASSIFICATION.—Uterine sarcomata may be classified according to the location of the growth in the cervix or in the body of the uterus; the latter being the most frequent. Sarcomata of the cervix may be further divided, according to their morphology, into two groups: (1) an indefinite group comprising the ordinary varieties of sarcoma; and (2) racemose myxosarcomata.

A. Sarcoma of the Cervix Uteri.—The cervix may be the seat of sarcoma at various periods of life; the majority of uterine sarcomata which occur in infancy and early life affect the cervix. Roger Williams believes that these are mostly of blastogenic origin, and calls attention to the frequency with which heterotopic elements are found. The growth may be polypoid and multiple, especially in children. Usually sarcoma of the cervix occurs as a diffuse infiltration, as a thickening of the mucous membrane, or as a circumscribed polypoid growth. It is rarely observed in the fibromuscular coat.

In the diffuse type the mucosa may be uniformly involved, although the vaginal portion shows the most extensive invasion. The cervix is generally greatly enlarged and infiltrated; its surface may be smooth or covered with irregular vegetations.

A circumscribed sarcoma, either sessile or pedunculated, may arise from the anterior or from the posterior lip. The sessile variety occurs in the form of an irregular, vegetating outgrowth, which has many points of resemblance to carcinoma; yet, as a rule, it is softer and more apt to attain larger size without necrosis than the more common carcinoma. The polypoid or pedunculated sarcoma of the cervix is probably the most common type of cervical sarcoma. It is seen as a more or less rounded tumor, which is attached to the portio vaginalis or protrudes through the cervix with a well-defined pedicle. The younger growths have a smooth surface, which consists of cervical epithe-

lium. With the further growth of the tumor more or less extensive degeneration may occur. The polypoid forms are soft and gelatinous in consistency
from œdema and myxomatous degeneration. They may be the seat of pseudo-
cystic or of cystic change. These growths are very malignant and recur soon
after removal.

The sarcoma which develops in the substance of the cervical wall is, as has
been stated, very rare, and may arise as a primary growth or as a malignant
degeneration of a pre-existing fibroid neoplasm. Histologically, the tumor
may be of the round-cell, spindle-cell, mixed-cell, or giant-cell type, all of which
forms occur with nearly equal frequency. The usual rule, that the round-cell
variety is the most malignant, holds good for these tumors of the cervix.

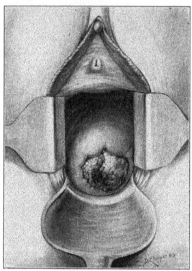

Fig. 278.—Sarcoma of the Cervix Uteri. (Original.)

The racemose myxosarcoma may be found at all ages. It resembles the
myxomatous grape-like sarcoma found in the vagina of infants. As is indicated by the terminology, its most striking characteristic is the development of grape-like clusters of round or oval polypoid growths. The tumor
begins as a polypoid outgrowth from the mucous membrane of the cervical
canal or from the vaginal portion of the cervix, and cannot be distinguished
from simple polyps of the mucosa without a microscopical examination. (Fig.
278.) The tumor grows slowly in the early stages, but, after a longer or shorter
period of quiescence, the characteristic masses make their appearance and
the growth proliferates with great rapidity. It soon becomes translucent
and myxomatous in appearance. As the disease progresses it invades the

vaginal vault by direct extension, and ultimately involves the uterine body, the parametrial tissues, and the vesico-vaginal and recto-vaginal septa. The pelvic lymph nodes may be invaded and metastases may be sent to distant organs. Under the microscope the growth resembles in appearance the myxosarcoma of the vagina; it may contain striated muscle and even hyaline cartilage. The free surface of the vegetation is partially covered with epithelium resembling that of the cervical canal, while other portions are covered with the stratified epithelium of the vaginal cervix.

Histologically, the structure varies somewhat according to the site of origin, yet it usually presents a central core developed from the cervical submucous tissue and of fairly dense structure. On the outside it is surmounted by œdematous tissue covered with epithelium. In the vicinity of the os, the polyp may be covered in part with cylindrical epithelium derived from the cervical canal, while another portion of the tumor may show the stratified epithelium characteristic of the portio vaginalis.

B. *Sarcoma of the Uterine Body.*—Sarcoma of the body of the uterus may be divided, according to its histogenesis, into three varieties: (1) that which originates in the deeper endometrium; (2) that which originates in the substance of the wall of the corpus uteri; and (3) that which develops from preexisting fibroids.

(1) Sarcomata of the corpus uteri originating in the endometrium are commonly found in

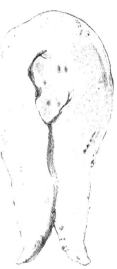

Fig. 279.—Round-Cell Sarcoma of the Fundus Uteri, Originating in the Endometrium. (From Veit's "Handbuch der Gynaekologie.")

adults, and are rare in early life. The new-growth may develop in the interglandular stroma, or in that part of the stroma which surrounds the blood-vessels and lymphatics. It develops as a diffuse infiltration of the mucosa, frequently forming irregular projections, in the form of nodes or polyps. (Figs. 279 and 280.) Sometimes these latter may project downward as elongated masses that reach as far as the vagina. The uterine body in such cases becomes markedly enlarged, and the cervical canal may be patulous. Inversion of the uterus, resulting from the paralysis of the normal wall, may be noted. The tumor may extend along the Fallopian tubes, or directly through the uterine wall. The growth is soft and very friable, and consists of a homogeneous vascular, brain-like structure. Some specimens may be so vascular that they resemble telangioma. Rarely does sarcoma of the mucosa remain localized for any considerable time: its tendency is to form polypoid projections or to invade neighboring structures. Necrosis is very common, and secondary invasion of the uterine wall with saprophytic organisms may follow. When the disease is secondarily complicated by hæmatometria or pyometria, pigment may be found in the cells. Instances of melanotic uterine sarcoma have been reported. The pelvic lymph nodes are usually involved early in the disease, and may be the seat of cystic degeneration.

Histologically these tumors may present any variety of the sarcomatous cell. After the growth is scraped away it recurs with great rapidity. It may become disseminated in the vagina and other pelvic tissues, or may be trans-

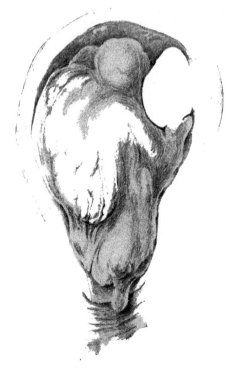

Fig. 280.—Polypoid Myxosarcoma of the Uterus, Beginning in the Endometrium. (From Veit's "Handbuch der Gynaekologie.")

mitted to distant organs, as the lungs, kidneys, bone, etc. Metastases occur through the blood most frequently and only rarely through lymph vessels.

(2) Sarcoma of the Corpus Uteri Beginning in the Muscular Wall.—This tumor, like that of the former class, is rarely found in early life. When it first develops this tumor manifests itself in the form of a circumscribed mass, which later may spread diffusely, especially when it originates in a myoma. It may become polypoid, however, and extend into the uterine cavity or outward to-

ward the peritoneum. A diffuse sarcoma of the parenchyma may invade the mucosa and project into the cavity of the uterus, when it is only with the greatest difficulty that one can differentiate it from a primary growth of the endometrium. Myxomatous degeneration and œdema of the tumor are common events, and the growth is prone to secondary infection, with a resulting slough which is sometimes so extensive as to resemble gangrene. Telangiectatic, lymphangiectatic, and cystic alterations are occasionally observed, although the latter are rare and are due in large part to localized degeneration and softening in the substance of the tumor. Unilocular or multilocular cysts have been described. These, according to some authorities, are probably derived

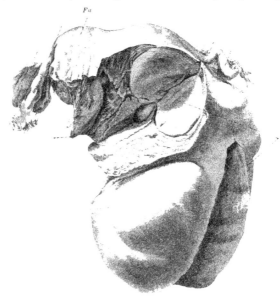

Fig. 281.—Sarcomatous Degeneration of Intraligamentous Fibroids. (From Martin und Jung, "Path. u. Ther. der Frauenkr.," 1907.) *Fu*, Fundus uteri.

from inclusions of the Wolffian body, but they may also come from the Muellerian glands, or from blood-vessels or lymphatics. Cystic sarcomata are usually subperitoneal and pedunculated. They may attain large size and are apt to become adherent to the neighboring organs.

(3) The sarcoma developing in a degenerating myoma is probably the most frequent variety of sarcoma of the uterine wal . The growth may be uninodular or multinodular, and may present all steps in the transition from a simple fibroid to a malignant sarcoma. (Fig. 281.) It is very difficult, in a given case, to say with certainty whether the growth began in the substance of the wall of the corpus or from a pre-existing fibroid.

METHOD OF GROWTH.—The disease early progresses by direct invasion, breaking through the limiting capsule that is sometimes present,. and invades the surrounding tissue in the same way as does a carcinoma. When it is incompletely removed, recurrence follows most rapidly. Metastases may occur through the blood or lymph channels and they frequently involve the lungs—the first filter through which the blood passes after it leaves the uterus.

SYMPTOMS.—The following symptoms are given as classic for the stages in which the patient seeks advice. As in carcinoma they usually represent an inoperable period of the disease. They may be enumerated in the following order: hemorrhage; absence of pain; a watery flesh-colored discharge; and cachexia.

The hemorrhage appears first as an increase in the menstrual flow, or as an irregular hemorrhage, usually resulting from overexertion or some trauma after the menopause. As the new-formation does not ulcerate as rapidly as the majority of carcinomata do, the increased menstruation is probably due to hyperæmia of the mucosa, as happens in fibromata. The loss of blood is not great when the growth breaks down.

Clay has commented on the absence of pain as a symptom in the early stages, and attention has also been called to this by A. R. Simpson. On the other hand, Gusserow mentions it as a fact that pain is frequently present, especially in the cases in which the growth develops in the substance of the uterine wall, and he states that, when the uterine cavity is rapidly distended by polypoid growths or by an accumulation of blood, the pain may become very intense, in the form of a uterine colic. In the late stages of this disease there is naturally much pain. The apparent discrepancy of opinion as to pain is best explained by the varying progress of infiltration. In carcinoma, for example, the pain is more severe when the disease extends upward and compresses nerve endings in the uterine wall and connective tissue; on the other hand, when the disease is localized in the lower cervix or manifests itself in the form of polyps in the vagina, there may be absolutely no pain.

The discharge has a slight odor, and resembles rice water in appearance; it is not often as offensive as that in carcinoma, owing to the facts that the sulci are less frequent, that external contamination is not so easily produced, and that there are not the same rapid ulceration and necrosis of tissue. Yet, when the disease has progressed to a considerable extent, the discharge may become equally fetid. The older writers called attention to the presence, in the discharge, of grayish-white shreds resembling particles of brain matter. Such shreds are undoubtedly diagnostic, but they occur late in the disease—i.e., at a time when the diagnosis should be plain.

Cachexia gradually develops in the late stages and is accompanied by loss of flesh, loss of appetite, and rapid failure of strength.

DIAGNOSIS.—On bimanual examination the uterus is found to be enlarged. If the tumor projects through the cervix, the diagnosis should not be difficult, as the examination will show that the mass is soft and pliable, and composed of polypoid masses. If the cervix is sufficiently patulous to admit the finger, irregularities in the cavity may be distinguished. Bleeding is in most cases easily produced. When the cervix is closed and there is no visible tumor growth, dilatation and curettage will enable one easily to secure tissue for microscopical examination. The uterus in the early stages is movable, but it soon becomes fixed. If a sound is introduced, the cavity of the uterus is found enlarged, and the procedure causes hemorrhage. The sound must therefore be used with extreme caution, if used at all. Frequently the condition is mistaken for a fibroid. Suspicion should be aroused by the presence of free or bloody fluid in the pelvis at the laparotomy. Not infrequently, in the past, this symptom has been disregarded at operation, especially when no pathological examination of the tumor has been made, and as a result the recognition of the true status of affairs has not been established until the advent of metastases or of a local recurrence.

There are many conditions, it must be remembered, that simulate sarcoma of the uterus, and in the great majority of cases the diagnosis will finally have to be made by the microscope; and even then it may not be possible to reach a sure conclusion. The disease must be differentiated from carcinoma, deciduoma malignum, interstitial or subserous fibroids, hemorrhagic endometritis, tuberculosis, and retained portions of the placenta. A microscopical study should be made of sections removed from different portions of the tumor, and the result of the examination should be considered together with the physical findings before a final opinion is given. When a fibroid undergoes a sarcomatous degeneration the occurrence of this change is not generally suspected in the early stages; indeed, it is commonly not recognized until the disease is far advanced. The chief changes which occur in the sarcomatous degeneration of a fibroid are the sudden increase in the rapidity of the growth of a tumor which previously had seemed to remain unchanged in size, the increased softness of the mass, and the development of ascites, metastases, and cachexia. And yet several of these symptoms may occur in fibroids in which no malignancy is present, as happens, for example, from twisting of a pedicle, etc. The microscopical examination of scrapings in such cases is often valueless from the diagnostic standpoint, because the disease may not yet have involved the endometrium.

PROGNOSIS.—The prognosis of uterine sarcoma is most grave in the rapidly growing forms, and yet, as in sarcoma of other organs, it varies somewhat according to the histogenesis of the tumor. The fibrosarcoma sometimes grows so slowly that the disease may continue for years before the fatal issue. The average duration is about three years; but the disease may continue for a longer period. Thus, Gusserow described a case in which the course was prolonged for ten years. The temporary relief afforded by removal of the growth lasts for a longer time, in most cases, than it does in carcinoma. But, when a recurrence takes place, the growth of the newer tumor is much more rapid than that of the primary one. Gessner reports that a recurrence followed the radical operation in 10 of 26 cases originating in the endometrium, and in the great majority it developed within a year. Sixteen cases were reported as cured, although only 5 were observed for more than five years. In 35 cases of sarcoma of the uterine wall, recurrence was noted in 14 cases, and in all of them within a year. The 21 remaining were accounted as cured, although only 5 had been followed throughout the five-year observation period.

TREATMENT.—Total extirpation of the uterus and adnexa, together with a wide removal of the parametrium, as is the practice in cancer, offers the only hope of a radical cure. There are on record but few cases of simple hysterectomy which have not been followed by a recurrence. When complete removal is impossible, palliative measures similar to those used for uterine cancer should be employed. Several variations have been noted as regards the earliness of recurrence after curettage, the differences seeming to depend upon the histological structure of the tumor. Generally speaking, the nearer the tumor approaches the round-cell type the greater the malignancy.

Endothelioma of the Uterus.—This extremely rare new-growth of the uterus arises from the endothelial lining of the lymph- or blood-vessels. Its rarity is attested by the fact that only ten or twelve cases have been described, thus far, in the medical literature, and, as regards some of these, there is the suspicion that they were in reality but atypical forms of other epithelial tumors, which were associated with lymph- or blood-vessel invasion. The first case was described by Amann, in 1892, in a woman thirty-one years of age. Pick described one in a patient fifty-two years of age, and Braetz noted one in a girl of eighteen years. The others were observed at or near the menopause. The tumor consists of an everting polypoid or papillary projection, or an infiltrating degeneration, which produces a dense induration of the surrounding tissue of the cervix. In its gross appearance the new-growth cannot be differentiated from a carcinoma, and the final diagnosis must be made with the aid of the microscope. With this aid the tumor is seen to be composed of an alveolar structure resembling, in general appearance, that of an adenocarcinoma. The cells are often very variable in shape and size, sometimes being flat or cuboid, while at other times they may have a cylindrical form. The alveoli may show a lumen which appears as a hollow cylinder lined with one or more layers of cells. In other places there are solid masses of cells, so arranged that they may be indistinguishable from those of an ordinary carcinoma. The diagnosis of this condition can be made with certainty only when the growth can be directly traced to the primary site of the proliferating intima of the blood-vessels or lymphatics. A probable diagnosis may be made when a tumor of the cervix, presenting the general characteristics described above, shows under the microscope an alveolar structure, together with an appearance as if an organic connection existed between the tumor cells and the surrounding stroma, provided that at the same time the epithelial elements of the organ are normal and have no evident connection with the new-growth.

Chorio-Epithelioma.—In 1888 Saenger directed the attention of the surgical and pathological world to a previously unrecognized tumor of the uterus. In the two cases which formed the basis of his report this form of new-growth followed pregnancy and rapidly led to a fatal issue through the development of metastases. As a result of his study, Saenger came to the conclusion that the growths developed from the uterine decidua and represented, therefore, an átypical sarcoma. (Fig. 282.) He gave to these tumors the name of "deciduoma malignum," and five years later collected in a monograph all that had been learned concerning this most interesting and fatal form of cancer. Later study has shown us that Saenger's conclusions as to the origin of the tumor cells are erroneous and that they arise from the syncytial and Langhans layers of the chorion. Consequently the term deciduoma malignum has been

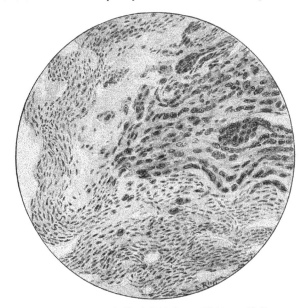

Fig. 282.—Section of a Chorio-Epithelioma. (Highly magnified.)

abandoned, and Marchand's suggestion of chorio-epithelioma has been accepted in its place as a more appropriate descriptive term.

ETIOLOGY AND PATHOLOGY.—The chorio-epithelioma is most prone to metastasize. As a rule, the primary uterine growth is of small size for one so rapidly fatal. It is observed in the form of a soft, dark or reddish nodule, resembling a hæmatoma. Vesicles like the beads of a hydatidiform mole are sometimes present. The metastases develop along the course of the venous channels and are thought to arise from the chorionic cells which have been detached from the placenta and swept into the circulation. Later, these cells erode and invade the blood-vessel wall. Out of 52 cases collected by Dorland, metastases were observed in the lungs in 78.3 per cent; in the vagina in 54 per cent; in the kidneys, spleen, and ovaries in 13.5 per cent; in the liver, broad ligament, and pelvis, respectively, in 10.8 per cent; and in the brain in 5.4 per cent. Vaginal metastases are of particular significance, and occasionally they are the only manifestations of the condition. In certain rare, but interesting, cases, the primary growth appears to have developed in the vagina, as in Schmorl's and Schmauch's cases; or there may be general metastases, without a hint of a localized tumor, as in cases described by Schmorl. In such cases it must be assumed that the primary growth was limited to the placenta, and that particles were cast off in the blood-stream, while the primary tumors were expelled with the afterbirth. Later, however, as the frequency of the normal deportation of chorionic villi became more fully recognized, it was assumed that metastases might be formed in any case in which the chorionic epithelium possessed malignant properties. Poten and Vassmer have reported a case in which the vaginal metastases appeared while a hydatidiform mole was still in the uterus.

As has been indicated, this growth originates from fœtal ectoderm, and the microscopic appearances vary considerably according to the distribution and relationship of the constituent cells. As a rule, there is a mixture of cells, derived from the syncytium and from Langhans' layer of the fœtal chorion. (Fig. 282.) The former type predominates in some cases, while in other cases the reverse is true. At the same time there have been described growths which consist entirely of syncytial elements. The syncytium is observed in the form of irregular masses of nucleated protoplasm greatly vacuolated, the nuclei being rich in chromatin, somewhat oval in shape, and with their long axis parallel with the edge of the mass. Mitoses are commonly seen in them. The cells derived from the Langhans layer are generally polyhedral, although they vary in size and shape. They appear clear and do not possess any intercellular connective tissue. The nuclei are round or oval, are larger than those of the syncytium, and stain less deeply. These cells contain glycogen. Extravasation of blood is found around and among the deeper growths. Degeneration and necrosis are frequently present in the tissue, and, for purposes of study, one must select the advancing edge of the growth. In another class of cases there have been found vacuolated buds or rings of epiblast filled with mucoid tissue and resembling early villi. These occur chiefly in cases in which the disease followed a hydatidiform mole. In metastases particles of the tumor are carried by way of the blood-vessels and rarely by way of the lymph channels.

RELATION OF THE DISEASE TO PREGNANCY.—The disease may sometimes begin during pregnancy, although it frequently begins a few days, weeks, or months after labor. MacKenna states that in the cases collected by him the average interval between labor and the earliest symptoms was ten weeks. It has been stated that rarely as long a period as one or two years may elapse. The growth may follow abortion, full-term labor, ectopic pregnancy, or hydatidiform degeneration of the chorion. There have been described a considerable number of cases in which the appearance of the tumor seemed to be a sequence of the last-named condition.

The view that chorio-epithelioma always follows a pregnancy and results from a special tendency of the epithelial layers of the villi to develop without purpose, received a shock in 1902, when Wlassow and Schlangenhaufer described generalized metastases following certain teratomata of the testicle which were composed of syncytium, Langhans cells, and even structures resembling chorionic villi. The observations of these authorities have been abundantly confirmed by Risel, Teacher, Frank, and others. To explain such cases the view has been developed that the trophoblast and its developmental layers preserve the faculty of proliferation, which is a peculiarity of all embryonic tissue during the whole of pregnancy, but which is displayed only in cases of certain changes in the maternal organism. Schlangenhaufer assumed that portions of fœtal membrane had been included in the teratoma and suddenly began to proliferate after lying dormant for years. Risel, on the other hand, holds that such an assumption is not necessary, and that a formation of the nature described may develop from individual portions of the fœtal ectoderm contained in teratomata. Tumors apparently identical with chorio-epithelioma have been reported as occurring in the testicle, in ovarian teratomata, and in the bladder of a virgin of seventy-five years of age.

CLINICAL FEATURES.—Ordinarily there is no suspicion of the existence of the growth during pregnancy, or even during the first few weeks after delivery. Hemorrhage, which is usually the first and most important symptom, may appear even in the latter part of the puerperium, although this symptom is usually lacking. The hemorrhage, at first, is irregular and later becomes more profuse and frequent. A dirty, watery discharge gradually makes its appearance. In more than one-half of the cases the first indication was the appearance of vaginal or vulvar metastases. These are not noted until some weeks or months after the puerperium, although in the case of Poten and Vassmer they appeared before the extrusion of the mole, and in J. W. Williams' case one week after labor at full term. The development of metastases in the lung is usually associated with pulmonary symptoms,—coughing and bloody expectoration,—although these are frequently lacking. Occasionally, as reported by Hoermann and others, the growth may perforate the uterine wall and give rise to fatal intraperitoneal complications. Other symptoms may be produced by metastatic developments in the kidneys, intestines, liver, brain, etc. Weakness and cachexia, due, in part at least, to the development of metastases, supervene. Pain is a variable feature, depending upon the parts involved by the secondary growth. As a rule, the tumor, unless removed by operative measures, rapidly causes death, and the majority of patients succumb within the first year. Indeed, it may be said that this is the most rapidly fatal malignant growth with which we are acquainted; and, although cases are occasionally encountered in which a permanent cure follows a simple curettage, such favorable results occur so rarely that it does not justify the postponement of a radical operation.

DIAGNOSIS.—In a considerable number of cases the diagnosis is not made until, after the lapse of a varying period of time after the puerperium, uterine hemorrhage occurs and necessitates currettage, and then the microscopical examination of the scrapings reveals the characteristic changes. In other cases, as has been indicated, the occurrence of vaginal metastases is the first indication of the existence of the new-growth. The probability of its development should always be borne in mind whenever a woman has expelled a hydatidiform mole, and the appearance of hemorrhage or of some obscure symptom should serve as an imperative indication for immediate curettage and the microscopical examination of the scrapings. When the disease begins in the uterus it forms a nodule in the mucosa, and this is soon followed by others. On palpation the uterus is found to be larger and softer than usual and is somewhat tender.

TREATMENT.—Only one form of treatment is to be recommended, viz., total extirpation of the uterus, provided the disease begins in this organ and curettage reveals the existence of the characteristic lesions. On the other hand, when vaginal metastases are present, the indication for the removal is less clear, as we know that in such cases the uterus may contain no growth, and that, in such a case, excision of the vaginal tumor may be followed by complete recovery. If these metastases are present, and if at the same time the uterus is the seat of a tumor, both the uterus and the vagina should be removed, although the chances for ultimate recovery are very slight. The operation should be done through the abdomen because the uterus may be removed with less trauma than when the vaginal route is chosen. It would appear that manipulation of the uterus is apt to force fragments of the uterine growth into the veins, thus increasing the risk of the development of metastases, unless the growth be approached from above. Therefore, the first step in the operation should be the ligation of the uterine and ovarian vessels before the uterus is subjected to manipulation. Eiermann has collected the statistics of thirty operative cases, six of which were free from recurrence after two or more years. The prognosis depends upon the malignancy of the tumor as well as upon the presence of metastases. Distant metastases indicate that the treatment can be only palliative.

XI. METHOD OF COMPARING THE RESULTS OF OPERATIONS FOR UTERINE CANCER.

There has long been the greatest difficulty in determining the results of the operative treatment of uterine cancer, owing in large part to a confusion of terms and to a neglect of a proper classification of material. With a common basis for the comparison of cases the results of the various clinics could be compared with some chance of arriving at the relative worth of the various types of operation. At the present time it is perfectly futile to attempt to compare the results secured by men who operate upon only ten per cent of the cases which come under their observation, with the results obtained by those who operate upon as many as five or six times this percentage—unless the cases are so tabulated as to admit of comparison without a careful sifting of the protocols. Naturally, the greatest misunderstanding has arisen from the grouping together of all uterine cancers, without any attempt to classify them according to the malignancy and the extent of the growth. Even though this is impossible in the strictly scientific sense, much can be done with a classification which separately considers cancer of the fundus, cancer of the portio vaginalis, and the carcinomatous growths of the intermediate part of the cervical canal. At the present time a growth which may not be removable by a simple vaginal hysterectomy, may *possibly* be removable by a more extensive operation. Consequently much of the confusion which is now resulting from the exclusion and selection of cases can be eliminated by an agreement as to what constitutes operability; also as to what shall be regarded as a cure. Of course there will be factors which we cannot hope to control and which will influence to a large degree the statistical results. Chief of these is the variation in the character of the cases applying for treatment in the various clinics. Thanks to the tremendous agitation of the cancer problem in Germany, both the laity and the profession are alive to the importance of early diagnosis and operation, and early cases are now common in the larger clinics. In this country early cases are the greatest of rarities. Moreover, there is much variation in the character of the material in the same clinic in different years, as may readily be seen by a study of Wertheim's report of cases in 1908. Given a disease such as uterine cancer, in which there may be the slightest line of demarcation between strictly operable and strictly inoperable cases, the clinic having the greatest proportion of early operable cases in which there is no question as to whether the case is inoperable or not, should present the best results.

Up to the present time the majority of investigators have agreed that the ultimate cures of the disease should be expressed in terms of the percentage of the total cancer cases under observation. There is little doubt, however, that the results will be more truly expressed in the percentage of cures of the cases treated by operation. Exclusion of cases can be prevented by a complete résumé of the whole material, classified according to definitions which are universally accepted. Thus, there must be agreement as to what constitutes the primary mortality, operability, limit of time which must elapse before an operated case may be regarded as cured, and how cases should be considered which succumb to intercurrent disease before the expiration of this time.

A number of postulates have been submitted by students of this question, chief among whom are Werner, Waldstein, and Winter. The methods of Waldstein and Werner demand that in order to make every phase of the report complete, an author publishing the statistics of his cancer cases should include:

(a) the total number of cases presenting themselves for treatment during a certain period, classified as cancer of the cervix, or as cancer of the body of the uterus;

(b) the number of cases selected from the total on which a radical operation was performed;

(c) the number on which a radical operation could not be performed;

(d) the total number and relative percentage of deaths following the operation, and

(e) the number of cases in which the patient is alive and free from recurrence five years after operation.

The formula given for expressing this result is

$$A = \frac{O \times D \times (100 - M)}{10,000}$$

in which formula O denotes the percentage of those seeking relief upon whom an operation was performed; D denotes the percentage of those who, after being subjected to operation, remained free from recurrence; and M denotes the percentage of primary mortality following the operation, either recent or remote.

Werner and Waldstein state that there are exceptions which can be made, and which agree in the main with the first set of postulates proposed by Winter. Thus, we should omit:

(a) the cases which are operable but in which the patient will not submit to the proposed treatment—for these cases should not be considered in the results any more than if the patients had not applied for treatment.

(b) cases in which the patient died, during the period of operation, of some intercurrent disease, as well as those which have been lost sight of.

Werner and Waldstein differ from Winter in emphasizing that all doubtful cases should be considered as recurrences for the reason that recurrence is much more frequent than cure. Werner insists that the following premises must be agreed upon if a proper classification is to be secured:—

(1) A case in which the patient has survived operation for five years and has presented no sign of recurrence during careful observation throughout this period, should be considered as cured, irrespective of future development of the disease, or whether the patient is subsequently lost sight of.

(2) When death results from intercurrent disease two years or more after operation, the case may be regarded as cured if no recurrence can be demonstrated in the scars and lymph nodes at a post-mortem examination conducted by a skilful pathologist.

(3) Cases should be classed as recurrent if death occurs before two years, irrespective of the fact that there were negative findings at the autopsy. Deaths from intercurrent disease within five years of the operation should be considered as recurrences, if the autopsy findings of a competent pathologist are not negative. In like manner, all cases lost sight of during the five-year period of observation must be classified with the recurrences. It is needless to say that the diagnosis of freedom from recurrence can be made only after the microscopic examination of serial sections of the suspected areas.

Statistics which comply with these postulates will be exempt from nearly all objections.

The radical operation is still in its infancy and has been adopted slowly, largely on account of the high mortality and because everywhere there are competent men waiting to learn the results obtained by others. Even at the present time there are few published results of great value, because common definitions have not been agreed upon, and the various Congresses have not seen fit to demand them. In February, 1908, Winter, seeking to obtain a basis for classification which would be acceptable to the various students in this field, proposed the following set of postulates, asking that those who are interested in the subject should inform him of their ideas concerning them.

WINTER'S TENTATIVE POSTULATES.

I. *Primary Mortality.*—Under this head should be included all deaths following the operation which would not have occurred had it not been undertaken. Thus, death from shock, cardiac paralysis, thrombosis and embolism, pneumonia, pyelitis, infection, etc., should be included in the primary mortality.

II. *Definition of Operability.*—All cases should be termed operable if a radical operation can be completely carried out. The term operable, therefore, should not be applied until the completion of the operation, as the opening of the abdomen first reveals the true condition of affairs. The defining of the term "radical" is a more difficult matter, yet at the present time the abdominal radical operation unquestionably consists of the following steps: (a) removal of the uterus and adnexa; (b) removal of the upper part of the vagina; (c) removal of both parametria; and (d) removal of the first or lower set of lymph nodes.

III. *The Permanency of the Cure.*—This must be based upon the fact that the patient has remained free from a recurrence for a period of five years.

IV. The following groups of cases must be omitted in computing the permanent cures: (a) those in which death results from the operation; (b) the cases which are lost sight of; and (c) all cases in which death takes place from some intercurrent disease within five years from the time of the operation, but in which, at the same time, no recurrence of the new-growth takes place. Deaths from some intercurrent disease before the lapse of the period after which the disease could be considered cured, should be omitted from the computation unless the case presented signs of recurrence. Even if the patient survived the operation for a period of three years without a return of the growth, it does not follow that the disease would not have recurred later. The fairest picture of ultimate results will be obtained if such is done, although the primary mortality may be slightly distorted. Deaths following the operation should be omitted in this section, because the patient would have died from the disease in all likelihood if the operation had not been performed.

V. The absolute cures are calculated from the total material after the following classes of cases have been omitted: (a) all patients who refuse operation; (b) all those who have been lost track of; and (c) all those who died of intercurrent disease before the end of the five-year period and in whom an autopsy has not demonstrated the existence of a recurrence. These cases should not be considered in the final computation, although record should be made of them.

In order to express the results clearly, the series should be arranged in such a manner as to show: (1) The number of cancerous patients who sought treatment during the series; (2) the number of those who refused operation; (3) the number of those who were found inoperable; (4) the number of those who died from the operation; (5) the number of those who could be accurately followed; (6) the number of those who were lost sight of; (7) the number of those who died of intercurrent disease during the five-year interval; and (8) the number of those in whom a recurrence was observed during this interval.

The percentage of absolute cures is made by determining the total number of those cases in which the patient died from the operation, of those in which a recurrence was observed, and of the inoperable cases, and then ascertaining the precise relationship which the cases that have survived the five-year period without recurrence bear to this grand total. Thus, for a certain five-year period two hundred cases applied to the clinic. Of these two hundred,

Refused operation .... 5 cases
Died from the operation .... 10 "
During the five-year period of investigation there were lost sight of .... 5 "
Died without autopsy· .... 5 '
Were found to have had a recurrence .... 50 '

In the calculation of the absolute cures we should subtract the following from our two hundred cases:

(a) Refusing operation .... 5 cases
(c) Lost from observation .... 5 "
(d) Dead of intercurrent disease, but without a careful autopsy .... 5 "
                                                                        ————
    Total... 15 cases

There remain, therefore, for the calculation of the absolute cures, one hundred and eighty-five cases, of which there were

(b) Dead as a result of the operation .... 10 cases
(e) Presenting recurrence .... 50 "
(f) Were found to be inoperable .... 90 "
(g) Alive and without recurrence five years after the operation .... 35 "

The percentage of absolute cures, therefore, is derived by dividing thirty-five by one hundred and eighty-five—i.e. (in round numbers) 0.19, or nineteen per cent.

The five-year limit is now generally accepted as the time at which freedom from recurrence shall be considered as an absolute cure. This period has been taken arbitrarily, just as, a few years ago, one of three years was accepted by the majority of investigators of this problem. Some indeed, at the present time,—as, for example, Lejars, Ott, and Martin,—favor a longer limit; for, unfortunately, it does not follow that death may not result from the cancer at a later period, even though a recurrence may not have manifested itself during the long observation-period of five years. Thus, in the case reported by Ries, which we have already once quoted, a recurrence manifested itself in the inguinal lymph nodes as late as nine years after the operation. However, the objections to extending the period of observation beyond the limit of five years, more than outweigh the recognized advantages. It is possible, of course, that the results of radical operations will show that late recurrences will be in the lymph nodes, as Mackenrodt and others have claimed, and that the five-year period will have to be extended, because it is based on the fact that the majority of the recurrences noted at the present time are local rather than regional. Yet there is to be considered the great practical difficulty of keeping cases under observation for more than five years, and all admit that statistics in which a considerable number of cases are lost sight of during the post-operative period of observation, are worthless. Moreover, the literature shows that only a small percentage of recurrences manifest themselves after five years. Thus Winter, in 1908, states that, of his three hundred and fifty cases, there were only two which certainly, and two which possibly, presented recurrences later than five years after operation, and that the literature shows that not more than ten in one thousand recurrences are first observed after this period. In Winter's series, five per cent of the recurrences were first noted during the third and fourth years after operation, and similar results are reported by others, these results depending somewhat upon the class of cases observed, as well as upon the type of operation performed. Thus Glockner noted 3 per cent, Thumin 3 per cent, and Hanisch 4.5 per cent in collected cases three and four years after operation, and Seitz found that 3 per cent of the recurrences from von Winckel's clinic were observed in the fourth year and the same percentage in the fifth year after operation. Similar findings may also be gleaned by a careful scrutiny of Wertheim's recent report.

XII. RESULTS OF RADICAL OPERATIONS UPON THE UTERUS.

At the present time there are few large series of cases showing the results of the radical types of operation upon the uterus, for the reason that it is now but thirteen years since the publication of Ries' classical paper and but seven years since the advent of Wertheim into this field. Ries has reported eight cases treated by his method of operation. Two of these patients died as a result of the operation, and six have survived the five-year test, although the earliest surviving patient manifested, nine years after the operation, evidences of a carcinomatous recurrence in the inguinal lymph nodes. Four of the six surviving patients were found, at the operation, to have involved lymph nodes, yet they survived for more than five years without local recurrence. Ries states (personal communication) that operable cases were the greatest rarity in his personal experience, and that he sought to operate upon all cases which presented any reasonable chance of being benefited by radical treatment. It is unfortunate that the investigator did not present his results so tabulated as to show the number of inoperable cases coming under observation, as it would serve to illustrate, in a most vivid manner, the rarity of operable cases in this country. There are no other published reports that show the results obtained by the advocates of lymph-node extirpation in this country. It is most unfortunate that Sampson's cases will not admit of tabulation, as his operation is one of the most complete hitherto described. His experience well illustrates the difficulty of following up the cases in which an operation has been performed, as he states (in a personal communication) that his correspondence directed to this end was most one-sided; the great majority of his clinic patients, having changed either their names or their addresses, were therefore often untraceable, while, in those who could be followed, recurrences were common. Although from the first he sought to operate upon all cases in which there was the most remote chance of completely removing the growth, he now, as a result of his experience, believes that the hope of effecting a cure can be entertained only in cases in which the disease is in a very early stage and the operation performed is of the most complete and radical character.

Wertheim, in 1908, reports the results which he obtained in a series of 120 patients upon whom he operated and who were followed for at least five years after operation. For this series the total number of deaths due to the operation was 27, representing a mortality of 22.5 per cent. Of these deaths 14 occurred in the first 30 cases (46.6 per cent), as contrasted with 13 deaths in the other 90 cases (14.5 per cent). The diminution of the mortality in the latter group is due in part to improvement in operative technique and also to the limitation of the use of the anæsthetic, but still another factor of some importance is to be found in the fact that Wertheim no longer employs the practice of systematically removing the lymph nodes. Included in this series of 120 cases, there were 3 patients affected with cancer of the uterine body, one with cancer of the vulva, and two others who died, during the period of observation, from carcinomatous disease which, as Wertheim states, was in no way related to the malignant disease of the uterus. Deducting these six fatal cases and the twenty-seven which resulted directly from the operation, we still have 87 cases, of which 51—or 58.6 per cent of the cases that survived operation—presented no sign of recurrence at the end of the five-year observation period. The operability during this period was 42.2 per cent of all cases applying for treatment, and the proportion of absolute cures is (according to Winter's older postulates) 24.7 per cent; or, according to Waldstein's formula $A = \dfrac{(O \times D \times [100 - M])}{10,000}$, it would be 19.16 per cent. This is slightly in excess of his previous reports of smaller series. Wertheim states that his operation cases now number over 400, and that in the last 158 cases there were but 12 which terminated fatally—a primary mortality of 7.5 per cent. No patients surviving operation have escaped observation.

Mackenrodt reported his experience at the German Gynæcological Congress in Dresden, in May, 1907. Unfortunately, his report is not complete in detail, although it is of the greatest interest. Of 144 patients who were operated upon by his radical method at dates varying from one and a half to six and a half years previously, 61.5 per cent are (at the time of the report) alive and without sign of recurrence. If the primary deaths following the operation are deducted from the table, the proportion of absolute cures is 70 per cent of those surviving operation. The operability of his cases during this period was 92 per cent and the percentage of primary mortality varied between 19 and 21 per cent. After deducting from his series 11 cases in each of which the patient died of some intercurrent affection without a recurrence of the cancerous disease, he gives his absolute cures as follows:

Period of Observation.	Percentage of Cures.
1½ to 6½ years	55.6
3½ " 6½ "	42.6
4½ " 6½ "	45.4
5½ " 6½ "	48.5
More than six years	58.3

It is unfortunate that his cases are not reported in detail so as to permit of comparison with Wertheim's. For comparison with this series he gives the results of igni-extirpation, in which 43 per cent remained free of recurrence for more than three and a half years. Yet, after six years this had decreased to 22 per cent, and after ten years to 12 per cent. The results, therefore, were not better than those obtained by the vaginal operation, as given by Olshausen. All his late recurrences resulted from involvement of the lymph nodes,—a fact which Mackenrodt considers as furnishing the strongest argument in favor of extirpation of these structures.

Bumm has, up to the present time, made no report of his results; he has given only a preliminary note in the description of his method which he published in 1905. In this he states that in 82 patients upon whom he operated there was a primary mortality of 22 per cent. The operability varied in his two clinics from 80 to 90 per cent. Of these patients 56 were operated upon more than a year previously, with the following results: the operative mortality was 17 per cent; 11 died of recurrence and 6 were living with recurrence; 6 were lost to observation, and 23, or 50 per cent of those surviving operation, were without return of the growth,—20 of them for a period of more than two years.

Gellhorn, in 1905, collected 225 cases in which the patient had been operated upon by the paravaginal method by Schuchardt, Schauta, and Staude, with a mortality of 12.4 per cent. The table which he gives is as follows:

Operator.	No. of Cases.	No. of Deaths.	Percentage.
Schuchardt	83	8	9.6
Schauta	91	11	12
Staude	51	9	17.6
Total	225	28	12.4

At the time when Gellhorn wrote, Schuchardt's cases alone were available for consideration, because the others had not yet passed the five-year limit. The series was small and included but twenty-five cases, representing 56 per cent of all cases seen. Forty per cent of the cases operated upon remained free of recurrence for five years. Calculated according to Werner's postulates, we obtain an absolute percentage of cures of 20.1 per cent.

Schauta, in 1908, reports a series of 258 cases operated upon by the paravaginal method, these cases constituting 48.7 per cent of the total cases applying for relief of cancer to the clinic. The operability varied during the six years, the limits being 33.3 per cent and 62 per cent. The primary mortality was 10.8 per cent, the limits varying from 3.4 per cent (one death in 29 cases) to 19.1 per cent (9 deaths in 47 cases). In the four other years, however, the mortality ran between 8.1 per cent and 12 per cent. Schauta's statistics for the cases observed for five years is as follows:

Total cases applying to the clinic during this series	116
Inoperable cases	60
Primary operation deaths	9
Died from intercurrent disease	4
Recurrence after operation	21
Patients lost from observation	0
Without recurrence five years after operation	13

The percentage of absolute cures, according to Winter's formula, is 12.6 per cent.

Staude, in September, 1908, reports the results of his experience with the extensive vaginal operation in cervical cancer. In contradistinction to the other advocates of this route, he employs a double-sided Schuchardt incision, which, in his judgment, gives far greater exposure of the parametrium than the incision of merely one side. His material consisted of 156 cases of cervical carcinoma, which were not further classified as to portio vaginalis or cervical cancers. He operated upon 104 of these with 21 deaths, an operability of 72.3 per cent, and a primary mortality of 20 per cent. Operation was refused in 13 cases. The greatest source of fatality was pelvic phlegmon, which arose from the vaginal-perineal incision and resulted in peritonitis with fatal issue in 9 cases. Other causes of death are given as follows: heart weakness, 3 cases; hemorrhage, 3 cases; sepsis, 1 case; Basedow's disease, 1 case; embolus, 1 case; ureteral necrosis, 1 case; not diagnosed, 1 case. The operative morbidity from injury to neighboring organs was 11.6 per cent and was divided between injury to the bladder, 6 cases, and injury to the ureter, 6 cases. At the time of his report there were 39 cases which were known to have had a recurrence. In the great majority of cases the recurrence developed in the scar in the vaginal vault or in the parametrium close to the scar. In 2 cases a recurrence was noted in the vaginal-perineal incision, and in only 3 cases was a recurrence found in the lymph nodes—once in the inguinal and twice in the iliac nodes. The reader should bear in mind that no attempt is made in this operation to remove the pelvic lymph nodes. As is generally the case, it was found that, in the great majority of instances, the recurrence took place in the first year after the operation. This was noted in 31 cases as opposed to 5 in the second year, 2 in the third year, and 1 in the fourth year. The number of absolute cures for five years, based upon Winter's classification, represents 23 per cent, and the number of cures for five years, based on the cases actually operated upon, represents 41.5 per cent. The oldest surviving patient in this series was operated upon twelve years previously, and the youngest at least

five years previously.   In this series are included 93 cases of cervical carcinoma,
tabulated as follows:

Operated... 58 cases.
Refused operation..... .... 11 "
Died of intercurrent affections .... 2 "
Lost sight of during the period of calculation .... 6 "
Died from the operation .. .. 9 '
Presenting a recurrence   .... 24 "
Inoperable cases... 24 '
Free from recurrence five to twelve years after operation .... 17 "

There is much confusion in the recent reports of results from vaginal hysterectomy and from the ordinary abdominal hysterectomy, because as yet various
authors have not followed closely either the Winter or the Werner postulates.
Thus, Hannes reports the cases of cervical carcinoma from April 1st, 1895, to
March 31st, 1901, in Kuestner's clinic. All the cases considered had been observed for five years or more after operation.   A total of 361 cases had been seen,
and of this number 145 were operated upon—99 by vaginal extirpations, and 46
by the Veit modification of Freund's abdominal operation.   This series includes all cancer cases operated upon by the older methods, for, since 1903,
the Wertheim abdominal method has been the routine of the clinic.   Hannes
shows a primary mortality of 8 per cent for the vaginal and one of 32.6 per cent
for the abdominal method; 15 per cent of the vaginal and 8.7 per cent of the abdominal cases were lost sight of.   In 24 of the vaginal cases the patient remained free from a recurrence of the disease for five years or more.   In 3 of
the abdominal cases the patient was known to be living and well, and in 3
others she was believed to be living and well.   He then states that the average
number of cures, according to Waldstein, amounted to 28.8 per cent for the vaginal cases and 14.3 per cent for the abdominal cases.   This, of course, is an error,
as such a differentiation cannot be made unless the vaginal operations were
performed exclusively during a certain definite period and the results calculated
from the total number of cancer cases in the clinic at that time.   The same
statement applies also to the abdominal series, and the absolute percentage of
cures cannot be computed except by combining both the abdominal and vaginal cases.

Doederlein reports the results obtained at his clinic from October, 1897,
to 1900.   There were 151 cases of uterine carcinoma during this period, and of
this number 73 were operated upon by the vaginal route, giving 48.3 per cent of
operability.   The primary mortality was 16.4 per cent, from which he calcu-
lates that 19.6 per cent were cured, according to the Winter postulates, and
15.8 per cent, according to the Waldstein postulates.   This material, however,
consists of both cervical and corpus cancers.   Doederlein states that 59 cases
(or 44 per cent of 134 cases of cervical carcinoma) were operable, of which number 14 still remained cured after the five-year observation period.   He states
that the absolute cures obtained by him amounted to 12.5 per cent, but, so far
as we can see, it amounts to only 10.4 per cent.   Since January, 1902, Doederlein
has adopted the method of Wertheim.   During this time there have been 175

uterine cancer cases, both cervical and corpus. Of these he has operated upon 115 (or 65.7 per cent), with a mortality of 16.5 per cent. Comparing the vaginal cases with those operated upon according to the Wertheim method, the mortality remains the same, yet the operability is increased from 44 per cent to 65.7 per cent.

Glockner reported the results of the operations performed during a period of fourteen and one-quarter years (to 1901) in Zweifel's clinic: 974 patients applied to the clinic, and of this number 260 were operated upon, with the hope of obtaining a radical cure (an operability of 26.69 per cent). The vaginal operation was done 225 times, or in 86.5 per cent of the operation cases. The total operative mortality was 8.46 per cent, and in nearly 82 per cent of these cases death was due to septic processes. Under observation for more than five years were 153 cases, and during this period 610 cancer cases came into the hospital; therefore, 25 per cent of all cases observed for more than five years were operated upon. Fifteen of the 153 patients died from the effects of the operation—a mortality of 10 per cent. One died from some other disease, 3 were lost sight of, and in one instance the finding was not verified. If these 21 cases are excluded, there remain 132 of which 85 were known to have had a recurrence, and 47 (or 35.6 per cent) in which it was known that the patient remained free from a recurrence of the disease. In this series, however, were included some cancers of the uterine body. The absolute cures, therefore, in the 610 cases, 25 per cent of which were operated upon, was 7.7 per cent, or, according to Winter's postulates, 9.72 per cent.

Hocheisen reviews a series of 1,706 cases of cervical carcinoma in the Charité in Berlin, between 1882 and 1903. The cases between 1882 and 1890 were collected by Gusserow, and after this period by Hocheisen. Of these, 1,538 were inoperable; 168 were operated upon by vaginal hysterectomy, with the following results: 23 died from the operation; in 94 a recurrence took place; 24 were lost sight of; and in only 27 was it known that a cure had been obtained. In 19 of the 23 primary mortalities death was due to some infective process.

Schindler gives the results of abdominal hysterectomy at Knauer's clinic in Gratz. The total number of cases observed was 588, and of these 117 were treated by abdominal hysterectomy. With one exception they were all cases of cervical cancer. The primary mortality of the entire series was 13.67 per cent, and the operability varied in the series between 22.8 per cent and 36.1 per cent. The absolute cures constitute 3.18 per cent, this estimate being based upon the total number of cases observed (588) and the total number of those living for five years without a recurrence.

Konrad, in 1908, reported the results obtained at Scabo's clinic, in Klausenburg, between the years 1894 and 1908; the results obtained previous to 1894 had already been reported by Akontz. During these fourteen years there were observed 544 cancer cases, which constituted 7.39 per cent of the total material of the clinic. These may be classified as follows: there were 377 cases of cancer of the portio vaginalis, or 69.3 per cent of all; 150 cases of cervical carcinoma, or 27.5 per cent of all; and 17 cases of corpus carcinoma, or 3.13 per cent of all.

The total operability in these cases was 4.41 per cent. Of the cancer material there were only 22 cases in which the time that had elapsed since the operation exceeded five years. During this time 386 cases were admitted to the clinic. The operability, therefore, was 5.7 per cent. Of the 22 patients referred to above, 15 remained cured for five years; a recurrence was noted in 6; and 1 died from the operation. Konrad figures his cures, according to Winter's postulates, as 3.54 per cent, and, according to those of Waldstein, as 3.53 per cent. Yet it will be seen that, of the 386 cases, only 15 were healed by operation, a pro-proportion which represents 0.41 per cent.

Zurhelle reported, in 1907, the results obtained at Fritsch's clinic in Bonn. During the year 1893 there were 253 cases of cervical carcinoma, of which 168 were inoperable. All of the 85 operable cases were treated by vaginal hysterec-tomy, with a primary mortality of 4 per cent. There were 178 cases between 1893 and 1902, of which number 117 were inoperable and 61 were operated upon by vaginal extirpation, with four primary mortalities. Of these, 25 remained free of recurrence for five years or more and were accounted cured; 28 were known to have had a recurrence; and 4 were lost sight of. The conclusions are as follows: The operability, for cervical cases which were operated upon sufficiently early to be observed for five years, was 33.2 per cent; the absolute cures, ac-cording to Winter's postulates, constituted 15.6 per cent, or according to Werner's rule, 14 per cent.

Olshausen, at the German Gynæcological Congress in Dresden, in May, 1907, stated that his operability once attained the high mark of 61.6 per cent and then fell again. The primary mortality reached 7.7 per cent, and in 1906 fell to 4 per cent; 24 of his deaths resulted from sepsis, 6 from embolism and second-ary heart failure and uræmia; 21 per cent of his cervical cases remained cured beyond a period of four years. He expressed the belief that not more than 10 per cent of uterine cancer cases can be cured by the vaginal operation.

EXTRA-UTERINE PREGNANCY.

By LEWIS S. McMURTRY, M.D., LL.D., Louisville, Ky.

UNDER normal conditions the human ovum is fertilized in the Fallopian tube and carried by ciliary movement into the uterine cavity for its future growth. It frequently occurs, however, that the ovum is fertilized and proceeds to partial or complete development at various points between the follicle in which it originated and the uterine cavity. This malposition of the fertilized ovum is known as "extra-uterine pregnancy." Since the fertilized ovum in some instances is implanted in that part of the Fallopian tube which passes through the wall of the uterus, the term "ectopic gestation" is used as having a synonymous but more comprehensive meaning.

Formerly this condition was regarded of interest only as a freak of nature, or as a pathological process, but since 1883, when Mr. Lawson Tait first operated for ruptured tubal pregnancy, it has become of the greatest practical interest. From a state of utter hopelessness as to treatment, it has been placed in that growing list of diseases in which surgery scores its most brilliant results. Up to 1883 ectopic pregnancy was regarded a very rare condition, but with improved knowledge, greater accuracy in diagnosis, and the facilities for increased observation afforded by the frequency of abdominal section, it is known to be of comparatively common occurrence. In the practice of the writer between four and five per cent of all abdominal sections have been for extra-uterine pregnancy.

VARIETIES.—With rare exceptions the ovum in ectopic pregnancy is implanted in the Fallopian tube. When in the middle portion of the tube, or ampulla, it is termed "ampullar"; when in the outer end of the tube-lumen or fimbriæ it is described as "infundibular"; and when in that portion of the tube which is situated in the wall of the uterus it is known as "interstitial." The term "primary" is applied to an ectopic pregnancy when the embryo or fœtus occupies the site of its original implantation; and when, by rupture or the process of development, the embryo takes a new situation it is called "secondary." Until very recently the existence of ovarian pregnancy was denied by the most competent observers. Many cases of so-called ovarian pregnancy were found upon careful dissection to be tubal primarily, with subsequent separation from their tubal attachment. The cases reported by von Tussenbroek, of Amsterdam, Thompson, of Portland, Me., and Webster, of Chicago, however, have established the fact that the ovum may be fertilized and developed to a greater or less degree in the ovary. These observations, accompanied by specimens, have become generally accepted and have put this long-mooted question beyond dispute. Ovarian pregnancy is so extremely rare that, for practical purposes, we may

690

regard all cases of ectopic pregnancy as tubal in their origin. The most common site of implantation and development is in the outer third of the tube. When the developing embryo penetrates and ruptures the tube, with partial escape of the ovum and retention of its placental attachment, it may continue to develop and then becomes an abdominal pregnancy. Since a recently fertilized ovum would be digested and absorbed if originally implanted in the peritoneum, it is only in this way that abdominal pregnancy can occur. Hence abdominal pregnancy is always secondary.

CAUSES.—Numerous explanations as to the etiology of extra-uterine pregnancy have been offered from time to time. An investigation of the various conditions which may favor the arrest and development of the ovum between the ovary and the uterus will almost inevitably lead to the conclusion that this accident is most probably the result of no one cause, but is due to various abnormal conditions. Mr. Lawson Tait attributed the arrest of the ovum to inflammatory changes in the mucous membrane of the tube (endosalpingitis), by which the ciliary movement of the epithelium was impaired or destroyed. The frequency with which ectopic pregnancy is preceded by a long period of sterility, and the wide prevalence of inflammatory disease of the tubes, give plausibility to this theory. The thickening and consequent narrowing of the lumen of the tube in endosalpingitis, with necessarily impaired peristalsis, tend to confirm this explanation. Such changes may impede and arrest the progress of the ovum in its passage, even if the ciliary movement of the epithelium is not destroyed. Tait's theory is not accepted by many authorities as the universal cause of ectopic pregnancy, but no other explanation has been offered which is in equal accord with clinical observation and histological investigation. With modifications, this etiological connection is adopted by most authorities, although both Hofmeier and Whitridge Williams have demonstrated that the cilia may be present and active in the pregnant tube. Other causes, which, by mechanically obstructing the lumen of the tube, may arrest the fertilized ovum therein, are adhesions, neoplasms, and congenital malformations.

COURSE AND TERMINATION.—The fecundated ovum may be implanted at any portion of the tube, when development will at once begin. The conditions here are very different from those afforded by lodgment within the uterine cavity. The glandular or lymphoid tissues, which play such an important part in forming a nidus for the ovum in the uterine mucosa, are absent in the tube. The ovum, however, as soon as it is implanted within the tube, begins to make its way through the tubal epithelium and comes to lie in the tissue immediately beneath. The proliferating ectodermal cells (trophoblasts) rapidly invade the surrounding tissues and penetrate between the fibres of the underlying muscularis. These trophoblastic cells have the power of rapid proliferation, and not only invade the tissues of the tube, but possess an erosive action by which muscle cells are destroyed and blood-vessels opened, forming numerous spaces in the maternal tissues filled with blood. In this way, by a process of erosion with hemorrhage, the ovum makes its way through the tissues of the tube. There is an effort on Nature's part for the development of the tubal tissues, but to a much less degree than in the uterus. As the ovum continues to develop the walls of the tube are stretched and thinned, but its rupture is caused more by the erosive action of the perforating villi and accompanying hemorrhage than by distention. The early stages in the formation of the placenta in both uterine and tubal pregnancy are identical, the microscopic structure of the fœtal portion being the same in both cases. The chorionic villi invade the wall of the tube, open up its blood-vessels, and at an early stage of development penetrate through to the peritoneum.

In the vagina and uterus changes take place that are similar to those which occur in normal uterine pregnancy. The walls of the vagina become lax and soft, the cervix uteri is softened, and the entire uterus is enlarged. The uterine mucosa becomes altered so as to present the condition found in the decidua vera of normal pregnancy. This decidua is usually cast off from the uterus soon after the death of the fœtus, and appears either in whole or in shreds in a bloody vaginal discharge. This is an important diagnostic sign. Being accompanied with contractile uterine pain it is often interpreted as an abortion.

Tubal Abortion.—Intratubal rupture, with consequent hemorrhage into the lumen of the tube, followed by extrusion of the ovum and blood-clot through the fimbriated opening of the tube, is known as "tubal abortion," and is the most frequent termination of tubal pregnancy when the original site of implantation is in the outer third of the tube. In the ampulla the tubal lumen is more patulous than in the isthmus, and in consequence expansion of the fœtal sac in the direction of the fimbriated opening is permitted. Tubal abortion is the result of perforation of the capsular membrane by pressure of the increasing fœtal structures, and especially of hemorrhage resulting from fœtal invasion of the tissues. This hemorrhage detaches, either completely or partially, the ovum from its bed, and gradually forces it by pressure from behind toward the fimbriated extremity, through which it may be extruded into the peritoneum, provided the separation of the ovum be complete.

If, however, the separation is only partial the ovum will remain in the tube and the hemorrhage will persist indefinitely. Under these latter conditions the ovum may increase in size as a result of infiltration with blood, and assume a structural state similar to that of the moles met with in uterine abortions. The blood will exude slowly from the fimbriated extremity, and form a large hæmatocele.

Tubal abortion may be followed by varied results, the severity of which depends upon the extent of the hemorrhage. The ovum may be completely or partially detached from the tube wall, the blood pouring through the fimbriated end of the tube. A large quantity of blood may be quickly poured into the peritoneal cavity, producing profound shock and endangering the patient's life; or a large hæmatocele may be formed, followed by a long period of convalescence; or a small hæmatocele only may result from moderate hemorrhage, to be promptly absorbed by the peritoneum. The ovum, too, is readily absorbed when expelled from the tube into the peritoneum, if this occurs in the early period of pregnancy. In this latter way many cases of tubal abortion terminate in spontaneous cure. Tubal abortion is most apt to occur during the first two months of gestation, before the fimbriated extremity has been closed with firm adhesions.

A common termination of tubal pregnancy is rupture of the tube. This may occur at any time between the third and the twelfth week after conception. The rupture may be complete or incomplete, intraperitoneal or extraperitoneal. The cause of rupture is the constant weakening of the tube wall by the embedded and developing ovum, with invasion of its tissues by ectodermal elements and later by the growing chorionic villi. An immediate cause of rupture may be overexertion, straining, a fall, or a vaginal examination. The rupture occurs most frequently at the placental site, and extrusion may take place into the peritoneum directly or between the folds of the broad ligament. The rupture

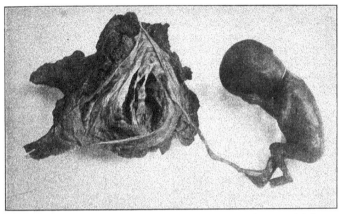

Fig. 283.—Fœtus, Fallopian Tube, and Tissues of Broad Ligament. Sac ruptured during operation, disclosing dead fœtus of four months' growth. (Case of Dr. A. B. Davis, Bulletin of New York Lying-in Hospital, 1909.)

at first may be a small rent or fissure, to be followed, after varying intervals, with renewed rupture and final escape of the ovum. (Fig. 283.) Profuse hemorrhage may occur from a small rent which does not permit the ovum to pass out of the tube. The rupture may at first be complete and permit expulsion of the entire ovum from the tube.

If expelled in its entirety the ovum will die, and, if the hemorrhage is not excessive, it will be absorbed. Should only the fœtus escape, however, and the placenta retain the greater part of its attachment, the fœtus may continue its development to full term and the placenta extend its peripheral attachment to the adjacent organs. Such result of rupture is exceptional, as the fœtus usually perishes as a direct result of separation of the placental attachment.

In a very small proportion of cases the rupture takes place in that part of the tube which is enclosed in the folds of the broad ligament and which is not covered by peritoneum. The ovum and accompanying hemorrhage are poured out in the loose areolar tissue between the layers of peritoneum forming the broad ligament and retained outside the peritoneal cavity. This results most frequently in the death of the ovum and the formation of a broad-ligament hæmatoma, which is the most fortunate termination—when Nature is unaided—of a ruptured tubal pregnancy. In a small proportion of cases the placenta is not completely detached from its tubal connections, and the fœtus may continue its development to full term. As the pregnancy advances the fœtal sac raises up the peritoneum from its parietal attachments, and forms an extraperitoneal pregnancy, or the broad-ligament sac may rupture and thus form a secondary abdominal pregnancy. This termination of tubal pregnancy was regarded by Mr. Lawson Tait as the only process by which the fœtus could go on to maturity. From my personal experience in operations for ruptured tubal pregnancy I am convinced that the frequency of rupture into the folds of the broad ligament has been greatly overestimated by writers upon this subject.

In interstitial pregnancy rupture may occur externally into the peritoneum, or the ovum may be extruded through the uterine opening of the tube into the uterine cavity. In the former event, on account of the vascularity of the structures, the hemorrhage is severe and often fatal; in the latter event the ovum may be thrown off from the uterine cavity as an abortion or continue its development as a uterine pregnancy.

In ruptured tubal pregnancy the life of the fœtus depends upon the extent to which placental attachment is retained. When the rupture occurs early and the ovum is entirely extruded from the tube, the fœtus is rapidly absorbed, as is proven by the fact that in many instances no trace of the fœtus is found in operations in these cases. It is a common observation to find placental tissue surrounded by blood-clot in a formless mass, and careful dissection will fail to disclose any remains of the fœtus. When, however, the attachment of the placenta is sufficiently preserved to maintain the life of the fœtus, the pregnancy proceeds under extra-uterine conditions. These conditions are fraught with constant danger to the life of both mother and child. The pressure of the developing fœtus, and the tension of the peritoneum covering the gestation sac, lead to partial detachment and hemorrhage. It is exceptional for the child of a full-term extra-uterine pregnancy which has been saved, to prove sound and vigorous. Such children are usually ill-formed and of feeble vitality.

When the fœtus survives primary rupture and the pregnancy advances to full term, there occurs, as a rule, what is known as "spurious labor." The pains resemble those of normal labor, and continue for several hours or even for days. The pains are due to uterine contraction, and are accompanied with a bloody discharge from the uterus. After spurious labor fœtal movements cease, showing that death of the child has taken place.

After the death of the fœtus, the liquor amnii is absorbed and the abdomen diminishes in size. If not removed by surgical intervention, the fœtus becomes enveloped in placenta and membranes, and may undergo any one of several changes in its form and structure. It may *mummify* by the absorption of fluids and shrinking of tissues. It may thus remain quiescent in the abdomen for a long time, extending over years. The fœtus may in other instances undergo calcareous change, by which process it is converted into a *lithopedion*. The calcified fœtus may be carried in the abdomen for years without harm. In a considerable proportion of cases, the fœtus and membranes are infected and *suppuration* takes place. Adhesions are formed around a huge abscess, which perforates in the direction of least resistance, discharges into the bowel, bladder, or vagina; and if the patient does not succumb from sepsis, bones are extruded through the rectum, bladder, vagina, or abdominal walls.

SYMPTOMS.—In ectopic pregnancy the early symptoms are those of normal uterine pregnancy. Usually the menstruation is suppressed, but this symptom is less constant than in normal pregnancy. There may be slight pain in one or the other ovarian region, but this is seldom heeded. If the fœtus dies at an early period, and rupture or abortion does not immediately occur, there is usually more or less uterine flow containing shreds and clots, which may be mistaken for an early abortion. Often the symptoms are so insidious that the patient does not consult a physician until tubal abortion or rupture takes place. Hence it often obtains that the first sign of an abnormal condition is when rupture occurs with severe hemorrhage into the peritoneum. The patient is suddenly seized with agonizing pain in the abdomen, followed by faintness and pallor. The pulse quickly becomes rapid and feeble, and may altogether disappear at the wrist; the lips are pale and a cold perspiration covers the surface of the body, with subnormal temperature. The patient may go into collapse and death ensue from the severe shock and hemorrhage; or, as more frequently occurs, the bleeding may be temporarily checked and reaction take place, to recur perhaps some hours later.. In other instances the initial symptoms of rupture are not so marked; the patient soon rallies, but will suffer a renewed and perhaps more severe attack later. In such cases the rupture consists of a small slit, followed later by a deep rent. If the symptoms of pain and hemorrhage are not pronounced, we may infer that the lesion is that of tubal abortion. In cases of rupture into the broad ligament the symptoms may be insidious and perplexing. Secondary rupture may occur at a later period in these cases, with severe hemorrhage and shock. In many cases of tubal abortion, and of early tubal rupture, the symptoms are not distinctive; the patient is relieved by an anodyne, and, later on, an operation will reveal the trouble to have originated in an ectopic pregnancy. Such are the cases formerly classified and treated as pelvic hæmatocele. Should the fœtus survive rupture and advance to full term, the symptoms are in the main those of normal pregnancy.

DIAGNOSIS.—While it is quite practicable to make a diagnosis of extra-uterine pregnancy prior to the time of rupture, as a matter of fact it is rarely accomplished. This is due, for the most part, to the fact that the physician is rarely consulted during the initial period before rupture or tubal abortion. When the patient is seen prior to rupture, a physician familiar with the history and symptoms so characteristic of ectopic pregnancy will have no difficulty in making at least a tentative diagnosis. When, with a history of recent pregnancy, one is confronted with the symptoms of agonizing pain in the pelvis and sudden collapse from internal hemorrhage, and finds upon vaginal examination a softened cervix with a fluid tumor within the peritoneum, the diagnosis becomes clear and unequivocal. When the child has survived rupture, unless a careful examination is suggested by the unusual history of the case, a correct diagnosis will rarely be made before the end of pregnancy. When rupture has taken place into the broad ligament, the diagnosis will be aided by finding, upon vaginal examination, a tumor upon one side of the uterus and intimately connected with it. The diagnosis of extra-uterine pregnancy at full term presents few difficulties. Vaginal examination will reveal the uterus but slightly enlarged and lying against the symphysis or low in the pelvis, while the outline of the child can be felt in the extra-uterine tumor.

In considering the diagnosis of ectopic pregnancy one must remember that both tubal and uterine pregnancy may coexist; also that repeated tubal pregnancy in the same individual has often been observed.

PROGNOSIS.—At every stage of its progress, extra-uterine pregnancy is one of the most perilous conditions which can assail a woman's life. As has been stated upon a preceding page, a considerable proportion of cases of tubal abortion and even of rupture terminate in hæmatocele which may result in spontaneous cure by absorption. But one must remember that no physician or surgeon, however skilled by study and experience, can separate by differential diagnosis these fortunate cases from those in which fatal hemorrhage may momentarily ensue. If the patient survives primary rupture, there remains the possibility of a secondary rupture, or the more common sequel of peritonitis with disintegrating and suppurating hæmatocele. If the fœtus survives rupture and goes on toward the full term of gestation, the life of both mother and child are constantly imperiled by the changes which must ensue in the abnormal environment, with spurious labor and its sequelæ at the end. Ectopic pregnancy, when left to Nature unaided by surgical intervention, presents a rate of mortality which is appalling. Schauta estimated the mortality at 68.8 per cent, this estimate being based upon the records of two hundred and forty-one cases, while Parry gives the same mortality as 67.20 per cent, in a series of five hundred cases. Of these, 52.88 per cent of the deaths resulted from rupture of the gravid cyst. These statistics do not, however, include that considerable class of cases of tubal abortion in which there are no severe symptoms and which end in recovery by absorption after a brief illness. With this class included the mortality would remain heavy. Under treatment by timely surgical intervention the mortality is less than five per cent.

TREATMENT.—In the present state of our knowledge concerning extra-uterine pregnancy, with the established results of surgical treatment before us, all so-called non-surgical methods of treatment are contra-indicated. These measures consist of evacuation of the liquor amnii, the injection of morphine and other substances to kill the fœtus, and the application of the galvanic current. Not only are these methods inefficient, but they beget dangerous complications and temporize with a condition which menaces life. Such methods of trteament are obsolete, and operative treatment is now generally accepted as the only rational and safe means of dealing with this serious condition.

The treatment may best be considered under the following headings:— (1) prior to rupture or abortion; (2) at the time of rupture; (3) after rupture; (4) in the advanced months of pregnancy; (5) after the death of the child.

(1) *Treatment Prior to Rupture or Abortion.*—As a result of increased familiarity with the symptoms and greater accuracy in diagnosis, cases in which the ovum is confined to its original site in the tube are recognized more frequently than formerly. An operation at this period prevents the serious consequences of rupture, is simple in character, and, with proper technique, is without mortality. The operation consists of abdominal section and removal of the tube in which the ovum is lodged. If the adjacent ovary and the tube and ovary of the opposite side are free from disease, these structures should be preserved. In one of the writer's recent cases, the right tube and ovary were removed at the time of rupture. Within a year the patient had a pregnancy in the left tube, which was recognized by her prior to rupture on account of the renewal of symptoms of her former illness. The enlarged tube could be felt by vaginal examination, and the symptoms and history were typical. At the operation the ovum was found to be situated near the fimbriated extremity of the tube. I trimmed away with scissors that portion of the tube which contained the ovum, stopped the bleeding with catgut suture, and preserved in a normal condition the major portion of the tube. With ne ovary and three-fourths of one tube preserved, the patient being a young and vigorous woman, free from any history or symptoms of infection, the expectation of normal pregnancy remains as a reasonable possibility. In operations before rupture the tube containing the fœtus will, as a rule, require to be removed in its entirety, and the tube and ovary of the opposite side should be brought into the incision and carefully examined. If the opposite tube is the seat of acute inflammation, or if the fimbriæ are destroyed and its lumen sealed by previous infection, it should be removed. In exceptional cases it will be necessary to remove the ovaries, but these organs should be preserved in whole or in part whenever practicable.

(2) *Treatment at the Time of Rupture.*—In the majority of cases of ectopic pregnancy the surgeon will be called in great haste to see the patient immediately after rupture of the tube has occurred. The patient will have been seized suddenly with intense pain in one or the other ovarian region, and will quickly show the characteristic symptoms of profuse internal hemorrhage already described upon a preceding page. It matters not how profound the shock and collapse, an effort must be made at once to save the patient's life. The abdomen must be opened and the bleeding arrested. Fortunately, when this is done with skill and expedition the effort will prove successful. Preparation for operation should be made rapidly, but with due care for asepsis and thorough work. A table should be improvised while assistants and nurse are being summoned, hot water obtained, and other needed preparations for operation hastened. While ether is being administered, an assistant should prepare salt solution for intra-

venous infusion. A full dose of strychnia should be given hypodermatically. In preparing the skin for the abdominal incision only the gentlest rubbing should be applied. As soon as the abdomen is opened, the operator should pass two fingers into the pelvis and bring up the uterus and its appendages. The ruptured tube will be readily recognized, and a clamp should then be placed upon the outer border of the broad ligament to compress the ovarian artery, and another clamp applied at the uterine end of the tube. The two clamps will arrest all hemorrhage, and the tube can be removed with scissors above the clamps and ligatures applied. The clots of blood may now be turned out with the hand, and one or two pitchers of warm salt solution may be poured into the abdomen, by which means the coagula will be more thoroughly removed. A liberal quantity of salt solution may advantageously be left in the abdomen, so as to liquefy the clotted blood and facilitate its absorption. It will also stimulate the patient and aid in refilling the depleted vessels. The abdomen should be closed without drainage. If the condition of the patient will permit, the opposite tube and ovary should be examined, but nothing not of vital importance should be done, and all unessential details of toilet and closure should be omitted. The patient should be placed quickly in a bed that has been previously warmed by hot water-bags and the foot of the bed should be elevated.

When profuse hemorrhage has taken place into the abdomen after rupture, and the patient is profoundly shocked and exsanguine, it is preferable to allow the patient to rally somewhat before adding the unavoidable shock of operation to the existing condition. Since a certain proportion of these patients die as a direct result of the continued hemorrhage, the decision to take this step is one of vital responsibility. The hemorrhage ceases as the heart becomes weaker and clot forms, and under stimulation the desired reaction usually occurs. After hemorrhage has ceased and reaction has been established, the operation will be borne without the extreme peril of additional shock. During the time of waiting for reaction, the preparations for operation should be in progress, the surgeon should be in constant attendance, and, upon finding undoubted evidence of returning hemorrhage, he should resort immediately to operation. It makes a marked difference in results, to operate during the ascending wave of reaction instead of during the descending current of increasing collapse.

The treatment of ruptured interstitial pregnancy and the treatment of ovarian pregnancy are practically the same as that of the tubal variety. In the former the sac and its contents are excised from the uterine wall and the incision closed by catgut sutures as after myomectomy. In ovarian pregnancy the ovary is removed entire and the pedicle secured as in other conditions.

(3) *Treatment after Rupture.*—There are numerous circumstances which may interfere with prompt surgical treatment at the time of tubal rupture or abortion. In a certain proportion of cases, especially of tubal abortion, the pain and shock may be of moderate severity, the hemorrhage being limited by the small size of the vessels opened. The diagnosis may not be clear, or a physician may not be consulted, and, after a few days' illness, the patient may be well.

These are the cases previously described as of tubal abortion, with moderate hemorrhage and spontaneous cure.

In other cases, after an illness more acute, the patient recovers, with an extensive hæmatocele. In another class of cases the shock and hemorrhage at the time of rupture may be extreme and severe, and for some reason operation is not done. In a goodly proportion of these cases the patient may rally and escape the immediate danger to her life, with a large hæmatocele, a lacerated tube, and the possibility of additional hemorrhage. When the rupture is extraperitoneal, in the folds of the broad ligament, the amount of pain and hemorrhage may not be great, and the patient will rally promptly and soon be apparently well. Even though the collection of blood be small, one must remember that the fœtus may survive primary rupture, and continue to grow and endanger the life of the patient later on. The formation of an hæmatocele after rupture is not a guarantee that active hemorrhage may not recur. On account of the proximity of the intestines, the blood-tumor is in constant danger of infection. Absorption is a slow process, and the patient is often confined to bed for weeks, with much discomfort from pressure. In the light of these facts, abundantly illustrated by clinical experience, the welfare of the patient in every variety and phase of ectopic pregnancy subsequent to rupture is best subserved by prompt resort to operation. The mortality of the operation is so slight, and the results so prompt and perfect, that it should be the invariable mode of treatment. Abdominal section in these cases eliminates all complications; removes the débris of tubal rupture, placental tissue, and clots; shortens convalescence, and leaves the pelvic structures in better condition in every respect than when the condition is left to Nature's unaided way. In the operative treatment of hæmatocele some surgeons have advocated the vaginal route as preferable to the abdominal incision for removal of the hæmatocele. In more than one instance, in the hands of skilled operators, when the clots were removed by vaginal incision, the hemorrhage was actively renewed, necessitating immediate resort to abdominal section. The abdominal incision alone gives access to the lacerated tube, and permits the operator to work with precision and make a complete operation. Adhesions to the intestines should be carefully separated, the coagula cleaned out, and the injured structures repaired.

(4) *Treatment in the Advanced Months of Pregnancy.*—When the fœtus survives rupture the placenta forms new and more extensive attachments, and progressive development ensues much in the same manner as in uterine pregnancy. After the beginning of the fourth month, until the end of the full term of pregnancy, the operation required is one of the most dangerous known to surgery. The danger lies in the capacity for hemorrhage of a quick and growing placenta attached to peritoneal surfaces. When the condition has been recognized in the early months of pregnancy there should be no delay in resorting to operation. Such delay adds to the risk of the mother. If, when the patient first comes under the surgeon's care, the fœtus has nearly reached the viable period, operation may be deferred a few weeks in its interest. The life of the mother is of prime consideration. Some operators have advised that the

operation be deferred until after the death of the fœtus, in order that the placental circulation may cease and lessen the danger of hemorrhage. Death has followed placental hemorrhage in operations performed several weeks after the death of the fœtus; and fatal complications, such as separation of the placenta, rupture of the gestation sac, and sepsis may occur at the termination of pregnancy. The writer operated in a case three weeks after spurious labor, and removal of the placenta was followed by such profuse and uncontrollable hemorrhage that the patient succumbed within twelve hours.

The operation should be performed in a well-appointed operating-room, with complete preparations to meet every emergency that may arise. As soon as the abdomen is opened, the sac should be carefully examined so as to avoid injury to the placenta. After the sac has been opened, the fœtus is delivered, the cord clamped, and the child removed and handed to an assistant. The next step is, whenever possible, to secure the ovarian and uterine arteries. Unfortunately, these vessels are not, on account of the altered anatomical relations, always accessible. The most difficult part of the entire procedure is the removal of the placenta. This can be more readily accomplished when it is situated in the pelvis. Whenever possible, the sac and placenta should be removed. In broad-ligament pregnancy this can more frequently be accomplished than when the sac is intraperitoneal. When hemorrhage is copious and uncontrollable by ordinary means, the aorta should be compressed by an assistant while a firm gauze pack is placed in the sac. When extensive adhesions and coils of intestines render extirpation of the sac and placenta impossible, the sac should be stitched to the abdominal incision and left open for drainage. The cord should, of course, be tied and cut off close to the placenta. Under these circumstances the placenta may gradually be cast off and come away in pieces.

Notwithstanding that primary laparotomy in advanced ectopic pregnancy with living child is followed by a mortality of about thirty-five per cent, the results are steadily improving under the modern operative technique.

(5) *Treatment after the Death of the Child.*—When death of the child occurs at any period of ectopic pregnancy, the circulation in the placenta begins a retrograde change. The placental bruit disappears, the vessels atrophy, and the entire placenta gradually shrinks away. For this reason, operation for complete removal of fœtus, sac, and placenta involves much less danger at this period than when the circulation is active in the placenta. The technique of the operation is in the main identical with that already described for advanced ectopic pregnancy with living child. When the fœtus has been dead for several weeks it will usually be found with skin macerated and disintegration in progress. The abdominal incision in these cases will necessarily be large, and the utmost care should be observed to protect the exposed peritoneum by gauze packing. The entire sac and its contents should be removed, and the abdomen closed without drainage, unless there should exist some positive indication to pursue a different course. When suppuration has taken place, the operation should be carried out with the same technique as would be observed in the removal of a suppurating ovarian cyst.

THE CÆSAREAN SECTION AND ITS SUBSTITUTES.

By LEWIS S. McMURTRY, M.D.. LL.D., Louisville, Kentucky.

THE Cæsarean section is an operation whereby the child is delivered from the uterus by abdominal section and incision through the uterine walls. The history of this operation dates from the earliest times, and it seems probable that it was rudely performed among some uncivilized races. The origin of the term is not clear. It has been claimed that Julius Cæsar was brought into the world by this means, and acquired his name from the manner of his birth (a cæso matris utero). This is not confirmed, however, by accurate historical data, and it is more probable that the name originated from the Roman law requiring this operation to be performed upon women dying during the last weeks of pregnancy, and known as the lex cæsarea.

The first treatise upon the subject was written in the sixteenth century by Rousset, a contemporary of Ambroise Paré, and the first operation done upon the living woman was probably done in 1610. With all the advances in surgery during the intervening years down to the last two decades of the nineteenth century, the operation was accompanied by such appalling mortality that it was seldom performed. It was not until the Listerian era, and after Porro and Saenger made their great contributions to the technique of the operation, that the Cæsarean section became established as a safe and beneficent procedure.

Indications.—It is customary to classify the indications for Cæsarean section under two heads—the absolute and the relative. The indication is absolute and the operation imperative when there is a living child in a deformed pelvis with a true conjugate diameter of 6.5 centimetres (two and five-eighths inches) or less. The indication is relative when there is a living child with a conjugate diameter of 7 centimetres, and a choice must be made between Cæsarean section and other procedures, such as pubiotomy, craniotomy, and other means of delivery. In view of the greatly improved results which now obtain after Cæsarean section, and its superiority over competing methods for preserving the lives of both mother and child, the scope of the operation has been very greatly extended, such extension depending, of course, upon the condition of the patient and the ability of the operator to command the proper facilities for performing a major surgical operation.

There are other conditions besides contraction of the pelvis which may cause such an insurmountable obstruction to labor as to necessitate the Cæsarean section. For example, a fibroid tumor in the lower segment of the uterus, or a prolapsed ovarian tumor with adhesions. may so block the pelvic canal

701

as to make the operation imperative. Before one resorts to the operation, however, in such cases, an effort should be made under anæsthesia to push such tumors upward and thereby free the canal. Carcinoma of the uterine cervix may render dilatation impossible, and become an indication for this operation. In performing the operation under the latter condition, the Porro-Cæsarean section, with total excision of the cervix, should be done if the disease has not advanced too far, and the patient's condition will permit. The Cæsarean section has been recommended by excellent authorities both in America and in Europe for certain cases of placenta prævia, also for eclampsia complicated by an undilatable cervix, but in the majority of such cases delivery may be accomplished by other and more conservative methods.

Choice and Time of Operation.—I have already alluded to the epoch-making contributions of Porro (in 1876) and Saenger (in 1882) to the operation under consideration. At that time all abdominal operations had a heavy mortality from septic infection, and the Cæsarean section, with a large wound in the uterus communicating with the uterine cavity, was especially prone to infection. Hemorrhage from the uterine incision added to the mortality. Porro gave to the operation the additional procedure of hysterectomy. After the delivery of the child through the uterine incision, the cord was clamped and divided, the placenta was allowed to remain, the uterine cervix was clamped and the uterus amputated, the pedicle being afterward fixed in the lower angle of the abdominal incision. By this operation the dangers, both of hemorrhage and of infection, were materially lessened. The result, so far as the woman is concerned, it will be observed, is quite different from that of the operation as previously done. By Porro's method the uterus is removed, and the possibility of future pregnancy is eliminated. Hence this operation is radical in its results.

Six years after the superiority of Porro's operation over the old procedure of abdominal section and uterine incision had been established, Saenger demonstrated the essential importance of suturing the uterine incision. Previous to this time the uterine walls, after incision and delivery of the fœtus and placenta, were left to the physiological contraction of the uterus, without sutures, for security against hemorrhage. As a result of Saenger's method and the simultaneous improvement in aseptic surgery, the Cæsarean section as thus modified was followed by unprecedented success and became the operation of choice. It will be observed that the result of this operation, so far as the mother is concerned, differs from the result of the Porro operation in that the uterus is preserved. Hence, the Saenger-Cæsarean section is known as the conservative operation, in contradistinction to the radical Porro-Cæsarean section.

In cases of deformed pelvis,—in fact, in the great majority of cases requiring delivery by abdominal section,—the conservative operation should have preference. It not only secures the desired results, but, in view of the fact that it can be performed in less time than the radical operation, it is to that extent a safer operation.

The Porro operation is the operation of choice when the uterus contains myomatous tumors, or when there is cancer of the cervix. Also in cases in which there is a strong probability of infection, the Porro operation should receive preference. As a determining factor in the result, the period of pregnancy or labor at which Cæsarean section is performed is of incalculable importance. It has been shown that, when skilfully performed in uninfected cases, and with favorable surroundings, the mortality is no greater than that of uncomplicated hysterectomy for uterine myomata. Thus, Olshausen reports sixty-five cases with a mortality of 4.6 per cent, and Reynolds, of Boston, reports thirty cases without mortality. When the operation, however, is performed upon infected patients by unskilled operators, with untrained assistants, and with inadequate hospital facilities, the mortality is heavy. The same may be said of the Porro-Cæsarean section, the mortality of which in uninfected cases, with the modern method of retro-peritoneal treatment of the pedicle, is about the same as in the case of other clean hysterectomies. With infected and exhausted patients, or when the operation is hastily and imperfectly performed amid unfavorable surroundings, the results are disastrous in the extreme.

Utilizing these facts, Reynolds divides cases of Cæsarean section into three classes: (1) Primary sections, performed before the beginning or at the onset of labor; (2) secondary sections, performed after a period of labor has demonstrated its inefficiency; and (3) late sections. When the operation is performed prior to labor, or at the beginning of labor, the best results are obtained.

In certain cases it is necessary for the patient to enter upon labor before a judicious decision of the question of delivery by section can be determined. In such cases vaginal examination should be made with sterilized rubber gloves and every other aseptic precaution, and repeated examinations should be avoided. With careful observance of such precautions, infection can be prevented and section performed with excellent results. But when the patient is exhausted by protracted labor, when there have been repeated attempts to deliver the child with forceps, and when examinations have been made by several attendants, all of these examinations being conducted with only a perfunctory observance of rules of asepsis, the Cæsarean section, however skilfully performed, offers only a forlorn hope of saving mother or child. To obtain the best results the physician should examine the patient in the early months of pregnancy, so that conditions pointing to obstructed labor may be recognized. Then the advantageous time for operation can be utilized. The responsibility thus placed upon the great body of the profession engaged in obstetrical practice is apparent.

Operative Technique.—The preparation of the patient for Cæsarean section is the same as for any abdominal section, and should be carefully made some hours in advance, if circumstances permit. The rigid observance, on the part of operator and assistants, of established rules with regard to asepsis, is of paramount importance. The abdominal incision should be made in the linea alba with the umbilicus as a centre, and should be long enough to permit delivery of the uterus. The uterus will be found immediately beneath the incision, and care must be observed not to wound that organ when the abdominal incision is made. An assistant should place his hands flat upon the abdominal wall, one on each side, and should make firm pressure throughout the operation, thus holding the uterus in position and keeping the abdominal wall and uterus in apposition. With the aid of strips of gauze, the peritoneum should be carefully protected from contamination by the uterine contents before the incision into the uterus is made. An incision corresponding in size and location to the abdominal incision is made in the uterus. If the placenta lies directly beneath the incision, as it does in a large proportion of cases, it should be cut through or quickly pushed aside, and the amnion punctured. The child is now grasped by both feet and lifted out; the cord is divided between two clamps; and the child is handed to an assistant. If labor has been in progress some time prior to operation, the head of the child may be fixed in the pelvis below the uterine contraction ring and require traction applied to the neck and shoulders, as well as to the feet, to dislodge it.

As soon as the child is removed from the womb that organ begins to contract firmly, and the hemorrhage is at once diminished. It was formerly customary, in order to control the hemorrhage, to tie an elastic cord around the cervix before incising the uterus, but this was found to produce atony of the uterus and a predisposition to post-partum hemorrhage. The method of manual compression of the uterine arteries in the broad ligament has also been abandoned, since such extensive exposure of peritoneal surfaces is required for this manœuvre. The uterus should not be brought out through the abdominal incision, and all unnecessary exposure and handling of peritoneal surfaces should be avoided. If the hemorrhage from the uterus is excessive after the delivery of the child, it can be effectually controlled by packing the uterus with a large gauze towel, and this can be gradually removed as the uterine sutures are introduced and tied. In operations of election, Olshausen advises the administration of a full dose of ergot hypodermatically just before starting the operation, to stimulate uterine contraction.

As soon as the uterus contracts after delivery of the child, the placenta and membranes will in most instances become separated and can readily be delivered. If not spontaneously freed, they should be peeled off with the hand, and thoroughly removed. The uterus will now contract more firmly, and be much d minished in size.

All superficial gauze and towels which may have been soiled in the preceding steps of the operation, are now removed and replaced by fresh towels. The sutures are then introduced to close the uterine incision. Silk, linen, and catgut have been employed for suture material, and all have served the purpose satisfactorily. With the improved methods of preparing catgut now in vogue, the chromicized suture of this material is preferable. It is sufficiently strong, will not come untied, and will remain in the tissues long enough to maintain apposition throughout the healing process. I have used size No. 2 with satisfactory results. The sutures are introduced (about one centimetre apart) from above downward, the entire thickness of the muscularis being included, but not the decidua. If necessary to control bleeding, each suture should be tied when passed. If oozing persists from the incision, a few moderately deep sutures may be placed between the deep ones. A superficial suture of catgut is now passed, the peritoneal covering of the uterus and a slight layer of the muscularis being grasped and the suture being drawn over the line of deep sutures along the entire length of the uterine incision.

All gauze and towels which were placed around the uterus are now removed and the omentum replaced. The abdomen is then closed in the usual way. The steps of the operation throughout should be performed with precision, and at the same time with all possible expedition. Unimportant details and refinements of technique should be omitted, and the operation completed in the quickest possible time compatible with thorough and accurate work.

The after-treatment is the same as that following other abdominal sections, a complete exposition of which may be found in another volume (Vol. VII.) of this treatise.

The Porro-Cæsarean section and the Saenger-Cæsarean section are identical in operative procedure up to and including the delivery of the child. As the body of the uterus is to be removed in the former, there is no contra-indication to placing an elastic ligature about the cervix prior to incising the body of the organ. For the same reason it is unnecessary to consume time with extracting the placenta and membranes. As soon as the cord has been secured and the child handed over to an assistant, the operator addresses himself to the modern operation for supravaginal hysterectomy with retroperitoneal treatment of the pedicle, which operation is fully described in one of the preceding articles of this volume. The Porro operation, performed in this way, is, of course, appropriate in cases of pregnancy so complicated by uterine myomata as to necessitate radical operative intervention. This operation may be indicated also in certain cases in which, for valid reason, it is desirable to protect the patient from future pregnancies. Sterilization of the patient, however, may be obtained, when the conservative section is done, by excision of a section of each Fallopian tube. Numerous cases are on record in which repeated Cæsarean section was performed upon the same patient. Leopold reports a case in which he performed the operation four times.

Vaginal Cæsarean Section.—In 1896 Duehrssen brought forcibly to the attention of the profession an operation for rapidly terminating labor, which has since been very generally applied, and is known as "vaginal Cæsarean section." It is especially applicable in cases in which labor is obstructed by a rigid and undilatable cervix, and in which it becomes necessary to terminate labor quickly. It is incomparably superior to the older methods of forcible manual and instrumental dilatation. It has its most appropriate application in cases of eclampsia with undilatable cervix. Increased experience with this operation has established its merits beyond question, and it is generally adopted as the operation of choice in the limited field in which it is applicable. Unfortunately, it requires special skill and at least three trained assistants for its performance, and hence is only exceptionally available in private practice.

Operative Technique.—The patient is prepared as for vaginal hysterectomy, and then, having been anæsthetized, she is placed in the lithotomy position and the Sims speculum introduced. The uterine cervix is next seized with traction forceps and drawn down toward the vulva, or strong traction sutures may be utilized for the same purpose. The vaginal wall is then incised from a point near the urethra to the anterior lip of the cervix uteri. A transverse incision is next made, and the bladder is dissected off the anterior surface of the uterus, the separation being mostly done by gauze dissection. The bladder

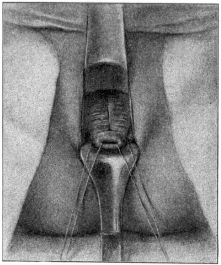

Fig. 284.—Vaginal Cæsarean Section. Exposure of the Cervix and Primary Incisions. (From J. Whitridge Williams' "Treatise on Obstetrics." D. Appleton & Co., Publishers, New York.)

is then drawn upward by means of a retractor in the hands of an assistant, and the anterior wall of the uterus thus exposed. (Fig. 284.)

If pregnancy has not advanced beyond the eighth month, or in cases in which the child is small at term, the cervix and lower segment of the uterus may now be incised in the median line of the cervix, the incision being from 8 to 10 centimetres in length. (Fig. 285.) Both retractor and speculum are now withdrawn, and the hand is introduced into the uterus. The membranes are then punctured, and the child turned and de vered.

If, however, the pregnancy has reached full term, the operation should begin with a posterior incision of the cervix, the peritoneum being separated from the posterior wall of the uterus to a distance corresponding with that already indicated for the anterior incision. After the posterior surface of the uterus is freed in this way, the anterior incision is made and the cervix is incised in the median line anteriorly and posteriorly to the required extent. When incisions are made both anteriorly and posteriorly, each incision, for obvious reasons, will be shorter than when the anterior incision alone is employed. After the child and placenta have been delivered, the speculum is replaced, and both incisions are closed with catgut sutures. When the uterine incisions are

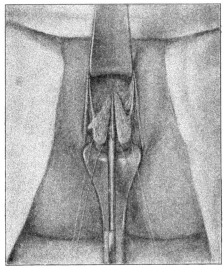

Fig. 285.—Vaginal Cæsarean Section. Incision of Anterior Uterine Wall after Separation of the Bladder. (From J. Whitridge Williams' "Treatise on Obstetrics." D. Appleton & Co., Publishers, New York.)

made as indicated, directly in the median line, the hemorrhage is not severe and can be readily controlled.

The after-treatment, in so far as the operation is concerned, is simple, and the same as is observed after plastic operations upon the uterine cervix.

Symphyseotomy and Pubiotomy.—Since both these operations are based upon similar principles and have identical indications for their application, it will not be inappropriate to consider both under one heading.

Symphyseotomy consists in division of the pubic joint, with the idea of thereby increasing the capacity of a contracted pelvis and permitting the delivery of a living child. This operation was in vogue in the eighteenth century, but, on account of imperfect technique, it fell into disfavor. After many years it was revived by Morisani in 1866, and since 1892 it has been practised considerably throughout Europe and America.

Operative Technique.—The patient, having been prepared for operation and anæsthetized, is placed upon the table lying on her back, with the buttocks brought down to the edge of the table. An incision is made immediately over the symphysis pubis, beginning just above its margin and extending to its lower border. After dividing the skin and subcutaneous tissues down to the fascia, the operator passes his finger behind the symphysis and frees the underlying tissues. The attachment of the clitoris to the symphysis is divided and a catheter passed through the urethra so that, by its aid, the latter may be pushed well below the line of incision. The pubic joint is then divided with a strong knife, the edge of the same being applied from without or the opposite, as may be preferred. Care should be observed to divide the subpubic ligament, whereupon the pubic bones will gape apart. The structure of the pelvis is such that, when the symphysis is divided, the ends of the bones gape to a distance of from 3 to 5 centimetres, and the innominate bones correspondingly tilt outward. As a result, the capacity of the pelvis is increased in its transverse and oblique diameters. A considerable venous hemorrhage usually follows the incision through the symphysis; it is best controlled by gauze packing. After the completion of the operation, the child is delivered by means of forceps or by version, as may be indicated. During the delivery of the child, firm pressure should be applied with the hands of assistants to the trochanters on each side to prevent too wide gaping of the pubic bones. By this operation the clitoris, bladder, and anterior wall of the vagina are deprived of their support, and in consequence are subjected to such tension during extraction of the child that these structures may be severely injured.

The wound is treated simply with sterile dressings. After delivery is completed, the thighs should be adducted, and a broad strong bandage, properly padded with cotton at the points where it passes over bony prominences, applied around the pelvis. This bandage should be secured snugly, so as to favor apposition of the ends of the pubic bones. The after-treatment is both tedious and laborious. Catheterization is usually required, the patient must be kept upon her back, and sand-bags are to be applied to the sides of the pelvis and thighs. In some hospitals a specially devised hammock-bed is used. As a rule, union of good strength is obtained in the severed joint, though it seems that, in a considerable proportion of the cases, there remains an appreciable increase in the size of the pelvis. While this does not seriously interfere with locomotion, it doubtless impairs to some degree the endurance of the woman. Injuries to the urethra and vagina are not uncommon, and require surgical repair later.

The maternal mortality of this operation in skilled hands is from five to eight per cent, with a fœtal mortality of at least ten per cent. From this it is apparent that the operation is inferior to the Cæsarean section so far as the mortality rate is concerned, and, when the prompt convalescence and perfect recovery of the patient in the latter operation are taken into consideration, the section is to be preferred. As a result of these facts, symphyseotomy has passed into disuse, being for the most part superseded by Cæsarean section and, in a small proportion of cases, by pubiotomy.

Pubiotomy.—This operation, known also as hebotomy, is based upon the same principles as symphyseotomy, with the important difference that the pubic bone is divided in its continuity on one side of the symphysis and that joint is not involved in the operation. It has the additional advantage that the incision is not in close proximity to the urethra and bladder, and hence injury to those structures occurs less frequently. This operation was recommended by Gigli, in 1893, and the bone is divided with the saw which bears his name. It is only since 1901 that the operation has been widely practised.

Operative Technique.—The preparation and position of the patient are the same as already described for symphyseotomy. With Gigli's method of operating the anterior surface of the bone was exposed by incision, but in 1904 Doederlein modified the operation by dividing the bone subcutaneously. This modification has been very generally adopted. An incision large enough to admit the index finger is made just above and parallel to the pubic bone on the left side, near the pubic spine. After the tissues have been divided down to the bone, the finger is passed into the wound and is made to separate the soft tissues from the bone. The periosteum is then incised with a blunt-pointed knife. A curved artery forceps, somewhat stronger than the average, is passed along the posterior surface of the bone until its tip end can be felt through the outer edge of the labium majus. There is now made, over the tip end of the forceps, a counter-opening which will permit its protrusion through the skin. The saw is next caught with the forceps and its end drawn out through the first incision. The saw will then lie behind and in contact with the bone. After the handles have been attached, the bone can be divided with a few strokes of the saw. When the saw is withdrawn, there will be some hemorrhage from the incisions, but this is readily controlled by gauze pressure. As a rule, the severed ends of bone separate to a distance of from 2 to 3 centimetres as soon as the saw is withdrawn, but sometimes this is prevented by the adjacent soft structures. The desired separation, however, will occur when traction upon the child is applied.

Should active hemorrhage occur from abnormal distribution of branches of the internal pudic artery, the entire wound should be laid open and the bleeding vessel secured. Should a large hæmatoma form later, it may become necessary to lay open the wound.

After the delivery is completed, the wound is dressed simply, and the bandage applied as previously described. A broad strip of adhesive plaster may also be first applied so as to make pressure over the pelvis.

Injuries to the urethra and lacerations of the vagina occur much less frequently in the course of this operation than in symphyseotomy. The union of the ends of the divided bone is usually strong, though it is perhaps more frequently fibrous than bony. The maternal mortality after this operation is about 2.5 per cent, as shown by reports of large numbers of cases. J. Whitridge Williams has reported twenty-five cases with no maternal, and three fœtal, deaths, only one of the latter being attributable to the operation.

The indications for pubiotomy are a living child and a moderate degree of contraction of the pelvis. It is especially applicable to the "border-line" cases in which it is necessary to test the second stage of labor in order to know that the head cannot pass the superior strait. In cases in which there is a moderate degree of pelvic contraction which has not been recognized beforehand,—cases in which labor has advanced and attempted instrumental delivery has failed,—pubiotomy may advantageously be applied in preference to the Cæsarean section.

PART XVII

THE LAW IN ITS RELATIONS TO THE PRACTICE OF SURGERY.

THE CIVIL OBLIGATION OF SURGEON AND PATIENT IN THE PRACTICE OF AMERICAN SURGERY.

By STEPHEN SMITH. M.D., LL.D., New York,

and

SIDNEY SMITH, LL.B., of the New York Bar.

I. **The Civil Obligation.**—ORIGIN OF THE CIVIL OBLIGATION.*—The civil obligation which the surgeon assumes when he undertakes the practice of the art of surgery, may be traced to remote antiquity, and its development has been along the lines of progress in the organization of civil government.

The first recorded method of treatment of the sick consisted in exposing them in public places in order that any passer-by, who had been affected with a similar disease and had been cured by some special remedy, could give the sufferer the benefit of his experience. At a later period those who had been cured of diseases were required to deposit in the temples where the sick more often gathered, a votive tablet, which contained a detailed account of the symptoms of their respective ailments, and a minute statement of the remedial agents which proved most beneficial. The collection of votive tablets in the temples became popular as records of a great variety of diseases which the sick could consult with the certainty that each would find his own case described and the appropriate remedy prescribed.

In the course of time it became apparent that the right and privilege accorded to every one to examine these records, and select remedies for his own disease, or that of an absent friend, were liable to great abuses. Too often the records were misinterpreted and remedies were misapplied to the detriment of the sick.

To correct this evil and preserve the useful features of the ancient custom, the records were withdrawn from public scrutiny, and placed in the exclusive charge and control of the priests of the temples. Thereafter the sick related their symptoms to these temple officials who recorded them in due form, and, after consulting the records, prescribed the appropriate remedies.

It naturally followed that, as the priests had the entire control of all the recorded facts and experiences in regard to the nature and treatment of the diseases of the people, they monopolized the practice of the art of medicine and surgery. This reform was a great advance in the progress of scientific medicine, for it not only secured greater accuracy of the records of the diseases

---

* Free use has been made, throughout this article, of the reports of medico-legal trials published from time to time in the Journal of the American Medical Association. (See also the Note printed at the end of this article.)—THE AUTHORS.

reported, but the treatment of the sick was more exactly in accordance with experience.

DEVELOPMENT OF THE CIVIL OBLIGATIONS.—In time these records became very voluminous and difficult of reference, and to simplify their use they were reduced to a system by collating the facts in the form of a code of practice. At a still later period these records, revised and collated, were regarded of such public importance as to be published under the title of "The Sacred Book." This book was the undeviating guide to medical practice for centuries, and some of its aphorisms have come down to our times. In that early period the practitioner who departed from its precepts did so at the peril of his life. All questions of practice were determined by this code and every violation of its sacred aphorisms was punishable with death.

It is not surprising that this code of rules governing the practice of the medical art was regarded with such veneration. It embodied the aggregate experience of centuries, being a faithful transcript of the phenomena of all known diseases, and the only guide to the proper use of remedies. It was a book of facts without a theory; a record of the unchangeable laws of nature in all that pertained to disease and its cure. To doubt its sacred precepts was an inexcusable heresy, and to violate them in practice was a criminal offence, punishable with the severest penalty in the penal code.

The influence of the "Sacred Book' can be traced through all subsequent ages. Nations have established standards of practice by which the civil responsibilities of those who publicly assume the functions of practisers of medicine and surgery can be judicially determined. These codes of laws are in accord with good public policy, as they are intended, as was the "Sacred Book," for the protection of the people against mere pretenders to a competent knowledge of the science and art of medicine. It is still held, nearly in the language of the ancient text, that any deviation from the recognized principles and methods of practice shall be deemed sufficient to charge the surgeon with malpractice in case of an injury arising to the patient. (Espinasse.) While this rule is designed to protect the patient from reckless experiments, it admits the adoption of new remedies and modes of treatment when their benefits have been demonstrated, or when, from the necessities of the case, the surgeon is left to the exercise of his own skill and experience. Carpenter vs. Blake, 60 Barb. (N. Y.), 488.

THE PRINCIPLE OF THE CIVIL OBLIGATION.—The principle upon which the civil obligation of the practiser of medicine was established by the ancients, was the standard of practice contained in the "Sacred Book." In effect, the obligation had as its fundamental principle the standard of practice of recognized authority at the time and place where the act was performed. Following this precedent all civilized governments have fixed as the basis of the obligation of the practiser of an art, the methods of procedure recognized and approved by competent authority at the time and place where the event occurred. By a standard of practice we understand that which is set up as a unit of reference; a form, type, example, instance, or combination of conditions accepted as correct; and hence as a basis of comparison; a criterion established by custom, public opinion, or general consent. (Century Dictionary.)

Some standard must be adopted by which to estimate the value and quality of the surgical treatment under consideration, otherwise experiments will take the place of skill, and the reckless experimentalists the place of the educated, experienced practiser. (Carpenter *vs.* Blake, *supra.*) But it is very evident that no kind of standard can have permanent value as a just criterion established by custom, public opinion, or general consent, for art is progressive and the principles which govern its practice must change from time to time with the advance of science and experience. These changes take place gradually, however, for alleged new truths do not establish a standard until they have received the approval of recognized authority in the particular department of science to which they are applicable. In order, therefore, to determine the standard of practice in surgery in any given case, it is necessary to consult the opinions of its acknowledged authorities and public exponents at the particular time, and in places similar to that, in question. On this fundamental legal principle rest the civil obligations and responsibilities of the Surgeon in the practice of his art.

II. Definition of " Surgeon," and the " Practice of Surgery."—SURGEON AND THE PRACTICE OF SURGERY DEFINED.—In European countries the term "Surgeon ' is applied to one who by education qualifies himself for the exclusive practice of manual operations on patients. In England, from which we have chiefly derived our professional customs, medical and surgical practitioners are distinguished by special titles. In this country the two branches of practice are not separated by any artificial distinctions. The terms "Physician" and "Surgeon" have been defined as follows: "A Physician is one who is versed in medical science, a branch of which is surgery, and a Surgeon is a Physician who treats bodily injuries and ills by manual operations and the use of surgical instruments and appliances." This is not only a proper definition of the terms, "Physician" and "Surgeon," in common parlance, but it places the two branches of medicine, as practised in the United States, in their true relations. While in the larger cities both medicine and surgery are in some degree practised as specialties, the great mass of physicians in this country are required to be versed in both branches of the medical sciences in order to be able to meet the emergencies of the communities which they serve. Recognizing this necessity, the statutes of some States define a physician as a person skilled in both medicine and surgery.

THE PRACTICE OF MEDICINE AND SURGERY.—If the definition of the word "Physician" includes the word "Surgeon," the definition of the phrase "The Practice of Medicine" must necessarily include that of "The Practice of Surgery," as understood and practised in this country. Accordingly, legislatures include both branches of practice under the one title, "The Practice of Medicine and Surgery," and in the details of the several provisions, the special methods of treatment by the Surgeon are included. The courts have held that the construction to be placed upon the phrase "The practice of Medicine and Surgery" must depend upon whether the statute of the State defines the phrase. When the statute does define the phrase, it is held that the courts of that State must define the meaning of the words in accordance with the statute and not place their own construction upon them, but in cases where the legislatures have not undertaken to define the meaning of the phrase it has been construed to be used in its ordinary and popular sense. The Supreme Court of Arkansas held, on appeal, that the trial court erred in giving its own meaning to these words, and in not defining them within the meaning of the statute of that State. Foo Lun *vs.* State Ark., 106 S. W. Rep., 946.

III. The Relation of Surgeon and Patient Must Exist to Constitute the Obligation.—The Surgeon May Accept or Decline Service.—The Surgeon is not under obligation to undertake the care of any person. (J. Ordronaux; J. J. Elwell.) He may accept or decline the service, however emergent the case may be. Wharton says, "No question can exist as to the legal right of a physician, unless he be an officer of government charged with specific duties which he thereby violates, to decline to take charge of a particular case." * It has been claimed that in extreme cases of emergency the Surgeon is under obligation to attend the patient, but the Courts have not sustained the contention. The Supreme Court of Indiana in a recent case of the arbitrary refusal of a physician to attend a sick person who died, as it was alleged, because the services of a physician could not be obtained, held that the act regulating the practice of medicine in that State "is a preventive, not a compulsory, measure. In obtaining the State license to practise medicine, the State does not require, and the licensee does not engage, that he will practise at all, or on other terms than he may choose." Hurrley Admr. *vs.* Eddingfield, 156 Ind., 416.

A similar case was recently tried in a court of France which gave the following opinion: "While the law of 1892 provides in a general way that every physician must respond to the requisitions of justice, a physician is absolutely free to refuse his services to any person whomsoever." (Dabon's case.)

The Obligation on Accepting Service Personal.—When the Surgeon actually undertakes the treatment of the patient the relation of Surgeon and patient is acknowledged and mutual obligations are established either in express or implied terms. On assuming the care of the patient the Surgeon is alone responsible for the details of treatment. Neither the attending physician who had charge, nor the consulting Surgeon who aids by counsel, assumes any responsibility for the treatment of the patient, unless they are professionally associated with him in the actual treatment of the case. If a Surgeon commences treatment and is discharged and another Surgeon assumes the treatment the former would be held responsible only for his own conduct, and not for those who succeeded him in the management of the case. Wood *vs.* Clapp, 4 Snead [Tenn. R.], 65.

The Consulting Surgeon not in the Relation of Surgeon and Patient. —The proper function of the Consulting Surgeon is to advise the Attending

* Wharton on Negligence (2d ed.), Sec. 731.

Surgeon and then retire from all connection with the case. The Attending Surgeon may accept the Consultant's advice and adopt the course of treatment which he recommends, when it becomes his own method for which he alone is responsible; or he may reject the advice altogether and pursue any other line of treatment according to the dictates of his own experience and judgment. The Consulting Surgeon assumes no liability for the results of the treatment which he recommends, as he has no part in its application, and hence does not sustain the relation of surgeon and patient as to such treatment.

SURGEON RESPONSIBLE FOR THE ACT OF HIS AGENT.—In Hancke vs. Cooper, 7 Carr & P., 81, a suit for alleged malpractice in venesection, it appeared that the operation was performed by the senior apprentice in the Surgeon's office. Inflammation of the wound followed with swelling of the arm. In reviewing the evidence, Tyndale, C. J., charged the jury that "The defendant is responsible for the act of his apprentice; therefore, the question is, whether you think the injury the plaintiff has sustained is attributable to a want of proper skill on the part of the young man, or to some accident. A Surgeon does not become an actual insurer; he is only bound to display sufficient skill and knowledge of his profession. If from some accident, or some variation in the frame of a particular individual, an injury happens, it is not a fault in the medical man. . . . The plaintiff must show that the injury was attributable to want of skill; you are not to infer it. If there were no indications in the plaintiff's appearance that bleeding would be improper, the defendant would not be liable for the bleeding not effecting the same results as at other times; because it might depend upon the constitution of the plaintiff. . . . The question is whether you think the plaintiff has proved that the injury resulted from the inexperience or want of previous knowledge on the part of the defendant's young man; if you do not, you will find your verdict for the defendant; if you do, you will find your verdict for the plaintiff, and give him such reasonable damages as you think him entitled to under all circumstances." There was a verdict for defendant.

The rule of law set forth in this decision is based on the elementary legal principle that one who acts through another acts for himself, but the evidence must establish the fact and relationship of agency.

LIABILITY OF PARTNERS IN THE PRACTICE OF SURGERY.—It is a principle of of law that copartners are generally responsible for the acts of each other, in the particular business of the copartnership. The application of this principle to copartnerships in the practice of surgery is defined in the case of Hyrne vs. Erwin et al., 23 S. C., 226, by the Supreme Court of South Carolina, as follows: "The law applicable to such cases, as we understand it, is the same as that which obtains in the general doctrine of agency; it applies, too, in the relation of master and servant, and like cases. It is this: In a partnership the parties associated are, in one sense, agents of each other, and the act of one within the scope of the partnership or business is the act of each and all, as fully so as if each was present and participating in all that is done. And each guarantees that within the scope of the common business reasonable care, diligence, and skill shall be displayed by the one in charge. Or at least that a failure on the part of one thus to exercise such reasonable care, diligence, and skill is a failure in law of each and all, and an injury resulting from such failure is the act of all. Where, however, the injury results from a wanton or wilful act of one of the parties committed outside of the agency or common business, and not from negligence or failure to bestow reasonable care, diligence, and skill within the agency, then a different principle applies, viz., that the party doing the act and causing the injury is alone responsible—the distinction between two cases growing out of the fact that the relation which the party doing the act bears to the others, is different in one case from the other. In the first his act being within the scope of the business, he acts both for himself and as agent for the others. In the other his act, being beyond and outside of the scope of the business, he acts for himself." *

THERE MUST BE A PREPONDERANCE OF EVIDENCE OF JOINT UNDERTAKING. —In Lower vs. Franks et al., 115 Ind., 334, it was held by the Supreme Court of Judicature of Indiana that, "Under the complaint, it must be shown by a preponderance of the evidence that the undertaking or contract was made jointly with both of the defendants for treating the limb. Such a contract may be implied from the conversations and conduct of the parties, and circumstances of the case, as well as by an express agreement. And, if you should find from the evidence that the defendants jointly undertook to treat the limb, each would be responsible for the acts of the other in treating the limb, and you would be warranted in finding against both the defendants if the evidence shows that any injury or damage resulted from the want of care or skill on the part of either or both defendants. On the other hand, if you should find that, by an express agreement or from the conversation and conduct of the parties and the circumstances of the case, as shown by the evidence, that the undertaking was separate on the part of each defendant, then each would only be responsible for his own acts in treating said limb and not answerable for the acts of the other."

SURGEON NOT LIABLE FOR ACTS OF AN INDEPENDENT PRACTISER.—The relation of the Surgeon in attendance to an independent practiser, whom he sends or recommends to his patient, has been much contested in the courts. It has been urged that the Surgeon holds the same relation to one whom he sends or recommends, though the latter is an independent practiser and may employ his own methods of treatment, as he holds to a partner or to an appointed agent. The decision of the court in the following case judicially determined this controverted question. Myres vs. Holborn, 53 N. J. Law, 193. Dr. M. engaged to attend the plaintiff's wife at her confinement. While the doctor was absent from home the event took place and Dr. P. attended the patient, representing Dr. M. In caring for the child Dr. P. severed the umbilical cord so close to the body that it was impossible to tie it, in consequence of which the infant died of hemorrhage. An action was brought against Dr. M., but the Court of Appeals of New Jersey, in the following opinion, held that there was no liabil-

* Am. and Eng. Ency. of Law, 2d ed., vol. 22, p. 805.

ity on the part of Dr. M.: "Dr. P. and the defendant were each of them prac-tising physicians of this State, having no business connections with one an-other, except that Dr. P. was attending the patients of the latter while he was temporarily absent. Even if it be admitted, therefore, that Dr. P. was em-ployed by the defendant to attend upon the wife of the plaintiff, that fact did not render the defendant liable for his neglect or want of skill in the perform-ance of this service, for an examination of the authorities will show that a party employing a person who follows a distinct and independent occupa-tion of his own is not responsible for the neglect or improper acts of the other."

EXAMINATION OF PATIENT WITHOUT TREATMENT MAY ESTABLISH THE RELA-TION OF SURGEON AND PATIENT.—The Supreme Court of Missouri held that it is not necessary in order to create the relation of Surgeon and patient that he should actually treat the patient. If the Surgeon makes an examination of the patient with the knowledge and consent of the latter, who believes that the examination is being made for the purpose of treatment, then the relation of Surgeon and patient is created by implication, and it is wholly immaterial what may have been the secret object of the examination. Smart *vs.* Kansas City, 105 S. W. Rep., 709.

A SURGEON DULY APPOINTED TO A HOSPITAL HOLDS THE RELATION OF SUR-GEON TO EACH PATIENT, ADMITTED FOR TREATMENT, OF WHOM HE ASSUMES THE CARE, EITHER PERSONALLY OR THROUGH HIS SUBORDINATES.—In discuss-ing the competency of two Surgeons as witnesses in the case of a patient treated in the hospital with which they were officially connected, the Supreme Court of Missouri says: "They were assistant surgeons in the hospital where the plain-tiff was taken for treatment, and they assisted in the treatment and amputation of the leg. Under and by virtue of their appointment, contract, or by what-ever arrangement they became assistant physicians in that hospital, that con-stituted them the physician and surgeon of each and every patient who entered that institution for treatment, and they had no legal or moral right or author-ity to view, treat, or operate on any of them, except by virtue of that appoint-ment or contract. Even their very presence there was traceable to and author-ized by that authority and none other. The relation of physician and patient is one of contract either expressed or implied, and can be treated in no other way. In cases of this character, the physician or surgeon, in accepting such a position, impliedly at least, agrees to treat such patients as are accepted into the institution, and when he assumes to examine them either by their express agreement, or by their implied or tacit consent, which may be inferred from the act of entrance into the institution, and which will be inferred in the absence of evidence indicating a contrary intention, the relationship of Sur-geon and patient is established. The same rule of law applies as fully and effectually to the assistant physicians and surgeons as it does to the physician or surgeon-in-chief." (Smart *vs.* Kansas City, *supra.*)

ASSISTING IN APPLYING DRESSINGS CONSTITUTES THE RELATION OF SUR-GEON AND PATIENT.—In Moran *vs.* Burnham, Mass., it was shown that the plaintiff had fractured his leg above and below the knee. The defendant was sent for, but, not being in town, a physician who rented a part of his office, reduced the fracture and dressed the limb with the assistance of another physician. The defendant was again sent for and requested to take charge of the case, but he declined on the grounds, 1, that the patient was not his; 2, because he had engagements out of the State for two weeks; and, 3, he was too sick to undertake such a case. He was then requested to assist in applying splints and bandages, to which he assented and did aid in the application of different dressings, using great care in readjusting the limb and making accurate measurements. The case was then left in the care of the physician, but eight days after, at his request, the defendant assisted in applying clean dressings. The defendant did not see the patient again for about eight weeks, the physician being in constant attendance. At the end of two and a half months it was found that the fracture was not united. The surgeons were discharged and subsequently the patient was operated upon in the Massachusetts General Hospital and recovered with a union of the bones, but with a much shortened limb. An action was begun against defendant for malpractice. The Supreme Court of Massachusetts held that the jury had two questions to consider: 1st, Was defendant retained and employed by the plaintiff? and, 2d, If so, was there any want of proper care and skill on his part in the management or treatment of the case by which the plaintiff had suffered damage? The Court ruled that defendant was retained and employed by the plaintiff and was responsible for the treatment throughout the whole time, and that the evidence showed no want of proper care and skill in the management of the treatment of the case. The verdict was in favor of the defendant.

This decision has been referred to as showing the liability of the Consulting Surgeon for the act of the Attending Surgeon. But this is a mistaken view of the facts. Though the defendant may have been called as a consultant he did not merely perform the duties of that office, which were simply to advise as to the treatment and then retire, leaving the attending surgeon to accept or reject his advice as his judgment might dictate; but he proceeded to direct and personally assist in the treatment and thus established the relation of Surgeon and patient, and became liable for the errors of treatment. The opinion of the court that defendant was "retained and employed" by the plaintiff rests on his consent, at the request of the patient, to assist at first in applying "different dressings," which he did, "using great care in readjusting the limb and making accurate measurements," according to his own statement. Eight days later, at the request of the attending physician, he assisted in applying "clean dressings," thus again assuming the relations of Surgeon and patient.

STATUS OF SURGEON WHEN SERVICES ARE REFUSED BY PATIENT.—In Meyer vs. Supreme Lodge Knights of Pythias, 178 N. Y., 63, the patient was in extremis and incapable of acting for himself, and a physician was called without his knowledge or consent to treat him. The patient ordered the physician to leave the room, saying that he did not want him, but he did not leave and remained to treat him as a physician. In order to treat him intelligently the physician sought information as to the nature of his illness and learned, partly through voluntary disclosures in answer to questions, and partly from observations of the physical symptoms, that the patient was suffering from arsenical poisoning. Thus informed the physician administered remedies. The patient objected and cursed the physician, ordering him from his bedside, but the latter refused to listen to the ravings of the would-be suicide, and continued to prescribe in order to relieve suffering and prolong life. The Court of Appeals of New York held that in all the physician did he acted in a professional capacity, even though it was done against the will and in spite of the remonstrance of the patient. When one who is sick unto death is in fact treated by a physician as a patient, even against his will, he becomes the patient of the physician by operation of law. The same is true of one who is unconscious and unable to speak for himself.

RESPONDING TO A CALL DOES NOT NECESSARILY CONSTITUTE EMPLOYMENT. —In Miller vs. Dumon, 24 Wash., 648, a Surgeon was called to a case of alleged fracture of the leg which one Dr. F. had been treating for ten or twelve days. On examination he decided that there was no fracture and retired from the case. Subsequently the patient began to use the limb, and while doing so the leg gave way in some manner, causing the patient much pain and suffering, and compelling him again to take to his bed. The Surgeon was sent for, but did not answer the call. The final result was a permanent injury to the patient's leg and an action for malpractice was commenced against Dr. D. The question as to the existence of the relation of Surgeon and patient was decided in the following instruction of the trial court to the jury which was sustained by the Supreme Court of the State: "The court instructs you that the fact that a physician responds to a call for his professional services does not necessarily constitute an employment unless some act is doné or advice given by the physician which indicates an intention on his part to enter upon the employment. He may absolutely refuse this employment if he sees fit. But when any act is done, or advice given, that may reasonably be construed into indicating an active entering upon the employment, then the liability of the physician attaches, and he may be held responsible for his negligence or lack of skill." Judgment was for the plaintiff which upon appeal was affirmed.

IV. The Civil Obligation a Contract.—THE CONTRACT DEFINED.—Blackstone defines a contract as "An agreement upon a sufficient consideration to do or not to do a particular thing." The contractural nature of the services of the surgeon is of modern construction, as formerly these services were gratuitous. Ordronaux says, "This doubtless reduces professions to the status of artisanships, and places them on a par with manual labor, conjoined to the special skill of a particular calling." The terms of this agreement may be expressed in writing or verbally, when it is called an *express* contract, or there may be no written or verbal form and no conditions specified under which the Surgeon assumes the treatment of the patient, but the relations of the parties to each other is such that the law recognizes by implication the existence of a valid agreement between them, known as an *implied* contract. The failure of Surgeons to realize the existence of the obligations of a contract whenever they assume the treatment of a case has often resulted in the neglect of details in its management that might readily have been avoided. This neglect becomes the basis of an action for malpractice. So much importance has latterly been attached to the contract as a protection against prosecutions, that Surgeons have been advised to adopt the practice of artisans, and in all severe and complicated cases make attendance contingent upon an express contract, written and signed.

THE EXPRESS CONTRACT.—This form of contract may consist of a written agreement in which all of the mutual obligations of the parties are determined and specified and to which their names are affixed. Such a contract is necessarily definite and precise in its terms and not liable to be misconstrued. Or the express contract may be oral, the terms being formulated verbally between the parties, either alone or in the presence of witnesses. Such an agreement is far less reliable than the written contract when its terms are contested in the courts, owing to the fallibility of the human understanding and memory of verbal transactions.

TERMS OF THE EXPRESS CONTRACT LIMITED BY PUBLIC POLICY.—While the terms of the express contract may include a great variety of details as to the obligations of the patient and Surgeon during the period of the attendance of the latter upon the former in a professional capacity, there are limitations to be observed when they conflict with public policy. The express contract may stipulate that the compensation of the Surgeon shall be contingent upon his effecting a cure, Smith *vs.* Hyde, 19 Vt., 54; Coughlin *vs.* N. Y. Cent. R. R. Co., 71 N. Y., 443; it may contain conditions relating to certain acts to be performed at certain times; it may provide that no other surgeon shall be employed without the consent of the one in attendance. But the Surgeon cannot stipulate that he shall not be held responsible for want of ordinary skill, for it would be against public policy if Surgeons were permitted "to contract for a release or escape from a liability rising out of their own negligence or wrong." (Becker.)

CONTRACT TO PERFORM AN IMPOSSIBLE ACT.—A further limitation to the terms of the contract occurs when the question of the impossibility of performing the act becomes an issue. According to Elwell * the Surgeon who contracts to do a thing that is absolutely impossible at the time of making such contract is not bound thereby, because no man can be compelled to perform an impossible act. But a distinction is made between a contract to perform an act which is accidentally impossible, and one which is absolutely impossible. In the former case the contract is binding notwithstanding it was beyond the power of the party to perform it, for it was his own fault that he did not provide against contingencies which he should have known might possibly occur. The performance, therefore, is not excused by the occurrence of an inevitable accident, though it was not foreseen by the party, nor within his power to control.†

THE IMPLIED CONTRACT.—Whoever undertakes to practise an art or pro-

* Malpractice & Medical Evidence, p. 20.   † Chitty on Contracts (Eighth Am. ed.), pp. 629, 630.

fession assumes an obligation, both civil and professional, which though implied, has all the force and validity of a formal contract. (Tyndall.) The obligations of the Surgeon under this form of contract have been variously defined by the courts, but the following judicial decision by the Supreme Court of New Hampshire concisely sets forth its principal features: "His contract, as implied in law, is, that (1) He possesses that reasonable degree of learning, skill, and experience ordinarily possessed by others of his profession; (2) That he will use reasonable and ordinary care and diligence in the treatment of the case committed to him; (3) That he will use his best judgment in all cases of doubt as to the best course of treatment." Leighton *vs.* Sargeant, 7 Foster (N. H.), 460.

CONTRACT UNALTERED WHEN SERVICES ARE GRATUITOUS.—The defence in suits for malpractice where the patient has been a charity case has been that the service on the part of the Surgeon was gratuitous, and hence that he should not be held to the same degree of responsibility. The courts uniformly rule that if a person holds himself out as a physician or Surgeon he must be held to ordinary care and skill in every case of which he assumes the charge, whether in the particular case he has received fees or not. McNevins *vs.* Lowe, 40 Ill., 209.

Justice Pryor, in an instruction to a jury in a case arising in the State of New York, thus forcibly explained the position of the courts when this question is before them: "It appears that the plaintiff was a charity patient; that the defendant was treating her gratuitously. But I charge you that this fact in no way qualifies the liability of the defendant. Whether the patient be a pauper or a millionaire, whether he be treated gratuitously or for a reward, the physician owes him precisely the same measure of duty and the same degree of skill and care. He may decline to respond to the call of a patient unable to compensate him; but if he undertakes the treatment of such a patient he cannot defeat a suit for malpractice nor mitigate a recovery against him upon the principle that the skill and care required of a physician are proportioned to his expectation of pecuniary recompense. Such a rule would be of the most mischievous consequence, would make the health and life of the indigent the sport of reckless experiment and cruel indifference." Becker *vs.* Janinski, 27 Abb. N. C. (N. Y.), 45.

V. The Obligation of Surgeon to Patient.—THE SURGEON MUST HAVE COMPETENT KNOWLEDGE OF THE SCIENCE AND ART OF SURGERY.—Discoveries in the natural sciences for the last half-century have exerted a sensible influence on all of the learned professions, but especially on that of surgery, the principles and practice of which have been relatively much enlarged through the studies and experiments of its professors. The patient is entitled to the benefits which the latest improvements in the practice of surgery would secure to him. The Surgeon who would not be found wanting in the emergencies of practice must apply himself with all diligence to the most accredited sources of knowledge. McCandless *vs.* McWha, 22 Penn. St., 261. The degree of learning and knowledge which the law requires is designated as "proper," "ordinary," "reasonable," and not "highest" nor "thorough." Regard must be had to the advanced state of surgical science, to the school of practice to which the surgeon belongs, and to the locality where he practises surgery, as will be further explained.

To insure the proper educational qualifications of Surgeons and physicians the laws of many States provide standards of medical education and boards of examiners, and licenses to practise are issued to those who pass a successful examination, and penalties are inflicted upon those who practise without a license. The possession of a diploma, or some other evidence of a proper knowledge of the medical sciences, should be required of every man who sets himself up as a "Doctor in Medicine," to treat diseases, or to act as an expert in a court of law where questions of skill in medicine and surgery are in issue. Courtney vs. Henderson, Marine Court of New York. The diploma of the college from which he graduated is the best proof of the Surgeon's education in his profession, but to be valid it must be proved that the college from which it emanated had corporate authority to grant degrees in medicine at the date of giving the degree, and, if the college of another State, its act of incorporation must be offered as proof of its authority to grant such a degree.*

THE SURGEON MUST HAVE THE REQUIRED DEGREE OF SKILL.—There has been much confusion in the opinions given on this question in the trial courts. Juries have been instructed that the Surgeon is bound to have such a degree of skill as will enable him to make a fractured limb "straight and of equal length with the other" (McCandless vs. McWha, supra); that the skill required must be "proportionate to the severity of the injury or disease," Utley vs. Burns, 70 Ill., 162; that reasonable skill is such as is ordinarily exercised by "thoroughly educated surgeons," Smothers vs. Hanks, 34 Iowa, 266. These instructions have been disapproved by the higher courts which have adopted rulings in accordance with the following opinion of Story.† ". . . In all of these cases where skill is required, it is to be understood that it means ordinary skill in the business or employment which the bailee undertakes; for he is not presumed to engage for extraordinary skill, which belongs to a few men only in his business or employment, or for extraordinary endowments or acquirements. Reasonable skill constitutes the measure of the engagement in regard to the thing undertaken."

This opinion is in accord with the leading English decision by Chief Justice Tyndall, which is as follows: "Every person who enters into a learned profession undertakes to bring to the exercise of it a reasonable degree of care and skill. He does not, if he is an attorney, undertake at all events to gain the cause, nor does a surgeon undertake that he will perform a cure; nor does the latter undertake to use the highest possible degree of skill, as there may be persons of higher education and greater advantages than himself; but he undertakes to bring a fair, reasonable, and competent degree of skill. And in an action against him by a patient, the question for the jury is whether the

---

* McClelland's Civil Malpractice; A Treatise on Surgical Jurisprudence, New York, 1877.
† Story on Bailments (5th ed.), p. 433.

injury complained of must be referred to a want of proper degree of skill and care in the defendant, or not. Hence he is never presumed to engage for extraordinary skill, or for extraordinary diligence and care. As a general rule he who undertakes for a reward to perform any work is bound to use a degree of diligence, attention, and skill adequate to the performance of his undertaking; that is, to do it according to the rules of art. . . . And the degree of skill rises in proportion to the value and delicacy of the operation. But he is in no case required to have more than ordinary skill, for he does not engage for more." Lamphier vs. Phipos, 8 C. & P., 478.

The doctrine more generally adopted in the decisions of the courts is thus stated: * "Although a physician or surgeon may doubtless by express contract undertake to perform a cure absolutely, the law will not imply such a contract from the mere employment of a physician. A physician is not a warrantor or insurer of a cure, and is not to be tried for the results of his remedies. His only contract is to treat the case with reasonable diligence and skill. If more than this is expected, it must be expressly stipulated for. . . . The general rule, therefore, is, that a medical man, who attends for a fee, is liable for such a want of ordinary care, diligence, or skill on his part as leads to the injury of his patient. To render him liable it is not enough that there has been a less degree of skill than some other medical man might have shown, or a less degree of care than even he himself might have bestowed; nor is it enough that he himself acknowledged some degree of want of care; there must have been a want of competent and ordinary care and skill, and to such a degree as to have led to a bad result. . . . But a professed physician or surgeon is bound to use not only such skill as he has, but to have a reasonable degree of skill. The law will not countenance quackery; and although the law does not require the most thorough education or the largest experience, it does require that an uneducated, ignorant man shall not, under the pretence of being a well-qualified physician, attempt recklessly and blindly to administer medicines or perform surgical operations. If the practitioner, however, frankly informs his patient of his want of skill, or the patient is in some other way fully aware of it, the latter cannot complain of the lack of that which he knew did not exist."

IF SURGEON CONTINUES TREATMENT HE MAY BE LIABLE FOR RESULTS.— If, however, the Surgeon continues in attendance upon the patient after he has declared his want of skill he may be held liable for unfavorable results. In Lorenz vs. Jackson, 88 Hun (N. Y.), 200, the plaintiff was struck by a fragment of steel which embedded itself in his left leg above the knee. He called Dr. J., who announced that the wound was of a serious nature and character, and that he did not regard himself as sufficiently experienced in surgery properly to treat the case, and advised that the services of a more skilled surgeon be secured. Pursuant to this advice Dr. B. was employed, the patient was removed to a table, and ether was administered by Dr. J., while Dr. B. probed for the piece of steel, widening the wound in the limb, and thereafter applied

* Shearman and Redfield, On the Law of Negligence, 5th ed. §§ 605–607.

bandages. **Dr. J.** remained with the patient through the night and administered to him hypodermic injections of morphine and atropia. This treatment continued for several days, until about the eighth day after the injuries were received, when it was found that dry gangrene had ensued. Another physician was then called, and it was finally determined that the limb must be amputated. An action was commenced against Dr. J. and Dr. B., and a verdict of three thousand dollars rendered. Dr. J. appealed from the judgment entered upon this verdict. The General Term of the Supreme Court decided, after referring to the rule mentioned above, as follows: "During the charge the trial judge recognized the rule stated in the citations just made, and carefully instructed the jury in respect thereto, and afforded the jury an opportunity to relieve the appellant from liability by the application of the rule if, in the judgment of the jury, the facts and circumstances disclosed by the evidence warranted its application. It must be assumed that the verdict of the jury, in regard to the branch of the case referred to, in the rule of law just mentioned, was found adversely to the appellant." The opinion also stated that after weighing the evidence which was very conflicting, the court was constrained to follow the rule that, unless the verdict is "against the clear weight of the evidence," it will not·be disturbed and the judgment against Dr. J. was therefore affirmed.

DEGREE OF SKILL AND CARE A MIXED QUESTION OF LAW AND FACT.—Becker * states that, "What constitutes reasonable care and skill is a mixed question of law and fact, like any other question of negligence. Where the evidence is undisputed and no conflicting inferences can be drawn from the facts presented, it is the duty of the court to determine whether or not there is sufficient proof of want of ordinary care and skill to be submitted to the jury. Where, however, the evidence is conflicting on that point, or the inferences to be drawn from the facts established might be differently drawn by different men having the same opportunity for observation, and the same circumstances before them, it is for the jury to say whether or not the defendant has exercised reasonable care and skill, guided by proper directions from the court as to the measure of skill required."

SURGEON MUST EXERCISE HIS BEST SKILL AND JUDGMENT.—In Patten *vs.* Wiggin, 51 Me., 594, it was held that the essence of the contract of the Surgeon with his patient as regards the employment of the skill which he possesses is that "he is to do his best—to yield to the use and service of his patient his best knowledge, skill, and judgment, with faithful attention by day and night as reasonably required, ... if he exercises his best skill and judgment with care and careful observation of the case, he is not responsible for an honest mistake of the nature of the disease, or as to the best mode of treatment, when there was reasonable ground for doubt or uncertainty." When a Surgeon is employed in difficult and emergent cases on account of his assumed or reputed high grade of knowledge and skill, he must bestow them to the full measure of his ability because his exceptional degree of knowledge and skill is the

* Med. Jurisp., Forensic Med., and Tox., vol. i., p. 83.

moving consideration to his employment.* If a case presents such complications that no recognized mode of treatment of any one of the conditions present will meet the exigencies of the case, the Surgeon is confronted with the requirement that "in all cases where there is room for doubt he must use his best judgment; . . . if he is possessed of proper skill, and, in the careful exercise of his best judgment, errs, such error will not involve him in legal liability." DuBois *vs.* Decker, 130 N. Y., 323. When, however, the case is one that involves doubt as to its nature and treatment, and the Surgeon does not believe that he is competent to treat it properly, it becomes his duty to advise the patient that he may secure the services of another surgeon. Pepke *vs.* Grace Hospital [Mich.], 90 N. W. Rep., 278; Jackson *vs.* Burnham, 1 Colo. App., 237.

BEST JUDGMENT ORDINARILY NO DEFENCE FOR NEGLIGENCE.—Ordinarily in an act for malpractice resulting from negligence it is no defence that a Surgeon acted according to his best judgment. The standard of careful conduct is not the opinion of the individual, but is the conduct of an ordinarily prudent man under the circumstances. Staloch *vs.* Holm *et al.*, 100 Minn., 276. To hold otherwise "would leave so vague a line as to afford no rule at all, the degree of judgment belonging to each individual being infinitely various." (Tyndall.)

LEARNING AND SKILL REQUIRED OF THE SURGEON WHOSE PRACTICE IS THAT OF A SPECIALIST.—As in all departments of science and art, so in the practice of surgery there is a growing tendency among junior surgeons to select a special branch of practice and devote themselves exclusively to it. A Surgeon who thus assumes the position of a specialist is employed because of his supposed special learning and skill in that branch of surgery, and hence his obligation to his patient is not measured by the same rule as that which is applied to the ordinary Surgeon. It is for the jury to determine, as a question of fact, whether the Surgeon, in a given case, holds himself out as a specialist. Murdock *vs.* Kimberlin, 23 Mo. App., 523. If he practises as a specialist, the standard of learning and skill required by the law is that ordinarily possessed by Surgeons who devote special attention and study to the particular disease, or class of diseases, which he has adopted as a specialty; thus, an oculist must exercise, in his treatment of a patient, the care and skill usually exercised by oculists in good standing. The specialist is "held to that degree of care, skill, and knowledge ordinarily possessed by practitioners devoting special attention and study to the same branch." †

In Baker *vs.* Hancock, 63 N. E. Rep., 323, the Supreme Court of Indiana held that if the practiser "possesses no greater skill in the line of his specialty than the average physician, then there should be no reason for his employment; possessing such additional skill, it becomes his duty to give his patients the benefit of it."

QUESTION WHETHER THE SURGEON WAS A SPECIALIST DETERMINED.—In

---

* Ordronaux, Jurisp. of Med.; J. J. Elwell, Med. Malpractice.
† The Law and the Doctor, vol. i., p. 11; Am. and Eng. Encyc. of Law, 2d ed., vol. 22, p. 802.

Rann *vs.* Twitchell, 71 Atl. Rep., 1045, the Supreme Court of Vermont says that a robust boy of thirteen years, on exploding a torpedo April 19th, was struck by a fragment under the inner corner of the right eye; the cut made in the lower lid was approximately an inch long, and at the upper end next to the inner corner of the eye the lid was cut off so that it hung down over the cheek, disclosing a wound under the eyeball into the socket of the eye. The physician who first had charge of him for a week became convinced that there was a foreign substance lodged in the eye or socket, and not feeling competent to operate, advised the employment of an eye specialist. The boy was accordingly taken to a hospital where the defendant undertook the treatment of the case. It appears from the evidence that the Surgeon-expert made no effort to learn the history of the case or its prior treatment, nor did he attempt to determine by probe or otherwise whether a foreign body was in fact lodged in the eye or its orbit, though it was plain that the use of a probe would have easily and safely discovered the piece of tin which was afterward removed. He gave the plaintiff's eye attention for a few days and then sent him home, assuring him that there was nothing in the eye and with instructions to the physician who first attended him as to its subsequent treatment. The eye grew steadily worse until July 18th, three months after the accident, when the first physician operated and removed from the orbit a piece of tin nearly an inch long and about one-half inch wide, which was buried in the tissue to such a depth that its nearest point was about a quarter of an inch from the surface.

This action for malpractice was brought against the defendant and the hospital jointly, but during the progress of the trial, at the plaintiff's request, the court ordered a verdict for the hospital and the trial proceeded against the defendant alone. At the outset of the discussion the parties disagreed as to the rule which was to be applied to the defendant to test the sufficiency of his diagnosis and treatment of this injury. The plaintiff claimed that the evidence was such that the defendant must be judged as a specialist, while the defendant insisted that there was no evidence to warrant the application of anything but the rule governing general practitioners. The Supreme Court agreed with the court below that the defendant must be judged in this case by the more exacting rule which applies to specialists. From his evidence the court learned that he had been a specialist for the twelve preceding years in the medical and surgical treatment of the eye; that in 1902 he was regularly appointed "ophthalmist"—which means an eye specialist—to the hospital mentioned; that at the time here involved he had charge of the eye, ear, and throat department of that institution. Moreover, the very circumstances in which he was employed in this case unmistakably showed it was the special skill that he was understood to have in the surgical treatment of the eye which alone induced the plaintiff to seek his aid, and it was perfectly plain that the defendant so understood it when the physician made the arrangement with him to treat this injury. So the court ruled that his professional conduct must be tested, not by the standard applicable to general practitioners, but by the stricter rule applicable to specialists.

In support of this ruling the court cited with approval the decision in Hawthorne vs. Richmond, 48 Vt., 477, and in a further discussion of the merits of the case held that one who holds himself out as a specialist in the treatment of a certain organ, injury, or disease is bound to bring to the aid of one so employing him that degree of skill and knowledge which is ordinarily possessed by those in the same general locality who devote special attention to that particular organ, injury, or disease, its diagnosis and treatment, having regard to the state of scientific knowledge at the time. The duty of exercising this degree of skill attached to this defendant at the time of his employment and was the measure of his responsibility in the diagnosis of the case to determine the nature and condition of the injury, as well as the proper treatment to be applied. He was not to be judged by the result, nor was he to be held liable for an error of judgment. His negligence was to be determined by reference to the pertinent facts existing at the time of his examination and treatment, of which he knew, or, in the exercise of due care, should have known. It might consist in the failure to apply the proper remedy on a correct determination of existing physical conditions, or it might precede that and result from a failure properly to inform himself of these conditions. If the latter, then it must appear that he had a reasonable opportunity for examination, and that the true physical conditions were so apparent that they could have been ascertained by the exercise of the required degree of care and skill, for, if a determination of these physical facts resolved itself into a question of judgment merely, he would not be liable for his error.

Tested by this rule, the evidence tended to show that the defendant's conduct did not measure up to its requirements. He had a fair chance to examine the eye, and, with the indications of the presence of the piece of tin so strong as the testimony of the first physician tended to show, it could not be said as a matter of law that the defendant in his preliminary examination to ascertain the essential data on which to predicate a professional opinion met the requirements of the rule above stated. The testimony tended to show that he did not, and the question should have been submitted to the jury, for the evidence showed that the tin ought to have been removed at the earliest possible moment. Wherefore, the Supreme Court reversed the judgment of the lower court in favor of the defendant specialist and sent the case back for a new trial.

DUTY TO INSTRUCT PATIENT AND NURSE.—In order to insure the successful issue of a case in surgery it is important to give proper and necessary instructions to the patient and nurse, not only during the treatment, but in the after-care. Beck vs. German Klinik, 70 Ill., 162; Pike vs. Honsinger, 155 N. Y., 203. In Carpenter vs. Blake, 60 Barb. (N. Y.), 488, the Supreme Court of New York said, "If in case of dislocation of the elbow joint, it is enough for the physician to replace the bones and put the arm on a pillow, with the part below the joint at right angle to that above it and directing the application of cold water, it would seem to be proper, if not necessary, that the attending Surgeon should inform the patient or those having charge of him or her, of the necessity of maintaining that position; and if there is a tendency in the limb to become straight, or if, in consequence of the severity of the injury to the ligaments above the joint, there is great pain, which renders the patient nervous and restless, thus increasing the tendency to relaxation, or to straighten, and, as a consequence to stiffen the joint, the danger should be disclosed, to the end that all proper precaution may be taken to prevent it. It is insisted that these dangers were imminent and yet no word was given. This was, in my judgment, culpable negligence; much of the suffering the patient has undergone, and much of the loss she has sustained, might have been prevented had the defendant done what it was clearly his duty to do, if he knew the consequences which might result from redislocating the joint or straightening the arm." Although upon appeal to the Court of Appeals of the State of New York this judgment was reversed, on a technical error in the charge to the jury by the trial justice (50 N. Y., 696), the language above quoted was approved in the subsequent proceedings in this case. Carpenter *vs.* Blake, 10 Hun, 358, affirmed by the Court of Appeals, 75 N. Y., 12.

DUTY TO GUARD AGAINST CONTAGION.—It is not only the duty of the Surgeon to protect his patient against the ordinary contagious diseases to which he is liable to be personally exposed, but it is his duty to protect his assistants, and the patient himself, from the contagion of the wound created by the injury, or in the operation.

Where a physician was employed to treat a wound which became an infectious sore and informed the patient's wife that there was no danger of infection, and on one occasion directed her to assist him in dressing the wound, whereby she became infected with septic poisoning, it has been held that such a state of facts was sufficient upon which to base a cause of action. The protection of the patient from infection by his own wound implies the proper and diligent use of antiseptic measures throughout the entire treatment of the case. If on account of ignorance or negligence the Surgeon fail to apply the proper and approved antiseptic remedies with reasonable care and diligence he would justly be responsible for any unfavorable results due to conditions which such remedies would have prevented. Edwards *vs.* Lamb, 69 N. H., 599; Harriot *vs.* Plympton, 166 Mass., 585.

In Piper *vs.* Manifee, 12 B. Mon. (Ky.), 467, an action for malpractice, it appeared from the evidence that a physician was warned by his patient's wife not to visit her husband if he attended a case of smallpox, to which he assented. She repeated her request on two different occasions to which he replied that he would not attend any smallpox patients. When the patient began to recover from the attack of typhoid fever, after three weeks' sickness, smallpox attacked him. The Court of Appeals of Kentucky held that upon the facts offered to be proved, and now to be taken as true, the physician was *prima facie* liable to an action. Even if there had been no warning it was his duty, in passing from his patients who were afflicted with an infectious and dangerous disease to others who were not so affected, to take such precautions as experience may have shown to be necessary to prevent the communication of the infection by his own visits. "Clearly the physician thus acting would be guilty of a breach of duty and of his implied undertaking to the patient."

CONSENT OF PATIENT TO THE INTRODUCTION OF A STRANGER INTO SICK-ROOM.—The obligation to protect the patient from the publicity of communications received in the discharge of professional duties extends to the introduction of a stranger, not a physician, into the sick-room. The consent of the patient or responsible person must first be obtained. Becker remarks: "The obligation to preserve inviolate a communication as a privileged communication, including in the meaning of the word 'communication' all knowledge or information received while in attendance upon a case, would be held to have been broken by the act of the physician (Surgeon) in bringing in a stranger who would not be privileged from testifying." *

In DeMay vs. Roberts, 46 Mich.; 160, a physician in attendance upon a woman in confinement allowed a man who accompanied him, as an assistant in carrying necessary articles, to remain in the room during the accouchement. Neither the patient nor her husband knew the "friend," but they supposed he was a physician or a medical student. There was but one room and the attendant conducted himself in a proper manner. A judgment was rendered against the physician and his friend, and the judgment was affirmed by the Supreme Court of Michigan, the Chief Justice writing the following opinion: "Dr. D. therefore took an unprofessional, young, unmarried man with him, introduced and permitted him to remain in the house of the plaintiff, when it was apparent that he could hear, at least, if not see, all that was said and done, and, as the jury must have found, under instructions given, without either the plaintiff or her husband having any knowledge or reason to believe the true character of such third party. . . . To the plaintiff the occasion was a most sacred one, and no one had a right to intrude unless invited, or because of some real and pressing necessity, which it is not pretended existed in this case. The plaintiff had a legal right to the privacy of her apartment at such a time, and the law secures to her this right by requiring others to observe it and to abstain from its violation. The fact that at the time she consented to the presence of S. (the 'friend'), supposing him to be a physician, does not preclude her from maintaining an action and recovering substantial damages upon afterward ascertaining his true character. In obtaining admission at such a time and under such circumstances without fully disclosing his true character both parties were guilty of deceit, and the wrong thus done entitles the injured party to recover the damages afterward sustained from shame and mortification upon discovering the true character of the defendants."

THE SURGEON MUST CONTINUE ATTENDANCE TO TERMINATION OF THE CASE.—Having undertaken the care of a case the Surgeon must give reasonable diligence in attendance until the condition of the patient requires treatment no longer. Of that condition the Surgeon is to be the judge, but in forming that judgment he is to exercise proper care, and is responsible for any injury which the patient might receive from too early discontinuance of at-

* Med. Jurisp., Foren. Med., and Tox., vol. i., 45.

tendance. Becker *vs.* Janinski, 27 Abb. N. C. (N. Y.), 45; Gerken *vs.* Plimpton, 62 App. Div. (N. Y.), 35. It has been held that if a Surgeon is called to attend in the usual manner, and undertakes to do so by word or act, nothing being said or done to modify this undertaking, it is quite clear as a legal proposition that not only reasonable care and skill should be exercised, but also continued attention so long as the condition of the patient might require it, in the exercise of an honest and properly educated judgment, and certainly any culpable negligence in this respect would render him liable in an action. Ballou *vs.* Prescott, 64 Me., 305. The Surgeon may cease attendance with the consent of the patient, or on giving the patient such reasonable notice as will enable him to secure the services of another Surgeon. Barbour *vs.* Martin, 62 Me., 536.

In Becker *vs.* Janinski, *supra*, it was held that a Surgeon becomes liable to an action for malpractice because of unreasonable delay in calling upon a patient; as where a Surgeon properly set a broken arm and at the time told the patient that he was going away on his vacation and would return in two weeks, and directed the patient to keep the arm in a sling. The Surgeon remained away five weeks, during which time the bones had slipped and so united as to cause permanent injury, and the Surgeon was held liable for damages.

As a corollary to the foregoing rule, it follows that the physician is the proper and sole judge of the necessary frequency of his visits to a patient so long as the latter is in his charge, and that upon bringing an action for such visits he is not required to prove them to have been necessary. Ebner Admx. *vs.* Mackey, 87 Ill. App., 306, affirmed 186 Ill., 297.*

VI. The Obligation of Patient to Surgeon.—THE PATIENT MUST GIVE THE SURGEON NECESSARY INFORMATION.—Essential to the intelligent and successful treatment of injuries and diseases is accurate knowledge on the part of the Surgeon of many facts relating to the physical condition of the patient, the circumstances attending the development of the disease, and the incidents on the occurrence of the injury. The patient is, therefore, under obligation to furnish the surgeon with full and accurate information to all inquiries as to the facts which throw light on the nature of the disease or injury. Becker says: † "The patient owes the duty to his physician of informing him fully of all the varied symptoms of his disease, or the circumstances attending his injury, and freely and with due confidence to answer all questions concerning his past history, which would tend to throw any light upon his present condition. To battle with the occult forces which play so important a part in determining the course or consequences of disease, it is absolutely essential that the physician should know all that is possible to be known of the patient's history, and of the history of the patient's family."

The patient is protected from any public exposure of facts in regard to himself or relatives that he may wish to conceal by the statutes of most of the States and the rulings of the Courts. These statutes absolutely forbid the Surgeon from divulging any information or communications which he obtains

---

* The Law and the Doctor, vol. i., pp. 13, 14, Wood on Master and Servant, § 177.
† Med. Jurisp., Forensic Med., and Tox., vol. i., p. 34.

in his examination or inquiries of the patient for the purpose of treating him professionally, except on the consent of the patient.

If the patient should give false information, or should wilfully neglect to give true information, the Surgeon would have the right, upon giving reasonable and due notice and opportunity to employ some one else, to discontinue his attendance and care of the case, and recover compensation for his services.

PATIENT MUST SUBMIT TO TREATMENT.—In Littlejohn vs. Arbogast, 95 Ill. App., 605, an action for alleged malpractice against a Surgeon who "negligently failed to discover and properly treat the dislocation (of the hip-joint), or, having discovered it, negligently failed to properly treat it," the Appellate Court of the State of Illinois gave the following opinion upon an appeal from a judgment in favor of the plaintiff: · "If the plaintiff in error (the Surgeon) was prevented from reducing the dislocation by the refusal of the defendant in error (the patient) to submit to an operation, he could not be held liable for damages resulting therefrom. It is the duty of a patient to submit to the necessary treatment prescribed by his physician or surgeon. If the patient is delirious, and cannot be made to understand the necessity of the treatment proposed, the physician or surgeon may co-operate with the patient's immediate family and resort to reasonable force. If the patient is in that condition and the members of his family having him in charge refuse to allow the proposed treatment, then the physician or surgeon would not be required to use force. Surely, he should not be held liable for injury to limb or health resulting from a failure to use the proposed treatment."

In Chamberlin vs. Morgan, 68 Pa. St., 168, another phase of this question was considered. This action was brought by Morgan, the father of a girl who sustained a dislocation of the arm, against the Surgeon, Dr. C., "for malpractice by which her arm that had been dislocated had become stiffened." After Dr. C. had treated the case for some time, the father consulted Dr. R., who proposed to administer an anæsthetic to the patient and reduce the dislocation, but the father refused to have the operation performed. The defendant, Dr. C., called Dr. R. as a witness and proposed to prove by him that "at his first examination of the arm of plaintiff, in the presence of and at the request of her father, he (Dr. R.) proposed to put plaintiff under the influence of an anæsthetic, and attempt to reduce it, and that Morgan (the father) replied in presence of plaintiff, 'that so long as she was improving so fast, as she had done since he came home, he should not have it disturbed,' and that the injury could then have been reduced." The offer was objected to by the plaintiff and rejected by the court. The verdict was for the plaintiff for $300. The defendant took a writ of error, and assigned the rejection of the above offer for error. The Supreme Court of Pennsylvania held this ruling to be correct, saying: "Had Dr. C. proposed this experiment there might be some reason to hold that he should have the opportunity of redeeming his mistake or even if he had called in Dr. R. to act in his behalf. Mr. Morgan merely requested Dr. R. to examine his daughter's arm and give his opinion about it. That did not oblige him to adopt his advice or to incur the hazard and expense of another operation. He owed no such duty to Dr. C."

PATIENT MUST CO-OPERATE WITH THE SURGEON.—In McCandless vs. McWha, 22 Penn. St., 261,. it was held that nothing can be more clear than that it is the duty of the patient to co-operate with his professional advisor, and to conform to the necessary prescriptions; but if he will not, or, under the pressure of pain cannot, his neglect is his own wrong or misfortune, for which he has no right to hold his surgeon responsible. No man may take advantage of his own wrong, or charge his misfortunes to the account of another.

This decision, sustained by competent authority,* makes the patient responsible for neglecting to conform to the necessary prescriptions even when under the pressure of pain he cannot. It is evident that the literal enforcement of such a rule by the Courts might relieve the Surgeon of all liability for unreasonable and impracticable demands upon the patient, and, by charging the latter with neglect to comply with his prescriptions, the Surgeon might conceal his own delinquencies.

This apparent defect in the decision of the presiding Judge (Woodward) was corrected in the opinion given by an Associate Judge (Lewis) of the same Court and on the same occasion. Without dissenting from the decision of Judge Woodward, Judge Lewis amplified the opinion of the former thus, "A patient is bound to submit to such treatment as his surgeon prescribes, provided the treatment be such as a Surgeon of ordinary skill would adopt or sanction. But if it be painful, injurious, or unskilful, he is not bound to peril his health, and perhaps his life, by submission to it. It follows that before the Surgeon can shift the responsibility from himself to the patient, on the ground that the latter did not submit to the course recommended, it must be shown that the prescriptions must be proper, and adapted to the end in view. It is incumbent on the Surgeon to satisfy the jury on this point; and in doing so, he has the right to call to his aid the science and experience of his professional brethren. It will not do to cover his own want of skill by raising a mist out of the refractory disposition of the patient."

PARENTS IN CHARGE OF PATIENT MUST OBEY DIRECTIONS OF THE SURGEON.— In Potter vs. Warner, 91 Penn. St., 362, an action for injury to a minor who was in charge of his parents, there was evidence tending to prove that all of the causes of complaint were produced by a neglect and refusal of the parents to follow the reasonable directions of the Surgeon. The Supreme Court of Pennsylvania held, that, if the jury found that the parents of the boy were in charge of and nursed him during his sickness, and that they did not obey the directions of the Surgeon in regard to the treatment and care of their son during such time, but disregarded the same and thereby contributed to the several injuries of which he complains, he cannot recover therefor. If the injuries were the result of mutual and concurring negligence of the parties, no action for the recovery of damages therefor will lie. A person cannot recover from another for consequences attributable in part to his own wrong.

* Hilliard's Law of Torts, 4th ed., vol. i., p. 240.

PATIENT MUST GIVE THE SURGEON PROPER OPPORTUNITY TO TREAT HIM.—
Although it is a legal doctrine that a patient is always at liberty to dismiss his
Surgeon at any time without notice, and without assigning any cause unless
there is a special contract that the service shall be rendered for a fixed period, the
patient must afford the Surgeon every reasonable facility for treatment during
the period of his attendance. In Dorris vs. Warford, 100 S. W. Rep., 312, an
action for damages for unskilful and negligent treatment of a broken arm, the
Court of Appeals of Kentucky reversed a judgment in favor of the defendant,
holding, that, if the jury believed from the evidence that the plaintiff was guilty
of negligence in failing to take proper care of herself, or to hold herself in readiness at reasonable times to be treated, and that such failure to take proper care
of herself or to hold herself in readiness to be treated was the proximate cause
of her permanent injury, and but for which negligence such injury would not
have resulted, then the law was for the defendant, and the jury should so find,
although it might further believe that the defendant was guilty of negligence
in the treatment of plaintiff's arm.

DUTY OF INJURED TO EMPLOY SURGEON OF ORDINARY SKILL AND EXPE-
RIENCE.—It is a rule of the Courts that an injured person, in order to be entitled
to damages, must have used reasonable care to effect a speedy and complete cure
of the injury. To that end he must employ a Surgeon of ordinary skill and
experience to treat him and use such other means as men and women of ordinary
judgment, under like circumstances, would exercise in the choice of a Surgeon
and the means to be used to effect a recovery. Chicago City Railway Co. vs.
Saxby, 213 Ill., 274, s. c. 75 N. E. Rep., 755. In Hooper vs. Bacon, 101 Me.,
523, s. c. 64 Atl. Rep., 950, a personal-injury case, the contention was that
the plaintiff's injuries did not receive proper surgical treatment, and that by
reason of want of proper care or skill on the part of the Surgeon employed
by the plaintiff, his injuries were greatly aggravated, and the consequences
much more serious than they would have been otherwise. The Supreme Judicial Court of Maine held that it was the duty of the plaintiff to use due care
in the selection and use of means for his recovery, and to that end to employ a
Surgeon of ordinary professional knowledge and skill, and to follow his necessary directions. If he did so he would be without fault in that respect himself,
and he would be entitled to recover compensation for all the damages sustained,
though the Surgeon may not have used the requisite skill, or may have erred in
judgment, and by unskilful treatment have prevented the plaintiff from recovery
from the injury as soon, or as perfectly, as he would have recovered under
skilful treatment.

PATIENT MUST PROCURE ASSISTANCE WHEN REQUESTED.—In Haering vs.
Spicer, 92 Ill. App., 924, a case of dislocated shoulder, the Surgeon was not called
to treat the injury until after the second day it was received. It appeared in
evidence that, owing to the inflamed and swollen condition of the shoulder, and
the resistance of the patient to tests applied by the Surgeon, it was difficult to
determine the extent of the injury. A more minute examination could have
been made by reducing the patient to unconsciousness by means of an anæsthetic,

but the testimony shows that would have been neither safe nor proper without the aid of a medical assistant. Though the testimony was conflicting as to whether the Surgeon declined further to treat the case without assistance of another physician to aid in administering an anæsthetic, and was refused, the court was led to believe, from a careful consideration of the evidence and corroborating circumstances, that such was the truth. The Appellate Court of Illinois held that, even if the Surgeon did make a mistake in diagnosing the case and said he did not think the shoulder was dislocated, he had the right to insist upon having aid as a condition to his further treating the case. The Court said, "It is the duty of a person who has called a surgeon to treat him for an injury to follow all reasonable advice prescribed, and if the surgeon requests needed assistance and the patient neglects or refuses to procure it, the surgeon cannot be held liable in damages for a permanent injury when the employment of assistance would have rendered the injury only temporary."

CONTRIBUTORY NEGLIGENCE OF PATIENT IN DELAYING TO CALL A SURGEON.—In Robertson *vs.* Texas and Pacific Railway Company, 79 S. W. Rep., 96, an action brought to recover for injuries from a red-hot cinder falling into the plaintiff's eye, there was a special plea of contributory negligence, on his part, in not having his injuries properly treated by a competent Surgeon until the injury was rendered more serious than it otherwise would have been.

The Court of Civil Appeals of Texas sustained the main charge to the jury, which was as follows: "If you should find that the plaintiff was injured by negligence on the defendant's part so as to entitle him to recover, but you should further find that the plaintiff was guilty of negligence, in delaying calling a physician and having his injuries treated, and that such negligence on his part aggravated his sufferings, and increased his injuries and the damages therefrom, you cannot, in such case, allow anything for such increase of his injuries or damages, but you can allow him for such damages as you find would have been sustained by him for his injuries, had he not been guilty of negligence in failing to obtain medical treatment for himself." The following special charge given the jury was also approved: "The law requires from one who receives an accident or injury to use the same degree of care and caution which a man of ordinary care and caution would use to lessen the effects of the accident, and make as light as practicable the injury."

VII. The Recognized Legal Requirements of the Surgeon.—RECOGNIZED METHODS OF PRACTICE MUST BE FOLLOWED.—In modern as in ancient times the Surgeon is held very strictly to the rule that his practice must conform to established rules and methods. The leading decision in this class of cases, and one which embodies correct surgical and legal principles, is as follows: Carpenter *vs.* Blake, 60 Barb., 488, 523. "Some standard by which to determine the propriety of treatment must be adopted; otherwise experiment will take the place of skill, and the reckless experimentalist the place of the educated, experienced practitioner. If the case is a new one, the patient must trust to the skill and experience of the surgeon he calls; so must he if the injury or the disease is attended with injury to other parts, or other diseases have developed themselves, for which there is no established mode of treatment. But, when the case is one as to which a system of treatment has been followed for a long time, there should be no departure from it, unless the surgeon who does it is prepared to take the risk of establishing, by his success, the propriety and safety of his experiment. The rule protects the community against reckless experiments, while it admits the adoption of new remedies and modes of treatment only when their benefits have been demonstrated, or when, from the necessity of the case, the surgeon or physician must be left to the exercise of his own skill and experience."

SKILL AND GOOD INTENTIONS NO BAR TO AN ACTION.—Jackson *vs.* Burnham, 20 Col., 533, was an action for alleged malpractice in the treatment of phimosis by the application of a flaxseed poultice by defendant. Gangrene ensued, followed by destruction of the member. On the trial it was proven that the flaxseed poultice was not a recognized remedy in this condition and that the unfortunate result was due to its use. Expert testimony described the ordinary and established practice in such cases to be incision of the foreskin so as to expose the glans and thus allow free circulation. The court charged the jury as follows: "If you find from the evidence that this defendant, in the treatment of the plaintiff, omitted the ordinary or established mode of treatment, and pursued one that has proved injurious, it is no consequence how much skill he may have, he has demonstrated a want of it in the treatment of the particular case, and is liable in damages." The Supreme Court of Colorado sustained this ruling in the following decision. "It therefore became a pertinent inquiry to be submitted to the jury whether the evidence showed an established mode of treatment in such a case, and, if so, whether defendant adopted some other mode, that proved injurious; and, if he did, it was immaterial how much skill he possessed, since his failure to use it constituted such negligence as would render him liable."

In Allen *vs.* Voje, 114 Wisc., 1, s. c. 89 N. W. Rep., 924, a case of curetting the uterus followed by tubo-ovarian abscess and removal of the right ovary and Fallopian tube, the verdict was for plaintiff, and damages were assessed at $300. On appeal the Supreme Court of Wisconsin affirmed the judgment of the lower court and sustained its charge to the jury, viz., "A departure from approved methods in general use, if it injures the patient, will render him (the Surgeon) liable, however good his intentions may have been."

In Paten *vs.* Wiggin, 51 Me., 594, the Supreme Court of Maine said, "If the case is such that no physician (Surgeon) of ordinary knowledge or skill would doubt or hesitate, and that but one course of treatment would by such professional men be suggested, then any other course of treatment might be evidence of a want of ordinary knowledge or skill, or care and attention, or exercise of his best judgment, and a physician (Surgeon) might be held liable, however high his former reputation."

THAT PATIENT RECEIVED INJURY FROM THE NEW METHOD OF TREATMENT PRACTISED MUST BE POSITIVELY PROVEN.—In Winner *vs.* Lathrop, 67 Hun (N. Y.), 511, where a surgeon, in connection with reducing a fracture of the patient's arm, had advised bathing the parts with a decoction of wormwood and vinegar, which the expert testimony condemned, the Court found, in view of the evidence, that such application could not have injuriously affected the desired cure, and held that such technical violation of the surgeon's duty could not avail the plaintiff where injury could not be directly traced to it.

LIABILITIES OF THE SURGEON WHO ADOPTS NEW METHODS OF TREATMENT. —How far this ruling of the Courts interferes with the progress of the art of Surgery, by rendering it dangerous for the Surgeon to resort to new remedies or operations, has created much discussion. In cases that have been brought to trial on this charge the Courts have been careful to discriminate between gross and obviously unscientific departures from the ordinary and established methods of practice, and those new methods which in the emergency which existed were deemed reasonable and necessary. The presumption of the law is in favor of the proper treatment by the Surgeon.

In Pratt vs. Davis, 224 Ill., 300, a case of operation alleged to be without consent, the Supreme Court of Illinois held that when unexpected conditions develop or are discovered in the course of the operation, it is the duty of the surgeon, in dealing with these conditions, to act on his own discretion, making the highest use of his skill and ability to meet the exigencies which confront him, and in the nature of things he must frequently do this without consultation or conference with any one, except, perhaps, other members of his profession who are assisting him. Emergencies arise, and when a Surgeon is called it is sometimes found that some action must be taken immediately for the preservation of the life or health of the patient, where it is impracticable to obtain the consent of the ailing or injured one or of any one authorized to speak for him. In such event, the Surgeon may lawfully, and it is his duty to, perform such operation as good surgery demands, without such consent.

PRACTICE MUST BE IN ACCORDANCE WITH THE RULES OF THE SCHOOL TO WHICH THE SURGEON BELONGS.—The principles of law governing the Courts in determining the questions arising in actions for alleged malpractice require that the rules relating to practice of the school to which the Surgeon belongs receive due consideration. The law, in the absence of a special statute, does not give exclusive recognition to any particular school or system of medicine, and the question whether or not a practiser in his treatment of the case exercised the requisite degree of care, skill, and diligence is to be tested by the general rules and principles of the particular school of medicine which he follows, not by those of other schools.*

In Patten vs. Wiggin, 51 Me., 594, it does not appear in the report what was the nature of the injury or disease, but the claim was malpractice in the treatment of the patient, and such ignorance, want of skill and judgment on the part of the Surgeon in managing professionally the case under his care, that the patient was more injured than benefited by his treatment. The following instructions to the jury by the trial Court were sustained by the Supreme Court of Maine: "If there are distinct and differing schools of prac-

* Am. and Eng. Enc. of Law (2d ed.), vol. 22, p. 801.

tice, as Allopathic, or Old School, Homœopathic, Thompsonian, Hydropathic, or Water Cure, and a physician of one of these schools is called in, his treatment is to be tested by the general doctrines of his school, and not by those of other schools."

In Force *vs.* Gregory, 63 Conn., 167, an action for damages for alleged malpractice in the treatment of a disease of the eye, the trial court charged the jury that the "defendant's negligence or want of skill in the treatment of the plaintiff's eye must be determined by all the evidence in the case; and if the defendant adopted the treatment laid down by one particular school of medicine and the medical testimony offered by plaintiff related to treatment prescribed by a different school, you will weigh the testimony, having regard to any bias or prejudice that might influence the testimony of those who belonged to a different school from that of the defendant." The Supreme Court of Connecticut held that the trial Court erred in not instructing as the defendant asked, in the words of the charge in Patten *vs.* Wiggin, *supra*, viz., that "If there are distinct and different schools of practice and a physician of one of those schools is called in, his treatment is to be tested by the general doctrines of his school, and not by those of other schools. The jury are not to judge by determining which school, in their own view, is the best."

A So-called School of Medicine Not to be Recognized if it Has Neither Rules nor Principles of Practice.—It follows that a School of Medicine, to be entitled to recognition under the preceding rule, must have rules and principles of practice for the guidance of all its members as respects principles, diagnosis, and remedies, which each member is supposed to observe in any given case. A class of practitioners who have no fixed principles or formulated rules for the treatment of disease must be held to the duty of treating patients with the ordinary skill and knowledge of physicians in good standing.*

Under this ruling suits for damages against irregular practitioners and pretenders have resulted in verdicts of incompetency and gross malpractice. Having no standard of practice, and no rules for their guidance, this class of charlatans has very justly been held to the exercise of the same degree of learning, skill, care, and diligence as is ordinarily possessed by physicians and Surgeons of similar localities.

In Nelson *vs.* Harrington, 72 Wisc., 592, an action to recover damages for malpractice in treating a case of hip-joint disease by a clairvoyant practitioner, the plaintiff secured a verdict for substantial damages, from which the defendant appealed. The Supreme Court of Wisconsin says, the defendant is what is known as a "clairvoyant physician," and held himself out, as other physicians do, as competent to treat disease of the human system. He did not belong to, or practise in accordance with the rules of, any existing school of physicians, governed by formulated rules for treating diseases and injuries, to which rules all practitioners of that school are supposed to adhere. The testimony shows that his mode of diagnosis and treatment consisted in voluntarily going into a sort of trance condition, and while in such condition to give a diagnosis of

* Am. and Eng. Ency. of Law (2d ed.), vol. 22, p. 801.

the case, and prescribe for the ailment of the patient thus disclosed. He made no personal examination, applied no tests to discover the malady, and resorted to no other source of information as to the past or present condition of the plaintiff. Indeed, he did not profess to have been educated in the science of medicine. He trusted implicitly to the accuracy of his diagnosis thus made and of his prescriptions thus given.

The defendant does not allege, nor was any evidence given or offered to show, that clairvoyant physicians, as a class, treat disease upon such principles, or that rules have been formulated which each practitioner is supposed to follow in the treatment of disease, as is the case with schools or systems of medicine such as the Allopathic or Homœopathic. The proposition that one holding himself out as a medical practitioner and as competent to treat human maladies, who accepts a person as a patient, and treats him for disease, may, because he resorts to some peculiar method of determining the nature of the disease and the remedy therefor, be exonerated from all liability for unskilfulness on his part, no matter how serious the consequences may be, cannot be entertained. It follows that the trial court properly refused to give an instruction to the jury, proposed on behalf of the defendant, in these words: "If the defendant was a clairvoyant physician, and professed and held himself out to be such, and the plaintiff and his parents knew it, and at the time he was called to treat the plaintiff both parties understood and expected that he would treat him according to the approved practice of clairvoyant physicians, and that he did so treat him, and in strict accordance with the clairvoyant system of practice, and with the ordinary skill and knowledge of that system, then the plaintiff cannot recover, and your verdict must be for the defendant." Instead of the words, "with the ordinary skill and knowledge of that system," employed therein, it should have read, "with the ordinary skill and knowledge of physicians in good standing practising in that vicinity."

STANDARD OF PRACTICE IN LOCALITY MUST BE CONSIDERED.—In determining whether a Surgeon brought to the treatment of a case "reasonable ". and "ordinary" learning and skill, his opportunities in the locality where he resides and practises must be considered. It is well stated that "it would be manifestly unfair to expect and require of a physician practising in a small country town, with no opportunities for experience in surgical cases save that usually had by country physicians, to have the same amount of knowledge and skill in matters of surgery as those physicians in the great cities, whose practice is more extended in its scope, and who have the opportunity of attending lectures and clinics, and of witnessing and taking part in operations requiring a high degree of skill and learning." * The following cases illustrate the rulings of the Courts.

In Small vs. Howard, 128 Mass., 131, an action in tort against a Surgeon for malpractice in dressing and caring for a wound of the wrist, it appeared that the patient's wrist had been cut through to the bone, severing all the arteries and tendons. Defendant, who had attended the case, was a physician practising in a country town of about twenty-five hundred inhabitants, and had no experience

* The Law and the Doctor, vol. i., p. 9.

in surgery beyond that usually had by country surgeons. Among the instructions which the trial judge gave to the jury was the following relating to locality: "The defendant, undertaking to practise as a physician and surgeon in a town of a comparatively small population, was bound to possess that skill only which physicians and surgeons of ordinary ability and skill, practising in similar localities, with opportunities for no larger experience, ordinarily possess; and he was not bound to possess that high degree of art and skill possessed by eminent surgeons practising in large cities and making a specialty of the practice of surgery." The Supreme Judicial Court of Massachusetts sustained this decision of the trial court, remarking, "It is a matter of common knowledge that a physician in a small country village does not usually make a specialty of surgery, and, however well informed he may be in the theory of all parts of his profession, he would, generally speaking, be but seldom called upon as a surgeon to perform difficult operations. He would have few opportunities of observation and practice in that line, such as public hospitals or large cities would afford. The defendant was applied to, being the practitioner in a small village, and we think it was correct to rule that "he was bound to possess that skill only which physicians and surgeons of ordinary ability and skill, practising in similar localities, with opportunities for no larger experience, ordinarily possess; and he was not bound to possess that high degree of art and skill possessed by eminent surgeons practising in large cities, and making a specialty of Surgery.'

In Ferrell vs. Ellis, 129 Iowa, 614, s. c. 105 N. W. Rep., 993, the trial court instructed the jury that: "The standard of skill and learning required in any case is that reasonable degree of skill and learning ordinarily exercised by the members of the profession at the time of the treatment in question, having regard to the advanced state of the profession at the time." This, the Supreme Court of Iowa held, was erroneous in not limiting the degree of skill and learning to that ordinarily possessed by physicians and surgeons practising in *similar* localities. The presumption that prejudice resulted was in no way obviated by the record, for no other physician than the defendant, resident in his village, testified, while several surgeons, of more or less experience residing in much larger towns, testified. The court decreed that for the error pointed out a judgment in favor of the plaintiff must be reversed.

DISTINCTION BETWEEN "PARTICULAR LOCALITY' AND "SIMILAR LOCALITY" AND BETWEEN "THE NEIGHBORHOOD" AND "THE SAME GENERAL NEIGHBORHOOD" OR "THE SAME GENERAL LOCALITY."—It is noticeable that in the preceding decision the ruling of the trial court was reversed because it did not limit the degree of learning and skill to that ordinarily possessed by physicians and Surgeons practising in *similar* localities. A distinction between "*similar* localities" and "the *particular* locality" is made, and the first form is that generally adopted for the following reason: "There might be but a few practising in the given locality, all of whom might be quacks, ignorant pretenders to the knowledge not possessed by them, and it would not do to say that because one possessed and exercised as much skill as the others, he could not be chargeable with the want of reasonable skill." Gramm vs. Boener, 56 Ind., 497.

The Supreme Court of Iowa thus states the rule: "But we are of the opinion that the correct rule is that a physician and surgeon, when employed in his professional capacity, is required to exercise that degree of knowledge, skill, and care which physicians and surgeons practising in *similar* localities possess." Dunbauld *vs*. Thompson, 109 Iowa, 199.

The terms "The Neighborhood" and "The same general Neighborhood" have been the subject of judicial comment. The Supreme Court of North Carolina held that "Skill and knowledge must be such as is ordinarily possessed by the average profession. It cannot be measured simply by the profession in the neighborhood, as this standard of measurement would be entirely too variable and uncertain. "Neighborhood" might be constructed into a very limited area, and is generally so understood, and that area might contain only one or two surgeons, and they might be of very inferior qualifications. It would be unjust both to the profession and its patients if, under such circumstances, these local surgeons assumed to be the standard of a learned profession and proved the standing of each by the ability of the other. The words "the neighborhood" are essentially different from the phrases, "the same general neighborhood," or "the same general locality." McCracken *vs*. Smathers, 122 N. C., 799, s. c. 29 S. E. Rep., 354.

Therefore, the standard is not the learning and skill of Surgeons of a particular locality, but that ordinarily possessed by Surgeons practising in similar localities, or neighborhoods.

REGARD MUST BE HAD TO THE ADVANCED STATE OF THE MEDICAL SCIENCES.— In judging the degree of skill which the Surgeon should bring to the discharge of his duty, regard is to be had to the advanced state of the medical sciences at the time. Discoveries in the natural sciences during the last half-century have exerted a powerful influence upon all the learned professions, but especially upon that of medicine. And of the medical sciences the most important discoveries have been immediately applicable to remarkable improvements in the practice of surgery. The standard of ordinary skill in surgery is therefore on the advance, and the patient is entitled to the benefits of these improvements. McCandless *vs*. McWha, 22 Penn. St., 261.

SURGICAL TREATISE DID NOT REPRESENT THE ADVANCED STATE OF MEDICAL SCIENCE.—In Peck *vs*. Hutchinson, 88 Iowa, 320, s. c. 55 N.W. Rep., 511, an action for damages arising from alleged malpractice, one charge was that the Surgeon "negligently and unskilfully undertook a painful operation on said eye without first giving the proper drug to render the patient insensible to pain." One of the errors assigned on appeal relates to this charge and the following is the opinion of the Supreme Court of Iowa: "Against the objection of the defendant, plaintiff was permitted to read to the jury from Wells' 'Treatise on the Eye' what the writer says as to the operation of 'iridectomy.' This evidence was objected to as incompetent, immaterial, and because the work was an old edition. The book was published in 1880, and states that chloroform should always be administered. It does not recognize local anæsthetic treatment; in fact, says nothing about it. The operation was performed in 1886, and it is claimed that after

1880, and prior to 1886, great changes had occurred in optical surgery; that, during that time, cocaine, a local anæsthetic, was discovered, and came into use, thus superseding the use of general anæsthetics in such cases. This may be conceded. The evidence, we think, preponderates largely in favor of the claim that in such cases the modern and better practice is to use local anæsthetics. Now that fact was fully shown to the jury, and from the evidence it appeared that the Wells book antedated the time when local anæsthetics first began to be used in this country."

LIABILITY FOR IMPROPER OPERATIONS.—If a surgeon is consulted in regard to the propriety or necessity of a given operation it is his duty, in the exercise of his required learning, skill and care, and his obligation in all cases to use his best judgment, to carefully discriminate as to the application of the proposed operation to the individual case. If, in his opinion, the operation would be injudicious, it is his duty to advise against it, and he would be liable if he failed to do so. If, however, the patient is of mature years and responsible for his acts, and insists upon having the operation performed after being fully informed as to its nature, whether unnecessary, or dangerous, or improper, the surgeon would be justified in performing it.* Gramm *vs.* Boener, 56 Ind., 497.

VIII. **Consent to Surgical Operations.**—GENERAL REMARKS UPON THE SUBJECT.—A surgical operation, however trivial, is always a new feature in the treatment of the case and may involve the most serious consequences, not only as it affects the immediate condition of the patient, but as it may have an influence upon his or her future. An anæsthetic administered for the purpose of puncturing an abscess may prove fatal, and the removal of organs, such as the ovaries, may destroy the most cherished hopes and anticipations of families. The fact that the Surgeon can never foretell the complications which may arise in the progress of an operation, nor the limitations of disease, renders it imperative for his own protection from censure that he should obtain the full and specific consent of the patient, or other person who may be responsible for his care, before undertaking the operation. A review of the cases brought into court for alleged malpractice shows that where specific consent is not obtained prior to the operation, authorizing the Surgeon to use his discretion in the treatment of unforeseen complications and conditions which may be met in the progress of the operation, the position of the operator may become exceedingly embarrassing. Consent may be express or implied.

THE EXPRESS CONSENT.—The express consent may be written or verbal, and in the latter form it may be made in the presence of the parties only, or it may be witnessed by a third party. The written form is the more reliable as the terms are specifically stated and there can be no mistake as to their meaning. The express verbal consent, whether made only by the parties present or in the presence of witnesses, is liable to the misunderstandings so common when testimony is based on the memory of the parties in interest. It is for this reason that the written express contract should be preferred.

In performing an operation under the express contract the Surgeon is bound

* The Law and the Doctor vol. i., p. 25.

to follow strictly its terms and limitations. Any deviation from the contract to meet unforeseen emergencies would render the Surgeon liable for injuries resulting therefrom to the patient. It is probable that neither the patient nor the courts would hold him strictly to the terms of the contract when a departure therefrom was satisfactorily proven to be necessary to save the patient's life, or even essential to his future health. But the Surgeon should fully understand the liabilities which he incurs when he departs from the terms of the consent.

The following cases illustrate the confusion and serious misunderstandings which are liable to occur when the consent is verbal.

Consent to Operate on Right Leg, but Surgeon Operates on Left Leg.—In Sullivan vs. McGraw, 118 Mich., 39, an action to recover damages for the wrongful operation by a Surgeon upon the patient—the claim was that the Surgeon was employed to operate on the right leg; that, after putting the patient under the influence of chloroform, the Surgeon wrongfully and carelessly operated upon the left leg, thereby causing the patient great pain and suffering. This case was tried before a jury, and the court directed the verdict in favor of the defendant. The plaintiff brought error.

The material facts in this case are as follows: The plaintiff testified that both legs had troubled him for several years; sores came out on the shin bone in 1893 and were healed; the right leg continued to be sore; in October, 1896, his right leg was very sore and he consulted the defendant who treated him, without improvement, for several months; defendant then advised him to go to the hospital and he would operate upon it; on May 11th, 1897, he went to the hospital, being very lame and using a pair of crutches, walking with them and using his left leg. The next morning the nurse prepared him for the operation by shaving his right leg from the knee down, as the operation was to be upon the shin bone; nothing was done with the left leg. The plaintiff testified that he never told the defendant, or any one else, that he wanted his left leg operated upon; that a week before the operation he showed defendant both legs so that he could compare them and that there had always been an enlargement of the shin of the left leg. The nurse testified that he prepared plaintiff for the operation; that he had a swelling of both legs, and witness asked him which leg was to be operated upon and he said the right leg, so he prepared that. A brother of the plaintiff testified that he was present at the operation and that when plaintiff was placed on the operating table both legs were exposed to the defendant who said, "See here! you fellows have made a mistake; you have prepared the wrong leg for operation." The defendant asked him which leg he wanted operated upon and the brother replied that he was confused and did not know, but he would telephone his folks so as to be sure; the defendant consented to wait, but the father came meantime and said it was the left leg. The father of the plaintiff testified that he arrived at the hospital after plaintiff had been put upon the operating table; that they showed him both legs, and defendant said, pointing to the right leg, "Is that the right leg?" "No," I said, "the other leg. I had my mind on that leg all of the time."

The court, at the request of counsel for defendant, directed the verdict in favor of defendant. The Trial Court stated to the jury, "It seems to me that this case turns upon the question of whether or not the doctor was negligent in operating upon the left leg, instead of upon the right leg. If I should leave this to you, I would have to say to you, if the doctor made these inquiries, and was told by the father that that was the leg to operate upon, that would justify him. Now, there is no doubt that he did; there is nothing to leave to you on the question of negligence, it seems to me. It is earnestly insisted upon the part of plaintiff that this case does not depend upon the doctor's negligence, but does depend upon the want of consent or absence of consent upon the part of the plaintiff. I do not so understand the law. Of course, if there had been no consent at all to any operation, it would have been clearly trespass to have touched the plaintiff's person. The plaintiff had gone there for the purpose of having an operation performed upon him. To touch his person was not technically a trespass; but in this case a mistake was made in the choice of legs to be operated upon. The liability, in making that mistake, must depend upon whether or not the doctor was negligent; and, as I say, there was nothing in this case which would warrant you in finding a verdict on that theory."

The Supreme Court of Michigan said, "There is no claim in the present case that the doctor did not have the skill and knowledge necessary for the operation. The declaration avers negligence on the part of the defendant in operating on the left instead of the right leg. We think the court below was not in error in saying that the only question in the case for determination was whether or not the defendant was negligent in operating on the wrong leg. We cannot, however, agree with the court below that there was no evidence tending to establish that fact. Plaintiff had put himself under the care of the defendant, and, as he says, for the purpose of an operation on the right leg. According to the plaintiff's statement, the doctor knew which leg was to be operated upon. The right leg was prepared by the nurse under the defendant's direction." After reciting further facts the court decided that the case should have been submitted to the jury for their determination, whether the defendant exercised that degree of care which, under the circumstances, he was bound to exercise and the judgment was reversed and a new trial granted.

REMOVAL OF BOTH OVARIES WITH CONSENT TO REMOVE BUT ONE.—In Beatty vs. Cullingworth, Q. B. Div., an English case, the judge instructed the jury that the plaintiff had tacitly consented to the operation, whereupon the jury gave a verdict for the defendant. The facts in evidence were that an unmarried woman who was engaged to be married when about to be operated upon, told the Surgeon that if he found both ovaries diseased he must remove neither, to which the Surgeon replied, "You must leave that to me." This reply the patient denied hearing. Both ovaries were diseased and were removed. Upon learning that both ovaries had been removed the patient broke her engagement and brought an action for damages. Upon the trial of the case the judge instructed the jury that the Surgeon had the patient's tacit consent to perform the operation, whereupon they rendered a verdict for the defendant. A Law Journal (44 Cent. L. J., 153) commenting on this decision remarked: "The action of the court in this case has met with very general criticism upon the ground that the facts, involving a direct prohibition, would seem to exclude the possibility of implying consent. As a contemporary says, it is one thing for a Surgeon to refuse to operate unless unlimited discretion is confided to him, and quite another thing to deliberately disobey instructions. Undoubtedly the defendant's wisest course would have been to refuse to operate unless the scope of his authority was agreed upon in advance."

CONSENT TO OPERATION ON RIGHT EAR, BUT SURGEON OPERATED ON THE LEFT EAR.—In Mohr *vs.* Williams, 95 Minn., 261, the plaintiff, a young woman, complained that the defendant, a surgeon, had been employed by her to perform an operation upon her right ear; but that after she was etherized he had operated upon the left ear, although she had never given her consent that any operation should be performed upon that organ. The defence appears to have been that although the original intention of the surgeon was to operate upon the right ear he discovered, upon the fuller examination which he was enabled to make when the patient was put under ether, that the left ear was the more seriously diseased of the two, and that he operated upon the left ear upon the understanding that the patient, by placing herself in his hands, had tacitly consented that he might do so if he deemed it advisable in the exercise of his best judgment. The judge who presided at the trial held that no such consent could be implied from the circumstances of the case, and that the defendant was at all events liable for a technical assault. The jury gave the plaintiff a verdict for more than $14,000. This judgment was reversed.

On a re-trial of the case (Mohr *vs.* Williams, 98 Minn., 494; 108 N. W. Rep., 818) the plaintiff again recovered a verdict, but this time for $3,500. The trial court granted the defendant's motion for judgment notwithstanding the verdict for the plaintiff, and from that order the plaintiff again appealed.

The Supreme Court of Minnesota, in reviewing the evidence brought out on the second trial, said in substance: The defendant does not question the propositions of law determined upon the last appeal, but insists that the evidence on the second trial, disclosed a condition of the left ear that demonstrated that the surgeon was justified in operating upon it as the only thing to do to relieve the plaintiff from a critical situation. But the Supreme Court was still of the opinion that the evidence did not conclusively establish the fact that the left ear was in such a serious condition as to call for an immediate operation. If the plaintiff placed herself in the general charge of the defendant, why did he not make an examination of the left ear as well as of the right ear? The defendant testified that he found an obstruction in the left ear when he examined her some three weeks before the operation. If the critical condition discovered at the time of the operation was such as to be reasonably anticipated from this obstruction, the delay of three weeks without giving it attention or treatment was suggestive of inattention and negligence. The judgment was therefore reversed and the case remanded for a new trial.

THE IMPLIED CONSENT.—Actions for malpractice in conducting surgical procedures without the consent of the patient occur for the most part under the implied consent. The prevailing opinion among Surgeons is that the fact of being employed by a patient is an implied consent on his part that the surgeon shall have full control of the treatment, including an operation, subject only to the general obligation that the Surgeon exercise reasonable and ordinary learning and skill, and his best judgment, and applies that learning and skill with proper care and diligence. It is apparent from a review of the decisions in actions involving these points that the Courts very critically consider all of the circumstances in each case and finally leave to the jury to determine the question of consent. The question to be decided in these cases when brought into court is as to whether, under the conditions which exist in each individual case, an implied consent was given. This is a question for the jury. The reported cases show that doubts and difficulties arise chiefly when the consent is verbal or implied and thus emphasis is given to the value of the written contract which has been advocated.

PATIENT'S CONSENT PRESUMED FROM CIRCUMSTANCES.—In McClallen vs. Adams, 19 Pick., Mass. 333, a woman suffering from disease of the breast was placed by her husband under the care of a Surgeon living at a distance. After ten weeks the Surgeon operated by removing her breast and she died at the end of one week. The husband refused to pay the charge for the amputation of the breast ($30), as it was claimed that the service was not performed at the request of the husband, and the surgeon commenced a suit for the recovery of his fee. The counsel for the plaintiff requested the trial judge to instruct the jury, "That as the defendant put his wife under the care of the plaintiff as a surgeon, he impliedly requested him to do for her what he should think necessary and proper, and as his wife must have assented to the operation, her assent must have been the assent of her husband, and therefore the defendant was liable to pay for this service." The judge refused to give this instruction, but instructed the jury as follows: "That as it did not appear that the wife had a cancer or cancerous humor when the defendant put her under the care of the plaintiff, the plaintiff was not authorized to perform the operation, so as to charge the defendant with payment, without proving to the reasonable satisfaction of the jury, that the operation was necessary and proper under the circumstances; and providing further that, before he performed the operation, he gave notice to the defendant, or that it would have been dangerous to the wife to wait, before he performed the operation, till notice could be given to the defendant; and as no evidence of this kind was given or offered, the jury would not be authorized to allow this item." The jury found for the plaintiff, but did not include the fee for amputation of the breast.

On appeal the Supreme Judicial Court of Massachusetts gave the following decision: "The court are of the opinion, upon the facts appearing by the bill of exceptions, that the defendant, by placing his wife under the care of the plaintiff, whom he knew, at a distance from his own residence, for medical and surgical treatment for a dangerous disease, impliedly requested him to do all acts, and adopt such course of treatment and operation, as in his judgment would be most likely to effect her ultimate cure and recovery, with the assent of the wife, and therefore that the operation in question was within the scope of the authority given him. They are also of the opinion, that the assent of the wife, to the operation, was to be presumed from the circumstances. Although it might have been an act of prudence in the plaintiff to give the defendant notice of the situation of the wife, and of his intention to perform a dangerous operation, yet we think he might safely trust to the judgment of the wife, to give her husband notice from time to time of her situation and intentions, and that it was not necessary, in point of law, for the plaintiff to give such notice, or have any new request, in order to enable him to recover a reasonable compensation for his services." The verdict was set aside and a new trial ordered.

SUBMISSION OF A CASE FOR JUDGMENT AND ACTION IS AN IMPLIED CONSENT.— An interesting phase of the implied consent from circumstances occurred in a case of alleged malpractice before the Appellate Division of the Supreme Court of New York, Second Department, in Brooklyn, New York. Wood vs. Wyeth, 81 N. Y. Supp., 1148. The plaintiff was the mother of a boy who had died under chloroform while submitting to an operation in a charity hospital. The mother contended that the boy was sent to the hospital to be examined and not for surgical treatment, and that the operation which was subsequently undertaken, and which resulted in his death, was performed without her consent or the consent of the maid whom she sent to the hospital with the lad. It did not appear, however, that the maid informed the surgeons at the hospital of any limitation upon her authority. She merely submitted the boy for their examination and, as they supposed, for treatment. Having ascertained that the boy was suffering from blood poisoning and that a simple operation was necessary for his relief, the surgeons proceeded to perform the operation with the result that their patient died from the effects of the anæsthetic. The contention of the plaintiff's counsel was that the surgeons ought to have informed the maid of their intention to perform the operation. The majority of the court voted for a reversal of the judgment and order dismissing the complaint, upon the ground that a technical error had been committed by the trial court in so doing, but the presiding justice and one other justice were in favor of affirming the judgment, and united in the following opinion:—"Under the facts here disclosed the defendants had a right to assume that the boy was there for treatment; that his case was submitted for judgment and action, and it would be contrary to law to hold that the fact that they did not disclose their intention of operating upon the boy, if this was a fact, to Agnes Evans, the maid who accompanied him, who does not appear to have suggested any limitation upon their right to treat the patient under their employment as alleged in the complaint, rendered them liable in an action of this character. We find no authority holding a contrary doctrine, and it would be holding the employees of a charitable hospital to a high degree of responsibility to say that they must notify the guardians of every patient brought to them for treatment before they can perform the simplest of surgical operations, under pain of being called upon to pay damages in the event of unexpected fatalities."

REMOVAL OF UTERUS—CONSENT ALLEGED AND DENIED.—In Pratt *vs.* Davis, 118 Ill. App., 161; Aff'd 224 Ill., 300, an important case arising in Illinois, the question of consent is very fully discussed. The trial was had before the court without a jury and resulted in a substantial award of damages to the plaintiff. The defendant appealed and the following statement of facts is taken from the report of the case in the Supreme Court of Illinois.

The plaintiff, a married woman about forty years of age, entered the sanitarium of the defendant for treatment of epilepsy with which she had been afflicted for a period of fifteen years. But she had been able to perform her domestic duties, and had borne three children since she had exhibited symptoms of epilepsy. The seizures had been increasing in frequency, and following each of them she would be very weak in body and dazed and uncertain in mind for several hours. The evidence of those who knew her in her daily life was generally to the effect that her mind, except during the periods immediately following these attacks, was normal.

The defendant made an examination of the pelvic organs, and found the uterus was contracted and lacerated, and that the lower portion of the rectum was diseased. On May 13th, 1896, he operated for these difficulties. She remained several weeks in the sanitarium without improvement and then returned home. On July 29th, following, her brother-in-law took her again to the sanitarium, at the request of her husband, and on the next day the defendant performed a second surgical operation upon her, and removed her ovaries and uterus. She remained at the sanitarium until August 8th, and then was removed to her home. Neither operation was successful in improving her health, but she grew gradually worse mentally, and on August 25th was adjudged insane and committed to an asylum. She was not a witness at the trial.

The cause of action was based on the removal of the uterus at the second operation; it was not claimed that the operation was unskilfully performed, but that it was performed without the consent or authority of the plaintiff and constituted a trespass to her person. The declaration averred that the plaintiff had placed herself under the care of the defendant and that he, without her consent or the consent of any one authorized to act for her, anæsthetized her and removed the uterus and ovaries.

On the part of the defence there was no pretence that the plaintiff herself consented to the removal of the uterus as a specific operation. The defendant testified that he told her just enough about her condition, and what he proposed to do, to get her consent to the first operation, saying:—"I worked her deliberately and systematically, taking chances which she did not realize the full aspect of, deliberately and calmly deceiving the woman; that is, I did not tell her the whole truth." Referring to the patient's consent to the first operation the defendant said:—"She knew that the womb was to be operated on, and she was willing that should be done. Consent for further work was not obtained." The defendant also justified his act by testifying that the plaintiff was mentally so unsound as to be incapable of consenting or of giving intelligent consideration to her condition, as to which, however, the evidence was conflicting.

The defence also contended that the husband gave an implied consent to the second operation, which the husband denied. The proof which the defendant gave that the husband did authorize it was that when the latter first brought his wife to the sanitarium "Davis said he was willing that I should do anything I thought necessary, only he made the request that I do as little as possible. The defendant then told Davis, in substance, that two operations might be necessary." The defendant also testified that while the plaintiff was at home her husband "told me she was no better. I told him to bring her back for the finishing work. I did not tell him what the finishing work would be. I had but one comprehensive talk with him. That was at the time he was there with the plaintiff." It does not appear that the husband denied that these conversations were had as related by the defendant.

The discussion of the question "What Constitutes Consent," by the Appellate Court, deserves special notice. In its preliminary remarks the Court says it thinks both Courts, it and the lower one, recognize adequately the great obligation to medicine and to surgical skill under which all civilized communities lie; but that, weighty as they are, they still do not confer on the physician or surgeon unlimited power to use his own discretion in the surgical or medical treatment of patients who, suffering from some bodily ailment, come to him for advice and assistance. Undoubtedly an implied license "to have," as the defendant's argument phrased it, "the proper remedial means brought to bear," often exists. The patient may, by his whole course of conduct, without any express language giving consent, evidently place his body at the disposal of the surgeon or physician whom he consults. And for a soldier to go into battle with a knowledge beforehand that surgeons attached to the army are to have charge of the wounded, might perhaps be considered an implied license for such operations as the surgeon afterward, in good faith, performed. Perhaps, too, the various cases which might be supposed of sudden and critical emergency, in which the surgeon would be held justified in a major or capital operation without express consent of the patient, might be referred to the same principle of an implied license. But the broad statement put forth by the defendant, as a correct proposition of law, that, "when a patient places herself in the care of a surgeon for treatment without instructions or limitations on his authority, she thereby in law consents that he may perform such operation as, in his best judgment, is proper and essential to her welfare," is not one to which this court can give assent. It does not hold, again to quote defendant's counsel, that there is " a universal acquiescence of lay and professional minds in the principle that the employment of a physician or surgeon gives him implied license to do whatever, in the exercise of his judgment, may be necessary." On the contrary, under a free government at least, the free citizen's first and greatest right, which underlies all others—the right to the inviolability of his person, in other words, the right to himself—is the subject of universal acquiesence, and this right necessarily forbids a Surgeon or physician, however skilful or eminent, who has been asked to examine, diagnose, advise, and prescribe (which were at least necessary first steps in treatment and care), to violate, without permission, the bodily integrity of his patient by a major or capital operation, placing him under an anæsthetic for that purpose, and operating on him without his consent or knowledge.

Counsel asserted that not a case can be found in the English or American reports where a Surgeon has been held liable for performing an operation without the consent of the patient. This is, perhaps, true. This Court has not been able, in its examination, to find such an one, but it by no means follows that the liability does not exist. It would rather indicate that, obedient to the law and the code of professional ethics as well, surgeons have abstained from actions from which the liability would accrue, or at least had not carried the contention that it does not exist into the courts of last resort. It was the court's opinion, except in cases where the consent of the patient is expressed or is implied by circumstances and occasions other than a mere general retainer for medical examination and treatment, and except also where there is a superior authority which can legally and rightfully dispose of the person of the patient, and which gives consent, a Surgeon has no right to violate the person of the patient by a serious major operation, or one removing an important part of the body. That the consent of the patient herself to such an operation as was performed in this case was necessary, if she was in a free condition and in such mental health as implied capacity to decide, it does not believe has been denied by any Court. And, in view of the testimony of both plaintiff and defendant, the Court held that the existence of any consent, express or implied, on the part of the plaintiff personally must be eliminated from consideration. The Court was also of the opinion that the preponderance of the evidence, with regard to the husband's consent, was that it was not given for the performance of the second or major operation. The judgment of the lower court was therefore affirmed.

The Supreme Court of Illinois, on appeal from the judgment of the Appellate Court, reviewed the facts and stated that it was not claimed that the operation was unskilfully performed, but that it was performed without authority or consent of the plaintiff and constituted a trespass to her person.

The Court, after careful consideration of the evidence, was satisfied that it did not tend to show that the husband had consented to the second operation. He testified that he did not and that, when he first took his wife to the sanitarium, the defendant told him the operation would be a trifling one and the defendant, while admitting that he may have said this, also testified to the conversations with the husband already detailed. The Court says these two conversations are relied upon by the defendant as the authority given by the husband for the second operation and they think it manifest that the authority given by the husband in the conversation first above quoted was exhausted when the first operation was performed and the patient taken away.

Although the defendant stated that he told the husband in that conversation that he could not determine the extent of the operation that would be necessary, and that the defendant gave him *carte blanche* to do whatever he thought proper, it was apparent that neither party then contemplated that the wife would be taken home after the first operation, and return to the sanitarium later for the purpose of undergoing a second operation. The Court thought it equally apparent from the defendant's testimony that, when the husband was directed to bring his wife to the sanitarium a second time for treatment, he did not understand that such an operation as the removal of the ovaries and the uterus was to be performed. The mere fact that after that conversation he had his brother take his wife to the sanitarium was not to be regarded as tending to show consent to an operation of that character.

In regard to the next point raised by the defence that, in the absence of express authority to remove the uterus, the law would imply the necessary consent from the fact that consent was, as the defendant said, obtained for the removal of the ovaries, the Supreme Court held that as there was no evidence which tended to show that any permission was obtained for the second operation, when the ovaries were in fact removed, there was nothing to raise the implication in question. Nor did the court think that consent was to be implied from the relation of the parties under the evidence in the case. The rulings of the trial and the appellate courts were left undisturbed and the judgment was affirmed.

CONSENT OF HUSBAND NOT NECESSARY IF WIFE IS COMPETENT.—In State ex rel. Janney *vs.* Housekeeper *et al.*, 70 Md., 163, a case in which an operation was performed upon a woman whose husband testified that he supposed the operation was to be for the removal of a tumor from her breast, and that he told the surgeon that if the formation was a cancer he objected to its removal, the trial resulted in a verdict for the defendants. The evidence was such that the jury might infer that the wife knew that the formation in her breast was a cancer.

The Court of Appeals of Maryland, commenting upon the evidence given and the law applicable to the facts shown, said, "When the doctors came to the house, she (the patient) had already prepared herself to undergo the operation. If she consented to the operation, the doctors were justified in performing it, if, after consultation, they deemed it necessary for the preservation and prolongation of the patient's life. Surely the law does not authorize the husband to say to his wife, 'You shall die of cancer; you cannot be cured, and a surgical operation, affording only temporary relief, will result in useless expense.' The husband has no power to withhold from his wife the medical assistance which her case might require." The judgment was affirmed.

In McClallen *vs.* Adams, 19 Pick., Mass. 333, the Supreme Judicial Court of Massachusetts gave the following decision: "The Court are of the opinion, upon the facts appearing by the bill of exceptions, that the defendant (the husband of the patient) by placing his wife under the care of the plaintiff (the Surgeon), whom he knew, at a distance from his own residence, for medical and surgical treatment, for a dangerous disease, impliedly requested him to do all acts, and adopt such course of treatment and operation, as in his judgment would be most likely to effect her ultimate cure and recovery, with the assent of the wife, and therefore that the operation in question was within the scope of the authority given him. They are also of opinion that the assent of the wife, to the operation, was to be presumed from the circumstances."

CONSENT OF WIFE TO OPERATION UPON HUSBAND.—Consent of the wife to an operation upon the husband is probably not necessary, if the husband is in a condition to give consent, and yet the Surgeon is more completely protected by obtaining her consent if any unfavorable result attends the operation.

CONSENT TO OPERATION UPON A MINOR.—In case of an operation upon a minor the consent of the parent or guardian should be obtained, except in an emergency where the life of the patient apparently depends upon immediate action. If the minor has arrived at years of discretion it will be proper to obtain his consent.

IX. Consent to Use of Anæsthetics and to Making Autopsies.—ANÆS-THETICS A NEW FEATURE IN THE PRACTICE OF SURGERY.—The employment of anæsthetics for the purpose of relieving pain is of comparatively recent date and the accidents which have occurred during their use have given rise to questions of liability of the Surgeon administering them. The sudden deaths that sometimes occur before the operative procedure has begun, have proved embarrassing to the Surgeon, although he may have obtained a satisfactory consent to the manual part of the operation. It is not usual, but quite exceptional, that a Surgeon informs a patient of the dangers of this initial stage of the operation, and the death comes as a surprise to the friends who are liable to regard it as proof that the accident was due to negligence, unskilfulness, or ignorance on the part of the Surgeon. The defence of the Surgeon to the charge of concealing the dangers of anæsthetics is that 1, these deaths are so rare as to be unworthy of notice among the dangers of the operation, and 2, experience proves that anæsthesia is more readily effected when the mind of the patient is undisturbed by fear or apprehension. He, therefore, avoids exciting the fears of the patient by every possible means and endeavors to create a feeling of hopefulness and security.

DEATH OF AN INEBRIATE FROM CHLOROFORM.—CONSENT NOT GIVEN.—MALPRACTICE ALLEGED.—In a case of death during the administration of chloroform in France, the trial court held that the Surgeon's technique was faultless, but that he had omitted to warn the patient and his family of the dangers of chloroform anæsthesia in general, and especially in persons more or less addicted to alcohol as was the case of this patient. The Court stated that as the operation was not undertaken for vital reasons, but merely for the reduction of a dislocated shoulder, the Surgeon should have explicitly informed the patient and his family, and have obtained their consent before undertaking the administration of chloroform for an operation that was not strictly necessary. In case of vital necessity the Surgeon has only his science and his conscience to consult, but in the case in question this does not apply.*

The Court of final appeal reversed this decision. Referring to the patient's alcoholism and tendency to syncope, the judge stated that all physicians are

* Gaz. Méd. Belge, Nov. 9th, 1905.

unanimous in declaring that alcoholism is not a contra-indication to the use of chloroform; injured workmen are frequently put under the influence of chloroform in the hospitals of Paris, even when they are drunk at the time, in order to undertake without delay some necessary operation. It is absurd to assert that anæsthetics should be used only when the life of the patient is in danger. Such a limitation would deprive the wounded and persons suffering from serious affections, requiring surgical intervention, of the relief offered by anæsthesia. Chloroformization reduces rather than augments the dangers resulting from operations; the frequently intolerable sufferings occasioned by an operation would certainly entail fatal syncope oftener than would the anæsthesia. The court denied the plea for damages on the ground, 1, that the chances of death by chloroform are very slight (1 in 2,000); 2, that the danger of sudden death under chloroform seems to lie more in the personal impressionability of the patient, and that this impressionability, and hence the danger itself, would be increased if he were informed beforehand of all the immediate and contingent perils to which the anæsthesia might hypothetically expose him; 3, that it is the duty of the Surgeon, on the contrary, to reassure the patient, to inspire his confidence, and to seek to dispel from his mind the apprehensions which can only be ominous for him.

DEATH FROM CHLOROFORM ADMINISTERED WITHOUT CONSENT OF PARENT. —Bakker *vs.* Welsh *et al.*, 144 Mich., 632, was an action brought by a father, as administrator of the estate of his son, seventeen years old, who had died on an operating table in a hospital while chloroform was being administered preparatory to the removal of a tumor from his ear.   As the record showed no want of skill in the operation, the principal point presented to the court was: Were the defendants liable in this action because they engaged in this operation without obtaining the consent of the father?   Counsel for the plaintiff stated that they were unable to aid the court by reference to any decisions in point, either supporting or opposing the plaintiff's contention, though they had devoted much time and research to the question.   They were content, therefore, to call the attention of the court to such general reasoning as led them to take the view presented.   The contention was that it is wrong in every sense, except in case of emergency, for a physician and surgeon to enter on a dangerous operation, or, as in this case, the administration of an anæsthetic, conceded to be always accompanied with the danger that death may result, without the knowledge and consent of the parent or guardian.   On the part of the defence it was contended, 1. Consent of the father was unnecessary; 2. The lack of consent was not the cause of the boy's death, hence not actionable; 3. That if it were, the action does not survive under the death act; 4. That the action, if any, is in the father, not in the administrator.   The trial judge directed a verdict in favor of the defendants.

On a writ of error brought by plaintiff the Supreme Court of Michigan said: "The record shows a young fellow almost grown into manhood, who has been for a considerable period of time, while living with his father, afflicted with a tumor.   He has attempted, while at home, to have it removed by absorption.

It does disappear, but after a time it reappears. He goes up to a large city and with an aunt and two sisters, all adults, submits to an examination, receives some advice, and goes back to his father with an agreement to return later to receive the report of the expert who is to make the microscopic examination. He returns accordingly, and with at least some of his adult relatives arranges to have a surgical operation of a not very dangerous character performed. Preparations are made for its performance. There is nothing in the record to indicate that, if the consent of the father had been asked, it would not have been freely given. There is nothing in the record to indicate to the doctors, before entering upon the operation, that the father did not approve of his son's going with his aunt and adult sisters, and consulting a physician as to his ailment, and following his advice. We think it would be altogether too harsh a rule to say that under the circumstances disclosed by this record, in a suit under the statute declared upon, the defendants should be held liable because they did not obtain the consent of the father to the administration of the anæsthetic." The judgment was affirmed.

EMPLOYMENT OF SURGEON HELD AN IMPLIED CONTRACT WHICH IMPORTED CONSENT UNDER THE COMPLAINT.—In Wood vs. Wyeth, *supra*, a boy was taken to a charity hospital by a maid, and on examination the surgeon decided that an operation was required; chloroform was administered and he died under its influence. The mother commenced an action and contended that the boy was sent to the hospital to be examined and not for surgical treatment; that the operation undertaken was without her consent or that of the maid. From a judgment and order in favor of the defendant obtained upon a second trial, plaintiff appealed. The Appellate Division of the Supreme Court of the State of New York, 94 N. Y. Sup., 360, affirming the judgment and order appealed from, held as follows. "The express allegation in the third subdivision that the said Robert Wood employed the defendants as physicians and surgeons to attend him and cure him necessarily implied that a contract to that effect had been made, or had arisen by operation of law, between the parents of the infant and the doctors; and it imported also that such parental consent had been given as was necessary to authorize the doctors to do whatever might be proper in the treatment of the patient for the purpose of bringing about the desired cure. With such an averment in the complaint, it was not necessary for the defendant to prove any further consent to the operation which was performed in order to justify a surgeon in performing that operation, provided only that it was proper and necessary."

CONSENT NECESSARY TO THE PERFORMANCE OF AN AUTOPSY.—This discussion of the civil obligations of the Surgeon in the practice of American surgery would not be complete without referring to the legal status of the dead body as regards the right of the Surgeon to make autopsies. The law provides the conditions under which autopsies may be made to meet the ends of justice, and the officials by whom such autopsies may be made, without the consent or even knowledge of relatives or friends. Autopsies made without consent, by other persons than such public officials, are illegal and the persons who make them are liable to actions for damages. In Foley *vs.* Phelps, 1 App. Div. (N. Y.), 551, it was held that "The right is to the possession of the corpse in the same condition it was in when death supervened," and that when this right is violated, such violation furnishes a ground for a civil action for damages. Taylor, in discussing this subject, gives the following as the order of succession of the relatives in whom this right vests, viz., first, the husband or wife of the deceased; second, if no husband or wife survives, then the children; third, if there is no husband or wife and no children, then, first, the father, second, the mother; fourth, after them the brothers and sisters of the deceased; fifth, after them the next of kin, according to the course of the common law, to the remotest degree, according to the descent of personal property.*

X. Violation of the Civil Obligation by the Surgeon Constitutes Malpractice.—MALPRACTICE DEFINED.—Malpractice in the practice of surgery is the bad professional treatment of disease, or bodily injury, from reprehensible ignorance or carelessness, or with criminal intent. A Surgeon, offering his services to the public as such impliedly contracts that he possesses and will use in the treatment of his patients a reasonable degree of skill and learning, and that he will exercise reasonable care and exert his best judgment to bring about a good result. A failure to perform this contract renders him liable for injuries caused to the patient thereby. The standard by which the degree of care, skill, and diligence required by surgeons is to be determined is not the highest order of qualification obtainable, but is the care, skill, and diligence which are ordinarily possessed by the average of the members of the profession in good standing in similar localities, regard being also had to the advanced state of medical science at the time. Unless it is so provided by an express contract, the Surgeon does not warrant that he will effect a cure, or that he will restore the patient to the same condition in which he was before the necessity for the treatment arose, or that the result of the treatment will be successful. The law, in the absence of a special statute, does not give exclusive recognition to any particular school or system of medicine, and the question whether or not a practitioner in his treatment of the case exercised the requisite degree of care, skill, and diligence is to be tested by the general rules and principles of the particular school of medicine which he follows, not by other schools. A class of practitioners who have no fixed principles or formulated rules for the treatment of disease must be held to the duty of treating patients with the ordinary skill and knowledge of Surgeons in good standing.†

WHAT MUST BE PROVED IN AN ACTION FOR MALPRACTICE.—In an action against a Surgeon for alleged malpractice the plaintiff must prove that the defendant assumed the character and undertook to act as a Surgeon without the education, knowledge, and skill which entitled him to act in that capacity; he must show that the Surgeon had not reasonable or ordinary skill, or he is bound to prove in the same way that, having such knowledge and skill, he neglected to apply them with such care and diligence, as, in his judgment, properly exercised, the

---

* The Law in its Relations to Physicians, pp. 323, 333.
† Am. and Eng. Ency. of Law (2d ed.), vol. 22, pp. 798–801 and cases cited.

case must have appeared to require; in other words, that he neglected the proper treatment from inattention and carelessness. Leighton *vs.* Sargent, 7 Foster (N. H.), 460.

MALPRACTICE FROM WANT OF A REASONABLE DEGREE OF LEARNING.— In Courtney *vs.* Henderson, Marine Court, New York, the plaintiff, a man fifty-seven years old, suffered from a disease of the eyes for which he was treated in the Eye Infirmary for several weeks with success. He left the Infirmary and placed himself under the care of defendant who operated on the eyes and made applications by which treatment the plaintiff lost his sight. The defendant's counsel contended that, "An error in judgment is not malpractice." The court held that to be good law when applied to a man skilled in anatomy, surgery, or physics, but that it had no application in this case; that the defendant, knowing nothing of anatomy, surgery, or physics, could have no judgment in the matter. The law contemplated a judgment founded upon skill and knowledge in these sciences. That man who would hold himself out to the world as a doctor and an oculist, without a diploma, without any knowledge of these sciences, and under such false pretences obtains a patient, and commences tinkering with the most delicate of all the organs, the eye, must be reckless indeed. An error in judgment, of a man skilled in a particular calling, is not malpractice, unless it is a gross error. But error in judgment in a science, of a man unskilled in that science (if such a thing can be), is malpractice. In other words, a person attempting to practise in physic or surgery, without first having obtained a knowledge of such science, is liable for all the damage that is the result of his practice. The court concluded, "I have no doubt the plaintiff lost his vision through the defendant's treatment, and that the treatment was the result of ignorance on his part." Judgment for the plaintiff for $500.

MALPRACTICE FROM WANT OF A REASONABLE DEGREE OF SKILL.—In Carpenter *vs.* Blake, 60 Barb. (N. Y.), 488, an action for damages for alleged malpractice in the treatment of a dislocation of the elbow-joint, it appeared that the plaintiff was thrown from a horse she was riding and her elbow-joint dislocated; the defendant, a practising physician and surgeon, was called to treat the injury; and the complaint was that the bones were never restored to their places, or, if they were, that proper measures were not taken to keep them there, and that the result was that the joint became stiff, and the arm useless. There was a verdict in favor of the plaintiff, on which judgment was rendered, and from that judgment the defendant appealed.

The General Term of the Supreme Court in the Fourth Judicial Department of New York (Mullin, P. J.) held that the plaintiff charged want of skill, as well as negligence. So far as the pleading could make want of skill material, it was done. The trial judge said, "I suppose it is entirely immaterial to the inquiry before you whether the defendant, at the time he undertook the reduction of this dislocation, was or was not reputed to be, or was or was not, a skilful surgeon. The question is, did he bring to that particular case the degree of skill to which I have referred?" The degree of skill to which he referred was that reasonable "degree of skill ordinarily possessed by the members of the profession to which he belongs—the average skill of his profession." By this language the court understood the trial judge to mean that, if the surgeon does not bring to the treatment of an injury, or of a disease, the ordinary amount of skill possessed by those in the same profession, it is immaterial how high his standing may be. If he has the skill and does not apply it, he is guilty of neglect. If he does not have it, then he is liable for the want of it. Whether, therefore, the surgeon possesses ordinary skill may be material in an action for malpractice, but not whether he possesses a higher degree of skill. That a Surgeon possesses skill may be shown by those of the same profession who can speak from personal knowledge of his practice. When the point in issue is whether skill was applied in a given case, the possession of skill without proof that it was applied would be no defence in a case of malpractice. When it is proved that the Surgeon has omitted altogether the established mode of treatment, and has adopted one that has proved to be injurious, evidence of skill or of reputation for it is wholly immaterial, except to show what the law presumes, that the defendant possesses the ordinary degree of skill of persons engaged in the same profession. In such a case it is of no consequence how much skill he may have; he has demonstrated the want of it in the treatment of the particular case. The failure to use skill, if the Surgeon has it, may be negligence; but when the treatment adopted is not in accordance with established practice, the case is not one of negligence, but want of skill. The New York Court of Appeals reversed this judgment (50 N. Y., 696), a bare majority of the court holding that the trial judge erred in charging the jury that it was entirely immaterial to the inquiry before them whether defendant, at the time he undertook the reduction of the dislocation, was or was not a skilful surgeon, evidence having been given upon the part of the defendant to show that he was reputed to be and was a skilful surgeon. With this exception the opinion of Judge Mullin was approved. (10 Hun, 12; 75 N. Y., 12.)

MALPRACTICE FROM NEGLIGENCE.—Whatever may be the special feature in the charge of malpractice, "negligence" is so uniformly alleged that its legal significance requires an authoritative definition. "Strictly speaking," says McClelland, "the term is limited in its application to carelessness in the performance of professional duty. Carelessness is its proper synonym. Duties performed without care, caution, attention, diligence, skill, prudence, or judgment, are negligently performed. Acts are so designated that are performed by one heedlessly, even where there is no purpose to omit the performance of duty. It is non-feasance, not mal-feasance. It is the omitting to do and not the ill-doing—this last being a want of skill." *

NEGLIGENCE IN THE USE OF THE X-RAY.—The use of this new agent in the practice of surgery has resulted in injuries to the persons which have been the subject of litigation. One of the first cases on record occurred before the trial term of the Supreme Court in the city of New York, but the case is not officially reported as there was no appeal. The treatment was for tuberculous glands

* Civil Malpractice.

of the neck and the charge against the physician was that he "unskilfully, carelessly, and negligently administered to the plaintiff what is commonly called or known as x-ray treatment, whereby the hair on the left side of the plaintiff's head was burned off, and her face and neck on the same side were greatly burned, hurt, and injured."

The court charged the jury upon the question of the physician's duty according to the familiar rule and held that the physician is not an insurer or guarantor, and in the use of the x-ray he does not insure the patient against a burn. The mere happening of an x-ray burn is not evidence of negligence. "If the jury find that the plaintiff received the burn of which she complains in consequence of the treatment by the defendant, they cannot infer that the defendant was negligent merely because the plaintiff afterward suffered from x-ray burn, for the cause of the burn may be beyond human knowledge, and even expert experience may not be sufficiently uniform to indicate a sure means of preventing it. Owing to the limitations of human knowledge, the exercise of every reasonable care does not always prevent accidents, and this is especially true in dealing with such comparatively little-known forces as electricity and x-rays. The jury cannot find the defendant guilty of the negligence alleged in the complaint unless it can find in the proofs some particular act of negligence which caused the burn. To punish the defendant because he cannot explain the cause of the burn is not necessarily to punish him because he has done wrong, but may be to punish him because he does not know something which science cannot find out, or has thus far been unable to find out. That would be manifestly unfair, and the law will not do it."

In Henslin vs. Wheaton et al., 91 Minn., 219, an action for negligence and unskilfulness in applying, to the body of the party suing, the device known as "Roentgen's x-rays" for the purpose of locating a foreign substance thought to be in his lungs, the plaintiff testified that the exposure of his person to the x-rays was made for too long a period of time, and that the tube or bulb through which the rays are generated was placed too close to his body. He testified to the number of times the x-rays were applied, and the length of time—from thirty to forty minutes on each occasion—and that the tube of the apparatus was placed within two inches of his person in each instance, except one. About two weeks subsequent to the application of the x-rays to his person there appeared upon his back what is termed an "x-ray burn." On the theory and claim that defendants were negligent and unskilful in applying the x-rays to his person, this action was brought to recover damages. The action was dismissed and a motion for a new trial was denied.

The Supreme Court of Minnesota, on appeal, said that the rule of liability is the same as that applied in other actions for malpractice, and one of ordinary care and prudence. This was the first case to come before it involving alleged negligence on the part of physicians in applying the recently discovered x-rays, and that no rule of care in such cases had been laid down. But there can be no doubt that the rule applicable to the care and skill required of physicians toward their patients in other cases applies. That rule was stated in Martin vs. Courtney,

87 Minn., 197, in the following language: "The legal obligation of the physician to his patient, where his conduct is questioned in an action of this character, demands of him no more than the exercise of such reasonable care and skill as is usually given by physicians and surgeons in good standing." The rule is one of ordinary care and prudence, and the question presented in this x-ray case was whether the evidence received and that offered on the trial tended to show a failure on the part of the parties sued to exercise such care.

In Shockley vs. Tucker, 127 Iowa, 456, an action to recover damages for injuries suffered by plaintiff by having his body burned by the use of an x-ray machine while being treated for appendicitis, the verdict and judgment were for plaintiff, and defendant appealed.

The Supreme Court of Iowa held that the allegations of the petition were broad enough to cover negligence in the use of the x-rays as a treatment for appendicitis, and also negligence in the method in which the x-rays were used. Evidence was introduced for plaintiff as to both forms of negligence. The complaint that the x-ray treatment was not proper for appendicitis was objected to on the ground that the witnesses did not belong to the same school of medicine as the defendant, but the case was submitted to the jury solely on the question whether the defendant had been negligent in his method of using the x-rays. The Court thought this was a question of science and skill, wholly independent of the methods of treatment of any school. That the plaintiff was severely burned in his abdomen by the use of the x-rays, and suffered great pain, and extended, if not permanent, disability therefrom, is clearly shown, and we hardly think it would be contended that such burning was proper treatment for any disease, or in accordance with the theories of any school. Judgment' reversed on a technical error.

NEGLIGENT MALPRACTICE IN LEAVING FOREIGN BODIES IN WOUNDS AFTER OPERATIONS.—In Samuels vs. Willis, 118 S. W. Rep., 339, the Court of Appeals of Kentucky state that the plaintiff charged malpractice in that the defendant negligently left or suffered to be left in her person after an operation for ovarian disease the surgical sponge, which irritated the intestines, causing them to ulcer- ate, creating a fistula which emitted fecal matter and noxious gases to the seri- ous impairment of her health, and causing her sickness and humiliation, mental and physical suffering for which she sought damages. The substance of the charge was that the Surgeon had negligently left a foreign substance in the plaintiff's abdomen after the operation, which had perforated her bowels, pro- ducing the effects specified. The charge that the substance left in the abdomen perforated the bowels was withdrawn and in lieu it was charged, first, that in the course of the operation the Surgeon negligently cut or perforated her intes- tines, and, second, that the sponge which he negligently left in her abdomen ulcerated her intestines, and "left an opening therein." The evidence failed to support the first charge, and the issue presented by the pleadings was the second charge. The evidence was conflicting whether the Surgeon left the sponge in the plaintiff's body, but its presence was not otherwise accounted for as he alone placed and removed the sponges that were used in the operation. Surgeons testifying in behalf of the defendant alleged that the best of surgeons left a sponge or some foreign substance in the bodies of their patients in performing similar operations. From this fact it was contended that, as the highest degree of skill and care are not exempt from the commission of such acts, a similar lapse by the defendant was not other than "ordinary care." But the court held that because all men are at some time careless does not relieve any man from the legal consequences of his careless acts; and that it was for the jury to decide whether the defendant exercised the degree of care in the case which ordinarily prudent and skilled surgeons, who practise in similar localities, usually exercise in such matters.

The trial resulted in a verdict and judgment for $3,500 for the plaintiff. The court decided that a statement of the case disposed of the claim that the damages were excessive, and it affirmed the judgment.

NEGLIGENCE IN LEAVING SPONGE IN WOUND.—DEFENCE THAT ITS REMOVAL WAS NOT PART OF THE OPERATION.—In Arkridge *vs*. Noble, 114 Ga., 949, the plaintiff was a charity patient on whom an operation was performed at a hospital conducted by the city of Atlanta, which furnished all of the preparations and the Surgeon performed operations free of charge. Judgment was for defendant and plaintiff brought error.

The complaint in this case was, in substance, that the defendant had performed a surgical operation upon her person which required an opening to be made in her abdomen, and that it was necessary, in the performance of the operation, to insert into her body, through the opening, certain sponges or pads, for the purpose of absorbing the blood and pus in the cavity, which sponges or pads should remain in the body while the operation was being performed, but should be removed therefrom before the opening was closed; that the defendant negligently and carelessly failed to remove one of these sponges, and closed the opening, allowing the sponge to remain in her body; that it remained there for more than a year, and finally passed out of her body through the rectum, having passed into the rectum through a fistula which the sponge had caused; that she suffered great pain during the time the sponge was in her body, and at the time it was being passed therefrom; that on account of the negligence of the defendant she is now and will always be a complete physical wreck.

The defendant testified positively that he removed all of the pads; that he reached down in the cavity as far as he could reach, searched all over, and removed all of the pads; that he knew he got them all out, because he went thoroughly through the cavity, and found nothing there; that he was satisfied he had found all that were placed therein. The testimony of numerous surgeons was to the effect that, if the pad had been left in the body as claimed by the plaintiff, it would have resulted in her death within a short time after the operation had been performed.

The defendant's counsel contended that the handling of these sponges or gauze strips was no part of the operation; that the rule of care and skill required of the surgeon in operating had no application to the case; the argument was to the following effect: "When a surgical operation of the character involved in the present case is about to be performed, the time when the skill of the surgeon is expected to become active is when the opening is made in the body, and continues while the sponges or pads are being in the body, but that when the affected portion of the body, whether it be an unnatural growth, or part of the human system, has been removed, and all precautions taken to prevent hemorrhage, and the moment arrives for the sponges to be removed, the operation is at an end, and no longer is the surgeon in a position where the knowledge or information which makes him a man of skill is required to be exercised, and that when the pads or sponges are being removed he is no longer the man of skill, exercising skill, but he is simply the ordinary man, and is required to exercise due care and diligence only."

The Supreme Court of Georgia held that the operation begins when the opening is made into the body, and ends when this opening has been closed in a proper way, after all appliances necessary to the successful operation have been removed from the body. From the time the Surgeon opens with his knife the body of his patient, until he closes the wound thus made, in a proper way, the law imposes upon him the duty of exercising not only due care, but due skill as well. During the entire time he must not only know what to do, but he must do it in a careful and skilful manner. It was conceded in the argument that the placing of the pads or sponges in the body required the exercise of skill. It seems to us that the removal of them from the body also requires some degree of skill. It at least requires a Surgeon to perform this service, and, if this is admitted, it is at the same time admitted that skill is required in the performance of the work. We do not suppose that any one would contend for a moment that a Surgeon would be authorized to leave this part of the work, even if not a part of the operation or necessarily incident thereto, to any one who was not skilled in the science of surgery. A knowledge of the human body is necessary in order to determine where these pads or sponges shall be placed when the operation is about to be performed. The Surgeon who testified in behalf of the plaintiff said during the course of his testimony: "It may seem strange, but it is a very difficult matter to find a sponge. It is an easy matter to overlook it." This testimony clearly shows that, in the removal of the sponges which have been placed in the human body, the person seeking to remove the same must be possessed of the requisite knowledge and information to find where they may have been placed, or may have gone during the performance of the operation and this knowledge or information on the part of the surgeon is what is called "skill." The removal of the sponges is a part of the operation; it is a part which requires the exercise of skill; and the charges complained of were held not to be erroneous. Judgment affirmed.

DAMAGE SUIT FOR LEAVING A COTTON SWAB IN WOUND; CHARGE OF MALPRACTICE NOT SUSTAINED.—The Swiss courts recently acquitted a Surgeon who was sued for damages by a patient on whom he had performed an operation for goitre and had left a cotton swab in the wound. Tedious suppuration and paralysis of the right vocal cord resulted and the patient claimed substantial damages. Drs. Burckhardt, of Basel, and Valentin, of Berne, testified that a wad of cotton soaked with blood resembles human tissue so closely·that, under the circumstances, its being overlooked should not be regarded as malpractice. The Surgeon was acquitted.

SURGEON NOT LIABLE FOR ERRORS OF JUDGMENT.—It is held by the courts that if a Surgeon is possessed of proper learning and skill he is not liable for a mere error of judgment, provided he does what he thinks is best after a careful examination. He does not guarantee a good result, but he promises by implication to use the skill and learning of the average Surgeon, to exercise reasonable care, and to exercise his best judgment in the effort to bring about a good result. MacKenzie vs. Carman, 103 App. Div. (N. Y.), 246, s. c. 92 N. Y. Supp., 1063; Pike vs. Honsinger, 155 N. Y., 201; Gerken vs. Plimpton, 62 App. Div. (N. Y.), 35.

In Eislein vs. Palmer, 7 Ohio Dec., 365, in which it was held that a Surgeon who, in repairing a laceration of the perineum, broke a needle, and, by reason of the patient's condition, was unable to make the necessary search to locate the fragment, but closed the wound with a part of the broken needle in the perineum and did not inform the patient of the accident, was not liable for his failure to impart such information. To have told her at that stage would only have endangered the success of the operation. Upon the discharge of the patient it would have become his duty to have apprised her of the accident, but just prior to the time the patient was dismissed the Surgeon was seriously injured by being thrown from his carriage, and on that account the patient did not learn of the presence of the broken needle until it was discovered and removed by another Surgeon at a subsequent operation. Upon the question of the liability of the Surgeon for his failure to apprise the patient of her condition at the time such information was due her, the court said, "Dr. P. did not have to anticipate dangerous and unavoidable accidents, but he had a right to expect that he would be able to attend Mrs. E. until she got well."

WHAT CONSTITUTES CRIMINAL MALPRACTICE?—In Gorden vs. State, 90 S. W. Rep., 636, the Criminal Court of Appeals of Texas held that to constitute "Negligent Homicide of the First Degree" there must be an apparent danger of causing the death of the person killed or of some other person. The want of proper care and caution distinguishes this offence from excusable homicide. The degree of care and caution is such as a man of ordinary prudence would use under like circumstances. The test of the offence seems to be that there must be an apparent danger of causing death. Without this it would seem this offence could not exist, or would not be made out. And the test of care or caution is that which distinguishes it from excusable homicide. The Court says that the question of apparent danger under the statute is perhaps one that may be fraught with more or less trouble when applied to surgical operations. Just how far the surgeon would be responsible for negligent homicide, where there is an apparent danger of causing death of the person on whom the operation is performed, the court does not here propose to decide. Whatever that responsibility is, and at whatever point it may occur, there must be an apparent danger of causing the death of the person on whom the operation is performed, and, of course, this must be viewed in the light of proper care and caution. Many of the operations that are performed to relieve suffering humanity are necessarily fraught with more or less danger, and this is as well understood by the patient, as by the operating surgeon. The Court is of the opinion that the statute never intended to hold a surgeon liable for a homicide in cases of this character, unless there was a want of proper caution and care in the operation, however dangerous that operation may be. It may be proper, perhaps, to state that, in some of the diseases for which these operations are performed for the relief of the patient, the chances are more than equally balanced against life that death will result. Under this character of case there would be an apparent danger of causing death, but in such case, before the surgeon could be held responsible for the homicide, there must be shown a want of proper care and caution in performing the operation. Of course, however dangerous the operation may be and however many ·may be the chances of producing death, the surgeon could not be held guilty, unless he acted without necessary caution and care.

In Hampton vs. State, 39 So. Rep., 421; s. c. 50 Fla., 55, the Supreme Court of Florida, discussing criminal malpractice from negligence, held that where the death of a person results from the criminal negligence of a medical practitioner in the treatment of the case the latter is guilty of manslaughter. This criminal liability is not dependent on whether or not the party undertaking the treatment of the case is a duly licensed practitioner, or merely assuming to act as such, acted with good intent in administering the treatment, and did so with the expectation that the result would prove beneficial. The real question on which the criminal liability depends in such cases is whether there was criminal negligence. Criminal negligence is largely a matter of degree, insusceptible of precise definition, and whether or not it exists to such a degree as to involve criminal liability is to be determined by the jury. Such criminal negligence exists where the physician or surgeon, or person assuming to act as such, exhibits gross lack of competency, or gross inattention, or criminal indifference to the patient's safety; and this may arise from his gross ignorance of the science of medicine or surgery, and of the effect of remedies employed through his gross negligence in the application and selection of remedies, and in his lack of proper skill in the use of instruments, or through his failure to give proper instructions to the patient or his attendents as to the use of the medicines. But where the person treating the case does nothing that a skilful person might not do, and death results from an error of judgment on his part, or an inadvertent mistake, he is not criminally liable.

LATER DISCOURTESY NOT PROOF OF MALICIOUS MALPRACTICE.—In Willard vs. Norcross, 79 Vt., 546, an action for alleged malpractice in the treatment of the plaintiff's wrists, there was a charge of intentional injury against the Surgeon. To prove the surgeon's animus the trial court admitted evidence that he treated the plaintiff discourteously after his attendance had ceased; his connection with the case having ended in January, while the incidents testified to occurred later than May. The discourteous acts consisted in an alleged effort of the surgeon to block the way of the plaintiff on three occasions when they met.

The Supreme Court of Vermont held that the admission of evidence of this discourteous treatment was error. It is true that evidence having a legitimate tendency to show a defendant's animus may be found in things subsequently said or done, but the court finds nothing in the cases to indicate that subsequent unconnected expressions of dislike are admissible as proof that an act in itself lawful was improperly done because of malice.

XI. Ordinary Procedure in Actions for Malpractice.—VERIFICATION OF THE CHARGE OF MALPRACTICE.*—In suits for malpractice against a Surgeon he is presumed at law, as defendant, to be competent for the task which he undertook, and that he discharged the duties which he assumed with fidelity and to the best of his ability. Haire *vs*. Reese, 7 Phila. (Pa.), 138. Therefore, the burden of proof that the Surgeon was guilty of malpractice in any form, rests upon the patient, as plaintiff, and it is incumbent upon him to make the charge of incompetency, want of skill, or negligence, as the case may be, and when issue is joined, to prove by proper evidence the truth of the allegations made. Chase *vs*. Nelson, 39 Ill. App., 53; Georgia No. Ry. Co. *vs*. Ingram, 114 Ga., 639; Winner *vs*. Lathrop, 67 Hun, 511; Styles *vs*. Tyler, 64 Conn., 432; Haire *vs*. Reese, *supra*.

The charge of malpractice is sometimes made by the patient in defence where the Surgeon has brought suit for the value of the services rendered. · In this case the Surgeon is not required, in the first instance, to prove that he exercised proper care and skill, but the defendant-patient who interposes this defence must sustain the charge by satisfactory proof. Robinson *vs*. Campbell, 47 Ia., 625. When a patient prosecutes an action against a Surgeon for malpractice, or to resist a demand for services rendered, and has proven, *prima facie*, his charges, the Surgeon proceeds to introduce evidence in rebuttal of the patient's charge, and it then becomes the duty of the jury, under proper instructions by the court, or of the court sitting without a jury, to weigh the evidence submitted by both parties and decide the questions at issue.

THE DEGREE· AND EXTENT OF THE PROOF REQUIRED ON THE PART OF THE PATIENT.†—It is stated, as a general rule, that the patient is required to prove his case by a preponderance, or greater weight, of the evidence. That is, if the Surgeon introduces évidence, which, in the opinion of the jury, counterbalances or outweighs that of the patient, the latter will have failed in the proof of his case. This rule is not peculiar in trials for malpractice, but obtains in all kinds of actions. Herrick *vs*. Gary, 83 Ill., 85. It is explained that by preponderance of evidence introduced by the patient to prove his contention, is not meant that the evidence must be so strong as to produce a clear conviction in the minds of the jury, or to satisfy them beyond all reasonable doubt, but it is sufficient if the evidence so far preponderates in favor of the patient that the jury may believe therefrom that the allegations made by him are true. Hoener *vs*. Koch, 84 Ill., 408. A case is referred to where an instruction to a jury to find for the Surgeon unless the patient shows by a preponderance of the evidence a state of facts from which no other "rational conclusion" can be drawn than that the Surgeon was unskilled, was condemned as requiring

* The Law and the Doctor, vol. i., p. 32.   † The Law and the Doctor, *supra*.

too high a degree of proof on the part of the patient. Pelky *vs.* Palmer, 109 Mich., 561; s. c., 67 N. W., Rep., 561.

EVIDENCE OF COMPETENCY OF SURGEON.*—It is held to be competent for the Surgeon to show that he has received a good medical and surgical education and that he is a regularly educated and skilful Surgeon (Leighton *vs.* Sargeant, T. Foster (N. H.), 460), but it is regarded as irrelevant to show by the general opinion of another physician whether the defendant is a skilful practitioner. Boydston *vs.* Giltner, 3 Or., 118; Williams *vs.* Poppleton, 3 Or., 139; Leighton *vs.* Sargeant, *supra.* The general rule is stated to be that, whenever the competency or skilfulness of the Surgeon is in issue, such evidence only is competent, or will be given any weight, as directly or circumstantially throws any light on that question, while matters which are collateral or remotely related are to be excluded. Illustrations of the rulings of courts as to the admissibility of remote facts are cited as follows:

In Baird *vs.* Gillett, 47 N. Y., 136, the court admitted evidence that the defendant, a physician, had not rendered a bill since his attendance upon the patient and a judgment of two thousand dollars was given in favor of the plaintiff. The Court of Appeals of New York reversed this judgment, holding that the question was entirely foreign to the issue; that by its admission the defendant was called upon to give explanatory or contradictory evidence by which the jury might be embarrassed in their deliberations; that they might be inclined to construe such forbearance on the part of the physician as an acknowledgment of his want of skill.

The testimony of a nurse, as to the difference in the method of treatment of the defendant from that of another surgeon, in a similar case, was excluded on account of its remoteness when the Surgeon was on trial for injuries alleged to be caused by unskilful practice. Challis *vs.* Lake, 71 N. H., 90.

The change of the course of treatment by a Surgeon, who succeeds to another in the care of a case, does not legally prove that the former method was not proper at the time. Weed *vs.* Baker, 49 Mich., 295.

It is pertinent for the patient to show in an action for damages for malpractice, by his own testimony or that of others, that the Surgeon was intoxicated, and what his appearance was at the time the service was rendered. Merrill *vs.* Pepperdine, 9 Ind. App., 416; s. c. 36 N. E. Rep., 921.

The question of the competency of a Surgeon as affected by engagement in other occupations has been differently decided. It has been held that evidence that he incidentally had the management of a farm which he owned had no tendency to prove general incompetency and was totally insufficient as a foundation of such an argument. In Mayo *vs.* Wright, 63 Mich., 32, the Supreme Court of Indiana, however, held that it was competent for the patient to show, as affecting the skill and knowledge of the Surgeon, that he was engaged in pursuits other than the practice of medicine and surgery. Hess *vs.* Lowery, 122 Ind., 225.

WHEN MALPRACTICE MUST BE SPECIFICALLY PROVEN.†—It is stated that

---

* The Law and the Doctor, *supra.*   † The Law and the Doctor, *supra.*

the rule is that the patient must distinctly and directly prove the specific charge of malpractice, as unskilfulness or negligence, and that the jury cannot, except in extreme cases, draw the conclusion of unskilfulness or negligence from mere proof of the result following the treatment. It would be an unjust rule that would infer that the Surgeon was necessarily at fault when the patient did not recover, or a cure was not effected, or even where serious illness or death followed the treatment. The following case is quoted in illustration:—Sims *vs*. Parker, 41 Ill. App., 284.

The patient went to a Surgeon, related his symptoms, was examined, and informed that he was ruptured. The Surgeon supplied him with a truss and applied it. The patient returned several times to the Surgeon and complained of severe pain; after wearing the truss about two weeks he became sick and an abscess appeared where the pad of the truss made pressure. The evidence showed that the patient suffered great pain from the abscess and was sick for a long time. The charge against the Surgeon was that the abscess was the result of too great pressure of the truss due to its improper adjustment. It appeared in the evidence of expert witnesses that there was in fact no rupture of the person of the plaintiff, and yet the Court held that a mistake in making a diagnosis, not shown to be the result of negligence or unskilfulness, did not give rise to a cause of action.

The Appellate Court of Illinois gave the following opinion in this case:— "While there is evidence tending slightly to support the contention that the abscess may have been produced by the pressure of the truss, there is absolutely no evidence that defendant was negligent or unskilful in his diagnosis, or in fitting the truss. Proof that he was mistaken as to the existence of a rupture, or that the abscess was caused by the pressure of the truss, was not enough to entitle the plaintiff to a verdict."

The following case is referred to by the same authority illustrating the point under consideration: *—

A school teacher had her left eye operated upon by a Surgeon for the cure of a strabismus. It was proved that before the operation her eye was strong and in good condition, except as to the strabismus. The operation resulted in relieving the strabismus, but she alleged that, after the operation, neither of her eyes was as strong as formerly, and that some time after the operation she suffered from a "spell of sore eye," that the lids were afterward inflamed and her eyes "watered" when they were exposed to the wind or to the cold; that she suffered from general weakness of the eyes. She was not allowed to recover on this evidence, the court holding as follows:—

"No proof was offered of the instruments used or the manner in which the operation was performed. No medical or scientific evidence was offered showing the cause of the present condition of the plaintiff's eyes, nor that the defendant was negligent or careless in the performance of the operation. . . . To maintain her action, she should have offered the evidence of skilled witnesses to show that the present condition of her eyes was the result of the operation, and that

* The Law and the Doctor, *supra*.

it was unskilfully and negligently performed." Pettigrew *vs.* Lewis, 46 Kan., 78; s. c. 26 Pac. Rep., 458.

WHEN MALPRACTICE FROM UNSKILFULNESS OR NEGLECT MAY BE INFERRED.*—There are cases which are regarded as exceptions to the rule that malpractice by the Surgeon must be affirmatively proven. In these cases the results, when proven, inferentially justify the conclusion that the Surgeon showed want of proper knowledge and skill, or of negligence, in his treatment.

In Richardson *vs.* Carbon Hill Coal Co., 10 Wash., 648, a Surgeon was found guilty of negligence in a case of fracture of the femur complicated with dislocation of the same bone at the hip joint. He discovered the fracture and reduced it, but did not discover the dislocation, though the displaced bone was pushed upward and backward, creating a large and easily discernible tumor. The Surgeon's attention was several times called to the fact that the patient's hip was painful, but he did not examine the part, always alleging that the pain was due to the fracture.

In Mitchell *vs.* Hindman, 47 Ill. App., 431, a case of Colles' fracture, the Surgeon applied a bandage so tightly to the hand and arm as to cause great pain and did not remove it until sloughs formed. On the trial the Court held that these facts were sufficient on which to base a judgment, though it was not shown that the fracture itself was not properly reduced.

THE RULE THAT MALPRACTICE MAY BE INFERRED IS LIMITED.†—The cases in which the conditions or circumstances justify the inference that the Surgeon has been guilty of malpractice in his treatment are comparatively few.

In James *vs.* Crockett, 34 N. B., 540, the Court refused to apply it where a Surgeon failed to discover that his patient's arm was dislocated, as he made more than one careful examination of the injured arm, and had called another Surgeon in consultation; hence there was no evidence of want of skill or negligence.

The position has been well taken‡ that a Surgeon may fail to discover the existence of a fracture and treat the injury as a bruise without becoming liable. Fractures in the vicinity of joints are often followed by such a degree of swelling of the soft parts before the Surgeon has an opportunity to examine them, that the existence of a fracture could not be discovered by the exercise of ordinary skill and care. The evidence must show that the condition of the patient was such as has been described at the time of the examination. Gedney *vs.* Kingsley, 16 N. Y. Supp., 792. The Surgeon should inform the patient that the conditions are unfavorable for determining the exact nature of the injury, and that other examinations will be required to make a correct diagnosis, for the patient may dismiss him from further attendance after the first examination, and the failure to give such advice might be considered as an act of incompetence or negligence by the jury.

LIABILITY SOMETIMES A QUESTION FOR THE JURY, THOUGH IMPROPER TREATMENT IS NOT SHOWN.§—There is a class of cases, according to the authority referred to, that constitute an exception to the rule that want of knowledge

---

* The Law and the Doctor, vol. i., p. 36.   † The Law and the Doctor, *supra.*
‡ The Law and the Doctor, *supra.*   § The Law and the Doctor, *supra.*

and skill or negligence must be affirmatively proven. They are cases where the evidence presented during the trial gives rise to a reasonable question, deducible from the results of his treatment, as to the Surgeon's skill or care. In Hickerson *vs.* Neely, 54 S. W. Rep., 842, the evidence showed that the patient suffered a fracture of the leg near the ankle joint; that the Surgeon was called on the day of the injury and undertook the treatment of the leg; that five days afterward he reset the bones and encased the limb in a plaster cast; that the plaster dressing was retained on the limb for about six weeks; that when the dressing was removed "the foot and ankle were crooked, and remained so, and were stiff." The verdict was in favor of the defendant (the Surgeon) in the trial court, but, on appeal, the Court of Appeals of Kentucky decided that the trial court erred in not permitting the question to go to the jury, to be determined from this and similar evidence, whether the Surgeon had been guilty of negligence in setting the broken bones. The higher court therefore reversed the judgment entered for the defendant by direction of the trial judge, and ordered a new trial.

In Griswold *vs.* Hutchinson, 47 Neb., 727, a Surgeon erroneously diagnosed a patient's case as ovarian tumor after an examination of about ten minutes, consisting in manipulating the abdomen and inserting the finger in the vagina, but he did not use a speculum, nor a uterine sound, and in consequence of a false diagnosis performed a needless operation. It was held that the facts presented were sufficient to take the question to the jury.

To Whom Cause of Action Accrues.*—The rule of the common law giving separate causes of action to the husband and father and to the wife and child for the same act of malpractice has been preserved in the jurisprudence of the several States and is now the law. Nixon *vs.* Ludlam, 50 Ill. App., 273; Stone *vs.* Evans, 32 Minn., 243; Long *vs.* Morrison, 14 Ind., 595; "Law in its Relations to Physicians," Taylor, p. 336. The principle underlying this law regards the family in certain respects as a single entity, the rights and liabilities being vested in the husband and father. If the wife suffers from the maltreatment of a Surgeon, the law regards the husband as injured in the loss of the services and society of his wife, and to recover this injury he sues alone. In addition, a cause of action arises in favor of the wife for the injury and the physical suffering to which she has been subjected by such maltreatment and upon this cause of action the husband and wife sue jointly at common law. In the States or jurisdictions where a married woman is permitted by statute to sue in her own name, the action is brought by the wife in her own name and on her own behalf. Practically the same causes of action arise when a child. suffers injury due to the malpractice of the Surgeon, viz., one to the father for loss of services and cost of care and treatment of the child, and one to the child himself for any pain and suffering and permanent injury beyond his minority. The suit for the child is brought by the father, or guardian, or by a third person called next friend.

Questions of Malpractice can be Litigated but Once.†—It is held that

*The Law and the Doctor. vol. i., p. 30.   † The Law and the Doctor, vol. i., p. 31..' ¹⁄

where these questions or issues have been raised between the parties and have
been judicially decided by a court of competent jurisdiction the questions so
decided cannot be again litigated between such parties. The doctrine is known
in the law as that of *res adjudicata*. In accordance with this doctrine it has
frequently been held by the courts that, in case a Surgeon has brought suit
against a patient for services rendered, and the case was tried, and decided in
the Surgeon's favor, the patient will thereafter be forever debarred from maintaining any action on account of malpractice in the treatment which constituted the basis of the Surgeon's claim, the theory being that all questions
pertaining to such alleged malpractice, having once been before the court,
cannot therefore be subsequently reopened between the same parties. Should
the patient fail to appear at the trial and thus allow a judgment against him by
default, the question has arisen, Will the judgment thus rendered against him
be likewise a bar? It is sufficient to state that the courts of several States have
given different opinions; viz., *affirmatively*, New York, New Jersey, Arkansas,
Gates *vs.* Preston, 41 N. Y., 113; Blair *vs.* Bartlett, 75 N. Y., 150; Bellinger *vs.*
Craigue, 31 Barb., 534; Ely *vs.* Wilbur, 49 N. J. L., 685; Dale *vs.* Lumber Co.,
48 Ark., 188; *negatively*, Indiana, Ohio, Wisconsin, West Virginia, Goble *vs.*
Dillon, 86 Ind., 327; Sykes *vs.* Bonner, Cinc. R. (Ohio), 464; Ressequie *vs.*
Byers, 52 Wis., 650; Lawson *vs.* Conway, 37 W. Va., 159.

XII. The Surgeon as a Witness.—SUGGESTIONS TO THE SURGEON AS A
WITNESS.—It has been truly remarked by Elwell * that the medical witness
rarely finds in works on medical jurisprudence those directions he needs to prepare him for the important duties of making up and giving opinions that are to
be received by a court and jury as facts, and that will warrant them in rendering
a verdict or judgment upon such opinions. The same authority also says,
"He who studies well the office of the professional witness,—combining, as it
does, the importance of the evidence, and the value of the position to the witness
himself,—will be impressed with the magnitude of the consequences involved,
and qualifications necessary for an easy and honorable, as well as pleasant
discharge of its functions."

PREPARATION OF WITNESS.—Elwell says that the medical witness can only
be prepared to do credit to himself, justice to the parties interested in the issues
of the case upon which he is called, and honor to the profession which he represents, by a thorough, well-ordered, well-digested knowledge and complete understanding of his profession, in all its extensive and intricate departments upon
questions in any of which he may be called to give an opinion. Professor
Coventry gives the following † advice to medical witnesses, "The medical witness
should have his mind fully prepared, before taking the stand, as to what he can
testify to, and his reasons, if they are required. He should, in his testimony,
avoid, as much as possible, the use of technical or professional terms, which
the jury would not be likely to understand; but if unavoidable, then their
meaning should be explained to the jury."

* A Medico-Legal Treatise on Malpractice and Medical Evidence, etc. By John J. Elwell,
M.D., p. 305 *et seq.*   † Report to the American Medical Association.

THE MANNER OF THE WITNESS.—Elwell states that if the witness proceeds in an equivocal, halting manner, not using affirmative terms, he will not receive that degree of credit that he would if he coolly, firmly, and candidly, without any real or apparent prejudice or hesitation, stated distinctly what he knows, and upon what his knowledge is founded. If the witness' manner is open, and free from that peculiar restraint and nervousness that usually characterize the interested or dishonest witness, and if he can give a clear and complete reason for his statement, then he will be believed. If, on the other hand, he is over-exact, or very loose in his statements, reluctant, or unable to give a good reason for what he says, he will be distrusted and discredited. Professor Coventry advises the witness, in giving his testimony, to keep cool and collected, and not permit himself to be irritated or confused by the counsel; he should avoid introducing any expression or opinion not immediately connected with the cause before the court.

AVOID DISCUSSION WITH COUNSEL.—Elwell says that the medical witness should never permit himself to be cunningly drawn into a discussion while upon the stand, either metaphysical or scientific; because it will always be carried on to disadvantage on his part. It is a discussion the court and jury can feel but little interest in, and the chances are that it will result to the discredit and discomfiture of the witness. The counsel being perfectly at home in the presence of the court, and the witness being placed in a new, and to him, perhaps, an embarrassing and awkward position, the former will, of course, have every advantage. The witness has done his duty when he has answered the question put to him, in as few words as will convey the sense he wishes to utter, with proper explanations, if any is needed. When he volunteers anything beyond this, not directly bearing upon the question at issue, he does it at his peril, and prejudices his position. While the witness has an undoubted right to clothe his ideas in his own language, and explain fully just what he means, let him study brevity, for he has no right to go out of his way, even to argue or defend his position, unless called upon so to do. After he has given an opinion and the grounds for it, whether right or wrong, it should be left there. The witness is entitled to the right—and should insist upon it—of having the question fairly and clearly stated, and he should not attempt an answer until he fully comprehends its bearing.

CARE IN ANSWERING CATEGORICAL QUESTIONS.—Elwell cautions the Surgeon as a witness to be careful as to categorical answers to questions, unless he completely comprehends the effect of such answers, and the extent to which they reach. Yes, or no, positively fixes the answer, and afterward it may be found difficult to qualify such answers. A witness may say yes, or no, to *facts* within his knowledge, but when the question involves several elements and various circumstances, as most professional questions do, these positive terms should be used cautiously and guardedly.

DIFFERENCE BETWEEN AN ORDINARY WITNESS AND AN EXPERT WITNESS.— In Sheldon *vs.* Wright, 67 Atl. Rep., 807, an action for alleged malpractice in the treatment of a fracture of the tibia, the Supreme Court of Vermont held that the ordinary witness testifies as to facts of which the jury have or should have knowledge of their own, but, nevertheless, they must apply their own good judgment to the testimony of such witnesses in determining what facts are proved. The expert testifies to facts of a different class, or to the interpretation of facts, for the most part about which the jury are not expected to have knowledge of their own.

SCIENTIFIC AND TECHNICAL KNOWLEDGE NOT WITHIN THE EXPERIENCE OF THE ORDINARY WITNESS.—In Rowe vs. Whatcom County Railway and Light Co., 87 Pac. Rep., 921; s. c. 44 Wash., 648, a personal-injury case, the principal issue at the trial was whether the plaintiff had curvature of the spine as a result of other injuries. Prior to the trial the court appointed three physicians to make a physical examination of the plaintiff at the request of the defendant who afterward called them as witnesses. These witnesses testified to certain tests which they applied to the plaintiff to determine whether he was suffering from curvature of the spine. The plaintiff called a medical witness in rebuttal who was not allowed by the trial court to answer the questions as to whether the tests were proper and fair. The reason assigned by the trial court for its ruling sustaining objections to these questions was, that the question whether the tests applied by the witnesses for the defendant were fair or proper, was for the jury.

The Supreme Court of the State of Washington held that in this the trial court erred. It ruled that the witness was asked his opinion on a matter involving scientific and technical knowledge, not within the ordinary experience of the witness or jury, and should have been permitted to answer. Certainly the ordinary juror is not qualified to determine whether any given test will disclose the presence or absence of curvature of the spine without the aid of expert or opinion evidence. Nor was there any merit in the claim that the testimony was not proper in rebuttal. While the witness had already testified that the plaintiff had curvature of the spine, stating fully the reasons for his conclusion, yet he was asked nothing concerning the test afterward applied by the defendant's witnesses and he could not be and was not required to anticipate the tests that might be resorted to.

ATTENDING SURGEON MAY TESTIFY AS TO PROBABILITIES.—In Vohs vs. Shorthill & Co., 130 Ia., 538; s. c. 107 N. W. Rep., 417, the Supreme Court of Iowa said, in a personal-injury case, that the rule as generally applied may be conceded to exclude medical testimony of merely possible or speculative results of the present condition of an injured party. But it is too well settled to require the citation of authorities that where an injury negligently occasioned is permanent or, if not permanent, recovery is not complete at the time of the trial, the injured party is entitled to damages already accrued, and such other damages also as the evidence shows him reasonably certain to sustain in the future. As bearing on that point it is certainly competent for a physician who has examined and treated him and knows his condition to express an expert opinion as to future consequences reasonably to be expected to follow the injury. And the court says of a certain physician that he was not asked to state results which were merely possible, but whether a given result was "likely," that is, probable, or reasonably to be expected. This the court thinks was competent within the rule. He was testifying from his personal examination, knowledge, and treatment of the plaintiff's injury, and there was no occasion for propounding hypothetical questions or to assume or state any special facts as a foundation for the inquiry to which answer was sought.

DISTINCTION BETWEEN EXPERT AND OPINION EVIDENCE.—In Schwantes *vs.* State, 106 N. W. Rep., 237; s. c. 127 Wisc., 160, the Supreme Court of Wisconsin holds that the scope of "opinion evidence" is not limited by the technical meaning of the term "science, art or skill." It says that the quoted expression, often found in decisions, in a view that might be taken thereof, conveys rather too narrow an idea of the scope of "opinion evidence." It may have no appreciable connection whatever with "science, art or skill," in a technical sense, and yet be admissible just as clearly as if it possessed such connection. All "opinion evidence" is not expert evidence in the general—the legal—sense of the term. The term "skill" as used in the quoted expression must be regarded in its broadest signification, not applied necessarily only to mechanical or professional knowledge. It includes every subject susceptible of special and peculiar knowledge derived from experience. The term "science, art or skill" as a limitation of expert evidence is more of a lexiconic than judicial origin. Webster defines the noun "expert" as "One who has skill, experience, or peculiar knowledge on certain subjects of inquiry in science, art, trade, or the like; a scientific or professional witness." That, strictly construed, is hardly a safe guide. The law writers define the term as "a person having special knowledge and skill in the particular calling to which the inquiry relates." The preliminary questions respecting "opinion evidence," that is, that of the competency of the witness, and that of whether the subject is within the scope of "opinion evidence," are in the field of competency, in which the judgment of the trial court is conclusive, unless shown to be clearly wrong.

EVIDENCE OF SURGEON AS EXPERT SHOULD BE UNBIASSED.—Although it is a truism to assert that the evidence of the Surgeon as an expert should be unbiassed, yet expert, or, as it is sometimes called, "professional evidence," has unfortunately fallen into such disrepute in the courts that we deem it important in this connection to counsel the Surgeon testifying as an expert, to preserve his mind in a completely unbiassed state in forming and expressing an opinion on the facts presented. The attitude of legal authorities and of the courts toward expert medical testimony justifies our cautionary advice.

In discussing this subject a noted author and distinguished jurist refers to the following cases: *

Lord Campbell in Tracey Peerage, 10 Cl. and Fin., 191, said that "skilled witnesses came with such a bias on their minds to support the cause in which they are embarked, that hardly any weight should be given to their evidence." Judge Taylor, in his work on Evidence (sixth ed.), p. 49, says, "Perhaps the testimony which least deserves credit with a jury is that of skilled witnesses; these gentlemen are usually required to speak, not to facts but to opinions;

* Thomas on Negligence (2d ed.), pp. 1208, 1209.

and when this is the case, it is often quite surprising to see with what facility and to what an extent, their views can be made to correspond with the wishes or the interests of the parties who call them. They do not, indeed, wilfully misrepresent what they think; but their judgments become so warped by regarding the subject in one point of view, that, even when conscientiously disposed, they are incapable of expressing a candid opinion." In Roberts vs. N. Y. El. R. Co., 128 N. Y., 464, the Court of Appeals, by Judge Peckham, said: "Expert evidence, so-called, or, in other words, evidence of the mere opinion of witnesses, has been used to such an extent that the evidence given by them has come to be looked upon with great suspicion by both courts and juries, and the fact has become very plain that in any case where opinion evidence is admissible, the particular kind of an opinion desired by any party to an investigation can be readily procured by paying the market price therefor."

These criticisms of expert evidence are undoubtedly severe, but there is sufficient justification for them to require a word of warning to Surgeons who appear in the courts as expert witnesses, especially in what are known as "personal-injury" actions. These cases now fill the court calendars, and are frequently brought and maintained by attorneys upon a contingent basis, relying upon a result favorable to the plaintiff for compensation for their services, and to meet the expenses of litigation including the fees of the Surgeons called as experts. When requested to testify as an expert the Surgeon should use discriminating judgment as to the merits and bona fides of the case in which his services are sought to be enlisted, and not allow himself to be drawn into any case the justice and fairness of which, from a professional standpoint, he himself is not reasonably well assured.

The Supreme Court of Pennsylvania very justly remarks in Huston vs. Borough of Freemansburg, 61 Atl. Rep., 1022; s. c. 212 Penn. St., 550, a personal-injury case, "In the last half-century the ingenuity of counsel, stimulated by the cupidity of clients and encouraged by the prejudices of juries, has expanded the action for negligence until it overtops all others in frequency and importance, but it is only in the very end of that period that it has been stretched to the effort to cover so intangible, so untrustworthy, so illusory, and so speculative a cause of action as mere mental disturbance. It requires but a brief judicial experience to be convinced of the large proportion of exaggeration, and even of actual fraud, in the ordinary action for physical injuries from negligence, and if the Court opened the door to this new invention the result would be great danger, if not disaster, to the cause of practical justice."

QUALIFICATIONS OF AN EXPERT.—In Macon Railway and Light Co. vs. Mason, 51 S. E. Rep., 569; s. c. 123 Ga., 773, the Supreme Court of Georgia held that nothing more is required to entitle one to give testimony as an expert than that he has been educated in the particular trade or profession; knowledge gained by consistent and close study of medical works renders one competent to testify as an expert concerning the matters of which he has thus learned; it is not necessary that he should be actively engaged in the practice of medicine;

nor is it essential that one who has a really scientific education on the subject should be a graduate of any medical college, or have a license from any medical board; what he knows is what really qualifies him to express an opinion as an expert, and a diploma or license is only important as furnishing satisfactory evidence of his competency as a witness.

COURT DECIDES AS TO QUALIFICATIONS OF EXPERT.—In Conley vs. Portland Gas Light Company, 58 Atl. Rep., 61; s. c. 99 Me., 57, the Supreme Judicial Court of Maine held it to be a universal rule that whether a witness called as an expert has the necessary qualifications to enable him to testify as such is a preliminary question addressed to the presiding justice, and his decision must be final and conclusive unless it is made clearly to appear from the evidence that it was not justified or was based on some error in law; expert capacity is a matter wholly relative to the subject of the particular question; a witness may be sufficiently qualified for one question and totally unqualified for the next; special skill and knowledge in regard to a particular subject can only come from experience or special study or both; mere casual observation, superficial reading, or slight oral instruction is not sufficient.

MATTERS FOR EXPERT MEDICAL TESTIMONY.—In Travelers Insurance Company vs. Thornton, 42 S. E. Rep., 287; s. c. 116 Ga., 121, the Supreme Court of Georgia held that an expert can testify as to what was the cause of death, or of an injury, or as to the effect of disease, or as to the effect of a blow on one sound or on one unsound; he can give his opinion on physical facts or as to the medical facts, but he cannot determine the legal classification of such facts. The expert may aid the jury, but he cannot act as a member of the jury; nor, while he is on the stand, can he transcend the functions of a witness, and under the guise of giving testimony state a legal conclusion.

In Taylor vs. Grand Ave. Ry. Co., 84 S. W. Rep., 873; s. c. 185 Mo., 239, the Supreme Court of Missouri held that it would be proper to state to the plaintiff's experts the nature and extent of the injuries received by the plaintiff as they appeared at the time of the accident, and then to ask them whether or not in their opinion such injuries might, could, or would result in paralysis. The experts having thus given an opinion, it would be for the jury to find the fact as to whether in this particular case the paralysis was caused as the plaintiff's experts said it might have been caused, or whether it was the result of other causes as the defendant's experts testified might be the case. There is a very essential difference between permitting an expert to give an opinion and permitting him to draw a conclusion. The one is the province of a witness; the other is, in the first instance, the special prerogative of the jury. When a witness is thus permitted by the court to invade the province of the jury, it goes to the jury with the endorsement of the court, and is calculated to make them believe that it was proper for the witness instead of the jury to draw the concluison.

WITNESS SHOULD BE PERMITTED TO EXPLAIN MEANING OF SCIENTIFIC OR TECHNICAL TERMS.—It was held to be eminently proper by the Supreme Court of Indiana in Swygart vs. Willard, 76 N. E. Rep., 755, that a witness dealing with scientific or technical terms, should, if possible, make his meaning more clear by reference to terms in common use. It was not improper for the same reasons to permit a physician to explain in this case the meaning of "Monomania" as used by him. He was rightly permitted also to explain the distinctive peculiarities of a mind suffering from insane delusions; the symptoms of dementia, and, on a hypothetical statement of facts showing some form of mental unsoundness, to testify under what class of unsoundness of mind the testator should be placed. A medical expert may also explain the effect resulting to the brain, nervous system, and body of a man from the excessive use of alcohol.

Inasmuch as an expert has the right to explain the reasons for his opinion, it was held to be competent for the witness to state an experiment in detail to fortify his opinion. Commonwealth, etc., vs. Tucker, 76 N. E. Rep., 134, 135. But the court said it is settled in Massachusetts that the rule allowing an expert to give the reasons for his opinion has its limitations, one of which is thus stated (citing from Hunt vs. Boston, 152 Mass., 168; s. c. 25 N. E. Rep., 82): "A party cannot put in evidence incompetent facts under the guise of fortifying the opinion of his witness, even if the evidence might have been properly admitted on the cross-examination of the expert." The experiment in question being incompetent as substantive evidence, the court properly excluded all evidence as to its nature, even whether made on a dead or living body, although offered under the guise of a reason for the opinion of the witness.

DEMONSTRATION OF INJURIES TO JURY BY EXPERT WITNESS.—Expert witnesses sometimes give their testimony with an air of authority offensive to the court. Their attitude is that of a professor giving a lecture to his class and in their excitement discuss matters foreign to the question at issue. Such exhibitions on the part of experts are under the control of the court, but they tend to impair the character and confidence of court and jury which an expert witness ought by his conduct to inspire.

In Rice vs. the Wabash Railroad Company, 74 S. W. Rep., 428, the Court of Appeals at St. Louis, Missouri, in a personal-injury case said that the company was loud and vehement in its complaint against what was termed the anatomical and surgical lecture of the suing party's expert witness in describing and illustrating, by reference to that party's nose, the nature of the injuries sustained. But, if the method adopted by the party suing in presenting such testimony was effective and potent, the court says, the presiding judge was clothed with broad discretionary authority in the proper course and seemly conduct of trials before him, and, in the absence of clear abuse of such power, the court is inclined to defer to his action, and assume that he properly controlled the management of the trial, and it was not disposed to hold that the manner in which the injuries of the party suing were demonstrated by the physician to the jury constituted reversible error.

ADMISSIBILITY OF EVIDENCE OF EXPERIMENTS BY EXPERTS.—In Commonwealth vs. Tucker, supra, a homicide case, one of the questions claimed to be material, was whether the azygous vein of the victim was severed by a stab in the back, the prosecution contending that it was and the defence that it was not. A medical expert testified on the part of the defence that, while it was barely possible that the vein was thus severed, yet it was highly improbable, and finally said that to him it seemed impossible; asked whether he had made any experiments for the purpose of "ascertaining that opinion," he replied that he had; asked whether he had made experiments on a body approximating the size of the victim in this case described by him, he said he had. Objection being made he was not allowed to show the nature of the experiment.

The Supreme Judicial Court of Massachusetts decided that the Court was fully justified in excluding the experiment and any inquiry into its nature. It says, the true ground of admitting the details and result of such an experiment is that it may be of assistance, but the question whether it may be, or whether it may not lead to too many collateral questions, is largely within the discretion of the court. The ruling was just in view of the nature of the question in dispute, viz., whether the azygous vein was cut by the stab in the back, taken in connection with the difference necessarily existing between the conditions in the case on trial and those under which the experiment was performed, and the obvious difficulty, if not impossibility, of ascertaining whether such difference had any material effect on the result.

EXPERT CANNOT BASE AN OPINION ON EVIDENCE OF OTHERS.—In Elgin, Aurora and Southern Traction Co. vs. Wilson, 217 Ill., 47; s. c. 75 N. E. Rep., 436, the Supreme Court of Illinois says a physician may testify as an expert from information obtained by a physical examination of the person who is the subject of the inquiry, but he should not be permitted to state his opinion based on the conclusion arrived at by himself made upon the evidence as he heard it and gave it weight. The proper course is to state hypothetically the case which the party producing the witness thinks has been proved, and to ask an opinion based on such hypothetical case. To permit the expert to base his opinion on the testimony as he construes it, and has weighed it, would be to permit him to exercise the functions of a jury, and, in a sense, decide the whole issue for them.

SIMULATION OF PAIN SUBJECT FOR EXPERT TESTIMONY.—In the personal-injury case of McGrew vs. the St. Louis, San Francisco and Texas Railway Co., 74 S. W. Rep., 816, the party suing had been thrown from a wagon in consequence of the frightening of a horse which she was driving. There was much evidence in the record to the effect that she was not injured to the extent claimed, and that some of her pretended injuries were feigned and simulated. One of the attending physicians who examined her injuries, and treated her for the same, testified that he had employed certain tests to ascertain whether she could feel pain in her limbs. He was asked whether or not she was simulating the absence of pain when the tests were applied.

The Court of Civil Appeals of Texas held that it was error not to admit this evidence, for the question asked, and the proposed answer thereto, were in its opinion the subject of expert testimony—a matter peculiarly within the province of the physician.

EXPERT EVIDENCE AS TO PERMANENCY OF INJURY.—In Hallum vs. Village of Omro, 99 N. W. Rep., 1051, an action brought to recover damages for personal injuries alleged to have been sustained on a defective sidewalk, the Supreme Court of Wisconsin stated that a surgeon had given his opinion as to the plaintiff's ability to control, normally, the action of her left limb from having observed her as she walked and had given opinion evidence as to the probable cause of such condition. The Court held there was no error in that. Again, the surgeon having knowledge as to what the plaintiff testified respecting her condition before and after the accident, was asked, on the hypothesis that her testimony was true, whether the injuries she was suffering from "were liable to be permanent." It was strenuously insisted that such testimony was conjectural and was erroneously received. The Court held that it is true that there can be no recovery, legitimately, for permanent impairment in a case like this in the absence of competent evidence warranting a conclusion, with reasonable certainty, that such impairment will exist as a result of the accident; but it is not necessary that opinion evidence should be confined to that high degree of certainty. Experts may properly testify to the mere probabilities of the case. It would ordinarily be very difficult to secure any more definite opinion evidence than that from a conscientious expert. An examination of the cases cited will show that "probable," "likely," and "liable" have been treated as synonymous, each dealing with reasonable probability, not with possibility; that what may probably or is likely or liable to be the future result of a personal injury is competent evidence to prove what is reasonably certain in the matter. That is according to lexical authority as to the meaning of the words. The better way, however, to provoke professional opinion evidence in such a matter is to ask for the expert's opinion, not using either term. But an interrogative as to what the probabilities are, or what is likely or liable to be the result as regards permanency of the injury, cannot be condemned as speculative or conjectural. This does not militate at all against the doctrine that the ultimate vital fact to be determined is what is reasonably certain to be the result. That is for the jury to determine from all of the evidence bearing on the question, including the opinion evidence as to what is probable, likely, or liable to be the result.

EXPERT TESTIMONY AS TO SUBJECTIVE SYMPTOMS NOT ADMISSIBLE AS EVIDENCE.—In Greinke vs. Chicago Railway Co., 85 N. E. Rep., 327, a personal-injury case, the Supreme Court of Illinois held that it is well settled that a surgeon when called as a witness who has not treated the injured party, but has examined him solely as a basis on which to found an opinion to be given in a trial to recover damages for the injury sustained by the injured party, cannot testify to the statements made by the injured party to him, or in his presence, during such examination, or base an opinion on the statements of the injured party. An expert witness called under such circumstances must base his opinion on objective and not on subjective conditions. The declarations of the injured party made to a surgeon, who has made an examination of such party with a view to qualifying himself to testify as a witness only, are not admissible.

The Court did not intend to hold that a surgeon may not be able, from an examination of an injured party, to form and express an opinion as to his physical condition and the probable cause which induced such condition, based on objective testimony alone, but what it intends to hold is that a surgeon who has not treated the injured party, but who has made an examination of the injured party solely with a view to testifying as an expert, should not be permitted to express an expert opinion to the jury based on subjective conditions, and then be allowed to fortify his opinion by stating to the jury acts of the injured party which could have been purely voluntary and under the control of the injured party, and which may rest on no other basis than the truthfulness of the injured party.

XIII. Compulsory Physical Examination of Plaintiff.—PHYSICAL EXAMINATION OF THE PLAINTIFF BY EXPERTS.—The right of the defendant to a physical examination of the plaintiff by experts in personal-injury cases is of importance to the Surgeon. Until a comparatively recent period it was held that the Court had no inherent power, and, in the absence of a statute conferring the right, might not, in advance of a trial of an action for personal injuries, compel the plaintiff on application of the defendant to submit to an examination of his person by surgeons appointed by the Court with the view of enabling them to testify on the trial as to the existence or extent of the alleged injury. This was the opinion of the Court of Appeals of the State of New York in the case of McQuigan vs. D. L. & W. R. Co., 129 N. Y., 50 (1891). This decision was notable as having reversed the first ruling affirming the power of the Court to order such examination which was made by the Superior Court of New York in 1868, and of a similar ruling by the special term of the New York Court of Common Pleas in Shaw vs. Van Rensselaer, 60 How. (N. Y.), 143.

THE ORIGIN OF COMPULSORY EXAMINATION.—The opinion of the Superior Court of the City of New York in Walsh vs. Sayre, 52 How. Pr., 334, is historical and should be quoted. The patient was a child suffering from a swelling in the left gluteal region. The Surgeon explored the swelling and finding pus he opened the abscess freely. In the discharge were shreds of dead cellular tissue, and one mass was so large as to require enlargement of the wound. The mother believing this mass was a portion of the child's flesh, became so excited that the child was dressed with difficulty. She was advised to return with the child on the following morning for treatment, but did not, and the Surgeon heard no more of the case until he was notified to defend himself in a suit for malpractice. It appeared that subsequently two surgeons had examined the wound and both alleged that the hip joint had been opened, and it was on their expressed opinion that the action was commenced. The Surgeon asked the court that a personal inspection be accorded him and other qualified surgeons, on the ground that the strongest evidence that could be brought forward to prove that the charge of the plaintiff was false would be the determination by surgical witnesses who were experts, as to the condition of the child with the cicatrix and of the joint at that time.

This "personal inspection" was objected to by the attorney for the plaintiff as a "personal trespass," and he would consent to nothing but an "oral examination." The Court sustained the objection on the ground that "there was no precedent allowing personal examination previous to the trial of the cause."

Upon petition, "the equity side of the court" recognized that there were other rights existing at the same time, side by side with those under the ordinary rules of law, and ordered that such an examination be made. The opinion of Judge Jones establishing this precedent from the point of view of the equity of the petition is a model of sound logic.

The Court said that, as the determination of the action depends on the judgment of skilled surgeons, the defendant will prosecute his defence under serious, if not disastrous, disadvantages if this motion be denied. For, in that event, he will have to combat the testimony of those surgeons who have already formed their opinions adverse to him, possibly under the influence of an unconscious bias and have not only so formed them but expressed them. There is no just reason why the defendant should be suffered to remain under this disadvantage when it can be easily avoided by a resort to the same means by which it was created. In a case where skilled surgeons may honestly differ in their views, it is not proper that the cause should be left to be determined on the evidence of two or three surgeons, selected by the plaintiff out of the whole body of surgeons, perhaps because their views are adverse to the defendant's; but it is eminently proper that defendant should have the benefit of the testimony of one or two surgeons of his own selection, and that these surgeons should have the requisite means of forming a correct judgment, one of which is an examination of the affected part.

In 1893 the Legislature of the State of New York enacted a law (Chap. 721) which authorized such examination upon application to the Court in the following terms (Code of Civil Procedure, Sec. 873): "In every action to recover damages for personal injuries, the court or judge, in granting an order for the examination of the plaintiff before trial, may, if the defendant apply therefor, direct that the plaintiff submit to a physical examination by one or more physicians or surgeons, to be designated by the court or judge, and such examination shall be had and made under such restrictions and directions as to the court shall seem proper . . . if the party to be examined shall be a female she shall be entitled to have such examination before physicians or surgeons of her own sex."

The constitutionality of this act and a similar one in New Jersey has been upheld by the courts of these States. Lyon vs. Man. R. Co., 142 N. Y., 298; McGovern vs. Hope, 63 N. J. L., 76. There has been constant progress in the recognition of the justice and equity of the ruling, in favor of "compulsory examination," by the higher courts of the States, and by the legislative bodies which have enforced the practice by law.

As early as 1877 the Supreme Court of Iowa in the case of Schroeder vs. C. R. I., etc., R. Co., 47 Iowa, 375, affirmed the power of the Court to compel examination of the plaintiff, and without reference apparently to the opinion of the Superior Court of New York in the case of Walsh vs. Sayre, supra. The plaintiff alleged that the injuries produced permanent disability. The defendant filed a written application requesting the court to make a proper order requiring the plaintiff to submit to a physical examination to determine the character and extent of the injuries. This application was denied by the trial court, it holding that it had no power to order such an examination. The Supreme Court reversed the judgment with the following remark, "To our minds the proposition is plain that a proper examination by learned and skilful physicians would have opened the road by which the cause could have been conducted nearer to exact justice than any other way. The plaintiff, as it were, had under his own control testimony which would have revealed the truth more clearly than any other that could have been introduced. The cause of truth, the right administration of law, demand that he should have produced it."

JUSTICE DEMANDS AN EXAMINATION.—In White *vs.* Milwaukee, etc., R. Co., 61 Wisc., 536, the Supreme Court of Wisconsin reversed the judgment of the trial court which had refused to grant an examination of the plaintiff in a personal-injury case on the ground that it had no authority to make such an order. The Court said: "On principle and authority we are satisfied this was error. The then condition of the injured limb had a most important bearing upon the question as to whether the plaintiff's injuries were permanent, and an examination at that time, the results of which would have been put in evidence before the jury, would in all probability have greatly aided them in determining the extent and consequences of the injury. It would be or might have been more satisfactory and conclusive evidence on that subject than the statements of the plaintiff or opinions of medical witnesses. The application for her examination contained in it every reasonable safeguard against offending the modesty or delicacy of the plaintiff, and although she might shrink from the examination, yet the ends of justice imperatively demanded that she should submit to it."

RIGHTS WHEN A PATIENT OFFERS HIS BODY FOR EXAMINATION.—In Pronskevitch *vs.* Chicago & Alton Railway Company, 83 N. E. Rep., 545, all of the plaintiff's clothes were removed from the upper part of his body, and his injuries were exhibited to the jury. The defendant requested the court to require him to submit to an examination by its physicians, in the presence of such witnesses as he might desire, in a private room or some place convenient to the courtroom. The plaintiff expressed a willingness to be examined before the jury by the physicians of the defendant, but not out of the presence of the jury. The trial court refused to compel the examination, and that ruling was assigned as error.

The Supreme Court of Illinois did not regard this ruling as error and held that its decisions have been that the court has no power to compel the plaintiff in a personal-injury case to submit to a physical examination. The plaintiff having offered his body voluntarily to the inspection of the jury, it then became a subject of examination under such reasonable restrictions as the court might see fit to require. Inasmuch as the plaintiff offered to submit to such an examination, in the presence of the jury, as the defendant might see fit to make, there was no just cause for complaint.

EXAMINATION OF A WOMAN.—The case of Alabama G. S. R. R. Co. *vs.* Hill, 90 Ala., 71, was one which involved the propriety of enforcing the rule of compulsory examination, when the plaintiff is a woman, in order to determine the dangerous and permanent character of her injuries. The examination required to be made of her person by an expert was of a kind most objectionable to a young woman of delicacy and refinement. The trial court denied the motion of the defendant for an examination of the plaintiff for want of power and the judgment was reversed on this ground. The Supreme Court of Alabama said, "We are satisfied from the evidence which was before the court when the last application was made, that such an examination would not have involved any ill consequences to the plaintiff. . . . Her delicacy and refinement of feeling, though of course entitling her to the most considerate and tender treatment consistent with the rights of others, cannot be permitted to stand between the defendant and a legitimate defence of a claim of a large sum of money. When it comes a question of possible violence to the refined and delicate feelings of the plaintiff on the one hand and possible injustice to the defendant on the other, the law cannot hesitate; justice must be done. Was it essential to the ends of justice that plaintiff should submit to this examination? We think it was.'

EFFECT OF VOLUNTARY EXHIBITION OF INJURED PART OR MEMBER IN OPEN COURT.—In Houston & Texas Central Railroad Co. vs. Anglin, 86 S. W. Rep., 785, the Court of Civil Appeals of Texas held that, whatever may be the rule in other jurisdictions, it regards it as well settled in that State that a court has no authority to compel a party to exhibit his person to a physician, or any other person, for the purpose of an examination; and the fact that he has done so once does not deprive him of the right to refuse to do so again. The Supreme Court of Texas reversed this ruling (89 S. W. Rep., 966) and held that as the plaintiff had voluntarily exhibited his injured chest to the court and jury it was an error to refuse to compel him to exhibit it to a physician called by the defense to prove that he had before examined the plaintiff and found his chest to be deformed.

REFUSAL TO SUBMIT TO AN EXAMINATION TENDS TO DISCREDIT CLAIM AS TO EXTENT OF INJURIES.—The Court of Civil Appeals of Texas, in Houston Electric Co. vs. Lawson, 85 S. W. Rep., 459, a personal-injury case, held that when a plaintiff in a case of this character refuses to submit to an examination, the fact of such refusal is a circumstance tending to discredit his claim as to the extent of his injuries, and is admissible in evidence for that purpose. Of course, there might in many cases of personal injury be reasons for a refusal by the plaintiff to submit to an examination which would greatly weaken, if not wholly destroy, the effect of such refusal as evidence; but the refusal, and the reason, if any, given therefor by the plaintiff, are facts to go to the jury, and must be weighed by them.

THE PRESENT POSITION OF THE QUESTION OF THE RIGHT OF COMPULSORY EXAMINATION.—At the present time it appears that the power of the trial court irrespective of statutory provisions to compel physical examinations of plaintiffs is *asserted* in the States of Alabama, Arkansas, California, Colorado, Georgia, Iowa, Indiana, Kansas, Kentucky, Michigan, Minnesota, Missouri, Nebraska, North Dakota, Washington, and Wisconsin, and is *denied* in the Federal courts, and in Illinois, Oklahoma, Massachusetts, Texas, and Utah.

XIV. Admissibility in Evidence of Pictures, Hospital Records, and Surgical Treatises.—PHOTOGRAPHIC PICTURES DULY AUTHENTICATED ADMISSIBLE IN EVIDENCE.—In State vs. Roberts, 82 Pac. Rep., 100; s. c. 28 Nev., 350, the Supreme Court of Nevada held that photography, engraving, and the art of picture making are important factors in our civilization, and the Courts in their search for truth should not be adverse to accepting the benefits which they bring. A glimpse at a photograph may give a more definite and correct idea of a building or of a person's features than the most minute and detailed testimony. When photographs are shown to be correct representations, and give a clearer and better understanding of relevant facts, it seems of reason and principle that their use as evidence should be favored.

In the same case the Court gave an instructive opinion as to the proper use of a photograph. It held that a photograph of a wound after it had been opened by the knife of a Surgeon was properly excluded by the trial judge, because the bullet hole was no longer in the condition caused by the accused. But it finds no error in the admission in evidence of three photographs, one of which showed the face of the deceased in the repose of death, in which a witness was able to recognize the features of the man picked up, while the others showed the entrances of the bullets on the arm and leg, and were illustrative and instructive in connection with the testimony of the physician and other witnesses. Some extreme cases were cited where photographs were rejected on the ground that witnesses had described what they would show, or that they would inflame or prejudice the jury—doctrines that this court is not able to sanction, and which are not supported by the weight of authority.

RADIOGRAPHS ADMISSIBLE ON THE SAME BASIS AS PHOTOGRAPHS.—In State vs. Matheson, 103 N. W. Rep., 137; s. c. 130 Iowa, 440, the Supreme Court of Iowa holds that the progress of x-ray photography is now as well established as a recognized method of securing a reliable representation of the bones of the human body, although they are hidden from direct view by the surrounding flesh, and of metallic or other solid substances which may be embedded in the flesh, as was photography as a means of securing a representation of things which might be directly observed by the unaided eye at the time photography was first given judicial sanction as a means of disclosing facts of observation; and for that purpose x-ray photographs, or skiagraphs, or radiographs, as they are variously called, have been held admissible on the same basis as photographs. The Court had no difficulty in holding that a radiograph admitted in evidence in this case, after proof that it was taken by a competent person, was admissible to show that there was in the body of the person of whom it was taken, some hard substance in the shape of a bullet, near the spinal column. There was no evidence that this object which was represented in the radiograph was a bullet, but it was proper for the jury to take the evidence for what it was worth as indicating that something in the shape of a bullet was lodged in the man's body. Whether it was in fact a bullet they must determine, just as they would have been required to determine the fact if the witness had testified that he saw something of the size and shape of a bullet. That was all he could have told simply by looking at it, if it had been exposed to view. Evidence as to the location of the bullet subsequent to that when it first lodged there after being fired would not be material in determining the course it took unless there was some reasonable ground for assuming that its location had not changed meantime. The Court thinks it can properly take judicial notice of the fact that a bullet embedded in human flesh usually becomes encysted, and does not change its location without external interference. The probability that the bullet when discovered by means of the radiograph was in the same position that it was when first lodged in the man's body was sufficiently strong to have warranted the jury in taking the information furnished by the radiograph for what it was worth, in their judgment, in determining what the course of the bullet was after entering the body.

PRELIMINARY PROOF OF THE CORRECTNESS OF THE PHOTOGRAPH REQUIRED.— In Chicago & Joliet Electric Railroad Company vs. Spence, 72 N. E. Rep., 796; s. c. 213 Ill., 220, a personal-injury case, it was insisted that the trial court erred in permitting the introduction in evidence of a skiagraph, or x-ray photograph, of a portion of the chest and body of the plaintiff. It was intended to show by the skiagraph that the party's heart had been displaced, that the walls of that organ had become thick, and that an abnormally heavy tissue had formed on the walls of the heart. The skiagraph was made by a person who testified that he was an x-ray expert; that he was regularly engaged in taking such photographs for physicians; that he took the negative from which the photograph was developed; that he developed the photograph and that it was an accurate and correct representation.

The Supreme Court of Illinois held that photographs taken by the x-ray process are admissible in evidence after proper preliminary proof of their correctness and accuracy has been produced; that the testimony of the x-ray expert who made the skiagraph was sufficient to justify the trial court in ruling that the picture should be admitted in evidence.

It appears that in the same case an expert on the part of the defendant gave testimony tending to show that the skiagraph had not been properly taken and expressed the opinion that the picture was of little or no value as a representation of the heart and other portions of the plaintiff. The trial court was not asked to exclude the picture on account of this adverse criticism, and the Supreme Court thinks that if the request had been made it should have been granted.

There was a similar ruling in Clapp vs. Norton, 106 Mass., 33, where it was held that before admission in evidence there must be a verification of the accuracy of the representation, and this is a preliminary inquiry to be made by the presiding judge whose decision is final. The testimony of the photographer is not required if the judge is satisfied by other evidence that the representations are substantially accurate. Commonwealth vs. Morgan, 159 Mass., 375; McGar vs. Borough of Bristol, 71 Conn., 652; Archer vs. N. Y., N. H. & H. R. R. Co., 106 N. Y., 589.

JURY MAY USE PHOTOGRAPHS IN THEIR DELIBERATIONS.—The Supreme Court of Illinois held that it was not error to allow the jury to take the skiagraph with them when they retired to consider their verdict. The practice act authorizes "papers read in evidence, other than depositions," to "be carried from the bar by the jury." "Papers in evidence" clearly embrace photographs or skiagraphs offered and received in evidence. Photographs or skiagraphs produced in evidence on a trial before a jury are, within this definition, "read" in evidence, and may be taken by the jury on their retirement to consider and determine the cause. Chicago & Joliet Electric Railroad Co. *vs.* Spence, *supra.*

THE X-RAY PHOTOGRAPHER MUST BE COMPETENT.—In Chicago City Railway Company *vs.* Smith, 226 Ill., 178; s. c. 80 N. E. Rep., 716, a personal-injury case, it was contended that error had been committed in admitting in evidence certain x-ray photographs taken by a physician for the purpose of showing the character of the plaintiff's injuries. Preliminary to the introduction of these photographs the physician testified that he was a post-graduate physician and surgeon and had had twelve years' experience in the practice of his profession in Chicago, and was experienced in the matter of taking x-ray photographs, and that he was competent to make x-ray views, and that he made the original negatives and the prints therefrom, and that the same were correct representations of what they purported to be. The Supreme Court of Illinois held that this preliminary proof was sufficient to authorize the reception of the photographs in evidence. What they proved or tended to prove, or whether they were impeached by the expert testimony introduced by the defendants, were questions for the jury. The testimony of the physician made a *prima facie* showing sufficient to justify the Court in admitting them in evidence.

AN EXPERT MAY USE AN X-RAY PICTURE TO EXPLAIN TESTIMONY.—In Sheldon *vs.* Wright, 67 Atl., 807, an x-ray picture of the plaintiff's leg was in evidence without objection. This was shown to one of the defendant's experts, and, under objection and exception, he was allowed, in substance, to state that the bearing of the two fragments of the broken bone as shown by the picture was not in exact line. The defendant's counsel claimed that this testimony was erroneously received, because the jury could decide about the matter as well as any expert. The Supreme Court of Vermont held that the surgeon was using the picture for the purpose of demonstration, and could rightly point out things which his practised eye discovered, so far as they were of significance. It was as though the expert had used the leg itself for the purpose of explaining its condition to the jury. The picture was referred to, and an examination of it was quite convincing of the propriety of medical testimony as to what it really showed.

HOSPITAL RECORDS NOT ADMISSIBLE AS ORIGINAL EVIDENCE.—In Griebel *vs.* Brooklyn Heights R. R. Co., 95 App. Div., 214, aff'md, 184 N. Y., 528, the Appellate Division of the Supreme Court of New York, Second Department, held that error was committed on the trial of a personal-injury case in receiving in evidence a paper containing certain so-called "bedside notes" alleged to have been made in a hospital in reference to the plaintiff while he was a patient there. They were introduced during the examination of a hospital nurse who was in the hospital at the time when the plaintiff was a patient in its wards. She described the paper as a "temperature chart," known in the hospital as "bedside notes," and said that such notes were taken in each case where a patient was brought to the hospital. Its contents related chiefly to the physical condition of the patient, specifying particularly the injuries from which he was suffering. The Court said that it was not aware of any rule of evidence which makes such a paper, offered under such circumstances, admissible. While it was clearly error to admit the document, the only portion thereof which could have been harmful to the plaintiff in this case was the following entry: "History, good. While getting on his wagon he slipped and his horses started up, the wagon passing over his right knee and across the abdomen." This appeared to have been written by one of the physicians of the hospital, from the statements made to him by the plaintiff, but this did not render the paper competent as original evidence.

HOSPITAL REGISTER MAY BE USED TO REFRESH MEMORY OF WITNESS.—In McMahon vs. Bangs, 62 Atl. Rep., 1098, a case before the Superior Court of Delaware, the head nurse of the hospital to which the plaintiff had been taken was produced by him as a witness, and after testifying as to his condition when taken to the hospital, was questioned as to a certain record of the case, which she testified was regularly kept by one of the nurses of said hospital, who had since been dismissed and was not present in court; said record was thereupon offered in evidence and was objected to by counsel for the defendant on the ground that the only person who could testify to said record, so as to make it proper evidence, would be the person who made it. The object of offering this paper in evidence, the court says, seemed to be to show pain and suffering. For that purpose the nurses themselves might be called, and under proper circumstances this paper could be used to refresh their memories. Beyond that the court thinks it was not admissible.

HOSPITAL RECORDS EXCLUDED AS "HEARSAY TESTIMONY."—In Price vs. The Standard Life and Accident Ins. Co., 90 Minn., 264; s. c. 95 N. W. Rep., 118, the Supreme Court of Minnesota held that a register of patients, kept at a hospital, naming or pretending to name the disease with which a patient was said to be suffering, is not admissible in evidence to show and establish the nature of the disease. The entries in the register in question were made by the Superintendent in charge, who was a female physician, in the usual course of business at the hospital, and showed when the patient entered, when he departed therefrom, and the nature of the disease from which he was said to be suffering. The Superintendent produced the register, and testified that the entries concerning the patient were made after the physician in charge had observed the case long enough and knew sufficiently about the patient to state the kind of disease, and were wholly based on information received by her from the doctor. The witness had no personal knowledge of the patient, and had no recollection of the case, apart from the record. Therefore, the court held that the entries amounted to nothing more or less than what the Superintendent wrote in the register, what the attending physician told or reported to her concerning the patient's illness. To permit these entries to be introduced in evidence was to disregard in a very noticeable manner the rule forbidding the introduction of hearsay testimony, as well as the spirit of the statute which prohibits the examination of a physician as to certain matters without the consent of the patient. The information communicated by the physician in charge to the Superintendent of the hospital was acquired by the former while attending the patient, and was necessary to enable him to prescribe or act for the latter. The physician would not have been allowed to make any such disclosure, and the statutory restriction on him could not be evaded by introducing in evidence testimony of a third party as to what the doctor said about the case. But the entries did not even rise to the dignity of a repetition of what the doctor said to a third party, for the Superintendent remembered nothing, except that she made the entries. This testimony should have been excluded.

HOSPITAL RECORD EXCLUDED AS PRIVILEGED.—In Smart *vs.* Kansas City, 105 S. W. Rep., 709, the Supreme Court of Missouri did not consider the records of the hospital admissible in evidence over the plaintiff's objection. It held that the diagnosis of the case was made by an examination of the patient and by interrogating her regarding the complaint. This is necessary to be known by the physician in order that he may prescribe the proper treatment, and when he once acquires that information the law declares it to be a confidential communication, and disqualifies the physician from divulging the same on the witness stand. The Court refers to Elliott's work on Evidence, and quotes from the discussion of such statutes the following: "It seems to be conceded by both opinions that hospital physicians, who attend such persons at the hospital, could not testify as to what they learned while so attending him." * The Court held this to be, undoubtedly, the rule as announced by all the authorities, and, that being so, it seems that it must follow as a natural sequence that when the physician subsequently copies that privileged communication on the record of the hospital, it still remains privileged. If that is not true, then the law which prevents the hospital physician testifying to such matters could be violated in both letter and spirit, and the statute nullified by the physician copying into the record all the information acquired by him from his patient, and then offer or permit the record to be offered in evidence containing the diagnosis, and thereby accomplish, by indirection, that which is expressly prohibited in a direct manner.

The mere fact that the ordinance of the city requires such a record to be kept is no reason why the statute regarding privileged communications should be violated. That record is required to be kept for the benefit of the institution, and not for the benefit of outside litigants. The object of the statute is to guarantee privileged communications between all patients and their physicians, and it is wholly immaterial whether they are in or out of hospitals.†

RULES GOVERNING THE ADMISSIBILITY OF SURGICAL TREATISES.—Surgical treatises have been used in trials, first, to test the competency of expert witnesses, and, second, as evidence. Under both circumstances there have been different rulings of the courts, but the weight of authority is in accord with the cases herewith cited.

* Elliott on Evidence, vol. i., Sec. 635.   † Jour. Am. Med. Assoc., Feb. 29th, 1908.

USE OF SURGICAL WORKS TO TEST THE COMPETENCY OF EXPERT WITNESSES.—
Beadle *vs.* Paine *et al.*, 46 Ore., 424, was an action to recover for injuries alleged
to have been sustained by plaintiff in the negligent treatment of his arm, by
defendants, which had been "broken, dislocated, and bruised." The result
of treatment was non-union of the bone. An expert witness testified that
"He had read the 'International Cyclopedia' somewhat, and pronounced the
work standard." The following question was put to the expert to test his
knowledge upon the subject, "I will ask you if it isn't stated in that work ('The
International Cyclopedia of Surgery'), page 43, volume 4, that cases occur of
persons—of a young man of fine, healthy condition—where the fracture remains
ununited at the end of the fifth or sixth month, and that, although the bones
are kept in apposition, and in every respect the treatment was correct " ? The
expert answered: "That is possible that this book says this, but I think that the
pathological condition, from what I have read and heard—that there must be
something lacking in the system, in the blood, that is not discovered." Exception was taken to this question.

On appeal, the Supreme Court of Oregon said, "It is difficult to see wherein
the answer was injurious to the plaintiff, or that the inquiry made tended
to weaken the witness' testimony in the least. But, however this may be,
counsel did not overstep the rule applicable. The witness was testifying as
an expert, and, his attention being called to the work, he showed some familiarity with it, whereupon he was asked if it did not state so and so touching the
subject in hand. The book was not offered, nor does it appear to have been
read from, and the sole purpose of the inquiry was to test the witness' knowledge
of the subject. We think it was proper."

Reference is made to the decision in Connecticut Mut. Life Ins. Co. *vs.* Ellis,
Adm'r., 89 Ill., 516, 519, "The witness had given the symptoms of the disease
with which the assured was affected, and pronounced it delirium tremens,
and, as a matter of right, plaintiff might test the knowledge possessed by the
witness of that disease by any fair means that promised to elicit the truth.
It will be conceded it might be done by asking proper and pertinent questions,
and what possible difference could it make whether the questions were read out
of a medical book or framed by counsel for that purpose? "

ADMISSIBILITY OF LEARNED TREATISES IN EVIDENCE.—Wigmore On Evidence,
Sec. 1690, Scope of Objections to Hearsay Rule, says: "More than one reason
has been advanced for prohibiting the use of learned treatises in evidence, but
the only legitimate one, and the one generally pointed out and relied upon
in judicial opinion, is that such an offer of evidence purports to employ testi-
monially a statement made out of court by a person not subjected to cross-
examination; that is, purports to violate the fundamental doctrine of the Hearsay rule. That this is the main objection is indicated in the following passages:
In Ware *vs.* Ware, 8 Me., 56, "These books do not come into court, as all
other evidence must, either by consent or under the sanction of an oath. Without such consent or oath, their contents are mere declarations and hearsay. . . .
The benefits of cross-examination would be lost by allowing books of such a

character to be evidence." In Ashworth *vs.* Kittredge, 12 Cush., 194: "The substantial objection is that they are statements wanting the sanction of an oath, and the statement thus proposed is made by one not present and not liable to cross-examination." In Brown *vs.* Sheppard, 13 R. C. Q. B., 179: "The opinions which are to be received upon which the jury is to deduce a certain fact, must be so given as to be subject to examination and cross-examination before the court and jury. Now it is obvious, if books upon skill and science are to be made evidence of themselves, the protection a person has of showing by an examination of the person advancing an opinion that it is improperly arrived at is quite destroyed." In State *vs.* Baldwin, 36 Kan., 17; s. c. 12 Pac., 318, it was held that "the great weight of authority is that they cannot be admitted, this upon the theory that the authors did not write under oath and that their grounds of belief and processes of reasoning cannot be tested by cross-examination."

TEXT-BOOKS ON SURGERY NOT COMPETENT INDEPENDENT EVIDENCE.—In Van Skike *vs.* Potter *et al.*, 53 Neb., 28, an action for damages in the treatment of a fractured patella by wiring the fragments together, and, during the operation, breaking a drill and leaving the fragment in the bone, the trial resulted in a verdict and judgment in favor of the Surgeons, to reverse which the plaintiff filed a petition in error.

The Supreme Court of Nebraska states that on the trial the plaintiff offered in evidence extracts from certain text-books on surgery; these offers of evidence the District Court excluded, and this ruling is an assignment of error. These text-books were offered for the purpose of showing the practice of reducing simple transverse fractures of the patella, and also of showing that the authors of the books offered in evidence condemn the practice of wiring, and that it should never be resorted to except in cases where the chances of life are equal to those of death; that it is dangerous, and that the results following in the greatest portion, and in far more than a majority, of the cases have proved fatal, and of very bad results. It is to be noted that these text-books were offered for the purpose of showing that, in the opinion of their authors, the wiring of the kneecap was not good surgery. They were not offered for the purpose of fortifying an opinion which had been expressed by an expert upon the witness stand, and whose opinion was predicated upon the text-books offered; nor were they offered for the purpose of showing that they contradicted the opinion expressed by such expert. But they were offered as independent evidence to sustain the plaintiff's contention that the wiring of the fractured kneecap by the defendants was not good surgery, and therefore negligence. Was this evidence competent? We think that the great weight of authority, both English and American, is to the effect that text-books of surgery, though standard authority, are not competent evidence.

In Railway Co. *vs.* Yates, 25 C. C. A., 103; s. c. 79 Fed., 584. the Circuit Judge, Thayer, stated the present rule of practice of the courts, thus, "The authorities, both English and American, are practically unanimous in holding that medical books, even if they are regarded as authoritative. cannot be read to the jury as independent evidence of the opinions therein expressed or advocated. One objection to such testimony is that it is not delivered under oath; a second objection is that the opposite party is thereby deprived of the benefit of a cross-examination; and a third, and perhaps more important, reason for rejecting such testimony, is that the science of medicine is not an exact science. There are different schools of medicine, the members of which entertain widely different views, and it frequently happens that medical practitioners belonging to the same school will disagree as to the cause of a particular disease, or as to the nature of an ailment with which a patient is afflicted, even if they do not differ as to the mode of treatment. Besides, medical theories, unlike the truths of exact science, are subject to frequent modification and change, even if they are not altogether abandoned. For these reasons it is very generally held that when, in a judicial proceeding, it becomes necessary to invoke the aid of medical experts, it is safer to rely on the testimony of competent witnesses, who are produced, sworn, and subjected to cross-examination, than to permit medical books or pamphlets to be read to the jury."

In MacDonald *vs.* Metropolitan Street Railway Co., 118 S. W. Rep., 85, the Supreme Court of Missouri, Division No. 1, says that in framing questions on the cross-examination of experts, counsel held in hand medical books and formulated questions from their language; the books were not read to the jury, but the jury could see that the examiner read from them. This method of examination was objected to, but counsel was permitted to adopt the scientific terminology of the author and put propositions to the witness obviously asserted by him, the jury being repeatedly cautioned that what was read from the book was not evidence and the jury should pay no attention to it; that the only thing they could consider was the evidence which fell from the lips of the witness along the line of verifying the propositions put by the examiner. It was held by the court that there was no error in this.

A STANDARD MEDICAL DICTIONARY RECEIVED IN EVIDENCE.—In State *vs.* Wilhite, 132 Iowa, 226; s. c. 109 N. W. Rep., 730, a medical witness testified that Dunglison's "Medical Dictionary," revised edition, is accepted by the medical profession as authority in the definition of words. Thereupon the definitions of "anatomy," "neurology," "ophthalmology," "pathology," and "physiology," contained therein were introduced in evidence over objection.

The Supreme Court of Iowa held that, even though the court might have taken judicial notice of the meaning of these words, it was not error to receive a standard medical dictionary in evidence as an aid to the memory and understanding of the court. Bixby *vs.* Railway Co., 105 Iowa, 293, and like cases were not in point. They hold that medical works, treating of the symptoms and cure of disease, are not admissible; not that standard authorities may not be received as proof of the meaning of medical terms.

XV. Exhibitions in Evidence Before Juries.—THE PRINCIPLE GOVERNING EXHIBITIONS BEFORE JURIES.—The tendency to employ exhibitions before juries in evidence has always been a subject for the exercise of the discretion of trial courts. The principle governing such exhibitions is the value and propriety of the special object to be exhibited in enabling the jury to arrive at the exact truth in regard to the matter or thing under consideration. Thus, the demonstration of injuries to the bones as fractures and dislocations by exhibition of the skeleton would give the ordinary juryman in a moment a more correct knowledge of the exact facts than he could possibly obtain by verbal descriptions. The same is true of the exhibition of injured limbs to prove the conditions which have resulted and to determine to what extent their usefulness has been impaired. It is in that class of cases where the signs and symptoms are objective that such exhibitions are most important and should be admitted. The objection to these exhibitions is in those cases where the symptoms are subjective and the jury is liable to be deceived as to facts, or to be unduly influenced by sympathetic appeals. To this class belong those persons who are "neurotic,' popularly "nervous." The effect upon the credibility of the testimony of such witnesses who have suits pending for alleged injuries, and are allowed to exhibit their ailments to juries, has not received the attention of Courts which its importance deserves.

Richardson, of Boston, in a recent paper * states that from a considerable acquaintance with personal-injury cases and an analysis of one hundred medico-legal cases, he is of the opinion that without the co-operative proof of objective symptoms, in a great majority of accident neuroses, physicians are justified in regarding the alleged injury as wilfully exaggerated, or as belonging to the so-called "litigation psychoses." He points out the possibility and importance of differentiating these litigation psychoses from what may be called true traumatic neuroses, thus avoiding the danger of contributing to injustice either to the claimant or to the defendant. He states also that litigation is undoubtedly a potent causative factor in the production and prolongation of functional neuroses, but those cases in which it is the chief present symptom are of a much milder grade and can usually be distinguished from those resulting from actual injury.

The rulings of the courts when the question of exhibitions before the jury has arisen are illustrated in the following adjudicated cases.

USE OF SKELETON TO ILLUSTRATE TESTIMONY.—In Chicago & Alton Railroad Co. vs. Walker, 217 Ill., 605; s. c. 75 N. E. Rep., 520, a personal-injury case, surgeons who testified on behalf of the plaintiff were permitted, over the objection of the defendant, to use the skeleton of a human foot in explaining to the jury the location of the various bones and ligaments of the ankles. The Supreme Court of Illinois held that the rulings in that regard were unobjectionable. It states that the skeleton itself was not offered in evidence, but was simply used by the expert witnesses to illustrate their testimony, and adds that the Court might, in its discretion, have permitted the plaintiff to exhibit her injured ankle to the jury and allow the surgeons to explain from it the nature and character of the injury. It was equally proper to use the skeleton for explaining the testimony. Moreover, even if the skeleton had been improperly used, no substantial injury could have resulted therefrom to the defendant, as its counsel had full opportunity to cross-examine the witnesses.

* Accident Litigation—" the Popular Graft." F. C. Richardson, Boston

ADMISSIBLE DEMONSTRATIONS BY SURGEON BEFORE A JURY.—In Stephens vs. Elliott, 92 Pac. Rep., 45; s. c. 36 Montana, 92, a personal-injury case, the surgeon, who attended the plaintiff at the time of his injury and for some two months thereafter, was permitted by the trial court, over the objection of the defendant, to make use of the plaintiff's arm to demonstrate his testimony. The reason urged for the objection was that the testimony already given by the plaintiff was to the effect that other physicians had operated on the injured arm after this one had ceased to give it his care and before the trial.

The Supreme Court of Montana says, conceding this to be true, the Court wholly fails to understand how it could affect the testimony of this physician in so far as his conclusions were based on facts obtained by him at the time of the injury, or why he could not by the use of the injured arm make his testimony all the more easily understood by the jury. Such an inspection of the injured limb in the presence of the jury is usually permitted; at least, the application to make such inspection is addressed to the sound, legal discretion of the trial court, and its ruling will not be disturbed except for a manifest abuse of such discretion. The Court failed to see wherein the trial court abused its discretion in this instance.

Another physician who testified on behalf of the plaintiff was also permitted to make an experiment, or rather demonstration, before the jury. He testified that the motor nerves of the plaintiff's right arm were entirely destroyed, and that in sympathy with this condition the sensory nerves, which controlled the feeling in the hand, had become so far paralyzed that the plaintiff had no feeling in his hand; and to demonstrate this he was permitted to stick a hypodermic needle into the back of the plaintiff's right hand.

The Supreme Court could not see any objection to the order of the trial court in permitting this demonstration before the jury. That such demonstrations are permitted is quite generally recognized by the courts and text-writers. The United States Circuit Court in Osborne vs. Detroit, 32 Fed. Rep., 36, held that, where the plaintiff claimed to be paralyzed by a fall, it was not error to permit a medical attendant, who had not been sworn, to demonstrate the loss of feeling on the part of the plaintiff by thrusting a pin into the side of the plaintiff claimed to be paralyzed.*

EXHIBITION OF AMPUTATED LEG TO JURY.—In Ford vs. Providence Coal Company, 99 S. W. Rep., 609; s. c. 30 Ky. L. R., 698, it was assigned as error that the trial judge refused to permit the plaintiff to exhibit his injured leg to the jury. The Court of Appeals of Kentucky held that, as the leg had been amputated, this ruling was not prejudicial. However, in the trial of personal-injury cases, the Court said, it is competent for the plaintiff to exhibit the injured member to the jury, and this he may do on the request of his counsel or of the adverse party—provided that the exhibition does not violate any rule of propriety or decency. Whether it does so or not is, of course, a question that must be left largely in the discretion of the trial judge. No objection of this kind could be urged in this case, as the exhibition of a man's leg that has been

* Jones on Evidence, vol. 2, Sec. 406; Wigmore on Evidence. Sec. 445 and Sec. 1160.

amputated could not be considered at all improper. Evidence of this character is really the best evidence obtainable of the extent and character of the injury that the person seeking damages has sustained, and the jury has the right to be aided in making up their verdict by a personal view of the injured member.

EXHIBITION OF INJURED MEMBER AS AFFECTING RECORD.—In Pittsburg, Cincinnati, Chicago & St. Louis Railway vs. Lightheiser, 78 N. E. Rep., 1033, a personal-injury case brought by the latter party, it appears that in the course of his testimony, and in explaining the character of his injury, the plaintiff exhibited his injured foot, and testified that it was stiff at the ankle joint, and by the movements of the foot showed the effects of the injury on his ability to use it. The defendant railway company insisted that it was error to permit this to be done, because it was thereby deprived of its ability to present a complete record. The Supreme Court of Indiana held that the company was not deprived of any substantial right by the action of the lower court, and the record was complete. This Court had previously held that such an exhibition of the injured limb was not error.

EXHIBITION OF A LIMB SHORTENED BY DISEASE.—In Fowler vs. Sargeant, I. Grant's Cases, 355, a case of injury to the hip joint by which the limb was shortened to the extent of two and a half inches, the plaintiff was allowed to exhibit himself to the jury that they might determine for themselves the nature of the injury received, and the surgeons were only permitted to examine him in the same way in which he was examined by the jury. The Supreme Court of Pennsylvania held that it was right to allow the plaintiff to exhibit the injured limb to the jury, because a sight is always better than a description, and the terms imposed upon the plaintiff by the court, were for the benefit of the defendant, of which he could not complain, unless he had asked for more and been refused.

EXHIBITIONS OF NERVOUS AFFECTIONS (LITIGATION PSYCHOSES) BEFORE JURIES.—In Clark vs. Brooklyn Heights Railroad Co., 174 N. Y., 523, a personal-injury case, the plaintiff was allowed by the Court to leave the witness stand assisted, and, at the request of his counsel, to exhibit himself to the jury in the act of writing his name and of taking a drink of water. The record represented him, through the stenographer's notes, as taking a glass of water with both hands, and as spilling the water, through the trembling of his hands, and as using his handkerchief in the same manner. The injuries received when his wagon and a street car collided consisted in the fracture of two ribs, and in various minor contusions, which did not prevent his leaving the hospital the day after. The plaintiff was a man fifty-seven years of age, and it was his assertion that, about two months after the accident, he was affected by a tremor, or a muscular twitching; and medical testimony was given to that effect, and of tests similar to the one described as made on the trial. He recovered a verdict of $10,000, and the Appellate Division affirmed the recovery, leaving the only question for the Court of Appeals, that arising on the exception of the company to the party being permitted to go through his performances before the jury.

The Court of Appeals of New York held that the object of this exhibition was to illustrate or emphasize the plaintiff's testimony that he could use his hands with difficulty either to hold things or to drink a glass of water; that the court should not have stretched its discretion to such an extent; and that, while it may not have been an abuse of judicial discretion, it was on the borderline of such an error. It is not objectionable, in these cases, that the evidence may go beyond the oral narrative, and may be addressed to the senses, provided that it be kept within reasonable limits by the exercise of a fair judicial discretion. It should be only of a nature to assist the jurors to an understanding of a situation or of an act, or to comprehend objective symptoms resulting from an injury. Examples of this class of evidence are frequent—in the exhibition of the person, and of the marks or obvious evidences of injuries sustained, etc. Personal injuries may be simulated and deception may be practised in such exhibitions, but that can no more be prevented than can perjury in testimony. When, however, proof is attempted to be made by allowing the plaintiff to act out on a judicial stage before the jurors what he or his physicians have testified to be some nervous affection resulting from an injury, the exhibition is improper, because unfair. As something under the sole control of the witness himself, it is beyond the ordinary tests of examination. Nor does such evidence allow of any record, beyond the reporter's notes of what he saw on the trial. It is intended to prejudice the minds of the jurors, and is calculated to affect the calm judicial atmosphere of a court of justice. The plaintiff in such cases has sufficient advantages without adding to them a spectacular illustration of his symptoms. The Appellate Division, in its general jurisdiction to review the proceedings on trials, might well have ordered a new trial, in the interests of justice. As it is, this court is compelled to affirm the judgment, with costs, because the matter was discretionary.

PATIENT ALLOWED TO WALK "THE BEST HE COULD" BEFORE JURY.—In Birmingham Railway, Light and Power Co. vs. Rutledge, 39 So. Rep., 338; s. c. 142 Ala., 195, a personal-injury case, the plaintiff was allowed to walk before the jury against the defendant's objection and was told to "walk the best he could." The Supreme Court of Alabama, reviewing the case, says it would be difficult, if not impossible, to reduce the result of that experiment intelligibly to paper, and no effort to that end was made; so this court was not advised whether he did his "best" in the way of walking, or, to the contrary, did his best in the way of impressing the jury that his powers of locomotion had been greatly impaired. Certainly there was temptation toward the latter course, and it would seem impracticable by any sort of "cross-exercise" to test the good faith of his gait. Ethically, there was grave doubt whether this man's physical organism should have been exposed to this temptation and to the strain necessarily incident to yielding to it, if he did, but on legal principle the evidence was on the same plane as that afforded the jury by a view of his person in repose, or by having him stand before them that one leg was longer than the other, were the shortening or elongation of a leg the thing complained of, or by exposing an arm to the jury on the invocation to do his best in bending at the joints, the claim being that it was stiffened.

XVI. What Constitutes Privileged Communications.—Privileged Communications Defined.—The patient is under obligation to give the Surgeon such information as may be necessary to enable him to treat the case intelligently. It follows that the patient may be required to divulge to the Surgeon facts in regard to his own habits and physical condition seriously reflecting upon his character and even upon the reputation of his ancestors. At common law such information on the part of the patient to his surgeon was not privileged, but in most of the States in this country it has come to be regarded as public policy that communications of such a confidential nature should be made privileged by law in the interests of the patient.

The Statutory Form of Privilege.—The State of New York was one of the first States to make statutory provisions defining and controlling privileged communications. Its law provides as follows: "A person duly authorized to practise physic or surgery shall not be allowed to disclose any information which he acquired in attending a patient in a professional capacity, and which was necessary to enable him to act in that capacity." Code of Civil Procedure, Sec. 834. Laws enacted by other States are very similar to this provision of the New York statute, the chief difference being in the forms of restriction. See "Medical Jurisprudence, Forensic Medicine, and Toxicology," Vol. I., for the laws of the States.

The interpretation of this statute by the courts is that, by "information," it means not only communications received from the lips of the patient, but such knowledge as may be acquired from the patient himself, from the statements of others who may surround him at the time, or from observation of his appearance and symptoms. Edington vs. Mutual Life Ins. Co., 67 N. Y., 185.

While the privilege is restricted to information necessary to enable the Surgeon to prescribe for, or treat, the patient, the tendency of the courts is toward a liberal construction, and the presumption is that the information would not have been imparted except for the purpose of aiding the Surgeon in prescribing for the patient. People vs. Coler, 113 Mich., 83; DeJong vs. Erie R. R. Co., 43 App. Div. (N. Y.), 427; Feeny vs. Long Island R. Co., 116 N. Y., 375.

Relation of Surgeon and Patient Must Exist.—The rule of the courts under which the statutes apply require that the relation of Surgeon and patient must exist, or at least that the circumstances are such as to impress the patient with the belief that it does exist.* Jacob vs. Cross, 19 Minn., 523. The privilege is created for the protection of the patient, and is personal to him, but he must establish the fact that between himself and the Surgeon the relations were confidential as the statute contemplates. People vs. Schuyler, 106 N. Y., 298; Eddington vs. Ætna Life Ins. Co., 77 N. Y., 564.

What Information is Privileged.—In general the rule extends to all information which is acquired professionally, that is, which is necessary for the treatment of the patient. It thus excludes from the evidence of the Surgeon such information however acquired, whether actually obtained from statements

* Amer. and Engl. Encycl. of Law (2d edit.), vol. 23, p. 84, and cases there cited.

of the patient or of others present at the time, or gathered from his observations and investigation of the case. The Surgeon will not be allowed to disclose the nature of the disease for which he treated the patient, and it has been held that his prescriptions could not be introduced in evidence, nor their ingredients explained. Nelson vs. Nederland Life Ins. Co., 110 Iowa, 600. The Surgeon cannot be allowed to testify as to his patient's previous state of health when he acquired the knowledge only from an inspection of, and conversations with, the patient as his professional attendant. Barker vs. Cunard Steamship Co., 91 Hun (N. Y.), 495, affirmed 157 N. Y., 693.

LIMITATIONS OF INFORMATION.—A recent authority discussing the limitations of the privileged information remarks: * "The limitation that the information shall be 'necessary to enable him to act in that capacity' has given rise to some conflict of authority. One line of decisions has been rendered holding that the information to be protected must have a direct bearing upon the condition for which the physician is attending the patient; that information as to the time of receiving a rupture for which the Surgeon was treating the patient was not necessary to enable him to act for the patient. Campau vs. North, 39 Mich., 606. Again, the obvious objective appearance of the patient, the inflamed face, the blood-shot eye, the fumes of alcohol, do not constitute information of the character protected by the statute. Linz vs. Mass. Mut. Life Ins. Co., 8 Mo. App., 363. The other and later line of decisions, which, it seems, represents the true doctrine, gives to the act a broad and liberal construction, and protects all information which necessarily comes to the Surgeon in the course of his professional intercourse with the patient, such as the appearance of intoxication, the presence of scars, defects, or marks of a loathsome disease appearing on a limb or a member of the body, disclosed upon baring such limb or member for professional treatment, Kling vs. City of Kansas, 27 Mo. App., 231; statements as to how the accident occurred which caused the injury for which the patient is treated—at least when such statements are elicited by the Surgeon for the purpose of ascertaining the character or extent of the injury, Raymond vs. B. R. & N. Ry. Co., 65 Ia., 152; statements by patients as to their condition of health prior to the time of rendering the professional services, Baker vs. Cunard Steamship Co., supra, such information coming within the protection of the statute. In fact, the courts in some cases have gone farther than this in protecting information obtained by Surgeons while professionally attending patients. In a case where the Surgeon attempted to disclose a statement made by the patient as to how he received the injury for which the Surgeon attended him, the Surgeon declaring that he elicited the information, not for the purpose of diagnosis, but of determining whether the railroad company was to blame, the court held such testimony inadmissible, and, quite justly it seems, rebuked the Surgeon for taking advantage of his professional relation to obtain information with which he had no professional concern. The Pennsylvania Co. vs. Marion, 123 Ind., 415."

SCOPE OF PRIVILEGE.—In McRae vs. Erickson, 82 Pac., 209; s. c. 1 Cal. App.,

* The Law and the Doctor, vol. ii., p. 20.

326, exception was taken to the exclusion of the testimony of a Surgeon as to a statement made to him by the plaintiff at the defendant's hospital to which he had been taken for treatment. It was contended that there was nothing in the record to indicate that the witness was acting professionally, or with a view to treating the plaintiff, or that the information was obtained with a view to treatment, and that the information was, in fact, not necessary to enable him to prescribe or act for the patient.

The Court of Appeals, Second District, California, held that the former point was obviously untenable. It held that the witness was a Surgeon, and as such was in charge of the defendant's hospital, and his services were remunerated by assessments on the wages of the men, so that he was, in effect, employed by the plaintiff. He examined the plaintiff as a Surgeon, and the plaintiff knew that he was examining as such, and the information sought was obtained from the plaintiff at the time he was examining, or some time during the day. The Court below was right in holding that the communication was made to the witness in the course of professional employment.

In regard to the second point, the Court says it was not informed as to the effect of the statement sought otherwise than by questions from which it could not be very clearly determined what the statement would have been. If it was as indicated by one question, asking if the plaintiff made a statement explaining how the rock fell, and how it hit him, the information sought was of a character necessary to the proper treatment of the patient; but information as to the direction or point whence the rock came, another question, would seem to have been unnecessary for such purpose; to this extent, if regard be had to the most obvious sense of the statute, the point raised would seem to have been well taken. But to give to the statute this narrow construction would equally exclude from its application many, if not most, of the answers to questions usually put, and properly and necessarily put, by competent Surgeons to patients of this kind, in order to enable them to act for their patients; this would be to defeat the obvious purpose of the act. Therefore, the Court was of the opinion that the view of the Court below was correct.

STATEMENTS AS TO HOW ACCIDENT OCCURRED NOT PRIVILEGED.—In Benjamin vs. Village of Tupper Lake, 110 App. Div. (N. Y.), 426, an action to recover damages for an injury alleged to have been sustained on a defective sidewalk, a Surgeon who had treated the plaintiff for the injury was called by the defendant and testified that he had a conversation with her as to the manner in which this accident occurred. He was then asked: "What did she tell you as to that?" Besides, he stated that "this talk was while I was making an examination of her in order to prescribe for her and as a part of my examination."

The Appellate Division of the Supreme Court of New York, Third Department, held that it was error to sustain an objection to the question. The witness nowhere stated that it was necessary for him to know how the accident happened in order to enable him to act for the plaintiff in a professional capacity, but it was apparent that it was not necessary for him to know how the accident happened in order to enable him so to act. It was sufficient for that purpose that he knew or was informed of the character of the injuries received and not as to how they were received. If the plaintiff in such talk made admissions to the Surgeon as to the manner in which the accident happened, it not appearing that the information so acquired was necessary to enable him to act in that capacity, such admissions were not protected by section 834 of the New York Code of Civil Procedure.

A NOVEL CASE OF BETRAYAL OF PROFESSIONAL CONFIDENCE.—The following case illustrates the extent to which the charge of betrayal of professional confidence may be made against the Surgeon. The remarkable feature of the case was that the confidential information was not conveyed to another person but to the Surgeon himself. It appeared that an English Surgeon's chauffeur was taken ill and entered an Infirmary where he came under the professional care of his employer. Examination revealed the fact that the man was suffering from aortic disease and was evidently unfit to have charge of an automobile. On the chauffeur's recovery the Surgeon, having betrayed the professional secret to himself, discharged his employee with two weeks' advance salary. The chauffeur commenced a suit against the Surgeon for betrayal of privileged information, but the court refused to grant a judgment in favor of the victim of misplaced confidence. London Letter.

XVII. Waiver of Privilege.—WHO MAY WAIVE PRIVILEGE.—The right to secrecy secured to the patient by legislative enactment involves as a sequence the right of the patient to waive that privilege at his discretion. The right is extended to the patient and not to the Surgeon and hence the former may waive the privilege and the latter would be compelled to testify. Johnson vs. Johnson, 14 Wend., 641. The effect of waiver does not cease at the death of the patient and the Surgeon is under obligation to secrecy as stringently after as before that event. Grattan vs. Met. Life Ins. Co., 80 N. Y., 281, 287. The right to waive after the death of the patient by one who lawfully represents him, and who stands in his place, is generally conceded. Such may be the wife of the decedent, Camp of Woodmen vs. Grandon, 89 N. W. Rep., 448; those representing the estate, State vs. Grinnell, 88 N. W. Rep., 342; the representative of the patient, Groll vs. Tower, 85 Mo., 249; or the executors named in the will, In re Hopkins Will, 73 App. Div. (N. Y.), 559. In case the patient is an infant the father as the natural guardian of his person has the right to waive the privilege though the guardian be a party to the action and interested in the disclosure, provided the disclosure will not be prejudicial to the infant's interest. Corey vs. Bolton, 31 Misc. (N. Y.), 138.

In this connection the question has been raised as to whom the right of objection to the admission of privileged communications pertains. Boston says, "it seems to be clear that the right to object differs from the right to waive, in that the latter is necessarily and logically dependent upon the relation between the patient and his representative, while the former is obviously suggested as the best method of enforcing the law." Medical Jurisp., For. Med., and Tox., p. 123. He concludes that it rests "with any party to raise the objection and assert the prohibition."

RELATION OF SURGEON AND PATIENT MUST EXIST.—This relation must exist to give legal effect to the waiver. Jacobs *vs.* Cross, 19 Minn., 523. To create this relation it is not necessary that the Surgeon should have been called by the patient himself, for the relation is created if the surgeon is summoned by the physician in attendance, or by friends, or even by strangers. Renihan *vs.* Dennin, 103 N. Y., 573. But the courts carefully distinguish between a visit of the Surgeon to obtain information concerning the patient and undertaking at such visit his treatment. In a suit for personal injuries, Weitz *vs.* Mound City Ry. Co., 53 Mo. App., 39, it appeared that the defendant sent his Surgeon to examine the plaintiff for the purpose of testifying as to the plaintiff's condition, but the Surgeon undertook the treatment of the plaintiff and thus created the relation of Surgeon and patient, and became incompetent to testify as to the information which he had gained.

THE EXPRESS WAIVER.—The express waiver may be in writing or verbal, and in either form the patient is under obligation to conform to its terms. In an application for insurance, Metropolitan Life Insurance Co. *vs.* Willis, 76 N. E. Rep., 560, the insured "expressly agreed and stipulated that in any suit on the policy any physician who had attended him might disclose any information acquired by him in any wise affecting the declarations and warranties" made in the application. But when a physician was called as a witness objection was made that he was not competent to testify and answer the question as to the disease that the insured was afflicted with when he was called to visit him because it was a privileged communication between physician and patient.

In a critical review of this case the Appellate Court of Indiana, Division No. 2, held that it was error to exclude the evidence. It says the rule is that such confidential relations will be protected by the courts except where the patient consents to their revelation by the physician. The court referred to the following decision in illustration, Penn. Mutual, etc., Company *vs.* Wiler, 100 Ind., 92. "Notwithstanding the absolutely prohibitory form of our present statute, we think it confers a privilege which the patient, for whose benefit the provision is made, may claim or waive." Here the assured, by an agreement in writing, waived this statutory privilege, and this Court has no doubt but that he had a right to do so. His waiver must operate as such to those claiming under him.

THE IMPLIED WAIVER.—The implied waiver grows out of the variety of conditions under which the Surgeon is liable to meet the patient. Although there is but one relation of the Surgeon and patient which renders the former incompetent as a witness, Fisher *et al. vs.* Fisher *et al.*, 129 N. Y., 654, viz., as professional attendant, the question constantly arises as to the proper construction to be placed on the character of his visit to the patient. He may visit the patient to obtain information which will enable him to appear as a witness, or to determine the sanity of the patient, or to learn the facts in regard to his injuries, or whether he has had syphilis. Under these circumstances he will be allowed to testify. But if during the visit he consents to undertake the treatment of the patient he becomes incompetent as a witness, for he has assumed the relation of Surgeon to the patient. To determine, therefore, the admissibility of the evidence of a Surgeon it is only necessary to learn positively whether he acted in a professional capacity in his relations with the patient, and whether the patient understood that this relation existed.

The question of waiver has also arisen in cases where patients detail the history of their injuries or diseases in their petition, complaint, or testimony, but the Courts have generally ruled that such proceedings do not constitute a waiver.

Is an Action for Personal Injuries a Waiver?—This question has excited much discussion in the courts. Wigmore says, "The whole reason for the privilege is the patient's supposed unwillingness that the ailment should be disclosed to the world at large; hence the bringing of a suit in which the very declaration, and much more, the proof, discloses the ailment to the world at large, is of itself an indication that the supposed repugnancy to disclose does not exist. If the privilege means anything at all in its origin, it means this as a sequel." *

The Decision of the Following Case is Important.—In Smart vs. Kansas City, 105 S. W. Rep., 709, the defendant took the position that the plaintiff by bringing the suit and asking damages for personal injuries thereby waived the incompetency of her physician and surgeon to testify regarding information acquired from her while attending her in a professional capacity.

The Supreme Court of Missouri, after quoting the Missouri statute which declares, as incompetent to testify, "A physician or surgeon concerning any information which he may have acquired and which information was necessary to enable him to prescribe for such patient as a physician, or do any act as a surgeon," the court says: The meaning of this section is not veiled in doubt; it disqualifies the physicians and surgeons from testifying to any information acquired by them while attending their patients in a professional capacity. Referring to Wigmore's opinion the Court says this is too narrow a view to take of the statute. If you could limit the inquiry to the particular injury sued for, there might be some apparent force in the contention for a waiver, but such injuries, when inflicted on weak and diseased people, will more than likely aggravate the previous ailments, and rather than disclose such troubles they might prefer to waive the aggravation and limit the recovery of damages to the apparent rather than to the real extent of the injury. Again a person might be suffering from some temporary loathsome disease at the time of the injury, and the one might have no effect on the other, or bear no relation whatever thereto. In either of those cases the court is unable to see any good reason for holding that he or she may not place the seal of secrecy on the lips of the physician or surgeon, who, through his confidential relation to the patient, has learned of those ailments, which, if made known, might and often do injuriously affect the business and social standing of such persons in the community where they reside. If it was not for this wise and beneficent statute, all the diseases to which the human flesh is heir could, and in many cases would, be uncovered and held

* Wigmore on Evidence. vol. iv., Section 2389.

up to public view, with no corresponding benefits to be derived therefrom, either as a defence to the case or in mitigation of damages.

The Court held that if the mere filing of the petition in the court in such cases waives the statutory privilege, then the statute quoted had no force or effect, and is an absolute nullity, because said section begins by stating "the following persons shall be incompetent to testify." If this statute is waived by the mere filing of the suit, then the patient cannot avail himself or herself of its provisions, and the disqualification of the physician and surgeon is removed, and they are thereby authorized to disclose all information acquired by them in the examination and treatment of their patients. If no suit is brought by the patient, there could be no occasion for the physician or surgeon disclosing the confidential communications; but the instant one is brought and trial had, and that being the only possible occasion on which the patient could avail himself of the statutory privilege, he is met with the proposition of implied waiver, and, as an inevitable result, the statutory privilege could not be invoked in that case, nor in any other. In other words, as long as a suit is not instituted the physician is disqualified by the statute, and in that case there is no express nor implied waiver, but under that condition he could not testify, because there is no case pending in which to testify. But if suit is instituted, that fact waives the statutory privilege, and he becomes a competent witness, and is authorized to disclose all confidential communications. Such reasoning leads to an absurdity, and totally emasculates the statute.

EXTENT OF WAIVER OF PRIVILEGE BY BRINGING OF ACTION FOR MALPRACTICE.—In Hartley vs. Calbreath, 106 S. W. Rep., 571, a case was brought before the Kansas City Court of Appeals where the question of the extent of waiver of privilege by bringing an action for malpractice was considered. It appeared that the plaintiff was thrown from a horse and dislocated his shoulder. The defendant was called and engaged to attend him. The evidence. tended to show that he reduced or "set" the shoulder, and pronounced it "all right," that he put the plaintiff's arm in a bandage or "sling" suspended from his neck, but he did not secure the arm to the body so as to prevent the upper portion from being free to move. He returned the next day, when the patient complained of severe pain. He then took off the bandage, or took the arm out of the sling and left it free. The plaintiff continued to suffer great pain, and, his shoulder not appearing to be doing well, he was at the defendant's office, and there, in the presence of another physician, the shoulder was examined and, not being thought to be in its proper place, another effort was made to reduce the dislocation. Subsequently still another effort was made by the use of "pulleys." According to the evidence in the plaintiff's behalf, the shoulder was not properly reduced or "put in place," whereby he lost much of the use of that arm and suffered great pain. The plaintiff's theory was that the defendant either failed to reduce the dislocation at first, or, if he did reduce it, that he left it so improperly bandaged and cared for that his arm had too much freedom of movement and the shoulder would not remain in place; that he was negligent and unskilful in not sooner discovering that the shoulder was not properly reduced and using immediate means to put it in proper condition. The defendant offered another surgeon as a witness, but on the plaintiff's objection he was not permitted to testify on the ground that whatever he knew about the case was privileged under the statute. It appeared that several months after the defendant's treatment of the plaintiff the latter called on the witness as a surgeon and was examined by him.

The Court of Appeals declares that there can be no doubt of the correctness of the lower court's ruling. It is true that in cases of this nature, the physician being a party, the necessity of the matter makes him competent to testify in his own behalf concerning communications between himself and his patient, notwithstanding the statute. Cramer vs. Hurt, 154 Mo., 112. This was placed on the ground that the plaintiff himself had removed the privilege of secrecy. Lane vs. Boicourt, 128 Ind., 420. But the witness offered in this case brought up altogether different considerations. He was in no way connected with the defendant's attendance on the plaintiff. He examined the plaintiff in his professional capacity with a view to seeing what could be done for him. The defendant did not answer this position by saying that the secrecy of the whole matter had been removed by the plaintiff bringing the present action and himself testifying, and by his having made it necessary for the defendant to testify and therefore the privilege did not longer exist; for the secrecy and privilege of the communications to the witness in question had not been removed.

It has been directly held by the Supreme Court of Missouri that a waiver as to one physician is not a waiver as to others who may have attended on the person making the waiver. The statute, says the court, "does not exclude the evidence by reason of its inherent character, but only when given by the persons within its purview." This court held, Arnold vs. Maryville, 110 Mo. App., 254, that the statute in privileging all necessary information and communications received by the physician from the patient did not apply to a physician who was called on, not with a view of giving the patient attention and relief, but for the purpose of qualifying himself as a witness. But in this case the trial Court and counsel first ascertained from the witness offered that nothing was said between him and the plaintiff about a suit, or his being a witness, but that he was consulted with a view to relieve the patient of his distress.

In regard to the opinion of Wigmore * that an exposure of the mere ailment, by bringing the action, is sufficient entirely to remove the bar of secrecy, the Court says that it regards his view as too much restricted. The object of the statute is not fully met in all cases by merely keeping secret the fact that a patient had a certain ailment. The primary object of the statute is the relief of the patient, and to that end it has made the way clear for him to permit a complete examination and to give full and free communication of everything connected with his ailment which may be necessary to enable the physician to prescribe for him. And those things are as securely included in the purview of the statute as the ailment itself, and an exposure of the ailment does not necessarily release secrecy as to them. The conclusion which the court reached was that the

* Wigmore on Evidence, vol. iv., Sec. 2389.

plaintiff by bringing the action waives the statute no further than the action discloses the ailment and its treatment by the physician or physicians therein named. He does not waive the privilege as to other physicians. If the privilege is waived as to other physicians called, as was the witness under discussion, disconnectedly from the defendant, it must be by some act of the plaintiff in himself disclosing what took place with such physician by calling it out in evidence. In this case the defendant and the consulting physician with him were permitted to testify, but when it came to the defendant's offer of the third physician, who afterward examined the plaintiff, there was no waiver as to him, and hence the court approved the trial court's ruling excluding him.

WAIVER OF PRIVILEGE BY STIPULATION IN CONTRACT.—The Supreme Court of Nebraska holds that it is not necessary that the waiver be made at the time of the trial, but it may be included in and made a part of the contract sought to be enforced in the action in which such testimony is offered. A stipulation in the contract of life insurance to the effect that the proofs of death shall consist in part of the affidavit of the attending physician, which shall state the cause of death and such other information as may be required by the insurer, constitutes a waiver and renders the attending physician a competent witness as to the confidential disclosures made to him by the assured concerning his last sickness. Western Travelers Accident Ass. vs. Munson, 73 Neb., 858; s. c. 103 N. W. Rep., 688.

WAIVER OF PRIVILEGE ON PERMITTING PHYSICIAN TO TESTIFY WITHOUT OBJECTION.—In Williams vs. Spokane Falls & Northern Railway Company, 42 Wash., 597; s. c. 84 Pac. Rep., 1129, a personal-injury case, the Supreme Court of Washington says that the plaintiff, no doubt, waived his privilege when he permitted a physician who had examined him in his professional capacity to give his testimony without making any objection.

CALLING ONE SURGEON AS A WITNESS IS NOT A WAIVER OF PRIVILEGE AS REGARDS ANOTHER SURGEON.—In Duggan vs. Phelps, 22 App. Div. (N. Y.), 509, a party suing for damages for personal injuries testified that after the accident he was taken in an ambulance to a hospital; that he left there the next day, and was then treated at home by his own physician, who testified in detail as to the injuries and treatment. The other party called the ambulance surgeon, who had charge of the party suing and treated him in the hospital. The Appellate Division of the Supreme Court of New York, Second Department, held that the calling of his own surgeon as a witness was not a waiver of privilege as to the ambulance surgeon; that it is held, Grattan, vs. Metropolitan Life Ins. Co., 92 N. Y., 274; Renihan vs. Dennin, 103 N. Y., 573, that what is seen by a surgeon in looking at the patient is within the privilege; that it is not necessary that the surgeon should be employed by the patient, or that there should be a contract relation between them; that the party suing, by calling his surgeon to testify as to his disease and its treatment, does not waive his objection to the evidence of other surgeons who had treated him at other periods, Hope vs. Troy & Lansingburgh Railroad Company, 40 Hun, 438, affirmed 110 N. Y., 643; that although a patient gives evidence as to his condition both before his entrance to a hospital and after he leaves it, he does not waive the privilege as to a surgeon who treated him in that interim. Baker *vs.* Cunard Steamship Company, 91 Hun (N. Y.), 495, affirmed in 157 N. Y., 693.

WAIVER OF PRIVILEGE IN OPEN COURT; WHAT CONSTITUTES SUCH WAIVER?— In the State of New York the waiver of privilege is governed by statute. Section 836 of the Code of Civil Procedure provides that unless the privilege is expressly waived upon the trial of an action, the surgeon or physician is precluded from testifying as to privileged matter. The section also provides as follows, "The waivers herein provided for must be made in open court on the trial of the action, or proceeding, and a paper executed by a party prior to the trial, providing for such waiver, shall be insufficient as such a waiver. But the attorneys for the respective parties may prior to the trial stipulate for such waivers and the same shall be sufficient therefor."

The construction of these provisions in the statute has recently been passed upon by the Court of Appeals of the State of New York in the case of Capron *vs.* Douglass, 193 N. Y., 11. As this decision embraces a discussion of the questions relating generally to waiver of privilege and may be considered as the latest authoritative judicial interpretation of their application, we quote it in full.

"This was an action brought to recover damages against the defendant, a physician and Surgeon, upon the ground that he was chargeable with malpractice in treating a fracture of the tibia and fibula of the plaintiff's leg. Upon the trial evidence was submitted by the plaintiff and his witnesses tending to show that on receiving the fracture the defendant was called as a Surgeon to attend the same; that he was negligent in reducing the fracture and in his subsequent care of the patient; that after several weeks there was no union of the bones and the plaintiff was removed to a hospital in the city of Utica where an operation was performed by Dr. G., aided by Dr. D., one of the Hospital Staff. The fractured bones united, but the usefulness of the leg was impaired.

"The defence was that the fracture was properly reduced and the fractured bones were placed in apposition, and that the cause of their failure to unite could not be determined by an external examination, but by an incision made at the place of fracture, as was done after his removal to the hospital, when it was discovered that some of the muscles of the leg intervened between the broken ends of the tibia, and a piece of bone between the ends of the fibula, thus preventing their coming together, a condition necessary to union.

"At the trial, Dr. G., who performed the operation and discovered the true cause of the failure of the bones to unite, testified as to the facts for the defendant without objection by the plaintiff. The defence then called Dr. D., the member of the House Staff who assisted Dr. G., but his evidence was excluded under Section 834 of the Code and an exception was taken. The trial court instructed the jury, 'If you find that the leg was properly set, the bones placed in apposition, at the time of the first operation by the defendant, and you find that muscular fibres prevented union of the tibia and that the loose fragment found at the place of fracture of the fibula prevented union of that bone and that such condition could not have been discovered except by the operation at the hospital requiring extraordinary skill, and find that the defendant was not guilty of negligence in failing to discover the condition of non-union prior to the time when he did discover it, then there is no liability and the verdict must be for the defendant.' At the request of the defendant the jury was further charged that, 'If the jury finds from the evidence that the fractured ends of the tibia were separated by tendon, muscle, or tissue, and for that reason could not have been made to unite without incision, and without the removal of the interposed substance, the plaintiff cannot recover for loss or damage resulting from delayed or non-union of such fragments by reason of the presence of such foreign substance upon the undisputed facts in this case.' The jury found a verdict for the plaintiff.

"It will therefore be observed that under the charge of the court the chief question of the fact involved was as to whether there were muscular fibres which intervened between the broken ends of the tibia which prevented its union and whether such a condition could have been discovered except by the operation which was made at the hospital requiring extraordinary skill. It is thus apparent that upon this issue the sustaining of the testimony of Dr. G. was of importance to the defendant, and, had he been permitted to avail himself of the testimony of Dr. D. who assisted Dr. G. in the operation, the result might have been different. We consequently cannot approve the ruling made upon the ground that the evidence was merely cumulative, for, being offered upon the trial to sustain the defendant's defence, he had the right to have it considered by the jury.

"The serious question presented upon this review calls for a construction of Sections 834 and 836 of the Code of Civil Procedure. Section 834, as far as material, is as follows, 'A person duly authorized to practise physic or surgery . . . shall not be allowed to disclose any information which he acquired attending a patient in a professional capacity, which was necessary to enable him to act in that capacity.' Section 836 provides, among other things, that the provisions of the Section apply to a Surgeon 'unless the provisions thereof are expressly waived upon the trial or examination of the person confessing, the patient or client.' . . . The waivers herein provided for must be made in open court, on the trial of the action or proceeding, and a paper executed by a party prior to the trial, providing for such waivers, shall be insufficient as such a waiver. But the attorneys for the respective parties may, prior to the trial, stipulate for such waiver and the same shall be sufficient therefor." There can be no question with reference to the discovery made by Dr. G. and Dr. D. in their operation upon the plaintiff at the hospital coming within the express language of the provisions of Section 834 of the Code, and the testimony, therefore, under ordinary circumstances would be privileged. But the question here presented is as to whether such privilege has been waived by the plaintiff upon the trial. He and his counsel sat by and permitted the testimony of Dr. G. to be given without interposing any objection thereto, thereby waiving the privilege which the plaintiff might have availed himself of had he seen fit. He has thus permitted the condition of his broken limb to be given to the public in an open trial, thereby forever preventing it and its condition from being a secret between himself and his physician.

"The intent of the Legislature in enacting the statute making such information privileged was, doubtless, to inspire confidence between the patient and his physician, so that the former could fully disclose to the latter all the particulars of his ailment without fear that he may be exposed to civil or criminal prosecution, or shame or disgrace, by the disclosure thus made, and thus enable the latter to prescribe for, and advise, the former most advantageously. As was said by Ruger, Ch. J., in McKinney vs. Grand Street P. P. & F. R. R. Co. (104 N. Y., 352), 'After its publication no further injury can be inflicted upon the rights and interests which the statute was intended to protect and there is no further reason for its enforcement. The nature of the information is of such a character that when it is once divulged in legal proceedings it cannot again be hidden or concealed. It is then open to the consideration of the entire public and the privilege forbidding its repetition is not conferred by the statute. The consent having been once given and acted upon cannot be recalled and the patient can never be restored to the condition which the statute, from motives of public policy, has sought to protect.'

"In the case of Morris vs. N. Y., Ont. & Western Railway Co. (148 N. Y., 88), it was held that when a party who has been attended by two physicians in their professional capacity at the same examination or consultation, both holding professional relations to him, calls one of them as a witness in his own behalf in an action in which the party's condition as it appeared at such consultation is the important question, to prove what took place, or what the witness then learned, he thereby waives the privilege conferred by the section of the code in question and loses his right to object to the testimony of the other physician if called by the opposite party to testify as to the same transaction. And in the case of People vs. Bloom (193 N. Y. 1.) which we have considered and determined in connection with this case at the present term, we have held that where the waiver of the privilege is by admitting the testimony of the physician without an objection in a civil action he cannot thereafter invoke the privilege by objecting to their testimony in a criminal action against him, in which he is charged with having committed perjury on the former trial. It would seem under the authorities alluded to, the plaintiff by admitting the evidence of Dr. G. to be given with reference to the discovery made at the operation, thereby also is deemed to have waived the privilege as to Dr. D. who was there assisting Dr. G. in the operation. But we prefer to rest our decision in this case on broader grounds.

"This action, as we have seen, is for malpractice. The plaintiff, both in his complaint and in his testimony, has fully disclosed all of the details of his affliction as it existed both at his home and at the hospital. He has given much in detail how the fractures occurred, how they were treated, his pain and suffering, and so far as he was able to comprehend, when not under the influence of anæsthetics, the particulars of the operation at the hospital. He himself has, therefore, given to the public the full details of his case, thereby disclosing the secrets which the statute was designed to protect, thus removing it from the operation of the statute. In other words he has waived in open court upon the trial all the information which he might have kept secret, by disclosing it himself. The character of the action necessarily calls for the disclosure of his condition and the treatment that was adopted by the defendant and those assisting him. To hold that the plaintiff may waive the privilege as to himself and his own physician and then invoke it as to the defendant and his physicians would have the effect of converting the statute into both a sword and a shield. It would permit him to prosecute with the sword and then shield himself from the defence by the exclusion of the defendant's testimony. It would enable the plaintiff to testify to whatever he pleased with reference to his condition and the treatment by the defendant without fear of contradiction. The plaintiff could thus establish his cause of action and the defendant would be deprived of the power to interpose his defence by reason of closing the mouth of his witnesses by the provisions of the code referred to. Such a construction of its provisions, we think, was never contemplated by the Legislature. It would lead to unreasonable and unjust results. Instead thereof a construction of the provisions of the code to the effect that when the privilege of the plaintiff has been once waived by him in court, either by his own testimony or by that of others given with his knowledge and consent, and his physical condition has been given to the public, the door is then thrown open for his opponent to give the facts as he understands them. This, to our minds, affords a more just and equitable rule and is the one evidently contemplated by the Legislature. Edington vs. Aetna Life Ins. Co., 77 N. Y., 564; Clifford vs. Denver R. G. R. R. Co., 188 N. Y., 349; Raub vs. Deutscher Verein, 29 App. Div., 483; Wigmore on Evidence, Sec. 2389 (and other references, which see).

"The judgment should be reversed and a new trial ordered."

XVIII. The Award of Damages.—THE PRINCIPLE GOVERNING THE AWARD OF DAMAGES IN SURGICAL MALPRACTICE.—It is the well-settled law, that if injury result to the patient of an attending Surgeon by reason of the want of ordinary skill or ordinary attention in the treatment of the former by the latter, the former may recover damages for the injury and such as are compensatory in their nature. These have been held to include both direct and indirect consequences, if referable to and resulting from the course of treatment complained of. Suffering also, which is produced in consequence of the acts in question, may be the subject of compensation; so also loss of time and actual expenses incurred in consequence of the fault, want of skill, or negligence of the Surgeon. Regard must also be had in such cases to the character of the resulting injury, as to whether it is temporary or permanent in its consequences. So also the situation and condition of the injured party may be considered. So also may be the effect of the injury in future upon the health of the patient, his ability to labor and attend to his affairs, and generally to pursue the course of life that he might otherwise have done. These elements are to be taken into consideration by the jury when the evidence tends to prove the existence of all or any of them. Carpenter *vs.* M'Davitt, 53 Mo. App., 393; Chamberlin *vs.* Porter, 9 Minn., 260; Tefft *vs.* Wilcox, 6 Kan., 46; Curtis *vs.* Railroad Co., 20 Barb. (N. Y.), 291.

DEFINITION OF DAMAGES.—The legal definition of the word "damages" is "the injury or loss for which compensation is sought" (Bouvier). Three grades of damages are recognized, representing the varying degrees of injury or loss, viz., 1, Nominal damages; 2, Compensatory damages; 3, Exemplary damages.

NOMINAL DAMAGES.—Nominal damages are awarded when the plaintiff or complainant has established his cause of action, but has not proved that he has sustained any injury or loss that can be measured by money value. In other words, a technical right has been invaded, but no pecuniary injury or loss has resulted to the complainant. The occasions when nominal damages might properly be given in actions for alleged malpractice are necessarily very rare, for if the surgeon is exonerated the verdict of the jury would be in his favor, while if the patient should establish his claim the jury would award him substantial damages. The following cases illustrate the conditions under which nominal damages were awarded in an action for alleged malpractice.

INJURY TO PATIENT FROM MALPRACTICE DOUBTFUL.—In Becker *vs.* Janinski, 27 Abb. N. C. (N. Y.), 45, the plaintiff had a miscarriage, and the evidence showed some improper treatment on the part of the defendant. It also showed that the patient's general health was impaired. On the part of the defendant evidence was introduced to show the injurious effect of a miscarriage upon the general health of the patient, and it was contended that the injury to her health, which was the subject of complaint, was the result of the miscarriage for which the defendant was not responsible; at least it was impossible to decide that the injury was due solely to the alleged improper treatment. The trial court instructed the jury as follows: "The defendant not being responsible for the miscarriage, he is not to be made liable for any of its consequences. If liable at all, he is liable only for the effects of the maltreatment of the plaintiff. So that, if you should find it impossible to distinguish between the consequences of the maltreatment—should you be unable to find upon the evidence that the plaintiff has suffered any injury distinctively due to maltreatment—you will award only nominal damages against the defendant."

WRONG APPLICATION TO THE EYE; NOMINAL DAMAGES.—In Stanley *vs.* Schumpert, 41 So. Rep., 565, and others, a Surgeon prescribed a mild solution to be applied to the eye of a patient under the direction of a trained nurse in a sanitarium. Another nurse, who happened to be in charge of the patient's ward, undertook to administer the solution, but negligently put the dropper into a bottle containing alcohol and applied this liquid freely to the eye. The application caused intense pain but the injury was very slight. An action for damages was brought against the lessee, and nominal damages of $25 were awarded for the suffering, though momentary, which the negligent mistake occasioned. The Supreme Court of Louisiana affirmed the judgment.

COMPENSATORY OR SUBSTANTIAL DAMAGES.—The legal principles and rulings of the courts governing the award of compensatory or substantial damages, when the patient establishes an ordinary case of malpractice against the Surgeon, and shows substantial injury therefrom, have been very compactly formulated as follows: * The measure of damages is the loss or injury directly or naturally resulting from the Surgeon's fault or negligence. Challis *vs.* Lake, 71 N. H., 90. The extent of the liability and of the damages recoverable depends in every case upon the particular circumstances. Tefft *vs.* Wilcox, 6 Kan., 46; Heath *vs.* Glisan, 3 Or., 64; Chamberlain *vs.* Porter, 9 Minn., 260. The jury are the sole arbiters of the amount which the patient should recover, unless the case is submitted to the judge without a jury and the principle governing the award is that it should represent, as nearly as possible, in dollars and cents the loss or injury sustained. In assessing damages due consideration is to be given to, 1. The pain and suffering caused by the malpractice, but the jury is cautioned to allow damages only for such pain and suffering as are directly attributable to the malpractice, carefully excluding such as are caused by the original malady or injury, Wenger *vs.* Calder, 78 Ill., 275; Carpenter *vs.* McDavitt, 53 Mo. App., 393; Gates *vs.* Fleicher, 67 Wis., 504. 2. The expense directly caused by the malpractice, particularly that incurred in the endeavor to be cured of the evil effects of the malpractice, allowance being made, however, for expense that is necessary and reasonable in amount only, Hewitt *vs.* Eisenbart, 36 Neb., 794. 3. The loss of time sustained by the patient, the reduction of his money-earning capacity, his disfigurement or impairment of senses or faculties, and, generally, all the detriments caused by the Surgeon's improper course.

SURGEON NOT LIABLE FOR SUFFERING FROM ORIGINAL INJURY.—In Wenger *vs.* Calder, *supra*, an action was brought against the Surgeon for alleged malpractice in the treatment of a dislocation of the elbow. The trial court instructed the jury as follows, "The rule of damages in this case, if you find for the plaintiff, is the pain and suffering undergone by the plaintiff and any permanent injury to the arm shown by the evidence, and consequent pecuniary loss, for life, after the time of the plaintiff's coming of age." The Supreme Court of Illinois held that, "This instruction was palpably erroneous. The injury which the plaintiff originally received to his elbow, was not produced by any agency or fault of the defendant, and there was no reason why he should be held to pay for the pain and suffering caused thereby. If there were any additional pain and suffering which the plaintiff underwent, because of the want of reasonable care and skill in the treatment, that might have been considered by the jury in assessing damages—nothing more. And there should have been the same limitation in the respect of any permanent injury to the arm."

LIABLE ONLY FOR INJURIES RESULTING FROM MALPRACTICE.—In Miller *vs.* Frey, 49 Neb., 472, a suit for damages alleged to have been caused by malpractice in setting and treating a broken arm, the plaintiff-patient recovered a judgment and the defendant-surgeon prosecuted the proceedings in error. The Supreme Court of Nebraska reversed the judgment of the trial court on the following ground, "It will be observed that several times in this instruction the

* The Law and the Doctor, vol. 1., p. 44.

court makes the test the loss sustained by reason 'of the injury complained of.' Elsewhere in the charge the broken arm is referred to in similar terms as 'the injury.' This instruction was misleading and erroneous. If the defendant was guilty of malpractice, he was not liable for all the injuries resulting from the breaking of the plaintiff's arm. He was liable only for such damages as resulted from his failure to exercise that degree of care and skill ordinarily exercised and possessed by physicians and surgeons in the treatment of such cases. That plaintiff suffered damages by reason of the breaking of his arm was indisputable. That some damages would have resulted from that injury in spite of the most skilful treatment is clearly unquestionable. The defendant, no matter how unskilful he may have been, was not liable for all the injuries resulting from the breaking of the arm. He was only liable for those resulting from malpractice; that is, for the damages accruing to plaintiff on account of the injury in excess of those which would have accrued to him naturally from the breaking of his arm had he been treated with that degree of skill ordinarily possessed by surgeons."

LIABILITY FOR LOSS OF EARNING POWER DUE TO MALPRACTICE.—In Froman *vs.* Ayars, 85 Pac. Rep., 14; s. c. 42 Wash., 385, a case of alleged malpractice in the treatment of a compound fracture of the bones of the leg about two inches above the ankle joint, it was contended by counsel for the defence that the case should be distinguished from one which is brought to recover for ordinary personal injuries where the injury is wholly due to the neglect of the defendant; in this case the primary cause of the result was the running away of the team for which the Surgeon was not responsible; the degree of his responsibility could not be as great as that of one whose negligence laid the first foundation of the injury.

The Supreme Court of Washington sustained the findings of the jury that the plaintiff would not have been deprived of a foot if the defendant had properly applied his learning and skill; the plaintiff, it is true, would have suffered pain and distress from the original injury, yet if the bones had properly united and the wound had healed, the suffering would have been temporary; now he must continue to suffer humiliation, inconvenience, and loss of earning power during his life. The issue before the jury was that the Surgeon did not exercise the degree of skill and care recognized by the standards of his profession as ordinary and reasonable, and that his failure in that regard was the responsible cause of the final and serious results to the plaintiff. The court did not think the award of $5,000 damages too large for the loss of a foot by a man forty-four years of age who had an expectancy of twenty-six years of life.

DAMAGES FOR UNAUTHORIZED EXAMINATION OF WOUND.—In South Covington & Cincinnati Street Railway Company *vs.* Cleveland, 100 S. W. Rep., 283; 30 Ky. L. Rep., 1072, an action brought by the latter party, who had been injured in a collision with an electric car, it was alleged that immediately after the accident she was carried into the house of a friend, and while there an inspector of the company, in pursuance of orders to investigate the accident, obtained admittance to the room where she was lying, without invitation or request, and roughly and rudely seized and took hold of her person and examined the wound she had received. For this indignity she asked $2,500. In respect to the conduct of the inspector, a preponderance of the evidence tended to show that the act was committed as claimed. The jury was told that if it believed that the inspector acted in the scope of his employment, and without the request or consent of the plaintiff, placed his hands on her person and examined her wounds, it would find for her in such sum as would fairly compensate her for the mental suffering and sense of shame or humiliation or wounded pride resulting from such action to which she was thereby subjected. The jury awarded her $500 for indignities. The Court of Appeals of Kentucky approved both the instruction and award by affirming the judgment of the lower court.

EXEMPLARY OR PUNITIVE DAMAGES.—While compensatory damages are estimated as an equivalent for the injury, exemplary or punitive damages are awarded, not as a mere reimbursement of pecuniary loss, but as a good round compensation and an adequate recompense for the entire injury sustained, and such as may serve for a wholesome example to others in like cases. There is no fixed and certain criterion of damages for personal injuries; the question as to their amount is within the sound and reasonable discretion of the jury; the damages given may be more or less exemplary, or otherwise, as the circumstances of aggravation or extenuation, characterizing each particular case, may reasonably require; whether exemplary damages should or should not be given, does not depend upon the form of the action, so much as upon the nature and extent of the injury done, and the manner in which it was inflicted, whether by gross negligence, wantonness, or with or without malice. Fleet & Semple vs. Hollenkemp, 13 B. Monroe (Ky.), 219.

CONDITIONS JUSTIFYING EXEMPLARY DAMAGES MUST BE STATED IN COMPLAINT AND APPEAR IN EVIDENCE.—In Baxter vs. Campbell, 17 S. D., 475, the complaint averred that the plaintiff suffered from a broken leg, between the knee and ankle, which the defendant treated so carelessly, negligently, and unskilfully, that he had been compelled to expend $200 for the services of another surgeon and had been damaged by his inability to work to the extent of $800, and also alleged "this plaintiff has suffered extreme pain, both of body and mind, and was greatly injured in bodily health, to his damage in the sum of four thousand dollars. Wherefore plaintiff demands judgment against defendant in the sum of five thousand dollars damages, as set forth in this complaint, for expenses, loss of time, and suffering." . . . The jury returned a verdict for $3,800 in favor of the plaintiff, and the defendant appealed.

The Supreme Court of South Dakota, on appeal, held that, while the complaint is limited to a claim of damages in the way of compensation for "expenses, loss of time, and suffering" arising from the alleged negligent and unskilful treatment of the case, and there is nothing in the testimony tending in the slightest degree to sustain an inference of malice, the court instructed the jury as follows: "Should the defendant's conduct show a wilful and malicious want of care and skill, the jury may allow as damages not only the actual damage proved, but such exemplary damages or smart money as, in their judgment, may be just and proper as a punishment to the defendant, in view of all of the facts and circumstances proved on the trial." Commenting on this instruction the Supreme Court held there was nothing in the conduct of the appellant from which malice may be presumed; to justify the imputation of malice, within the rule of punitive damages, the injury must have been conceived in a spirit of mischief, and partake of a criminal or wanton nature; under the pleadings and the proof, there was nothing to warrant exemplary damages, and it was erroneous to give an instruction upon so dangerous a proposition not in the case; there being nothing in the complaint or evidence from which malice may be presumed, the instruction authorizing the imposition of exemplary damages was seriously prejudicial to appellants. The judgment appealed from was reversed.

GROSS NEGLIGENCE AND EXEMPLARY DAMAGES.—In Brooke vs. Clark, 57 Tex., 105, a Surgeon was charged with gross negligence in placing a ligature around the penis of the appellee at his birth instead of around the umbilical cord, destroying most of the glans. Fifteen days after the birth of Henry N. Clark, suit was brought by his next friend in his behalf to recover damages of Dr. J. B., the accoucheur, which resulted in a verdict of the jury in favor of Clark for $5,500.

On appeal the Supreme Court of Texas held that the criminal indifference of the defendant to results was a fact which the jury were at liberty to infer from the gross mistake which he either made or permitted to be made, and the grievous injury which was liable to result and did result therefrom. If there was other evidence tending to negative any wrong intent or actual indifference on his part, still the existence or non-existence of such criminal indifference was a question of fact for the jury, and was rightly submitted to them. If the conduct of the defendant in the discharge of his duty as accoucheur was so grossly negligent as to raise the presumption of his criminal indifference to results, the Court very greatly doubted whether it should avail to exempt him from exemplary damages, for him to show that he had no bad motive, and that he acted otherwise in a manner tending to show that he was not, at heart, indifferent. Where the act is so grossly negligent as to raise the presumption of indifference, evidence that in other matters connected therewith he had shown due care, and that actual indifference would have been in fact indifference to his own interest, should, they thought, not be allowed for any other purpose than to be considered by the jury in fixing the amount of exemplary damages. The judgment was affirmed.

EXCESSIVE DAMAGES.—The question as to amount of damages belongs to the jury, and the general rule has been that a new trial will not be granted in an action for excessive damages, unless they are so clearly excessive as to indicate that the jury acted from passion, prejudice, partiality, or corruption, or were misled as to the measure of damages. Kelsey vs. Hay, 84 Ind., 189. Honest well-meaning men are liable to be led astray by strong feelings of sympathy, arising from a narration of painful and protracted sufferings, and while thus excited often inflict upon the author of them a severer punishment than he deserves. Howard vs. Grover, 28 Me., 97.

In Olwell vs. Skobis, 105 N. W., 777; s. c. 126 Wisc., 578, an action brought to recover damages for an injury to one of the eyes of the plaintiff necessitating long and painful treatment, three operations thereon, and its removal, the Supreme Court of Wisconsin said, there is no exact rule for estimating damages in such a case. In certain cases in other jurisdictions verdicts of from $2,000 to $5,000 for the loss of an eye have been held not to be excessive. In this case the jury assessed the damages suffered by the plaintiff, a woman amanuensis and bookkeeper, by the injury referred to, at $12,000; but this court is constrained to hold, for the purposes of a new trial of the case, that a verdict for more than $6,000 on substantially the same evidence as to damages as in this case would be deemed to be excessive.

In Leeson vs. Sawmill Phoenix, 83 Pac., 891; s. c. 41 Wash., 423, a jury brought in a verdict of $5,500 damages for an inguinal hernia on the right side caused by a blow on the abdomen from the handle of a chisel thrown back by an alleged defective machine. The plaintiff, who was about forty-seven years of age, was said by all physicians who testified in the case to be in a healthy normal condition, with the exception of the hernia. There was also testimony that he could probably be cured by an operation which would cost in the neighborhood of $200 or $300. The Supreme Court of Washington holds the award under these circumstances excessive, and that $3,500 would be ample compensation. An excessive verdict in a case like this, it says, is not only an injustice to the defendants, but it is a menace to the welfare of the state, and should not be upheld.

WHEN MENTAL SUFFERING IS AN ELEMENT OF DAMAGES.—In Manser vs. Collins, 69 Kan., 290, the negligence charged in the petition against the Surgeon was that he failed and neglected to ascertain the dislocation of the right arm and shoulder and left elbow, when the same was easily discoverable by the exercise of ordinary care and attention and that he wholly failed to treat said injuries, and that the dislocations were not discovered until another physician was called. The answer on the part of the Surgeon was a general denial, with an allegation of contributory negligence on plaintiff's part. The jury found that the nature and extent of plaintiff's injuries could have been determined and discovered by a physician of ordinary skill and ability at the time the Surgeon was called, May 18th, 1900, and at any time thereafter up to June 9th, 1900; that if the nature and extent of the injuries had been discovered by the Surgeon they could have been cured, or remedied so that her condition would have been improved, and she would have been relieved of bodily pain. In answer to the question, what sum would compensate the plaintiff for the mental anguish suffered by her by reason of the failure of the defendant to discover the injury to her right shoulder, the answer was $250, and in answer to a similar inquiry as to the compensation for mental anguish from the Surgeon's failure to discover the injury to her left elbow the award was $200.

The Supreme Court of Kansas, reviewing the case in error, held that where mental suffering is an element of physical pain, or a consequence of it, damages for such mental suffering may be recovered; mental suffering, however, resulting from the injury which arises in the mind, but is not a part of the pain naturally attendant on and connected with the injury, cannot be regarded as an element of damage.

ALLEGED MALPRACTICE AS DEFENCE IN ACTION TO RECOVER FEES.—Cases frequently occur where the patient refuses to pay the Surgeon, alleging malpractice on the part of the latter. The law implies a promise on the part of the Surgeon that he has ordinary skill, and that he will execute the business entrusted to him with ordinary care and skill; if he fails in this duty he is guilty of default in his undertaking, and cannot collect the pay for his services, but is liable in damages to the person who employed him. Bellinger vs. Craigue, 31 Barb. (N. Y.), 534. The law would not on the trial presume that the Surgeon had neglected his duty and made default of his undertaking, for a breach of duty, or negligence, or fraud is not to be presumed. Starr vs. Peck, 1 Hill (N.Y.), 270. The burden of proof is therefore cast upon the defendant-patient to disprove the allegation of performance in such complaint.

CONTRIBUTORY NEGLIGENCE AS IT AFFECTS THE AWARD OF DAMAGES IN ACTIONS FOR MALPRACTICE.—In prosecutions for alleged malpractice the defence is often made that the patient or plaintiff contributed to the injury by his failure to comply with the directions of the Surgeon or defendant. It is a well-settled principle of law, that a party seeking to recover for an injury must not have contributed to it in any degree, either by his negligence, or the disregard of a duty imposed upon him by a party who, by his negligence or want of care or skill, may also, in some degree, have contributed to the injury. Smith vs. Smith, 2 Pick. (Mass.), 621; Hibbard vs. Thompson, 109 Mass., 286. This grows out of the doctrine that a party who has directly, by his own negligence or disregard of duty, contributed to bring an injury upon himself, cannot hold other parties, who have also contributed to the same, responsible for any part thereof, nor does it make any difference that one of the parties contributed in a much greater degree than the other: the injured party must not have contributed at all. Griselman vs. Scott, 25 Ohio St., 86. An authority thus states the law, "Contributory negligence on the part of the plaintiff, who complains that he has been damnified by the negligence of the defendant, is in general an answer to the action, on the ground that a man cannot complain of that which he himself has helped to bring about." * Proof of the commission by the defendant, or his servants, of the injury of which the plaintiff claims, very generally carries with it *prima facie* proof of negligence, and it is for the defendant to show that the injury was the result of inevitable accident, or that it was occasioned by the negligence or misconduct of the plaintiff himself.

In these suits the plaintiff is required, as a general proposition, to prove that the immediate cause of the injury complained of was the wrongful act of the defendant, to which his own wrongful act did not immediately contribute. Hence, it has been held that the complaint must show by averments that he was not at fault. Scudder et al. vs. Crossan, 43 Ind., 343.

* Addison on Torts.

No Damages Allowed if Injury by Neglect of Patient cannot be Separated from that Caused by Surgeon.—In Hibbard *vs.* Thompson, 109 Mass., 286, an action for alleged malpractice in which contributory negligence on the part of the patient was charged by the defence, the trial judge instructed the jury as follows:—"The burden of proof is on the plaintiff to show that all the injuries for which he seeks damages proceeded solely from want of ordinary skill and care on the part of defendant. If it be impossible to separate the injury occasioned by the neglect of the plaintiff himself, from that occasioned by the neglect of the defendant, the plaintiff cannot recover. If, however, they can be separated, he may recover for such injury as the plaintiff may show thus proceeded solely from want of ordinary skill or ordinary care of the defendant. In the present case, the plaintiff claims damages of the defendant for want of ordinary care and ordinary skill in the treatment of him by the defendant, by which, as he says, first a bed sore was caused, and second, after the bed sore was caused, it was improperly treated, and neglected. If the plaintiff should fail to satisfy you that the sore was caused by neglect of the defendant for this damage of course he could not recover, but he might still recover for the injury occasioned to him solely by the subsequent negligence of the defendant in not taking proper care of it (should he prove such neglect), even if the sore was occasioned by the plaintiff's own carelessness. If, however, in the case last supposed, injury has resulted to the plaintiff not solely from neglect in the subsequent treatment of it by the defendant, but also from his own subsequent neglect, and the jury are not satisfied but that both causes have combined to produce the subsequent injury, the plaintiff cannot recover for it. While on the one hand the defendant would not be released from his duty to exercise ordinary care and ordinary skill in his subsequent treatment of a disease because at a previous stage of it the plaintiff had himself been negligent and had thus contributed to the condition in which he was, on the other hand it would be for the patient to show, if he seeks damages for want of ordinary care and ordinary skill on the part of the defendant in his subsequent treatment, that it proceeded solely from this, and not from any subsequent neglect on his own part."

The Supreme Judicial Court of Massachusetts sustained this ruling and remarked that, "The first part states the ordinary rule as to the negligence of the plaintiff; the second states the proper limitations of the rule. It is an important limitation; for a physician may be called to prescribe for cases which originated in the carelessness of the patient; and though such carelessness would remotely contribute to the injury sued for, it would not relieve the physician from liability for his distinct negligence, and the separate injury occasioned thereby. The patient may also, while he is under treatment, injure himself by his own carelessness; yet he may recover from the physician if he carelessly or unskilfully treats him afterwards, and thus does him a distinct injury. In such cases, the plaintiff's fault does not directly contribute to produce the injury sued for."

Plaintiff Having Recovered Damages cannot Institute Another Suit for Same Act of Malpractice.—The plaintiff's cause of action includes the right to recover for damages past, present, and future * and hence a patient having once recovered and collected a judgment from a Surgeon for a given act of malpractice, such judgment is a complete satisfaction of all damages which may have resulted, or which may thereafter result, from such act of malpractice, and no further action can be brought to recover for further injurious results as they may subsequently manifest themselves.† The law will not tolerate a multiplicity of suits, but always compels a party litigating to enforce his whole right in a single suit, when the right is of such a nature as to render that possible. Howell vs. Goodrich, 69 Ill., 556.

DAMAGES FOR CERTIFYING THAT PATIENT HAS GONORRHŒA.—A Surgeon wrote on a certificate the fact that a member of a club was suffering from gonorrhœa and gave the certificate to the secretary of the club. The member brought an action for libel and slander. The surgeon pleaded that the communication was privileged, but the jury decided against him and awarded $750 damages to the plaintiff. The solicitors of the association state, in commenting on the case, that when a Surgeon in the course of his duties has to fill a certificate of this kind relating to the health or sickness of a person, and the ailment is one the disclosure of which would constitute a libel, he ought to give the certificate to the patient, and not to a third party. (London Letter.)

In McDonald vs. Nugent, 98 N. W. Rep., 506; s. c. 122 Iowa, 651, the Supreme Court of Iowa held that to charge another with being afflicted with venereal disease is slanderous per se (by itself). From an early date in the development of the common law of slander and libel, a charge made by one person that another is infected with a venereal disease has been held to constitute one of the few exceptions to the general rule applicable to oral slander—that, to be actionable per se, the words must impute some crime to the person defamed. The theory on which questions like this are held maintainable is not that the slanderous words impute a crime, but that the charge made, if true, or if generally believed to be true, would necessarily exclude the person thus impugned from the benefits of decent society. A charge of crime in the ordinary sense of the word is a mild and harmless imputation, when compared with words which brand a man or woman as a leprous outcast, and it is a healthful doctrine that which holds to strict accountability any one who indulges in such injurious reflections on another. When slanderous words, whether oral or written, are actionable per se, proof of the speaking or publication is all that is required. Malice in such cases is presumed without other evidence.

XIX. Explanatory Remark; Attitude of the Courts; Concluding Suggestions.—SCOPE OF ARTICLE.—In the preparation of this article the authors have endeavored to state in as precise and comprehensive form as the limited space would allow the civil obligations which the Surgeon assumes who undertakes the practice of American surgery. These obligations have been largely increased during the last half-century by the great advance of the medical sciences, the enormous expansion of industrial enterprises with the attendant injuries to

---

* Taylor's The Law in its Relations to Physicians, p. 392.
† The Law and the Doctor, vol. i., p. 47.

operatives, and the vast movements of the people by improved methods of public transportation and the attendant accidents to persons. While formerly the Surgeon was rarely summoned to testify in courts except in occasional actions for alleged malpractice, he is now a conspicuous witness in the "Personal Injury" and "Litigation Psychosis" cases which burden the calendars of the courts. In the trial of these actions new questions, both surgical and legal, are constantly occurring which require the most discreet consideration on the part of expert witnesses and the courts for correct judicial determination. The scope of this article has therefore been enlarged so as to include some of the more important features in the trial of cases, other than those for malpractice, in which the Surgeon is called to testify.

In order to give to the text the highest authority on the subjects treated the decisions of the higher courts of the States have been selected, and the language of the original decisions followed, with such abbreviations without impairing the meaning, as our limits required. These decisions in their connections have a twofold value, for while they establish the laws in their special jurisdictions, as regards the particular matter at issue, they throw a much-needed light upon those purely legal questions which are still of doubtful interpretation. Even the number of citations of these decisions has been limited to those believed to be most authoritative in order to avoid repetition.

In the classification of subjects for discussion the legal rather than the surgical order has been followed. A critical examination of the cases applicable to the subject-matter of the article and the decisions of the courts thereon, clearly show that the rules of law governing the qualifications and duties of the Surgeon, and the conduct and liabilities of both Surgeon and patient are of general application. The legal principles governing the rulings of the courts are illustrated by cases of alleged malpractice in every branch of the practice of surgery, and they are found to be the same, whether the case be in operations, or in the treatment of fractures or dislocations, or the injuries and diseases of any organ or part of the body. Though different cases must necessarily present for judicial consideration marked differences in details peculiar to the subject-matter from which the cause of action arose, yet the final disposition of all questions occurring in the course of litigation will in general be in accordance with the legal rules established by the authorities cited.

ATTITUDE OF THE COURTS.—There is a widespread sentiment in the medical profession that the courts show but slight appreciation of the peculiarly difficult conditions under which the practisers of that art are compelled to perform their duties, and that the legal rules governing the trial of cases of alleged malpractice are applied with marked discrimination against the physician or surgeon. We are persuaded that a judicious review of the preceding pages will convince an unprejudiced mind that this sentiment has no just foundation. It has its origin in an unfamiliarity with, or a misconception of, the rules governing the admissibility of evidence which have had the sanction of the most noted jurists for years. On the contrary, there is ample evidence that the Courts have uniformly recognized the medical profession as devoted to the most sacred of callings—the relief of human suffering—and have shown a proper appreciation of the manifold difficulties which daily beset the Surgeon in the discharge of his duties. When through some unfortunate circumstance his professional acts have been the subject of critical review in legal tribunals, judges have shown commendable judgment in protecting him from hostile treatment, provided it appears from the evidence that he has brought to the treatment of the case ordinary learning and skill and has exercised proper care and diligence in applying that learning and skill. It is equally true that these decisions show that the Courts have judiciously discriminated between the legitimate practiser of surgery and the mere pretender, and that charlatanism in every form has received stern rebuke when its practices have come within the purview of legal tribunals. "The law has no allowance for quackery."

The charge of a trial judge to the jury in a suit for alleged malpractice which held that a Surgeon "was accountable for damages just as a stone-mason or bricklayer," received the following criticism from the highest court of the State of Pennsylvania: "He (the Surgeon) deals not with insensate matter like the stone-mason or bricklayer, who can choose their materials and adjust them according to mathematical lines; but he has a suffering human being to treat, a nervous system to tranquillize, and a *will* to regulate and control. The evidence before us makes this strong distinction between surgery and masonry, and shows how the judge's inapt illustration was calculated to lead away the minds of the jury from the true point of the case." McCandless *vs.* McWha, 22 Penn. St., 261.

The Supreme Court of Pennsylvania, in Richards *vs.* Willard, 176 Penn. St., 181, commenting on the fact that the suit was brought against a Surgeon who gave his services gratuitously, said, "If such gentlemen are to be harassed with actions for damages when they do not happen to cure a patient, and are to incur the hazard of having their estates swept away from them by the verdicts of irresponsible juries, who, caring nothing for law, nothing for evidence, nothing for justice, nothing for the plain teachings of common sense, choose to gratify their prejudices or their passions by plundering their fellow-citizens in the forms of law, it may well be doubted whether our hospitals and other charitable institutions will be able to obtain the gratuitous and valuable services of these unselfish and charitable men."

Perhaps a more striking illustration of the appreciation by the Courts of the difficulties which the modern Surgeon encounters in his practice and their efforts to secure an impartial judgment from juries when his alleged errors are the subject of judicial determination, is found in the opinion of the Supreme Court of the State of Georgia in the case of Arkridge *vs.* Noble, 114 Ga., 949. The action was for negligence in leaving a sponge in the patient's body. The Court said, "Reasonable or ordinary care is not an absolute term, and has no arbitrary meaning. If the care and skill required of him in doing this thing was not measured by the reasonable care and skill of a surgeon, what was the measure of it? Was it that of an upholsterer stuffing or removing the stuffing of furniture? Or that of a railroad employee operating a train? Or that of a master toward his servant? Or what was it? It may seem at first blush, as perhaps it has impressed counsel, that, if the surgeon put the sponges inside of a patient's body, care would require him to take them all out. But when we remember that abdominal surgery, as now practised, is largely a matter of a few years' growth, that until quite a recent period it was considered that an incision or wound which penetrated the abdominal cavity was certainly fatal, and that now such operations are very frequently performed; that the surgeon must make a small incision, not over a few inches in length; must insert and properly place a number of sponges or gauze pads, sometimes as many as a dozen as the evidence discloses; must, partly by sight and partly by feeling, reach the seat of the trouble and cut away the necessary parts; must tie up the loose ends, remove the sponges, and close and sew up the opening, arranging for proper drainage; and all this with the utmost promptness, for sometimes a slight delay may mean death,—circumstances and surroundings must be considered in measuring duty. Some of the witnesses in this case testified that, with the surgeon's mind and attention riveted on the delicate and dangerous work before him, it was very difficult, if not impossible, to keep in his memory the exact number and placing of these sponges; that he must needs rely somewhat for the count upon another; that he exercised such care and skill as he could in finding and removing the sponges, and then had the operating nurse to aid him by keeping count of them; and one or more said that, if the surgeon should stop at the critical moment to count sponges before closing the wound, the patient might die. This system may be imperfect. What system is not? But certainly it would never do to turn juries loose to fix some arbitrary standard—each jury for itself—of how abdominal surgery ought to be performed, regardless of how the surgeons had found it safest and best to do, nor, which would amount to the same thing, to say whether a method of performing an operation, even if universally adopted by the most skilful surgeons, seems reasonable to the jurors' mind or not. This is especially true where the practice of surgery is permitted only by those who have studied the recognized methods, and have had certain training, and have been found to be sufficiently proficient, and have been licensed. If the practice of surgery were thrown open to everybody to act on his general judgment, without skill or training, perhaps the rule might be different. The average juror might in such a supposed state of affairs, if it can be supposed, be able to judge of the mode of performing operations as well as the practitioner, of whom no training, skill, or knowledge was required. If all surgeons had perfect reason and perfect skill, there should be no failures. Medical and surgical science must advance gradually. It has its errors and its failings. But it would hardly do for every doctor who gives a prescription, or every surgeon who performs an operation, to do so at the risk that, if the result is not good, a jury may mulct him in damages, if they should think the method of treatment or of conduct was unreasonable, although it was the well-recognized and universal method."

CONCLUDING SUGGESTIONS.—A review of the preceding discussion of the civil obligations which he assumes, on undertaking the care and treatment of a patient, must impress the conscientious surgeon with the value of a knowledge of the rulings of the higher courts of the country, on the complex questions which have arisen in actions for alleged malpractice. Their decisions teach him that to avoid censure by the courts his conduct should be characterized by fidelity to the patient throughout the entire case, for failure at any time to meet the ordinary indications or emergencies vitiates the entire attendance, as the obligation is continuous to the termination. Bellinger *vs.* Craigue, 31 Barb. (N. Y.), 534.

It is apparent that he should endeavor to forecast every possible source of failure and thus be prepared for every emergency, for he is best prepared to assume responsibilities, and bear them lightly, who can most accurately estimate the risks and difficulties which he is to incur (Paget). In diagnosis, prognosis, operation, and after-treatment, his opinions should be formed, and his course of procedure deliberately taken and followed, without being unduly influenced by the solicitation of patient or friends, or the suggestions of consultants. Every step should be taken with such deliberation and care as to preclude the possibility of a charge of neglect in the diligent application of learning and skill. Thus the Surgeon not only secures that confidence of patient and friends so necessary to success at every stage of progress and especially in critical emergencies, but he fulfils the just requirements of the civil obligation.*

Note.—The authors desire to acknowledge their indebtedness in the preparation of this article to the series of "Medico-legal" trials reported in the *Journal of the American Medical Association.* Without the aid of these carefully prepared reports, which reflect great credit upon their authors, it would scarcely have been possible, within a reasonable length of time, to treat the subject of the relations of the Surgeon to the law except in a very imperfect manner. Credit is also due to the excellent work of Prof. Martin J. Wade, entitled "A Selection of Cases on Malpractice of Physicians and Dentists" (St. Louis, Medico-Legal Publishing Company, 1909).

* "Principles and Practice of Operative Surgery," by Stephen Smith, M.D., 1887.

PART XVIII.
ADMINISTRATIVE SURGICAL WORK.

HOSPITALS AND HOSPITAL MANAGEMENT, MORE PARTICULARLY WITH REFERENCE TO THE SURGICAL NEEDS OF THESE INSTITUTIONS.*

By CHRISTIAN R. HOLMES, M.D., Cincinnati, Ohio.

Introductory Remarks.—The earliest hospitals were the temples of the god Æsculapius, to which the sick came, or were brought, to learn by dreams or other signs how they might recover from their illness. The patients lay in the temple court or in huts clustered about the sacred edifice. In the days of Hippocrates the ministration of physicians took the place of the orphic utterances of the gods. With the decay of Greek civilization medical and surgical knowledge, what little was left, took its flight from Europe to Asia Minor and the northern coasts of Africa, to reappear, only after the lapse of many centuries, in the persons of the Arabian physicians in the Iberian peninsula. Among the Romans there does not seem to have been much distinction between a hospital and an inn, and our word "hospital" is derived from the Latin hospitalia, a guest house. Mediæval Christendom made use of the monasteries for hospital purposes, just as they were also used as shelters for travellers and as sanctuaries for the oppressed; and the oldest European hospitals of to-day betray, in their architecture, their traditions, and some of their customs, their monastic origin. The materialistic eighteenth and nineteenth centuries, however, in this as in so many other matters breaking with tradition, applied themselves diligently to the solution of this definite problem—How may we best take care of the sick and injured?—and attempted, with a fair measure of success, to make use of all the improvements in architecture and engineering that distinguished that remarkable period.

The size, arrangement, and shape of hospital buildings have undergone much variation in the course of the last two centuries, and have been the subject of much discussion. At first, we had the "block hospital" where the entire institution was included within four walls and under one roof. This was the first step in the evolution of the mediæval fortress-monastery into the modern hospital. Some of the most famous hospitals of France and England, of ancient foundation, preserve this type, or some slight modification of it, to this day.

* The writer has found it impracticable, within the comparatively narrow limits prescribed by the editors, to discuss more than a few of the aspects of the broad subject of hospitals and their management; and even these few topics have necessarily, for the same reason, been treated by him in a somewhat superficial manner. He has also found that it was not possible, in describing the construction and management of a large general hospital, to develop as fully as he would wish those aspects of the problem which are of special importance to the surgeon.

823

(Figs. 286 and 287.) As the medical profession steadily advanced in its study and comprehension of disease it recognized that various evil conditions afflicting the sick (and even sometimes the well, the hospital servitors) frequently arose within the walls of the hospitals themselves, and to these conditions was given the comprehensive term of "hospitalism." It is extremely interesting to note that each of the great wars of the latter quarter of the eighteenth century and the first three quarters of the nineteenth added extensively to the knowledge of hospitalism and brought forth valuable suggestions as to the manner in which

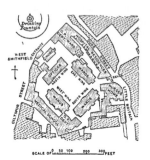

FIG. 286.—Ground Plan Showing the Distribution of the Different Buildings of St. Bartholomew's Hospital, at Smithfield, London, England.

it should be combated. Without going into detail it is sufficient to note that it was recognized that the massing together of large numbers of sick and wounded under one roof was extremely harmful, and that both medical and surgical patients very frequently got along better in the open air of the country regions, even when exposed to inclement weather, than did similar patients who were confined in the warmer, sheltered, but oftentimes dark and ill-smelling wards of the old-established hospitals of the cities. After the war of the American Revolution Dr. Tilton wrote: "It would be shocking to humanity to relate the history of our general hospitals in the years 1777 and 1779, when within their walls was swallowed up at least one-half of our army, owing to a fatal tendency in the system to throw all the sick of the army into the general hospitals; whence crowds, infections, and consequent mortality too afflicting to mention." Dr. Jones, also, who had "walked the hospitals" of England and France before the outbreak of the Revolution, wrote, concerning his own experiences in the field, "that in the cold weather of winter the best hospital he ever contrived was upon the plan of an Indian hut. The fire was built in the midst of the ward, without any chimney, and the smoke, circulating round about, passed off through an opening about four inches wide and a few feet long in the ridge of the roof." After the Crimean War Macleod, in his "Notes on the Surgery of the Crimean War," said: "If properly constructed and erected on suitable ground, there are no structures better adapted for the hospitals of an army in the field than wooden huts or canvas tents. The dreadful epidemics which have so frequently pursued armies, and the mortality which has attended their wounds, have in not a few instances been due to the employment of stone buildings as hospitals. The ventilation is more apt to be deficient or to become deranged in them than in huts or tents, and hence the effects of overcrowding become the more pernicious." "It was often proved in the history of the late war," says Jackson in his work on the economy of armies, "that more human life was destroyed by accumulating sick in low and ill-ventilated apartments, than by leaving them exposed in severe and inclement weather at the side of a hedge or common dyke." Writing a few years later, Miss Florence Nightingale said: "The reason why agglomeration of a large number of sick under one roof leads to disaster, is to be found in the simple fact that agglomeration argues either stern necessities of another kind or great ignorance and danger of misman-agement; and, besides all this, it argues unforeseen events and altogether such a deficiency in the general administrative arrangements as is sure to be accom-panied by want of proper ventilation, want of cleanliness, and other sanitary defects. If anything were wanting in confirmation of this fact, it would be the enormous mortality in the hospitals, which contained perhaps the largest number of sick ever present at one time under the same roof, viz.: those at Scutari. The largest of these too notorious hospitals had at one time 2,500 sick and wounded under its roof, and it has happened that, of Scutari patients, two

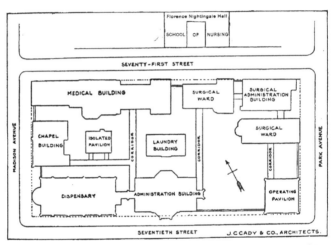

FIG. 287.—Block Plan of the Presbyterian Hospital, New York City. (By courtesy of the of the hospital authorities.)

out of every five have died. In the hospital tents of the Crimea, although the sick were almost without shelter, without blankets, without proper food or medicines, the mortality was not above one-half what it was at Scutari; but these tents had only a few beds each. Nor was it even as high as this in the small Balaklava General Hospital which had part of its sick placed in detached wooden huts, while in the well-ventilated detached huts of the Castle Hospital, on the heights above Balaklava, exposed to the sea-breeze, the mortality among the wounded, at a subsequent period, did not reach three per cent."

The logic of these experiences of the metropolitan and military surgeons was evidently that only a moderate number of cases should be gathered under one roof, that each patient should have abundant floor space and breathing space, and that a generous supply of fresh air was absolutely necessary. These things were being vehemently urged by the leaders of the medical profession in France and England at the period of the American Civil War, and the experiences of that war gave additional weight to their arguments. The movements of enormous armies over large areas in which there were but few cities and towns of considerable size, resulted in the evolution of the huts and tents of the American Revolution and the Crimean War into the Barrack and Tent Hospitals of the American Civil War. Long wooden wards were constructed on the style of the barracks, or hospital tents were put together end to end so as to make long wards. These were plain, cheap, clean, of open construction, easily and quickly put together or as rapidly taken down, and capable of almost indefinite expansion in times of emergency; and they yielded better results than any previous military hospital had ever done—or, indeed, than did the military hospitals of the crowded cities of Europe in the Franco-Prussian War, fought six years later. A consideration of all these facts, therefore, led some of the extreme advocates of the pavilion system, as it had come to be called, to lay it down as a law of hospital construction that "all hospitals should be pavilions of a temporary character, to be used only ten or fifteen years and then replaced by new buildings, as the only safe method for the prevention of 'hospitalism.'" As a matter of fact, some pavilions of this character were added to the hospital establishment of some of the oldest foundations in America. Meanwhile, the true nature of "hospitalism" was being elucidated by the development and demonstration of the germ theory of disease by Tyndall and Pasteur, and it was made evident, not only that Florence Nightingale was justified in demanding non-absorbent materials for the interior finish of wards, but that the use of non-absorbent materials and the exercise of a new cleanliness—surgical cleanliness—in all parts of the hospital would obviate the necessity of destroying old wards and building new ones every fifteen years. This new surgical cleanliness, however, with its dramatic possibilities of controlling zymotic diseases and of performing surgical operations as yet undreamed of, concentrated attention upon only one aspect of the functions of a hospital, and in some minds reduced the institution almost to the level of a factory wherein only the environment and adjustment necessary to mechanical perfection of production were to be considered. That very much more than this is necessary, all of those physicians who visit the sick in their homes of various degrees of mental and moral as well as of physical comfort, will agree. The whole environment, mental and moral as well as physical, must receive the careful attention of those who plan, build, and manage hospitals. Any hospital that fails in the first two requirements is not doing as much as can be done in the third. For the best results and for completeness of results it is absolutely necessary that the whole environment of the hospital patient shall be cheerful and that the personnel of those attending him shall be of the highest standard. That the pavilion hospital is the best form of hospital from every point of view is now almost universally conceded. That single-story pavilions are, theoretically, the most correct from a strictly scientific standpoint, may be admitted. It is now, however, possible to say— from what we know of the causes of disease, of the science of ventilation, and of the principles and materials of construction—that it is permissible to build pavilions of two or three stories when the site of the proposed hospital is salubrious and the area to be devoted to it is of generous proportions. Pavilion hospitals of all these types are being constructed now. The magnificent new National Hospital at the city of Mexico has one-story pavilions. The recently completed Chester Park Hospital—the contagious diseases department of the Boston City Hospital—has two-story pavilions admirably arranged for carrying out the work of the department; and the newly planned Cincinnati General Hospital, situated on one of the highest points of the city and surrounded by a park of twenty-seven acres, is designed for three-story pavilions. Pavilions of more than three stories are certainly to be condemned, "most of them being," as Cowles says, "but a modification of the old block plan." For several years past there has been an energetic advocacy of the "sky-scraper" hospital—an earnest attempt to induce hospital builders to return to the block hospital plan of the eighteenth and early part of the nineteenth century. The attempt has not met a very cordial reception at the hands of hospital architects and managers, but the literature in its favor is so voluminous and has been distributed so widely that it is necessary to examine the arguments. They are found to be as follows:—

1. The site "should be as high as possible, near a park, river, or lake, in as quiet a location as available, away from the street cars or railroad tracks and still easily accessible to the patients and their friends. The larger the grounds the better it is for the institution." * All of these desirable attributes are sought for pavilion and corridor hospitals as well, and therefore it is evident that economy of space, so far as the hospital grounds are concerned, is not to be urged as an argument in favor of the new type of block hospital.

2. "At that time" (the date of the building of the Johns Hopkins Hospital) "observation had demonstrated the fact that if one patient in a given part of the hospital became infected the other patients were likely to suffer in the same manner, and that patients in another building at a distance might remain free from the infection. Consequently it seemed wise to separate as much as possible the patients in separate pavilions. At the present time we know that the infection was carried from one patient to another through the ignorance of the attendant who manipulated all the patients in the same pavilion, but could not contaminate those with whom he did not come in contact." Such pathological heresies as this can be denied at once and in toto. Thirty-five years ago John Tyndall wrote his famous paper on "A Struggle with an Infected Atmosphere," and every year, almost, has yielded us fresh information on this important subject —the last valuable contribution being that made by Dr. E. C. Rosenow (American Journal of Obstetrics, Dec., 1904) on the subject of "Streptococci in Air of Hospital Operating Rooms and Wards during an Epidemic of Tonsillitis." Rosenow, by microscopic examination and by culture experiments by the method of exposed plates, demonstrated the existence of the same organism in the

* This and the following arguments for the "many-storied hospital" and against the "low hospital buildings" are taken from numerous papers in the recent work of Dr. A. J. Oschner on "Hospital Construction and Management," Chicago, 1907.

tonsils of those attacked by the angina, in the air of the wards and operating rooms, and in the infected peritoneal cavities of women who had been subjected to laparotomy during the progress of the epidemic.

3. The third argument, however, distinctly admits the facts of air-borne contagion. It does not fit with the second and is stated in this way: "Ever since Pasteur's observations determined the presence of micro-organisms in the ordinary air and their absence on high mountains, it has become more and more apparent that the air near the surface of the earth contains more micro-organisms than that higher up. This is especially true in cities, in which the street dust is laden with germs and is much thicker at the level of the first than at the level of the higher stories. . . . This fact must condemn low hospital buildings." It is obviously absurd to compare the sixth floor of a city building to a mountain top. The air of a mountain top is germ-free because it rests upon snow fields, bare rocks, and undisturbed forests, and cities, travelled roads, the domestic animals, and men are noticeably absent. The two skyscraper hospitals put forward as models—the Augustana and St. Mary's Hospital,

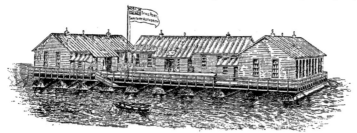

Fig. 288.—Floating Hospital on the River Tyne, England.

Chicago—contain wards on their second and third stories just as do pavilion hospitals, and no evidence is brought forward to show that the patients which these second and third stories shelter do not thrive as well as the patients in the upper stories. The patients in the upper stories are private patients, the patients in the lower stories are ward patients. The plans of the two hospitals show wards, private rooms, operating rooms, pantries, and kitchens on the top floor—the sixth floor.

4. The next point is that "the building can be set back from the street, which will still further lessen the amount of street dust. It will also lessen the disturbance caused by the street noise." This, of course, cannot be made to apply only to tall buildings. If the proper amount of space is allotted to a hospital—and its construction should be undertaken on nothing less than the proper amount of space—all buildings, be they one or many, can, and should be, set back from the street.

5. "If land can be secured overlooking a park or any other attractive landscape, the higher the building the more patients can obtain a view of this landscape." To this it may be replied that if a hospital is set in a park, as it should

be, all the patients can enjoy and be much benefited by the beauty of their surroundings, and they should, when possible, be taken directly into the open air.

6. "The building can be more easily placed so that every room and every ward secures sunlight during some portion of the day. With low buildings one is constantly compelled to infringe upon the sunlight in order to secure a sufficient amount of space for the number of beds required." The answer to this is that the problem for the six-story hospital and that for the pavilion hospital are exactly the same, and that, in the case of low buildings, one is not compelled to infringe upon the sunlight at all. The space between buildings—twice the height of the nearest building, for hospitals in this latitude—is abun-

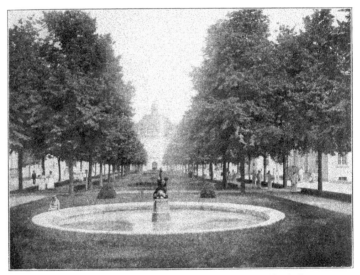

Fig. 289.—Park-like Grounds of the new Rudolph Virchow Hospital, of Berlin, Germany.

dant to procure for every room and every ward of the one-, two- or three-story pavilion as much sunlight as can be procured for the six-story block hospital. These indefinite propositions are not enough to shake the conclusions arrived at, and the laws of hospital construction laid down by Florence Nightingale, Sir James Y. Simpson, Mr. Erichson, the great French surgeon Tenon, the Johns Hopkins Hospital Commission, and Sir Henry Burdett. Air-borne contagion is a fact; it is wrong to put a large number of sick and wounded under one roof; the ventilation of tall buildings is complicated and made difficult by the necessity of a number of elevator shafts and chutes of various kinds; it is practically impossible properly to isolate contagious cases and their nurses and attendants when there is such easy access to the other parts of a large hospital; and, finally, in its suggestion of the office building or the factory, there must always be wanting in such a structure that function of the hospital which can be described as a homelike shelter for the sick. As for the question of saving time for the visiting staff, this argument is not very forcible; most of the visiting staff have but two or three wards to visit daily, and it is not asking too much, in return for the great privileges they are accorded, that they yield the welfare of the patient the first place.

In rare instances a small town may be so situated that it can advantageously

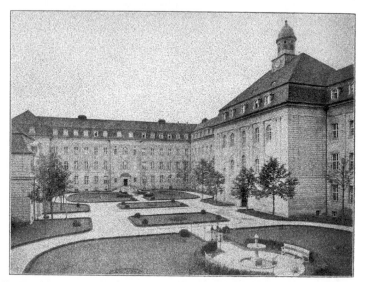

Fig. 290.—Mass Composed of the Principal Buildings of the Rudolph Virchow Hospital, of Berlin, Germany.

adopt the plan of a floating hospital, a model of which is shown in the accompanying figure. (Fig. 288.)

The Modern Metropolitan Hospital.—Before entering into a detailed description of the component parts of a great urban hospital it would, perhaps, be well to describe one such institution as a type of our modern conceptions of hospital design, thereby facilitating subsequent analysis and minuter descriptions of various buildings and departments, and rendering comprehension of detail more rapid and exact. The Rudolph Virchow Hospital, of Berlin (Figs. 289–302), is perhaps the most famous of the most recently completed European hospitals, and a description of its arrangement and buildings will enable the reader to compare it with the hospitals of what may be called the American type, that will be alluded to and described in this article. The Rudolph Virchow Hospital covers an area of 25.7 hectares or 63.5 acres. Its capacity is

2,000 beds, divided among the various services as follows: internal medicine, 500 beds; surgery, 564 beds; obstetrics and gynæcology, 220 beds; infectious diseases, 178 beds; nervous diseases, 18 beds; male skin and venereal diseases, 374 beds; and female skin and ·venereal diseases, 146 beds. Of physicians, nurses, and administrative employés there are 700. Residences are provided for the Superintendent, the Medical Director, the Surgical Director, and the Director of Obstetrics. In all, residences or suitable suites of apartments are provided for twenty-five married employés. This provision for

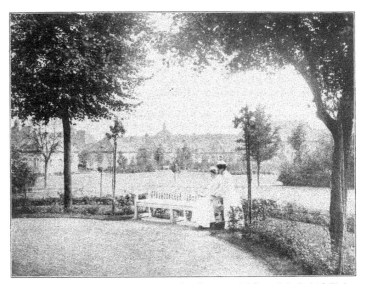

Fig. 291.—A Distant View of Some of the Less Important Buildings of the Rudolph Virchow Hospital, of Berlin, Germany. The park-like character of the grounds is well shown in this and the preceding photographs (Figs. 289 and 290).

married employés assures a stability of service that American hospitals would do well to note and copy. The entrance to the hospital is through a two-story porter's lodge, beyond which is a garden court formally laid out with walks and planted with lawns and trees. (Figs. 289 and 291.) This is closed in front, on both sides of the lodge, with one-story buildings containing the administrative offices on the left and the waiting and examination rooms for men and women on the right. The garden court is surrounded, on the other three sides, by an imposing mass of buildings (three stories and an attic in height). (Fig. 289.) The wing on the left is the Nurses' Home; that on the right is the residence of the unmarried physicians; and, northwest of this, in a semi-detached building, is a casino for the medical staff. The central mass of the western side of the court is occupied in front by an imposing and architecturally beautiful double stairway leading up to a hall to be used for meetings of physicians, Christmas celebrations, and other festal occasions.   Laterally from this central mass the obstetrical and gynæcological departments extend out toward the left and the right.   These three-story buildings contain general administrative rooms, consultation and examination rooms, warming kitchens and sculleries, a Director's room, physicians' service room, apartments for an Assistant Physician, a Volunteer Physician, and Midwives, operation, narcosis, and delivery rooms, as well as bath-rooms and toilets.   There are also isolation rooms, with forty-three beds.   Four two-story pavilions, each containing two twelve-bed wards with their accessories, project from the western front of the gynæcological-obstetrical department into the upper park-like end of the great *Mittelallee*.

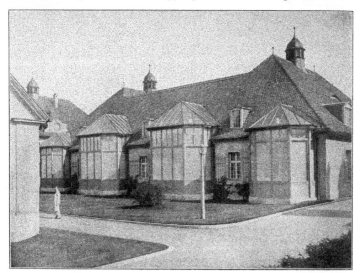

Fig. 292.—Photograph of the Front of the Building Devoted to Operative Work; the Rudolph Virchow Hospital, of Berlin, Germany.

This *Mittelallee*—or boulevard, one might almost call it—stretches away 425 metres (about 1,380 feet) and forms the East-West axis of the hospital grounds and of the building plan.   Two rows of trees, with a walk between, border the central lawn on both sides,—a fine bronze fountain is placed where the North-South axis cuts the *Allee*,—and the tower of the chapel closes on the west what is a most beautiful vista.   (Fig. 289.)   It may be well to remark here that these grounds were laid out and planted some seven years before the buildings of the hospital were finished; the result being that the completed and newly inhabited hospital found itself in a garden of rich, well-rooted turf and well-grown trees, that made it a most pleasant place of residence to those serving it and agreeable to the tired senses of the unfortunate sick.   On both sides of the

Mittelallee stretch the two-story pavilions of the Departments of Surgery and of Internal Medicine—eleven pavilions for the former, on the south, and ten pavilions for the latter, on the north. Provision is made for bringing patients, even bed patients, out into the *Allee* where they can lie in the open air in intimate contact with the grass and trees. On the south of the fountain, where the south-north axis of the hospital cuts the east-west axis on the *Allee*, is the Pharmacy Building, and south of this, again, the Surgical Building or Operating Pavilion. (Figs. 292 and 293.) The plans of this latter show, on the ground floor, four large operating rooms, with large bays on the north side. It will be observed that each has its own Instrument room and Sterilizing room. (Fig. 294.) Across a wide corridor are four "preparation rooms," etherizing rooms,—one for each operation room,—and, behind these, dressing rooms. A small interior court gives additional light and air to this main part of the building, and a larger court in the rear gives beauty, light, and air to the accessories of the operating pavilion arranged on both sides and at the end of the court in the order named—viz.: linen room, plaster-bandage room, microscopical

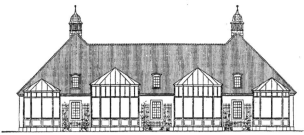

FIG. 293.—Schematic View of the Front of the Building Devoted to Operative Work; the Rudolph Virchow Hospital, of Berlin, Germany.

laboratory, utensil room, physicians' room, Director's room, and servants' room. Behind the Operating Pavilion and across a wide avenue, is a separate building devoted exclusively to Roentgen-ray work and photography. On the south-north axis, north of the *Mittelallee* and separating the Internal Medicine Pavilions for men from those for the women, lies the Bath and Medico-mechanical Department. (Fig. 299.) Like the Surgical Pavilion it contains a central court with grass and trees. It is a one-story building, surmounted by the usual steep attic roof. In the centre, opening on the garden court, is a disrobing room; behind this are a rest room and, at the rear of the building, the cold-water baths. In front of the garden are a series of rooms for individual tub-baths, and, on the front of the building, a large hall for the mechanical apparatus. Along the west side of the building, from front to rear, in the order named, are rooms for the physician, a room for a private patient, two rooms for the Head Nurse, a dining room, a linen room, an electrical-apparatus room, a carbonic-acid bath, an electric bath, a vapor bath, a warm-air bath, and a hot-air bath. On the eastern side of the building, from front to rear, we find an examination room, two private rooms, a utensil room, a linen room, two Inhalatoriums, toilet rooms, a long room for sand baths, and a room for steam baths. At the western end of the *Mittelallee* stands a structure containing the Pathologico-Anatomical Institute and the Chapel. The Chapel faces a wide, park-like entrance to the hospital grounds, and, to those who approach it from the avenue on the north, there is no suggestion of the scientific uses of the further end of the building. Except for the Chapel, which is of a conventional ecclesiastical architecture, the building consists of one story with a well-lighted basement. The Chapel itself occupies the central mass of the western extremity of the building. On the right, is the room for the clergyman; on the left, is that in which the body is prepared for burial. Behind the Chapel are the rooms for the family and intimate friends of the deceased. The janitor's room is at the rear of the right wing. The rest of the building encloses three courts, as is shown in the figure, and the offices are arranged as follows:—On the northern side, from the Chapel east, in the order named, are found the Histological Laboratory, two autopsy rooms —one containing three tables and the other four,—and two rooms for the Prosector. On the southern side, from the Chapel eastward, are the Bacteriological Laboratory, the culture room, the photographic studio, a little room for the chemical balances, and a large apartment for the Chemical Laboratory. Beyond a small office is a service room for the physicians and a servants' room. The first cross corridor separating the western from the central court contains

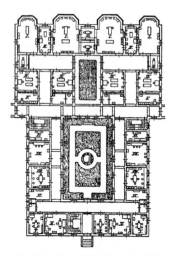

Fig. 294.—Ground Floor Plan of the Building Devoted to Operative Work; the Rudolph Virchow Hospital, of Berlin, Germany.

I, I, I, I, Rooms for operations; *II, II,* sterilization rooms; *III, III, III, III,* rooms for instruments; *IV, IV, IV, IV,* preparation and etherization rooms; *V, V,* rooms in which the surgeons and their assistants may change their garments; *VI, VI,* lavatories; *VII, VII,* rooms in which plaster-of-Paris bandages are prepared; *VIII, VIII,* rooms for microscopic work; *IX, IX,* rooms for storage of utensils, etc.; *X, X,* rooms for the surgeons; *XI, XI,* rooms for the directors; *XII,* room for the attendants.

Two inner courts aid in furnishing light and ventilation.

a washroom for the Histological Laboratory, a preparation room, and an incubating room. The other corridor has provision for two rooms for chemical balances and an office. Under the Chapel, in the basement, is a large store-room for coffins. To the left of this are two rooms—one for the public, and a small special room for the viewing of infectious bodies behind a glass partition. On the right is a museum. On the north of the enclosed courts are found, in the following order: a dressing room, two morgues, and a refrigerator; and, on the south side, two rooms for museum purposes, a workshop, a glassware room, a room for vivisection, and two rooms for disinfection. At the eastern end of the building are a maceration room and a room for the animals intended for experimental purposes. The cross corridors contain rooms for reptiles, servants' rooms, and bath rooms for the physicians. The Power House, Kitchen, and Laundry, each occupying a separate structure, take up the major part of the triangular space to the north of the pavilions for Internal Medicine; and three pavilions (for skin and venereal diseases of men), with their connecting corridor, lie to the north of the Administration Buildings on the east front. The smaller pavilions, for skin and venereal diseases of women, lie south of the Obstetrical Department. The Department for Contagious Diseases lies at the south end of the south-north axis of the hospital plot. It consists of six pavilions, each surrounded by wide open spaces, as can be seen in the figure. The floors of these pavilions are divided up into single and double rooms and small wards containing from three to five beds—an arrangement which allows of a most careful classification of cases of each disease. The southern pavilion is for quarantine purposes, and is divided into a number of sections containing rooms for one bed, two beds, three beds, etc., so that even whole families can be properly segregated here. The eastern pavilions are for measles and scarlet fever in females, and the western pavilions are for the same diseases in males. The central pavilion is for diphtheria.

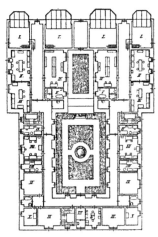

Fig. 295.—Second Floor Plan of the Building Devoted to Operative Work; the Rudolph Virchow Hospital, of Berlin, Germany. The four front rooms (I, I, I, I) are devoted to operative work; and the remaining rooms on this floor are utilized for a variety of purposes—the making of plaster-of-Paris dressings, the storage of collections of pathological specimens, accommodations for the Nursing Sisters, cooking, etc.

Finally, there is a beautiful and well planted Recreation Park which occupies the southwestern portion of the grounds and is of about eight acres in extent. The cost of the buildings and ground was 16,323,000 marks ($4,080,750). The cost of the equipment 2,745,000 marks ($686,250). The cost per bed was—without equipment, 8,162 marks ($2,040.50), with equipment, 9,534 marks ($2,383.50).

The Proper Location for a Hospital.—Modern methods of transportation have contributed as much to the present method of taking care of the sick and injured as any one of the innumerable factors that have enabled us to reach our present state of perfection. The electric tram car (Figs. 303 and 304) and the automobile ambulance (Fig. 305) have brought the suburb with its grass and trees and pleasant open spaces within a few minutes' travel of the crowded city's centres of commercial and industrial activity. This allows of the placing of hospitals in the most salubrious situation and does not bind them of necessity, as formerly, to nearness to the residences or work places of the hospital population. It is no longer necessary that hospitals should be near congested centres of population any more than that workmen should live near their work or professional and business men near their offices. Cities are expanding and the residence sections are becoming attenuated. The movement

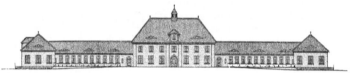

FIG. 296.—Schematic View of Front of the Pavilion for Medical Patients; the Rudolph Virchow Hospital, of Berlin, Germany.

of the latter is toward the open spaces. Enlightened hospital designers all over the world are taking part in the movement. Holding to the dictum "the greatest good to the greatest number," and recognizing that the greatest number are not the emergency surgical cases, but are those in which pure air and sunlight are prime requisites, the men who have the deciding of such questions are sending most of the new hospitals of the present time to locations where they

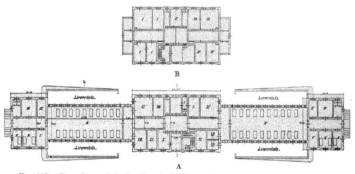

FIG. 297.— Floor Plans of the Pavilion for Medical Patients; the Rudolph Virchow Hospital of Berlin, Germany.
The following are among the principal rooms of the ground floor (*A*) of the pavilion:—*I, I*, reception rooms; *II, II, II, II*, main and smaller wards; *VII*, treatment room; *IX*, room for the Nursing Sisters; etc.
On the second floor (*B*) of the central building there are bedrooms for the physicians, the Nursing Sisters, and the house servants.

will have pure air and sunlight. Emergency hospitals in factory districts and near railroad yards will sometimes be necessary, but the patients in these will be immeasurably benefited by transference to the suburban hospital as soon as they are able to stand the transportation. Sir Henry Burdett, in a recent article, says: "I realize, as the medical profession is realizing, that the atmosphere of a great city grows less and less suitable to the rapid and complete recovery of patients who may undergo the major operations or be suffering from severe and acute forms of disease. Asepsis, it is true, has reduced the average residence in the best hospitals from thirty-five days to less than twenty days. It has thereby added one million working days, each year, to the earning power of the artisan classes in London alone. Medical opinion is more and more favoring the provision of suburban or convalescent hospitals to which patients suffering from open wounds may be removed from the city hospitals. This course is advocated to overcome the difficulty arising from the fact that, in many cases, patients cease to continue to make rapid progress toward recovery after the seventh or ninth day's residence in a city hospital. A change, in such

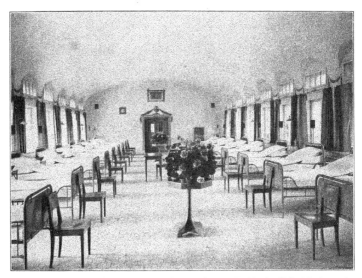

Fig. 298.—Photographic View of One of the Main Wards in the Pavilion for Medical Patients; the Rudolph Virchow Hospital, of Berlin, Germany.

cases, to the country restores the balance and completes the recovery, with a rapidity often remarkable. Thinking out the problem here presented in all its bearings, realizing the great and ever increasing cost of sites for hospitals in great cities, the heavy consequential taxes and charges which they have to meet there, and all the attendant disadvantages and drawbacks, I venture upon an anticipation in regard to the future of our hospitals. Why should we not have, on a carefully selected site, well away from the contamination of the town and adequately provided with every requisite demanded from the site of the most perfectly modern hospital which the mind of man can conceive, 'the hospital city'? Here would be concentrated all the means for relieving and treating every form of disease, to the abiding comfort of all responsible for their adequacy and success. Necessarily, the means of transit to and from the hospital city and its rapidity would be the most perfect in the world, and therefore the members of the medical staff, the friends of the patients, and all who had business in the hospital city would find it easier and less exacting in time and energy to be attached to one of the hospitals located therein than

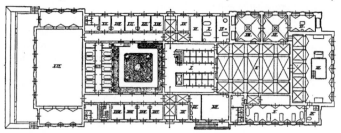

Fig. 299.—Ground Floor Plan of the Bathing Establishment and Medico-Mechanical Institute of the Rudolph Virchow Hospital, of Berlin, Germany.
The following are among the more important rooms in this large building (over 250 ft. in length):—
I, dressing rooms; *II*, resting room; *III*, cold-water baths; *IV*, steam-bath cabinet; *V*, sand baths; *VI*, hot-air bath; *VII*, warm-air bath; *VIII*, steam bath; *IX*, electrical baths; *X*, carbonic-acid bath; *XI*, room for electrical treatment; *XII*, inhalatorium; *XIV*, medico-mechanical apparatuses; etc. Near the centre of the building is a single inner court.

to one situated in the centre of a big population in a crowded town. To provide for the urgent and accident cases, a few receiving houses or outpost relief stations would be situated in various quarters of the working city, where patients could be temporarily treated, and whence they could be removed to the hospital city by an efficient ambulance service. I can see the Hospital City established,

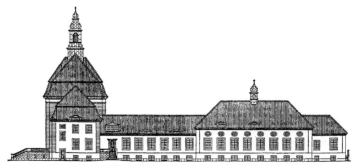

Fig. 300.—Schematic Profile View of the Pathologico-Anatomical Institute and Chapel of the Rudolph Virchow Hospital, of Berlin, Germany.

and I can realize the comfort it will prove in practice to the medical profession, to the patients' friends, to those who have to manage the hospitals and train the medical and nursing students, and, indeed, to all who may go there, as well as to the whole community. The initial cost of hospital buildings would be reduced at once to a quarter or less of the present outlay. The money spent on administration and working must be everywhere reduced to a minimum. The hygienic completeness of the whole city here contemplated, its buildings and appliances, must expedite recovery to the maximum extent. In all probability, the removal of the sick from contact with the healthy would tend in practice so to increase the healthiness of the town population, of the workers in the city proper, as to free them from some of the most burdensome trials which now cripple their resources and diminish materially the happiness of their lives. I hope, therefore, that the United States (where a city has sometimes sprung up in twelve months) may be the home where this ideal of mine may first find its realization in accomplished fact. I may never live to see such a city in actual working or in its entirety, but I make bold to believe that its adoption will one day solve the more difficult of the problems involved in the curing of the sick in crowded communities." It is frequently pointed out that

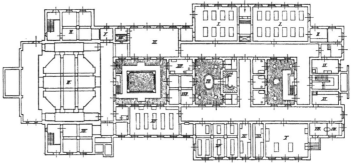

Fig. 301.—Basement Plan of the Chapel and Pathologico-Anatomical Institute of the Rudolph Virchow Hospital, of Berlin, Germany.
Some of the more important rooms are the following:—*I*, *I*, cellars for preservation of dead bodies; *V*, room where the bodies of persons dying of infectious diseases may be inspected; *VIII*, *VIII*, disinfecting rooms; *X*, room for vivisection purposes; *XIV*, room in which the collections of specimens are kept.

some of the largest and most famous of the older hospitals—indeed, almost all of them—are situated near the centres of cities or in crowded residence or industrial districts. (Figs. 306 and 307.) The truth about most of our downtown American hospitals is that originally they were situated in the suburbs,—sometimes in the face of the protest that they were remote and inaccessible,—and that the rapidly growing city has flowed past and beyond them, hemming them in and demonstrating the want of foresight of their founders in not acquiring an adequate site. In the case of some cities, fortunately rare, the problem of location is complicated by the unfortunate geographical location of the city itself. New York, for instance, lies on a long and narrow strip of land which is so densely covered by residences and business houses as to preclude the securing of large tracts of land for hospital purposes. The city has grown with extreme rapidity, and perforce in one direction only, so that open spaces, not occupied by houses, are now extremely remote from the densely populated portions of the city. This is, however, in a measure compensated for by the extensive water front of the city, which permits the island to be swept by currents of air from the bay and the North and East Rivers. The atmospheric conditions there are entirely different from those of inland cities, In these latter every effort should be made to remove the hospital to the large open spaces of the suburbs.

The Hospital Unit.—To the ward and its immediate accessories has been given the technical name of "the hospital unit"; and, to understand the hospital, a perfect understanding must be had of the hospital unit. In discussing this we are brought back at once to a discussion of the principles that underlie all hospital construction. The object of the hospital is to take care of sick and injured human beings. While they are within its care the hospital must discharge for them all the functions of a home. It must furnish shelter and at

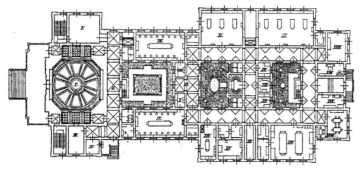

Fig. 302.—Ground Plan of the Chapel and Pathologico-Anatomical Institute of the Rudolph Virchow Hospital, of Berlin, Germany.
The more important parts are the following:—*I*, chapel; *V*, room where the dead bodies are exposed; *VII*, histological work-room; *IX*, bacteriological work-room; *XI, XI*, dissecting rooms; *XV*, room for photographic work; *XVI*, chemical laboratory. Three inner courts aid in furnishing light and air for some of the rooms.

the same time an abundance of light and fresh air. In cold climates it must furnish warmth during the rigorous months of the winter. It must furnish for each inmate a bed and an abundance of clean bed-clothes, which implies a sewing room, a linen closet, and a laundry. It must furnish efficient means for the disposal of waste and the maintenance of cleanliness. It must furnish supplies of food and proper means of cooking and serving them. It must furnish the physicians and surgeons who daily visit the sick with facilities for the proper exercise of their art, and it must furnish to those who nurse the sick all the necessary space and equipment for carrying out the orders given by the medical attendant. Especially important is it that it should furnish the cheerful surroundings necessary for the mental welfare of the sick, which means the shunning of buildings and surroundings which even remotely suggest the sky-scraping office building, the crowded and evil-smelling tenement, or the noisy factory. Therefore to the hospital there must always attach those features which are inseparable from a properly arranged home—bedroom, bathroom, sitting room, dining room, kitchen, pantry, laundry, heating and ventilating equipment, and—last but not least—garden. These are modern ideas; in the monastic days of the hospital they did not obtain.. Regarded in this way the principles of hospital construction are simplicity itself and may be applied with equal facility to the cottage hospital of a village or to the immense institu-

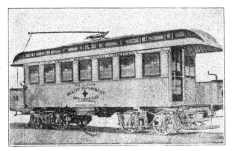

Fig. 303.—Ambulance Car of the St. Lou's Health Department.

tions of a modern metropolis. It is in the development of these principles, however, in order that they may meet the particular requirements of climate or population, of prevailing diseases or accidents, or of special classes of cases, that

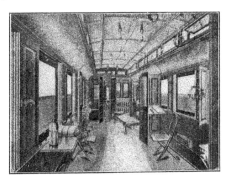

Fig. 304.—Interior of the St. Louis Ambulance Car. (Designed by Dr. Geo. Homan.)

the resourcefulness, skill, and foresight of the designer of hospitals are put to the test.

Bearing the basic principles of hospital construction in mind,—that the hospital is the home of the sick and must discharge all of the functions of a home, —we can conceive a mental picture of the simple arrangements and equipment of the average home and expand and differentiate it until we have arrived at the hospital unit of the modern municipal hospital. Let us take up, at first, the hospital unit as it has been developed to-day for the large municipal hospital. The plans of the new Cincinnati General Hospital (Figs. 317–320 and Plate D) have been evolved after a personal inspection of many of the leading hospitals of Europe and America, and after the original sketches had been submitted to a number of leading hospital superintendents of America, to Architect F. Ruppel, designer of the Hamburg-Eppendorf Hospital. and to Sir Henry Burdett, of London.   It may, therefore, be claimed, with some degree of justice, that these plans represent the prevailing ideas of hospital experts at the beginning of the twentieth century.   A description of a typical ward pavilion (Plate D) is as follows:—

The pavilions lie directly north and south, and on their northern ends the basements of the pavilions are connected by a covered passage; the upper part

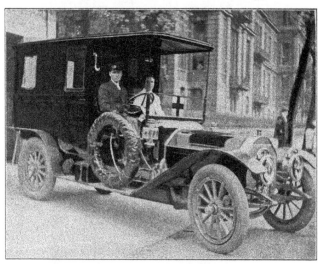

Fig. 305.—Automobile Ambulance of the Cincinnati Hospital.

of this passage, or half-tunnel, is from three to six feet above grade level, and is so constructed as to give ample light and ventilation.   The grade of the floor of the basement passages is one in one hundred, permitting a patient to be wheeled from one end of the extensive grounds to the other without the use of inclines or elevators.   Above the basement corridor is an open colonnaded porch one story high.   The floor of this porch, and the roof of the same, which has a width of fourteen feet, will be used for the open-air treatment of patients whose beds can be rolled out upon them through the central corridors from the wards.   To the right of the door entering the central corridor from the porch a door opens into a space communicating with the stairs and elevator. This space is called the "Fresh Air Cut-Off" (7' 0" x 19' 0"), the object of which is to prevent the air from the basement and from the other stories entering into direct communication with the ward. The fresh air enters this space from the door or transom and is exhausted through the ventilating shaft near the elevator. This fresh air cut-off also permits the complete isolation of the first floor from those above, as all supplies, etc., can be brought directly into the first ward from the porch. The elevator carries patients and supplies from the basement to the three floors of the pavilion and to the roof garden, where there are also a small serving room, a toilet, and an observation room. The food is delivered from the central kitchen by trucks, each carrying supplies for three wards. During its passage from floor to floor the truck remains on the elevator; the attendant, after pressing a button to notify the nurses that the food is being delivered, opens, near the elevator, a small door that communicates with the serving room, places the cans and metal boxes containing the food and drinks on a Tennessee marble slab just within the serving room, closes the door, and,

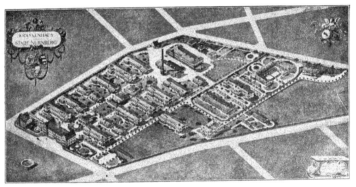

FIG. 306.—Bird's-Eye View of Hospital at Nuernberg, Germany.
The institution has accommodations, in its numerous one-story and two-story pavilions, for 990 patients, as follows: medical cases, 529; surgical cases, 252; genito-urinary cases, 121; cases of skin disease, 45; cases of mental disorder, 43. The small square building near the center of the left end of the oblong plot, and with large open spaces at both ends, is devoted exclusively to surgical operations.

starting the elevator, proceeds to the next floor without delay. Next to the door through which the food is passed, there is another small door through which the refrigerator is supplied with ice. The elevator, which is run by electric power, is automatic. The bench in this hall is for the use of students awaiting the arrival of the staff officer,—or for messengers, and others who have no business to enter the central corridor.

The central corridor (8′ 0″ x 67′ 0″) is lighted by large glass-panelled doors and transoms at both ends, and also by light coming through the transoms above the doors of all rooms opening into the hall. Near the north end of the corridor will be a bench where the convalescent patients may meet their friends; this arrangement giving them greater privacy than in the ward and avoiding any unnecessary disturbance of the other patients. A sanitary drinking fountain is also placed in the corridor near the visitors' bench.

The food coming from the central kitchen enters the serving room or diet kitchen (13' 6" x 15' 9") through the pass-door described above, and is here divided, and, if need be, re-heated, for ward and dining-room distribution. The food for the ward, together with all the dishes, etc., is put in bulk on a small truck, and the patients are served, right and left, as it passes down the ward.

Both in the interest of economy and in that of the convalescent patients themselves, the latter eat their meals in the dining room for convalescent patients, a room which measures 14' 9" x 15' 9". This room can also be used as a day room should the overcrowding of the ward demand the use of the ward solarium for bedridden patients.

The bath-room (9' 6" x 15' 9") will have a portable and a stationary bath-tub. The latter will be set so that the nurses can have access to it on three sides. Here will also be stationed a lavatory truck which the writer has designed. It will hold hot and cold water tanks above and a slop tank below, and will have racks for wash-basins, towels, etc. It will be used after the manner

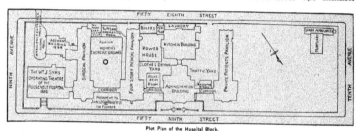

Plot Plan of the Hospital Block.

Fig. 307.—Plot Plan of the Roosevelt Hospital Block, New York City. (By courtesy of the hospital authorities.)

of the food-truck, thus doing away with all necessity for the nurses to run back and forth with the wash and waste-water basins.

The sink-room measures 9' 2" x 17' 2". Much thought has been bestowed on this very important place, both as to arrangement and as to location. In order that no odors may pass from it into the hall and ward, this room is connected with a separate exhaust and ventilating system; the foul air being exhausted through the enemata stack. In this sink-room we find the customary sink and a Washburn sterilizer made entirely of metal, porcelain not being sufficiently durable where steam-pressure is used. Into this sterilizer the stools from the bedridden patients are emptied, after they have first been disinfected by steam, and then the bed pans and urinals, after they have been emptied, are put into another sterilizer and disinfected by steam under pressure. They are then placed in the bed-pan rack, which is made of pipes through which hot water is constantly flowing—an arrangement which insures a constant supply of warm and dry vessels. There is also an enemata stack, in which stools or urine to be saved for the physician's inspection are placed upon enameled-iron-bar shelves, there being a separate stack for each floor.

The sanitary and economical handling of the soiled linen in a ward is a problem of some importance. In most hospitals in Europe and in many in this country, there is provided a room where soiled linen is permitted to accumulate until it is carried to the laundry, by way of the stairs or elevator, in baskets, bags, or cans. To avoid this laborious and uncleanly way, there was introduced by the writer (in 1905) a very simple and sanitary clothes-chute, which extended from each floor to the basement. This chute was made of 15-inch glazed sewer pipes embedded in concrete. The upper part is covered with a metal cap, and is provided inside with a perforated ring connected with the water supply, so that the interior of the chute can be flushed as often as may be thought desirable. If, at any time, because of some special infection, a more complete disinfection be thought necessary, formaldehyde can be applied from below.

From the sink-room a door leads into the nurses' work room (8' 0" x 10' 0"). This latter room serves the double purpose of a fresh-air cut-off between the ward and sink-room, and of a place where the nurse can prepare poultices, fill hot-water bags, etc. Here, also, is kept the case containing poisonous drugs. The work room is connected with the ward by an open arch, so that the nurse can, even if at work, see the red lamp flash at her desk at the entrance to the corridor. All stools and urine from the bedridden patients in the ward are carried through this room into the sink room, which is much more desirable than to have them carried through the corridor by which all the food enters, and through which visitors, physicians, and patients are passing to and fro. At the entrance from the corridor to the ward is placed the head nurse's desk, protected from draughts by wooden panels below and plate glass above; this arrangement giving her an unobstructed view of every bed in the ward; and beyond into the solarium, as well as throughout the whole length of the corridor. The wall within the enclosure for the head nurse's desk is recessed down to the floor; the lower part is filled in with a small closet thirty inches high, with shelves and doors in front. This is covered with a marble or enameled top and contains a small bowl with hot and cold water faucets; and above this is placed the medicine case. Above the nurse's desk is a Sturm relay annunciator. From any bed in the ward or in any of the small rooms, a patient, by simply pressing an electric button, causes the large red electric light to flash over the head nurse's desk, and a smaller light to flash over the bed in the large ward or over the door of the small room. These lights continue to burn until the nurse has responded to the call and has pressed a button which extinguishes the signal.

Let us now examine the rooms to the left of the corridor, beginning at the main entrance from the porch.

The first room encountered is the urinalysis, treatment, and class-room, which measures 9' 0" x 15' 0", exclusive of the bay window. The door leading to this room is extra wide, so as readily to permit the patients to be taken into the room in their beds, either for the purpose of making special dressings or examinations, or for that of exhibiting them, as a means of instruction, before a small class of students. Here also all routine urine, sputum, and other tests for the patients in this ward are made by the resident physician. A sink with hot and cold water, gas, and electric light attachments, a slate-top table, and a recessed, glass-shelved implement case, complete the equipment. During the last few years the advanced physicians and surgeons, both in this country and in Europe, have been clamoring for more small rooms in connection with the large wards,—rooms where noisy, dying, or ill-smelling patients, or those manifesting special pathological features, may, both in their own interest and in that of the larger number of patients in the open ward, be taken. For this reason, one two-bed and three single rooms have been placed in these pavilions. In order that the various kinds of services may have the size of the combined treatment and lecture room adapted to their special needs, this room has been so planned that the partition between it and the two-bed ward (10′ 10″ x 16′ 9″) can be placed as shown in the first small drawing on the left of the larger plan (Plate D), thereby enlarging the lecture and treatment room and reducing the two-bed to a one-bed room. By the placing of a door in this partition, there are provided desirable arrangements for the gynæcological service, or delivery rooms for the obstetrical service. The room in question being so far removed from the general ward, the noises incident to the obstetrical service would not disturb the patients in the ward. Immediately after delivery or after the performance of an operation, the patient can be placed in one of the small quiet rooms (9′ 2″ x 15′ 0″) until it appears desirable to move her into the open ward. The door leading into each one of the small rooms will have a peep-hole covered with a movable metal plate, so that the nurse, as she passes down the hall, may inspect the room without disturbing the patient. If the ward should be assigned to surgical cases, it might be desirable to have the combined treatment and lecture room so enlarged as to permit of its being used also for making minor operations, such use being facilitated by the abundance of north light which the room possesses. By the omission of the partition between it and the two-bed ward, there will be provided a room like that shown in the second small figure. (Plate D.) The window frame in the first single room from the porch is to be furnished with iron fastenings so placed that a wire screen can readily be put in position, thus making this a strong-room—one so guarded that a delirious patient would not be able to escape through the window during the absence of the nurse.

Beyond the small rooms, there will be seen, in the plan, the hot closet. A four-shelved metal rack on rollers fits into this space, the back wall of which has a coil of heating pipes. Here is kept a constant supply of warm blankets for immediate use in cases of shock, etc. Next comes the drying-room in which rubber sheets, blankets, etc., may be promptly dried. This room receives indirect light from the linen room; and the latter room is supplied with extra heating coils in order that the linen may be perfectly dry and warm when used.

A small, well-lighted supply closet adjoins the linen room. In this closet the executive nurse can keep all extra ward supplies locked up. Near it, is located the nurse's toilet (N. T.). The small square place adjoining is the vent and pipe stack.

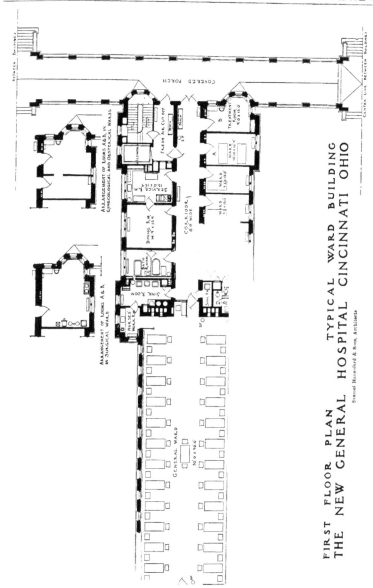

FIRST FLOOR PLAN
THE NEW GENERAL HOSPITAL CINCINNATI OHIO
TYPICAL WARD BUILDING
Samuel Hannaford & Sons, Architects

At the end of the corridor, on the left, is a large closet for ward maid's slop-sink, buckets, brooms, and vacuum cleaning tools. It receives indirect light from the patients' toilet room, and its ventilation is effected by way of the adjoining ventilating stack.

Passing through the door from the corridor we enter the ward. Then, turning to the left, we encounter a double-swinging, glass-panelled door, which admits us, through a fresh-air cut-off (8' 6" x 6' 8"), to the patients' toilet room (9' 0" x 14' 0") in which are two wash-stands, with hot and cold water, and three toilets. The lids of the latter are weighted so that, when not in use, they always stand vertically. The bowl of the closet serves also as urinal, it having been proven by experience that any and all of the regular forms of urinals become, in time, offensive. This room is also connected with the special exhaust ventilating system.

The Ward.—The inside measurements of the ward are 90 x 30 x 13 feet. It contains twenty-four beds, giving 112½ square feet of floor space, and 1,462½ cubic feet of air space, for each bed. Every bed stands between two windows, the latter extending to the ceiling. The upper part of each window is fitted with a hopper-transom that opens inward. The heating is by means of two-and-a-half-inch hot-water pipes, and by indirect method through openings at both ends. At the southern end of the ward, on one side of the door leading into the solarium, there is a sanitary drinking fountain, and on the other side there is a wash basin. The presence of the latter convenience is due to the fact that a physician or surgeon, after examining a patient at this end of the ward, will not infrequently need to wash his hands and he will thus be saved the necessity of making a special trip to the other end of the ward. The partition at the southern end of the ward has two large swinging windows for admitting plenty of sunlight—and, if desired, fresh air from the solarium. The door, also, has large glass panels, and above it is a large tilting transom. The solarium measures 14' 9" x 32' 6". On one side is placed a small, well-lighted, and well-ventilated toilet room, and on the other side there is a sink-room. These are very useful under all conditions, and are especially so for the feeble convalescents and the crippled patients who will spend much of their time in the solarium. Should the ward become overcrowded, a number of beds can be put in the solarium. Under such conditions, the presence of the toilet and sink would greatly simplify matters, and correspondingly reduce the labors of the nurses.

The Solarium.—Of late years the value of fresh air and sunlight in the treatment of many conditions, notably the various infections, is beginning to receive the recognition that has always been its due. The solarium is now a recognized adjunct of the ward, and open spaces with grass and trees and flowers about the pavilions are a part of the hospital. Recently the roof garden has come into use. It was first adopted by the older institutions of the eastern American cities, which were hemmed in on all sides by closely built-up and very valuable ground; but there is no reason why it should not be used on a large scale even in pavilion hospitals, which have an abundance of park space about them, for bedfast cases which can be benefited by exposure to fresh air—such as cases of pneumonia and other infections of the lungs, of surgical tuberculosis, of the different forms of anæmia, of puerperal infection, etc. In a description of the Roof Garden and Solarium of the "Lying-In Hospital of the City of New York" (Fig. 308), Dr. James W. Markoe says: "As in all institutions built in large cities, that cannot spread out owing to the extreme cost of land, it was found that the pavilion plan so largely in vogue abroad was not feasible, making it necessary to construct the wards one upon another. By this construction the ideal method of having the open-air piazza directly next to the ward was impossible for many reasons, thus leaving the roof the only available place, and even this had its drawbacks, for the very changeable and

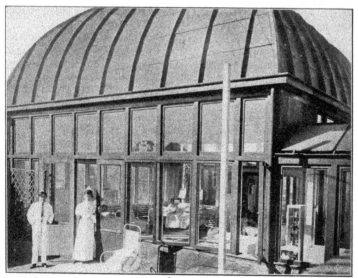

FIG. 308.—Solarium of the Lying-In Hospital of the City of New York. (By courtesy of Dr. James W. Markoe.)

severe climate of New York made it necessary for part to be under cover, thus reducing the space available for entire open-air treatment. Devoted to this purpose is an area of 2,744 square feet, having a central Solarium entirely enclosed in glass but with windows that can be opened on all sides; these are always open except in very cold or inclement weather, and even then not all are closed, while on either side there are two roof-spaces with tile floors and side walls sufficiently high to prevent any patient getting over. These are directly open to the air and sunshine and are made more attractive by boxes of growing plants around the edges. . . . A ward organization has been instituted and the results have been so uniformly good that the Solarium is usually occupied to the limit of its capacity." In Markoe's service the following classes of cases are sent to the Solarium or Roof Open-Air Ward. (1) Normally pregnant women during the day. (2) Abnormally pregnant women are frequently kept there both day and night. (3) Such cases as those of placenta prævia and those in which the hæmoglobin is below normal, the object kept in mind being to continue pregnancy until a viable child can be delivered. (4) The varied cases of toxæmia of pregnancy, except eclampsias in the convulsive stage. (5) Cases which call for surgical operations either during or after pregnancy. Such patients do distinctly better during their convalescence if they are kept on the roof for several days, or for as long a period as possible, before operation, and are returned to the roof as soon as the first effects of the anæsthetic have passed off. (6) Post-partum cases of exhausted vitality or complicated by infection.

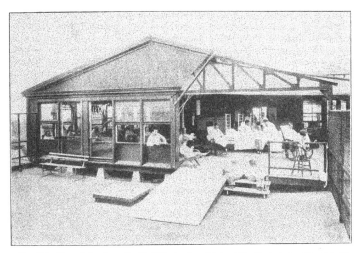

Fig. 309.—One of the Open-Air Roof-Wards, Completed, of the Presbyterian Hospital, New York City.
(Figs. 309–313, 322, 323, and 326–329 have been copied through the courtesy of the hospital authorities.)

That a hospital must have either an abundance of surrounding park space or Solaria, or both, is further emphasized by a recent communication from Halsted, of Johns Hopkins, who shows that many tuberculous affections, which were formerly believed to be curable only by extensive surgical operations, may, in fact, be entirely cured by continuous living out of doors in a suitable climate.

In the accompanying illustrations (Figs. 309–313) are shown several instances of the open-air ward as established in other hospitals in the city of New York. The excellent results obtained in the treatment of various diseases, by the establishment of these relatively inexpensive roof wards, have more than justified the wisdom of the method. In the new Agnes Memorial Sanatorium near Denver, Colorado, extensive piazza spaces, connected with the wards of both the first and second floors, have been provided.   These may readily be utilized as open-air wards.   (Fig. 314.)

Light.—The problem has always been to furnish artificial light that is bright yet diffuse, and that does not shine directly and glaringly into the eyes of the patients.   Some form of portable light is also desirable.   This should be of such a kind that a bright light may be directed where needed without disturbing others in the same ward.   Every hospital of considerable size should have an electric lighting and power plant, consisting not only of the proper number of dynamos, but also of a large storage battery of as many cells as may be necessary.   The advantage of this storage battery is that, after a certain hour in the evening,—say, for instance, ten o'clock,—light, elevators, and all electric appliances can

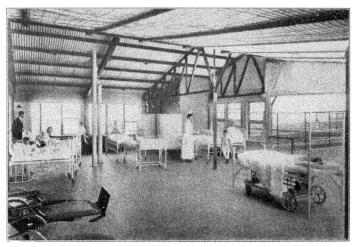

Fig. 310.—Interior View of One of the Roof Wards of the Presbyterian Hospital, New York City. The photograph was taken when the awnings were down.

be switched on to the battery, thus doing away with all vibration from engines and dynamos, and also saving labor and fuel.   The question of furnishing the diffuse light for the wards without glare is met in some institutions by so placing the lights above a conical steel or opal glass shade that the light is reflected upward against the white ceiling and thence diffused throughout the ward.   This, its advocates claim, gives a light closely approximating sunlight and without glare.   The ward lights can also be regulated by "dimmers," or by an apparatus so arranged that the light can be diminished at will by the turning of a thumb-screw at the switchboard on the side wall.   At the head of each ward bed there should be a socket into which can be inserted a plug with a portable light which has also a steel shade that reflects the light in only one direction.   This is used for light in applying dressings and giving night medication.   It has also been suggested that small—say, four-candle-power—lamps might be placed at the head of each patient's bed, so that he may read at night, if permitted, without unduly annoying those in neighboring beds; or that the modern "high low," of which there are now many ingenious styles on the market, might be installed in a little cabinet next the bed, as is done in the berth of a sleeping car.*

What is technically known as "vapor lighting" has recently been perfected sufficiently to be applied to practical commercial uses. Vapor lighting is dependent upon the physical fact that an electrical current passing through a tube containing rarefied air or the vapor of some of the metals will produce incandescence. Up to the present time the incandescence produced in glass tubes containing the vapors of the metals has produced such a disturbance of color values, especially among the reds, that its use in hospital work is out of the question. Rarefied atmospheric air is as yet the only gas which gives good results, and what is known as the Moore Light (the tubes of which contain rarefied atmospheric air) has been subjected to the test of actual use for commercial purposes and has proven itself highly satisfactory, as it perfectly imitates natural light, and all colors and shades of colors are seen as by daylight—a condition not as yet attained by any other artificial light. (Fig. 316.) The inventor claims the following advantages:—"The cost of an installation, due to its being construction work, varies with its location, the length of the tube, its shape, the intensity of the light required, the kind and number of fixtures desired, and other local conditions, but it is already less than the cost of a first-class incandescent lighting system with its necessary wiring, and eventually it will be far cheaper. . . . The Moore tube supplants both the lamps and the wiring

* There has recently appeared (November 14th, 1907) the " Report of the Committee of Oculists and Electricians on the Artificial Lighting and Color Schemes of School Buildings " (Boston School Document, No. 14), and their observations on the general subject of lighting are very comprehensive and thoroughly practical. The report (see p. 27), which is signed by Jas. E. Cole, Dr. Geo. S. Derby, Robert H. Hallowell, Dr. F. I. Proctor, and Dr. Myles Standish, advocates the employment of the tungsten lamp. "The direct light [from the tungsten lamp] is greater than that obtained from the standard fixture. . . . It will be seen that the fixture is extremely simple, consisting merely of a rod or chain, from which is suspended a shade holder, shade, and lamp socket. (Fig. 315.) The shade is open at the base, is made of clear glass, with the inner or outer surface enameled in a manner to give an appearance of frosting, and the outer surface fluted in a manner similar to that of the ordinary prismatic shade. The extreme simplicity of the fixture reduces the cost of keeping it clean. . . . The comparative current-consumption of a school room lighted with nine 40-watt tungsten lamps, nine 100-watt G. E. M. lamps, and the present standard lighting with indirect clusters, is as follows:

9 Tungsten 40-watt lamps . . . . 360 watts.
9 G. E. M. 100-watt lamps. 900   "
6 Indirect Clusters (present standard two 8-candle power and two 16-candle
    power each). 960   "

" The saving of current by the substitution of nine G. E. M. lamps for the present standard clusters is not great, but the increase in illumination is considerable, as the average candle foot from the present standard clusters, when clean, is about 1.5, as against 2.5 from the G. E. M. lamps and shades as just described. The saving by substitution of tungsten lamps is 62.5 per cent in current-consumption, which, applied to the entire school lighting bill, would amount to a considerable sum. From this sum, however, should be deducted the cost of lamp renewals, after which deduction the apparent saving is about 45 per cent. This saving could not be obtained, however, without discarding or remodelling the standard clusters now in use."

of the old systems. . . . The cost of operation is considerably less than that of the incandescent electric lamp system. An average installation pays for itself several times over during the first year, due to the amount it saves on current. . . . In many instances the replacing of long lines of incandescent lamps by a long Moore tube reduces the current bill more than three-quarters for the same amount of useful light. . . . The Moore light has twice the illuminating power of six-glower Nernst lamps and six times the value of incandescent lamps. . . . The intensity of the Moore light can be regulated from a faint glow to twenty or more candle-power per foot, producing an extremely brilliant illumination, yet with the great advantage of low intrinsic intensity—a condition which is recognized as ideal by the highest authorities on illumination.

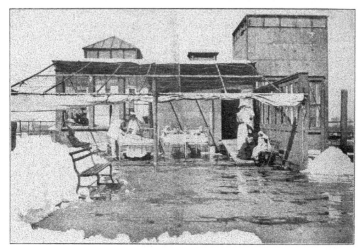

Fig. 311.—View Showing Partial Utilization of the Roof of One of the Presbyterian Hospital Buildings, New York City, as a small open-air ward.
The view was taken after a heavy fall of snow.

The eye suffers no inconvenience whatever after staring at the Moore light. . . . The Moore light automatically and continuously feeds itself from the atmosphere; therefore the life of the Moore light is practically unlimited. . . . It is a wireless light that eliminates about ninety per cent of the dangerous, costly, and objectionable concealed wiring. . . . The heat of the Moore tubes is much less than that of any other light. It is the coldest light known. . . . The color of the light may be made anything desired, from a perfect duplication of daylight to the special tints most suitable for photographic purposes, etc. Perfect diffusion is obtained for the first time. . . . The light radiates from such an extremely large area as compared with all old-style spots or points of light that the result is a shadowless light not producible by any other means."

Window Shades, Screens, etc.—Among the minor accessories of the ward none is more important than the window shade. From some hospitals the roller window curtain has been abolished as a dust collector which distributes its accumulations whenever it is rolled up or down, and reliance is placed altogether upon inside shutters. These latter cannot altogether escape criticism on the same ground. The problem has been very cleverly solved for one hospital—the Lying-In Hospital of New York—by means of the use of outside roller window shades designed by Dr. Markoe and made of heavy duck. These roll up and down on guides and are said to be very satisfactory. These outside shades, however, are adapted only to a clean atmosphere. They probably could not be used with any satisfaction in the soot-laden atmosphere of our

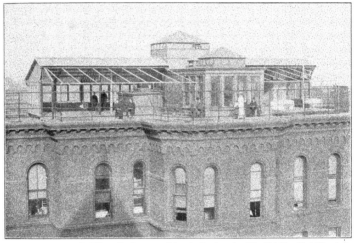

Fig. 312.—Steel Shed Recently Constructed for the Presbyterian Hospital, New York City, to be used as an open-air ward.
The photograph was taken almost immediately after the completion of the structure, and while the equipment was in progress.

western cities, where soft coal is used and our manufacturers have not yet learned how thorough combustion of the carbon is accomplished.

Now that we know something concerning the rôle played by the housefly and the mosquito in the spread of disease,—and the culpability of these and other insects is probably greater than has as yet been definitely fixed,—it is incumbent upon us to screen thoroughly every hospital door and window, not alone for the sake of the patients, but also for the sake of the health of the community at large. Horses, whose manure is the breeding-place of the Musca domestica, Stomoxys calcitrans, and other flies that visit houses, should not be allowed about a hospital. Stables and horse ambulances should be abolished and garages and automobile ambulances substituted in their stead. Not only should the hospital itself render itself blameless in this respect, but municipal ordinances should require that every horse and cow stable within the municipal limits should render their manure cellars and manure piles innocuous, as far as the breeding of flies is concerned, by treating them at intervals with residuum oil mixed with earth, lime, and phosphates, as is done in France. This same residuum oil mixed with water is also used in the treatment of privies and cesspools. "Two litres of the oil per superficial metre of the pit is mixed with water, stirred with a stick of wood, and then thrown into the receptacle. It is said to form a covering of oil which kills all the larvæ, prevents the entrance of flies into the pit, and, at the same time, the hatching of eggs. It makes a protective covering for the excrement, and this is said to hasten the development of anaërobic bacteria, as in a true septic pit, leading in this way to the

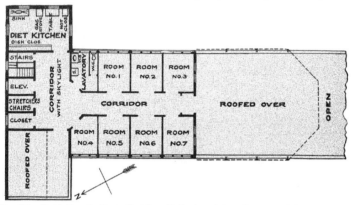

Fig. 313.—Sketch Plan of a Nearly Ideal Open-Air Roof Ward, from the plan made for the Roosevelt Hospital by the late W. Wheeler Smith, architect. (By courtesy of the hospital authorities.)

rapid liquefaction of solid matters and rendering them much more unfit for the development of other bacteria."

In every hospital in a tropical or a subtropical country, where there is frequent necessity of contending with infectious diseases, such as malaria and yellow fever, that are carried by winged insects, a number of portable isolation rooms should be provided. These are made of light metal or wooden frames on which is stretched wire screening with a mesh of about 0.06 of an inch, preferably of copper wire, so as to withstand the corrosion of a damp, warm atmosphere. The "room" is just large enough to contain a bed, a small table, a commode, and a chair,—i.e., is about nine feet nine inches in length, the same in width, and eight feet in height. The interior is approached through an anteroom of the same wire screening, with an inner and outer door closing promptly by means of strong springs, so that one coming from the outside must pause a moment in this vestibule before entering the apartment of the patient. This can be easily and quickly erected over one bed in a general ward if need be, and a suspected case could be thus watched with perfect safety to the surrounding patients and attendants until such time as a correct diagnosis could be made and a proper disposition made of the case. During an epidemic of yellow fever the bed of every fever patient should be screened in this way, as it is the only safe and efficient manner of isolating the cases from the contagion-carriers.

Heating and Ventilating.—The question of heating and ventilating hospitals is one of supreme importance, both from the standpoint of mechanical engineering and from that of administrative expense. The results of Pettenkofer's experiments on respiration show that, when the CO_2 is maintained at $\frac{2}{10000}$ in excess of what is found in the outer air, the ventilation is at least good; in which case there will have to be admitted into any building 3,000 cubic feet of fresh air per person per hour while in repose, 4,500 cubic feet for persons at gentle exercise, and 9,000 cubic feet for persons at hard work. It is customary in hospitals to provide for a minimum admission of 3,000 cubic feet of air per bed per hour, with mechanical means of increasing the admission to 6,000 cubic feet of air per bed per hour when it is deemed necessary. This amount of air seems to cover the contingencies, and insures a standard in which the excess CO_2 will be about $\frac{2}{10000}$. Taking this minimum of 3,000 cubic feet of fresh air per hour per bed and applying it to a 36-bed ward of a hospital, we shall find that it will be necessary to pass through the ward 108,000 feet of air every hour and 2,592,000 feet every twenty-four hours. With coal at $5 a ton of 2,000 pounds (a fair average for the whole United States), it will require 20 cents per hour for fuel to maintain the warmth of every one million cubic feet of air passed through a building, taking one day with another throughout the winter. In the case of hospitals in which the heating is to be maintained day and night,—say, through 180 days of a year,—the cost of fuel

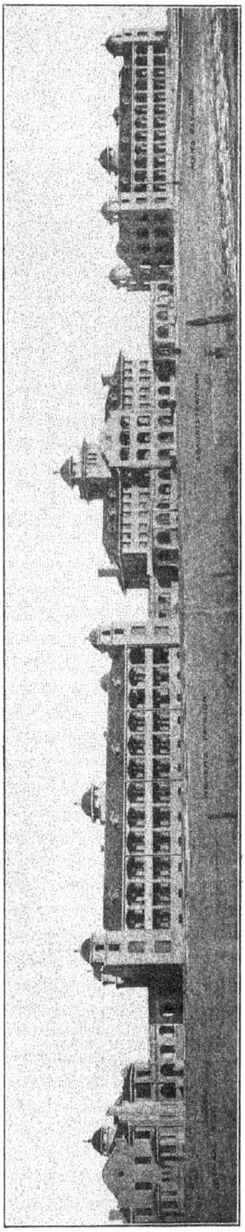

Fig. 314.—The Agnes Memorial Sanatorium, near Denver, Colorado. (By courtesy of the hospital authorities.)

for the same time will be $864 for every 1,000,000 cubic feet of air passed in an hour throughout the season. This, of course, does not include interest on the plant, labor, service, etc., which increases it to about $2,000 per season per million cubic feet of fresh air passed into the building every hour. As the plant grows larger this can be reduced to probably $1,500 per year for each additional million cubic feet of air admitted per hour.

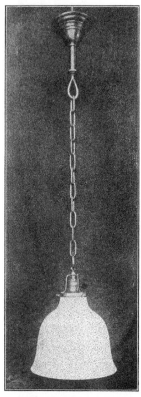

Broadly speaking, there are two principal methods of ventilation in use in hospitals. One of these is the aspiration system, in which the vitiated air is sucked out of a building through vents which are warmed sufficiently to create a draught out of each room or ward through them, the aspirated air being replaced in the building by fresh air which is brought in through ducts and warmed or not by steam or hot-water radiators as may be required by the season. The other system is that of the "blower" or "forced draught" system, which is divided into the "exhaust method," where a fan is employed to exhaust the air from the building, and the "plenum method," where a fan is employed to drive the air into the building. It will be observed that the principles of the exhaust method and of the aspiration system are the same, except that the means for aspirating the air from the building are in one case thermal and in the other mechanical. We will take up first the plenum system, a system which is now being installed in a very large number of the hospitals, schools, libraries, churches, factories, and theatres throughout the country. We will then observe with some minuteness its mode of action and will consider the theoretical and practical objections to its use. The name of the system —"plenum" meaning full—implies that the air of the ventilated building is to be kept somewhat under pressure,—that the air is to be forced through. A large open window, or air-intake, is left in the wall of the building, or a tall stack like a smoke stack is run up above the roof so as to take the air from some distance above the ground. The fresh air enters here, is caught by the fan, which is the mechanical factor of the "draught system," and is blown across a system of heaters and water

Fig. 315.—Tungsten Lamp Shade, and Supporting Fixture, as recommended by the Committee of Oculists and Electricians for Adoption in the Public Schools of Boston, Mass.

pans and thence into a system of flues which carry this warmed and moistened air to the various rooms of the building, entering them through openings in the walls about eight feet above the floor. From thence it is taken, still under pressure (for the doors and windows are all kept shut), into vents or foul air shafts which conduct the vitiated air from the room at the floor level. This latter arrangement is the reason why this system is frequently known as the "down-draught system," because the air enters the rooms at a comparatively high level and leaves them at a low level, the draught being, therefore, down. The varying exposures of the rooms of a hospital, or other building similarly occupied, require that more heat shall be supplied to some than to others. With a constant and equal air-supply to each room it is evident that its temperature

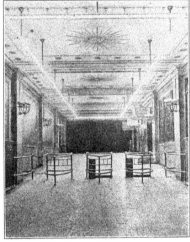

Fig. 316.—The Moore System of Lighting Large Rooms by Means of Glass Tubes Containing Rarefied Atmospheric Air through which an Electric Current is Passed.

must be directly proportional to the cooling influences within and around the room, and that no building of this character is properly heated and ventilated where the temperature cannot be varied without affecting the air-supply. To this end, air of a given temperature may be conducted to the base of each flue and there tempered to a degree suitable to the requirements of the room supplied. The air is heated to the maximum required for maintaining the desired temperature in the most exposed rooms, while variety in temperature of air supplied to the other rooms is secured by mixing with the hot air a sufficient volume of cold air at the bases of the respective flues. Here is placed a mixing damper, so designed as to admit either a full volume of hot air or a full volume of cold air, or to mix them in any desired proportion without affecting the resulting total volume delivered to the room.—The damper should be operated by a thermostat in the room with which the flue connects. The warm air, as it leaves the register, is supposed to rise to the ceiling, expand, flow out under it, strike the windows on the sides of the room, cool and sink to the floor, and then, under the pressure of the incoming air, to return along the floor to the outlet on the same side of the room as the register. In this estimate of the movement of the air, it is held that each patient in the hospital ward is also a factor in setting up air-currents which rise from about the warm body and from the warm lungs to the ceiling, spread to the walls with their contained windows, become cooled at the cool window panes, and sink to the floor to be withdrawn through the vents. One engineer, who is evidently a warm advocate of this system, says, in discussing this point in connection with school rooms: "It may be said that the child is breathing the floor air which is passed to the ceiling over its body, and this is to a great extent true; but it is utterly impracticable to bring fresh air directly to the lungs of each child in a crowded room, and therefore all that can be done is to secure a dilution or standard of purity which is reasonably good." It may be said, in conclusion of this part of our subject, that those who most favor this system say that the whole matter cannot be better expressed than in the words of the late Robert Briggs, of the American Society of Civil Engineers, in an address on the superiority of forced ventilation: "This mooted question will be found to have been discussed, argued, and combated on all sides in numerous publications, but the conclusion of all is that, if air is wanted in any particular place, at any particular time, it must be put there, not allowed to go. Other methods will give results at certain times or seasons or under certain conditions. One method will work perfectly with certain differences of internal and external temperature, while another method succeeds only when other differences exist. One method reaches to relative success whenever a wind can render a cowl efficient. Another method remains perfect as a system if no malicious person opens a door or window. No other method than that of impelling air by direct means with a fan is equally independent of accidental natural conditions, equally efficient for a desired result, or equally controllable to suit the demand of those who are ventilated."

Having examined the plenum or down-draught system, let us consider some of the theoretical objections to its use, and endeavor, if we can, to see how it has worked in practice in the types of buildings which are the subject of our study. The most elaborate report that I have been able to find on the subject is that of the Woodbridge Commission on the ventilation of the Capitol at Washington. Among other things they say: "The relative merit of the upward versus the downward system of ventilation may be estimated from the following considerations: 1. The direction of currents of air from the human body is, under ordinary conditions, upward, owing to the heat of the body. This current is an assistance to upward and an obstacle to downward ventilation. 2. The heat from all gas flames used for lighting tends to assist upward ventilation, but elaborate arrangements must be made to prevent contamination of air by the lights if the downward method be adopted. 3. In large rooms an enormous quantity of air must be introduced in the downward method if the occupants are to breathe pure fresh air, or about three times the amount which is found to give satisfactory results with the upward method. 4. In halls arranged with galleries the difficulty of so arranging downward currents that, on the one hand, the air rendered impure in the galleries shall not contaminate that which is descending to supply the main floor below, and that, on the other hand, the supply for the floor shall not be drawn aside to the galleries, is so great that it is almost an impossibility to effect it. Perfect ventilation cannot be obtained by the downward method, for this would only provide for the dilution of the impure air, while in perfect ventilation the impurities are not so diluted, but are completely removed as fast as formed, so that no man can inspire any air which has shortly before been in his own lungs or in those of his neighbor. For these and other reasons the board thinks that the upward method should be preferred." The argument that, because carbonic acid gas is fifty-two per cent heavier than air, it is therefore desirable to ventilate by the downward current in a room, rather than by an upward one, cannot be considered a valid one for the very apt reason that Woodbridge gives: "The carbonic acid gas yielded by respiration from the lungs and by transpiration through the skin is as thoroughly diffused in the warm-air currents rising from the body as is the same gas made by a candle or gas flame in the air currents ascending from those flames. It is plain that gas, when once diffused in air, can, because heavier than air, no more settle downward out of the air and occupy the lower stratum of a room, than the salt, because heavier than water, can settle out of the sea to its bottom. Carbonic-acid tests made of the air in two theatres and a music hall in Boston, with upward ventilation, clearly show air of remarkable purity at the floor or breathing plane and a quick transition from that purity to impurity at a plane at the balcony level, and a further vitiation at the gallery level."

I find in one of the treatises, in advocacy of the plenum system, the following significant admission: "The point of discharge should be at least eight feet above the floor, and the air movement should be directed toward the outside walls. The ventilation register should be in the same inner wall as the supply opening, but close to the floor. There is thus induced toward this outlet a return flow of the air in a well-distributed mass. The currents are in reality stratified, the lower one serving to take up the emanations from the lungs of the occupants as it sweeps slowly across them directly toward the ventilating register." So much for the theoretical objections to the "forced draught" or "down draught" system. I have observed, in my reading on this system, that it is sometimes necessary to supplement its heating powers by a direct radiation system. Moreover, one of its advocates, in discussing the fresh-air supply, makes the following admission: "In hospitals, from a theoretical standpoint, too much air cannot be supplied—in practice, it frequently runs up to 100 cubic feet per minute and over. In the hospital of moderate size the plenum system will meet all requirements, but under certain circumstances, in more complicated structures, it becomes desirable to assist its action by exhaust fans." The Houses of Parliament in Berlin were also originally equipped with the down-draught system, but the sanitary engineer in charge of the work, being doubtful of the efficiency of the method, planned and provided for an up-draught system also. After a practical trial of the down-draught system, it was considered eminently unsatisfactory for heating and ventilating the parliament chamber; so the up-draught system already installed was brought into use, and at present it seems that the down-draught system is used for one hour, before the assembling of the members at the parliamentary sessions, for the preliminary warming of the chamber, and afterward the up-draught system is used during the sittings to preserve the freshness of the air and to maintain a satisfactory temperature while the chamber is occupied by members and spectators. Sir Douglas Galton, F.R.S., in his "Report of the Barracks and Hospital Improvement Commission," says: "The writer has visited, on several different occasions, three of the important hospitals in Europe and the United States of America in which the ventilation depended on propulsion, and on every occasion the propulsion happened to be out of use for the time."

All things being taken into consideration, it is probable that the most satisfactory and by far the cheapest method of heating and ventilating hospital wards in this climate is by direct radiation. If we do not use the down-draught system,—if we do not use a fan either for the impulsion of fresh air into a building or for the extraction of foul air from it,—there are but two methods left that we can choose from. One is to bring the cold air into the building through a short duct, convey it to a radiator where it may be heated, and then allow it to pass off through an upcast shaft through or near the ceiling. The second alternative is the natural method of ventilation, to which reference is made a few lines further on.

Billings says: "The proper position of the foul-air registers depends on the purpose of the room and on the season. In large assembly halls and especially where it is desired to provide for respiration air as pure as possible, instead of foul air diluted to a certain standard, the discharge openings should be above. . . . When we come to deal with rooms having a large floor area in proportion to the height and containing fifty or more persons whose heat-production is a factor that must be taken into consideration, there is some danger that, in the down-draught method, there will be an unsatisfactory distribution of the fresh air when the temperature of the external air is not below 50° F." It is held that it is frequently necessary to aid the extraction of the vitiated air by placing small radiators in the extracting shafts, so that the air in these shafts shall be heated and shall thereby acquire an upward movement. It is pointed out that this is a waste of heat, for the radiated heat subserves no other purpose than that of warming the air in the shaft and is an expensive motive power. This may be admitted, but it is probably balanced by the necessary overheating of the very much larger quantities of air required to be delivered by the plenum system. In many structures these vents can be run to the smoke stack from the fire boxes of the boilers and will there be heated sufficiently to maintain a good up-draught. One of the most reasonable methods that I am acquainted with is that of an English engineer who has planned what he calls a " natural method of ventilation," although this term is usually applied to ventilation by means of doors and windows, which the sanitarians consider as no ventilation at all. In this Boyle system the heating and ventilating systems independent. Radiant heat is used. Boyle thus describes his system and points out its advantages:—"Natural ventilation properly applied is the most constant and reliable. It requires little or no attention, is always in action, and cannot get out of order or break down, as so often happens in mechanical ventilation. Care should be taken, in the employment of ventilators, that they are of correct construction and that both the outlets and the inlets are sufficient in size and number and so placed as effectively to accomplish the work they have to do. The outlet ventilators should be fixed on the highest part of the roof, clear of all obstructions, so that the wind can reach them freely from every quarter. The fresh-air supply should be properly proportioned to the extraction. The combined area of the inlets should in all ordinary cases be at least equal to that of the outlet shaft. Main exhaust shafts should be at least of equal area to the combined area of the branch pipes. Branch pipes should have as great an upward angle as possible and should never enter the main shaft at the same level unless when parallel. All pipes should be made of metal and should be circular in shape, to reduce friction. The vitiated air should be extracted at the ceiling, to which point it naturally ascends. The fresh air should be admitted directly through the walls, at a low velocity, in an upward direction through a number of small inlet brackets or tubes distributed around the walls to secure more complete diffusion and an equable movement of the air in all parts of the building. Air never should be admitted in cold weather in a horizontal direction, as a disagreeable draught would result. The velocity of the air-supply should not exceed two feet per second. The inlet channels should communicate directly with the outer air, be as short as possible, and easy of access for the purpose of cleaning. Long inlet channels are objectionable, as they harbor dirt and are difficult of access. Where simple tubes or brackets are used, the tops should be about 5 feet 9 inches above the floor. Where the air-supply is warmed it may be delivered at a lower level—that is, where it passes through radiators in entering the room. The inlets should be fitted with regulating valves to control the air supply. The fresh-air supply should not be overheated, as its hygienic properties are thereby seriously impaired. Heating a building by hot air should, therefore, be avoided, as injurious to health. Radiant heat is the healthiest and most effective. Where open fires are used they should have a separate air supply led directly to them from the outside air through a three- or a four-inch pipe, to prevent them drawing the hot vitiated air from above down into the breathing air, thus creating draughts and unduly affecting the ventilating arrangements."

The Administration Building.—This, the great office and official residence building, where the representatives of the hospital, both medical and lay, come in contact with the general public, must be carefully planned and must have abundant space for the transaction of the complicated businesses that have to be despatched day after day without intermission. To the hospital officers these important affairs become matters of daily routine; to the friends of the patients and the public at large they are unusual happenings, often fraught with highly emotional interests. Hence, agreeable physical surroundings and arrangements for transacting these matters decently and with a proper regard for reasonable privacy and the feelings of the visitors will go far toward establishing a cordial understanding between the citizens of a community and their hospital. The plans of the Administration Building of the Cincinnati General Hospital (Fig. 317) show a building two hundred and seventeen feet long, with a maximum depth of sixty-seven feet and a minimum depth of fifty-six feet. The entrance, through the centre of the eastern front, is through a porch and a tiled lobby to the central corridor, which occupies the long axis of the building. On the right of the lobby is the entrance to the general office. North of the office, on the eastern front, are a vault, a file room, and a bookkeeper's office. Across the corridor from the general office are Registration and Consultation Rooms for the Visiting Staff. At the north end of the corridor is an Assembly Hall with a seating capac-

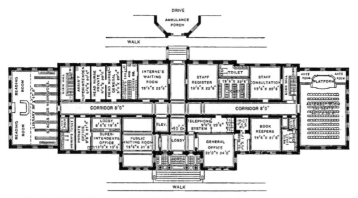

Fig. 317.—Plan of First Floor of the Administration Building, Cincinnati General Hospital.

ity of two hundred. This can be used for the meetings of medical societies and conventions. Clinical material from the wards of the Hospital and specimens from the Pathological Institute can be easily brought to these meetings without discomfort to patients or inconvenience to Curators. To the left of the entrance lobby, on the east front, is a waiting room for the general public. Across the corridor to the west is a waiting room for the internes, with a locker and toilet room adjoining. Next to these waiting rooms are, on the east, the Superintendent's Office, and on the west the office of the Superintendent of Nurses. At the southern end of this floor is a Library containing a stack room for 45,000 volumes and a reading room twenty feet by forty-seven feet. In the basement are file rooms for the statistical department of the hospital and billiard rooms and a swimming pool for the internes. The second and third floors provide fifty-four sleeping and sitting rooms for the resident physicians, internes, and officers of the hospital.

The Receiving Ward.—The receiving ward of a general municipal hospital is too often inadequate in size and equipment, and in the future it should receive more consideration at the hands of hospital designers. Under ordinary circumstances there are needed a waiting room, where applicants for admission can await their turn for examination, and an examination room equipped with such simple means of diagnosis as are necessary to determine to which one of the classified services the patient is to be assigned. These apartments should be in duplicate—one set for the men, another for the women. Children are brought for examination to the women's side of the department. In addition to these there should be some other rooms. A small operating room is a necessity, as numbers of cases are daily brought to the municipal hospital to have wounds closed and dressed, abscesses opened, fractures set, dislocations reduced, etc., and, after the necessary attention has been paid to their ailments, they insist upon going to their homes. Sometimes children are delivered, and emergency tracheotomies made, in receiving wards, and adequate facilities should be provided for all such work. This necessarily involves the presence of a small ward of two or three beds, where patients may be temporarily accommodated until they can be assigned to the proper hospital service or sent to their homes. It is necessary that certain classes of cases receive immediate intelligent treatment upon their arrival at the hospital and without the delay incident to the usual bath and history-taking before they are transported to the wards assigned to the ordinary patients. The most numerous of these classes are the poison cases and the severe burns. The initial treatment of both these conditions involves haste, the active employment of several persons besides the medical officer, and a certain amount of "messiness,"—the latter being dependent upon the necessity of washing out the stomachs of probably unconscious poisoned persons, and upon the prevalent use of "carron oil" as an application to burnt surfaces. All of this can best be done in the receiving ward under the immediate direction of the receiving physician, while the interne in charge of the service acts as assistant and removes the case to the ward when it is proper so to do. The sunstroke cases constitute another class of cases that need immediate attention. Since the improved management of these cases, introduced into the sugar refineries of Philadelphia some fifteen years ago, a very large proportion of these patients who used formerly to be lost, are now saved, and it is incumbent upon all hospitals in those parts of the United States where sunstroke is prevalent in summer, to make the special provision that is necessary for the proper care of these cases. As a room attached to the receiving ward of the new Cincinnati General Hospital has been especially designed for this service, the floor plan is here reproduced (Fig. 318) to facilitate an understanding of the subject. This method of treatment does away with the old method of packing the patient in ice in a bath tub and substitutes a fine spray of ice-cold water with which to whip the entire surface of the body, and a frequent washing-out of the lower bowel—also with ice-water. The character of this work, which must sometimes be kept up for a considerable length of time, necessitates, as will be readily seen, a chamber whose floor can be flooded with water without danger to neighboring floors or underlying ceilings. An additional reason why such cases as those enumerated above should be treated in the receiving ward is that their initial emergency treatment in their own wards would disturb the peace of that ward and occasion a degree of excitement that could not but be bad for some, if not all, of the other patients in the ward. This applies particularly to medical wards, to which most of these

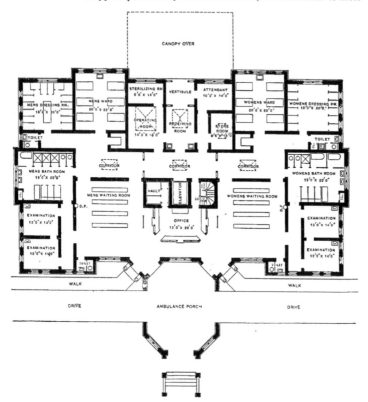

FIG. 318.—Plan of the Receiving Ward of the Cincinnati General Hospital.

patients would be assigned. Finally, the whole building should be so arranged that, in case of need, all of these rooms could be thrown into one great hall. This need comes when a great public calamity befalls the community, such as a fire panic in a theatre or hall, a railroad accident, the collapse of a crowded building or a hotel or asylum fire. Public opinion, always critical of hospital management, is at such times excited and irritable and demands instant and humane attention to the suffering victims. This cannot be given if the receiving ward is small or is cut up into a number of small rooms by immovable partitions. The available space must be large enough to hold as many stretchers as can profitably be used in transporting cases by the elevators to the proper wards, and as many beds as possible, so as properly to secure the comfort of those patients who must await transportation until an empty stretcher returns. Bungling, due to overcrowding at such a time, produces an ill effect both on the minds of the hospital attendants who are working at a disadvantage and on the minds of that portion of the public who happen to see it, instilling into the latter a suspicion that the hospital management is inefficient; while a smooth and rapid disposal of all cases, even when the number is large, and possibly exaggerated in the public mind, fills the hospital men and women with a sense of duty well performed, and engenders in the public a feeling of confidence in that institution which, they see, is built and equipped for any emergency. There is another important class of cases that must be provided for in the receiving ward. It not infrequently happens, especially at night, that men or even women who have been drinking, but are not necessarily intoxicated, have been found by the police or citizens lying in an apparently helpless condition on the street or in some building. They are brought to the hospital, as their helplessness indicates, and sometimes it is a very nice question to determine whether or not a real injury is present or whether their stupid, incoordinate condition is only due to some ingested alkaloid or to alcohol. The frequently reported cases of partially intoxicated persons who have been rejected by the hospitals and have died a few hours later in a police station, will at once occur to the reader, and those who have had experience in receiving wards can testify to the difficulties of diagnosis and the heavy sense of responsibility that come with these cases. There must therefore be provided means of housing these cases for a few hours, so that they can be watched and their physical condition determined by a properly prolonged period of observation. When the diagnosis is properly made the cases may be transferred to a hospital ward, allowed to go to their homes, or turned over to the police, as the case may be. At any rate there will then be no excuse for serious error on the part of the receiving physician. He will have been provided with the proper facilities for humanely and reasonably protecting the interests of the possible patient and of the hospital, and he will not need to worry over possible blunders on his own part. Furthermore, many seriously injured persons will be relieved of the charge of alcoholism or drug addiction, and will be spared the stigma of the police station. To this end there have been placed in the Receiving Ward of the Cincinnati General Hospital two "temporary wards"—one for men and the other for women and children. Each ward contains eight beds. As indicated before, these wards will serve a variety of useful purposes. Not only will they assist in determining the character of these doubtful cases, but they may also be used for poison cases, for emergency operative and obstetrical cases, and as rest rooms for those who insist upon going to their homes after the dressing of wounds, fractures, dislocations, etc. They will also accommodate most of those cases received after nine o'clock in the evening,—as no cases will be admitted to the general wards of the hospital after that hour, except in case of urgent necessity. The receiving ward of the Cincinnati General Hospital is contained in a one-story building one hundred and thirty feet long and seventy-seven feet deep. It is situated immediately behind the Administration Building in the front centre of the hospital grounds. Entrances both for foot-passengers and for ambulances and patrol wagons are on the eastern and western fronts. These give access to waiting rooms for men and women on both sides of the clerk's office where the names and addresses of the patients are taken. On the southern side of the building is the men's department. After having had their admission histories taken at the clerk's office, they will be seated in the waiting room until such time as the receiving physician summons them to the examining room. If they are accepted as patients, the attendants take them to the toilet room where they receive their baths and hospital clothes before being taken to the wards. The dressing room in the southwest corner is used by outgoing patients in laying off their hospital uniform and donning their street clothes. The clothes of all patients that seem to need it are taken from the toilet room, where they are laid off at the time of admission, to the disinfecting station, and, after having undergone the process of disinfection, are sent to the clothes room in the basement where they are hung upon a numbered rack in a numbered clothes bag, not to be taken from thence until the patient is discharged from the hospital or dies. Across the corridor from the men's dressing room is a small disinfecting room for the prompt treatment of verminous clothing—which must always be fumigated as soon as the individual divests himself of it, and not handled or transported by the clean attendants, as vermin are very actively mobile. On the western side of the men's wing, next to the outgoing dressing room, is the men's temporary ward containing eight beds, the function of which has been previously described.

In the centre of the western front is, on one side of the entrance corridor, an operating room for emergency cases, with its accessory sterilizing room, and on the other side there are a room for the ward attendant, and a store-room. The women's side of the building is a duplicate of the men's side.

When accepted into the hospital by the receiving physician, the patients are given a cleansing bath in the toilet room, are clothed in fresh hospital uniform, and are taken to their assigned wards on foot, in rolling chairs, or on stretchers, as their condition demands, through the passage or tunnel which leads to every building on the grounds, and which leaves the receiving ward through the lobby. Immediately outside the entrance to the receiving ward, on both the east and the west fronts of the building, and opening to the north and south, are "portes cochères," or ambulance porches, measuring twenty-seven feet by thirty-four feet, with an entrance twelve feet wide guarded by sliding doors so arranged that they may be opened by means of a cord hanging over the driveway within easy reach of the ambulance driver. In the basement of the building, in addition to the clothes-rooms already referred to, will be the "sunstroke room." Here are all the special conveniences for managing cases of sunstroke by the methods previously described. It must not be supposed, however, that the treatment of sunstroke cases is to be the only function of this apartment. Here is where all the acute poisoning cases, whether from alcohol, one of the alkaloids, Paris green, carbolic acid, or what not, can have their stomachs and intestines washed out with the greatest efficiency and the minimum of discomfort to the hospital attendants. Here also maniacal and noisy lunatics, who are frequently brought in an emergency to general hospitals, may be held, without annoyance to the sick, until the proper disposition can be made of them and their transference to an asylum effected. In fact, a number of emergency uses of such an isolated apartment will suggest themselves to the practical hospital superintendent or receiving physician.

The Surgical Pavilion.—Since the introduction of Listerism so much thought has been given to the method and the proper environment of surgical operations that some recent examples of the surgical operating amphitheatre and its accessories may rightly be considered as wellnigh perfectly adapted to the present status of operative surgery. The shape and the arrangement of any

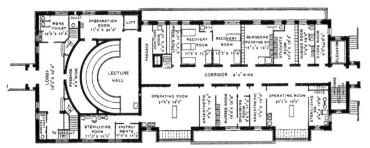

Fig. 319.—Plan of First Floor of the Surgical Pavilion, Cincinnati General Hospital.

given surgical building will depend of course to a great extent upon the space to be allotted to it in any given plan, and to the size and requirements of the hospital for which it is to be built; but it is possible to make a catalogue of the requisites of such a service as a guide in the planning of a surgical pavilion for any hospital. (Fig. 322.) If the hospital in question conducts a clinical school of surgery the principal operating room will serve at the same time as the pit of an amphitheatre of greater or less extent according to the prospective number of students. The operating room proper and the amphitheatre will be constructed on the general surgical principles of simplicity of lines and surfaces and amenability to thorough cleansing by flushing with water—possibly with antiseptic solutions—and, if necessary, by disinfection effected through the generation or liberation of antiseptic gases. The risers of the amphitheatre should be high so as to allow, to each row of spectators, an unobstructed view of the operating table. Light should be had by skylight and abundant window space with northern exposure. Some surgeons have made a plea for additional skylights and windows facing south (to be screened during the hours of active

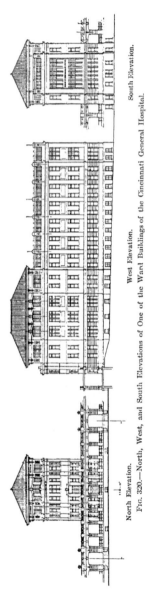

South Elevation.

West Elevation.

North Elevation.

FIG. 320.—North, West, and South Elevations of One of the Ward Buildings of the Cincinnati General Hospital.

use of the room) on the ground that the flooding of the theatre with sunlight, whenever this is possible, is one of the best safeguards against infection. In addition to the operating amphitheatre it will be necessary to have one or two smaller operating rooms according to the size of the hospital, one of which rooms should be reserved for pus cases—such as the opening of abscesses and infected joints. Some hospitals include among the apartments of the surgical pavilion a laboratory or workshop and a small operating room for the orthopedic surgeons, where, after tenotomies, transplantations, or osteoclasis, they may apply plaster of Paris bandages—or, indeed, use plaster in any of the great number of conditions in which they find it useful. If this plaster room is not assigned to the surgical pavilion, provision must be made for it in or near the surgical wards to which the orthopedic cases are assigned. Conveniently near the operating rooms must be etherizing rooms provided with all the necessary paraphernalia of the anæsthetist. At least two such etherizing rooms should be allowed to four operating rooms. Similarly, recovery rooms should be provided in the same proportion, where patients can recover from the disagreeable after-effects of anæsthesia and not be returned to their beds in their wards in a condition which would disturb those seriously ill or would terrify those yet to undergo operation. As modern operative conditions demand that those in contact with the patient lay aside their outer cloth garments before entering the operating room, dressing rooms (with such accessories as toilets and shower baths) should be provided for the surgeons and their assistants and for the nurses. These should be spacious and should have plenty of locker room. They must be of the type of bath-room that can be thoroughly flushed and cleaned. If the hospital be a large one, in which much operative work is done, it would be well to have separate dressing rooms for the visiting staff and for the house staff, as they would have to accommodate a large number of individuals in fairly rapid succession. The nursing force is usually constant in numbers and personnel during the whole day. These dressing rooms must be furnished with everything requisite to allow those using them to become surgically clean before entering the operating room. The burden of a very large proportion of the work and the responsibility for a very large proportion of the success of the operative service of any hospital fall upon the clinic nurse and her assistants, and the designer of the surgical operating pavilion must, therefore, bear in mind all the necessities of this service. In the first place, this nursing force, under the direction of their chief, must cut, shape, and prepare all dressings, pads, and bandages and must do up in packages for sterilization and subsequent use these dressings and bandages and, in addition, towels, napkins, caps, gowns, sheets, leggings, blankets, etc. Therefore there must be provided a large workroom, furnished with tables and the proper shelving where gauze and muslin

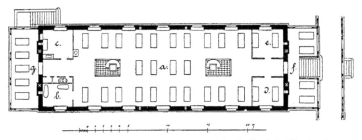

Fig. 321.—Plan of Ground Floor of One of the Pavilions of the City Hospital at Dresden, Germany. (From Ruppel: "Anlage und Bau der Krankenhaeuser," Jena, 1896.) a, Main ward; b, bath-room and two closets; c, tea kitchen; d, room for patients who are very ill; e, nurses' room; f, room for convalescents; g, small ward for use in the summer season; h, passage-way. The numbers in the scale refer to metres.

in rolls may be received from the store-room, where the other articles may be received from the laundry, and where all can be properly prepared for sterilization and for use in the operating room. The dressing and toilet room for the nurses has already been spoken of. The sterilizing room must have in connection with it a room for the care and storage of instruments, and also one for the storage of packages of sterilized dressings, gowns, etc. The sterilizing room is furnished with sterilizers, several designs of which made in standard sizes by manufacturers of hospital furnishings are on the market. (See Vol. I., Part IV.) These, of course, derive the steam used in them from the power plant, and they are so designed and constructed that the articles placed in them can be subjected to a steam pressure of several hundred pounds, the exact amount being indicated and regulated by a gauge and safety valve. Sinks and tables in this room afford facilities for the washing and other care of instruments before they are sterilized and put away. In each of the operating rooms—in view of the not infrequent necessity of operating at night—there should be ample provision for electric illumination, both stationary and portable, and electric plugs should also be conveniently placed in the walls nearest the operating tables, to afford power for dental engines, cauteries, or other electrically energized instruments or mechanical appliances. This latter matter is becoming increasingly important, as the use of electricity in the surgical arts is more and more developed.

As a concrete example of the most modern design in the way of surgical pavilions I call attention to the recently completed plan of the ground floor of the Surgical Pavilion of the new Cincinnati General Hospital (Fig. 319), which shows a building one hundred and fifty feet long and fifty-one feet wide, with two bays, each projecting five and a half feet on the north side. These bays correspond to the position of operating rooms. (See also Figs. 322, 323, and 325.)

Along the south side of the building extends an area way, to give light and abundant ventilation to the basement rooms on that side. A large room in

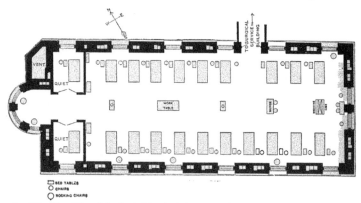

Fig. 322.—Plan of One of the Surgical Wards of the Presbyterian Hospital, New York City, showing disposition of beds and ward furniture.

the southeast corner of the basement is intended for use as a students' waiting, locker, and lunch room. Next to this, in a westwardly direction, is a kitchen for the lunch counter and a large unassigned space. On the north side of the corridor, the easterly room is a toilet for the servants, and the space under the amphitheatre is occupied by a fan and heater room. A small room next to this is a storage room for the orthopedic surgeons and will contain an iron platform on rollers holding two small iron barrels for plaster of Paris, all necessary apparatus for suspensions, splints, supplies of metal rods and bands, and all other desiderata for this special work. The larger room west of this will be devoted to the application of plaster of Paris in those cases in which a cutting operation does not immediately precede the use of the plaster. Strong iron hooks are embedded in the ceiling and walls in convenient situations for vertical suspension and for the use of hammocks. Next to the orthopedic room is a waiting room, and then follow three rooms for the x-ray department—for the arrangement of which the reader is referred to the section which treats of that special department. (Vol. I., Part III.) The western end is occupied by the elevator and stairways.

The first-floor plan shows, on the south side of the building, the students' entrance leading into the lower lobby of the surgical amphitheatre. Stairways lead up, right and left, to small lobbies on the second floor, which are the entrances proper to the students' seats. The small room to the east of the lower lobby is a toilet for women.

The surgical amphitheatre, with a capacity for seating two hundred and fifty persons, occupies the major portion of this end of the building, and has as its accessories a preparation room and an elevator. It will not be used for operations, but only for the demonstration of cases which do not involve the making

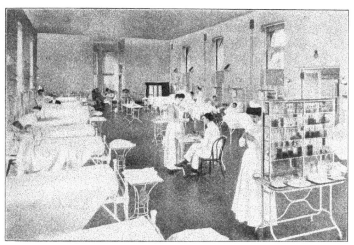

Fig. 323.—Interior View of the Men's Surgical Ward, Presbyterian Hospital, New York City.

or dressing of wounds. Operative work is provided for by the presence, in the building, of five operating rooms, two of which, lighted by bays, occupy the east side of this first floor with their rooms for instruments and for sterilizing and anæsthetizing purposes. The nurses' dressing rooms separate the two operating suites. On the west side of the central corridor are found, in the order named, a janitor's sink room, a warming closet and linen room, two recovery rooms, a surgeon's dressing room, a room where the students can leave their coats, wash, and be put in spectators' gowns, a nurses' toilet, and a store room. Operations will be witnessed by the students in these small operating rooms, from movable platforms which can be shifted from place to place so as to enable them to obtain the best point of view. The south end of the second floor contains the upper part of the amphitheatre. The eastern side of the building contains two general operating rooms, with their sterilizing rooms, a nurses' dressing room, an anæsthetizing room, and a special ophthalmic operating room. The western side contains surgeons' preparation rooms, anæsthetizing and recovery rooms, a nurses' toilet, and a large nurses' work room, where pads, dressings, and bandages of all kinds can be cut, folded, and done up in packages for sterilization. The multiplicity of operating rooms in this building lends itself easily to a proper and safe classification of operative surgical cases, and insures that at least two shall be constantly kept for "clean cases."

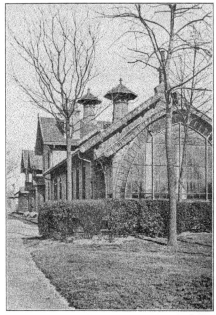

FIG. 324.—View of the Exterior of the Boucicaut Hospital, at Paris, France. (Note how little the architecture of this building suggests the ordinary hospital structure.)

Large operating amphitheatres are provided in several of the leading hospitals of the United States,—as, for example, in the Roosevelt Hospital, the Presbyterian Hospital (Figs. 326–329), and St. Luke's Hospital, in New York City, as well as in some of the other large cities.

The Medical Pavilion.—Until very recently, in the majority of American hospitals those members of the staff who devoted themselves to internal medicine (such as the internists, the gastro-enterologists, and the pediatrists) had a just cause for their complaint that the surgical features of the hospital were developed to a very high degree at the expense of the less theatrical necessities of the medical service. The advances of modern medical therapeutics, however, as distinguished from operative surgery, have assumed such importance that the claims of these men can no longer be disregarded. It certainly is curious that, in a country supposed to be pre-eminent in the mechanical arts, the mechanical department of therapeutics should have developed itself on the operative surgical side alone. The European hospitals and the hospitals of the Latin-American nations have been wonderfully progressive along these lines, while we unfortunately have singularly neglected a multitude of mechanical, electrical, and hydro-therapeutic measures which, in the hands of others, have proven themselves to be of the greatest value. It is probably because of the prevailing lack of knowledge of, or lack of interest in, these subjects on the part of the average American physician, and the lack of equipment in almost all American hospitals, that certain sanatoria, which make these measures a

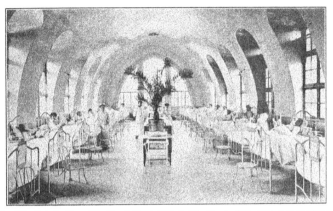

Fig. 325.—Interior View of the Female Surgical Ward of the Boucicaut Hospital, at Paris, France.
(Note the pleasant effect made on the eye by the vaulted ceiling of the room.)

very prominent feature in their management and in the treatment of certain chronic internal derangements, have obtained such a vogue among the people and such a reputation among certain classes in the profession, as well as among large numbers of the laity, for their "cures." Our medical schools must, in the future, supply instruction in these arts, and our hospitals must equip themselves with every tried and proven therapeutic device. Every modern hospital, therefore, even though of modest dimensions, should have its departments of mechanico-therapy, electro-therapy, and hydro-therapy. As provided for at present, sometimes these departments are given separate buildings, as in the Mexican National Hospital mentioned on page 827; but it seems to the writer that it would better subserve the convenience of the service, especially in such a climate as we have throughout the major part of the United States, if all of these departments were housed in a single building easily accessible from all the medical wards. This mechanico-electro-hydro-therapeutic pavilion,

as it might be called, would be the proper place for the amphitheatre in which
would be delivered all those clinical lectures of the hospital curriculum which
did not necessitate the use of either the surgical or the pathological amphitheatre—such, for example, as the lectures on internal medicine, on nervous
diseases, on diseases of children, etc. And in the same amphitheatre could be
demonstrated to student classes the use of the various apparatuses employed
in modern mechanico-electro-hydro-therapeutics. If it seemed necessary,
the space required for the attainment of the latter object could be obtained
by the construction of a small balcony in each of the rooms devoted to a special
purpose,—a balcony such as would hold a dozen or fifteen persons,—just as is
now frequently done in many of the operating rooms of private or semi-public
hospitals, such as St. Mary's, of Rochester, Minnesota, where Drs. W. J. and
C. H. Mayo hold their clinics. If, however, the floor space provided were gen-

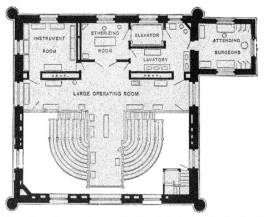

Fig. 326.—Plan of Main Floor of Operating Pavilion of the Presbyterian Hospital, New York
City. The theatre has a seating capacity of 120 persons.

erous, there would be no objection—in fact, there would be a decided advantage
—if the students were taken directly upon the floor and thus brought in close
contact with the patients and the therapeutic apparatus. The equipment in
any given hospital will, of course, depend upon the judgment and desires of the
medical staff; but, in general, it may be said that the mechanical outfit should
at least comprise: (1) One gymnasium equipped with its proper complement
of horses, rings, bars, weights, ladders, etc., and means for the thorough employment of that system of exercises which is known as the Manual Swedish Movements or Medical Gymnastics. (2) Mechanical apparatus intended for the
application of mechanical passive exercise. Certain forms of passive exercise
may be administered by machinery far more effectively than by hand. The
rapid, steady, and prolonged movements which can be administered by machinery cannot, so far as efficiency is concerned, be even approximated by

the human hand. Certain kneading and percussion movements may also be administered more effectively by mechanical means than by the manual method. Bed patients from the wards will frequently be brought to the medical pavilion for this purpose. (3) A special form of the application of mechanics to exercise is found in what are known as vibrators. Special forms are designed for use for the hands and arms and for the feet, and there are also vibrating stools, vibrating tables, vibrating chairs, and sets of vibrating chairs in which several patients may be treated at once. The hospital designer should provide space and electric power for these devices. (See Fig. 330.)

The department of hydro-therapeutics should offer facilities for the use of a number of the various forms of baths. In the first place, there should be provided a swimming pool. The value of this form of exercise in water is universally recognized and nowhere disputed. The tank should be situated where it may have a solid foundation, i.e., on the ground floor or in the basement, but direct sunlight—through a generous window space or skylights—

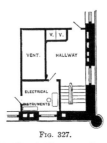
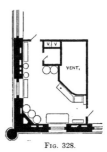

FIG. 327. FIG. 328.

FIG. 327.—Electrical Instrument Room under Theatre Seats of Operating Pavilion Shown in Fig. 326.
FIG. 328.—Sterilizing Room under Theatre Seats of Operating Pavilion Shown in Fig. 326.

should have abundant access to all parts of it. Should there be plenty of space for such an arrangement it would be well to have two tanks—a larger one with the water at a temperature of about 74° F., and a smaller one with the water at a temperature of about 60° F. There should be apartments and equipment for Turkish baths and Russian baths. There should be tubs for tub-baths of varying temperatures, and specially constructed small tanks for electro-hydric baths. Appropriately shaped tubs will provide for Sitz, half-, foot-, leg-baths, etc., and curtained closets should be furnished for showers, douches, jets and sprays, and for vapor or steam baths. As necessary adjuncts to the various uses of water there should, of course, be provided space for the accommodation of rest couches and massage tables, and for the beds, rolling chairs, etc., necessary for the transportation of those patients who are unable to walk from the wards to the hydro-therapeutic department.

Electro-therapeutics will not demand as much space nor as elaborate arrangements as do mechanico- or hydro-therapeutics; still, as the use of electricity is in demand by many departments of medicine, and as it is frequently made use of in conjunction with the other physiological remedies (water and exercise), it is well to provide for a large proportion of the hospital population. This subject is so familiar that it is unnecessary to do more than mention the various forms of electrical current to be provided for—sinusoidal, galvanic, faradic, static, and high-frequency. A fairly large hall with alcoves suggests itself as the best form of room in which an electrical department can be accommodated. Of late years phototherapy has claimed increasing attention and, for obvious reasons, naturally demands a place in the electro-therapeutic department. Given an exposure to the south, with properly arranged windows or skylights, a room devoted to this department would furnish solar light, whenever it was available, and at the same time would have current and place for the use of

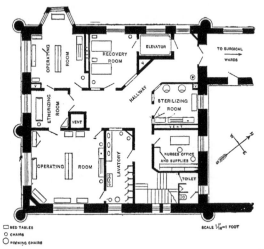

Fig. 329.—Ground Floor Plan of the Operating Pavilion, Presbyterian Hospital, New York City.

the photophore, the incandescent electric-light bath, and the arc-light bath, various forms of which seem to be coming into quite extensive use.

Medical Photography.—The aid of the camera in recording cases will be sought to a greater or less extent by every service in the hospital, and therefore there should be established, in some central location, a photographic department equipped with the best possible portrait camera and a number of good portable cameras which can be taken to the wards when occasion requires. Probably the best place for this department (with its well-lighted studio and its dark rooms) would be the building containing the medical departments. If the size of the hospital justified it, there might be another photographic department in the surgical pavilion. In any event, there should be a photographic department in connection with the pathological service, and it should be reserved exclusively for the use of the latter. No apparatus from the pathological department should be allowed to enter any other part of the hospital. The building requirements of studios and dark rooms demand that these departments be well provided for ih the working plans of the hospital, as attempts to utilize, for this highly special purpose, rooms not originally designed therefor, is emi_ nently unsatisfactory both as regards the comfort and efficiency of those who have to work therein and as regards the results achieved. The whole process of photography, depending as it does upon the abundance and the quality of diffused daylight at one stage, and its absolutely complete absence at another, renders it necessary that the studios should be assigned a situation where they can be given an extensive northern exposure by skylight, while the dark rooms must be provided for in such a way that they can be freely ventilated during

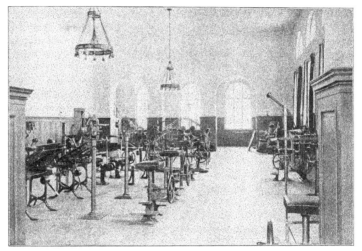

Fig. 330.—View of a Room Equipped with Mechanical Apparatus for Therapeutic Purposes.
(Rudolph Virchow Hospital, Berlin, Germany.)

any number of consecutive hours. All plates taken by the photographic department should be the property of the hospital and be filed away carefully in suitable receptacles. They are as much part of the record of a case as is the history written in the wards *intra vitam* or the specimen taken for the museum after the patient's death. Prints may be given to all those interested in the case, but the plate should be carefully preserved at the hospital studio. The modern hospital bed—known as the "blacksmith bed" and made in one solid piece without joints—can be picked up and clamped in a rolling carriage, so that any patient may at any time be transported to a photographic studio, an x-ray room, or any other part of the hospital without the body being disturbed. These rolling carriages or trucks are perhaps more frequently used in carrying patients from the wards to solaria or open-air porches, in order that they may obtain the benefit of sunlight and fresh air.

The Roentgen-Ray Department.—The requirements of Roentgen-ray work are of such a unique character as to demand a special arrangement and special construction of the quarters assigned to this department, not only for efficiency in conducting it, but also for the protection of the operator against the dangers of over-exposure. The recent progress in x-ray technique and the widening of its field of applicability render the Roentgen laboratory an indispensable adjunct to a modern hospital. The fact that the x-ray department will receive cases, not only from the surgical wards, but from practically every ward in the hospital, with the possible exception of the obstetrical wards, makes it essential that the Roentgen laboratory be centrally located and of easy access to patients in wheel chairs and on stretchers. The amount of x-ray work to be done in a general hospital is very large and is constantly increasing. Much work may also be referred from the receiving ward and from the out-door department, if there be one attached to the hospital. The amount of floor space should, therefore, be ample.

In accordance with the suggestions of Dr. Sidney Lange, it may be laid down as a general rule that not fewer than from four to six rooms are necessary, namely:—(1) A waiting room for patients. In this room the patients may be prepared for examination—may dress and undress; bandages and dressings may be removed before the examination or treatment and readjusted afterward; anæsthetics may be given to those patients who are to have a fracture set or a foreign body removed under the x-ray, or to children to keep them quiet during the examination. (2) A director's or operator's room and skiagraphic Library. In this room the records may be kept, and large specially constructed wall cases for the proper filing and indexing of the x-ray plates should find space here. This room should have a northern exposure, the window panes being made of ground glass, to provide the soft, diffuse light necessary to the display and study of the x-ray plates. For the protection of the operator, this room should be separated from the adjoining room, in which the x-ray apparatus is located, by a wall in which sheet lead is incorporated. A switch-board placed against this wall will enable the operator to control from this room the apparatus in the x-ray room proper, while a small window in this wall, covered with ray-proof glass (the so-called lead glass), will enable him to watch the x-ray tube in operation, and the patient. This arrangement offers complete protection to the operator. (3) The x-ray room proper should be well-lighted, but capable of being instantly darkened for fluoroscopic work. It must be able to accommodate, in addition to the rather bulky x-ray apparatus and patients on stretchers, a group of physicians or a class of students witnessing a demonstration. It must be so arranged as to be converted on short notice into an operating room for such minor surgery as demands the use of the x-ray. If much therapeutic work is to be done, necessitating the use of the x-ray for several hours each day, a separate room should be provided, preferably on the opposite side of the operator's room and separated from it by a sheet-lead wall.

It should contain a small apparatus (specially adapted for therapy) which is controlled by a switch-board placed in the operator's room. Treatments and examinations could thus go on simultaneously. (4) A photographic dark room, well ventilated from the outside by curved air-passages which will admit air but not light. The room should adjoin the x-ray room proper, so as to admit of the immediate development of the plates. It should be of ample size to permit of the handling of large plates. Where plenty of space is available, the library or collection of skiagraphs may be placed in a separate room. The collection of plates grows rapidly and becomes very bulky. The practical value of the x-ray department depends in a measure upon the size, nature, and proper indexing of the collection of plates available for comparison and study. If an orthodiagraph, for the measurement of the heart and the study of the lungs, is to be used, it should be placed in a permanently dark compartment (without windows), partitioned off from, or adjoining, the x-ray room proper. Two rooms would thus be added to the previous estimate, making seven rooms in all. (See also the article on Radiographic Work in Vol. I., Part III.)

Chapel, Morgue, and Pathological Laboratories.—In accordance with the rule that the surroundings of the patients should be made as cheerful, if not as beautiful, as possible, the building containing the morgue, the pathological department with its autopsy rooms, and the chapel should be so placed that neither it nor its approaches can be seen from the windows of the wards. This can the more easily be done because the morgue should be in the vicinity of the refrigerating plant, which will bring it in the neighborhood of the power building, which is always, if the shape of the hospital lot allows, behind the ward buildings and at the back of the lot. Every hospital, whether small or large, should be a school of pathology to its medical staff and their associates and students. To this end the greatest care should be bestowed upon the arrangement and equipment of the pathological department. In metropolitan hospitals the morgue, the autopsy rooms, the pathological laboratories and museums, and the chapel are grouped in one building which is usually known as the Morgue and Chapel, or as the Pathological Building. (Figs. 331–334.) In most provincial hospitals provision for a museum and a chapel will probably have to be omitted. When brought from the wards of the hospital the bodies of the dead should be placed in the sliding racks of the refrigerator, which can easily be regulated to almost any desired degree of coldness. Here they can be kept in a practically perfect condition until such time as they are autopsied or claimed by friends and delivered to an undertaker for burial. On account of the character of the work conducted in the autopsy rooms the ceilings of these rooms should be very high,—at the least, sixteen feet,—and, if necessary, exhaust fans should be provided near the ceiling to assist the ventilation. These rooms should be abundantly lighted from above by skylights, and most generous provision should be made for electric illumination for work at night or on dark winter days. Autopsy tables of slate or marble, preferably the latter, specially grooved on their surface for the proper conduction of fluids to a sink, are made by manufacturers of hospital equipment. Water must also be brought down from above for the purpose of flushing the parts under examination, and these water pipes may conveniently be combined with the electric light conduits in one fixture. It goes without saying that the walls and floors of such rooms should be finished in some adamantine material that will not crack nor wear rough under frequent flushing and scrubbing. In all hospitals where a systematic school of pathology is conducted for medical students, an amphitheatre must be provided, and the pit of this amphitheatre should be constructed upon the model of an autopsy room and equipped with a suitable autopsy table. It is true that not all demonstrations before the class are actual autopsies,—possibly, only a small percentage of lectures will be of this character; but the autopsy table will serve equally well for the exhibition and demonstration of wet and preserved specimens. For this reason the museum, with its refrigerator for fresh specimens and its equipment for mounting and preserving both wet and dry specimens of all kinds, should be convenient to, and open directly into, the amphitheatre. The pathologist's working laboratories should be in close connection with the autopsy rooms,—not necessarily with the museum,—and should be so disposed in the building as to command a northern exposure with abundance of light. There should also be a photographic studio and dark room. It should not be forgotten that a large hospital accumulates valuable pathological material rapidly, that these specimens need large and heavy jars with an abundance of preserving fluid for their proper care, and that this means a generous allowance of space and the need of a correspondingly strong floor. The architect should therefore be informed of these requirements beforehand, in order that he may rightly apportion his space and calculate correctly the necessary supports. In connection with the morgue there should be a room for undertakers, where they can embalm bodies or otherwise prepare them for burial. This undertakers' room should be a large one,—and, if the hospital be one of five hundred beds or more, it would be wise to make provision for two rooms of this character. The part of this building intended for the use of the public as a chapel, in which funerals can be held, should have a separate entrance of its own remote from the entrance to be used by the pathologists, hospital servitors, and medical students. About this part of the building there should be nothing to suggest the medical school or the autopsy room.*

* The chapel need not be large (30 feet by 30 feet is sufficient), but it should have certain accessories to add to the comfort of those using it—such, for example, as a waiting room for the family of the deceased (with a toilet for women), one for the officiating minister who may have to don ceremonial robes, and one for the undertaker and his assistants. From the peculiar relation which this department of the dead holds to the scientific work of the hospital and to the families of the patients, it behooves the hospital designer to bestow especial care upon its planning and construction. The plans of the Chapel, Morgue, and Pathological Institute of the Cincinnati General Hospital show a building 120 feet long, with a maximum width of 62 feet and a minimum width of 54 feet. At the north end of the basement, immediately under the chapel, is placed the special and accessory heating apparatus for the building, this apparatus being necessitated by the imperative demand for increased ventilation. The character of the work to be carried on and the certainty of a great volume of evil odors attending this work render it necessary that an especially large volume of properly heated air should pass through the building at all times, so as to keep the atmosphere in a proper condition for the laboratory workers and the students. The room containing this apparatus is twenty-eight feet by thirty-five feet. On each side of it

The Kitchen and Service Building.—The details of the Kitchen and Service Building should receive the most careful consideration from the hospital designer, for upon the more or less successful solution of its arrangement depends the more or less successful prosecution of its daily task—that is, the dispensing abundantly and promptly, and without confusion or friction, of a vast quantity of domestic supplies, including properly cooked and heated food, to the large hospital population, both patients and attendants, who depend upon it, not only for their daily but also for their hourly needs. These problems have of late years been well worked out, especially in connection with the activities of hotels and hospitals; and the practice of domestic science, which includes the study of such engineering and architecture as applies to buildings devoted to the art, has risen to the dignity of a profession. (Fig. 335.) And it is a highly significant and important fact that it has risen to this dignity inasmuch as it affords some guarantee that henceforth the character and the preparation of the food, the methods of cleansing, lighting, and ventilating, and the details of the store-room, the kitchen, and the sleeping room will have intelligent and educated supervision—something which hitherto they have sadly lacked. Unfortunately, my relatively small allowance of space compels me to abstain from entering into the details of this branch of our subject.

The Management of Hospitals.—The schemes of management of hospitals are many and of a most diverse character. The hospitals of the Catholic Church,

is a students' toilet room. On the west side of the building we find a cold-storage room large enough to contain thirty bodies, and from this room an elevator ascends to the undertaker's room on the first floor and the amphitheatre on the second floor. Next to the cold-storage room is a room for the coroner's official post-mortem examinations, when this official wishes to make an autopsy himself or delegates some physician other than those attached to the hospital to make one. In this room will be a large tub where bodies can be placed and thoroughly cleansed after autopsy. On the east side of the basement are two store-rooms, an incubator room, a sterilizing room, and a room for the preparation of culture media. These latter are generously supplied with vents, as much of this work gives rise to disagreeable and penetrating odors. At the southern end of the building are elevators, toilets, and stairways.

The chapel, thirty-five feet by twenty-eight feet, occupies the major portion of the eastern end of the first floor. To the south of the chapel we find the undertaker's room, opening both into the corridor and into the chapel, and a large laboratory, forty-six by twenty feet. On the north side of the corridor, which leads west from behind the altar of the chapel, we find two laboratories, a library, and a custodian's office, in which latter the records of the reception and the disposition of the bodies are kept. The second-floor plan shows, at the eastern end above the chapel, a laboratory and the amphitheatre of the Pathological Department, constructed and arranged in such a way that in it post-mortem examinations may be made before the class. The elevator from the cold-storage room opens into the amphitheatre. The corridor behind the amphitheatre gives access to a large laboratory (twenty feet by fifty-one feet) on the south side of the building; and, on the north side, to a laboratory, a secretary's office, the Pathological Director's study and his private laboratory. On both sides of the amphitheatre are extra autopsy rooms, carried up two stories for the sake of perfect ventilation. The third-floor plan shows the upper part of the amphitheatre at the east end, and three laboratories on the south side. Three small laboratories and a large laboratory occupy the north side of the corridor. It is intended that ultimately the larger part of the fourth floor shall be occupied by a museum. The northern side of this floor on the western end will be occupied by the photographic department, with special provision for microphotography. On the south side will be the Curator's work room. On the roof will be covered pens and open yards for animals, with all the necessary accessories for properly taking care of them.

for instance, are under the care of the various sisterhoods and are governed by the rules of those orders. Until recently the entire personnel of these hospitals, except the medical staff and the necessary mechanics, was drawn from the ranks of the sisters. Latterly, in recognition of the demands of modern medicine and surgery, training schools for nurses have been established, and the nursing has

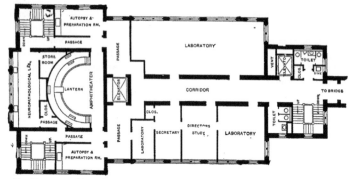

Fig. 331.—Plan of Second Floor of the Pathological Building, Cincinnati General Hospital.

been done by the modern trained nurse. Hospitals of the Protestant Churches and of the various benevolent orders are usually governed by boards of trustees who are elected by the governing bodies of the churches or orders, or by the contributors to the support of the hospital. State Hospitals are governed by boards of trustees appointed by the governor of the State, and Municipal

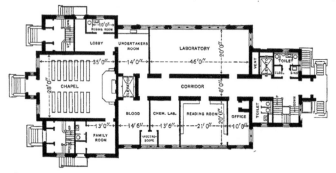

Fig. 332.—Plan of First Floor of the Pathological Building, Cincinnati General Hospital.

Hospitals are governed either by boards variously appointed, or directly by some department of the city government, such as the Department of Charities and Corrections, when there is one. The various churches and charitable organizations have probably adopted what is to each of them the best and most convenient form of hospital management. Therefore, the large problem in which every one as a citizen is vitally interested, is: How shall we manage our public hospitals, both municipal and State, so as to secure the greatest efficiency? The general answer is that these institutions must be committed to the care of men whose qualities and training are a guarantee that their trust will be discharged with an eye only to the public good, and whose tenure of office will not depend upon the uncertainties of partisan politics.   It is true that the American people are slowly learning to allow common sense instead of partisanship to guide them in their conduct of municipal and State affairs, and it is also true that in one instance an American municipality of the first rank has elected and again and again re-elected one of the most efficient men in the public service as head of the city's charities and corrections notwithstanding the fact that his national politics are opposed to the politics of a very large majority of his fellow-citizens.   For all this, however, it were better to remove all these positions that guide the policies and control the appointment of the executive staffs of

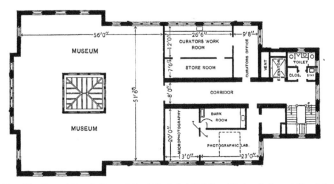

Fig. 333.—Plan of Fourth Floor of the Pathological Building, Cincinnati General Hospital.

these institutions, beyond the reach of party managers, so that the patronage will not tempt them, in times of political stress, to subordinate the interests of the sick and injured to the possible advantages of themselves and their friends. It is therefore better that a hospital be governed by a board appointed by some responsible elective official such as a governor or a mayor.   The board should consist of not more than seven members (five or even three is indeed a better number) the terms of whose service should be of such length as to secure the retirement of one member each year, with the appointment of a new member or the reappointment of the old one.   The question of compensation is an important one.   If salaries are paid they are but small, as the service does not take much of the time of the board of members; but, if a small salary is attached, small politicians are likely to seek the positions for the sake of adding that much to their annual incomes.   Therefore it is better to pay no salaries and to give the appointments to public-spirited citizens who are willing to give of their time to this worthy department of the public service.   At the same time these citizens should have an absolutely free rein in the management of the hospital; they should have the appointment of all employés in all departments and should alone direct and be responsible for the expenditure of the moneys allowed them from the taxes. They should be chosen from among those citizens who have evinced an interest in the charities of the city or State, and they should not be asked to divide their authority and thereby weaken the efficiency of their administration. To the appointing power, of course, should be reserved the right of calling these managers strictly to account for any proven dereliction of duty, publicly inquired into and established, and of removing them from office; and also the right of appointing others to take their places. The superintendent appointed by this board should be a physician. It was very generally asserted, in years gone by, that physicians were lacking in the executive ability necessary to the successful management of large affairs and that a hospital could be managed only by a business man. It is only necessary, in order to refute such a

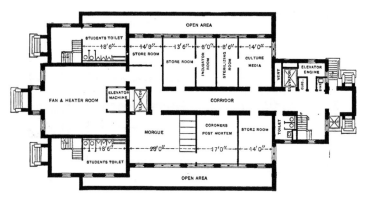

Fig. 334.—Plan of Basement of the Pathological Building, Cincinnati General Hospital.

foolish assertion, to call attention to the fact that the hospitals of the United States Army, Navy, and Marine Hospital Service are, and always have been, under the superintendence of medical men, and that their management has been uniformly and conspicuously successful. The insane asylums of almost every State in the union are also under the care of physicians, and, where these latter have not been interfered with by incompetent boards of trustees, their service has been eminently satisfactory. Of late years the largest and best hospitals of the country, both those of municipal foundation and those erected and maintained by private charity, have been under the care of medical superintendents; and it is a most noteworthy fact that, wherever this has been done, there is no further discussion as to the relative merits of physicians and laymen as hospital superintendents and no suggestion that any of the latter be chosen as successors to any of the former. In smaller communities where it would be difficult or impossible, on account of the expense, to secure the services of a physician as a superintendent, it will be found that there are, among our trained nurses, many women excellently well qualified to fill the combined positions of superintendent and head nurse. No nurse should be chosen for such a position unless she has already served in some large hospital as head nurse and in that manner been tested in the management of subordinates. The medical knowledge of these women and their intimate acquaintance with the working details of large institutions make them most competent and successful managers of the class of hospitals referred to,—in several of which they have for many years filled these positions. In the larger institutions, where organization is most thorough and division of labor necessary, the superintendent will have as his assistants a chief clerk in charge of accounts, a head nurse in charge of the nursing department, a matron in charge of the kitchen and house-cleaning departments, and an apothecary in charge of the drug department. These officers should be appointed by the board on the recommendation of the superintendent. If the board should see fit to reject some of his nominees it should

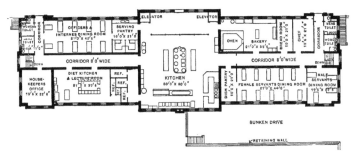

Fig. 335.—Plan of First Floor of the Kitchen and Service Building, Cincinnati General Hospital.

invite him to make other recommendations, as it is most important that the superintendent should have subordinates that he can trust and that the subordinates should understand that they have been selected by the superintendent before appointment by the board and not appointed by the latter independently of the judgment or wishes of the former. In this way, too, the heads of departments will understand that they must satisfy the superintendent in the discharge of their various duties; and, as the latter is responsible to the board for the conduct of the institution, the satisfaction of the superintendent is a matter that precedes the submission of any question to the board. The heads of the various departments make daily reports of the conduct and of the needs of their departments to the superintendent, and in this way he is kept in constant touch with the details of management. The superintendent is theoretically the officer who admits and dismisses all patients in the hospital, and this power should never be taken away from him; otherwise the maintenance of discipline among the patients is impossible. The actual routine work of the examination and admission of patients is, in the larger hospitals, delegated to an admitting physician, and the dismissal of patients—except for infraction of the rules, when the superintendent exercises his full authority—is done by the superintendent on the recommendation of the medical staff; the latter stating that the patient is well, has recovered sufficiently to be sent to his home, or, being incurable, is incapable of further improvement under hospital treatment and should be removed to an infirmary or home for incurables. The matter of an appointment of an admitting physician for the larger hospitals should receive more consideration than is usually given to it. It has been the almost universal custom to choose for this position an interne on service in the house or one whose service has just expired. The service, however, should be a permanent one and should be given to a man who has had experience in general medicine and surgery and who is tactful and resourceful. The admitting physician is the one hospital medical officer who is called upon to meet great emergencies. He must treat acute poisoning cases, sunstroke cases and labor cases, and must sometimes rapidly dispose of great numbers of those injured in some great calamity such as a fire or a collision. It must also be remembered that a considerable number of men and women who are taken to metropolitan hospitals suffering with wounds, fractures, or dislocations, insist upon going to their homes after having their injuries attended to in the receiving ward, and it is imperatively necessary that these citizens should be given the services of a skilled and experienced man whose qualifications shall command the respect of the public and the press and whose advice will carry weight with the patient and his friends. A hospital in which only 2,500 new cases or less per annum are examined in the receiving ward, will need only one receiving physician; but, where the new cases exceed that number, two men are needed properly to attend to this work, as the night work entailed by the increased number of cases will be more than one man can attend to and remain in the proper physical condition intelligently to meet the emergencies that are constantly arising both day and night. The division of time could be made into three eight-hour periods per day, or into two periods of twelve hours each; the night and day work alternating between the two physicians by months. These men should be well paid. In fact, the pay should be sufficient to attract men of superior professional qualifications, so that presently this responsible position shall appeal as a career to interested and properly equipped men, and the professional receiving physician or resident physician of a hospital would emerge on a plane with the new professions of hospital superintendent and professional anæsthetists—two careers that are abundantly justifying their existence before a world that is constantly demanding specialization and greater efficiency.

The Organization of the Medical and Surgical Staff.—New hospitals are being organized every day and old institutions frequently change their methods and form of government. The division of privileges and duties among the consulting and visiting surgical and medical staff and the assignment of services and responsibilities among the house staff are frequently matters of extended discussion, developing radically divergent views and leading to more or less unsatisfactory experimentation. A certain general uniformity prevails in these matters in the various hospitals of the United States, modified here and there by local custom and tradition. As it is well, however, to have, for our guidance, some standard that has been approved by long use in an intelligent community, I will give here a few abstracts from some of the more important regulations governing the organization of one of our oldest hospitals, and will add such comments as the various subjects seem to demand.

Superintendent.—"The trustees shall annually . . . elect by ballot a superintendent, who shall also be the resident physician and whose term of office . . . shall continue one year, and until his successor shall be elected." (By-Laws of the Cincinnati General Hospital.) In metropolitan hospitals the superintendent delegates his duties as resident physician to a salaried medical officer chosen for that purpose, who, indeed, frequently bears the title of Resident physician, and this officer performs, in the name and by the authority of the superintendent, all the medical and surgical duties assigned to the latter officer. This arrangement relieves the superintendent of the routine medical and surgical work which would devolve upon him as resident physician, while it secures to him authority and control over every department of the hospital. This is the reason why, in large municipal hospitals, at any rate, the superintendent should be a well-qualified medical man. The titles and numbers of the visiting medical and surgical staff should depend upon the size of the hospital and the various services that it is divided into.

The Staff of Visiting Physicians and Surgeons.—In the majority of hospitals in this country the members of the visiting staff receive their appointment from the trustees or governors of the institution; their nomination, in most instances, emanating from those who are already members of the staff. The number of those constituting either the medical or the surgical staff varies, as a matter of course, a good deal in the different hospitals. In one case, for example, there will be a single surgeon at the head of the surgical department of the hospital, and under him there will be several assistant surgeons, the number varying according to the average number of patients requiring surgical treatment. This, I believe, is the plan adopted at many of the hospitals in Germany. In another institution, the service will be divided among as many as six surgeons, all of them of equal rank and authority, and each one of them serving for from two to six months continuously according to the manner in which the service is subdivided. Twenty-five or thirty years ago this was the almost universal custom among the large metropolitan hospitals in the United States. At the present time the tendency is so to organize the service of the attending medical men, both physicians and surgeons, as to render this service as attractive and as instructive as possible to those in charge.

Formerly, it was a very common practice for the attending physicians and surgeons to draw lots for the purpose of determining the particular periods of the year during which each one should be on regular duty; and doubtless this or some similar method is adopted at the present time in all hospitals in which the attending staff consists of four or more members. In those hospitals in which the work is so organized that the attending surgeons or physicians have a continuous service, it is provided that one of the assistant surgeons shall take the place of the chief during periods of illness, vacation, etc.

The remarks of Dr. A. J. Ochsner, of Chicago, in relation to this matter of the visiting staff of a hospital are so instructive and of such a practical nature that I shall make no apology for quoting them here somewhat fully:—*

"The visiting staff of a hospital containing not more than four hundred surgical beds should never consist of more than four attending or visiting surgeons, in order that the patients may be directly under the care of men who have a sufficient amount of work in the institution to make it worth while to take a desirable amount of responsibility. If each surgeon's division contains more than thirty beds, it is well to conduct it as a separate unit with a separate assistant visiting surgeon and a separate resident surgeon for each unit, because this number of patients is sufficient to keep one resident surgeon reasonably engaged, and because, by making a separate department, there is a possibility of thorough systematizing. . . . The service of members of the visiting staff should be continuous, in order that a uniform system may be developed. During the vacations of the visiting surgeon, the assistant visiting surgeon will naturally continue the system of his chief, so that there will be no interruption in the development.

"In each department the responsibility should rest on the visiting surgeon, who should personally visit every patient three times each week at least, and should invariably examine every patient within forty-eight hours after admission, and as much earlier as possible. Either he or the assistant visiting surgeon should personally examine every patient who enters the hospital seriously ill at once upon admission and before an operation is performed or active treatment is begun. In case neither of these surgeons is obtainable, then a visiting surgeon from another department should be called, who should take charge of the case temporarily in case an immediate operation must not be performed. In case an immediate operation is indicated by the existing condition, then the patient should remain permanently under the care of the surgeon performing the operation, in order to make the after-treatment accord with the conditions required, as indicated by the conditions found and corrected at the time of the operation. . . . In order that the duty of visiting the serious cases personally may not become too burdensome to the members of the visiting staff, the following system has been employed with great benefit. If there are four visiting surgeons, one treats all cases that come to the hospital directly,—i.e., without being referred to the service of any particular surgeon,—which are admitted from the first to the seventh of each month inclusively. The second surgeon treats all that are admitted from the eighth to the fifteenth inclusive. The third treats those which are admitted from the sixteenth to the twenty-second inclusive, and the fourth surgeon those admitted from the twenty-third to the end of the month. . . . Each surgeon can then be prepared to respond to emergency calls during his active period. He can arrange his other work

* "The Surgical Organization of a Hospital," by A. J. Ochsner, in Keen's " System of Surgery," Philadelphia, 1909.

accordingly. During the time he is not on active duty he can complete the treatment of the cases admitted during his active period. He can operate on the cases referred to him personally and on those sent to the hospital by himself. This plan greatly reduces the wear and tear, and still the service remains continuous and enables the surgeon to establish a reasonable system, and at the same time the patients can be certain of competent care."

Farther on, in the same article, Dr. Ochsner states that the following scheme represents what he considers to be an ideal organization of the surgical staff of a hospital:—

1. "Visiting surgeon—in control of the entire department; continuous service; period of service not to exceed twenty-five years.

2. "Assistant visiting surgeon—in control of entire department during vacation of visiting surgeon. First assistant in all important operations. In charge of night work and emergency cases when the visiting surgeon is not available. Continuous service. Period of service not less than five nor more than ten years. Appointed by visiting surgeon. Must have served as externe and as resident surgeon.

3. "Resident surgeon—one for every thirty patients; serves as second assistant for a period not less than one and one-half nor more than three years.

4. "Externes—each resident surgeon should have one or two assistants, serving for a period of three, four, or six months. These young men should be recent graduates or senior students in some recognized medical school. They should serve as clinical assistants to the resident surgeons, without responsibility. They should not be permitted to administer any treatment independently. . . . If there is an out-patient department, this may be placed under the care of the assistant visiting surgeon, who may choose his assistants from the resident and externe staff. This makes the out-patient department permanently subordinate to the hospital proper."

The Nursing Department.—The number of nurses necessary for the proper equipment of a large municipal general hospital is variously stated by various authors. Some fix the number as high as one nurse to three patients, but the proportion generally accepted as sufficient by most of the large American hospitals to-day is one nurse to five patients; the actual distribution of the nurses in the hospital varying from a very small allotment, in the case of such departments as the obstetrical service, to a very large allotment in the medical service. In considering the nursing force and its distribution throughout the hospital, and estimating the requirements present and future of the nurses' home, we must bear in mind the dual character of the hospital nurse—as nurse and as student—and the peculiar division and subdivision of the nursing force as a working organism. In the one case the nurse as a student must be assigned successively to all or almost all the regular services in the hospital, and, while in those services, she must acquire certain experiences by having charge of certain definite kinds of work. For instance, in the medical service the pupil will be giving plunge or sponge baths this week, will be superintending the preparation and distribution of food next week, and will be preparing and administering medicines the week after, and so on. On the other hand, it is evident that, from an educational standpoint, the pupil must not be advanced too rapidly, lest she miss the substantial groundwork of her profession, and lest a responsibility beyond her educational qualifications be thrust upon her, to the possible

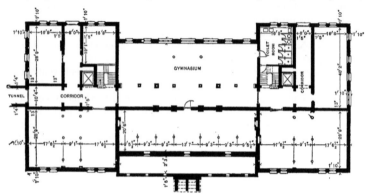

Fig. 336.—Plan of Basement of the Nurses' Home, Cincinnati General Hospital.

injury of a patient. In the second place, the nurses are subject, as before stated, to various divisions and subdivisions. Primarily, there is the division into the day and night force; secondarily, there is the division of these two forces among the various hospital services in the proper proportion; and, thirdly, there is

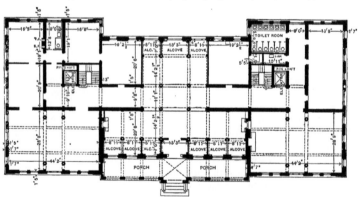

Fig. 337.—Plan of the First Floor of the Nurses' Home, Cincinnati General Hospital.

the frequent necessity of assigning to serious cases, in almost every service of the hospital, special nurses who are to devote their attention exclusively to one particular case. As these latter considerations have to be governed to a very great extent by the former, it will be seen that the management of the nursing force in every large hospital calls forth the best executive ability and resourcefulness of the superintendent of the training school for nurses.

The work of nursing being a severe strain both on mind and body, the nurses' home should have a comfortable interior and pleasant surroundings. It should, if possible, be cut off from the rest of the hospital buildings by trees and shrubbery, and should be furnished within with possibilities both for recreation and for exercise. The physical and mental excellence of the nursing staff is one of the best possible assets of a hospital, and nothing should be neglected that tends to conserve these valuable qualities. If the nurses are afforded abundant opportunities of enjoying themselves in their own home, they will not be so strongly tempted to seek that enjoyment outside.

Another even more important matter is the food supply. While many institutions have an evil reputation in this respect, it is highly probable that

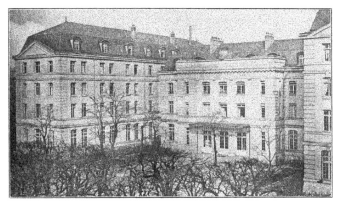

Fig. 338.—School for Female Nurses at Paris, France; under the Management of the "Assistance Publique."

the fault lies more in the manner in which the food is cooked and served than in the food supply itself. A great variety of good and nutritious food is procurable in all markets at reasonable prices, and a good cook can make the simplest fare appetizing. It will certainly pay any hospital management, therefore, to engage thoroughly competent cooks at liberal wages and thereby secure the contentment of its working force while maintaining their digestions and their vigor unimpaired. It is usual in most hospitals for the superintendent of the training school to take her meals with the other heads of departments in an "officers' dining room." When we consider, however, that it is her duty to train nurses, not only for the technical duties of their profession but in all the amenities and qualifications that go to the making of a good nurse, not only in a hospital but in the homes of a refined and educated class of the population, it is to be seen that it is her duty to preside at the meals of her nurses and to inculcate manners and lead in topics of conversation that will give to her graduates the refinement that should be the possession of every member of this delicate and peculiar vocation. Such a motherly familiarity will make it the more easy to establish and maintain the honor system, both in conduct and in school work, which should prevail in every training school.

The plans of the Nurses' Home of the Cincinnati General Hospital were submitted to superintendents of training schools and to others familiar with institutional work in many hospitals, before the work of construction was begun and it is believed that they represent the highest standards of this character of building. These plans (Figs. 336 and 337) show a building one hundred and sixty-five feet long, fifty-eight feet deep through the centre, and seventy-six feet deep through each wing. On the basement floor provision is made, in the west centre of the building, for a gymnasium seventy feet long and thirty-one feet wide. This is lighted by four single windows and three double windows

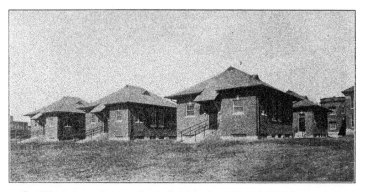

Fig. 339.—One-story Structures for the Isolation of small Groups of Miscellaneous Contagious Diseases and Mixed Infection that cannot be placed in the General Wards; Philadelphia Hospital for Contagious Diseases. (By courtesy of the hospital authorities.)

in the western wall. On the north the gymnasium opens into a toilet room containing the usual shower baths. In the northwest corner is a room to be fitted up as a private laundry for the nurses, where they may themselves wash and iron such articles as they are unwilling, for any reason, to send to the general hospital laundry. The rest of the abundant space on this floor is to be utilized as trunk rooms, store rooms, etc. The first-floor plan shows the main entrance to the building through a porch and vestibule opening into the main reception hall. This is a large handsome space shaped like an inverted T or Greek cross, the horizontal arm of the cross measuring seventy feet and the vertical arm fifty-three feet. On the east wall of this hall are placed, on each side of the main entrance, three alcoves, each seven feet deep by nine feet wide, and on the west wall there are three more alcoves of a similar shape and of similar measurements. In these alcoves the nurses may entertain their visitors with a reasonable degree of privacy,—a fact which will add very much to the home-like features of the place. The northwest corner room (40 ft. x 17 ft.) of this floor is the library, and the northeast corner room (44 ft. x 29 ft.) is a lecture room, where the pupil nurses will receive their instruction from the Superintendent of the Training School and from the members of the hospital staff.

Some idea of the importance attached abroad to the practice of giving nurses such a systematic course of training that they shall be thoroughly well fitted to take care of the sick in the community at large may be formed from the accompanying illustration (Fig. 338), which is copied from a photograph of the School for Female Nurses at Paris, France.

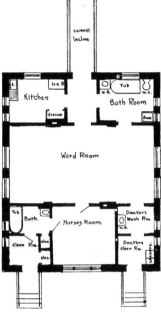

Fig. 340.—Floor Plan of One of the Small Isolation Hospitals Shown in Fig. 339.

Special Hospitals.—As general medicine and surgery have become specialized there has arisen a demand for special hospitals, and therefore we find to-day an ever-increasing number of hospitals devoted to special departments of medicine and surgery. As might be expected in populous, wealthy, and highly civilized communities, these varieties of hospitals represent all the specialties in medical and surgical practice, and we find in a single city,

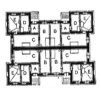

Fig. 341.—Ground Plan of Observation Pavilion in Vienna—a small hospital for the care of cases in which more time must elapse before the diagnosis of an infective disease may safely be excluded. A, A, Entrances; B, B, rooms for the nurses; C, C, rooms for patients; D, D, teakitchen; E, E, bathrooms. (From "Das Wiener Versorgungsheim.")

in addition to the great national or municipal general hospital, ophthalmic hospitals, hospitals for women and children, surgical hospitals, hospitals for diseases of the chest, lying-in hospitals, orthopedic hospitals, hospitals for contagious diseases, hospitals for nervous and mental diseases, hospitals for diseases of the nose, throat, and ear, and emergency hospitals for the prompt care of acute disease or accident in the congested centres of industrial activity. In addition to these are the great institutions for those unfortunate conditions which are regarded as essentially chronic and in a great majority of cases incurable. It is easy to see that almost all of these varieties of hospitals present special problems of their own in the matters of location, construction, and management. The ophthalmic hospital, for instance, having of necessity a large out-patient department, should have a location central to the residence district that it serves and easily accessible from the homes of its prospective patients.

Hospitals for Contagious Diseases.—Hospitals designated by this title are those which are planned for and used for the reception of cases of the ordinary contagious diseases of children, viz., diphtheria, measles, and scarlet fever. Hospitals for the other contagious diseases such as consumption and smallpox are always set off by themselves in selected locations and are not grouped with nor classed with the others. One of the best-known hospitals for contagious diseases in the United States is the Chester Park Hospital of Boston. It is the contagious-diseases department of the Boston City Hospital, and was designed by the Architect Wheelwright and Dr. Rowe, the Superintendent of the Hospital.

If the plans of any of the older hospitals for contagious diseases are compared with those of quite recent date,—as, for example, those of the Philadelphia Hospital for Contagious Diseases, which was completed in 1909 (Figs. 339 and 340), and that of an observation pavilion in Vienna (Fig. 341),—one will scarcely fail to observe an evolution from the complexity of a decade and a half ago to the greater simplicity of these recent buildings. This greater simplicity has been found perfectly compatible with the proper management of the cases and the arrest of the spread of contagion, and, of course, it makes at the same time for greater efficiency by reducing the amount of detail work required from the physicians and nurses.

MILITARY SURGERY.

By Major CHARLES LYNCH, Medical Corps, U. S. Army.

THE special lesions which military surgeons encounter particularly from the nature of their calling are ably discussed elsewhere in these volumes. The present article will be devoted, therefore, to questions of organization and administration affecting the medical department of the army which physicians in the service are called upon to solve, but which should be of interest to all medical men as patriotic citizens with special knowledge of the requirements of medicine and surgery.

Military sanitation has loomed so large, from the recent experiences of armies at war, that the suggestion has been made that medical officers should be styled military sanitarians rather than military surgeons. Both terms are misleading, however. The military medical officer, as a matter of fact, is neither exclusively a surgeon nor a sanitarian. An efficient army is one which preserves its own strength at the maximum while at the same time it is prepared to inflict the maximum injury on the enemy. The medical department should participate in the attainment of both these objects; that is to say, the medical department should be such as will most promote the efficiency of the army of which it forms a part. In order that it may accomplish this, it is evident that the professional talent available must be so organized and administered that maximum results shall be attained. Ability to do this constitutes the specialty of the military medical officer. Nor can this be effected solely by good sanitation. The latter, it is true, will result in many men being found on the firing line instead of in hospitals at the rear. But good surgery is potent in effecting the same result. By good surgery, in this connection, good surgical technique is not meant; perhaps it may be best described as surgery appropriate to the time and place.

Appropriate surgery in war means, first, such surgical assistance at all points as is most effective from the patriotic standpoint,—that is, which will add most to the efficiency of the army; and, secondly, that which is best for the individual. Not infrequently in war the interests of the individual must be sacrificed to those of the nation. Good surgical assistance in war strengthens the army at the front by increasing the morale of troops, which is always impaired if the needs of the wounded are not given prompt attention. In furtherance of the same object the wounded must be promptly removed from the vicinity of their comrades. At the same time, no wounded should be permitted to go further to the rear than their condition demands, and this devolves on the medical department, as does also fitting the wounded for prompt return to the ranks through efficient surgical treatment. Humanity also demands that, as soon as the opportunity offers on the way from front to rear, but especially at the rear where it can be made of most use, there shall be available to the individual soldier the finest surgical skill in the nation, with the best facilities for exercising it.

In this discussion it is not possible to describe surgical organization and administration exclusively. The organization of the medical department of an army does not permit this. It will, therefore, be necessary to discuss the organization and administration of the army medical department as a whole, and only occasionally to give consideration to questions of a purely surgical nature. The general principles governing the operations of the medical department must, of course, be the same in all armies, but as this article is intended mainly for American readers it is thought best to discuss these principles in connection with the United States Army. This will, therefore, now be done without further preamble, beginning with a study of the general organization of that Army.

General Organization.

1. The organized land forces of the United States consist of the Regular Army and of the organized militia when called into the military (land) service of the United States.

2. In peace the Army of the United States consists, ordinarily, of the Regular Army; but whenever the United States is invaded or in danger of invasion from any foreign nation, or of rebellion against the authority of the Government of the United States, or the President is unable with the regular forces at his command to execute the laws of the Union, he may call into the military service of the United States all or any part of the militia organized as a land force.

In war, or when war is imminent, the Army of the United States, after the organized militia has been called into service, may be further augmented by the employment of volunteers.

3. The Regular Army of the United States consists of general officers, the General Staff Corps, the Adjutant General's Department, an Inspector-General's Department, a Judge-Advocate-General's Department, a Quartermaster's Department, a Subsistence Department, a Medical Department, a Pay Department, a Corps of Engineers, an Ordnance Department, a Signal Corps, the Military Academy, chaplains, regiments of cavalry, field artillery, and infantry, a Coast Artillery Corps, and such other officers and enlisted men as are provided for by law.

* * * * * *

After January 21st, 1910, the organization, armament, and discipline of the organized militia in the several States, Territories and the District of Columbia will be the same (with some minor exceptions) as that which is now or may hereafter be prescribed for the Regular Army. (Field Service Regulations.)

The following table refers to the regular establishment and is quoted from the Army List and Directory of Officers of the Army of the United States, dated June 20th, 1910, at the Adjutant General's Office:—

AUTHORIZED STRENGTH OF THE ARMY.

	Major generals.	Brigadier generals.	Colonels.	Lieutenant colonels.	Majors.	Captains.	First lieutenants.	Second lieutenants.	Chaplains.	Total commissioned officers.	Enlisted men.
General officers	6	15								21	
Adjutant General's Dept.	1	1	5	7	10					24	
Inspector General's Dept.		1	3	4	9					17	
Judge Advocate General's Department		1	2	3	6					12	
Quartermaster's Dept		1	6	9	20	60				96	200
Subsistence Department		1	3	4	9	27				44	200
Medical Department		1	15	21	102	110	a396			a645	(b)
Pay Department		1	3	4	20	25				53	
Corps of Engineers		1	10	16	32	43	43	43	1	189	2,002
Ordnance Department		1	6	9	19	25	25			85	720
Signal Corps		1	1	2	6	18	18			46	1,212
Bureau of Insular Affairs		1	1		1					3	
Fifteen regiments of cavalry			15	15	45	225	225	225	15	765	12,775
Six regiments of field artillery			6	6	12	66	78	62	6	236	5,220
Coast Artillery Corps		1	14	14	42	210	210	167	14	672	19,321
Thirty regiments of infantry			30	30	90	450	450	450	30	1,530	25,231
Porto Rico Regiment of Infantry						11	10	10	1	32	576
Military Academy			4	2						6	500
Recruiting parties, recruit depots, and unassigned recruits											8,000
Service — school detachments											546
United States Military Prison guards											320
Indian scouts											75
Total Regular Army	7	27	124	146	423	1,270	1,455	957	67	4,476	76,898
Additional force: Philippine scouts						52	64	64		180	5,732
Grand total	7	27	124	146	423	1,322	1,519	1,0²1	67	4,656	82,630

a Includes 221 first lieutenants of the Medical Reserve Corps on active duty.

b Under the act of Congress approved March 1st, 1887 (24 Stat. L. 435), the enlisted men of the Medical Department (Hospital Corps) are not to be counted as part of the strength of the Army. The authorized strength of the Hospital Corps is 3,500 enlisted men.

The Organized Militia.—The strength of the Organized Militia, as reported by the officers of the Regular Army after the annual spring inspections, is 118,926 officers and enlisted men. This is an increase of 7,985 over that reported last year. This total strength is distributed among the infantry, cavalry, and artillery arms, as follows:

Infantry:

Regiments	141
Separate battalions	9
Separate companies	8
Cavalry, troops	69
Field artillery, batteries	48
Coast artillery, companies	88

Since the spring inspection reports there have been organized 31 additional companies of Coast Artillery, and plans have been made in the several seaboard

States and the District of Columbia for the organization of 19 more during the ensuing year, making a total of 138 companies of Coast Artillery which will probably be in existence by the end of the fiscal year 1910.

As showing clearly the aims and objects of the War Department authorities in regard to the organization of our land forces the following quotation is made from the most recent report of the Secretary of War:—

Military Policy for Defence of the United States.—The military system of the United States contemplates a correlation of the Regular Army with the National Guard. It necessarily follows that the organization of the Regular Army and the militia in combination should be such as to permit them to cooperate and practise together in time of peace under conditions similar to those which would obtain in time of war.

For several years, and more particularly since 1903, the War Department and the National Guard organizations have been working together in great harmony and with increasing effectiveness toward this end.

Joint camps of instruction and manœuvres in which the army and national guards have taken part have been held biennially since 1903 in different parts of the country which have been of pronounced benefit to all the troops engaged. The participation of the National Guard in these manœuvres has given to the Regular Army the inestimable advantage not otherwise obtainable of experience in the manœuvring of large masses of men under conditions of service assimilated so far as practicable to the actual conditions that may be expected when war is on. The National Guard, in addition, had the opportunity to acquire military experience in association with professional soldiers. The number of men, Regular Army and National Guard combined, participating in these different manœuvres has ranged from 30,000 to 50,000. Recognizing the fact that Congress was not likely to authorize in time of peace so large an increase in the seacoast artillery as is necessary for the complete manning detail for all the guns of the coast defence of the United States, the plan has been inaugurated and put in successful operation of relying on the militia of the seacoast States to furnish a part of the remainder. The time has now arrived when a rational plan should be devised for a similar cooperation of the army and the militia with respect to the mobile army.

In order to put such a plan in operation and permit of practice under war conditions in time of peace by the Regular Army and the Militia in combination the United States should be divided into a number of territorial and tactical districts, so that the organized militia of the States comprising such districts may be conveniently combined with the Regular Army stationed therein into permanent brigades, divisions, and corps for instruction and tactical organization. It will probably be found desirable to have in each State in such district at least one military post, the said posts to be occupied by troops of the different arms of the service in such numbers that when the troops from all the posts included in the district are assembled they would constitute a division, including the proper proportion of all arms and branches of the regular service. This regular organization should be the educator and assistant of the militia forces of these States and should be the centre from which general instruction could be given. No post smaller than a regimental one is of real value from a military standpoint, so far as education, discipline, and drill are concerned.

The present system of departmental military government should give way to an organization tactically correct for war purposes; that is, these various troops, both regular and militia, gathered together, should be permanently designated in name and organization, with all the attendant system which would be in existence in time of war, so that when the troops retire to their proper stations they will not lose their brigade or division organization and will be controlled by their proper commanding officers, stationed within the district.

In each tactical corps or division district a central point for a camp site should be selected, with a view to the convenience and economy of easy concentration of both the regular and militia forces in such district. The regular and militia troops should be concentrated for instruction at these points. Such camps will answer the purpose of permanent brigade posts, so far as instruction is concerned, and the marching to and fro from the regimental stations to such points will bring the army before the people and more or less in contact with them.

Should such plan be carried out it would be possible to concentrate about eight army corps—possibly somewhat imperfect and incomplete. In case the Regular Army alone should be required it would be practicable to concentrate at least eight complete divisions at eight different points, each division complete in itself for any possible use as an expeditionary force. Should a larger force be required, then the militia composing the other organizations of each corps could be quickly assembled at the concentration points with the Regular Army. Every State should have a young and active officer of the Regular Army detailed at headquarters, who should report direct to the corps commander and have general supervision, under the militia authorities, of the instruction of the militia. There should be on the staff of each corps commander an officer of the army, who should have entire charge of all militia affairs in the corps district. The commander of each district, in addition to the Regulars under his control, should have general supervision of all the National Guard troops of the States included in his district, and, while in time of peace he has no power to issue orders, he could, however, by his interest and suggestion, be of great value to the militia. He should be given the power to supervise the equipment and instruction of the troops of his district and held responsible for their mobilization and general condition.

In time, at the points of concentration in each corps district, there should be established supply depots, so planned that upon the assemblage of the corps or divisions there would be available such equipment as might possibly be lacking in the various States for the equipment of their organizations, although it is contemplated that the States should themselves carry all that is necessary for at least the minimum strength required. At such depots could also be carried the supplies for any additional volunteer force, up to a moderate number, which might be deemed necessary to complete in its entirety the organization of any one of the various corps.

What is greatly needed is a decentralization of the powers of supply and initiative. The present centralization always breaks down the moment it is put to the test, and the peace organization of the army as it stands to-day is incomplete and improper for military purposes.

It is proposed to submit such plan of organization to the governors of the States, asking their assent thereto, as all this system, so far as the National Guard is concerned, must be voluntary. Upon receiving such assent from the governors, the War Department should designate in each district the exact organizations, assigning the various branches of the service to their proper brigades or divisions. While this will necessarily result in an incomplete organization, as there will be lacking in all branches certain organizations both in the Regular Army and in the militia, still it will be the first step toward carrying out this proposed creation.

There is a shortage of various militia organizations to complete the proposed corps. In order to obtain these necessary organizations the various States should be urged to add to their national guard such organizations as would be required in each district.

The question of coast defense and of utilizing the militia in connection with the coast artillery has been so far developed that it may be assumed that the present system will be continued until perfected, and it is therefore not considered at all in the foregoing, which relates only to the mobile army.

As noted above, in war it is intended that the army be supplemented by the employment of volunteers. At the present writing, however, no law exists for the organization of a volunteer army. What the Chief of Staff lately had to say on this subject is as follows:—

A most important matter for the general welfare of the country is the passage of a comprehensive measure for the organization of a volunteer army, to be raised only after Congress has made a declaration of war. Such a measure would not cost a dollar in time of peace, but would be of inestimable value if the country ever engages in another war. The passage of such legislation will permit of the preparation in peace of all the necessary plans for the organization, equipment, and supply of such a force and the selection of places of mobilization. Without the necessary legislation all such matters must be deferred. The necessity for this legislation should be again urged upon Congress.

For the purposes of this article a more careful and detailed study of the organization of the medical department of the army is demanded.

Organization of the Army Medical Department.

The Medical Department, under the Act of Congress approved April 23d, ·1908 (35 Stats. 66; G. O. 67, 1908), consists of the Medical Corps, the Medical Reserve Corps, the Hospital Corps, the nurse corps, and dental surgeons; to which may be added the contract surgeons employed by virtue of the provisions of the Act of February 2d, 1901 (31 Stats. 752; G. O. 9, 1901) and other civilians employed from time to time under the authority of the annual appropriation acts.

Medical Corps.—Extract from the Act of April 23d, 1908:—

Sec. 2. That the Medical Corps shall consist of one Surgeon-General, with rank of brigadier-general, who shall be chief of the Medical Department; fourteen colonels, twenty-four lieutenant-colonels, one hundred and five majors, and three hundred captains or first lieutenants, who shall have rank, pay and allowances of officers of corresponding grades in the cavalry arm of the service.

Sec. 3. That promotions in the Medical Corps to fill vacancies in the several grades created or caused by this Act, or hereafter occurring, shall be made according to the seniority, but all such promotions and all appointments to the grade of first lieutenant in said corps shall be subject to examination as hereinafter provided: *Provided*, That the increase in grades of colonel, lieutenant-colonel, and major provided for in this Act shall be filled by promotion each calendar year of not exceeding two lieutenant-colonels to be colonels, three majors to be lieutenant-colonels, fourteen captains to be majors, and of the increase in the grade of first lieutenant not more than twenty-five per centum of the total of such increase shall be appointed in any one calender year: *Provided further*, That those assistant surgeons who at the time of the approval of this Act shall have attained their captaincy by reason of service in the volunteer forces under the provisions of the Act of February second, nineteen hundred and one, section eighteen, or who will receive their captaincy upon the approval of this Act by virtue of such service, shall take rank among the officers in or subsequently promoted to that grade, according to date of entrance into the Medical Department of the Army as commissioned officers.

Sec. 4. That no person shall receive an appointment as first lieutenant in the Medical Corps unless he shall have been examined and approved by an army medical board consisting of not less than three officers of the Medical Corps designated by the Secretary of War.

Sec. 5. That no officer of the Medical Corps below the rank of lieutenant-colonel shall be promoted therein until he shall have successfully passed an examination before an army medical board consisting of not less than three officers of the Medical Corps, to be designated by the Secretary of War, such examination to be prescribed by the Secretary of War and to be held at such time anterior to the accruing of the right to promotion as may be for the best interests of the service: *Provided*, That should any officer of the Medical Corps fail in his physical examination and be found incapacitated for service by reason of physical disability contracted in the line of duty, he shall be retired with the rank to which his seniority entitled him to be promoted; but if he should be found disqualified for promotion for any other reason, a second examination shall not be allowed, but the Secretary of War shall appoint a board of review to consist of three officers of the Medical Corps superior in rank to the officer examined, none of whom shall have served as a member of the board which examined him. If the unfavorable finding of the examining board is concurred in by the board of review, the officer reported disqualified for promotion shall, if a first lieutenant or captain, be honorably discharged from the service with one year's pay; and, if a major, shall be debarred from promotion and the officer next in rank found qualified shall be promoted to the vacancy. If the action of the examining board is disproved by the board of review, the officer shall be considered qualified and shall be promoted.

Sec. 6. That nothing in this Act shall be construed to legislate out of the service any officer now in the Medical Department of the Army, nor to affect the relative rank or promotion of any medical officer now in the service, or who may hereafter be appointed therein, as determined by the date of his appointment or commission, except as herein otherwise provided in section three.

Section five above was modified by proviso in the Act approved March 3d, 1909 (a), reading as follows (35 Stats. 737):—

Provided, That any major of the Medical Corps on the active list of the army who, at his first examination for promotion to the grade of lieutenant-colonel in said corps, has been, or shall hereafter be found disqualified for such promotion for any reason other than physical disability incurred in the line of duty shall be suspended from promotion and his right thereto shall pass successively to such officers next below him in rank in said corps as are, or may become, eligible to promotion under existing law during the period of his suspension; and any officer suspended from promotion, as hereinbefore provided, shall be re-examined as soon as practicable after the expiration of one year from the date of the completion of the examination that resulted in his suspension; and if on such re-examination he is found qualified for promotion, he shall again become eligible thereto; but if he is found disqualified by reason of physical disability incurred in the line of duty, he shall be retired, with the rank to which his seniority entitles him to be promoted; and if he is not found disqualified by reason of such physical disability, but is found disqualified for promotion for any other reason, he shall be retired without promotion.

Reference to the table giving the authorized strength of the army will show the number of medical officers actually in service.—It will be noted that a considerable number of medical officers are still required to attain the strength contemplated by the Act in force at present.

Medical Reserve Corps.—Extract from the Act of April 23d, 1908:—

Sec. 7. That for the purpose of securing a reserve corps of medical officers available for military service, the President of the United States is authorized to issue commissions as first lieutenants therein to such graduates of reputable schools of medicine, citizens of the United States, as shall from time to time, upon examination to be prescribed by the Secretary of War, be found physically, mentally, and morally qualified to hold such commissions, the persons so commissioned to constitute and be known as the Medical Reserve Corps. The commissions so given shall confer upon the holders all the authority, rights, and privileges of commissioned officers of the like grade in the Medical Corps of the United States Army, except promotions, but only when called into active duty, as hereinafter provided, and during the period of such active duty. Officers of the Medical Reserve Corps shall have rank in said corps according to date of their commissions therein, and when employed on active duty, as hereinafter provided, shall rank next below all other officers of like grade in the United States Army: *Provided*, That contract surgeons now in the military service who receive the favorable recommendation of the Surgeon-General of the Army shall be eligible for appointment in said reserve corps without further examination: *Provided further*, That any contract surgeon not over twenty-seven years of age at date of his appointment as contract surgeon shall be eligible to appointment in the regular corps.

Sec. 8. That in emergencies the Secretary of War may order officers of the Medical Reserve Corps to active duty in the service of the United States in such numbers as the public interests may require, and may relieve them from such duty when their services are no longer necessary.

Provided, That nothing in this Act shall be construed as authorizing an officer of the Medical Reserve Corps to be ordered upon active duty as herein provided who is unwilling to accept such service, nor to prohibit an officer of the Medical Reserve Corps not designated for active duty from service with the militia, or with the volunteer troops of the United States, or in the service of the United States in any other capacity, but when so serving with the militia or with volunteer troops, or when employed in the service of the United States in any other capacity, an officer of the Medical Reserve Corps shall not be subject to call for duty under the terms of this section: And *provided further*, That the President is authorized to honorably discharge from the Medical Reserve Corps any officer thereof whose services are no longer required: And *provided further*, That officers of the Medical Corps of the Army may, upon the recommendation of the Surgeon-General, be placed on active duty by the Secretary of War and ordered to the Army Medical School for instruction and further examination to determine their fitness for commission in the Medical Corps: And *provided further*, That any officer of the Medical Reserve Corps who is subject to call and who shall be ordered upon active duty as herein provided and who shall be unwilling and refuse to accept such service shall forfeit his commission.

Sec. 9. That officers of the Medical Reserve Corps when called upon active duty in the service of the United States, as provided in section eight of this Act, shall be subject to the laws, regulations, and orders for the government of the Regular Army, and during the period of such service shall be entitled to the pay and allowances of first lieutenants of the Medical Corps with increase for length of service now allowed by law, said increase to be computed only for time of active duty: *Provided*, That no officer of the Medical Reserve Corps shall be entitled to retirement or retirement pay, nor shall he be entitled to pension except for physical disability incurred in the line of duty, while in active duty: And *provided further*, That nothing in this Act shall be construed to prevent the appointment in time of war of medical officers of volunteers in such numbers and with such rank and pay as may be provided by law.

In addition to the 216 officers of the Medical Reserve Corps given as on active duty in the tabular statement of strength, 239 officers are on the inactive list of that corps. Many on the latter list are specially distinguished in their profession and are of more than national reputation. Their services could naturally be made of the greatest value in the event of war, though generally these officers have received no military training.

Hospital Corps.—Extract from the Act of March 1st, 1887 (24 Stats. 435):—

That the Hospital Corps of the United States Army shall consist of hospital stewards, acting hospital stewards, and privates; and all necessary hospital services in garrison, camp or field (including ambulance service) shall be performed by the members thereof, who shall be regularly enlisted in the military service; said corps shall be permanently attached to the Medical Department, and shall not be included in the effective strength of the Army, nor counted as a part of the enlisted force provided by law.

  *   *   *   *   *   *

The Act of March 2d, 1903 (32 Stats. 930), defines the present status of the corps as follows:—

That hereafter the Hospital Corps of the United States Army shall consist of sergeants first class, sergeants, corporals, privates first class, and privates; the rank of sergeants first class, sergeants, and privates first class shall be as now provided by law for hospital stewards, acting hospital stewards, and privates of the Hospital Corps. That the Secretary of War is authorized to organize companies of instruction, ambulance companies, field hospitals, and other detachments of the Hospital Corps as the necessities of the service may require.

Acting cooks, Hospital Corps, under the act approved May 11th, 1908, are authorized as follows:

One to each post or station where a hospital is conducted and whose garrison is equal to two companies or more but less than a regiment or its equivalent; one to each transoceanic transport; two to each Hospital Corps company of 100 men or less, and an additional one where the strength is greater than 100 men; two to each general hospital (one of them to be the special diet cook) recruit depot, and post having a garrison of a regiment or more where a hospital is conducted.

* * * * * *

Lance corporals may also be appointed in the Hospital Corps, but no detachment is permitted to have more than one non-commissioned officer to four privates.

The Hospital Corps is now always kept at approximately full strength, 3,500. In fact, this number is not sufficient to permit the regulation allowance in peace at the various posts, etc.

Contract Surgeons.—Extract from the Act of February 2d, 1901, Sec. 18:—

That in emergencies the Surgeon-General of the Army, with the approval of the Secretary of War, may appoint as many contract surgeons as may be necessary, at a compensation not to exceed $150 per month.

Few contract surgeons are now employed, their services being utilized only at arsenals, at very small posts, or in case of temporary emergency.

Dental Surgeons.—Extract from the Act of February 2d, 1901:—

That the Surgeon-General of the Army, with the approval of the Secretary of War, be, and he is hereby, authorized to employ dental surgeons to serve the officers and enlisted men of the Regular and Volunteer Army, in the proportion of not to exceed one for every one thousand of said Army, and not exceeding thirty in all.

* * * * *

Extract from Act of March 2d, 1907 (34 Stats. 1163):—

That hereafter the number of dental surgeons authorized by law shall be thirty-one, of which number one shall be detailed to the United States Military Academy.

The dental corps is kept constantly at the maximum number, 31.

Nurse Corps.—Extract from the Act of February 2d, 1901:—

Sec. 19. That the Nurse Corps (female) shall consist of one superintendent, to be appointed by the Secretary of War, . . . and of as many chief nurses, nurses, and reserve nurses as may be needed. Reserve nurses may be assigned to active duty when the emergency of the service demands.

* * * * * *

The number of women nurses now fixed by the Secretary is 100. The number actually in service averages between 90 and 100.

The regulations governing the Army Nurse Corps are also applicable in general terms to male nurses under contract.

No male nurses are employed in time of peace.

The employment of male nurses, of female nurses not in the Nurse Corps, of cooks and of other civilians necessary for the proper care of sick officers and soldiers is authorized in the annual appropriations for the "Medical and Hospital Department," under such regulations fixing their number, qualifications, assignment, pay and allowances as may be prescribed by the Secretary of War. The pay of other civilian employés, such as clerks, messengers, watchmen, packers, laborers, etc., in the administrative offices and supply depots of the Medical Department is provided for in the same appropriations.

The latter class varies somewhat in numbers from time to time. Shortage in the clerical force sometimes occurs, but, generally speaking, the needs of the medical department in the direction of the personnel in question are adequately met.

Organized Militia.—It has been stated above that the organization of the militia now corresponds to that of the regular establishment. While this is true in the meaning of the paragraph cited, it should be noted that the militia, generally speaking, so far as the medical department is concerned, has only a few administrative medical officers and the medical officers attached to troop units. A few field hospitals are now being established, but, so far as known at present, these do not exceed three or four for all the States. The medical personnel of the militia, too, is wholly confined to medical officers and hospital corps men. The total number of the former is approximately 674 and of the latter 2,240.

National Aid Volunteer Associations.—The American National Red Cross is the officially recognized voluntary aid association of the American people. This association was reorganized in 1905 and it is now in close touch with the War Department. Three or four Red Cross Relief Columns have been started in various parts of the country, but have not yet been placed on the definite status occupied by similar organizations in other countries. A limited number of women nurses and a very few physicians have also been enrolled. At present, therefore, our Red Cross has almost no trained personnel from the military standpoint.

REWARDS IN THE ARMY MEDICAL SERVICE.

Pay of Medical Officers.—The medical corps of any army must compete with the civil profession and with other governmental services for candidates; therefore it is necessary to examine with some care into the relative rewards.

The pay of medical officers of our service is the same as for other officers of like grade, and is as follows: (See page 906 for table.)

Medical officers, as well as other officers in our service, receive certain allowances in addition to their pay, and these are on a fairly liberal scale. Each medical officer has quarters, fuel, and lights, or commutation therefor provided. He may obtain forage for two horses, if such horses are actually kept.

TABLE OF PAY ALLOWED BY LAW TO OFFICERS OF THE ARMY, ANNEXED TO THE ARMY REGISTER CONFORMABLY TO THE RESOLUTION OF THE HOUSE OF REPRESENTATIVES OF AUGUST 30TH, 1842.

GRADE.	PAY OF OFFICERS IN ACTIVE SERVICE.					
	PAY OF GRADE.		MONTHLY PAY.			
	Yearly.	Monthly.	After 5 years' service.	After 10 years' service.	After 15 years' service.	After 20 years' service.
			10 per ct.	20 per ct.	30 per ct.	40 per ct.
Lieutenant General	$11,000.00	$916.67	....	....	....	....
Major General	8,000.00	666.67	....	....	....	....
Brigadier General	6,000.00	500.00	....	....	....	....
Colonel	4,000.00	333.33	$366.67	$400.00	$416.67	$416.67
Lieutenant Colonel	3,500.00	291.67	320.83	350.00	375.00	375.00
Major	3,000.00	250.00	275.00	300.00	325.00	333.33
Captain	2,400.00	200.00	220.00	240.00	260.00	283.00
First lieutenant	2,000.00	166.67	183.33	200.00	216.67	233.33
Second lieutenant	1,700.00	141.67	155.83	170.00	184.17	198.33

GRADE.	PAY OF RETIRED OFFICERS.					
	PAY OF GRADE.		MONTHLY PAY.			
	Yearly.	Monthly.	After 5 years' service.	After 10 years' service.	After 15 years' service.	After 20 years' service.
Lieutenant General	$8,250.00	$687.50	....	....	....	....
Major General	6,000.00	500.00	....	....	....	....
Brigadier General	4,500.00	375.00	....	....	....	....
Colonel	3,000.00	250.00	$275.00	$300.00	$312.50	$312.50
Lieutenant Colonel	2,625.00	218.75	240.62	262.50	281.25	281.25
Major	2,250.00	187.50	206.25	225.00	243.75	250.00
Captain	1,830.00	150.00	165.00	180.00	195.00	210.00
First lieutenant	1,530.00	125.00	137.50	150.00	162.50	175.00
Second lieutenant	1,275.00	106.25	116.87	127.50	138.12	148.75

NOTE.—The highest grade in the medical department is that of Brigadier General.

Below the grade of major a government horse and horse equipment are provided when required for official duties. Each officer is also permitted to buy certain articles of food from the subsistence department at wholesale prices, and he receives travelling expenses at the rate of seven cents per mile while travelling on duty. The medical officer has all his books and instruments provided by the government. It is estimated that these various allowances amount to from $1,200.00 in the lowest grade, to $1,800.00 in the upper grades. All officers are retired on three-quarters pay if they become disabled as an incident of service. It should be remembered, however, that all physicians in the army have expenses incident to service which their brothers in civil life can escape.

The question of promotion is a no less important one in contrasting relative rewards. By the recent act to increase the efficiency of the medical department, service in the grade of first lieutenant was reduced from five to three years. Promotion to grades above that of captain depends wholly on the occurrence of vacancies, and there is no selection except for Surgeon-General. On account of the great number of original vacancies created by the act in question, promotion occurs at the present time at a relatively rapid rate. Some medical officers have reached the grade of major with a total service of less than ten years. In the nature of things this is but a temporary condition, however, and, as soon as the original vacancies created by the act have been filled, attainment of the grade of major will require seventeen or eighteen years, or even a longer service, as was formerly the case. The new act will also serve to promote some majors to the grade of lieutenant-colonel after a service of less than twenty years. This period will, however, just as for the promotion of captains, be considerably lengthened in the near future. The last officer promoted to colonel had served for about thirty years, although, for the reasons stated above, this period is considerably less than that usually required.

As compared with civil practice it will be noted that the rewards are much larger at the outset, but that the higher grades of the medical corps are not characterized by emoluments comparable with those of the successful practitioner in civil life. As compared with the line of the army, promotion in the medical corps is rapid up to the grade of lieutenant-colonel. After that, the advantages are with the line, and this is especially marked for the rank of general officers. Any line officer with creditable service stands a fair chance of appointment to one of the many vacancies which occur in this grade. With the medical corps, however, the chance for any individual to be appointed Surgeon-General is decidedly remote.

While the material rewards have been given precedence it is undoubtedly true that they alone do not operate to induce physicians to enter the medical corps of the army. The notable achievements of some of the members of that corps during and since the Spanish-American War have acted as a considerable incentive in attracting candidates. Then besides, the military spirit is no less in the medical profession than in other walks of life, and a few physicians would select the army as a career no matter how bright prospects they might have outside it. Tradition and family association with the service also influence some men to choose it by preference.

Pay of Medical Reserve Officers.—Officers of the Medical Reserve Corps receive the pay of first lieutenant, with the usual allowances and increase for service. They are not eligible for promotion except when they change their status by entering the medical corps from the medical reserve corps.

Pay of Militia Medical Officers.—Medical officers of the Militia receive the same pay as do other officers when in the service of the United States. Promotion varies so much in the different States and from time to time that it is impossible to discuss it. Generally speaking, such promotion depends upon the occurrence of vacancies.

Pay of the Members of the Hospital Corps.—The Hospital Corps rates of pay are as follows: (See page 908 for table.)

Pay of Dental Surgeons and Nurses.—Dental surgeons receive $150.00 per month, with certain allowances. Nurses receive $50.00 per month, with certain increases for length of service and for foreign service. Chief nurses receive addi-

Rank.	1st enlist-ment.	2d enlist-ment.	If re-enlisted within three months.				
			3d enlist-ment.	4th enlist-ment.	5th enlist-ment.	6th enlist-ment.	7th enlist-ment.
Sergeant first-class	50	54	58	62	66	70	74
Sergeant .... } Acting cook	30	33	36	39	42	45	48
Corporal	24	27	30	33	36	39	42
Private first-class	18	21	24	27	30	33	36
Private	16	19	22	23	24	25	26

tional compensation up to $30.00 per month. The pay of the Superintendent is $1,800.00 annually. Nurses also have fairly liberal allowances.

As the efficiency of the medical department must naturally be dependent on the character and attainments of the individuals composing it, and as these must in general terms depend on the rewards offered, careful study of this subject is demanded. Until the passage of the recent act to increase the Medical Corps it may be stated, without fear of contradiction, that these rewards were too low. At the present time they would appear to be adequate, as there were 250 applications for examination last summer, and sixty candidates were obtained for the Army Medical School. It should also be noted that the pay of the army was increased at about the time when the medical department bill was passed. In time to come, when promotion in the medical corps again becomes very slow, especially if the cost of living continues to increase, the medical corps will undoubtedly again suffer from a lack of candidates. Even under present conditions it must be realized that the vacancies created have not, up to the present time, been filled.

National Guard medical officers, as has been previously stated, receive the same rewards when actually in service as do other medical officers. So the remarks previously made apply equally to the former. Under present conditions, however, a much larger sacrifice of time is demanded of militia medical officers than was formerly the case, and it is quite within the bounds of possibility that at some time in the not distant future, it will become increasingly difficult to keep up the strength of the National Guard so far as medical officers are concerned.

From what has already been said in reference to the compensation of officers of the Medical Reserve Corps it will be realized that the rewards in this corps are notably lower than in the Medical Corps proper, as there is no promotion in the former. Under present conditions it is possible to get the few physicians required for active service in the Reserve Corps. This corps was created by giving a new status to physicians who were serving as contract surgeons—that is, to those who were recommended therefor. So far as known, all these gentlemen accepted their commissions in the Reserve Corps. Nearly all, however, regard this employment as of a temporary character and so drop out when the opportunity offers to better themselves in civil life. The attractions of the Reserve Corps are not to be despised by the young physician who desires temporary employment. Some of the older men in the Reserve Corps are so wedded to the service that they do not desire to return to civil practice. The rewards of this corps are of course totally inadequate for the distinguished physicians on its inactive list. These gentlemen, however, only accepted commissions therein with the understanding that they would be employed solely when their country demanded their services, and therefore, so far as they are concerned, the question of compensation does not enter.

Relatively, the compensation of the Hospital Corps was notably decreased, as compared with the rest of the army, by the recent bill providing for increase of pay. This has caused the Hospital Corps to be regarded as less desirable. Applications for transfer from Hospital Corps to Line were formerly very rare. In the fiscal year ending June 30, 1908, thirty-six such transfers were made, and last year these increased to sixty-seven. Moreover, it is becoming increasingly difficult to enlist good men for the Hospital Corps. The natural tendency, unless the pay is increased, must be toward a less efficient corps.

No great difficulty has been experienced in obtaining a sufficient number of dental surgeons to keep that corps at its maximum. This has not been true of the Nurse Corps which has continually been about ten per cent short of the maximum number. An act which has recently been approved, should serve to remedy this condition.

ADEQUACY OF PERSONNEL.

Another most important question in this connection is whether the allowances, as regards numbers, of the various classes of medical personnel are adequate for the needs of our service. To determine this, it is first necessary to study what these needs are. It is scarcely necessary to state that the organization of any army should be based on its requirements for war. Our practice, contrary to that of every other nation, so far as the medical department is concerned, has been to disregard the possibility of war and to supply a personnel less numerous than is required in peace. I am informed that a careful study of the requirements of our medical department based on the necessities of war, but demanded in peace if an efficient war organization is to be built up, shows that there should be a regular establishment of one thousand medical officers. This estimate is reached in the following manner:—In the event of war with a first-class power we should require four hundred thousand men at once. For the proper care of this number a medical department personnel of forty thousand (ten per cent of the total) would be needed. Ten per cent of the total forty thousand should be medical officers. Japan, from her recent vast experience in war, estimates that all medical officers in a war army should have received military training. In fact, that nation found that only such officers could be depended upon for efficient service in the Russo-Japanese War. In Great Britain, which (with the exception of our own country) is at the other end of the scale, the military authorities state that, with fifty per cent of trained officers of the regular establishment, they would be in a fairly satisfactory condition.

It will be seen, therefore, that one thousand medical officers for the regular establishment is a more modest estimate than would be made by any other nation. This number has been reached, however, by several specially well-informed medical officers who have taken into account all the positions which, for satisfactory service in our four-hundred-thousand war army, would have to be filled by trained officers of the regular establishment. From what has been said the impression should not be gained that the training conferred by service as a medical officer in the National Guard is not appreciated. On the contrary, the special ability acquired through such training by medical officers of the National Guard has been taken into full account in the estimate in question.

Before we conclude this subject it will be well to point out that, so far as medical officers of the regular establishment are concerned, we are the only civilized nation which has failed to provide at least sufficient medical officers for the needs of the peace army. During the present period of peace, we are compelled, owing to the shortage of officers of the Medical Corps, to employ approximately one hundred and fifty officers in the Medical Reserve Corps. This number is exclusive of candidates for the Medical Corps commissioned in the Medical Reserve Corps for instruction at the Army Medical School.

It may be appropriate here to devote a few words to the consideration of the number of medical officers of the National Guard generally esteemed necessary as an adequate preparation for the organization of our army in war. As already noted on an earlier page, very few States have as yet provided field hospitals and ambulance companies. It is thought that the National Guard should provide enough medical officers for all the organizations at the front. In most nations the needs of the line of communications of war armies have been partially provided for by the Red Cross, by the organization of relief columns. As stated, we have only begun the creation of similar voluntary aid organizations.

On the basis of a ten-per-cent medical personnel for a four-hundred-thousand war army approximately thirty-two thousand Hospital Corps men would be required. It is assumed that the difference between thirty-six and forty thousand,—the thirty-six thousand being composed of four thousand medical officers and thirty-two thousand Hospital Corps men,—would be filled by dental surgeons, women nurses, and civilian employés. It being assumed again that special military training is as requisite for the Hospital Corps as for the Army generally, six thousand Hospital Corps men in peace would be required as a framework for the thirty-two thousand required for the war army. As noted elsewhere, the present allowance for the regular establishment is thirty-five hundred Hospital Corps men. This number does not meet the peace requirements of the Army at its present strength on the basis of the allowance set by the regulations. For these, about forty-one hundred Hospital Corps men are needed. It is believed that the requirements of the National Guard, so far as the Hospital Corps is concerned, should be based on those for the organizations of the front, as already noted in connection with medical officers.

No discussion is required on the subject of the creation of a corps of civilian employés for war, as this naturally could be provided for at the time, in accordance with the special needs of the military and medical situation. It is also believed that the dental surgeons required for the increased needs of a war army could be got by the employment of civilian dentists. It seems to be the general opinion, however, that thirty-one dental surgeons, the number at present in the service, do not meet the requirements of our regular army in peace. The Surgeon-General, in his last report, stated that to give each man in the service one treatment a year would require a corps of sixty dental surgeons, and he recommended that this number be allowed. As no recommendation for increase of the Nurse Corps is to be found in this report it is presumed that the present number is considered sufficient for the needs of the service.

QUALITY OF THE PERSONNEL.

In the organization of any medical corps quality is scarcely, if at all, less important than quantity. The standard set for the Medical Corps of our army has always been a high one, and searching examinations are required for entrance into the corps and afterward for each promotion up to the grade of lieutenant-colonel.

Appointments to the Medical Corps of the Army are made by the President after the applicant has passed the prescribed examination and has been recommended by the Surgeon-General.

(a) The examination will consist of two parts—a preliminary examination and a final or qualifying examination with a course of instruction at the Army Medical School intervening.

.   .   .   .

An applicant for appointment in the Medical Corps of the Army must be between twenty-two and thirty years of age, a citizen of the United States, and a graduate of a reputable medical school legally authorized to confer the degree of doctor of medicine, in evidence of which his diploma will be submitted to the board at the time of his preliminary examination.

Hospital training and practical experience in the practice of medicine, surgery, and obstetrics are essential, and an applicant will be expected to present evidence that he has had at least one year's hospital experience, or the equivalent of this in practice.

The preliminary examination will be as follows:

Physical: The physical examination must be thorough and will conform in all respects to that required of candidates for commission generally. Each applicant will also be required to certify that he labors under no physical infirmity or disability that can interfere with the efficient discharge of any duty he may be called upon to perform.

Written examination on the following subjects: Mathematics (arithmetic, algebra, and plane geometry), geography, history (especially of the United States), general literature, Latin grammar, and the reading of easy Latin prose. English grammar, orthography, and composition will be determined from the applicant's examination papers.

This examination may be omitted in the case of applicants holding diplomas or certificates from reputable literary or scientific colleges, normal schools or high schools or of graduates of medical schools which require an entrance examination satisfactory to the faculty of the Army Medical School.

Written examination in the following subjects: Anatomy, physiology and histology, chemistry and physics, materia medica and therapeutics, surgery, practice of medicine, obstetrics and gynæcology.

.   .   .   .

. Applicants who attain a general average of not less than eighty per cent in the written examinations will, upon pledging themselves to accept a commission in the Medical Corps, if found qualified in the final examination, and to serve at least five years thereunder unless sooner discharged, be appointed to the Medical Reserve Corps with the rank of first lieutenant and ordered to the Army Medical School, Washington, D. C., for instruction as candidates for admission to the Medical Corps of the Army. If, however, a greater number of applicants attain the required average than can be accommodated at the school the requisite number will be selected according to relative standing in the examination.

.   .   .   .

The final or qualifying examination will be held at the close of the term of the Army Medical School and will be conducted by at least three members of the school board. It will comprise, first, a thorough physical examination; second, the regular school examination; and third, a clinical examination. .A candidate claiming a knowledge of ancient or modern languages, higher mathematics, or scientific branches other than medical, may be given a special examination in the same. Proficiency in such special examination will receive due credit in determining the candidate's relative standing.

The searching character of the preliminary examination for entrance into the Medical Corps may be appreciated from the fact that about one out of every three candidates who present themselves for examination, is accepted. A few more are rejected at the final or qualifying examination. This year (1909–1910), for the first time, a mid-year examination has been held at the Army Medical School; it is understood that two candidates were dropped as the result of this examination.

Appointments in the Medical Reserve Corps are made by the President after the applicant has passed the prescribed examination and has been recommended by the Surgeon-General. ·

The physical examination will conform to that of the Medical Corps.

The professional examination will consist of an oral examination in the following subjects: practice of medicine; surgery; obstetrics and gynæcology; and hygiene.   ·

Should the oral examination in any subject be unsatisfactory, the applicant may be permitted to take a written examination on that subject.

(Manual for the Med. Dep't.)

Medical Reserve Corps officers have no examinations after they enter that service.

The examinations for the medical officers of the organized militia are, in very general terms, based on those for medical officers of the regular establishment. They are regulated, however, by the various States concerned, and naturally they vary very widely in different parts of the country. Generally speaking, States with strong militia organizations demand an adequate and satisfactory examination for medical officers, and States with weak National Guard organizations require little or no examination for entrance into their Medical Corps, and no examinations thereafter. In this connection it is very encouraging to note that, in recent years, examinations for the Medical Corps have been made much more searching in the States as a whole.

In the regular establishment members of the Hospital Corps who are enlisted for, and permanently attached to, the medical department have the same physical examination for enlistment as that required for soldiers generally, and they must satisfy the requirements of all soldiers in reference to enlistment. No examination is required for promotions to the grade of corporal, lance corporal, and private first class. For the grade of sergeant the candidate must pass a satisfactory examination under the direction of the Surgeon-General or the chief surgeon of a division or department; for sergeants first class, an examination is given under the direction of the Surgeon-General.

In nearly all the States candidates for the Hospital Corps have a physical examination on entering the service. Their examinations for promotions vary widely in different States.

Candidates for the position of dental surgeon are required to pass a rigid physical examination, and those who do not possess the required physical qualifications will not be permitted to enter upon the professional examination. The latter examination embraces both theoretical knowledge and practical operative and prosthetic dentistry; particular stress being laid upon clinical examination in practical work. (Manual for the Med. Dep't.)

No examination other than that on entrance is required from dental surgeons.

Candidates for the Army Nurse Corps are required to pass a satisfactory professional, moral, mental, and physical examination. No examination other than that for entrance is required, except for promotion to the grade of Chief Nurse.

DUTIES OF THE MEDICAL DEPARTMENT.

The duties of the medical department, as defined by Army Regulations, are as follows —

The Medical Department is charged with the duty of investigating the sanitary condition of the Army and making recommendations in reference thereto, of advising with reference to the location of permanent camps and posts, the adoption of systems of water supply and purification, and the disposal of wastes, with the duty of caring for the sick and wounded, making physical examinations of officers and enlisted men, the management and control of military hospitals, the recruitment, instruction, and control of the Hospital Corps and of the Army Nurse Corps (female), and furnishing all medical and hospital supplies, except for public animals.

EDUCATION AND TRAINING.

For the performance of these duties a special education is required. Contrary to the custom in a number of other services our medical officers are all graduated physicians when they enter the Medical Corps.

The Army Medical School, which is located in Washington, D. C., is conducted for those candidates for the Medical Corps who have passed the preliminary examination, for older medical officers who obtain permission to attend, and for medical officers of the organized militia. As a matter of fact, few students are found there except from the first class, although in almost every school course are one or two medical officers of the organized militia. In the nature of things it is not probable that great numbers of such officers will ever find the time necessary for attendance upon this school.

The object of the Army Medical School is to train the students therein in such subjects as are appropriate to the duties which a medical officer of the army is called upon to perform.

The course of instruction shall be both theoretical and practical, and shall embrace a period of eight months, commencing on the 1st of October.

The course of instruction shall embrace the following subjects:—(1) Duties of medical officers, Medical Department administration, and customs of the service; (2) military hygiene; (3) clinical microscopy and bacteriology; (4) military surgery; (5) military and tropical medicine; (6) sanitary chemistry; (7) hospital corps drill; (8) operative surgery; (9) ophthalmology and optometry; (10) x-ray work; and (11) equitation.

(Manual for the Medical Department.)

It will be noted that this list of subjects contains a number which would be studied as a matter of course in any medical school. In practice it has been found, however, that this is necessary in order to qualify medical officers for all their duties in the service. This also seems to be the practice in similar schools in other countries, though a number of such schools devote considerably more time relatively to military instruction. It is noteworthy that most military medical schools are increasing their courses on the subject of map reading, and it certainly seems essential, in these days of large armies, that medical officers should be proficient in this and other military subjects to a greater extent than has been the case with us in the past.

In the regular establishment all service constitutes, or should constitute, a course of post-graduate instruction. The searching examinations for promotion which have been previously mentioned render it necessary that all medical officers should keep abreast of the times in medicine as well as in their military duties if they wish to avoid the risk of failing for promotion or even of being separated from the service.

Tropical service also presents its special problems, and service in the field in a tropical country is now by no means unusual. Manœuvres on a great scale, such as are held in the more military nations, have not been available to us until within the last few years. Nor as yet do they compare favorably, in respect to the questions presented for solution by large bodies of troops gathered together on a war footing, with the grand manœuvres conducted by a number of countries. Moreover, shortage in personnel and transportation, which always exists in the medical department in our manœuvres, makes the lessons to be learned from them by that department of much less value than they would be if provisions could be made to put it actually on a war basis at such times. As a matter of fact, until the summer of 1909 no complete field hospitals and ambulance companies had been assembled since the Spanish-American War. In the interim the organization of these two units had been considerably changed, and consequently there was only theoretical knowledge of how they would actually be operated. In 1909, however, three camps for the instruction of militia medical officers were established. Each of these camps had a complete field hospital with an ambulance company. They were so successful in all respects that, it is presumed, they will be established every other year in the future, the general manœuvres being held in the intervening years. The difficulties encountered in organizing complete field hospitals and ambulance companies for the camps in question have led to an increased sentiment, on the part of many officers, that a few of these organizations should be maintained at all times. Nothing has yet been done in this direction.

As is true in other respects, the education of medical officers of the organized militia varies to a considerable extent in the different States. In some, correspondence schools are in operation; in others, medical officers are gathered together at more or less frequent intervals for study and discussion of their special problems; and, in still others, practically no instruction of this character is given. All medical officers of the organized militia now have some experience in examining recruits, which unquestionably benefits the service as a whole, though it is extremely burdensome and time-consuming for these physicians, who, as a rule, are busily occupied with their own private practices. These medical officers also have the opportunity for drill presented by the medical departments of the organizations to which they belong. Summer camps and manœuvres afford them practice in military sanitation. It is the universal opinion, however, that the camps for instruction for militia medical officers established in 1909, which have been mentioned above, afforded the best opportunity that has yet been presented for the instruction of such officers.

Since the immediately preceding paragraphs were written another long step in advance has been taken in methods for educating medical officers. This is described as follows in a general order issued July 11th, 1910:—

1. A field service school for medical officers is established as a part of the Army Service Schools at Fort Leavenworth, Kansas.

2. This school will be known as the Army Field Service School for Medical

Officers. Its object is the preparation of officers of the medical corps and of medical officers of the organized militia for the better performance of their duties as administrative and staff officers on field service and to make research into such subjects as may concern medical officers under field conditions.

3. The commandant and the secretary of the Army School of the line will be the commandant and secretary, respectively, of the Army Field Service School for Medical Officers. The assistant commandant will be an officer of the medical corps with grade not lower than that of major.

PERIOD OF INSTRUCTION.

4. The course of instruction will cover a period of not less than six weeks, beginning about April 1st of each year.

STUDENT OFFICERS.

5. Selection of student officers will be made as follows:

(a) The Surgeon General will submit to the Adjutant General of the Army, not later than January 1st of each year, the names of not less than four nor more than eight officers of the medical corps whom he recommends for detail for instruction in the school.

(b) Medical officers of the organized militia who may apply for entrance and whose admission may receive the approval of the Secretary of War, not to exceed a total of six in any one session, may also be detailed for instruction in the school, subject to the provisions of paragraphs 6, 11, 13, 14, 15, 16, and 17, General Orders, No. 69, War Department, 1910.

The details will be announced in orders from the War Department.

COURSE OF STUDY.

6. The course of study will be conducted under the three existing departments of the Army Staff College as follows:

I. The Department of Care of Troops.
II. The Department of Military Art.
III. The Department of Engineering.

I. Department of Care of Troops.

The course will comprise the following subjects or fields of inquiry:

(a) Duties of the medical department in the field; general sanitary organization; the details of organization of the various sanitary units; the functions of administrative medical officers; sanitary equipment and supply; the transportation service of the front; range of modern weapons; battle casualty percentages; location and function of mobile relief organizations during action; sanitary service of the line of communications and of the base; the use of the Red Cross and other voluntary aid associations.

Instruction will be by lectures, conferences, problems, terrain exercises, and the practical use and direction of organized field sanitary units.

(b) The civil function of the medical department in occupied territory.

Instruction will be by conferences and problems.

(c) The preparation of a scheme for the organization, equipment, and supply of the medical department of a large military force, either expeditionary or on the defensive.

Instruction will be by conferences and problems.

II. Department of Military Art.

The course will comprise the following subjects:

(a) Organization and administration of troops in the field; orders; the elementary principles of tactics; staff administration and supply.

Instruction will be by lectures, demonstrations, tactical and staff rides.

(b) In co-operation with the department of care of troops there will be at least one manœuvre on map or terrain to illustrate the relation of the sanitary service to the military forces as a whole.

III. Department of Engineering.

The course will comprise theoretical and practical work in the following subjects:

(a) Military topography, map reading; the principles and practice involved in the use of all classes of maps for military purposes.

Instruction will be by lectures, conferences, practical examinations, and studies of terrain.

(b) Military topography, sketching; the principles and practice involved in the rapid making of simple road and position sketches.

Instruction will be by lectures, conferences, and brief field practice.

CO-OPERATION.

7. The student officers of the Army Field Service School for Medical Officers and the organized sanitary units located at Fort Leavenworth will be used with the several service schools in terrain exercises, manœuvres, and staff or tactical rides, to the end that the student officers of all these institutions may obtain the maximum benefit from the exercises prescribed.

CERTIFICATES OF PROFICIENCY.

8. Student medical officers who complete the course satisfactorily will receive certificates setting forth that fact.

NEGLECT OF DUTY.

9. Should any student officer neglect his studies or other military duties he will, upon recommendation of the academic board, approved by the commandant, and by authority of the Secretary of War, be relieved by the commandant from duty at the Army Field Service School for Medical Officers and sent forwith to join his proper station.

REPORT ON QUALIFICATIONS.

10. At the end of the course of instruction the academic board will report upon the qualifications of each student officer for the performance of medical staff duties.

Each report will be forwarded by the commandant, with such remarks in the case as he deems proper, to the Adjutant General of the Army for file with the personal record of the officer concerned.

ORDERS TO GOVERN.

11. So far as they do not conflict with this order the provisions of General Orders, No. 69, War Department, 1910, will govern.

By another general order of approximately the same date an Army Field Service and Correspondence School for Medical Officers has been organized at Fort Leavenworth, Kansas, and has been designated as one of the Army Service Schools. At present it is realized that only a small number of medical officers will find it practicable actually to go to Leavenworth. For this class the "correspondence school" is designed. Students of this school will be given practical problems for solution from time to time. The solutions will be returned to Fort Leavenworth within a specified period and will then be commented on by the medical officer in charge of this special branch of the work. The "correspondence school" is already in operation. The thirty ranking majors of the medical corps in the United States who have not been examined for promotion have been designated by the Surgeon General as students for the first course. The first problems have been solved by these officers and returned to Leavenworth.

Some years have now elapsed since the first company of instruction for the Hospital Corps of the regular establishment was created. Four such companies are now in existence. As far as possible all men entering the Hospital Corps are sent first to such companies. I quote the following from the regulations on this subject:—

The length of the course of instruction for recruits is four months and in addition to discipline covers the following subjects: (1) Duties of a soldier; (2) bearer drill; (3) first aid and personal and camp hygiene, including the sterilization of water and disinfection; (4) anatomy and physiology; (5) diet cooking; (6) nursing, including bandaging and the use of Medical Department appliances; (7) materia medica and pharmacy; (8) care of animals, and equitation; (9) clerical work; (10) field work.

Instruction in clerical work, materia medica, and pharmacy will only be given to men of sufficient intelligence and aptitude.

Selected men who have completed this course of instruction may be given two months additional instruction in one or more of the following subjects: Pharmacy, clerical work, and cooking. Instruction for non-commissioned officers including candidates for that position, covers the following subjects: Elementary hygiene, minor surgery, army regulations, mess management.

Besides the instruction given to Hospital Corps men of the regular establishment, at the companies of instruction, every Hospital Corps detachment under its senior medical officer is also given courses of instruction both in winter and in summer: these courses being appropriate to the different seasons. Non-commissioned officers and men of this corps are also continually practised in their duties in garrison and in the field. Manœuvres are of value to them just as they are to medical officers.

No such elaborate course of instruction as that outlined above can of course be given to the Hospital Corps of the National Guard. As a general thing, it is only practicable to teach these men discipline, drill, and first-aid, nor do they have much practice in caring for sick, for at the annual encampments and manœuvres, the only time when they could have sick to care for, serious cases are promptly sent to hospitals or to their homes. In a few States, in a very few organizations, schools for non-commissioned officers of the Hospital Corps are conducted. At the general manœuvres members of the Hospital Corps of the organized militia get the benefit of practical experience in the performance of their duties in the field.

Dental surgeons hardly require instruction in military duties, nor do they receive it. Members of the Army Nurse Corps are invariably sent on appointment to a large military hospital, where they can learn the military routine before going to the tropics or elsewhere.

It will be noted that nothing has been said in reference to instruction of officers of the Medical Reserve Corps, nor is there any general system for this. At present, newly appointed officers of this corps on the active list are usually assigned to a large post where they can be initiated in their duties by a senior medical officer. Officers on the inactive list are supplied by the Surgeon-General's office with the more interesting publications which appear from time to time on the medico-military service.

Aside from formal courses of instruction the closer affiliation of recent years between medical officers of the regular establishment and those of the National Guard has been of considerable educational value to both classes. A society, The Association of Military Surgeons of the United States, is also available to both. This society publishes monthly a journal to which National Guard and Army medical officers both contribute. The annual meeting of the association permits the interchange of views and experiences.

The distribution of an army in time of peace is of course a matter of very considerable importance in regard to the effectiveness of its training for war. This applies to the medical department as well as to other parts of the army, though this is sometimes forgotten. In a word, there is no question but that any army which in time of peace is organized as nearly as may be as it would be in war enjoys a considerable advantage when war comes. The opposite condition has been the bane of the American army ever since its creation. Not so many years ago the presence of hostile Indians in our Western country necessitated the maintenance of many small garrisons, and similar conditions are true in the Philippines to-day. It is obvious that an army so distributed is totally unable to make a practical study of the problems connected with serious warfare. While present conditions would permit our army to be gathered into large garrisons within the limits of the United States proper, we nevertheless still maintain considerably over a hundred small posts. A number of these, it is true, are coast artillery posts, which must be maintained in any event. The report of the Secretary of War, quoted at length above, shows that the War Department is quite aware of this unfortunate condition of affairs.

Without further discussion of this subject we may now consider the effect which these numerous small posts have on the medical officers of the regular establishment. It is believed that they tend to exert a dwarfing influence, both from the military and from the medical standpoint. From the military standpoint the small post presents very little opportunity for practical instruction. From the medical standpoint conditions are not very much better, as the opportunities for medical practice are necessarily limited. Moreover, a wholly false sense of proportion is created as to military and medical duties, the latter being given far too much prominence. It is not too much to say that, in the past at any rate, the status of the medical officer was fixed wholly in the minds of most people by his success as a family practitioner in garrison. It is almost needless to point out that this was in no sense the measure of his value as an army medical officer. What has been said does not mean that it would be desirable to subordinate the doctor to the officer. Quite the contrary, he should be a good doctor when he enters the service and should continue to be so, giving all his patients the care and attention to which they are justly entitled; but at the same time this should not be permitted to take all his time nor to interfere with his preparation for war, which is as essential to him as to any other officer. In the later years of the medical officer's service it seems essential that the administrative part of his work should replace to a considerable extent the medical. To be sure, it seems a great pity that medical experience should be sacrificed by such a plan. It is impossible to escape from it, however, if we are to have an efficient medical service in war, the goal for which we should all be striving. This fact seems to have been recognized in our service by the character of the examinations which are now prescribed for promotion to the grade of lieutenant-colonel in the Medical Corps. Knowledge of medicine alone is not sufficient to enable the officer to pass these examinations, nor—as has been previously stated—should this be the case if we are to have an efficient medical corps in war and, so far as this conduces to that result, an efficient army. In considering this question it will be well to look at the other side of the picture. In reading the history of the Civil War it will be found, in numerous instances, that eminent civil practitioners commissioned as medical officers, without previous experience to fit them therefor, and placed in positions of great administrative responsibility, disregarded their responsibilities in this respect and devoted themselves to professional attendance on individuals. Some of these gentlemen have recorded with great pride the number of amputations they made, and undoubtedly made well according to the teachings of that time, but at the same time they were wholly unmindful of the measures which they should have taken as medical officers to promote the efficiency of the army of which they composed an important part. Contrast this condition of affairs with that which existed in the well-organized Japanese Army during the Russo-Japanese War. In that army it was fully realized that, in the interests of the service, as well as in those of the individual, there must be competent direction. This the trained medical officers of the higher grades furnished, thus insuring at all points the surgical skill available to those who needed it, without themselves attempting individually to operate.

Besides the small garrisons which have been mentioned above, a certain number of medical officers in time of peace are stationed either in the Surgeon-General's Office as assistants or as chief surgeons of departments. All these positions imply a considerable administrative responsibility. Our four general hospitals serve as excellent schools for instructing medical officers in administrative work on a scale much larger than that of post hospitals. The general hospitals also give excellent professional advantages which are extended under the policy of the present Surgeon-General to the maximum number of medical officers. A few medical officers are detailed at supply depots, the various schools, etc., and a few have done extremely creditable service as sanitary administrators in Cuba, the Canal Zone, and the Philippines. A very small number are assigned as attending surgeons in cities. The general policy in assigning attending surgeons has been to afford them an opportunity for medical study. Shortage in personnel, however, has made this almost a "dead letter," and, although the advantage of the German plan of assigning medical officers to civil hospitals has been recognized for many years, our corps has never been large enough to permit such a scheme to be put into practice.

As is generally known, medical officers of the National Guard in time of peace devote but a small portion of their time to their military duties. The high grade of efficiency demanded of such officers in recent years has imposed increased sacrifices on their part, and, under present conditions, it is believed that they are devoting as much time as could be possibly expected of them, due account being taken of the fact that nearly all of them must meet the demands of an active civil practice.

The remarks made above in reference to the medical officers of the regular establishment apply with almost equal force to the Hospital Corps. There is, however, one very important difference between the regular medical officers and Hospital Corps men: the former are well qualified in their professional duties on entering the service, while the latter have everything to learn. It is essential, therefore, that Hospital Corps men receive instruction in the actual care of the sick before they are perfected in their military duties; on the other hand, it is desirable that they obtain a certain amount of military knowledge before they are assigned to duty in hospitals. Provision is usually made for both under present arrangements. For example, the ordinary garrison hospital enables Hospital Corps men to learn how to care for the sick, and—as their duties are much less complicated than those of medical officers—they have an opportunity to gain at manœuvres an amount of military experience which is almost if not quite sufficient to enable them to perform such duties well. It is certainly essential, in the training of these men, that everything should tend to develop the military spirit. Under modern conditions of warfare the medical personnel is exposed to such grave risks that every one of their number should be taught to be a good soldier.

Dental surgeons are employed in peace just as they would be in war. The ideal arrangement for the members of the Army Nurse Corps would be to create in peace an organization of which each member would be competent to assume important administrative duties in the event of war. Their employment in peace is intended to promote this object. As will be readily appreciated, however, administrative talent is comparatively rare; hence it is only with a nurse corps of the very best class that this could be accomplished. Employment of the Army Nurse Corps in peace should, without question, help toward the development of the administrative faculty, and administrative positions, with increased pay, are always open to nurses as soon as they manifest that they are capable of filling them.

SUPPLIES.

As previously noted, the medical department is charged with the duty of furnishing all medical and hospital supplies except such as are needed for public animals. This includes medicines, dressings, surgical instruments, operating-room equipment, hospital furniture, the pouches carried by Hospital Corps men, the various medical and surgical chests, those for hospital messes and for food, etc. In addition, a part of the litters and all the travois are provided by the medical department. The equipment of men and horses comes from the Ordnance Department, the food from the Subsistence Department, and the Quartermaster's Department furnishes clothing, tents, animals, wagons, ambulances, etc., as well as sterilizers for water and incinerators. This department also constructs hospital buildings. In time of peace no great difficulty is experienced in obtaining all the various supplies required by the Medical Department. Campaign, or even field, service presents a very different condition, however, and there is much to be said in favor of the opinion expressed by many medical officers that, as a correct principle of administration, the Medical Department should supply all articles used exclusively by that department. The experiences of the Spanish-American War showed that, in the midst of very complex duties, it was extremely difficult for the Quartermaster's Department to give attention to the clamorous needs of the Medical Department. In war the needs of the Medical Department are so enormous that, in the belief of many officers, these needs will never adequately be provided for during peace unless the responsibility for accomplishing this be entrusted to the department itself. What has been said is not intended to maintain, however, that any one department should attempt to be complete in itself so far as supplies are concerned. This is impracticable in any army. An army is in fact very like a chain the strength of which depends on the weakest link; that is to say, no matter how strong our medical department might be, if the other departments were weak the former could not perform its duties properly. The question is often asked: "Was not the Japanese medical department in the Russo-Japanese War very competent and efficient?" It certainly was, but its efficiency was dependent, not on itself alone, but on the fact that it was a part of an extremely well-balanced and well-organized army, in which every other department performed its full part. It is equally certain that, in the event of another war, if this does not prove to be the case with us, the Medical Department will again suffer from criticism which will not be wholly deserved. So far as the medical supplies furnished by the Medical Department itself are concerned, we are now much better prepared than at the time of the Spanish-American War, as such supplies are on hand in sufficient quantities to equip eight divisions. Moreover, tentage for this purpose has been obtained from the Quartermaster's Department and is available for issue with Medical Department units.

Since the passage, some years ago, of the Dick Bill, which requires that the equipment of National Guard organizations be the same as that of the regular establishment, many medical supplies have been issued to the medical department of the guard. Most of this property has been that which pertains to regimental organizations. As noted above, very few Organized Militia field hospitals have yet been created, and therefore naturally there has been little call on their part for equipment. So far as known, no Organized Militia regiments have full medical equipment for either the regimental infirmary or the hospital, but a number have a sufficient amount of such equipment to enable them to take the field for a short period. More or less tentage is also on hand in the regimental medical departments of many States. Transport is generally lacking or is present in very meagre amount.

From what has been said it is apparent that the Medical Department of our army is not wholly prepared for war. It is only fair to point out, however, that conditions in this respect have improved infinitely within the past few years. Before the Spanish-American War there were comparatively few men within the Medical Department itself who realized what the demands of war would be. In the army at large, at that time, it is safe to say that there were not half a dozen officers who had seriously studied the needs of the Medical Department as part of an army in war, and there was no public sentiment in favor of the creation of a medical department nucleus from which could grow a strong body that would support the weight of war. Now the Medical Department itself is clearly aware of what it must have if it is to play its proper part in war; and a large number of officers outside of that Department realize its necessities very nearly as well as does the Department itself. The question is one of a complicated character and not easy for everybody to understand. Its satisfactory solution may be looked for only in the remote future, when a public sentiment shall have been created in favor of making the expenditures necessary to the building up of a Medical Department framework strong enough to stand up under the heavy load that will be placed upon it during war. Some such public sentiment was manifested by the passage of a bill in 1908 to increase the efficiency of the Medical Department of the Army. Other countries have made much progress in bettering the organization of their medical departments, and it therefore behooves us as a nation, if we would not fall behind, to give the most serious consideration to this subject.

Organization in Time of War.—While the organization provided for our army in time of peace is totally different from that provided for any other army, it may be said, in general terms, that the war organizations of different countries (our own included) do not vary except in minor details. Just at present our War Department is making some radical changes in organization and administration. These are embodied in the new Field Service Regulations and the new Manual for the Medical Department. The latter has not yet been published It is believed, however, that the text as it now stands in the MS. will not be materially altered before it is set up in type, and that I may therefore safely refer to it here as something definitely settled. It is evident that, with radical changes so imminent in the Manual, any discussion based upon the statements made in the older text would be obsolete almost before his article is printed.

Before I proceed to discuss the Medical Department particularly it will be necessary for me to describe the organization of our war army as a whole. The following paragraphs are taken from the new Field Service Regulations:—

UNITS OF ORGANIZATION.

The company and regiment are both administrative and tactical units; the battalion and brigade are, as a rule, tactical only. The division is the great administrative and tactical unit and forms the basis for army organization. A *separate brigade* is a command designated as such in orders from competent authority.

Permanent brigades and divisions are created by the War Department. A brigade normally consists of the headquarters and three regiments of infantry. It is the appropriate command of a brigadier general.

For the purposes of instruction at field exercises, manœuvres, etc., temporary brigades and divisions may be formed, and the necessary staffs provided.

DIVISION.—A division normally consists of—

TROOPS
Headquarters
3 brigades
1 regiment of cavalry
1 brigade of field artillery, 2 regiments
1 pioneer battalion of engineers
1 field battalion of signal troops
4 ambulance companies
4 field hospitals

SERVICE OF SUPPLY
Officers and assistants
1 ammunition train
1 supply train (including sanitary reserve)
1 bakery train
1 pack train. Unless detached therefrom, the pack train accompanies the supply train

A division is the appropriate command of a major-general.

A *cavalry brigade* consists of the headquarters and two or more cavalry regiments, three being the normal organization. When the brigade acts independently, horse artillery is attached.

A *cavalry division* consists of—

TROOPS

Headquarters
2 or more cavalry brigades, 3 being the normal cavalry component
1 regiment of horse artillery
1 pioneer battalion of engineers (mounted)
1 field battalion of signal troops
2 ambulance companies
2 field hospitals

SERVICE OF SUPPLY

Officers and assistants
1 ammunition train
1 supply train (including sanitary reserve)
2 or more pack trains. Unless detached therefrom, the pack trains accompany the supply train
A light bridge train is attached when necessary

FIELD ARMY.—A command composed of two or more divisions, and the necessary auxiliary troops, constitutes a *field army*. It receives a numerical or territorial designation, and is the appropriate command of a lieutenant-general. The auxiliary troops forming part of a field army ordinarily consist of—

1 cavalry division or brigade
1 brigade of heavy artillery, consist-
    ing normally of 1 regiment for
    each division in the field army
1 pontoon battalion of engineers
1 aero-wireless battalion of signal
    troops
1 ammunition train
1 supply train
1 ambulance company
1 field hospital

⎫
⎬ Auxiliary Division
⎭

For purposes of administration, marching, and camping, the auxiliary troops (less the cavalry) of a field army are generally united in rear of the divisions and when so united form the "auxiliary division." To this division may also be attached siege artillery and an engineer park, according to the nature of the operations, and a guard of infantry or cavalry when necessary. As far as practicable, the auxiliary division is maintained near the head of the line of communications.

Divisions or brigades operating independently have the necessary auxiliary troops attached. Detachments may also be organized, the composition and staffs being determined by the duty to be performed.

ARMY.—A command composed of two or more field armies constitutes an *army*. It receives a territorial designation and is the appropriate command of a general. Field armies and armies are created only by authority of the President.

Divisions, including cavalry divisions, receive numerical designations in the order of their creation. Brigades are designated First, Second, etc., in each division.

LINE OF COMMUNICATIONS.—For each field army or important expeditionary force about to take the field, a *base* is selected and equipped and a service of the *line of communications* established, both under the control of the commander of the field army or expeditionary force, unless otherwise ordered by the War Department.

MEDICAL DEPARTMENT.

The Medical Department consists of the surgeon-general, and of the commissioned and enlisted personnel, nurses and dental surgeons, authorized by law for that department. The personnel of the department and all other persons assigned to duty with that department, are collectively called *sanitary troops*.

For duty in the field, sanitary troops are divided into (1) those assigned to regiments and other units, and (2) those formed into independent sanitary units, such as ambulance companies and field hospitals.

The following table (on page 927) shows the distribution of the sanitary troops forming part of a complete division. In this distribution the troops assigned to the infantry are divided pro rata among the regiments of that arm. A like distribution is made of the sanitary troops assigned to the cavalry and artillery. The injured of commands having no sanitary troops seek the nearest medical service available.

Auxiliary division of a field army:
1 major, chief surgeon
1 major, inspector   } Headquarters
1 sergeant, 1st class (mounted)
4 privates, 1st class, and privates (mounted)
1 ambulance company
1 field hospital
The personnel attached to the organizations.
Headquarters of a field army:
1 colonel, chief surgeon
1 colonel, inspector
2 majors
2 sergeants, 1st class (mounted)
9 privates, 1st class, and privates (5 mounted)
1 ambulance
1 wagon
The sanitary personnel of the headquarters of an *army* is prescribed when the army is organized.
Line of Communications
For each division at the front:
1 transport column
1 sanitary supply depot
2 evacuation hospitals
1 base hospital
1 base depot
Such other sanitary formations as may be necessary.

Further details in reference to the organization of our medical department for war are contained in the following paragraphs (page 928). It is presumed they will be incorporated substantially as written in the new Manual for the Medical Department.

SANITARY PERSONNEL

DIVISION

	PERSONNEL									MOUNTS AND TRANSPORTATION									Remarks
										MOUNTS			Ambulances	TRANSPORTATION				Total Animals	
	Lieutenant-Colonels	Majors	Captains & Lieutenants	Total Commissioned	Sergeants 1st Class	Sergeants & Corporals	Privates 1st Class and Privates	Total enlisted	Grand Total	Officers	Enlisted men	Total		Wagons	Draft Animals	Pack Animals	Total draft and pack animals		
Division Headquarters	1	1	1	3	1		6	7	10	5	5	10						10	One led horse for each officer above the grade of captain.
Inspection	1			1		1		2	3	2	2	4						4	
Infantry, nine regiments		9	27	36	9	27	180	216	252	45	72	117		9	36	9	45	162	
Cavalry, one regiment		1	3	4	1	3	20	24	28	5	22	27		1	4	1	5	32	
Artillery, two regiments		2	4	6	2	4	36	42	48	8	38	46		2	8	2	10	56	
Engineers, one battalion			3	3		3	4	6	12	3	6	9						9	
Signal, one battalion			2	2		2	6	9	8	2	4	6						6	
Supply train		1	2	2	1	1	3	8	10	2	4	6						6	
Ambulance companies (4)		5	20	21	8	1	281	4	5	1	54	3	48	12	240	16	256	3	
Field hospitals (4)			16	21	12	29	193	318	339	22	34	76		32	128		128	332	
*Reserve supplies			1	1	1	25	9	230	251	26	3	60		6	24		24	188	
						1		11	12	1		4						28	
TOTAL	2	19	80	101	35	97	745	877	978	122	246	308	48	62	440	28	468	836	

CAVALRY DIVISION

	Lieutenant-Colonels	Majors	Captains & Lieutenants	Total Commissioned	Sergeants 1st Class	Sergeants & Corporals	Privates 1st Class and Privates	Total enlisted	Grand Total	Officers	Enlisted men	Total	Ambulances	Wagons	Draft Animals	Pack Animals	Total draft and pack animals	Total Animals	Remarks
Division Headquarters	1	1	1	3	1		6	7	10	5	7	12						12	One led horse for each officer above the grade of captain.
Inspection	1			1		1		2	3	2	2	5						5	
Cavalry, nine regiments		9	27	36	9	27	180	216	252	45	216	261		9	36	9	45	306	
Horse Artillery, one regiment		1	2	3	1	2	18	21	24	4	20	24		1	4	1	5	29	
Engineers battalion, mounted			3	3		3	6	9	12	3	9	12						12	
Signal battalion			2	2		2	4	8	10	2	8	10						10	
Ammunition train			1	1		1	6	8	8	2	4	6						6	
Supply train			1	1	1	1	3	4	5	1	2	3						3	
Ambulance companies (2)		2	10	10	4	14	140	158	168	10	26	36	24	6	120	8	128	164	
Field hospitals (2)			8	10	6	12	96	114	124	12	28	28		16	62		64	92	
*Reserve supplies			1	1	1		11	11	12	1	3	4		6	24		24	28	
TOTAL	2	13	57	72	23	64	469	556	628	87	314	401	24	38	246	18	266	667	

*With supply train.

ORGANIZATION

SANITARY UNITS

AMBULANCE COMPANY

Personnel:
5 medical officers.
9 non-commissioned officers.
70 privates first class and privates.
    Total personnel 84.
Transportation:
. 12 ambulances.
3 four-horse wagons.
4 pack animals.
Mounts:
4 officers.
13 enlisted men.*

FIELD HOSPITAL

(Capacity 108 beds)

Personnel:
5 medical officers.
9 non-commissioned officers.
3 sergeants first class.
6 sergeants.
48 privates first class and privates.
    Total personnel 62.
Transportation:
8 four-horse wagons.
Mounts:
6 officers.
8 enlisted men.*

RESERVE MEDICAL SUPPLY

Personnel.
2 medical officers.
2 non-commissioned officers.
9 privates first class and privates Hospital
    Corps.
    Total personnel 12.
Transportation:
6 four-horse wagons.
Mounts:
1 officer.
2 enlisted men.

EVACUATION HOSPITALS

(Capacity 324 beds)

Personnel:
14 medical officers.
24 non-commissioned officers.
8 sergeants first class.
16 sergeants.
129 privates first class and privates.
    Total personnel 167.
Transportation:
2 four-horse wagons.
3 ambulances.
Mounts:
30 officers.
4 enlisted men.

BASE HOSPITALS

(Capacity 500 beds)

Personnel:
20 medical officers.
1 dental surgeon.
24 non-commissioned officers.
16 sergeants.
129 privates first class and privates.
Nurses (female) 46.
    Total personnel 220.
Transportation:
3 ambulances.
2 four-horse wagons.
Mounts as required.

BASE MEDICAL SUPPLY DEPOT

(For a division)

Personnel:
2 medical officers.
15 enlisted men.
12 privates first class and privates.

HOSPITAL SHIP

(200 beds)

Personnel:
5 medical officers.
5 non-commissioned officers.
35 privates first class and privates.
    Total personnel 45

* In each division the director of ambulance companies and of the field hospital, and
majors, have each one sergeant and one private first class, or an ordinary private in additi
Mounts: 2 officers and 2 enlisted men.

† For each additional division there should be two sergeants and eight privates.

TRANSPORT COLUMN

Personnel:
  2 medical officers.
  10 non-commissioned officers
  32 privates first class and privates.
    Total personnel 44.
Transportation:
  12 ambulances.
  1 wagon.
Mounts:
  3 officers.
  7 enlisted men.

HOSPITAL TRAIN

(A hospital train is made up of ten cars, eight of which are assigned to patients, and will carry 200 men.)

Personnel:
  3 medical officers.
  3 non-commissioned officers.
  24 privates first class and privates.
    Total personnel 30.

The allowance of personnel and material for the Sanitary Squads and other medical department field units is not fixed, but is dependent on the special circumstances.

Before proceeding to the discussion of the operation of the Medical Department in the field it is thought best to quote a few paragraphs referring to the Medical Department from the proposed text for the new Manual and from the Field Service Regulations:—

OBJECTS.—1. Preservation of the strength of the Army in the field.

(a) By the necessary sanitary measures.

(b) By retention of effectives at the front and sending of ineffectives to the rear without interference with military movements.

(c) By prompt succor of wounded on the battlefield, thus promoting the morale of troops and preventing losses to the firing line by line soldiers accompanying wounded to the rear.

2. Treatment of ill and injured. (Med. Dep't Manual.)

PERSONNEL.—In time of war the Sanitary Service includes:

1. All persons serving or employed by the Medical Department, including officers and men temporarily or permanently detailed therein.

2. Members of the American National Red Cross Association assigned to duty with the Medical Department by competent authority.

3. Individuals whose voluntary service is duly authorized. (Med. Dep't Manual.)

Organized Voluntary Aid.—The American Red Cross incorporated by Act of Congress (January 5, 1905), to furnish volunteer aid to the sick and wounded of armies in time of war, is therefore the reserve emergency organization of the American people in time of war. All volunteer aid from any society or association must be furnished to the army through the American Red Cross.

The personnel of the American Red Cross may be employed for service with the army in time of war with the authority of the Secretary of War on recommendation of the Surgeon-General. No one will be so employed unless he or she be physically qualified for service.

   *   *   *   *   *   *

Except in special emergencies Red Cross organizations shall be used only on the line of communications and base and at home.

In general terms the sphere of the work of the Red Cross personnel in war, and of their preparation and training in peace for war, should be as follows:

(a) Organization, training, and equipment of *relief columns* to assist in the care and transportation of sick and wounded.

(b) Organization and training of *hospital detachments* composed of groups of physicians, nurses, pharmacists, cooks, etc., to at once replace the regular service or act as auxiliaries in military hospitals.

(c) Organization and training of other recognized Red Cross columns, detachments, etc.

(d) Taking over certain special branches of hospital work, such as laundry, repair of linen, diet kitchen, etc.

(e) Establishment of rest and food stations.

(f) Collecting, storage, and distribution of Red Cross supplies of all kinds.

(g) Collecting and forwarding gifts.

(h) Formation of information bureaus to keep relatives and friends advised of the location and condition of sick and wounded and prisoners of war.

(i) Providing and equipping hospital ships and trains, automobile ambulances, and other means of transportation.

(k) Providing and furnishing convalescent homes and special hospitals. (Med. Department Manual.)

Independent Voluntary Aid.—Upon the recommendation of the Surgeon-General, and with the authority of the Secretary of War, the chief surgeon of an army in the field, of a division, or of the line of communications or a department, or the commander of a general hospital may use the services of civilian physicians, nurses, male and female, litter-bearers, cooks, etc., voluntarily offered, and will assign such persons to duty as may be most expedient for the good of the service.

(a) As a rule such voluntary aid will be used only at home and base hospitals, or on the line of communications. In emergency the services of physicians and litter-bearers may, however, be utilized with the advance.

(b) Persons whose voluntary services have been accepted will be under the orders of the officers commanding the hospital, etc., to which they may be assigned.

(c) The voluntary services of no person will be accepted unless he is physically sound and otherwise qualified for effective service. (Med. Dep't Manual.)

TRANSPORTATION AND SUPPLIES.—During a campaign transportation which properly pertains to the medical department is assigned to that department and will not be diverted therefrom by commanders subordinate to the one by whom such assignment was made, nor by officers of other staff departments. This includes ambulances, wagons and animals with their personnel, hospital trains, ships and boats, together with the crews for working such trains, ships and boats.

Transportation for the temporary use of the medical department, including wagon and railway trains, boats, etc., is reported by the officer in charge to the senior medical officer, under whose orders such transportation remains until the special work for which it was assigned is completed. The movements of sanitary trains and transports conform to schedules established by the commander of the line of communications.

Medical and other supplies for the use of the sick and wounded are transported, so far as possible, by the medical department with its own transportation. Supplies which cannot be thus transported are invoiced to the Quartermaster's Department for transportation, and their shipment is expedited as much as possible, ammunition and rations alone, as a rule, having precedence.

When necessary, members of the Hospital Corps are detailed to accompany medical property.

When not otherwise provided for, repairs to transportation and the shoeing of animals are done by the Quartermaster's Department on request from the proper medical officers.

The medical department provides each company unit with a litter; on the march these litters are carried on the combat train or by men detailed for that purpose. (Field Service Regulations.)

DUTIES.—The medical department is charged with the *administration of the sanitary service.* Specifically its duties are:

1. The initiation of sanitary measures to insure the good health of troops.

2. The direction and execution of all measures of public health among the inhabitants of occupied territory.

3. The care of the sick and wounded on the march, in camp, on the battle-field, and after removal therefrom.

4. The methodical disposition of the sick and wounded, so as to insure the retention of those effective, and relieve the fighting force of the non-effective.

5. The transportation of the sick and wounded.

6. The establishment of hospitals and other formations necessary for the care of the sick and injured.

7. The supply of sanitary material necessary for the health of the troops and for the care of the sick and injured.

8. The preparation and preservation of individual records of sickness and injury in order that claims may be adjudicated with justice to the government and to the individual.

In addition to caring for the sick and wounded, medical officers act as sanitary advisers of commanders and instruct the troops in personal hygiene. Beginning with camp sites and the water supply, they continue their supervision of these and other sanitary matters to the close of the campaign.

(Field Service Regulations.)

CONTROL.—The senior medical officer of an army or smaller command is charged with the general control of the sanitary troops serving therewith, and commands the independent sanitary units. He may be authorized by the commander to make assignments of the personnel, and in emergencies the entire sanitary service of the command may be placed at his disposition.

(Field Service Regulations.)

INSPECTIONS.—Before troops are sent to camps of mobilization they are carefully examined to detect the presence of contagious disease, especially typhoid fever. Such examinations are made by medical officers of the regular army when practicable, otherwise by militia or volunteer medical officers, and the subsequent movements of the troops examined are contingent on the results of such examinations. Similarly before taking the field the troops are again examined, and those physically unfit are excluded.

In campaign *sanitary inspectors*, on the recommendation of the Surgeon-General, are assigned as follows: One to each division and as many as may be necessary to the line of communications, base of operations, and home territory.

(Field Service Regulations.)

The Medical Department in campaign operates in three zones. These three divisions are home territory, the line of communications, and the front. The two latter are considered together here, as in our service both are under the general direction of one administrative medical officer. Home territory includes all medical department organizations at home as well as all which are directly administered under home authorities. In an over-sea expedition the sea separates home territory from the line of communications. In continental warfare the line of communications may begin at the edge of home territory or may even include some of that territory. The line of communications is best described as the zone lying between the base of operations and the front; the latter term is self-explanatory. It is hardly thought necessary, for the purposes of this article, to discuss the differences which exist in different armies in regard to the organization and administration of these various zones.

The following scheme (on page 933) shows the organization of our Medical Department in campaign.

In connection with this table it may be desirable to explain that each of the administrative medical officers, except the Surgeon-General, represents the Medical Department on the staff of his commander. In like manner the Surgeon-General is the representative of the Medical Department at the War Department. In our organization, however, all of these medical officers, except the chief surgeon of the field army, have certain medical department organizations directly under them.

In studying the work of the Medical Department in war one must remember that it runs in two channels—the stream of wounded from the front, eventually coming to home territory, and a stream in a contrary direction, viz., that of supplies coming from home territory. Both of these streams are temporarily blocked here and there in their course and then are again increased in volume. (See Plate LVI.)

Home Territory.—The organization of the medical department of an army in campaign of course starts in home territory, and is then advanced to the front as the troops advance. In this description, therefore, it is thought better to start in home territory with the outbreak of a war. Just as with every other army, our troops must then be mobilized. The practice will probably be, as was the case in the Spanish-American War, to mobilize troops from the various sources at large camps of mobilization. Troops of the regular establishment would naturally come from the various posts. These, therefore, need not be discussed here until they have actually arrived at the camps of mobilization. The Organized Militia would first be assembled in state camps, as would also state volunteers. National volunteers, if such volunteers are organized, would be gathered into regimental camps at various points throughout the country. The medical department organization for such camps would be simple. Regimental infirmaries and hospitals conducted by the regimental officers would be sufficient to care for ill and injured. At this time the duties of the medical officers should consist principally in preventing epidemic diseases in their organizations. Almost universally in the Spanish-American War troops

EXPLANATION OF PLATE LVI.

Scheme showing Medical Department Organizations from Front to Rear in Battle.

At the top of the plate are seen cavalry, infantry, and artillery in action. These constitute the great part of the normal division. Immediately in rear are the Regimental Aid or First-Aid Stations. One or more of these stations has been established for each arm. This is not true of the Division Stations, however, only three of which are illustrated for the entire division. A method to be commended where practical, in order to concentrate medical personnel and supplies.

The green dotted lines leading to the Station for Slightly Wounded give the course ~f wounded who are not severely hurt and are able to walk toward the rear. The red dotted lines show the course of severely wounded toward the rear. The transport of these wounded devolves on the Ambulance Companies until the Field Hospitals are gained and afterward on Transport Columns till they reach an Evacuation Hospital.

A Collecting Station for Slightly Wounded, Field Hospitals (including one in reserve), a Transport Column, and Evacuation Hospitals are all shown. A Rest Station on the route of ₽ Transport Column is also illustrated as well as a Rest Station for walking wounded coming from the Station for Slightly Wounded. The Reserve Medical Supply is located in a village near the front, and two Evacuation Hospitals in a village further to the rear. From the Evacuation Hospitals wounded are carried to the base by a Hospital Train. At the latter a Base Hospital, a Convalescent Camp, and a Base Medical Supply Depot are all illustrated. Water transport from the base to a home port is provided by a Hospital Ship, which is shown.

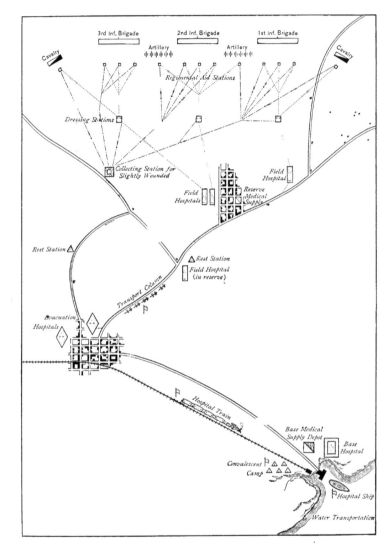

SCHEME SHOWING MEDICAL DEPARTMENT ORGANIZATIONS
FROM FRONT TO REAR IN BATTLE

(Reproduced by permission of the author, Major Paul F. Straub, Medical Corps (General Staff), U. S. A.)

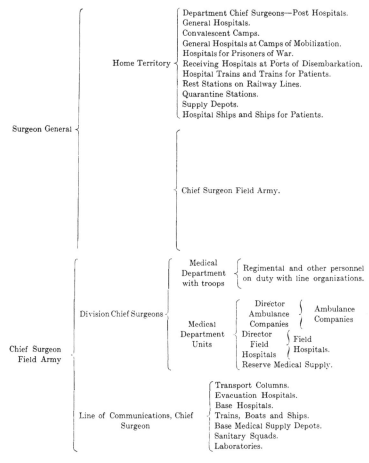

Surgeon General
- Home Territory
  - Department Chief Surgeons—Post Hospitals.
  - General Hospitals.
  - Convalescent Camps.
  - General Hospitals at Camps of Mobilization.
  - Hospitals for Prisoners of War.
  - Receiving Hospitals at Ports of Disembarkation.
  - Hospital Trains and Trains for Patients.
  - Rest Stations on Railway Lines.
  - Quarantine Stations.
  - Supply Depots.
  - Hospital Ships and Ships for Patients.
- Chief Surgeon Field Army.

Chief Surgeon Field Army
- Division Chief Surgeons
  - Medical Department with troops
    - Regimental and other personnel on duty with line organizations.
  - Medical Department Units
    - Director Ambulance Companies — Ambulance Companies
    - Director Field Hospitals — Field Hospitals.
    - Reserve Medical Supply.
- Line of Communications, Chief Surgeon
  - Transport Columns.
  - Evacuation Hospitals.
  - Base Hospitals.
  - Trains, Boats and Ships.
  - Base Medical Supply Depots.
  - Sanitary Squads.
  - Laboratories.

going from state camps to the general mobilization camps brought typhoid fever with them. The purpose of the paragraph in the Field Service Regulations which provides for sanitary inspection of troops which are to be sent to the general camps of mobilization is, so far as may be possible, to prevent infective diseases from being carried to the latter. Many of the medical officers at the smaller camps would doubtless have some medical supplies, and these should be supplemented, or the required amount should be obtained when necessary, by requisition on the Surgeon-General. The sick, except those with minor affections, should not accompany the troops to which they belong to the general camps. Some of them could be transferred to post hospitals and to

general hospitals, while provision for others, at least for a time, would necessarily be made in civil hospitals of their vicinity.

The discussion of this subject will be mainly confined to the mobile army
in campaign, but it would be well to remember at this time that, in war, our
territorial departments as well as many of our posts, would probably still be
maintained. Moreover, in a serious war it would be necessary considerably
to augment the medical department at the coast artillery posts, which would
have to be increased in strength. The majority of the sick and wounded of
the coast artillery could be cared for in the post hospitals of the various garrisons, unless there is a likelihood that these might be so exposed to fire that
they would have to be abandoned. In this case it would be necessary to establish hospitals at less exposed sites. In any event some coast artillery patients
would be transferred to general hospitals. Except so far as the establish-

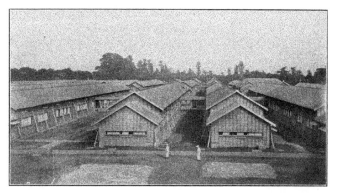

Fig. 342.—Reserve Hospital, Hiroshima (Corresponding to our General Hospital).

ment of new local hospitals is concerned, medical department organization for
the coast artillery in war would present slight difficulties. Locally the conditions
at each garrison would have to be considered by themselves. Prompt succor
of the wounded would always involve the presence of the medical department,
both officers and men, with the troops. After first-aid had been given, the
wounded, when opportunity offered, would be taken to a place sheltered from
fire somewhere in the rear of the works. Questions relating to sanitation would
naturally be solved much as they are at posts in peace.

Returning to the medical department organizations in home territory these
will now be discussed in some detail.*

* All cuts except the chart showing the organization of the medical service of an American
division in battle (Plate LVI) are reproduced from photographs secured personally by the author
during the Russo-Japanese War. The slight differences which exist in organization of the medical department of our army as compared with that of the Japanese are not material in this
connection. The latter too is the only army which has had experience in war in the operation
of a medical department conforming to the present accepted standard.

General Hospitals.—In our service the hospitals directly under the Surgeon-General are called general hospitals (see Fig. 342). In peace only four such hospitals exist in the United States. In war the general hospitals would have to be considerably augmented in numbers. The one at the Presidio, San Francisco, and the one near Washington, D. C., could also be increased in size. So many factors have to be considered when we undertake to determine the proper size and accommodations for such hospitals in war that it is difficult to state even approximately the number of beds which should be provided for them. With an army of four hundred thousand in the field and fairly good communication between the field army and home territory, not far from ten per cent of this number, or forty thousand beds, would be required for the general hospitals. This num-

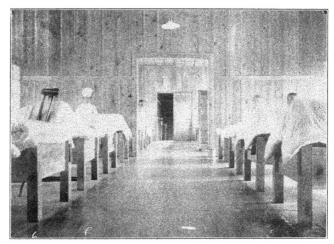

Fig. 343.—Ward Reserve Hospital, Tokyo.

ber would naturally be somewhat diminished if patients from the field army were treated in post hospitals or elsewhere than in general hospitals at home, or if circumstances necessitated the treatment of many patients for long periods on the line of communications. The estimate of forty thousand beds might, it is true, prove to be excessive at times, but of course in war there is no way by which every bed in every hospital can be occupied; therefore, some margin of safety must always be provided. The general hospitals should be provided with the highest surgical and medical skill available in our country and should be as well equipped in all respects as are our best civil hospitals. (Fig. 343.) In fact, these are the only war hospitals which are intended to give definite and final treatment to all cases requiring it. In these hospitals, situated as they would be at or near the large cities, in order to facilitate administration, the skill of the distinguished surgeons of the Reserve Corps could best be utilized. Some of these gentlemen would of course wish to go into the field, but it would be practicable for relatively few to do this, and the patriotism of those remaining at home could be made of the greatest value in the general hospitals. (Fig. 344.) In the majority of instances such hospitals would be entirely separate, one from another, and their individual commanding officers would be directly responsible to the Surgeon-General. Detailed plans for the construction of such hospitals may await the advent of war. It is interesting to know, in this connection, that the Japanese, who have such hospitals at each of their division districts in Japan, make yearly contracts for any construction which they think will be likely to be required during the coming year. In the event of war the contractors are called upon to erect the needed buildings. In some instances in the Russo-Japanese War such hospitals were erected and ready for occupancy within forty-eight hours after the contractors were called upon to construct them. They were rough, it is true, but

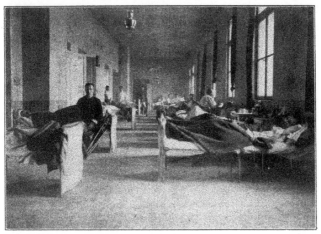

FIG. 344.—Russian Red Cross Hospital, Port Arthur.

were far better than tents which we have relied on to a considerable extent for this purpose in the past.

Convalescent Camps.—In war there are always numbers of patients who no longer require hospital treatment, but who are not yet strong enough to return to duty with their organizations. For them, in our service, as well as in most modern armies, convalescent camps are established. (Fig. 345.) Each such camp is made a branch of a general hospital, in order to facilitate administration, the commanding officer of the former being responsible for conducting the camp. The number and size of such camps would necessarily depend on the special circumstances.

General Hospitals at Camps of Mobilization.—One of the most important lessons of the Spanish-American War was that, if disease is not to spread widely in our troops, the sick must be promptly separated from the well at the camps of mobilization. Moreover, at this time it is absolutely unjustifiable to utilize the Medical Department organizations belonging to troops for the care of the sick. On the contrary, all such Medical Department organizations must be held in readiness to accompany their troops. On these accounts it has been determined to organize general hospitals at mobilization camps. It is intended that such hospitals be housed in buildings, and plans for such buildings have been prepared. The number of these hospitals would also depend on the special circumstances, but it is not probable that any mobilization camp could afford to be without one. The new Medical Manual will provide that, if the Surgeon-General does not establish such hospitals, this shall be done by the chief surgeon concerned.

Hospitals for Prisoners of War.—Provision is made that such hospitals be

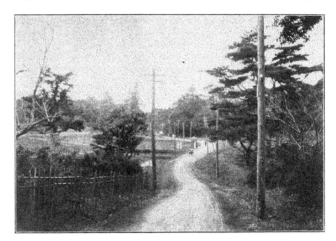

Fig. 345.—Convalescent Camp, Atami.

provided by the War Department at such points and of such capacity as may be required.

Receiving Hospitals at Ports of Disembarkation.—These hospitals are also established on recommendation of the Surgeon-General; they, as well as convalescent camps, are made branches of general hospitals, whenever possible. Their name almost describes their special function. It is of course essential that patients debarking from a ship be sheltered and cared for until some arrangements can be made for their permanent disposition. The size and capacity of such hospitals will depend on the special circumstances.

Hospital Trains and Trains for Patients.—Hospital trains have a fixed material and personnel, but trains for patients have neither, and are in fact made up of the railroad transport at hand. Both classes of trains operate under the orders of the Surgeon-General and each is commanded by a medical officer. Both classes of trains might of course operate in other than home territory; in which case the chief surgeon involved would assume the position of the Surgeon-General. During the Spanish-American War hospital trains were made up of tourist sleepers with a diner attached; this arrangement was not wholly satisfactory, but, on the whole, proved fairly so. (Fig. 346.) It is possible that some of the kitchen cars constructed on recommendation of the Subsistence Department would be available to the Medical Department in time of war. We have

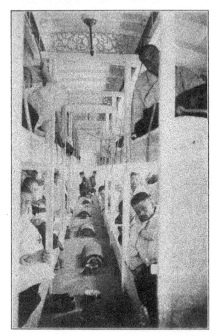

Fig. 346.—Interior of Japanese Hospital Car: a third-class coach, adapted for hospital purposes.

lately begun to secure excellent apparatus with which to fit baggage cars for the transport of patients. At the time of the Civil War we accomplished a good deal in this direction, but since then, and even up to a quite recent date, other more military nations have far surpassed us in this respect. This is an activity which presumably belongs with special appropriateness to the Red Cross. The number of hospital trains and trains for patients could only be determined in accordance with special needs.

Rest Stations on Railway Lines.—These stations, though they have been provided for by other nations, have never heretofore been described in our regulations. It is intended that they shall be organized by the Surgeon-General at points on the railway lines where attention can best be given to the sick and wounded *en route*. It is also intended that, so far as may be possible, the personnel of each such station should be obtained locally and should be furnished by the Red Cross. Presumably rest stations would be organized on the general plan followed by the Japanese in the Russo-Japanese War, which plan comprehended two sections for each station. These were called the nursing section and the comfort section. The first gave to the ill and injured such medical aid as was necessitated by their condition; the second cheered the soldiers on their way to the front and comforted them on their return. It should be noted that, for the latter section, no technical knowledge is required.

Quarantine Stations.—The necessity for the establishment of such stations

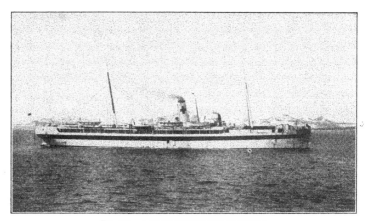

FIG. 347.—Japanese Hospital Ship near Dalny.

would of course be dependent upon the special conditions under which a war was conducted. It would devolve on the Army to prevent the introduction of disease by returning troops, though it might be possible for all such quarantine work to be done by other agencies as in time of peace. From what has been said it will be apparent that neither the number, the personnel, nor the material of such stations can be fixed.

Supply Depots.—It would probably be necessary, in the event of war, to establish new medical supply depots and to augment the size of some of those now in existence. The number and size of such depots would of course depend upon the special necessities of the case.

Hospital Ships and Ships for Patients.—Both of these classes of ships would operate between home territory and some station of the army over sea. They are discussed here because they would be under the jurisdiction of the Surgeon-General and would therefore form a part of the Medical Department organization of home territory. Just as is the case with hospital trains, hospital ships have a fixed material and personnel, while ships for patients have neither. The latter consist of any ships available for the temporary use of the Medical Department. (Fig. 347.) Both hospital ships and ships for patients are commanded by medical officers. On account of our national lack of a merchant marine, and because of the many demands which would be made upon it in a war over sea, it is probable that it would be exceedingly difficult for us to obtain suitable vessels for this purpose in the event of war. Moreover, in a great war over seas the demand for ships for the ill and injured would be very great. For example, in the Russo-Japanese War the Japanese operated about twenty hospital ships, besides a half-dozen ships for carrying the less

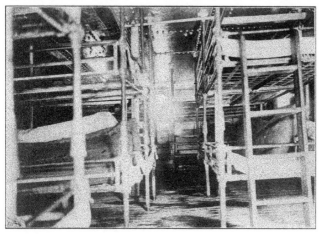

Fig. 348.—Ward in Japanese Red Cross Hospital Ship. The fittings are removable and are stored by the Red Cross in time of peace when the vessel is used for commercial purposes.

severely afflicted patients. (Fig. 348.) The American Red Cross has, through its War Relief Board, obtained some important data on the subject of merchant vessels which might be made available for hospital purposes in time of war. So far as known, this is all which has been done in this direction, though the experience of a number of medical officers who served on hospital ships during the Spanish-American War could be made of considerable value.

Field Army.—As shown in the table on organization (page 933) the principal medical officer of a field army is called "Chief Surgeon, Field Army." Immediately subordinate to him, so far as the medical service is concerned, are the division chief surgeons, and the chief surgeon of the line of communications. It is thought that, if a detailed statement is given of the duties of the first-named, it will hardly be necessary to discuss those of the other chief surgeons. It will be understood that the chief surgeons of divisions and of the line of communications perform duties very similar to those of a chief surgeon of a field army, with certain modifications necessitated by the peculiarities of their services, all of which will be discussed in their proper places. (See Plate LVI.)

The Chief Surgeon, Field Army, has general charge of the sanitary service of the army and is held responsible for the proper and effective management of the same. He exercises general supervision over sanitation and over the care and treatment of the sick and wounded; to his judgment is left the question of retaining effectives at the front and of sending ineffectives to the rear; and it is his duty to see that medical supplies be on hand in sufficient quantities. He has his headquarters with the Commander-in-Chief, to whom he acts as sanitary adviser, and whom he keeps informed on the work of the medical department, always consulting him on matters of importance. He issues, or requests the issue of, orders containing general instructions on personal hygiene and camp sanitation. He exercises general supervision over the instruction of the army in hygiene and first aid. He controls the distribution, instruction, employment, and professional supervision of the entire sanitary personnel of the army. He directs Red Cross personnel on duty with the army, and decides whether voluntary aid individually offered is to be accepted and directs how it shall be employed. He exercises general supervision over the provision of necessary transport, supply, shelter, camps, etc., for sick and wounded. He is the custodian of funds and property contributed for the use of patients, supervises the expenditure of funds pertaining to the medical and hospital appropriation, and holds and distributes a general hospital fund. He partially occupies the position of the Surgeon-General so far as the army is concerned in matters relating to repair of hospitals. He communicates with the Surgeon-General in reference to the medical arrangements necessary for the transport of patients from the army and for sanitary personnel and supplies to the army. He has general charge of the movement of sick and wounded from front to rear, and their removal from the base, and the removal of supplies from base to the front. He co-ordinates the sanitary service of the front and the line of communications and keeps himself informed as to their efficiency. Whenever the sanitary situation is so serious at any point as to demand his presence he requests the necessary orders to enable him to perform the duty required. The chief surgeon of the field army arranges for medical attendance at army headquarters. In order that he may act intelligently he should obtain copies of all orders which affect the work of his department. He may be authorized to make assignments of the medical department personnel and to issue orders and instructions "by order" of the general commanding when authorized to do so. When no chief surgeon of the line of communications is detailed the chief surgeon of the field army performs his duties.

As noted above, the duties of the division chief surgeon are of a character very similar to those which have just been described. Naturally, however, the division chief surgeon belonging to a smaller command is enabled to take much closer personal direction of the medical department. Over the medical department in the division, too, the division chief surgeon exercises quite a different character of control, depending on whether the organizations in question consist of those with troops or of medical department units. The former are a part of the command of line officers, while the latter are commanded by the division chief surgeon himself.

Regimental Medical Department.—The regimental medical department is responsible for the execution of sanitary measures in connection with the regiment and for the temporary treatment of sick and wounded, with all the duties which such responsibility implies. In common with nearly all modern armies our organization contemplates that only temporary treatment shall be afforded the ill and injured at their regiments. This is essential, as the establishment of regimental hospitals would necessitate such an enormous personnel that a condition impossible for war would be created.

Division Medical-Department Units.—The very large size of the present division and the large amount of ground which it must cover, especially in battle, has led to the creation of two new medical department officers in our service. They are called the director of field hospitals and the director of ambulance companies. Each, as a representative of the division surgeon, directs and co-ordinates the medical-department units under him. They are also expected to keep in close touch with the other medical department organizations which are in the immediate vicinity and which form part of the chain of medical relief.

The duties of the field hospital are so concisely described in the Medical Manual that it is impossible to abridge that text; it is therefore quoted in full:—

The principal function of the field hospital is to receive wounded from the firing line, the first aid station and the dressing station, and after necessary treatment to transfer them to the rear. Other uses of field hospitals are wholly subordinate to this. They may, however, be used under orders of the division chief surgeon for temporary or cantonment hospitals or some of their personnel and supplies may be used for these same purposes. In such cases they must always be prepared to advance with their division on the receipt of orders.

This paragraph establishes one of the most important principles in medical-department field administration, viz., that field hospitals are part of the front and should under all circumstances be ready to accompany their troops.

Ambulance companies occupy an even more advanced position than field hospitals, and their principal function is to open dressing stations in the rear of the firing line and to collect and transfer wounded after giving the necessary treatment.

The last medical-department organization under the division surgeon is the reserve medical supply, one of which is assigned to each division. This is stationed well up toward the front, so that the divisional medical organizations may be promptly resupplied with all articles issued by the medical department.

Line-of-Communications Medical-Department Units.—To quote again from the proposed text for the Manual of the Medical Department:—

The service of the line of communication includes the evacuation of the field hospitals, establishment and operation of evacuation and base hospitals, casual and convalescent camps, transportation of patients, return to the front of men fit for duty, transfer to general hospitals or home stations of men gravely or permanently incapacitated, and the procuring and forwarding of medical supplies.

A new organization in the line of communications, so far as our service is concerned, is the transport column. This organization, and one is organized for each division, transfers patients from field to evacuation or base hospitals or to stations on the railway or boat landings, and furnishes the necessary care *en route.* In order to accomplish the latter purpose rest stations are established when the length of the transfer renders such action necessary. Transport columns would appear to offer a particularly good field for Red Cross activity and it is anticipated that the personnel of this association will be used for that purpose in our service.

Two evacuation hospitals will be mobilized for each of our divisions. These organizations are not new to us, but are the old stationary hospitals renamed. They are intended to replace field hospitals, so that the latter may accompany their organizations, or to receive patients from them with the same object in view. So far as it does not interfere with this function evacuation hospitals are used for ordinary hospital purposes on the line of communications.

One base hospital is mobilized for each of our divisions. These base hospitals receive patients from evacuation and field hospitals and from the line of communications and the base; they give definite treatment to a certain number of ill and injured and send further to the rear those patients whose condition is such that they may be regarded as either permanently disabled or as likely not to recover for some time. Naturally, however, the treatment accorded patients in base hospitals would depend to a considerable extent on a number of factors, the most important of which are ease of transportation to home territory and the facility with which patients can be supplied at the base.

Convalescent camps are sometimes established in connection with base hospitals, just as they are with general hospitals.

Casual camps are also sometimes made use of at the base. They are designed to receive arriving and departing medical-department personnel and to facilitate the distribution of both officers and men.

Base medical-supply depots are always required in war, and, when it appears necessary, our regulations provide that branches of such depots may be established at appropriate points on the line of communications.

Two other new organizations are contemplated for the line of communications of our service; these are sanitary squads designed to execute hygienic measures at the various posts on the line of communications, and laboratories in which may be carried out such investigations as are necessitated by the special sanitary situation. The organization of sanitary squads, as stated in the table of organization, has not yet been fixed. The personnel of line-of-communications laboratories is the subject of recommendation by the chief surgeon to the commander.

Medical-department trains and ships have already been alluded to in another connection, and, as previously stated, they may also be required in the line of communications. Their employment and the personnel and supplies for them, and likewise for hospital boats, are the subject of report by the chief surgeon of the line of communications to the commander. Under certain circumstances, especially after a great battle, it may be necessary for the Medical Department to take advantage of all rail and water transport returning from the front in order that the wounded may be carried further to the rear.

ADMINISTRATION.

All the medical-department field organizations have been described, and it now becomes necessary to discuss their operation and administration under the varied conditions of war.

Camps of Mobilization.—Camps of mobilization have been previously mentioned, and it is believed that it is already clearly understood that such camps are to be located where our war army is first concentrated prior to encountering the enemy. It has also been shown that, during the Spanish-American War, these camps constituted veritable hotbeds of disease. The two measures of greatest importance for preventing such a condition of affairs in any future war would be to exclude men suffering from typhoid fever from such camps and to isolate, at the earliest moment practicable, cases of typhoid appearing in the assembled troops. The importance of general hospitals near the camps in the accomplishment of the latter object has already been discussed. As previously stated, it is intended that all troops at state and similar small camps shall be examined for typhoid and other infective diseases before being sent to camps of mobilization, and that their transfer to the latter shall be contingent on the results of such examination.

From what has just been said it will be obvious that there should be no great number of sick in our camps of mobilization, and this is almost essential if medical officers are to be afforded an opportunity for instruction at this time. Even under the best possible conditions a large percentage of the medical-department personnel at the camps of mobilization must be destitute of the slightest military training, and it will therefore be necessary to devote a great deal of time to instructing them in their military duties. Instruction in personal hygiene and first-aid will also have to be imparted by the Medical Department to the army personnel generally if it is to be capable of protecting itself from disease under field-service conditions and of mitigating the effects of wounds received in future battles. It will likewise be necessary to complete the equipment of the Medical Department and to exercise the personnel of that department in its use. All such work should be carried on by the various medical officers involved under the direction of the chief surgeons of the camps.

No new principles are involved in the movement of troops from camps of mobilization to the field. The most important duty devolving on the Medical Department at this time will be guarding against the inroads of disease.

Marches.—The proposed text for the new Medical Manual provides that, on the march, the chief surgeon of the field army and the division chief surgeons shall accompany their respective staffs and acquaint themselves with the topography of the country so far as it affects the care, shelter, transportation, etc., of the sick and wounded.

Ordinarily regimental medical officers march, the senior with the regimental commander, and one in rear of each battalion unit. Each regiment is followed by an ambulance from the ambulance train. Unless otherwise ordered, these ambulances rejoin their trains at the beginning of an engagement. If a regiment operates alone, it is accompanied by three ambulances.

The ambulance companies and field hospitals of a division generally march in rear of the division field train as follows:

Ambulance companies.

Ambulance company trains (in order of their companies).

Field hospitals.

If an engagement is imminent, these organizations usually precede the division baggage train, and one ambulance company (less ambulances and wagons) or detachments thereof, follows each brigade. For smaller commands the march of the sanitary troops is similarly conducted.

Circumstances may require the first ambulance company with part, or whole, of its train to be placed immediately in rear of the advanced guard so as to provide for that formation. (Field Service Regulations.)

The sick and wounded who fall out during a march are placed in the regimental ambulance, and when this is filled they are assigned to the ambulance train or other transport at the rear. Weak and footsore men are relieved of their equipment and permitted to march in the rear of the regimental ambulance.

On the march in a campaign, it is essential that the ill and injured (except the trivial cases, which will recover promptly) be separated from their organizations. On halting for the night, therefore, it is contemplated that all but the trivial cases be transferred to a field hospital or otherwise disposed of. Unless it is clearly impracticable to adopt this course the sick and wounded should be sent promptly to the line of communications, as otherwise they would tend to immobilize field hospitals which is absolutely inadmissible, as these hospitals must accompany the troops to which they belong. Even if such patients must be temporarily cared for at field hospitals, they should be promptly transferred to the rear, and the sanitary personnel accompanying them should immediately rejoin their troops. On the march, at the halt for the night, arrangements for the care of the sick and wounded devolve on the division surgeon, who should communicate as promptly as possible with the line-of-communications chief surgeon in order that the latter may relieve him of his patients. The use of the personnel and supplies of a field hospital for the establishment of a temporary hospital, while the troops are on the march, is permissible under the regulations, but it is also provided therein that this should never be done if it can be avoided; and, in this event, the field hospital should be quickly replaced from the line of communications.

Camps.—It is not intended that regimental hospitals be used in campaign.

Their employment is only permissible in the military occupation of a country. In camps, therefore, regiments must rely on their infirmaries for emergency cases and for the treatment of the slightly sick or injured, serious cases being promptly transferred to hospitals. In camps at prolonged halts in the field, cantonment hospitals are established by the division chief surgeon with the authority of the division commander. One of the most important duties of the division surgeon at a prolonged halt is to prevent unnecessary loss of men from service at the front, and he does this by close supervision over cantonment hospitals. He should only permit patients who are permanently incapacitated, or who are likely to be disabled for a long time, to be sent to the rear. In all other cases the patients should be retained and treated. The personnel and supplies of field hospitals and ambulance companies are used for cantonment hospitals and for the transport of patients to the rear, but they must be replaced from the medical department of the line of communications prior to a movement of the division in ample time to allow them to accompany their troops. Isolation hospitals are sometimes made branches of cantonment hospitals.

Combat.—The following scheme taken from the proposed text for the new Medical Manual shows clearly the organization of the Medical Department in battle:—

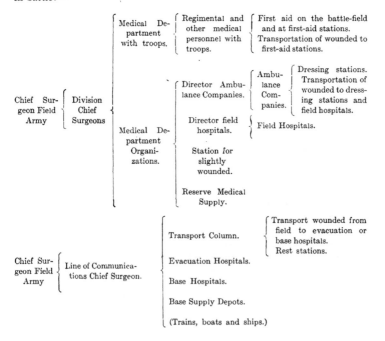

It is regarded as absolutely essential that chief surgeons be informed in advance of contemplated movements of the organizations to which they belong; otherwise no proper preparation can be made for the work of the Medical Department in such movements. The regulations in different armies vary considerably in respect to the obligations of commanders in this particular. Our own Field Service Regulations read as follows:—

"As far as practicable, commanders keep their senior surgeons informed of contemplated movements in order that the sanitary service may make proper preparations."

The Japanese, who certainly have had large experience in war, provide that army and division chief surgeons shall have the right to know all orders affecting the movements of their commands in order that they may make preparation for the participation of the medical department therein. Whether medical officers below the grade of chief surgeon know anything in reference to the movements of the troops would appear to be immaterial, as direction devolves on the latter. Our new Manual will provide further that chief surgeons should make every proper effort to secure from their commanders information in regard to intended military movements.

In combat it is intended that the chief surgeon of the field army co-ordinate the sanitary services of the divisions and that of the line of communications so that wounded may be promptly removed from the front and medical supplies be furnished thereto ·as required. It is essential that, prior to a battle, the army chief surgeon arrange that all medical-department organizations be freed of patients as far as possible. Such organizations will include all those at the front and the most advanced ones of the line of communications. The army chief surgeon must also concentrate medical supplies immediately in rear of the mobile army. In battle the line-of-communications chief surgeon replaces division medical organizations promptly, receives patients from them, and replenishes the supplies of the reserve medical supply. He also is in charge of the transportation of sick and wounded in the line of communications and of the work of furnishing them supplies. Division chief surgeons exercise a general supervision over the medical-department organizations at the front and over the work of furnishing them supplies.

From what has been said, it is obviously essential that, before a battle, all these administrative medical officers fully inform themselves on the condition of their medical departments, in order that they may promptly repair any deficiencies in personnel and material. They should also arrange for extra supplies if they are likely to be required, and for extra transportation and personnel. Such measures are contemplated by our regulations. It is also obvious that the closest co-operation between the chief administrative medical officers is essential to effective medical service in combat. Previous arrangements should be made by these officers to cover all points involved in the movement of wounded to the rear and of supplies to the front. Division chief surgeons are required, by the use of maps and personal exploration of the terrain, to determine in advance, so far as is practicable, the best situations for dressing stations, field and evacuation hospitals, rest stations, and for reserve supply depots. Moreover, they are expected to inform the chief surgeon of the field army, and the chief surgeon of the line of communications of the result of this study so far as it concerns them. Senior surgeons with troops are expected to ascertain, before a battle, that their equipment is complete and that each man has his first-aid packet in serviceable condition.

Immediately prior to an engagement the division chief surgeon, usually with the authority of the division commander, makes the detail of personnel for the collecting station for slightly wounded and directs where its supplies should be obtained. The battle order usually designates the place of assembly of the sick on the morning upon which a battle is expected. They are ordinarily sent to the station for slightly wounded nearest to an evacuation or base hospital, or to a transport column. Our new Manual will require that due notification of their destination be given the chief surgeon of the line of communications. During an engagement the division chief surgeon is habitually found with the division commander whom he consults when practicable as to the location of dressing stations and field hospitals. He is permitted, however, when such a course seems necessary, to locate them himself, afterward reporting to his commander. Orders in reference to them are sent to their respective directors, and the opening and closing of field hospitals are reported to the chief surgeon of the field army, and, when necessary, to the line-of-communications chief surgeon.

The following paragraphs are quoted from the Field Service Regulations:—

Unless duly detached all sanitary troops accompany their units into battle. During battle, however, the chief surgeons of divisions, subject to the approval of their commanders, make such assignments of the division sanitary troops as the situation requires. One surgeon from each regiment is generally attached to an ambulance company or field hospital.

By direction of the regimental commander, the band may be assigned to duty with the sanitary service.

In the absence of medical assistance the wounded apply their first-aid packets if practicable. With this exception the care of the wounded devolves upon the sanitary troops and no combatant unless duly authorized is permitted to take or accompany the sick or injured to the rear.

Diagnosis tags are attached to all wounded and killed as soon as practicable.

At the beginning of an engagement the wounded are cared for by the regimental sanitary troops. Those able to walk are directed to the rear; the others are taken to sheltered places as soon as possible, out of the way of the advancing troops.

As soon as warranted by the situation, the following stations from front to rear are established for the care of the sick and wounded:

1. First-aid stations—generally one for each regiment (Fig. 349);
2. Dressing stations—generally one for each brigade (Fig. 353);
3. Field hospitals—set up as required (Fig. 357);
4. Station for the slightly wounded—generally one for each division.

While during an engagement, as a rule with foot troops, the wounded are treated at certain established stations, with mounted troops only rarely can such stations be established early, and not infrequently their establishment must await the conclusion of the combat.

Regimental Medical Personnel.—The manuscript of the new Medical Manual defines the duties devolving on the regimental medical personnel in combat as follows:—

First aid to the wounded on the battle-field; removal and direction of wounded to places of comparative safety near the firing line; establishment of a first-aid station; removal of and direction of wounded thereto, likewise simple treatment thereat; direction of wounded to the dressing station and also under exceptional circumstances transportation of wounded to this station.

In this connection it should be noted that in the new Field Service Regulations our regimental medical personnel has been considerably augmented in strength. Similar action has been taken by a number of other nations as a result of the lessons of the Russo-Japanese War. Without question the additional men were required in our service, the more so as we do not employ company bearers who are detailed from the troops in most armies. We do, however, contemplate

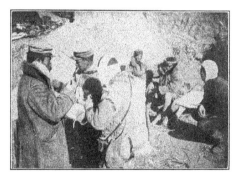

Fig. 349.—Japanese First-Aid Station; Battle of Mukden.

using the band, though whether members of such organizations will be of much value is problematical. It is contemplated that, on advancing into battle, the medical personnel and the band, if present, will march immediately in the rear of its unit with the supplies (including at least eight litters) carried on their persons by officers and men, and that the remaining supplies intended for the first-aid stations will be transported by pack animals. (Figs. 350 and 351.) As stated above, it is not contemplated that these stations shall be established until this is warranted by the situation. If they are established when troops are advancing, they will soon be left behind and so will be in great part useless. Their establishment, therefore, which is determined by the regimental surgeon, should not take place until the number of casualties is considerable,—that is, until the firing is so heavy that shelter must be obtained for the regimental medical per-

sonnel. The distance of first-aid stations from the firing line has been the subject of an animated discussion in all services; nor is it likely that anything
definite will be determined in reference to this subject. Modern warfare, with
the increased range of small arms, with the employment of machine guns, and
with the increased use of artillery, has added immeasurably to the difficulties
of the medical department at the front, and nowhere more so than in the location of first-aid and dressing stations. If the former are to be of any use they
certainly must be close to their troops and yet in open ground this can only
result in heavy losses to the medical personnel and ineffective shelter for
wounded at the station. The only conclusion that can be reached, therefore, is
that the regimental surgeon must exercise his best judgment in respect to the

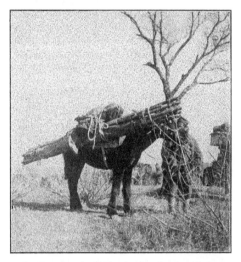

FIG. 350.—Battalion Medical Supplies, Battle of Mukden.

location of the first-aid station and that the choice of a location must depend
on the availability of a place where fair shelter from fire can be obtained.
Our new Manual contemplates that the senior medical officer of the regiment,
with his first assistant, three non-commissioned officers, and seven privates,
shall take post at the first-aid station, while the junior assistant, with a
non-commissioned officer and the remainder of the detachment, shall keep in
touch with the firing line, attending to the needs of the wounded so far as
possible and removing the helpless to the station. The band, if present, will
be in part detailed as bearers, while those not so employed will remain at the
station. Whether it is desirable for a medical officer to be stationed with
the firing line has also been the subject of much discussion. It is true that
in this part of the field there can be no picking out of bad cases, nor will

it be possible for the medical officer to move freely from point to point. It is now generally believed, however, that even with these disadvantages, and at the risk of the loss of a medical officer whose services may be very badly needed later, when it will be impossible promptly to replace him, it is essential for the purpose of maintaining the morale of the troops, that a medical officer should accompany them. It has been the general experience that soldiers fight better when they know that, if they are wounded, every provision is made to give them skilled surgical attention as promptly as possible. Moreover, a medical officer on the firing line will occasionally be able to care for a severe case of hemorrhage which requires prompt treatment of such a character that it could not well be given by a comrade or a hospital corps man.

The bearers, taking advantage of shelter, of lulls in the fight, and of darkness, bring to the first-aid station as many wounded as they can reach without subjecting themselves or their patients to greater risks than those to which the combatants are exposed. (Fig. 352.) If the firing should be very heavy, it may be

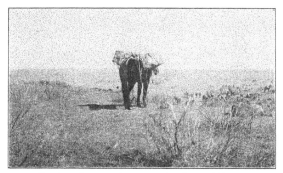

Fig. 351.—Battalion Medical Supplies, Battle of Mukden.

necessary for the bearers to drag wounded into trenches, ravines, or other inequalities of the ground where they are left till darkness permits their removal to the station. In combat all wounded who can walk must be compelled to do so, the litters being reserved for those whose injuries make it necessary for them to be carried. Examination of the figures furnished by equally competent observers as to the percentage of wounded who can be expected to walk to the rear, shows the widest discrepancies. My own experience inclines me to believe that these discrepancies are at least partially due to differences in classification; that is to say, some observers seem to count as wounded requiring transportation all those who must be transported at any point from front to rear, while others take into account the battle-field only. Seventy per cent has been given by some writers as the number of wounded which would require transportation, while others have given an estimate as low as fifteen per cent. In my opinion 85 per cent is not far from correct for the number of wounded who will be able to get back by themselves from the firing line to the first-aid station. This percentage will then be somewhat decreased when from this number are subtracted those who have to be transported from the latter to the field hospital. The final subtraction of those who have to be transported still greater distances will doubtless bring the number of the wounded, who require transportation from the front to the rear, up to the seventy per cent named above. Again, in respect to the percentage of the wounded who will require transportation from the firing line to the first-aid station, it should be remembered that the distance between the two should rarely exceed a thousand yards, and in broken country may be considerably less than this; and, further, that the effect of wounds on soliders in battle is usually to induce them to leave the point where the wounds have been received no matter how severe they may be, for a place at the rear—unless, of course, the wounds are of such a nature as absolutely to incapacitate them from doing so.

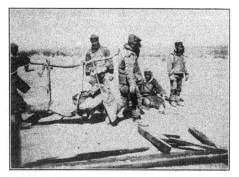

Fig. 352.—Bearers Removing Wounded from Firing Line to First-Aid Station, Battle of Mukden.

Our regulations provide that only members of the sanitary service shall be permitted to accompany wounded to the rear; and, as the regimental medical personnel must at all times retain close touch with the troops, no one belonging to it or assigned thereto is permitted to go further to the rear than the regimental aid station, except by the authority of the regimental or division surgeon. This brings up another question regarding the rôle of the medical department in promoting the efficiency of the army. With a medical department adequate in size and in close touch with troops in battle, and with troop commanders who are very strict disciplinarians, few losses should be sustained at the front from unhurt men accompanying their wounded comrades to the rear. If, however, the wounded are not promptly succored by the medical department, human nature will assert itself in the face of the most stringent measures adopted to prevent unwounded line soldiers from accompanying the wounded to the rear. This fact was observed again and again in the Russo-Japanese War, and has been commented on by Russian as well as by other observers. On numerous occasions the indulgence in this practice on the part of the Russians cost them so dearly that the Japanese found a very decided lessening in resistance at the points where this occurred. My own observation during the war in question is confirmatory of the correctness of this statement. For example, in one of the hard-fought battles on the Russian right, at Mukden, I am certain that the loss of Russian bayonets at the front contributed greatly to the Japanese success at this particular point.

From the first-aid station the wounded are sent promptly to the rear as soon as possible, and this station should never be permitted to become over-crowded. The wounded who are able to walk are directed to a dressing station, to a field hospital, to a collecting station, or simply to the rear. The wounded who are unable to walk are delivered to the bearers of the ambulance company as soon as they arrive.

First-aid stations are closed finally, or are closed temporarily and then

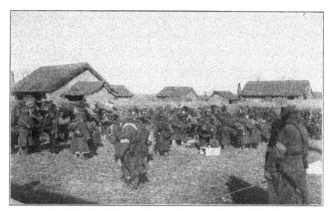

FIG. 353.—Establishment of a Dressing Station, Battle of Mukden.

advanced, as directed by the regimental surgeon. In reaching his decision the latter must always regard the primary necessity of keeping in touch with his regiment. If night falls before a battle is decided, the regimental medical personnel, with the bearers of the ambulance company, take advantage of the darkness to reach advanced positions in searching for the wounded. The hours of darkness are also utilized for clearing first-aid stations of wounded.

Let us next consider the character of surgical assistance which is appropriate for regiments in battle. Under conditions of modern warfare, this must be of a very simple nature. At or near the firing line little more can be done than to apply the first-aid packet, and frequently the wounded man must do this himself or have it done by a comrade who happens to be near him. Fractures should, if possible, be immobilized here and dangerous hemorrhage checked. Not much more can be accomplished at first-aid stations. Here, dressings should be inspected and readjusted if necessary, and restoratives and analgesics should be administered as required. No operations are performed. This represents the possibilities under the general conditions which obtain at first-aid stations. In exceptional cases, however, more extensive surgical work may be done— as, for example, when the enemy retires quickly and lack of further resistance permits the regimental medical personnel to remain stationary. Under such circumstances the facilities for doing clean surgical work become the most important factor in determining the procedure. Even then insufficiency of equipment and lack of facilities for obtaining water, etc., will limit operative work at the first-aid station to the minimum.

From what has been said above in reference to surgical assistance at the front it is clear that the ultimate results of wounds must depend to a great extent on a good first-aid packet, well applied by unskilled but trained hands. It is believed that the present United States Army first-aid packet is the best which has as yet been devised. It consists essentially of two long gauze bandages

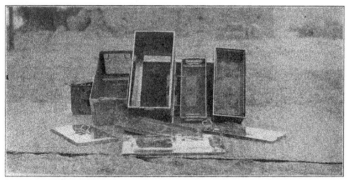

FIG. 354.—Japanese Field Sterilizer for Instruments and Dressings.

with a compress sewn in the centre of each. The compress may be easily applied to the wound without being touched by the hand or anything else, and then the ends of the bandage are wrapped around the part and tied firmly so as to hold the compress in proper position. One bandage with its attached compress is used for one wound, and the other for a second one. The contents are enclosed in a metal case that absolutely protects them from contamination until it is opened, which can be done easily even by a seriously wounded man. Our regulations provide that in war all soldiers shall be instructed in the proper use of the first-aid packet. Neither of the combatants in the Russo-Japanese War profited from the benefits of a good first-aid packet skilfully applied. Every Japanese soldier carried a packet, but the type used was one that could not well be applied without soiling it in handling. The Russians had a better packet, but it was not carried by a large percentage of their men.

The Ambulance Company.—The duties of the ambulance companies in our service are:—(1) To establish and operate the dressing stations; (2) to assist the regimental personnel at the front; (3) to carry the wounded (on litters) to the dressing stations and thence (in ambulances) to the field hospitals.

Dressing stations are established by the ambulance companies under instruction from the division chief surgeon. (Fig. 353.) As soon as the advance ceases preparations are made to open these stations. It is contemplated that the ambulance company with its pack transportation shall follow the brigade to the point selected by the division surgeon for the dressing stations. No general rules can be formulated for the location of these stations. They should if possible be beyond the range of rifle fire and be well protected from artillery fire, and it is desirable to have them as near the regimental aid stations as practicable in order to save the bearers and the walking wounded. An accessible road for ambulances from the rear to the station possesses obvious advantages, as does also a good water supply. The director of ambulance companies

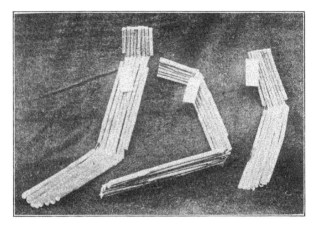

FIG. 355.—Kaulyang Splints.

directs the opening of dressing stations and reports their opening to the division chief surgeon. The bearers proceed to the front as soon as the station is opened. When practicable, they are divided into as many parties as there are regimental aid stations. The bearers direct the walking wounded to the station for slightly wounded, and then transport the other wounded to the dressing station; when practicable, too, they assist the regimental medical personnel in succoring the wounded at points in advance.

Meanwhile, the commanding officer of the company, who remains at the station, makes ready for the reception of wounded there. In order that these may be complete he notifies, when practicable, the wheeled transportation in the rear to report promptly at the station with wagons and ambulances. The following departments are prescribed for our dressing stations:—Dispensary; kitchen; receiving and forwarding department; department for the slightly wounded;

department for the seriously wounded; and mortuary. The names of these departments are regarded as sufficiently descriptive without detailed explanation. One of the most important departments is the kitchen, for here the wounded must be given hot and stimulating foods in order that they may recover from shock and be fortified for the journey to the rear. The slightly wounded, as soon as they have been given attention, must be sent promptly to the rear, in order that the dressing station may be freed for the oncoming wounded. The regulation transport provided for wounded from a dressing station to the rear consists of ambulances. Our regulations contemplate that these shall reach dressing stations promptly, even at the risk of losses; they also contemplate that, in case the ambulances prove insufficient for the wounded, the division surgeon shall request from the division commander the use of all returning transport of the division. (Fig. 356.)

This brings up one of the most important questions which the medical depart-

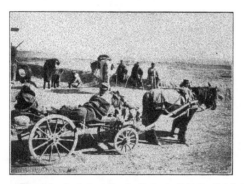

FIG. 356.—Japanese Wounded en Route from Dressing Station to Field Hospital, Battle of Mukden.

ment is called upon to solve under modern battle-field conditions, viz., the problem of clearing the field quickly after an engagement. In a great battle it must be obvious that the personnel and means of transportation of the medical department cannot be adequate for this. Under such circumstances, therefore, every possible measure must be taken by division surgeons to supplement it; one of these—that of securing all returning transport—has just been mentioned. This was adopted by the Japanese in the Russo-Japanese War, but they also made use of hundreds of hired bearers in the great battles of that war. The fact that we have ambulances while they have none, would, it is true, help us out to some extent, but in great battles we should also have to hire bearers whenever they could be obtained. To my mind the achievement of the Japanese, day after day, in the battle of Mukden, of clearing the field within twelve hours of all wounded except those in the most advanced positions, was the most notable performance in this respect which any army has yet achieved.

During the day-time, when a battle is still in progress, it will rarely be possible for ambulances to advance further than the dressing stations; after night-fall it will sometimes be possible for them to go further to the front, and when a battle is concluded they can be made of great use in collecting wounded at advanced points on the battle-field.

Orders for ambulance companies to close a dressing station or to close and advance come from the division chief surgeon, who obtains the authority of the division commander when practicable, but otherwise acts on his own initiative. Under exceptional circumstances the director of ambulance companies is permitted to act on his own initiative. In both cases a report should be promptly made to the higher commander. In case of retreat, when it is impossible to evacuate the wounded, they are left with a sufficient personnel to care for them. On the conclusion of an engagement the dressing stations are closed as promptly as possible and report of the fact is made to the division surgeon, who will ordinarily use the personnel at field hospitals or elsewhere.

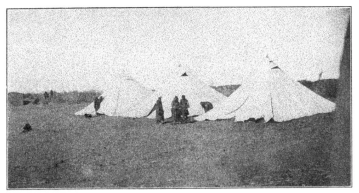

Fig. 357.—Tents of a Japanese Field Hospital in Advance, Battle of Mukden.

The number of dressing stations is dependent on circumstances; ordinarily however, one will be required for each brigade.

A few words must be said in reference to the character of the surgical assistance to be given at dressing stations. One should remember, in considering this question, that dressing stations, to be efficient, must be well toward the front and not any too well sheltered from the enemy's fire. Moreover, while conditions in them are somewhat better for clean operative work than they are in first-aid stations, they are still by no means ideal. It is also true of dressing stations that the wounded must be hurried back from them in order to make room for more wounded. The rule that we have established, therefore, is that at dressing stations only such rare operations are to be performed as may be immediately required to save life or to permit further transportation. Permanent occlusive dressings may be applied if time permits. The conclusion in regard to this question is that no operative interference should be permitted when the surroundings, with respect to the conditions of asepsis or antisepsis, are unfavorable, and that no wounded for whom transportation is available should be unnecessarily delayed at the dressing station. Under exceptional conditions the wounded may sometimes be given more definite treatment at dressing stations, just as is done at times at the first-aid station.

Certain facts brought to light by recent experience in regard to field equipment are of special interest in their bearing upon the dressing stations. It is realized, of course, that the surgical equipment for such stations should be simple and compact. The Japanese sterilizer for instruments and dressings is one especially adapted for use at both dressing stations and field hospitals, although, as might be expected, they used it to a much greater extent at the latter. This sterilizer weighs very little and can be packed in an extremely

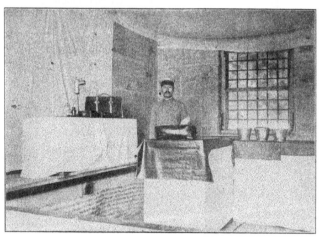

Fig. 358.—Operating Room, Japanese Field Hospital.

small space, so that it may be transported on a pack animal; it possesses a further advantage of utilizing almost any kind of fuel to be found in the field. (Fig. 354.) An ample supply of rubber gloves is essential for both field hospitals and ambulance companies. Under the conditions of field service surgeons' hands become extremely rough, so that they cannot be made surgically clean. Moreover, for obvious reasons, in dressing large numbers of wounded an ample supply of gloves is highly desirable. The Russo-Japanese War again emphasized the necessity for a most liberal supply of litters and splints at the front. The Japanese more than doubled their litters in this zone, often improvising them from any materials that happened to be at hand. They also resorted to many expedients to make splints from materials which could be obtained locally. An ingenious splint of this type is illustrated. (Fig. 355.)

Before leaving the subject of dressing stations I may be permitted to comment briefly on the subject of the protection afforded the medical personnel by the Red Cross emblem. While, as far back as the field hospital, this emblem may under certain circumstances result in protection from the enemy's fire,—though it by no means always does so,—its use at the front in battle carries absolutely no protection. In this connection it should be remembered that in the Japanese Army, during the Russo-Japanese War, the losses of the infantry were highest, and, so far as the front was concerned, the losses in sanitary personnel came second on the list. This argues no inhumanity on the part of the Russians; they utilized their fire as appeared to them best for the defeat of the enemy, and the distance to which their projectiles carried was so great that they did not know whether or not sanitary personnel was in the line of fire. It is probable that, in future wars, other nations will acquiesce in the conclusions of the Japanese, viz., that in battle it is best not to display a Red Cross flag at first-aid or dressing stations, as it can only serve to attract fire.

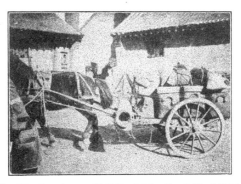

Fig. 359.—Some Japanese Field Hospital Supplies, Battle of Mukden.

Field Hospitals.—In combat the duties of our field hospitals may be enumerated as follows:—

Opening and in some cases replacing dressing stations.

Preparations for the wounded, including the arrangement of an operating room.

Reception of the wounded.

Providing shelter for the wounded for a longer or shorter period.

Providing food.

Supplying extensive and—in many instances—definite treatment.

Sending selected cases to the rear or delivering them to another organization.

Closing stations.

In general terms, the provisions for the establishment of field hospitals and for closing them, etc., are similar to those for dressing stations. If possible, field hospitals should be centrally located, so that they may easily be reached from front and rear, and yet they should not be on the main road. An ample supply of good water is necessary, and suitable buildings are very desirable. The ideal situation for a field hospital in battle is just beyond the limit of artillery fire. If the enemy retires promptly, field hospitals may replace dressing stations to manifest advantage, as this obviates a transfer of wounded. Only one field hospital should be opened early in the battle, and in appropriate cases the director of field hospitals may instruct those in the front to transfer all their patients to the hospitals established further to the rear. (Fig. 357.)

The following departments are described as belonging properly to a field hospital:—a dispensary; a kitchen; a receiving and forwarding department; a department for the slightly wounded; a department for the seriously wounded; an operating room; a mortuary; and a transportation department.

As was true in the case of the dressing stations, the names of these depart-

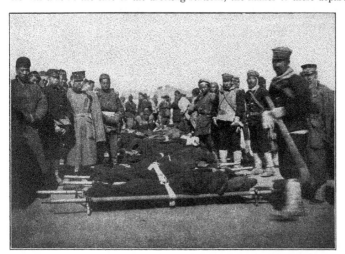

FIG. 360.—Japanese Transport Column, Battle of Mukden.

ments are sufficiently descriptive without detailed discussion. In a field hospital it is just as important to provide for the feeding of patients as it is at a dressing station, and, while at the latter the conditions require that easily prepared stimulating foods be administered to the wounded, at the field hospitals more elaborate meals may be served to advantage. The wounded who are able to walk and those with trifling injuries should be sent to the rear as soon as possible, under the charge of that one of their number who ranks highest as an officer or a non-commissioned officer. (Fig. 360.) The transportation department of a field hospital is intended for the convenient assembling of all transport at one point. Under ordinary circumstances during a battle the wounded who require to be transported will be sent to the rear as promptly as transportation is available for them. On the conclusion of an engagement, however, a field hospital may be temporarily immobilized; in which case it will provide for patients as do other permanent hospitals. In combat a field hospital uses all of its own transport for sending the wounded to the rear, and may also obtain some of the returning transport of the division for this purpose, just as is done in the case of the dressing stations. While field hospitals should, if possible, free themselves of wounded so as to be prepared to advance with their division, this will sometimes be impracticable; in which case, under orders of the division surgeon, all wounded will be concentrated in one or two field hospitals, so that the others may advance to provide for the subsequent needs of troops.

Before dismissing the subject of the operation of field hospitals in battle I must devote a few words to the manner in which the patients should be cared

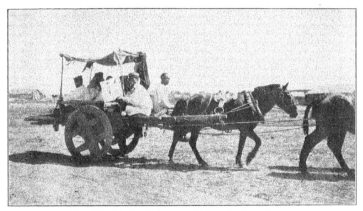

FIG. 361.—Bringing Patients to a Railway Station at Tieling.

for in those hospitals. From what has already been said it will be noted that field hospitals in combat are the first places where the wounded, on their way from the front to the rear, are safe from the fire of the enemy. Moreover, under ordinary conditions the field hospital will be the first place to which it is possible to bring adequate supplies for operations, etc. At the same time it is not intended that the field hospital in battle shall serve as a permanent hospital for wounded; it simply represents one of the stopping-places in the journey from the front, and, as it is compelled to move with its division, can retain the wounded but a comparatively short time. These conditions will limit operative procedures to those necessary to fit the wounded for transfer to the rear. Operations will be rare, but many extensive dressings will be required under all circumstances. (Fig. 358.) Occasionally, of course, much more complete treatment may be given in field hospitals. On account of the conditions in the field the greatest care should always be taken to dress cases in such a manner that they will not require re-dressing for some time. (Fig. 359.)

Due consideration having now been paid to the principal field medical organizations at the front which are directly concerned in the care and treatment of those who are wounded in battle, it may be well to pause at this point for a moment to refer to subjects concerning medical organizations at the front as a whole. First, in reference to cases of hemorrhage which may come under observation:—With the modern small-calibre rifle but few severe hemorrhages may be looked for. Wounds from artillery projectiles are more serious in this as in other particulars, but even so the experience of recent wars, in which

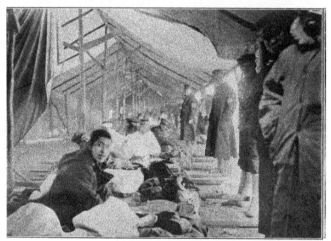

Fig. 362.—Rest Station, Mukden.

artillery and the frightfully mutilating hand grenades were largely emp oyed, demonstrates the fact that relatively few cases of hemorrhage fall into the hands of the military surgeon at the front. The subject of the treatment of abdominal wounds has attracted a great deal of attention in recent years because of the notable success obtained from prompt operation upon these cases in civil practice. From what has been said it should be clear that, in battle, the conditions —so far as they relate to the opportunities offered for operating on abdominal wounds—are wholly dissimilar from those which exist in civil life. At the front, therefore, it is certain that one will only in very few instances be justified in operating on an abdominal wound. Another question to which much attention has been devoted, is the transportability of the wounded in battle. This is believed to be a military rather than a surgical problem. All the wounded, except those who are moribund, should, as soon as this can be done, be sent as far to the rear as the field hospital, nor is it permissible to retain them even there. In practice it will as I believe be found better to take long chances in getting all the wounded away from the field to a hospital where they can receive more suitable treatment and where they may be permitted to remain for some time.

Station for the Slightly Wounded.—This station is new, so far as our service is concerned. It is designed to relieve dressing stations and field hospitals from the care of the slightly wounded who can walk and who require but little attention. It is intended that all the wounded who arrive at the station shall be allowed to rest, that their wounds shall be dressed or re-dressed as may be necessary, and that restoratives and easily prepared food shall be given them. From time to time parties of wounded will be despatched to the rear as opportunity offers. The personnel for the station is provided from the different regiments

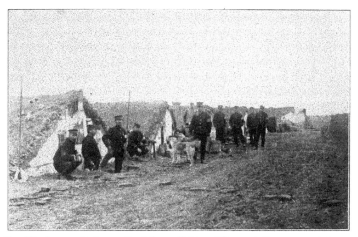

Fig. 363.—Japanese Stationary Hospital near Mukden. This organization corresponds to our evacuation hospital.

by the division chief surgeon. It will, as a rule, consist of one medical officer, two non-commissioned officers, and eight privates. Ordinarily, this station will be at a point about as far in advance as that at which the most advanced field hospital is located. The description of the station indicates clearly what surgical assistance should be given there.

Service of the Line of Communications in Combat.—The following Medical Department organizations under the chief surgeon of the line of communications are concerned in the transportation and treatment of the wounded in combat:— Transport Columns; trains, boats and ships; evacuation hospitals; and base hospitals.

Transport Columns.—Reference to the table on Medical Department organization will show that only a small amount of transport is allotted to a transport column. It is intended, however, that this shall be largely augmented when circumstances require, and especially before a battle, from the local resources of the country. This is a subject for recommendation by the chief surgeon of the line of communications. (Fig. 361.)

Just before a battle, transport columns should be advanced well toward the front.

The duties of transport columns are described as follows:—

The removal of the wounded from field hospitals to hospitals further to the rear, or, more rarely, from evacuation to base hospitals; the necessary care and treatment of the wounded *en route;* the establishment of rest stations when this is necessitated by the distance of field hospitals from hospitals in the rear or by other circumstances.

It is expected that, as soon as the division chief surgeon becomes aware that he will have many wounded, and after he has established a field hospital, he will request the chief surgeon of the line of communications to send a transport

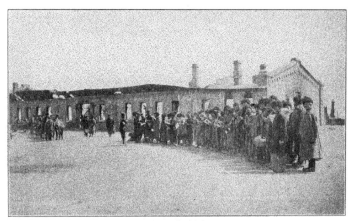

Fig. 364.—Slightly Wounded Russians being Assembled at Mukden after the Battle.

column to it. This same authority will determine the destination of the column on its return. Unless the distance from the field hospital in question to the destination of the transport column is more than a day's march the column will ordinarily proceed directly and as promptly as possible from one to the other. If, however, the distance is greater than this it will usually be necessary for the transport column to establish a rest station at some intermediate point *en route,* where the wounded may be given temporary attention and care. The destination of a transport column in battle will vary according to circumstances. It may be a hospital in the immediate vicinity on the line of communications, or a railroad station or boat landing. If it is one of the latter it will often be necessary to establish a rest station at this point. (Fig. 362.) Part of the personnel and supplies may be left here when the column returns to the front for other wounded. The surgical procedures which may be carried out while the wounded are in charge of a transport column will necessarily be wholly of an emergency character.

Transport columns are also sometimes used for carrying patients from evacuation to base hospitals, to railway stations, or to boat landings. It is not intended, however, that they shall ever be deflected from the front for this purpose if they are required there.

Evacuation Hospitals.—The prescribed duties of evacuation hospitals in combat are as follows: the establishing or the replacing of one or more field hospitals, when necessary; the hospital treatment of a more or less definite character for all the wounded received; the preparation of patients for transportation, and their despatch to base hospitals.

Emphasis has already been laid upon the necessity of having the medical

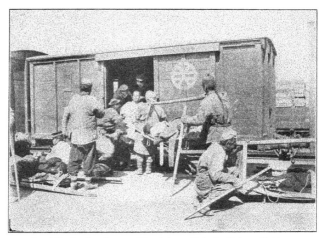

FIG. 365.—Loading Japanese Wounded on a Train for Patients, Mukden.

department organizations of the line of communications relieve those at the front of their patients, in order that the latter may accompany their troops. Evacuation hospitals are most important in effecting this purpose. Before a battle they should be located at convenient advanced points in the line of communications, in order that they may supplement the service of field hospitals. While they are not mobile in the sense that the latter are mobile, nevertheless they are not fixed in position like base hospitals. Evacuation hospitals have almost no transport of their own; hence, when it is necessary to move them, the chief surgeon of the line of communications must procure transport for them. In combat their site should not be changed except when the battle has moved so far from them that the distance is too great for moving wounded, when the field hospitals are overwhelmed with wounded, and when the convenient route for the evacuation of the wounded no longer passes through them. (Fig. 363.) At the conclusion of an engagement it will often be advantageous to have evacuation hospitals replace one or more field hospitals in order to give better treatment to patients than the more limited facilities of the latter afford. The departments described for a field hospital are likewise those of an evacuation hospital.

Although evacuation hospitals will be expected to do any necessary operating, the character of the surgical treatment given in them will vary widely according to the special conditions existing at the time. During a big battle, when great numbers of wounded are being received, it will not be practicable to do more than emergency operations and to prepare patients for further transport. Under such circumstances the wounded must be hurried to the rear, so that room

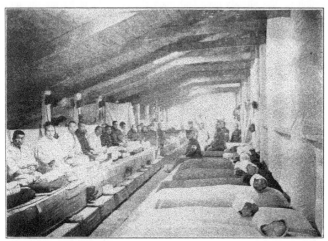

Fig. 366.—Japanese Line-of-Communications Hospital, Mukden. This corresponds to our base hospital.

may be made for oncoming cases. (Fig. 364.) Under opposite conditions, however, complete treatment should be given at evacuation hospitals, but always, in order to free the front, patients permanently incapacitated should be sent to the rear when their condition permits. Evacuation hospitals should not permit the front to be depleted, and minor cases should be returned thence to the front. Patients are sent from evacuation hospitals to the rear under arrangements made by the chief surgeon of the line of communications. Ordinarily, he should obtain the personnel for accompanying parties from a source other than the evacuation hospital, as personnel can rarely be spared from the latter.

Trains, Boats, and Ships.—The subject of trains and ships has already been discussed in connection with home territory; boats in the line of communications are ordinarily administered like ships for patients. The only point which it is desired to make here, in connection with these organizations, is that in battle the chief surgeon of the line of communications must be prepared to make use of them if the necessity arises. (Fig. 365.)

Base Hospitals.—On the eve of a battle the chief surgeon of the line of communications will be compelled to increase his base hospitals near the front or to augment the personnel and supplies of those in existence there. Base hospitals near the front should also be freed of patients before a battle, in order to make room for the wounded. Base hospitals will not be moved in battle, but new ones may be established when those already in existence are too far separated from the army, when they are needed to supplement the more advanced hospitals, or when new sites will be more convenient for handling the wounded. (Fig. 366.)

In battle the wounded from the more advanced base hospitals will necessarily

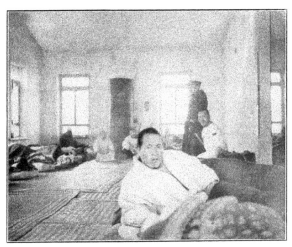

FIG. 367.—Line-of-Communications Hospital. Dalny. This corresponds to our base hospital.

be sent to the rear in case more wounded from the front must be provided for. Parties to accompany the wounded will be provided by the chief surgeon of the line of communications, and should usually come from base hospitals far to the rear, where the demands for personnel will not be so urgent as they are toward the front.

Base hospitals are provided with the necessary facilities for doing all surgical work, and under ordinary circumstances there would be no object in postponing the necessary surgical procedure till a later stage in the journey of the wounded man from front to rear. (Fig. 367.) Usually, however, the wounded who require very long treatment in hospitals had best be sent home when their condition justifies such a step. Similar action should always be taken with the wounded who are permanently incapacitated for service. In order not to deplete the front the wounded who have sufficiently recovered should be returned from base hospitals to the front as promptly as possible.

Furnishing Supplies to the Medical Department in Battle.—Attention has already been invited to the fact that, in war, two currents exist in the administration of the medical department: one of patients from the front, and the other of medical supplies from the rear. In battle the flow of both of these currents is necessarily more rapid than at other times. Preliminary to a battle the chief surgeon of the line of communications is expected to obtain, by requisition or by local purchase, all the medical supplies required both for the front and for the line of communications at this time. Supplies for the former should also be brought into advanced positions in the line of communications. (Fig. 368.) From these supplies division chief surgeons will be expected to stock their

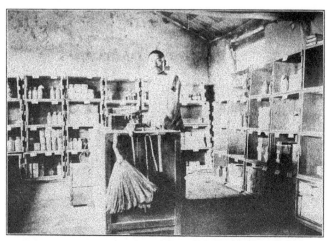

FIG. 368.—Japanese Medical Supply Depot at Tieling.

Reserve Medical Supplies very completely. Furthermore, division chief surgeons, in preparation for a battle, should require field hospitals, ambulance companies, and troops to procure all the medical supplies which they will require from the Reserve Medical Supply. Like action should be taken by the chief surgeon of the line of communications to outfit his medical department organizations from supply depots in the line of communications. It will always prove much easier in battle for medical department organizations on the line of communications to replace their medical supplies than it will be for those at the front. When the opportunity offers, division surgeons should move up medical supplies to points from which they may conveniently be conveyed to the front.

In battle regimental medical organizations will usually be compelled to depend on their own medical supplies, which rarely may be replenished from the reserve stock. Under exceptional conditions they may be allowed, on the authority of the division surgeon, to secure supplies from an ambulance company or a field hospital. In combat a field hospital, replacing a dressing station in order that the ambulance company may advance to establish another dressing station, will replace all supplies which have been used by the ambulance company. Similar action will be taken by evacuation hospitals which replace field hospitals. Supplies for the station for slightly wounded will come from the Reserve Medical Supply or from a field hospital.

NAVAL SURGERY.

By SURGEON-GENERAL CHARLES FRANCIS STOKES,

United States Navy.

NAVAL surgery is defined as the branch of surgery dealing with those wounds and accidents incident to service on a naval vessel in peace and war which, by reason of their frequency or the unique character of the agents producing them, may be regarded as peculiar to the environment. It comprehends further all problems of organization, transportation, and equipment related to the care of the injured.

Many operations for disease are undertaken on naval ships, but such practice is not essentially different from that obtaining in all civilized communities and so does not call for mention in a special treatise. It will be noted, too, that surgical states arising under the typical conditions of land warfare are not given place in this definition. These latter are excluded on the ground that naval surgery, as defined, can justly claim recognition as a specialty. For the purpose of adjusting the terminology to this distinction, the writer would restrict the application of the term "military surgery" to the surgery practised by land forces, and in addition begs to offer a generic term which shall include both specialties—the "Surgery of Warfare." Until comparatively recent times, the fighting personnel in naval warfare was composed of land forces embarked for an expected engagement, and, as a consequence, naval surgery presented no separate development. Even so late as 1798, the framers of our own government provided that the duties of the War Department should include supervision of naval affairs. Thus, naval surgery has emerged so recently from a subordinate position that the term "military surgery" has been expanded to embrace the surgery of ships, but it will be conceded that the distinction drawn is justified, when due weight is accorded the highly specialized development of the modern battleship, the peculiar character of wounds and accidents encountered, and the unique nature of the surroundings in which battles are fought at sea.

Duties of Medical Corps.—A medical officer may be assigned to navy yards, hospitals, ships, recruiting offices, and various special duties. In these places he may be suddenly called upon to pass judgment on any subject falling within the broad domain of medicine, since all matters relating, however remotely, to the health of the personnel are referred to him. His services may be required to-day in obstetrics, in legal medicine, or for the examination of suspected water; to-morrow, in a surgical emergency, in the treatment of wounds by venomous

970

fish, or in the handling of a yellow-fever epidemic. Consultants and reference libraries are often far away, and, from his stock of assimilated knowledge, he must make decision and assume sole responsibility for his judgment. It is possible, however, that the extent of this diversity of practice will be restricted at certain stations by the specific character of the duties assigned or the proximity of expert aid.

At a navy yard * the nature of the clinical work done is much like that in a civilian out-patient department. The sick and injured of the Navy and Marine Corps are treated, and civil employees, who may number several thousand, receive first-aid. Careful records must be kept, not only for medical purposes but also to preserve data by means of which subsequent claims for pensions may be decided. Families of officers furnish cases similar to those met with in civilian practice, and, in addition, medical services may be furnished a large native population, as is done in certain of our island possessions. Sanitary and quarantine responsibilities round out a list of duties most unusual in their range.

Service at a home hospital is comparable to that at any first-rate civilian hospital, except that all administrative affairs are under the immediate control of a commanding officer. Under him there are a supervising or executive surgeon and a number of junior officers who are generally assigned to specific duties. At a hospital outside our continental limits, the character of cases received is altered by the large proportion of tropical diseases or other affections peculiar to the country.

There are also certain general duties concerned with the conduct of the naval organization which devolve on medical officers. The character of these may be sufficiently indicated by the mention of certain of them: The care of all kinds of property; the upholding of discipline; the instruction of subordinates; duty on courts-martial and boards of examination or survey; and such sanitary and emergency work as exigency may require.

Recruiting is entitled to individual mention. It is in the recruiting office that the enlisted personnel is born, and the standard of excellence adhered to there fixes permanently the standing of our Navy, since laxity in recruiting can be only slightly compensated by subsequent rigidity of training. In every war, the losses by disease—at least in land operations—far exceed those inflicted by the engines of warfare,† and it may safely be affirmed that incompeteney in the medical department can inflict more damage on a fighting force than the most egregious blunders of the commanding officers. Resistance to disease and the manifold effects of injuries can be predicted only in a hardy physique, and the issue of any military enterprise thus becomes largely dependent on the manner in which the duties of the medical corps have been per-

---

* "Some Features of the Medical Department of the Navy in Peace and War," by C. F. Stokes, Medical Record, New York, August 14th, 1909.

† A few brief references to conditions in recent wars will amply substantiate this statement: See ref. Spear—Seaman, J. Assn. Mil. Surg., xvii., 500. Longmore: "The records of battles for the past two hundred years show that there has rarely been a conflict of any duration in which at least four men have not perished from disease for one from wounds."

formed. One of the chief contributions of the corps to military success—the bringing of every man to his post of battle in a state of the highest vigor—is possible only when the fundamental work of wise selection is well done in the recruiting office

In the Crimean Campaign, the Allied Forces lost 50,000 from disease and 2,000 from bullets. "Who'e regiments died away from disease without having seen the firing line.'"

In the French Campaign in Madagascar, 14,000 men were sent to the front; 29 were killed in action and 7,000 persihed from preventable disease.

Reliable figures are wanting for the Russo-Japanese War. It is acknowledged that the conduct of medical affairs by the Japanese was unique in its success, and yet the deaths from disease probably amounted to over twice those due to wounds.

On September 14th, 1905, there were in the Russian army east of Lake Baikal—

	Officers	Men
Wounded	34	746
Sick	1,129	30,035

Accidents and Wounds in Time of Peace.—The injuries to which seafaring men are exposed have always been of a specialized character. Formerly naval ships used no steam at all, or drew their fires when clear of port, and the accidents then were almost altogether due to the handling of sails and tackle in all weathers. With the transformation which ships have undergone (Fig. 369), there has been a correlated change in the men who work them and in the accidents that prevail. Seamen have passed with sails. They are now become gunners, firemen, machinists, electricians, and mechanics. The injuries sustained comport with the new type of activities. They are the accidents that take place in every industrial centre multiplied in frequency by the concentration of the various kinds of machinery in a space in which the utilization of every cubic inch has been contrived with the greatest ingenuity. Machinery is exploited for every purpose. It manipulates guns and handles ammunition; it raises and lowers boats, causes ponderous turrets to revolve, drives the cranes, and drops and weighs anchors. Even in the smaller matters of work in the galleys, automatic meat-choppers, dough-mixers, and bread-cutters add to the chances of injury. There are great boilers and extensively ramified steam-pipes located in closed compartments where the dangers of escaping steam are intensified. Powerful explosives are stored and handled in large quantities at times when the stimulus of competition tends to disregard of due precautions. Passages, hatches, and ladders are a prolific source of falls, especially when the ship is rolling and pitching at sea. Although these traumatisms of a general character are in nowise peculiar to naval life, yet their occurrence is so favored by conditions on board ships of war that, in few other places, are they met in such number, and they come to fill a large place in naval practice. Some injuries, such as ordinary wounds, contusions, and fractures, require no comment here; others merit more extensive notice.

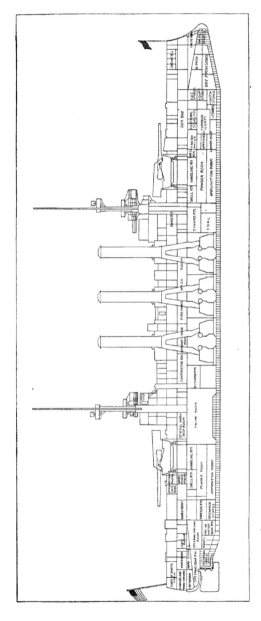

Fig. 369.—Inboard Profile of a Battleship.

Wounds by Bites and Stings.—Wounds are occasionally inflicted by dog-fish, pike, and sharks. They are much more infrequent than might be expected in view of the number of predaceous fish present in tropical waters.

Sailors and marines, in common with all who frequent tropical regions, are exposed to the bites or stings of noxious insects, scorpions, myriapods, reptiles, and other animals. These are not peculiar to naval life and, in fact, they are almost always the accidents of land operations. The wounds made by *venomous fish*, however, are almost exclusively seen among seafaring men, including sailors and fishermen.* In this connection we do not speak of those fish which, when eaten, cause an alimentary intoxication, but only those which possess a venom sac in conjunction with some defensive weapons, usually one or more spines. Such fish are not numerous and the association of any species with the wound can rarely be determined, so that extended description is unnecessary.

Of the symptoms produced by these fish, pain is the most characteristic. With certain species it is excruciating and radiates throughout a limb. The agonizing character of the pain is evinced by the maniacal symptoms it produces and by the observation that rats, experimentally inoculated, frequently amputate their own limbs. There are also general symptoms—muscular in-co-ordination, weakness, a feeling of deep anxiety, vomiting, and a slowing of the heart. There is local paralysis of both motor and sensory nerves. Death is not commonly the result of the wound, but it may occur promptly in syncope or later as the result of complicating tetanus or septicæmia. Local gangrene is the rule after wounds by the more poisonous species, eschars being thrown off slowly and healing long delayed.

Treatment.—The wounds, when first seen, should be freely incised to allow copious bleeding, thoroughly washed out, cupped, and cauterized. The pain is combated by moist dressings and morphia. Constitutional symptoms may require stimulants.

Landing parties are subject, in certain countries, to wounds by *poisoned weapons*. Most tribes use a vegetable extract, but some dip their weapons in putrefying meat or tetanic earth. The nature of the poisons varies so greatly that no general rules of treatment can be laid down.

Venomous Marine Snakes † are very common in all tropical waters. Most of them belong to the suborder, Ophidia colubridæ, family Hydrophinæ. The hydrophinæ are viviparous and rarely come on shore. All are poisonous and vicious. The symptoms following their wounds are suggested by a mention of the active principles of the venom: 1, a thrombin; 2, a hemorrhagin; 3, a hæmolysin and an agglutinin; 4, a polyvalent cytolysin; and 5, a principle which attacks the central nervous system.

The venom of most of the hydrophinæ contains a large proportion of neuro-

---

* See: Gatewood, "Naval Hygiene"; J. M. Rogers, R. N., "W. I. Poisonous Fishes"; U. S. Fish Commission Bulletins; Rochard and Bodet; "Traité d'Hygiène"; Pellegrin: "Les Poissons Vénéneux"; and the article by Major Mason in Vol. III. of this series.

† Stejneger; Noguchi; Calmette; Mason; et al.

toxin, and hence œdema and ecchymosis are not noticeable characteristics of the wounds which they inflict. Stupefaction, paralysis, dyspnœa, and cessation of respiration form the usual train of symptoms. When death is delayed, there is generally a diminished proportion of neurotoxin, and the local symptoms are consequently more pronounced. Death may occur in a few minutes. In patients who recover, the loss of the bactericidal properties of the blood is manifested by the frequency of secondary infections.

Non-specific treatment is concerned (1) with retarding and intermitting absorption by means of a tourniquet, and (2) with removing or destroying the free venom. Excision, cupping, and sucking are useful measures. Permanganate of potassium and chromic acid are remedies, either of which may be used, in one-per-cent solution, for local injection. Many drugs—strychnine (Mueller), morphine, nicotine, curare, alcohol, coffee and tea—have been recommended by various authors, but their employment has resulted in doubtful benefit, and has even, in some cases, hastened death. Salt solution may be of advantage. Artificial respiration should be kept up for one hour, or at least for as long a time as the heart continues to beat.

Specific antivenine is almost never at hand and not much work has been done leading to the production of a polyvalent serum.

Scalds.—Burns by hot water and steam are very common among the engineer force. Bursting pipes or valves permit the sudden escape of large volumes of steam under pressure into small compartments. Long ladders confine the men as in a trap, since it is impossible to find the way out in the midst of scalding vapors, or, indeed, to survive the attempt. The action of the steam, although brief, is intense. The vapor is superheated at the moment of its escape and the high temperature combines with the specific heat of steam to inflict terrible scalds.

"At the moment of explosion (of the boilers) men rushed on deck panic-stricken, mutilated, and crying horribly. Some tried to throw themselves into the sea; others sank to the deck without voice or power of movement, overcome by the agony and dying quickly. Some of the unfortunates were entirely stripped of their skin. The nails hung dangling from the extremities of the fingers and toes. One saw large surfaces quite denuded where removing the clothing had torn away great masses of tattered skin. The features were quite unrecognizable. The skin was pale, flabby, without elasticity, white as if boiled, the eyes alone appearing animated, lit with an expression of despair. Most of the men, however, died asphyxiated. The inspired steam had penetrated quite to the bottom of the bronchioles and obstructed them with masses of detached epithelium mixed with the products of the plastic exudate. These men succumbed in paroxysms of horrible suffocation, spitting up with difficulty the lining membrane of the tongue and mouth." (Saurel.*)

As a part of first-aid instruction, men should be warned that escape from the compartment is not to be thought of. The vapor tends to rise, and hence let them be taught to lay hold of some covering, throw themselves flat on the

* "Traité de Chirurgie Navale."

deck, face down, shut the eyes, hold the breath and wait. The time will not be long, for condensation will be completed in a few moments at most.

Of a different character are the burns due to explosion of smokeless powder. In these, the lesion results from exposure to an intense flame of short duration.

"Flarebacks" * are made possible by the admixture of a limited quantity of air with explosive gases remaining in the breech of the gun and they may lead to the explosion of powder charges in the turret or near the gun. Devices to prevent the occurrence are now installed on ships, but such accidents have been not infrequent in all navies.

We may take a report † of one of these accidents as typifying what may be expected. Out of thirty-five persons exposed directly to the flame, thirty-two perished. Three charges of three hundred and sixty pounds each were ignited, one in the turret and two in the handling room. The bodies of the unfortunate victims showed no lesion suggestive of the disruptive action of exploding powder. The lesions were those to be expected as a result of exposure to sudden and intense flame of short duration. The time of exposure is estimated at one to three minutes, the integument of their whole bodies being hardened, charred, and split open in places. They lived four hours, however, and were conscious until the end. Many of the victims showed a peculiar, hardened, blanched, and waxy appearance of the exposed skin and mucous membranes, with charring only of the hair.

It is of interest to note that it was impossible to utilize board stretchers in the removal of the injured men from the turret, nor was it advisable to tolerate the delay incident to fastening straps. A blanket was used to lower the men from the turret and it proved satisfactory.

Irrespirable Gases.‡—Burns are not the only result of powder explosions. Intoxication, asphyxiation, and acute respiratory lesions are seen in connection with them. Symptoms may also develop under various conditions of gun practice, especially where a breeze carries back into the ships the fumes from the guns.

Smokeless powders consist of nitroglycerin, nitrocellulose, guncotton, and metallic nitrates, or other deterrents, such as urea and vaseline. Picric acid is used in some European powders. Guncotton and nitrocellulose yield, when detonated, large amounts of carbon monoxide. When the powder is not exploded, but burns as it does in modern firearms, a considerable quantity of the oxides of nitrogen is given off.

The toxic action of these gases has been frequently reported. Spear § states that the fumes from the Japanese Shimose shells caused nausea, weakness, and sometimes unconsciousness, and that recovery in some cases required several days. Urie ‖ reports that "the gases generated penetrated the different

* Gatewood : "Naval Hygiene."
† J. F. Urie, Surgeon, U. S. N., "Report of the Surgeon-General of the Navy," 1904.
‡ Spear, R., Report to Surgeon-General of the Navy on Russo-Japanese War; Keiffer, J. A. M. A., "Smokeless Powders," with references.
§ Op. cit.
‖ Report to the Surgeon-General of the U. S. Navy, 1904.

parts of the ship in the vicinity of the explosion. The composition of the gases is not accurately known. The vapor from the muzzle of the gun after discharge has a distinctly reddish tint and the odor of nitrous acid. Carbon monoxide and marsh gas are said to be generated. A number of officers and men were variously affected by inhalation of the gases. An exhilaration was experienced at first, followed in a few cases by a partial loss of consciousness. Other effects of the inhalation of the products of combustion were those caused by the irritative action of gases on the lining of the respiratory tract."

Experiments by Keiffer give the characteristic symptoms: The pulse rose to 118–128 and became arrhythmic and dicrotic. The subjects complained of angor cardii, great distress in the chest, a feeling of oppression in the head, smarting of the eyes, and dryness of the throat. There was marked loss of hearing, amounting to one-half; acuity of vision was diminished $\frac{5}{20}-\frac{7}{20}$, and mental confusion was apparent. A headache of great violence appeared early and lasted twenty-four to forty-eight hours. An initial flushing of the face was succeeded by a peculiar turgescence. There was an average fall in the blood-pressure of 50 mm. of Hg. Locomotion and co-ordination were markedly affected. Free nitrates could be demonstrated in the urine.

The presence of NO_2 in the products is evidenced by the acrid, reddish fumes whch are so irritating to the fauces and conjunctivæ. When present in large amounts, nitrogen peroxide causes severe and perhaps fatal pulmonary irritation. "The NO_2 (or the nitrites) converts the hæmoglobin into a mixture of methæmoglobin and nitric-acid hæmoglobin." Thus we have most of the symptoms due to the permanent binding of the hæmoglobin with CO and NO_2, and its partial reduction to methæmoglobin. In addition, the NO_2 has on the lungs an intensely irritating action which may prove fatal. The treatment of these cases would be similar to that for poisoning by illuminating gas, with direct transfusion of blood occupying a prominent place.

In the late Russo-Japanese war, hand grenades filled with chemicals producing noxious or irrespirable gases made their reappearance. It is very improbable that these will play a part in ordinary naval warfare, but they may find employment under special circumstances. No forecast can be made as to the nature of the substances to be used.

In the Battle of Tsushima Straits, the distribution of groups of cases of asphyxiation demonstrated that the crew was more subject to this accident in the better ventilated compartments. During battle, a ship is apt to be enveloped in gases arising both from the discharge of its own guns and from the bursting of the enemy's shells. It is inevitable that these gases should be drawn in by the blowers and distributed throughout the ship. Prolonged stoppage of the blowers is impracticable, although, during a short and severe engagement, air from the outside may be supplied to the fire-room only. But even if the blowers stop, the enveloping gases may find their way in by penetrating shell tracks, hatches, or other adventitious openings, and exploding shells may spread fumes into neighboring compartments. To meet this situation, Bastier * suggests that air may be stored under pressure so that compartments can be occasionally cleared. The value of this suggestion is shown by an experience † of the Russians, when the complete medical force attached to a dressing station was rendered unconscious by the fumes from the Shimose shells.

Asphyxiation.—Asphyxiation is of common occurrence. Submersion every year leads among the causes of lethality, it having furnished, in 1909, fifty-one deaths out of a total of two hundred and eighty-six. Accidents of this general character may always be anticipated among divers and the crews of submarines; and on surface craft, also, men are sometimes overcome in double bottoms or other compartments which have been deprived of their oxygen by paint and other reducing substances. Submarines, at least, should be supplied with some form of oxygen-generating apparatus.

If the asphyxiation is due to submersion, the patient should be placed in the prone position and rhythmically suspended by the hands of the manipulator clasped about the abdomen, in order to clear the respiratory passages. Artificial respiration is best maintained by the Brosch-Sylvester method. It is described by Keith ‡ as follows:

"In 1897 Brosch modified the Sylvester method as follows: 'He raised and extended the arms by the patient's head exactly as Sylvester recommended, but in place of stopping the movement after the first degree of traction had been exercised, he used a considerable degree of force to continue the movement until the arms actually touched the table or ground on which the supine patient was placed. At the end of this movement the body is arched upward so that it rests on the ground only at the shoulders and at the heels. The spine is overextended. With the withdrawal of the operator's force the body recoils on the ground, and the chest at the same time begins to collapse. The expiratory movement is completed by forcing the patient's arms against the chest, not toward the lateral aspects as advised by Sylvester, but directly over the sternum and yielding costal cartilages which are forced inward so as to compress the lungs and heart. Meyer and Loewy have recently (1908) carried out experiments on the efficiency of the Brosch-Sylvester method. They found that they could fill the lungs with from 1,000 to 3,000 c.c. of air with each movement (Schafer's method, 300 to 400 c.c.) and effect a respiratory exchange varying from 7,000 to 16,000 c.c. per minute, while Schafer finds that he can produce a respiratory change (per minute) of 5,850 c.c. with his method, an amount which he regards as amply sufficient for the purpose of resuscitation.'"

In connection with Crile's studies on resuscitation, it is interesting to note that both the above methods furnish a rhythmic, although slow, compression of the thorax, and that Crile's chief measure of injecting adrenalin centripetally is practicable at the same time. A sterile irrigating apparatus, a sterile saline solution, and a hypodermic syringe may easily be kept ready at all times.

*Arch. de Méd. Nav., No. 12, 1908.
† Braisted, op. cit.
‡ The Lancet, London, March 13th. 20th, 27th, 1909.

Damage Done to the Ears.—When a large piece of ordnance is discharged, the gaseous pressure within the tube is communicated to the atmosphere in the neighborhood with its degree diminished proportionately to the expansion which the gas has undergone. The onward movement of the blast and the oscillation of the gaseous medium tend to replace this sudden high pressure with a vacuum, characterized by equally abrupt onset. The effect of this and succeeding rapid alternations of positive and negative pressure is seen in the vasomotor system and the tympanum.

The general agitation, together with the compression and suction applied to the abdomen, brings on nausea, giddiness, and fainting; but these transitory effects appear insignificant when we turn to the permanent damage often done to the auditory apparatus.

Ordinary gun practice brings about in many individuals a degree of deafness which is apparently a simple suspension of function. These cases may be regarded as analogous in origin to instances of temporary blindness, anuria, or other examples of inhibition of epithelial structures. Complete restoration of hearing shortly takes place. Deafness that is permanent may, however, result and be unaccompanied by any demonstrable lesion. The nature of such changes is not known. They may be scleroses of the middle ear, minute hemorrhages, or injuries sustained by the auditory mechanism of the internal ear.

These injuries are apparently more common when a rigid attitude of expectancy, which favors bone conduction, is assumed at the instant of discharge. Bone conduction is frequently lost as a result of gun-firing, and we know that violent driving inward of the stapes sets up vibrations of the endolymph and perilymph which may be of such intensity that the auditory nerve terminals are affected. So it is at least probable that, apart from the injuries inflicted upon the membrana tympani, the nervous mechanism of the internal ear is the part most commonly damaged. It is not altogether clear to what extent the occurrence of these lesions is influenced by opening the Eustachian tube at the moment of the blast. This expedient is intended to equalize the pressure on each side of the membrana tympani, but it fails signally of its purpose. The tortuosity of the internal approaches delays the pressure wave from one to four seconds, it is said. Moreover, the delayed positive wave may reach the inside of the tympanic membrane at the precise instant that a negative oscillation acts on the outside, thus doubling the aural effects of the blast. The Germans believe that the first atmospheric blast is what commonly ruptures this membrane, bursting it inward, but they mention not infrequent cases of patulous Eustachian tube, in which the rupture occurred outward, presumably from the augmentation of the negative wave just described.

Headache, pain, tinnitus aurium, and partial deafness are such common accompaniments of gun-firing that little notice is taken of them unless the hemorrhage is considerable, in which case an aural examination will usually show single or multiple tears of the membrana tympani. In these cases the drum membrane heals promptly under simple methods of treatment; but many cases are not reported until otitis media or other complication drives the individual to the medical officer.

Any officer or man, incapacitated by reason of deafness, is lost to the service as truly as if deprived of a limb, and prophylaxis demands our attention. Plugging the external meatus has proved an efficient means of protection, but has not yet come into general use for several reasons. The chief objection to the procedure is that verbal or telephonic communication is hindered by plugging the ear, although this statement loses much of its weight when it is remembered that defective hearing is apt to result from failure to use these devices. Another objection, not less real, is that the enlisted men are indifferent, or they consider it effeminate to adopt elaborate precautions against what seems only a trifling discomfort. Refusal on the part of the personnel to avail themselves of protection for such reasons should not be tolerated when the loss to the active service and the unnecessary increase of the always large retired list are given due reflection. It is, therefore, believed that ear protection should be made mandatory.

The selection of the best means of protection then becomes necessary, and the choice is difficult, since no device yet suggested is free from defects. Absorbent cotton and shredded wool have been tried and have been found to afford considerable protection to the anatomical structures of the ear and freedom from symptoms, without materially interfering with audition. They also keep the meatus clean, and accidents, if they occur, are less likely to be followed by septic complications. On the other hand, cotton is liable to be sucked out unless well placed, and there is some danger attending the practice of instigating unskilled men to force cotton into their ears with a match. The cotton may also require removal by a medical officer, or be forgotten until a purulent discharge leads to its discovery. Modelling clay, wax, paraffin, and other plastic materials have given satisfaction. They are molded closely to the meatus, and, like wool, mitigate aural shock without totally interrupting hearing. It is said that such substances are more effective when worked up with cotton or wool into a strongly cohesive mass.

Perhaps the most satisfactory solution of the problem is furnished by an instrument invented by Elliott. (Fig. 370.) It consists of a ball with which to plug the meatus, and a wing which serves to engage the auricle and hold the apparatus in place. A canal, which perforates the instrument throughout its length, provides for hearing, while the tortuous course of the channel diminishes the aural effects of an explosion to limits which can be borne without injury.

A perfect fit is, of course, indispensable, and, to insure this, a great number of the instruments would be required in a large assortment of sizes. It has been suggested that each man be furnished with one pair as a part of his outfit; but, if that were done, the small implements would be continually mislaid or lost altogether. The English Admiralty has recently investigated the subject of ear protection, and has decided to leave the choice of means to the individual. Much ear trouble seen in the Navy results from high diving, and some aural injuries produced by gun-firing are not discovered until an otitis develops after swimming, so that it is often hard to verify the origin of a ruptured tympanic membrane.

Space Allotted the Medical Department on a Battleship.—Having reviewed the special accidents which may happen on a modern battleship, we may now turn to consider what provision has been made for meeting this formidable array of surgical emergencies, for nursing the cases of disease that may develop, and for curtailing the epidemics that may break out from time to time. When one bears in mind that the offensive and defensive resources of the ship cannot be materially sacrificed to humanitarian motives, it is remarkable what complete facilities exist on board naval ships for coping with every medical situation. Such facilities as we possess are not a concession to the Medical Department, but betoken a recognition of the unity of aims pervading all branches of the service.

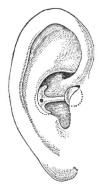

FIG. 370.—Elliott Ear Protector.

It will be seen by references to the plan (Fig. 371) that the space allotted to the Medical Department consists of an examining room, a ward, a dispensary, an operating room, an isolation ward, and a bath-room (Fig. 372) with closet. In the large ships (Fig. 373) about twenty-eight beds are provided for the sick, and these suffice to accommodate about three per cent of the total rated complement. Under ordinary circumstances, the average number of sick on a cruising ship will amount to 1.75 per cent of the complement. Additional beds are, however, needed over this flat average, in order to provide for an increase in the number of sick due to accidents, epidemics, or a lack of opportunity to transfer men to a hospital. Also, better discipline is maintained in the sick bay if the members of the Hospital Corps are berthed there and kept apart from the crew. So, to the number of beds required for the average sick list, there should be added a marginal provision for unusual conditions and berthing facilities for the Hospital Corps. On the other hand, cruising ships rarely have a full complement, and there will be some sick on the list who do not require a bed in the sick bay, so that an allowance of beds on a basis of three per cent of the complement should suffice for the needs of the Medical Department.

The isolation room contains at least two beds, though usually four are provided. This room is of the utmost value in limiting the spread of infections and also in caring for the very sick when relative quiet is important.

The dispensary (Fig. 374) contains primarily a stock of all drugs and supplies that are ever used by the medical officer on duty: if his practice requires the use of preparations not regularly supplied, they can nearly always be obtained. A chemical equipment is furnished for clinical examinations, analysis of water and foods, and determination of poisons. In this room is kept the microscope also, with such bacteriological accessories as are required for the examination of smears, maintenance of cultures, and the preparation of vaccines. Roentgen apparatus is not at present supplied to ships of war, but attention is being given now to the selection of a type adapted to the peculiar demands.

Although a discussion of the structural details of a sick bay, and of much of the equipment, belongs more properly to a treatise on naval hygiene, we may speak here of certain requirements intimately concerned with the practice of surgery. Cubic space is always limited and adequate artificial means must be provided for the frequent renewal of air. In the absence of such provision, cases of shock, hemorrhage, and gas poisoning are deprived of the oxygen they need, and volatile anæsthetics may reach a concentration at which they are explosive and productive of physiological effects on the operators.

The walls of the operating room (Fig. 375) are of steel, heavily painted or covered with cork paint, and the floor is of mosaic tiling. All these surfaces permit satisfactory cleaning of the room. Steam from the boilers is used in the

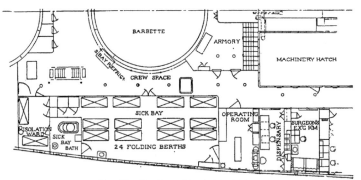

Fig. 371.—Sick Bay on Board a Battleship.

sterilizing apparatus (Fig. 376), which consists of a pressure chamber and instrument and utensil boilers, with tanks for hot and cold sterile water. Tables, sinks, and other accessories are of the most approved type.

Artificial lighting must be relied on exclusively. The choice of lighting units is restricted by the prevalence of excessive vibrations from the engines and during gun-fire, so that lamps having fragile filaments cannot be used. Although possessing certain defects, the Nernst form of electric glow lamp is perhaps the best adapted to surgical purposes, since it is the only small unit lamp that gives white light and at the same time is sufficiently resistant to jarring vibrations.

Although the sick bays on our recent ships are small, they are equipped for every kind of work, and during a cruise the equipment is sure to be tested in the most diverse ways. It will be seen that nothing essential is lacking for the diagnosis and successful treatment of disease, but there are, outside the sick bay, certain influences which are potent in restricting practice.

These hindrances are inseparable from the environment. There will be much incidental noise and bustle when there are a thousand men living within a small space. That noise will be increased by the fact that the dwelling is a busy machine shop as well, and there will be, while at sea, some vibration from the

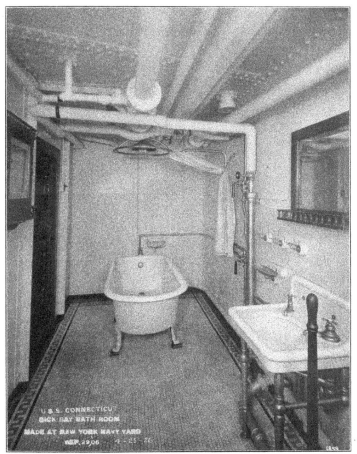

Fig. 372.—Sick Bay Bath Room, U. S. S. *Connecticut.*

engines and perhaps violent pitching and rolling of the ship. These conditions do not contribute to the successful conduct of either medical or surgical cases. Therefore, we hold it as a guiding principle that the care of no serious case should be undertaken on a fighting ship when it can be avoided. There will, notwithstanding, arise emergencies in which postponement of operation or transfer of a case to a hospital is impossible. Then the surgeon may proceed with full assurance that, so far as the facilities of the sick bay are concerned, he may expect an ideal result.

Anæsthetics.—It has been found that the methods of administering anæsthetics need not be altered to suit climatic conditions. Even the open drop method of giving ether is practicable in the high temperature of the tropics. Indeed, it is the custom to keep American operating rooms at a temperature quite equal to that prevailing in tropical countries, and the anæsthetist accustomed to work in our amphitheatres will discover that hot climates entail no

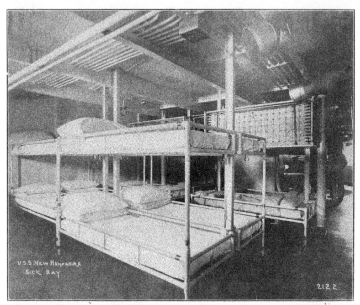

Fig. 373.—Portion of Sick Bay, U. S. S. *New Hampshire*, Showing Superposed Folding-cots.

departure from familiar practice. The choice of anæsthetic will depend upon the preference of the individual medical officer, but bulky anæsthetics like nitrous oxide can rarely have a place. Ether and chloroform soon fill a small room with vapor which, as has been mentioned, may reach such a concentration that the operator is affected during prolonged exposure, and, too, explosive mixtures are formed,—a point of practical importance, since a chance shell may destroy the electric wiring and a candle or lantern will then be required. Further, the operating room of a sick bay is not remotely situated. It is in the midst of all the sick. The odors and noises incident to a chloroform or ether narcosis add to the distress of the injured who are awaiting their turn and who may well be completely unnerved by the presence in the next bed of a shipmate in the throes of recovery. Should there be a collision, or should fire break out, orders may have been issued to throw overboard all explosives and inflammables, thus in a moment depriving a medical officer of all his ether, chloroform, and ethyl chloride. Moreover, there is often great difficulty in finding experienced attendants for the overwhelming number of cases that may accumulate. Local anæsthetics are not open to these grave objections,—they do not affect the operator, are not liable to explode, are not inflammable, occupy little room, and are not attended by disagreeable after-affects. They lessen the number of assistants and nurses required, and their physiological "blocking" action

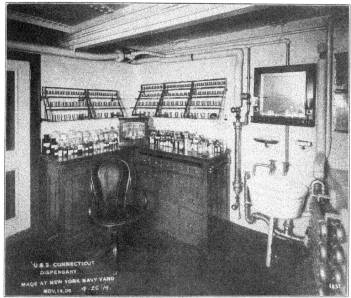

Fig. 374.—Dispensary, U. S. S. *Connecticut.*

is of the utmost value in that it permits one to operate early in spite of existing shock. Venous and terminal arterial anæsthesia are particularly adapted to certain injuries, and spinal anæsthesia deserves wider employment under conditions of naval warfare when broad considerations may justify the routine adoption of methods which, under normal circumstances, are restricted in their application to special cases. It is, then, imperative that the naval medical officer should perfect himself in the various uses of cocaine and its substitutes.

General Surgical Technique.—General surgical technique differs in no respect from that practised in shore hospitals, although, where a choice of methods is sanctioned by good practice, preference should invariably be given to the simpler. For example, if it becomes generally accepted that two applications of tincture of iodine constitute a safe method of sterilizing the skin, it should be forthwith adopted as being superior to procedures which involve the tedious application of successive solutions that are difficult to prepare and yet more difficult to store in sufficient quantities. Attention will be directed later to novel considerations arising from the havoc of battle and imposing new guides for our conduct, so that it is neither desirable nor possible to prescribe uniformity in practice. The pressing demands of hundreds of wounded, the possible de-

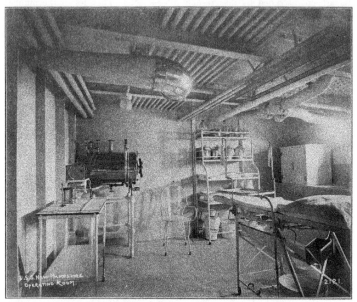

FIG. 375.—Portion of Operating Room, U. S. S. *New Hampshire.*

struction of all our carefully planned provisions and other unforeseen factors, may, indeed, force us to depart widely from all accepted practice and assume risks that would be unjustifiable under less extraordinary circumstances.

Duties of the Medical Corps with Reference to Battle.—Having passed briefly over the organization of the Medical Department and its activities in times of peace, we may now with propriety treat at some length its functioning in relation to battle. While it is true that, in the main, our active part in influencing the issue of a conflict will have been terminated before the day of battle, yet there are many specific preparations to be made when a battle is impending,—measures designed to relieve suffering, sustain naval effectiveness, and contribute to prompt recuperation from the effects of the engagement. These preparations, together with the duties of the Medical Department, may be conveniently assembled for purposes of description under three chronological headings, namely, Before, During, and After Battle. The first group is concerned, as has been said, in making such preparations as may tend to minimize the damage inflicted by the enemy, support courage, lessen suffering, preserve life, and restore naval efficiency. The second group falls in a period of time corresponding to the course of the action, and, from the circumstances attending a naval battle, the duties embraced may be very limited, both in number and in scope. The third group involves restoring the crew as promptly as pos-

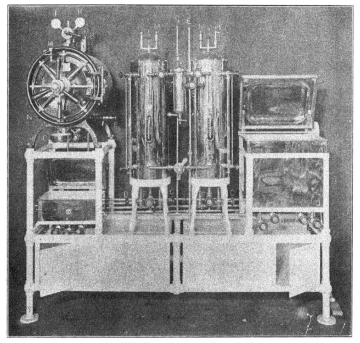

Fig. 376.—Steam-Pressure Sterilizing Outfit.

sible to its normal pitch of effectiveness, lessening suffering, and preserving life and future industrial usefulness.

1. BEFORE THE BATTLE.

A. Maintenance of a State of Preparedness.—Both matériel and personnel must be kept in a high state of preparedness, and their condition attested by periodic inspections. Anæsthetics, gauze, antiseptics, ligatures, instruments, splints, and other supplies must be at hand in sufficient quantity and variety;

for, although it may be possible to recruit these materials from a station or hospital ship, the cruising ship may be acting as an independent unit remote from such assistance, and hence the equipment should be collected without reference to the possible neighborhood of reserve supplies.

Identification Tags.—It is not uncommon for the dead to be unrecognizable. Under certain circumstances, it may be impossible to say who are dead, and who have escaped to other ships or been captured by the enemy. Our responsibil:ty for a man does not cease with his death; we must care for his body, when possible, and forward a report of his death, so that both the Department and the man's family may have authentic information concerning his fate. Some means, then, of insuring identification should be provided. The method most in favor is to suspend from the neck, by a light metal chain, an aluminum disc on which is stamped the wearer's full name and rate.

Dressing Tags.—In each hospital corps pouch there is to be found a package of linen dressing tags, conspicuously multi-colored. These, when properly used, are of invaluable assistance in the methodical handling of the wounded. The member of the Medical Corps who first sees a patient estimates his condition as accurately as possible and leaves attached to the primary dressing information as to the severity of the wound, urgency of the need of further attention, what transportation may be endured, the nature of the treatment already given, and at what time the dressing was performed. The ready legibility of the information is assured by colored detachable coupons. For example: if both coupons are detached, the plain white card signifies that the patient is able to walk, the presence of the blue coupon indicates that transportation is required, the retention of the red coupon denotes a serious condition in which life would be jeopardized by transportation.

First-aid Instruction.—In the press of work following battle there will be no opportunity for instruction or even supervision. Therefore, the members of the Hospital Corps must be so saturated with an understanding of their duties that the performance of them becomes automatic and may be relied on in the midst of the most perturbing surroundings. Such familiarity comes only from long experience or unremitting drill. The members of the Corps must be taught the art of nursing, they must be proficient in the management of the general types of injuries and post-operative cases, they should be familiar with the phenomena of anæsthesia, and they should be able to prepare, store, and handle the special material of surgical practice.

These men must be taught their duties as carriers—how to estimate the urgency of various injuries, how to control hemorrhage, perform artificial respiration and apply temporary splints; how to handle a man with due regard to the requirements of his injury, manage transportation in the face of formidable obstacles, and aid men prostrated with burns, scalds, or shock. Finally, they must be imbued with a spirit of serene confidence in their own resources. This temper will not only sustain them when in trying situations and at the head of independent posts, but also will give fresh heart to their despairing charges.

The training we have outlined should not be confined to the Hospital Corps. The difficulties under which the Medical Department labors during battle will be dwelt upon at greater length in another place, and it will be seen that many groups of men are removed from the possibility of outside assistance for considerable periods of time. The aid which they receive must be given by their combatant companions, and it will devolve upon the members of a gun crew to pull a wounded comrade off to one side and perhaps to staunch a smart hemorrhage. Such ministrations are not primarily humane in purpose. They are chiefly undertaken in order that the helpless and the dead shall not be left under foot to unnerve the gunners by their cries and groans or the mute eloquence of their plight. Wounds are rendered less terrible when every man may enter into action borne up by the certainty that should he fall he will receive the succor that his sacrifice merits. So, from these points of view, the training of the whole personnel in the principles of first-aid becomes of great military importance.

Yet, men are apt not to appreciate the importance of the subject, and they remain indifferent until the presence of an enemy brings them face to face with the hazards of combat. Moreover, they are totally lacking in any general information which might help them to understand the principles involved. This indifferent attitude, and the defects of early training, require that the instruction imparted be in the nature of simple demonstrations and practical exercises, given as frequently as possible to small sections of the crew, and made interesting. The scope of such first-aid instruction is not fixed, but it is generally agreed that the subjects treated should include: artificial respiration; immediate care of cases of burns, scalds, and shock; handling and transportation of the wounded; application of first-aid dressings; and control of hemorrhage. It has been found that the occasional demonstrations allowed medical officers do not suffice to teach the subjects thoroughly, and one of two courses should be adopted, to wit: either the number of hours allotted to first-aid teaching by medical officers should be largely increased; or midshipmen at the Naval Academy should be so thoroughly schooled in the principles and practices of first-aid that, when commissioned, they are qualified to teach it to their divisions as a routine drill. The latter course is demanded by the naval importance of adequate instruction in the subject.

B. *In Expectation of Immediate Battle.*—Before proceeding to plan our preparations for battle, it will be necessary to forecast, so far as we may, the circumstances which battle may develop. We ought, for instance, to get some idea of how many wounded there may be, the damage which may be done to the decks and passages and particular localities by gun fire, the nature of the projectiles in use, the character of the wounds encountered, and other contingencies with reference to which our scheme of first-aid must be designed.

The Number of Wounded.—Contrary to general expectation, apparently there has not been an increase in the loss of life on board ships during recent battles. Gun fire has become enormously more destructive, but means of defense have been to a corresponding degree elaborated, and the range at which battles are fought has been steadily increased, so that the number of casualties necessary to compel acknowledgment of defeat, the number for which we must provide, remains remarkably constant.

In former times, every man was, on occasion, a member of a gun crew. In these days of specialization, the proportion of fighting men is necessarily smaller. Few members of the special branches can leave their own duties to replace gunners who have fallen, and we may reckon that, when one-half the ship's complement is disabled, it is no longer possible to fight the ship. Therefore, we may say that, when the casualties on a ship amount to one-third or one-half of the complement, she will drop out of action; and that, in the event of greater loss of life, the mortality in the medical department, the destruction of supplies, and the local conditions will make the rendering of any aid quite impossible.

Of the total number of casualties, we can dismiss almost one-half from our consideration; that is, the dead and slightly wounded require no special provision. We may, then, expect a list of seriously wounded, who will require immediate treatment and subsequent care, comprising one-sixth to one-fourth of the complement. Therefore, we should proceed with our preparations on the assumption that, on a battleship, we must afford facilities for the surgical treatment, nursing, and feeding of two hundred wounded.

As bearing further on this subject, a few statistics from the most recent war are instructive:

From the Japanese* side we have the following figures for the whole Russian war:—

Total killed and wounded	3,674
Dead at once	1,887
Dead, after being wounded	116
Recovered; sent to duty	1,408
Recovered; invalided	34
Patients remaining	229

It is noteworthy that over half the total number of killed and wounded were killed outright, and that few (150) of the wounded subsequently died or were invalided, but on the contrary most of them (1,408) were later returned to duty.

The mortality, according to rank, was:—

Commissioned officers	304
Warrant officers	86
Petty officers and men	3,219
Employés	65

Statistics on which percentile calculations could be based are lacking.

The fleet at the Battle of Tsushima suffered (according to the reports made public by Admiral Togo) the following casualties:—

Killed	113
Severely wounded	101
Wounded	317
Total	531

*Surgeon W. C. Braisted, U. S. N., Report to Surgeon General, 1905.

"On the Russian ships, however, the loss of life was so great in some cases and the wounded so numerous that the surgeons, I am told, were completely paralyzed and unable, not only to perform operations, but even to make the necessary dressings. The Russian casualties were estimated at from 5,000 to 8,000." *

"The rate per cent (as gathered from the study of a large mass of statistics) of killed and wounded for each class, under the heads of officers, seamen, combatants and non-combatants, shows that surgeons and medical attendants have the largest rate; next, officers and seamen, engineers and stokers having the smallest rate."†

At first glance, this mortality among those of the hospital branch is very surprising, but there is a reason why the distribution of casualties should be as stated. Armor furnishes protection against the direct flight of shells, but does not shelter the personnel from the fragments of shells which have exploded above or which have dropped in their flight behind the armor. The hospital corps men are exposed equally with all others who are stationed above the protective deck, and, in addition, the nature of their duties, unless all activities are suspended during battle, leads them to seek out places where, for the moment, the injured are most numerous and the danger greatest.

Character of Present-Day Warfare.—In the contest of development which is always being actively waged between the offensive and defensive powers bestowed on ships, the offensive qualities have generally been in the lead. This has resulted in a tendency to depend largely on distance for defence and to let the effects of long-range gun-fire decide the contest. Out of this tendency we have seen the "all-big-gun" ship evolved. Combat between ships of this description will be fought at long ranges and by guns upward of ten inches in calibre.

The duration of battle will depend on many factors. Between ships equally matched in speed and offensive power, there is no reason to believe that the contest will be short, since the increased destructive power of the guns is offset by the number of misses and decreased effectiveness of fire at the long ranges. When, however, by reason of any circumstances, an overwhelming fire is concentrated on one ship, the ensuing carnage and structural damage entail a brief action.

Nature of Missiles.—Because of the great distances which will separate the ships and also on account of the general distribution of armor, small arms will ordinarily play no part in a naval engagement. Even the use of secondary batteries—usually of six-inch guns—is becoming restricted to defence against torpedo craft. Consequently the projectiles of present-day naval warfare will probably be exclusively 10-inch to 14-inch shells. A ship of the *Michigan* class, mounting eight 12-inch guns, is able to throw seven tons of metal a minute, with a muzzle velocity of 2,700 D feet. The shells are of steel, conical in shape, adapted to penetrate armor, and are furnished with a detonating mechanism

---

*Braisted, loc. cit.
† P. M. Rixey, in Keen's "System of Surgery," 1908, vol. iv., p. 1027.

designed to ignite the contained charge of explosive after the interior of the ship has been gained.   When a shell explodes, the disruptive action of the powder is so modified by the onward momentum of the mass that the area of damage from the fragments forms a cone with its apex coinciding with the point occupied by the shell at the instant of disruption.   (See Fig. 377.)   It happened on the *Texas*, at Santiago, that a gunner standing in the neighborhood of *a* (Fig. 377) was severely burned by the flash of a bursting shell and yet entirely escaped injury by fragments.   A glance at the diagram will make it evident that the

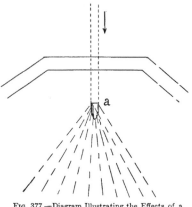

FIG. 377.—Diagram Illustrating the Effects of a Bursting Shell.

men on the engaged side of a vessel are less dangerously situated than those on the unengaged side.   The necessity of protecting the men on the unengaged side is at once apparent.   On some of the later vessels each gun crew is enclosed in a small armored compartment, but in other ships the crews of the secondary battery are without protection from their rear, so that, as shown by the record, one shell may disable sixty men. When each crew is not sheltered in its own miniature fort, it becomes our duty to give the crews such individual protection as may be possible.   Both the Russians and the Japanese * regarded limiting the danger zone as most important, and they utilized for this purpose hammocks, festoons of chains and cables, sand-bags retained by torpedo wire netting, or mattresses.   The Russians had great confidence in the protective power of coal, and exploited the bunkers whenever that was possible.   Woodwork gives rise to flying splinters, and all that is movable should be thrown overboard before action, stored in an unoccupied compartment, or enclosed in nettings.

The character of the injuries encountered has been already foreshadowed. Intact shells may leave only scattered fragments of a man or may cleanly amputate a member.   Bursting shells spread their pieces broadcast, so that an individual may be shredded if near, or sown with scraps if more distant.   Splinters from woodwork inflict all sorts of acerated and punctured wounds.   Cut steam pipes fill compartments with scalding vapor.   Exploding shells fill the spaces with noxious gases, and perhaps ignite powder charges which, in turn, envelop men in flames and add to the poisonous fumes.

Local Conditions.—Although these terrible injuries imperatively require immediate attention, little assistance can be given during the progress of the battle.   The very dangers of which we have spoken—the flying missiles and

* Braisted, Spear, op. cit.

splinters, spreading gases, fire and explosion—require that each part of the ship be isolated, to the end that the damage following any one shot may be circumscribed. Battle hatches are battened down, and most apertures in the honeycomb of bulkheads are fast closed. Even the few passages that remain open are liable to be obstructed by buckled iron work and débris. So the impossibility of intercommunication between the different parts of a ship effectually precludes any extensive exercise of our functions during battle. (Fig. 378.)

How, then, shall we organize to render what little aid we can, in view of circumstances so beset with difficulties? Perhaps this phase of our subject can best be unfolded by taking up in order the selection of posts for the wounded,

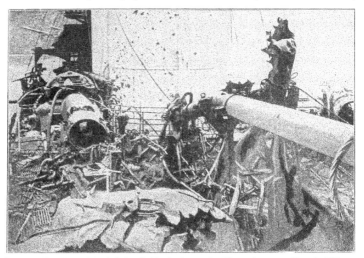

Fig. 378.—Boat Deck of the *Orel* after the Battle of Japan Sea. May 30th, 1904; to Show the Difficulty of Giving First-Aid to the Wounded. (From Braisted.)

the distribution of matériel, the stationing of personnel, and the transportation of the injured.

Posts for the Wounded.—In describing our dressing stations we shall be guided largely by a scheme which is capable of being applied to shore conditions without material alteration. The reasons why the constitution and equipment of naval forces should, so far as is practicable, conform to those of the military forces of a nation, have their basis in the frequency of landing parties. When a landing party is thrown on shore without warning, the excitement and disorder which follow do not favor the successful operation of a staange system suddenly put into practice under novel surroundings. We shall escape much confusion if our familiar system can be landed with us, for it will be readily granted that in any stress, a system is less likely to break down the more automatic has become the practice of its principles. In the event of war, the number of newly enlisted men may be in excess of trained men, and, at best, there may be neither time nor opportunity for adequate drilling to insure the mastery of a system of first-aid adapted only to naval employment. This difficulty is not lessened if teaching another system for landing parties be attempted. Moreover, in combined operations with the Army, harmony of action, transportation of supplies, and replacement of equipment are greatly facilitated by the suggested uniformity, which should be extended to embrace details of organization, equipment, and perhaps nomenclature.

In conformity with the idea, the parallelism of naval and military schemes for furnishing aid will be indicated.

Military.	Naval.
Base Hospital	{ Sanitary Base. { Hospital Ship.
Stationary Hospital	Secondary Station.
Field Hospital	Primary Stations.
Field Dressing Stations	Relief Stations.
Regimental Aid	Relief Parties.

As a preliminary to any remarks on the selection of dressing stations, it may be pointed out that it is impossible to present any schemes of first-aid except in the most general way, since there will be required in each case of attempted application more or less extensive modifications which can be determined only after careful study of the ship for which the scheme is to be appropriated. The regular sick bay must generally be abandoned. In our more recent ships it is situated on the gun deck where the maximum of air, light, and space is obtained, but it gains those desirable endowments at the sacrifice of protection, since its position above the armor belt renders it very liable to be gutted during action. So, if we place the sick bay on an upper deck for the sake of securing light and air during the many years of peace, we must make up our minds to abandon it, and all its fixed equipment, without compunction during the brief period of battle when protection becomes of paramount importance. For, the stations which are to serve as centres for the collection of the wounded must, first of all, afford reasonable security. Secondly, the stations must be accessible, and hence are to be located with reference to ladders and hatches—particularly those which are apt to remain open during battle. Thirdly, there must be sufficient space for the performance of dressings and operations and to accommodate the accumulated wounded.

The Secondary Station.—The primary station is, above all, a reserve station, in which the medical supplies are secured against destruction. Here are stored all supplies remaining after issue for immediate use during the progress of the battle has been made. Volatile anæsthetics are gathered here in metal lockers, quantities of sterile gauze are accumulated, and instruments are kept in readiness for such operations as may be imperative. The senior surgeon will have his post at this station and will direct, so far as may be possible, the conduct of his department.

From this brief review of the services required of the secondary station, the necessity of a secure location is obvious. A place below the protective deck should be chosen, and a station located there for use as storeroom only. The space, however, beneath this deck is in great demand. So much room is required for the motive power, magazines, and other equipment or gear that are rightly regarded as vital parts of the ship, that it may prove impossible to create a post there. If so, a position behind armor can be obtained, and it should be carefully surveyed in order to take advantage of coal bunkers or other fortuitous means of added protection. In such case, it can be merged with one of the two primary stations.

The neighborhood of hatches which will be kept open is essential if this station is to be the seat of any surgical work during action; but its function as a hospital is so much less important than its use as a place of safe storage, that the latter consideration should guide us in our choice if both requirements cannot be fulfilled. Again, it is pointed out that, if we would not be left without material when the need is greatest, the choice of a reserve station must be wisely made, and, if two suitable localities are available, our stores should be divided between them for greater precaution against destruction.

Primary Stations.—The primary stations should be located behind armor on the berth deck, one forward and one aft. With these, absolute protection is less essential. Yet, much material will be gathered in them. They will serve also for the detention of many wounded, and members of the Medical Department will be there in number. Therefore, a degree of protection should be sought; but, if the secondary station is fortunately situated below the protective deck, the matter of accessibility of the primary stations becomes of equal importance with that of their safety.

It is important that there be an unobstructed passage-way between the two primary stations, so that attendants, supplies, and patients may be easily transferred from one to the other as the needs of the moment may dictate. Circumstances can easily be imagined—as when a shell has wiped out one station, when one station is swamped with patients while the other is idle, or when the approach to one from the upper deck is obstructed—in which ready communication would be required.

The scope of relief offered by the primary stations will vary according to circumstances and according to the precise plan of aid adopted by the senior officer, but, in any case, it seems not advisable to make large collections of wounded at these poorly protected points, since the slight benefit to be gained thereby will rarely justify the attendant risks.

Relief Stations.—Through men at the relief stations the system of first-aid is first brought into contact with the crew. These stations filter out the slightly wounded, dress them, and send them back to their guns; and serious cases are passed along, correctly tagged, to the primary stations, or are retained in small groups until opportunity for transport presents itself. These stations are distributed in such number and localities as may be practicable, due consideration being always had to the number of men capable of the work and the necessity of preserving them for later and more important service. One station, at least, should be established where it is most accessible to the fire-room force. It should be specially prepared to treat cases of scalds, heat exhaustion, and asphyxiation.

It is probable that the advantage which would accrue from the protection that might be given these stations after the manner indicated for gun crews,— viz., heavy tarpaulins, nettings, mattresses and such materials, sometimes recommended to be used to limit the flight of splinters and shell fragments,— would be overshadowed by the danger from fire, which must always be seriously considered.

The effective prosecution of the duties belonging to the relief stations will be served by avoiding too great fixity of station. Free mobility will permit men to go wherever need arises, adjust themselves to the frequent shifting of a crew, and maintain a proper regard for their own safety. Means of telephonic communication should be established, if possible, in all stations.

To recapitulate: the relief and primary stations may be regarded as sieves of increasing fineness, which pass the cases according to their gravity. At the relief stations, a temporary dressing will be applied and the man, if slightly wounded, will be returned to his post. If his injury precludes further service during the engagement, he may be made comfortable where he has fallen, or moved on, when occasion offers, to a primary station where he is more sheltered from the effects of gun fire, can receive a more elaborate dressing, and be given a resting-place. If, however, hemorrhage or obstructive asphyxiation demands immediate interference, he may be operated on in this station.

The arrangement of stations may be shown in a tabular form:—

1. Secondary station, principally a secure store-room, but also an equipped operating-room, situated either—a, below, the protective deck, in which case no work could be done there during action; or b, on the protective deck, behind armor, for both storage and active work, in which case it would be merged with one of the primary stations.

2. Primary stations, one forward and one aft, on the protective deck behind armor.

3. A number of relief stations.

Syncope would seem too slight an affection to deserve specific mention, but the cases are rather common. They arise from fright and ungrounded apprehension regarding the seriousness of wounds. Pain may require anodynes, not only for its alleviation, but also to suppress its disquieting effects.

Very numerous psychoses seem to develop under the conditions attending warfare. The immediate results of battle are hysterical excitements and confused states. These usually clear up in a few days, but irritability, fearfulness, and emotional instability remain for weeks. It may be that prolonged exertion, deprivations, loss of sleep, hunger and thirst play as important a rôle in the causation of these states as the psychic trauma of battle. The psychoses may develop *de novo*, or in combination with certain intoxications, or on the basis of a special neuropathic constitution. In any case, the circumstances of war stamp them with a depressive character such as is not noticed in times of peace. The number of mental diseases in the Russian Army is estimated at possibly 3,500 in the three years of the war.*

There are also three points of surgical practice which deserve mention in connection with first-aid. First, tourniquets should not be widely distributed, since they are rarely necessary, are frequently applied irrationally, and are often overlooked and left in place twenty-four hours. Many medical officers feel, therefore, that they are productive of more harm than good. Second, hypodermic syringes are very apt to be used without discrimination. Except morphia, hypodermic medicaments rarely do good and frequently hasten death, and their employment ought to be rigorously restricted to medical officers. Third, antiseptic solutions are bulky, difficult to handle and store, and their usefulness is much less than is generally supposed. For the disinfection of skin surfaces, tincture of iodine is peculiarly adapted to our purposes. Its employment cannot be attended by any seriously harmful results. Very small quantities are required; its action is rapid, two "paintings" being sufficient without preparatory or adjuvant treatment of the skin, and no solutions, which inevitably wash extraneous dirt into the wound, are used. The use of chemical antiseptics on open wounds is deprecated, unless the infection require actual cauterization of the tissues by Harrington's solution, phenol, or tincture of iodine.

Matériel.—In the preparation of material, we are to bear in mind that supplies must be sufficient for dressing 200 men; that every one of these will require two or more dressings daily; that the size of the wounds and their infected character call for bulky dressings, and that we must provide against the total destruction of our sterilizing plant. Hence, an enormous amount of gauze is to be prepared, in small packets for dressing stations, and in large packages or drums for continuous use during the hours of operating after engagement. Quantities of sterile water and solutions should be stored in enamelware or glass containers enclosed in a strong mesh. The frequency of burns and scalds requires a large supply of ointment and picric-acid solution. The preparation of other material needs no special mention.

At the relief stations we shall place first-aid packets, shell packets, tourniquets, splints, adhesive gauze, and bandages. At the primary stations we shall place these same materials, and in addition an outfit for a few operations —such, for example, as tracheotomy and ligature of vessels. At the secondary station few, if any, dressings will be done, but a few operations may be performed. This station is sure to be well supplied, since it is the storage place; but, in order to prevent oversight, some of the supplies needed may be detailed:—

Dressings: Gauze, bandages, safety-pins, drainage tubes, and adhesive plaster.

Instruments, ligatures, sutures, and needles.

Sterile water and salt solution.

* See Richards, in Journal of Military Surgeons, February, 1910.

Chemicals: Tincture of iodine, Harrington's solution, phenol, bichloride, liquid soap, and picric acid.

Hypodermic syringes, solutions of morphine, and solutions for local anæsthesia.

Infusion apparatus for rectal, hypodermic, and intravenous use.

Accessories: Basins, trays, buckets, pitchers, lanterns, candles, and matches.

Dry-goods: Sheets, towels, gowns, aprons, sleeves, and gloves.

Operating and dressing tables.

Sand-bags for the splinting of fractures.

Since steam and water are shut off from the pipes above the protective deck,

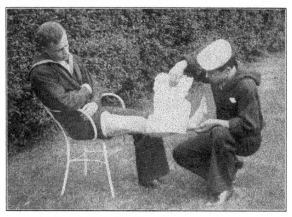

FIG. 379.—Stokes' Shell-Wound Packet being Applied.

electric sterilizers are very useful, although their value is lessened by the possibility that, at any time, the current may be interrupted.

The reader may not be familiar with the "first-aid" and "shell-wound" packets. The first-aid packet, as adopted by a joint Army and Navy Board, is composed of gauze compresses, bandages, and safety-pins, all enclosed in a water-tight metal case, with instructions for its proper use. These packets, intended for the small perforating wounds of small-calibre fire-arms, can have very limited use in naval warfare. Of far more value is a dressing of the character of the Stokes' "Shell-Wound Packet." (Figs. 379 and 380.) This is described as follows:—

"A piece of No. 16 galvanized wire gauze is shaped into a parallelogram 8 inches by 6; a piece of gauze, 4 feet in length, is cut off the roll, is folded lengthwise, and is securely stitched to one 8-inch side of the wire form. The wire frame is filled with cotton in the form of a compress and the gauze is folded over it and is stitched to the frame for security. The remainder of the fold of gauze still attached is snugly wound about the rigid compress. A piece of unbleached muslin, 4 feet long and 9 inches wide, is then stitched to the free end of the gauze and it, too, is made to encircle the form. Its free end is nicked with the scissors at several points so that the whole dressing may be easily secured by splitting and tying the muslin. Three safety-pins fix the muslin at the sides and ends."

This dressing can be made on board ship, with wood or bamboo if wire is not at hand. It is sterilized, enclosed in a small, individual muslin bag, and issued. The correct application of these packets is simple and the crew should receive thorough drilling in handling them. "Dummy" dressings can be kept on hand by the Medical Department for issue to the various divisions during their first-aid drills. It is desirable to attach one of these bags to the person

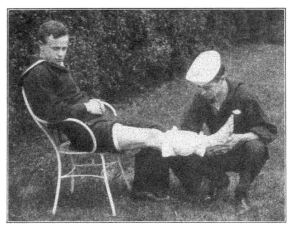

FIG. 380.—Stokes' Shell-Wound Packet Applied.

of each member of the crew, and also to distribute numbers of them widely about the ship, particularly in the turrets and other places likely to be isolated during action.

Spear's shell-wound packet (Fig. 381) embodies a coaptation splint of wood. It is described as being capable of repeated sterilization by either steam or solutions. It supports a single member and attaches it to the trunk or opposite member, is quickly applied, and is applicable to all sites. The Hodgen (Fig. 382) and the Cabot (Fig. 383) splints are very valuable for treating wounds of naval warfare.

Mattresses are useful for couching the wounded while awaiting opportunity for transporting them. Life-preservers also may be hung here and there as a precautionary measure. The Russians possessed cork mattresses which saved many lives among both the well and the wounded when the ships had to be abandoned.

Each member of the Hospital Corps is to be equipped with either a large or a small pouch. A list of their contents indicates their range of usefulness:—

Large Pouch.	Small Pouch.
Bandages.	Bandages.
Pocket case.	Pocket case.
Chloroform.	
Catheter.	
Diagnosis tags and pencil.	
First-aid packets.	First-aid packets.
Folding lantern and candle.	
Gauze.	Gauze.
Jack-knife.	Jack-knife.
Ligatures, catgut and silk.	
Mist. chloroformi et opii.	
Pins and safety-pins.	
Adhesive plaster.	Adhesive plaster.
Rubber bandages.	Tourniquet.
Scissors.	
Spt. Ammon. Aromat.	Spt. Ammon. Aromat.
Wire gauze (for splints).	Wire gauze.
Hypodermic syringe.	
Hypodermic solutions.	

Personnel.—In the description of the distribution of the personnel, it will be noted that the plan provides for a continuous first-aid service during the progress of battle. This outline of activities may here be qualified by certain affirmations, which will be laid down without further elaboration at present:—

Extensive first-aid is impossible and undesirable.

Multiple relief stations afford all the assistance possible.

Most first-aid will be impromptu.

No organizing for transportation is possible or desirable.

For the performance of the duties expected, we have on a battleship two, perhaps three, medical officers, one hospital steward, two first-class hospital apprentices, and four to six hospital apprentices of the ordinary grade.

Three medical officers are needed on a battleship. If we are to attempt much in the way of first-aid during battle, the limited means of communication require that a fourth officer be stationed on the gun-deck; but, since it is generally accepted that medical officers should remain at the dressing stations, where they receive the wounded as they come, the fourth officer is not essential. The number should not, however, be less than three. Each of the principal stations should be furnished with an officer, although, if there are only two officers, one may have his post in the secondary station and the other must then divide his attention between the two primary stations. It must be anticipated that accidents may disable one or more officers; and, when it is borne in mind that, allowing an average of ten minutes for a dressing, thirty-three hours of actual work will be required to complete the dressing of the wounded, and that incidental demands will consume much time in the first hours after an engagement, thus delaying further the prompt rendering of assistance, it will be seen that at least three medical officers should be attached to each battleship.

Hospital Corps.—The hospital steward is placed at the central dressing station where he is first assistant to the senior medical officer in whatever activities are carried on at the station. He serves, in addition, as a means of communication, by which the senior officer receives reports of affairs at the subsidiary posts and issues new or modifying orders.

The two hospital apprentices, first class, are divided between the two primary stations, where they likewise become first assistants to the junior officers. The other hospital apprentices, perhaps six in number, are distributed according to the judgment of the senior officer. One, at least, will be needed

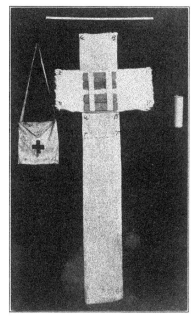

FIG. 381.—Spear's Shell-Wound Dressing.

at each of the principal stations. Two would be desirable, but we are then confronted with the situation that there remain no Hospital Corps men for duty at the relief stations. The services offered by the relief stations can not be entirely withdrawn; and since we have at most three hospital apprentices for this duty, we are driven to turn to other branches for assistance in the carrying out of our scheme.

To what branches shall we look to furnish this special detail? Japanese ships were over-manned, so that a sufficient number of bandsmen, yeomen, and messmen were assigned to this single duty. But, whatever complements may be embarked on our ships in time of war, all our vessels now show a deficiency in their quotas, and every man, whatever his rate, who is not specifically enlisted in the neutralized Hospital Corps, contributes in some way to the fighting of the ship. Bandsmen and others are employed in the passing of ammunition, or other occupations below decks, in which their co-operation is needed, and, therefore, when the medical officer requests a temporary detail, he is met by the assertion that men cannot be spared.

Naval exigencies rightfully dominate any situation arising from conflict of interests, but it is usually possible to effect a compromise. The number of men required for first-aid and transportation is now computed at 5 per cent of the complement; that is, 50 men out of a crew of 1,000—a proportion which, as the experience of the Japanese shows, is not excessive. But, a point of equal importance with the number of men to be requested is that we should endeavor to obtain the same individuals on all occasions, in order that we may train these men for the proper performance of their duties. So, what with the conflict of interests and the necessity of training, it may be necessary to cut the estimate just given down to fifteen or twenty men. This reduction can be conceded the more willingly when the limitations of activity suggested in the beginning of this section are borne in mind.

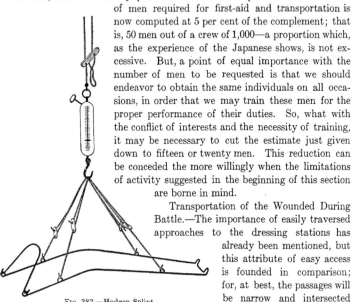

Fig. 382.—Hodgen Splint.

Transportation of the Wounded During Battle.—The importance of easily traversed approaches to the dressing stations has already been mentioned, but this attribute of easy access is founded in comparison; for, at best, the passages will be narrow and intersected with bulkheads, and the communication between decks will be by ladders or hatches which are not superimposed. Very little methodical handling of the wounded will be possible, and, for the most part, the comrades of the fallen man will pull him to one side where he will lie until after the battle.

It is conceivable that, if a gun crew in a turret were wiped out by a shell, or if the disabled should interfere by their number with the working of the guns, the hatch might be opened and the men dropped out on the unengaged side. The central dressing station would then be notified by telephone, and the men reclaimed by the carriers if possible; but the advisability of such procedure is open to grave doubt.

C. Prophylaxis.—There still remain to be made a few final preparations which tend to minimize the damage suffered.

It will be remembered that the wounds of naval practice are prone to suppurate and frequently harbor fragments of clothing. The number and severity of septic cases may be greatly lessened if the men are compelled to bathe just before action and put on clean clothes. Sterilization of underclothing is practicable on board ships which possess a large disinfecting chamber, and, if put into practice, promises a further protection from infection.

Supplies of drinking water ought to be placed in convenient locations. The extreme thirst accompanying hemorrhage and shock is familiar, and, when further intensified by the smoke and acrid fumes of gun fire, it is rightly described as a torture, for which we should not fail to provide relief. Cold water serves another useful purpose. It is a most effective stimulant to wearied men, invigorating their bodies and sharpening their dulled faculties.

If some more elaborate method of ear protection is not adopted, the use of cotton should be made compulsory. It is of distinct value in affording protection from the effects of gun-fire and, should accidents occur, its use lessens the likelihood of complications. Dryness of the eyes, a sequel of exposure to the fumes of smokeless powder, is very annoying and, in a short time, impairs vision. The Japanese found that buckets of boracic-acid solution, conveniently located for quick rinsing of the eyes, were of great benefit.

Action having been taken to make the skin as clean as may be, the excessive mortality of abdominal wounds, and the futility of operation, prompt us to attempt

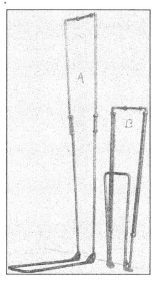

Fig. 383—Modified Cabot Posterior Wire Splint.

some measure calculated to render the intestinal contents innocuous. Naturally, the wholly successful methods familiar in gastro-intestinal surgery are not practicable, but nevertheless some real lessening of intestinal toxicity may be brought about by such simple measures as we can employ. The amount and variety of intestinal flora can be greatly diminished by a diet which both can be and is completely absorbed. Not only are the results of abdominal wounds mitigated when the intestine is empty and comparatively free from organisms, but the course of wounds other than abdominal is favorably influenced when the intestines are not loaded with putrescent material, and the body is not surfeited with food. It may, then, be worth while to restrict diet before battle, so that digestion may be perfect, absorption complete, and assimilation not beyond physiologic needs. A mild cathartic is a further means to this end.

2. During Battle.

The reader will have been struck with the limited activities of the Medical Corps during battle, as indicated by the slight provision for the transportation of wounded and for operative procedures. This is not due to a lack of earnest desire to ameliorate suffering or even to a well-grounded distrust in the results of surgical interference under conditions imposed by battle. On the contrary, the most potent checks on our activity are broad considerations of naval efficiency. "The Navy is created to fight. Every part of its organization ought to further that end,—all should be sacrificed to it. The succor of the wounded, whatever be its importance from a humanitarian view, should not entail the least hindrance to manœuvring and naval action." * Here we see our course indicated. So far as we may aid the wounded. let us do so; but let us never attempt that which might impair the safety of the ship, or jeopardize the fortune of the fleet and the triumph of the larger interests at

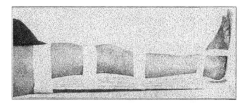

Fig. 384.—Cabot Splint in Use.

stake. If the sight and sounds of wounded men undermine courage, the injured should be removed; but, if their removal entails open hatches, which may be a source of danger, then the injured must lie where they have fallen. Many parts of the ship are so cut off that access to them is impossible. For instance, the turrets have but one interior opening and that is sacred to the raising of ammunition, a function with which we cannot interfere. In the balanced turrets there is a hatch in the overhang, but the maintenance of positive air pressure within the turret—to prevent flarebacks—renders it necessary that the hatch be kept closed during action. Bulkheads must be kept closed to limit the spread of all destructive agencies. Open hatches permit the entrance of shells, and, therefore, cannot be tolerated. So, considerations affecting the structural integrity of a battleship effectually inhibit our activity during the progress of an engagement.

Prompt removal of the wounded is not imperative, not even of moment. While the courage of the crew may be supported by the certainty of attention in case of injury, there are instances in history which prove that a crew may fight on, deluged in blood, until scarcely a man is left on his feet. The French have found that, if supplies are at hand. the members of a gun crew never fail

* Bremaud: "Étude sur le Service Médical à Bord," 1897.

NAVAL SURGERY. 1005

to apply a dressing to a wounded companion and then to pull him to one side. And there is not good reason why he should receive further attention, since those who have fallen on board a ship are not liable to be trampled on by subsequent cavalry or artillery charges. They are in reasonably clean surroundings and in a tolerable temperature. They face no possibility of being abandoned or left for hours to lie without protection on a battlefield, tormented with insects and thirst, or slowly freezing, and the duration of uninterrupted battle is bound to be short, so that in the pause the wounded can receive all reasonable attention without undue delay. Moreover, the wounded, by reason of their injuries, are not absolved from further obligations to their ship, fleet, and country. They must continue to serve with fortitude until the end of battle. Indeed, under these circumstances, we meet some of our most inspiring examples of heroism. Finally, by a merciful provision, a state of apathy is induced by shock and wounds from fire-arms, so that insensibility persists for a long time. This anæsthesia is so marked that, in former times, military surgeons seized the opportunity it afforded for the performance of major operations. We may fairly conclude that leaving the wounded until the end of battle is far less cruel than at first appears.

Reference to the preceding tables will make clear another point bearing on the advisability of not attempting aid during battle. The great majority of casualties are slight, or else result in immediate death. The latter class of injuries we cannot help. The former seek us out at our stations. and, if we remember that naval surgery must be guided by the principle of the greatest good for the greatest number, it may well be doubted whether it is the part of wisdom to risk our trained carriers in removing a small part of the wounded to a place in which they are neither more comfortable, more safe, nor better cared for, and then possibly find that, as a result, proper attention cannot be given the mass of wounded after battle because of casualties in the medical department.

Apprehension need not be felt by the medical officer if provisions promise to be inadequate for the relief of the wounded during battle, nor need he entertain regrets if he perforce becomes a passive onlooker. He is compelled to wait by constraints which he cannot break, and his zeal should be restrained until after engagement.

The far-reaching effects of the recent revolution in battleship construction are not yet fully realized. In the present ships, building and projected, the guns of the main battery are mounted in turrets, and the small guns of the secondary battery are not manned, unless to repel an attack by torpedo craft. A prudent commander will keep all his men, except the gun crews in the turrets, in the most protected locations below. A recent report * states that "there will be only four persons exposed above armor—two at the range-finders and two on the fire-control mast." To these may be added the travelling inspection parties whose duty is to discover fire. So, practically the whole crew will be divided into three groups according to location:—those in the turrets, those

* A. M. D. McCormick.

between decks and behind armor, and those below the water line and the impervious protective deck. Now, practically no one can enter or leave the turrets during action. The engineer force and stokers, below the protective deck, cannot receive aid even from primary stations, since the space below this deck cannot be traversed because of the closure of bulkheads and the formation of water-tight and forced-draft compartments, and the reserves are held behind armor as much out of danger as the dressing stations themselves can be. Thus, more and more, with each advance in battleship construction, do our activities during engagement become curtailed.

The scheme at present in general use is incapable of application, and can result only in a useless loss of life among those whose services can ill be spared. Notwithstanding this, the writer has presented that scheme of first-aid in detail, because it is one that has received sanction in the past, has been tested in action, and is applicable to many ships still in commission. But it is now obsolescent, passing with the type of ship for which it was designed; and it may be confidently asserted that hereafter our preparations for battle will be confined to the establishment of a safe store-house, locating a few relief stations, and distributing ample supplies in the turrets, fire-room, and between decks. In brief, our activities will begin at the close of the battle.

Transportation During a Lull in the Battle.—At any time there may occur, from one cause or another, a suspension of battle. Hatches and bulkheads may then be safely opened, turrets can be entered, and carriers may expose themselves without risk. It is not to be doubted that, after the heat of action has passed, the sight of dead and horribly mutilated comrades, lying in apparent neglect, has a seriously depressing effect on the remainder of the crew, and we should seize the opportunity to accomplish what we can.

Our general dispositions are not at all those which will be outlined for use after battle, because, if we expect that the conflict will be shortly resumed, our real work cannot yet commence, nor can we freely choose new dressing and operating stations. Our original battle stations will be retained, and we are to confine endeavors to removing all the wounded from their posts and assembling them in localities chosen primarily for the protection they afford, and secondarily for space, air, and easy access. The place selected will necessarily be behind armor, probably on the berth deck at one of the regular dressing stations. It is true that the most pressing cases will be dressed also, so far as time permits, but nevertheless it is chiefly our resources of transportation which will be exercised. The system of raising and transporting the wounded is not different in its operation during a lull than after action, and its description in this connection will serve for both occasions.

In planning the details of any system of transportation, we should remember that moving individuals in safety and comfort is not our sole aim. We must strive for the complete relief of all the wounded in the least time, and, in consequence, the injured must be considered collectively. Hence, it follows that we must devise measures for meeting two requirements, namely, speed and safety. Speed will be gained by distributing carriers and arranging their respective duties so that a wounded man shall traverse the passages with the least delay. Safety will be served by employing proper stretchers and by training the carriers to handle men with due regard to their injuries.

From the point of view of transportation, the wounded may be divided into four groups:—

(a) Those who can present themselves at the dressing stations;

(b) Those who require the assistance of one or two men;

(c) Those who need to be carried in arms, and

(d) Those who require stretchers and the utilization of hatchways.

The first and second groups of cases offer no problem. These men will find their way to the dressing stations, either unaided or with such assistance as may be improvised by their companions. But the cases included under "d," cases of men whose extensive maiming permits no such impromptu expedients, require an apparatus which shall safely transfer the sufferer in the recumbent position. The men, also, who need to be carried in arms, escape much discomfort if they are put at once in a stretcher, which shall serve both as a litter and as a bed until there is opportunity for transfer to a hospital ship.

We have estimated the wounded at two hundred. About one-half of these will fall in groups "c" and "d"; and, therefore, we should be provided with means for transporting one hundred wounded in an expeditious manner. There will not, however, be sufficient stretchers for this number, and it is therefore fortunate that some cases are of such a character that the injured man may be transported when laced up in a hammock and mattress, thus relieving somewhat the stringency in the supply of stretchers.

The passages which must be traversed by the wounded are horizontal, inclined, and vertical. To these may be added a fourth—aerial—which appertains more particularly to the transference of cases, either by whip or by the aerial cable, from the battleship to a dock, lighter, or hospital ship. This method will, therefore, be described later. It is to be remembered that all passages will present difficulties far greater than are incidental to their design. The destruction wrought by gun-fire will encumber decks and passages with obstacles and débris that offer serious impediment to transportation, and will have to be reckoned with. (See Fig. 378.)

Horizontal passages ordinarily offer little difficulty, although they may be narrow and tortuous, and even totally impassable after a severe engagement. The patient is to be lifted on a stretcher and then carried or slid along the deck from the place where he fell to the dressing station or hatchway. The carriers having been trained in the execution of their duties, no supervision is necessary, unless to pass judgment on the advisability of moving a man who is threatened with hemorrhage or in whom the injury consists of an evisceration.

If the dressing station is not on the same deck, vertical or inclined passages will next be employed to reach the lower deck on which the station is located. Whether the patient is lowered obliquely along a ladder, or horizontally through a hatchway, he must be secured against falling. Even though the maintenance of a horizontal position is premeditated, the hatch is apt to be small, and the ropes may not be perfectly adjusted, so that the patient has to be passed through on end. Hence, the possibility of his slipping out must be obviated, whatever the mode of transport designed.

It may be necessary to traverse several hatches which are not superposed, and thus there is required a stage of horizontal transport in the midst of the vertical. Certainly, some horizontal transport will be required from the land-

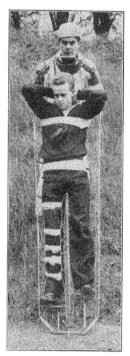

ing place to the dressing station. As will be seen, therefore, horizontal and vertical or oblique passages usually alternate in the course followed by the wounded man on his way to the dressing station.

The character of the duties of the carriers is now apparent. To accomplish the transference with the least delay, it is probably best to divide the duties of the carriers, one set collecting the wounded and delivering them at the hatchway, a second set lowering the stretchers either by hand or by whip, and a third set removing them from the landing on the lower deck to the appointed place. It is likewise evident that specially trained men are required only to select cases, according to the urgency of their condition, and place them in stretchers with due regard to the nature of their wounds. Further transfer can be accomplished by any of the crew, and, during a lull or after the battle, plenty of men can always be impressed for this service. It may be anticipated that four or five minutes will generally be consumed in the complete conveyance.

Means of Transportation.—Stretchers.—A great number of stretchers have been devised for use on ships of war, but very few fulfil the numerous requirements. A stretcher must be rigid, yet simple; it should permit the recumbent position;

FIG. 385.—Stokes' Splint Stretcher. it should be safe and comfortable; it should be adapted to all the vicissitudes of transportation on board ships; it must be non-inflammable and not give rise to splinters; it should be capable of use as a bed; it must take up little room; it must not add to the injury; and should give reasonable splinting.

The use of blankets, hammocks, and other materials which are always at hand, will suggest itself to every officer, and our description of devices will be limited to the "Stokes Splint Stretcher," which is officially adopted in the U. S. Navy.

The "Stokes Splint Stretcher" is a wire basket (see Fig. 385) conforming roughly in outline and dimensions to a man's body—80 x 20 x 8 inches. The free border of the basket is finished with half-inch galvanized steel. Two longitudinal braces of the same material add strength and rigidity, and serve further as runners. The frame has handles which are used as hand-grips and for the attachment of ropes. From the frame is suspended the basket of galvanized wire netting. The wire is heavy enough to give firm support, yet pliable enough to be moulded to an extremity and thus act as an efficient splint. One end is divided into gutters for the legs, an arrangement which facilitates splinting of the extremities. Additional fixation can be obtained by bandages run through the mesh. The weight of the body is kept off the perineum by two adjustable foot pieces. The body is secured in the stretcher by straps which encircle the thorax and pelvis. These retention straps also act to protect the perineum when both limbs are injured or the patient is unconscious. A sanitary opening is designed for cases in which it may be necessary to retain the wounded man in the stretcher for hours or days. The stretchers may be nested in lots of three.

A glance at the illustrations (Figs. 385 and 386) will make the description clear. The reader will readily perceive, without further details being supplied, what are the capabilities of the device and that it fulfils our above-mentioned requirements.

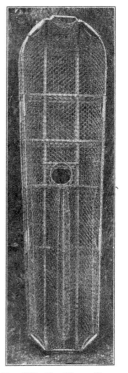

3. AFTER THE BATTLE.

Mention has not heretofore been made of a necessity which will arise at the close of battle, that is, the prompt evacuation of the stations which were selected for the period of combat. They were located primarily in view of the protection afforded, which was deemed of paramount importance during battle; but, now that the necessity for protection has passed, the disadvantages inseparable from a safe location lead us to seek new quarters. The battle stations are more or less inaccessible and small, and have become overheated, encumbered,

Fig. 386.—The Figure Shows Three Stokes' Stretchers Nested.

and charged with foul air. The continuous administration of volatile anæsthetics is dangerous in such a confined, poorly ventilated space, and it is unsurgical to attempt operative procedures until a favorable site has been fixed upon and occupied.

In the selection of a new station we may be seriously hampered by the effects of gun-fire. The superstructure may be extensively riddled, perhaps totally untenantable. The upper decks may be in a disordered or even chaotic state, so that we shall be forced to content ourselves with a position on the lower deck at one of our battle stations. The ward room is well adapted to our use, and it may happen that the regular sick bay, having escaped being gutted, can be occupied, in which case our task is much lightened. If not so fortunate, we should strive to secure some accessible location which is spacious, unencumbered, well-ventilated, and well-lighted.

This new post becomes our hospital and is the centre of all subsequent work. All patients will be congregated there—not only for dressing, but also for retention afterward; and, hence, we must now assemble there every resource the ship affords for the care of the injured.

While the carriers are engaged in the transportation of the wounded, a number of our men will be busied in bringing equipment from the abandoned stations and the reserve store-rooms. All our instruments will be needed, since the regional distribution of injuries may compel us to attack nearly every structure and tissue of the body. Two tables, at least, will be required for simultaneous operating, and a copious supply of cold and hot water is important, particularly if water and steam remain shut off because of damage to the piping.

The space reserved should be so divided—nominally, at least, if not in fact—that it will be practicable for us to follow a fixed program. There should be a gathering place, or receiving room, to which all patients are first brought. There they are inspected carefully and labelled, according to their requirements, for one of two destinations—either the main operating-room or the space set apart for minor dressings. After receiving treatment, the patients are removed to the recovery room or to berthing space. The reality of this division of space will depend on the deck plan, but adherence to the principle involved will add to the speed and smoothness with which we accomplish the work. Rapidity in handling cases is necessary, not only to give attention to each sufferer as soon as possible, but also because the physical strength and mental energy of the operators are not inexhaustible.

The allotment of duties corresponds to the division of space. A junior officer should remain in the recovery room and inspect cases as they arrive, decide whether an operative or simple dressing is required, and tag the individual for his proper destination. He should also estimate accurately the requirements of each case, so that injuries may be dealt with in the order of their urgency. He is aided in the exercise of this function if he be guided by a sequence which is accepted as justified by universal experience. Threatened hemorrhage furnishes the most insistent class of cases, and these are given priority. Severe wounds of the abdomen come second; then perforating wounds of the joints; and, lastly, large wounds complicated by fracture, with or without comminution of the bone. Since some of the injured may have to wait several hours, it is obviously most important that their relative urgency be nicely appraised.

The hospital steward is qualified to apply dressings and carry out all necessary procedures at the station for minor dressings. In the operating station, the senior officer and one junior will be separately occupied in the performance of operations and more complicated dressings. Even here, regard for the common good leads us far from the ideal treatment of the individual. The immobilization of simple fractures, for example, is much less important than haste, and is, therefore, to be postponed. It is certainly unwise, also, to indulge at this time in prolonged search for suspected foreign bodies, although when the first rush of work is over their possible presence should never be lost sight of. Primary capital operations are not justifiable; failures quickly cause their abandonment and it is regarded as axiomatic that we should operate only when intervention is unavoidable and then do the least possible. Rochard expresses the same idea:—"We should not risk losing many wounded whom we might save, in attempting to save a very few whom almost surely we shall lose."

The utilization of the hospital apprentices will be, in part, such as seems best at the moment, but it is well to have most of them assigned to specific duties. Some may be used to undress the patients and prepare their injuries for examination. One can be employed in rendering the field of operation sterile with an iodine swab, two may administer anæsthetics, and others may have charge of post-anæsthetic nursing. One should give his whole attention to sterilizing instruments,—a difficult matter in the absence of steam and hot water. The galley, however, will be turned over to us, although its remoteness may make carrying hot water and sterile instruments a tedious process. Some apprentices must act as assistants, and one should have sole charge of sterile instruments, dry-goods, and ligatures. This last man can keep himself apart from the operations and hand over materials as they are called for from the general supply. A clinical clerk is a necessity. Many considerations oblige us to keep accurate records of persons and casualties. With the aid of the identification tags, the name, rate, and injury of every man reaching the receiving room, even the dead and unconscious, can be entered on a card. During examination and treatment of a patient, the examiner should dictate to the recorder an accurate description of the injury and details of treatment. Outline charts of the body are very helpful. The office of the recorder is permanent so long as any of the wounded are retained on the sick-list. It is quite possible that none of the Hospital Corps can be spared for this duty, and a member of the yeoman branch may then serve. He should be a skilful stenographer.

Surgical technique, under the circumstances, cannot be perfect, although, by assigning specific duties to each man, we may be reassured that details will not be overlooked. Only a few suggestions regarding technique need be added to what has already been said. By using rubber gloves, detached sleeves, and aprons, we can save much time that would be otherwise consumed in scrubbing the hands and changing gowns. Instruments and needles should be washed and returned in carbolic solution to the appointed apprentice under whose charge they remain, immersed in the solution, until called for. Other points will suggest themselves. Orderly management and painstaking observance of details are indispensable; yet, however faithfully we compass these requisites, we may be certain that our resourcefulness will be severely tried, and that success will depend far more on personal adaptiveness than on equipment or system.

Our responsibilities do not yet cease with the completion of an operation, for the patients must be berthed and nursed until transfer is possible. Our facilities for berthing the wounded are poor. Hammocks are not well adapted. They impose a flexed position, uncomfortably restrict movement, and compress the limbs. Stretchers will be few in number and will be required in continuous transportation. Hammock mattresses scattered about the deck are objectionable, in that they allow patients to roll about with the motion of the ship, to the detriment of their wounds and at the cost of much suffering. In spite of their drawbacks, however, these mattresses must usually be our chief resource. The twenty-two beds in the sick bay, if perchance they have escaped destruction, will be invaluable at this time, and the carpenter may be able to help us further by converting a number of hammocks into rigid hanging-cots.

For the nursing of the wounded, the corps men are to be apportioned to watches, for active and rigorous surveillance of the patients, so that we may deal promptly with secondary hemorrhage or other complications. All the bed cases must likewise receive sanitary attention, for the most part from attendants slightly acquainted with their duties, so that careful oversight is obligatory. In addition, the numerous patients must be fed,—no small undertaking in itself where there exist no conveniences for serving food. It is evident that these duties will occupy our regular corps men, and also a large additional detail, for many days.

The hygiene of the sick bay should not be lost sight of in the press of curative measures. During the early hours, we must obviate the concentration of anæsthetic vapors. Later, how to provide sufficient fresh air and how to prevent overheating and undue humidity, become real problems, particularly if the system of ventilation has been ruined by gun-fire.

It can be prophesied with assurance that all wounds will inevitably suppurate, but we cannot, for that reason, neglect measures designed to limit the spread of infections. The prevention of gangrene and erysipelas especially requires thorough methods of disinfection. On no account should we allow the dressing stations to become littered with soiled dressings. Such material is best deposited directly in large bags of paraffined paper which should be tied up when full and thrown into the furnaces. There is no occasion for rehearsing further minutiæ of aseptic and antiseptic procedure, but they should not, for that reason, be the less esteemed.

The ship, as a whole, likewise demands notice. To illustrate to what a state the ship may have been brought, Spear * says: "The *Rossija* was covered with flesh and blood, and, despite frequent washings and disinfections

* Op. cit.

by formalin, the stench of decomposing tissues remained on board for two months. Shortly after the fight it was almost unbearable." * There remains only the question of the disposal of the dead. The Russians summarily threw the killed overboard, and it was the opinion of the officers that this was the only practical method of disposing of the dead while active fighting was going on. If the loss of life be great, this course must be followed, but it should not be countenanced otherwise. Those who die on our hands, or who reach us already dead, ought to be unobstrusively diverted to a side room where they are removed from sight. A special detail party can be employed to collect the dead in a place set apart for use as a morgue, until opportunity for burial presents itself. This party need not be recruited from the Hospital Corps, but should, nevertheless, be supervised, in order that the absence of life may be determined beyond doubt. Keeping careful lists of the killed, as well as of the wounded, is very essential to the Pension Commissioner to help him decide claims for pensions, and is also a duty we owe the families of the deceased. It is not possible to embalm the dead for return to their relatives, and a burial at sea is the most they can receive.

Wounds of Naval Warfare.—The wounds of naval warfare have already

* Since writing the foregoing, further study of naval conditions has led me to arrive at conclusions which should be embodied in this article, in order to bring it up to date. They deal with the monster problem that will confront us after battle, which has, up to this time, in my opinion, remained unsolved. If the battle organization be sixteen ships, then we shall have approximately 16,000 men engaged and must provide for the care of from 4,000 to 5,000 killed and wounded of our own and possibly as many more of the enemy.

This great responsibility presents military and humanitarian difficulties that only thorough preparedness can satisfactorily meet. Among the military features may be mentioned the imperative necessity for the immediate removal of the killed and wounded, in order that the fleet may, if required, again engage in battle. The knowledge of the fact that both officers and men will· be cared for promptly by skilled surgeons, equipped with every device and appliance that the necessities of the situation may demand, will be comforting to those about to engage in battle, tending to uplift the spirit and morale of the command.

How are we to remove from the ships these scattered and maimed thousands of fighting men? The success of the fleet may depend upon this very manœuvre. The difficulties of hastily transferring from ship to ship an equal number of uninjured people at sea is, in itself, a large problem. What are we to do with them after we have taken them out of the ships? This leads us to the consideration of the establishment, as a war measure, of a great medical base, to be located either in the Pacific, or in the Atlantic, depending on the probable field of operations. Upon the completeness with which the organization and equipment of this great plant is prepared and its personnel drilled, will depend its success or breakdown in time of war.

If it were possible, which is not the case, it would not be advisable to scatter our wounded here and there through the civil hospitals of our cities. We must keep them together, as far as expedient from the "firing line," until they are finally disposed of. It is probable that a great hotel for administrative purposes, and accommodating the wounded, with its grounds for expansion under canvas, can be made use of. One only of our naval hospitals has a suitable environment and is so located that it could be utilized as the heart of a great sanitary base.

How are we to give the wounded prompt and efficient treatment, identify and tag them,—in other words, give them the care along humanitarian lines which their great sacrifice merits? It is obviously advisable that they should be ministered to by the same hands that first cared for them at the "firing line," until they are finally disposed of at the sanitary base.

I have devised a plan which it is believed will meet the complicated difficulties of the great problem that has been outlined, removing the wounded promptly, giving them excellent care received considerable incidental notice in other connections, but a general review may not be out of place. (See Figs. 387 to 393 inclusive.)

Some wounds, although not many, are caused by intact shells which have failed to explode. These may still have undiminished velocity, or may have expended most of their energy in piercing armor and thus be "spent." They may also have been deflected by angular impact on some resistant surface and thereby have acquired extreme gyratory motion. But even if the velocity of these missiles has been reduced, their weight is still often sufficient to shear off a member cleanly (Fig. 388), or mutilate a body beyond recognition.

Hemorrhage, of course, furnishes the prime indication for interference in these cases. The shock and previous loss of blood will usually be so considerable that amputation is not justified for some hours at least, and all that can be done immediately is to catch and tie the bleeding points, or, if necessary, ligature in continuity.

Bursting shells bring about diverse results. They may cause severe injury by their concussion-blast, their flame may produce extensive burns, and their fumes may be overpowering. Actual wounds are inflicted by the fragments, and by splinters to which has been communicated the nature of missiles. The

with continuous treatment at the hands of the same group of medical officers until they are finally disposed of at the base. It is fully appreciated that conditions may arise which will necessitate a modification of these methods of meeting the peculiar exigencies of unexpected situations.

It should be understood that this scheme is purely a war measure, and that, under the articles of the Geneva Convention and Hague Conference, the necessary ships may be procured anywhere, may coal and provision in any port, being neutralized under the Red Cross, and are, consequently, not likely to be an encumbrance to the fighting forces.

It is probable that Congress will, in the near future, authorize the establishment of a Naval Medical Reserve Corps, without which the proposed plan will not be feasible. Only those of the highest professional attainments should be commissioned in the Reserve. They will be quartered, in time of war, on great ships capable of carrying a thousand wounded each; they will not be exposed to gun-fire or capture; they will be able to serve their country along humanitarian lines, bringing their great professional skill to bear upon the Navy's wounded and leaving the medical officers of the regular establishment free to stand side by side with their combatant confrères, centring their efforts on keeping as many men at their stations as possible.

Briefly stated, the plan is as follows:—Four ships, capable of caring for 1,000 wounded each, will be required for 16 battleships. Each of these ships will carry a few necessary regular medical officers, and in addition there will be one regular medical officer for each ship of the battle fleet, and under him at least 5 medical reserve corps officers and 25 hospital corpsmen, representing the unit for a single ship. Behind this unit will be such dressings and appliances as may be necessary for a first dressing and preparation for immediate transport. Each one of the four sanitary ships will, during a lull, or after an action, care for the wounded of four battleships, which comprises a division in the battle fleet. The humanitarian units will go to their respective ships, taking along with them their necessary paraphernalia; will take charge of the wounded, look to their immediate removal, and will follow them along to the base. The flow of wounded to the sanitary ships will be continuous and uninterrupted, and the desirable details heretofore outlined can be carried out.

The medical officers attached to the fighting ships, who have participated in the hazards of battle, would probably not be physically fit to attend the scores of wounded that would surround them, nor is their equipment sufficient for the needs of such an occasion. With the proposed plan in operation, these medical officers on the fighting ships would be relieved of this great responsibility, and the wounded would be better cared for, which would lead to a lessening of suffering and better end-results.

size of fragments is variable (Fig. 387), depending somewhat on the design of the shell, but mostly upon the primary shattering power of the explosive used. The more violently explosive is the powder employed, the smaller and more numerous are the fragments, and the greater the number of the injuries which they inflict,—injuries, however, which, individually, are less grave. Whatever the size and number of the fragments, they all possess the extreme irregularity of shape which would be expected in view of their origin.

The wounds resulting from bursting shells are most diverse in character. They vary, not only with the tissue involved, but also with the size, shape, velocity, and gyrations of the fragments or splinters causing them. Sometimes an individual will actually be sown with fifty or more small pieces (Fig. 389),

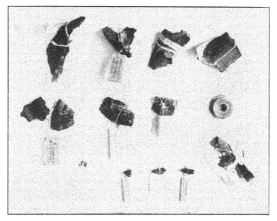

Fig. 387.—Shell Fragments Removed from Patients.*

* Figs. 387-393, included, are taken from specimens and photographs presented to the President of the United States by Surgeon-General Suzuki, of the Imperial Japanese Navy.

and yet escape fatal injury. The pieces often possess no great powers of penetration and are very likely to be found embedded in the superficial tissues, or even just under the skin. All sorts of complications, involving bones, organs, vessels, and nerves, are seen, and many interesting sequelæ follow.

There is a growing tendency to get rid of all woodwork on board ships of war, because, in the past, flying splinters have caused more damage than projectiles. The splinters acquire a velocity nearly equal to that of a shell, and, on account of their bizarre shapes, exhibit very irregular flights and inflict strange wounds.

Until recently, there has existed no classification embracing the relative frequency with which the parts of the body are struck in naval warfare, although military surgery abounds in such statistics. The Japanese made a beginning after the Chinese war, and doubtless their forthcoming figures for the Russian war will give us information which will be of invaluable aid in making our preparations for battle. Suzuki records the parts wounded in the Chinese war as occurring in the following order of frequency: the head, lower limbs, upper extremities, abdomen and lumbar region, thorax and back, and, lastly, the neck. Preliminary reports from the Russian war are quite different.* The order is: lacerated flesh wounds; wounds of extremities, with or without fracture; head; vessels and nerves; thorax, and abdomen (rare). A complete classification of wounds received in naval warfare is obviously beyond the scope of this article. There is space only for a few general remarks in connection with their regional distribution.

Wounds of the head are of all degrees, from slight abrasions to complete pulpefaction of the cranium. The face suffers many injuries, the features sometimes being horribly mangled by large projectiles,—a type of injury which is less apt to be fatal to its possessor than to undermine the courage of his com-

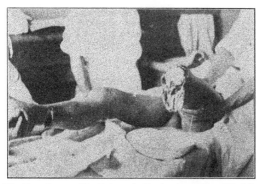

Fig. 388.—Russo-Japanese War Photograph, Showing Amputation of Limb by Shell.

panions. The frequency with which the eye is affected may be judged by the fact that fifty eyes were enucleated in one Japanese hospital. Fractures of the cranium are likewise very common. Treatment of these cases should be confined at first to stopping hemorrhage and elevating depressed fragments. Later, drainage of sterile or infectious abscesses is often required. Symptomatic measures, such as lumbar puncture and cerebral decompression, may prove extremely useful on occasion, especially since there will be no opportunity for refined diagnostic procedures and we may be able to say only that compression exists without being at all prepared to specify the precise cause. One sometimes sees the so-called "gutter" fractures, in which a furrow is made in the outer table alone, and it must be remembered that, conversely, the inner table may be fractured and bulge inward, with no apparent damage to the outer.

It has been found not expedient to treat gunshot wounds of the cranium expectantly. The external wound rarely affords a clew to the extent of the injury, and symptoms are fallacious guides when prolonged and attentive

* Braisted.

observation is quite out of the question. It is therefore held that every case of cranial injury, on its arrival at the operating station, should be subjected to formal exploratory operation, and the pathological indications followed. Even with this precaution, most head injuries will prove fatal. The marked lethality following gunshot wounds of the skull during the Revolutionary war, led to very extensive trephining, and reports of that operation furnish material for one of the most interesting chapters in the history of military surgery.

Shell wounds involving the spinal column and cord are apt to imply a poor prognosis. Large segments of the cord may be carried away, or destroyed by disseminated fragments of bone. The hopeless character of the injury denies these cases early attention, but, when service is possible, a laminectomy for the relief of all pressure should be undertaken.

Wounds of the extremities may be immediately fatal from hemorrhage, but this is quite uncommon by reason of the fact that the usual crushing and

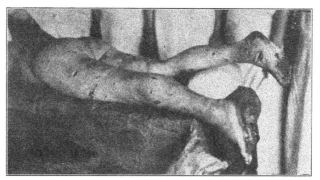

FIG. 389.—Russo-Japanese War Photograph, Showing the Multiplicity of Wounds from Shell Fragments.

searing character of the injury effectually closes the blood-vessels. The wounds are so varied that they defy brief description. Tissues are lacerated and contused so that they appear simply as a bloody mass of pulp. (Figs. 390 and 391.) Fragments of flesh hang by shreds. Muscles lose their tone and remain as swollen and inert masses protruding from the wound; or, on the other hand, they may be carried away in mass, leaving large gaps in the limb. (Figs. 392 and 393.) Bones may be cleanly fractured or extensively comminuted with fragments widely scattered throughout the soft parts. Blood-vessels and nerves do not escape the general destruction.

Ablation of a member necessarily involves a surgical amputation. Injuries short of ablation should be treated with the one idea of saving all the tissue possible. Considerations of practical functioning have no place on a battleship. They are reserved for a subsequent time when the wound has healed and interference may be adventured with good assurance of the ultimate results to be attained. Fortunately, injuries of the abdomen are rarely

seen among the wounded, perhaps, in part, because they are apt to be immediately fatal.* They are serious, in that a viscus is usually injured and peritonitis naturally results. Very few laparotomies should be undertaken, although
progressive hemorrhage may demand action. By far the larger number of
patients will recover if the details of the Ochsner and Murphy treatment of
peritonitis be rigidly heeded. Secondary abscesses and particular injuries, like
rupture of the urinary bladder, are treated along general surgical lines.

Wounds of the chest, also, are best treated expectantly. On a ship there
can be no pressure chambers for operations on the thorax, and it is far wiser
to wait until secondary complications require treatment. However, execs-
sive dyspnœa from accumulations of blood and air in the pleura, or threatened
exsanguination, may make the risk of operation justifiable.

Blood-vessels and nerves are subject to very interesting injuries. Not

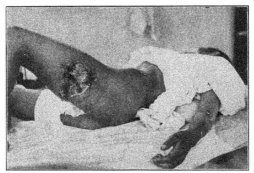

Fig. 390.—Russo-Japanese War Photograph, Showing Large, Lacerated, Contused Shell Wound.

only may they be severed by a missile, or imperiled by a spreading infection,
but their integrity suffers from the passage of a missile in their vicinity. When
a large projectile inflicts a wound, there ensues commonly a peculiar condition
which has already been described. A coagulation necrosis, like that following a
burn by a hot-water bag, affects the tissues in the neighborhood of the tract.
This necrobiotic process results in a sloughing wound, sluggish repair, secondary
hemorrhages, physiological severance of nerves, and late aneurysms. The
frequency of these traumatic aneurysms may be inferred from the report that
in one hospital a Japanese surgeon had operated on one hundred and ten cases
during the war. The suture of cut nerves is indicated as an early procedure;
later, nerve anastomosis or transference should be tried.

Foreign bodies are so frequently met in wounds that very careful search
is demanded. Shell fragments escape notice in the most surprising fashion.
They make their way by pushing the body structures aside, and often no trace
of their passage remains in the bruised and swollen tissues. An example may

* Braisted, op. cit.

be cited of a case which presented, on inspection, what seemed to be a simple abrasion of the skin over the knee that had become covered with a dry crust. Influenced by experience, the Japanese surgeon carried out an exploratory operation. It developed that a large shell fragment had fractured the patella, penetrated the knee-joint, and disorganized it, without causing external evidences. Splinters of wood easily escape detection, especially after they have been macerated by several days' retention. The wood becomes pulpy and the soft chips are not recognized in the profuse purulent discharge. Pieces of clothing are very frequently carried along with the missile. They, likewise, often elude our search.

Suppuration.—Practically all shell wounds suppurate, and the factors which lead to this state seem unavoidable. The wounds are mostly of large size and

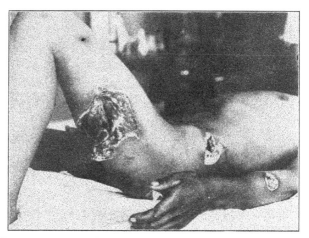

Fig. 391.—Russo-Japanese War Photograph, Showing Multiple, Lacerated Shell Wounds.

smeared with the grime and sweat of battle; dressings will often be applied by unskilled hands under perturbing surroundings, and the tissues are so contused and coagulated, as by a burn, that they are devitalized and thus afford a fit soil for infection. Consequently, under the most favorable facilities for treatment, suppuration will be universal. When the Medical Department is overwhelmed, as may happen, the condition of the wounded men becomes horrible, rivalling in luridness the pictures of pre-antiseptic days. So far as treatment is concerned, the principal point is to see to it that drainage and counter-drainage become routine measures.

Shock.—It is evident that such severe traumatisms united with hemorrhage will present us with many cases of severe shock. The symptoms of the two conditions are blended here as elsewhere, so that they may be indistinguishable, and it is fortunate that similar methods of treatment are indicated for both conditions. The need of fresh air merits first mention; and that means not only the supply of sufficient oxygen, but the elimination of the noxious powder gases which form a stable union with hæmoglobin. There may not be much opportunity for intravenous infusion, but subpectoral infusion and proctoclysis should have extensive employment. Transfusion can have no place in the early hours succeeding battle, unless the casualties have been very few. The use, in true shock, of so-called stimulants is mentioned only to be discouraged,

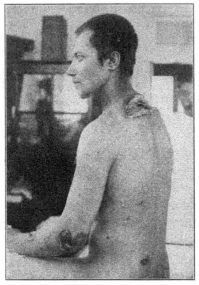

Fig. 392.—Russo-Japanese War Photograph, Showing Multiple, Lacerated Shell Wounds. Note loss of tissue.

although they may be extensively employed in restoring the numerous cases of syncope.

Hospital Ships.—If one fact stands out clearly from the foregoing review of our duties in relation to battle, it is that every consideration demands the removal, from a fighting ship, of all who are unable to render unimpaired service. The removal of the sick before an engagement frees them from the hazards of a naval battle, releases a certain number of attendants, and leaves additional space at our disposal. After a battle, early transference of the wounded is necessary, not only to furnish them with attention which they can receive only imperfectly on a battleship, but also to disencumber the fighting vessel of its wounded, restore the attendants to their naval duties, and remove a prolific source of bad morale.

Although humanitarian considerations need not be slighted, the most potent motives prompting us to disencumber battleships are purely naval, and in laying out our plans to care for the wounded, we shall have to keep before us our aims, and our limitations as well. We are to further the naval efficiency of each ship and bestow on the wounded every attention that may conduce to their comfort and recovery, yet we must recommend no procedure which is likely to affect the mobility or integrity of the fleet.

For the attainment of our ends, the utilization of a shore hospital first suggests itself. However, since we cannot recommend that the fleet abandon

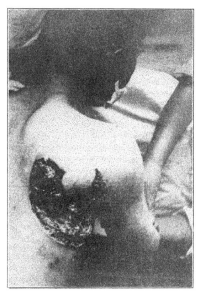

FIG. 393.—Russo-Japanese War Photograph, Showing Extensive Lacerated Shell Wounds.

a strategic position, or that ships be detached for ambulance service, this will be possible only if the fleet withdraws to a naval base, and even then there may be a hurtful delay before shore is reached. Thus we can never expect to be in a position to depend on our naval hospitals to meet the immediate needs arising after battle.

Civilian hospitals, either domestic or foreign, have serious drawbacks, even when near the place of battle. Our wounded become liable to capture by the enemy; they pass from under naval control; they rarely can be returned to duty, and their records are often not obtainable.

We expect that, at the outbreak of hostilities, a number of ships will be commissioned for ambulance service. These ships are very useful to disembarrass the vessels of the line and convey the wounded to the nearest base hospital, but they are, nevertheless, a half-way measure, inasmuch as the injured are without proper treatment during the days consumed in passage.

The only entirely satisfactory means of accomplishing our aims is by attaching one or more hospital ships to each fleet. They join naturally the train of the fleet, which then consists of ammunition, supply, repair, "mother," ambulance, and hospital ships, and are in every way subject to the same administrative control. Like shore hospitals, the hospital ships are under the command of a medical officer, except that navigation is in charge of a civilian sailing master.

Personnel.—The medical personnel of a hospital ship should include surgeons, dentist, pharmacist, hospital stewards, hospital apprentices, and nurses, —all in sufficient numbers for the needs of peace. In time of war, the quota should be greatly augmented, not only in view of the increased amount of work, but also to fill vacancies caused by casualties among the medical officers attached to the fighting ships.

Services Rendered.—The hospital ship is a store-house from which supplies and personnel may be recruited. It is equipped with every facility for ambulance service at sea. It is not only able to gather the wounded from the fleet, but it can give them every advantage accruing from elaborate equipment, so that they may be retained on board while incapacitated, or transferred to a shore station, as may be required by the number of the wounded, amount of supplies, nearness of base, and accumulation of men incapable of further service. Its speed enables it to accompany the fleet during all manœuvres, and be present at all times. Thus the hospital ship, and it alone, is capable of dealing with the problem of what to do with the wounded after battle.

In times of peace, the duties of a hospital ship are hardly less important. Some of the smaller craft have no sick bays, and those on the larger ships, although they suffice so long as the number of patients does not rise much above the average, may become totally inadequate at any time. These circumstances are not even disquieting, if there is at hand a hospital ship prepared to receive all cases, and particularly those which require isolation, surgical operation, or special treatment of any sort. Such a ship is also fitted to carry out any process of disinfection, make laboratory examinations, take Roentgenograms, and, in fact, undertake any species of medical activity that might be expected of a large shore hospital. It may be further employed in taking the sick from tropical stations for short sea-voyages.

The value of a hospital ship as a graduate school is not inconsiderable. It enables the personnel to become familiar with all their duties which appertain to battle, and also enables medical officers who are remote from medical centres during their cruise, to attend clinics on board the hospital ship and become acquainted with the medical and surgical material of the fleet.

Functioning.—Before battle, the hospital ship is expected to distribute supplies to the ships about to enter action and remove the sick from them, so that they can then begin fighting with every man at his post.

Its duties during battle are perfectly clear, but any method of accomplishing them must be tentatively adopted. In the first place, the neutral character of a hospital ship constrains us to give aid to friend and foe without discrimination, and this obligation may entail difficulties in deciding what course to pursue in a given case. Secondly, there is the question of how near the scene of battle shall the hospital ship remain. We know that battleships may sink in a very few minutes, and the hospital ship, if distant, can give no aid. On the other hand, self-protection requires that a hospital ship be removed from the possibility of injury by long-range gun-fire. Situations must be met according to their individual requirements, but in general it may be said that hospital ships can remain in view of the combatants and approach disabled vessels after they drop out of the line of battle. The writer, during fleet manœuvres, made certain observations on this point. It was found that flag signals were not visible at the distance maintained for safety, and that it was possible to keep in clear view only the masts, stacks, and smoke of the fighting ships. A

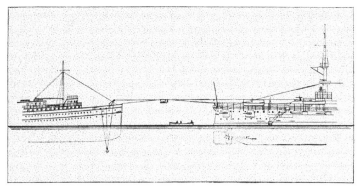

Fig. 394.—Stokes' Apparatus for Transferring the Wounded at Sea.

wireless apparatus is indispensable to keep the hospital ship properly informed of need for its services.

The course to be followed after battle is clearly defined. First, the ambulance service should be embarked, and all the wounded, except perhaps the moribund and the very slightly injured, should be collected and brought to the hospital ship where the entire personnel stands in readiness to receive and distribute the wounded in accordance with the scheme already outlined for use on battleships. No difficulties will arise in berthing and treating the wounded if the capacity of the ship is not exceeded. However, if the number of wounded in the fleet exceed the accommodations of the ship, it must then serve as an ambulance, carrying the more seriously wounded to the nearest base hospital, giving them, on the way, such treatment as they require, and returning immediately to the fleet to pick up the remainder of the wounded. The keeping of medical and surgical records as material for a medical history of a war is incumbent on the staff of the hospital ship, and there are usually enough men on board so that verbatim records can be transcribed, Roentgenograms made, and photographs of interesting lesions taken.

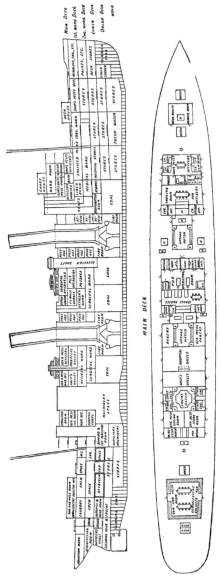

Fig. 395.—Ideal Hospital Ship; Inboard Profile and Main Deck.

The Hague conferences, subscribed to by nearly all countries, insure the immunity of hospital ships so long as they do not violate the obligations of neutrality. Although they are allowed unrestricted action, it is always at their own risk, and they should exercise every precaution to keep from between combatants and to remain outside the range of missiles during action; for no service can be rendered during battle that would in any way justify exposure to gun-fire. Judging from events of recent wars and the trend of present preparations, naval battles of the future will be attended by at least one hospital ship, with its attendant medical transports. Whether these are controlled by the Army, Navy, or relief societies, they are all bound, in return for immunity

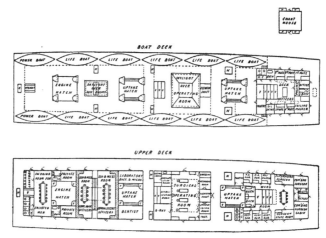

FIG. 396.—Ideal Hospital Ship; Boat Deck and Upper Deck.

granted, to observe the rules of conduct laid down, more or less precisely, by the articles of the Hague Conferences.

Transportation.—It here becomes necessary to speak of new methods of transportation, in addition to those already described, for patients must now be transferred from ship to ship. We have for this service ambulance boats and an aerial cable-way. The Japanese employed any boats that were at hand, but, when the weather permitted, they preferred to use flat-bottomed boats on which was laid a platform for stretchers. Patients were lowered by whip from the deck to the ambulance boat, towed to the hospital ship, and hoisted to a side port. The inswing of the davit was made feasible by an ingenious hatch, cut in the deck above. The Russian hospital ship *Mongolia* lowered two large wooden platforms over the side by steam cranes, and boats came alongside. The device was not tried in rough water, but generally gave very satisfactory service. It may be noted, in passing, that some method of transportation is possible in any sea in which guns can be fought.

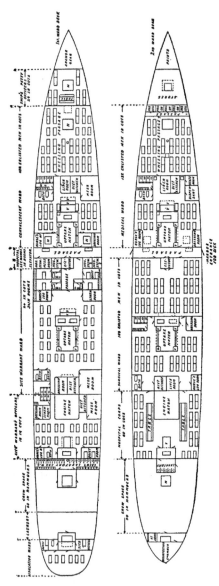

Fig. 397.—Ideal Hospital Ship; First Ward Deck and Second Ward Deck

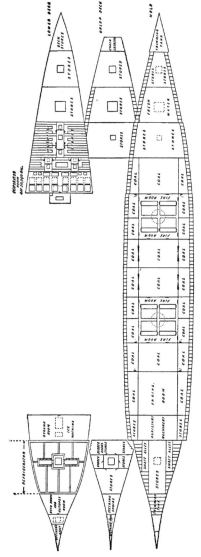

Fig. 398.—Ideal Hospital Ship; Lower Deck, Orlop Deck, and Hold.

To supplement the method of using boats and to expedite the transfer, in April, 1898, the writer devised an apparatus (Fig. 394) which consists roughly of a steel hawser made fast to the fighting ship, a weight let over the side of the hospital ship sufficiently in excess of the weight of the hawser, the patient, and the transferring car, to keep the line taut and clear of the water while effecting the transfer. This type of apparatus can be used in any sea-way in which the guns can be fought, and the ships, while the transfer is being accomplished, lie dead in the water. The splint stretcher can be used as a transferring car, or a chair carriage devised by the writer may be employed. This apparatus differs from all coaling devices that the writer has seen and suits the purpose better than any that he knows of.

It is not possible, within the scope of this article, to cite at length the structural specifications and equipment of an ideal hospital ship. A few requirements may, however, be noted.

The ship should have a displacement of about ten thousand tons and be of dimensions which will insure both speed and stability. Bilge keels are an aid in securing steadiness. It is important that the ship should have a speed of twenty knots, in order to keep with the fast divisions of the fleet, give assistance expeditiously, and carry patients to a shore station with little delay.

Oil-burning engines will obviate the abundant deposit of coal dust during "coaling ship" and will prevent the settling of cinders and soot in the tuberculosis and isolation wards on the upper deck. Large side ports are a help in handling the wounded.

The medical and surgical features are, essentially, those designed for any general hospital, with certain modifications necessary to adapt them to ships. The five hundred beds desired will be distributed in the various wards according to the number of patients expected in each class—that is, surgical, medical, contagious, etc.

The writer has designed a ship with reference to these needs and others not specified. A study of the appended plans will give a very accurate idea of the points to be observed. (Figs. 395–398.)

Landing Parties.—It frequently happens that ships, squadrons, or fleets are under the necessity of landing a number of men for the purpose of effecting a surprise, seizing a position, or punishing uncivilized tribes. In fact, shore expeditions are more common than formal naval battles. This survey of Naval Surgery cannot, therefore, be concluded without touching upon our duties relating to land operations, although they will be discussed very briefly, since our problems on shore are nearly identical with those confronting the Army surgeon, and they have been treated at length in the article on "Military Surgery." The resemblance of our scheme of first-aid to that of the Army has already been explained, together with the ready practicability of putting the naval system in practice on shore without essential modification. Our equipment, too, is adapted to the needs of landing parties; some parts of it, as the first-aid packet and the Hospital Corps pouch, being even more suitable for use on shore than on ships.

The personnel of the Hospital Corps should, if possible, comprise two per cent of the expeditionary force, it being unfortunately out of the question to stipulate the five per cent required by the Army organization. The hospital apprentices will each be supplied with the pouch described on page 1000. These pouches, with the addition of a few light litters, will suffice unless the size of the expedition and its expected duration warrant the planting of a Field Hospital, in which case we shall have to carry also the Field Hospital outfit which is issued to flagships.

So far as the size of the expedition requires and the number of hospital apprentices permits, stations will be established precisely as on board. There will be mobile relief parties (regimental aid) near the firing line, relief stations (field dressing stations) in the rear and out of the danger zone, but as near as is consistent with safety, and secondary stations (field hospitals) farther in the rear and centrally located. The ship itself may be considered the primary station (or stationary hospital). The ambulance service will be difficult, because of the lack of carriers and wheeled litters. This is not, however, a serious matter during action and, afterward, carriers can be detailed.

Our men will usually be either attacking fortifications, or both forces will be mobile as in the ordinary field battle. In either case our functions here will be inhibited by much the same influences as on board ship. Sometimes it will happen, when the men fall back after an advance, that the wounded will be left lying between the lines where assistance is impossible; or it may be simply that the wide danger zone of modern fire-arms compels the Hospital Corps to keep behind cover, or out of range, and renders it much safer for the wounded man to remain flat on the ground than to be lifted up for transport. Our duties, then, will begin here, as on board ship, after the battle.

Attention must be called to the different character of weapons used in land warfare. Ninety per cent of the wounds met are caused by small-bore, jacketed bullets, which generally show a tendency, at the usual distances, to perforate cleanly. The first-aid packet is well adapted to these wounds and may answer as a permanent dressing, since there is not the proneness to suppuration that we see in shell wounds.

The Army finds that "with mobile troops in action against a mobile army in the field, the most difficult problems of surgical assistance are presented." How much greater will be the difficulties to be overcome by a naval force lacking the transportation facilities of an army on the march! The situation must be dealt with as best it may. Carts may be seized by the belligerents, navigable streams utilized, and extra details for stretcher service obtained. But, whatever devices be exploited, the means of transporting the wounded to the rear, and then back to the ship during retreat, will remain a source of serious concern to the Medical Department.

The writer takes pleasure in acknowledging the valuable services rendered by Passed Assistant Surgeon Harold W. Smith, U. S. Navy, in the collection of data and in the preparation of the illustrations for the text.

ADMINISTRATIVE RAILROAD SURGERY.

By JAMES ALEXANDER HUTCHISON, M.D.,
L.R.C.P. and S. (Edin.), Montreal, Canada.

Introductory Remarks.—Railroad surgery may be considered that branch of general surgery which has to deal with the care of persons injured in any of the manifold operations of a railroad.

While primarily this had to deal with injuries received on, or by, moving trains, for obvious reasons it has been forced to extend its sphere to any injuries received in any situation incident to railroad operations. The large number of injuries resulting from the operation of railroads has brought about the necessity for a special organization. From the records of the Interstate Commerce Commission, we find that over one hundred thousand persons are killed and injured in railroad accidents yearly, and that this appalling number continues to increase from year to year. With the development of railroads, the management of the better class of roads soon realized that the best interests of all required that men accustomed to dealing with such cases be constantly in close touch with the railroad executive.

It is the duty of the railroad company which undertakes to transport passengers, to do so with reasonable safety, and at the present time a railroad is held by the courts to be responsible if its passengers are not carried in complete safety to the end of their journey. Public opinion demands, in addition to the safeguarding of the passenger or other person, prompt attendance and subsequent care of the injured.

The responsibility of the railroad does not end with the safety of passengers, but includes the protection of its employees against the various hazards of their occupations. Here again, in many instances, the law, and practically in all instances public opinion, permit no excuse for the lack of prompt relief and care of injured employees.

The frequent introduction of new methods in railroad transportation, developed by new appliances, by modifications of speed, by the great increase in the weight and size of locomotives and rolling stock, and by new forms of motive power, such as electricity and compressed air, continually alters the nature of the most frequent accidents.

While the development of systems for the care of injured passengers and employees was primarily the result of humane motives, other reasons of expediency and financial interests were quickly recognized.

It is clearly to the advantage of the railroad to have injuries put under the most favorable conditions for a rapid repair and recovery, that the period of disability may be reduced to a minimum, permitting the return to duty of experienced and valued employees with the least possible loss of time, thus diminishing the cost of the accident to the railroad and to the injured individual. The hazard of further accident is also lessened, as it is a well-known fact that, where an experienced and competent employee is withdrawn from a special duty, it is not always possible to have his place supplied with an equally trained servant, the inexperienced man being frequently the victim or unwitting cause of further accident.

The question of compensation in railroad injuries looms so large that special attention has to be directed by railroad managements to this aspect of the injury. Whether the injured person be an employee of the railroad or not, it is equally to the interest of the company to have the period of disablement not an unduly prolonged one. For these reasons it has become necessary to provide surgeons who have been trained for the treatment of the special features presented by the surgical conditions met with in railroad work. This has resulted in the formation of a distinct specialty. The surgical conditions met with differ in no way from those met with in ordinary general surgery. The specialty is almost entirely concerned in the administrative features involved. The writer proposes therefore to deal with these special features, and will avoid the consideration of the scientific aspects of the surgery involved in a railroad injury, in the belief that these conditions have already been fully dealt with in the foregoing articles in this system.

Historical Notice.—The first railroad development having taken place in Great Britain, it was in that country that the first provision was made for the hazards arising out of the new form of locomotion. Measures for the care of persons injured on or by railroads were early provided, ultimately developing into relief organizations. At the very outset fears were entertained that this new invention would be accompanied by extreme dangers and by all manner of maladies. We find it gravely stated, for example, in a leading periodical in 1825, that railroad travelling would be as safe as being fired out of a rocket. It is a lamentable fact that the opening of the Liverpool and Manchester Railroad on September 15th, 1830, was attended by the death of a leading citizen.

Among the earliest organizations providing for the care of the injured on railroads, was that of the London and North Western Railroad of Great Britain. This was quickly followed on the continent of Europe, France and Germany leading. In the United States one of the first was that of the Pennsylvania Railroad Company, soon after followed by the Baltimore & Ohio Railroad Company, the Missouri Pacific Railroad Company, and many others. Several important roads in the East, however, have no definite provision in the form of an organization. In Canada, as early as 1873, the Grand Trunk Railway Company had an organization which provided for the care and relief of employees injuried on duty.

Two distinct groups of conditions obtained, and still obtain, in North America.

In the East the railroad is tributary to a well-organized community, having a dense population, with towns only a few miles apart. General hospitals are numerous, and experienced medical practitioners are within easy reach. Thus the railroad can command, at a moment's notice, all necessaries for the care of the injured.

In addition to caring for surgical emergencies arising out of accidents, railroad managements early had to consider the necessity of meeting conditions which owed their origin to old age, sickness, and improvidence, conditions which unfortunately prevail in all densely populated districts. These special conditions led the railroads of the Eastern States and of Canada to provide, in addition to surgical attendance for injuries received on duty, attendance for surgical accidents occurring when off duty, medical attendance during sickness, special allowances in the form of sick and injury benefits, and various forms of relief insurance, the same conditions having already determined the larger scope of relief organizations in Europe. The older the railroad, the more necessary it appears to be to make these special provisions.

In the western portions of the whole of America, conditions were entirely different. The railroad spread out over the uninhabited prairie and population followed. Those engaged in railroad building and operations, were, for the most part, young and vigorous men. The absence of towns, hospitals, and medical practitioners made it necessary for the railroad management to provide accommodation for the sick and injured. The hospital system thus grew up in the West, and there reached its highest state of development. The conditions in the West are rapidly approaching those of the East, and the hospital system must eventually be succeeded by the relief department of the East.

Organization of the Relief Work.—To speak more particularly of the methods for the relief of the sick and injured, there are four principal types in operation at present:—

> 1. The Relief System.
> 2. Surgical service without a Chief Surgeon.
> 3. Surgical service with a Chief Surgeon.
> 4. The Hospital System.

The Relief System.—This system is in operation in many of the large eastern railroads, and is gradually being extended to the west. It differs in many respects in the different railroad systems. In some railroads it is maintained as a department of the Company, in others, jointly by the railroad and its employees, or entirely by the employees. Membership may be either voluntary or compulsory, and may include temporary as well as permanent employees. Membership is dependent on a monthly assessment, varying according to the age, the hazard of employment, or the salary.

When joint management obtains, a Committee of Management, consisting of representatives elected by the members and officers nominated by the railroad executive, controls affairs; in some cases executive control is vested in trustees appointed by the courts.

The benefits to be obtained by membership in the relief system vary in many respects. Among the more important features are daily compensation, for limited periods of time, for injury and sickness occurring on or off duty, surgical and medical attendance during periods of disability, hospital mainten-ance, benefits in case of permanent disability.　In addition, some relief systems include elaborate features covering pensions for old age, bank savings, building and loan departments.　The Baltimore & Ohio Railroad Company is an example of the latter.

The present high standard of development of relief systems has been attained in the face of many obstacles and often in spite of great opposition from those for whom the organization was created.

The many mutual benefit organizations throughout the country offered what seemed to the railroad employee more advantageous terms in benefits to be ob-tained in return for the monthly assessment.　Experience has shown, however, that many of these societies were not founded on actuarial figures, and thus, in time, they either became insolvent or were obliged to increase their rates.　It was then appreciated that the railroad relief organization, with its assurance of financial assistance from the parent company, had always been on a sound basis.

The Pensylvania Railroad and the Grand Trunk Railroad are examples where the railroad absolutely guarantees the relief organization against any annual deficit.

Surgical Service without a Chief Surgeon.—Although this method has ob-tained for many years, it must be looked upon as an evolution up to one of the more highly developed organizations.　It cannot be doubted that this manner of medical administration offers many disadvantages.　Under this system, medical officers are appointed at various points on the railroad, and they report either directly to a divisional officer or to the executive of the road.　Systematic medical supervision of the work of local surgeons cannot be maintained without a medical executive.

Surgical Service with a Chief Surgeon.—At the present time there is practically no question as to the advantages of having a Chief Surgeon in charge of the medical work of a railroad.　It has been frequently pointed out that, where it was possible for the Chief Executive of a small railroad to be in charge of every department, he was able to have personal knowledge of the medical as well as other affairs of that railroad; but, with the combination of small roads into large ones, resulting in the present railroad systems embracing thousands of miles, the necessity for subdividing responsibility became apparent, and in course of time the Chief Surgeon became the Head of the Medical Department, practically becoming the professional adviser of the executive on all medical affairs of the railroad.　In order to have a uniform policy in medical adminis-tration, there must be a medical executive, thus securing systematic care of the injured on all parts of the railroad.　He is in a position to consider the various new methods suggested from time to time and to bring them to the attention of the railroad executive.　Not infrequently these suggestions are the result of the experience of a local surgeon, whose ideas, however good they may be, would have very doubtful chances of being considered by the executive without the intervention of a Chief Surgeon or other medical arbitrator.

The personal knowledge which a Chief Surgeon acquires in the routine administration of a railroad, and contact not only with members of the profession throughout the territory through which his railroad operates, but also with the railroad officials, enable him to see the point of view of both sides and thus to prevent much misunderstanding. The Chief Surgeon should assume the responsibility of determining matters of ethics, and explaining to the Management the duties the local surgeon owes to the patient and to his profession.

Not long ago, a Local Surgeon was requested, by the railroad official in charge of his district, to visit at their homes several men who claimed to be unfit for work by reason of various minor injuries. The Local Surgeon, believing that it was his duty to obey the request, at the same time recognized that he had no right to visit these men and demand the privilege of examination to enable him to comply with the official's orders. The matter was then referred to the Chief Surgeon, who decided at once that the Local Surgeon should not be asked to visit the employee's house, but that the employee must present himself at the office of the official or surgeon for examination. This simple point caused much controversy, and, without the intervention of the Chief Surgeon, the Local Surgeon would have been obliged to offend the official or commit a breach of medical ethics. The knowledge on the part of the Local Surgeon that there is a Chief Surgeon to supervise him, is an incentive to do the best type of work.

Incompetent surgical work can be best recognized by an experienced Chief Surgeon; the laity is, and must always be, incompetent to judge.

The Chief Surgeon becomes familiar with local conditions. In course of time his knowledge extends beyond an appreciation of the standard of work done by the local railroad surgeon. He learns, for example, what are the qualifications of the neighboring general practitioner, who may from time to time be called in an emergency, and as a result he is perhaps able to stimulate this practitioner to acquire further knowledge, or, if he finds that nothing can be accomplished in this direction, he will at least be able to protect the railroad employee by not permitting this man to be called even in an emergency.

The Chief Surgeon of any large railroad soon becomes familiar with the standard of work done in various parts of the country, and, if medical appointments are under his control, it is possible by careful selection to create a standard of work much above that done in the same community by others. In this lies the chief value, not only to the railroad, but to the medical profession, of a competent, experienced Chief Surgeon.

The railroad is being called upon with increasing frequency to defend itself against claims for compensation. In order that the Claims Department may obtain the most satisfactory results, it is absolutely essential that it should co-operate actively with the Medical Department. Such co-operation is best obtained through a Chief Surgeon. It is hardly necessary to add, that the office of the Chief Surgeon should be at headquarters.

As all railroad surgery carries with it important financial considerations, the Chief Surgeon must always be the best judge of the financial value of services rendered. No fee bill or schedule of charges can ever be framed which will meet the conditions of all cases, and, where the decision rests with an officer other than a medical man, dissatisfaction must follow from time to time. Again, the value of services varies much in different parts of the country, and, in city and country districts, only a medical man can familiarize himself with the varying conditions prevailing.

Surgical expenses are a steadily increasing charge on all growing railroads, and to have these charges under the control of one official who is familiar with, and in constant touch with, the various officials primarily responsible for authorizing the service, is a distinct economy.

Even in legal cases, the Chief Surgeon should be more familiar with the special features of each claim than any other official, and thus be able to determine, in a particular district, who, of the various surgeons, can offer the fairest evidence. Unfortunately, local interest not infrequently influences the judgment of a particular medical witness. Under these circumstances the Chief Surgeon or his representative, usually a Division Surgeon, is the only official familiar with these conditions, having gathered them in his intercourse with local and other surgeons by attending the various medical meetings in different parts of the country. Again, he is the only official of a railroad who can possibly recognize this partisan spirit. He is able to recognize the expert whose evidence is influenced by the remuneration which he receives. It is the duty of the Chief Surgeon to eliminate this unsatisfactory element, and much benefit has already been obtained by the refusal to continue this type of witness who, while representing the railroad, brings it into disfavor. The railroad lawyer not infrequently uses this type of men for the immediate advantage that may be gained, without regard for the future evils which such a course brings on the whole medical profession. The Chief Surgeon has been a great factor in educating the Local Surgeon and others to appreciate the fact that he is never expected to depart from a strictly honorable course.

The Hospital System.—The hospital system is essentially an American plan and is not in existence in Europe. It was evolved out of the rude temporary hospital provided during the construction of the railroads in the far West. The value and benefit of a hospital close at hand, in districts far removed from the ordinary evidences of civilization, were beyond dispute. On the completion of the railroad, the need for hospital accommodation continued as great as during the construction period, and it was this need which resulted in the development of the modern system. Though the first hospital established in the United States for the treatment of injured employees alone, was established on the Lehigh Valley Railroad by Judge Asa Packer, at his own individual expense, this action was not followed by the establishment of a hospital department on that railroad; and it was not until 1868 that the Central Pacific Railroad created a hospital department. Its first hospital building was opened for patients in 1869 at Sacramento, California. The cost, for building and land, was $64,000. It had accommodation for one hundred and twenty patients, and contained a number of private wards. It was maintained at first by voluntary contributions of fifty cents a month, but as this did not produce sufficient revenue, it was followed by a compulsory fee from all employees including the General Manager and all officers.

The first railroad hospital on the Missouri Pacific Railroad was built at Washington, Missouri, under the auspices of the late Dr. John W. Jackson, in 1879.

This continent owes a debt of gratitude to Dr. Warren B. Outten, the Chief Surgeon of the Missouri Pacific Railroad, for the active work he has done in developing the highest ideals in the railroad surgeon, and in the establishment, on a firm basis, of the hospital system for those parts of the country which have need for such a system.

The general plan of the hospital system provided one or more hospitals situated at convenient points along the line of the railroad, to which all cases of sickness and injury arising among employees may be taken. In many of these hospitals provision is made for injured passengers. Private wards are also provided. On Southern railroads separate wards are provided for colored employees.

Not infrequently, the principal hospital of the railroad is so situated that the Chief Surgeon is Surgeon-in-Chief of that hospital. If such a hospital is situated in a large city, all of the various branches of medicine, as well as the specialties, are represented on the staff, each medical officer taking charge of a department. One or two of the senior medical officers may devote their whole time to the hospital service, the remaining members being in private practice and visiting the hospital from time to time as may be necessary.

In this central hospital there may be provided office accommodation for the business staff which directs the finances and other details of the whole department. Such a hospital may accommodate two hundred or more patients.

The smaller or subsidiary hospitals on the same railroad—hospitals which provide for from twenty to seventy-five patients—are, in some instances, under the charge of one or more resident medical officers who devote their whole time to the service; or, again, they may be in charge of a medical officer who is engaged in private practice. In such a hospital there may be a junior resident medical officer who has immediate charge of the hospital. In the case of a very small hospital in some distant part of the railroad, such a staff may be able to care for the ordinary conditions of injury, but, where all surgical cases are treated to a conclusion, much that might be beneficial to the patient is lacking. To refer to only one detail, one might mention the lack of a pathological or a bacteriological department. When such an organization acts as a temporary hospital, forwarding important cases to a larger hospital that is fully equipped, it is a desirable establishment.

Under the hospital system it is usual to appoint, at different places along the railroad, local surgeons who render immediate aid to the injured and who arrange for transportation to the nearest railroad hospital of the Company. Should the patient prefer to remain at his home, he is obliged, in the case of certain railroad systems, to provide, at his own expense, any further medical attendance that may be required. This causes a break in the chain which must lead to many disadvantages. From the surgical point of view, for example, the patient may lose the service of an experienced surgeon, and, from the railroad point of view, there is a probability that he will lack the assistance which the hospital department is able to give in the form of friendly surroundings and in warding off unwise advice as to the railroad's responsibility for the accident —advice which may lead to much unwise litigation in which the patient is often the greater loser.

Shortly after hospitals were established, the employees were in doubt as to the wisdom of the arrangement, they believing that their interests would be better served if they were quite independent. This view obtains to a small extent even at the present time. It is generally conceded that their individual rights are safeguarded in the hospital. This has been brought about by the large army of conscientious surgeons who have followed the advice so often given, that the railroad surgeon is to act in the best interests of the patient at all times, and not as part surgeon and part claims agent. At the present time there is no difficulty of this kind where the hospital is properly equipped, not only with hospital accommodation and appliances, but with properly chosen surgeons.

In some instances the hospital of one railroad system arranges for the admission and care of employees of another railroad, either by assigning a portion of the building to the medical control of the surgeon of that railroad, or by admitting them without distinction at a specially fixed charge. Another arrangement is for the hospital department of a railroad to take over a certain number of beds in a general hospital, retaining the medical control, but leaving the maintenance, service, etc., with the hospital management.

Where private wards are available to other than passengers and employees, the conditions under which they may be occupied differ in different hospitals. In some cases, for example, they are limited to the families of the employees, in others to the patients of members of the medical staff. The latter plan is open to criticism, and leaves too much to the judgment of the staff.

In some hospital systems it is the practice to allow the dispensary attached to the hospital to supply dressings and medicine, to employees not resident in the hospital, on the prescription, not only of the Local Surgeon, but also of general practitioners who are not connected with the hospital.

There is a wide difference of opinion as to the merits of the railroad hospital system as against the use of city general hospitals. While admitting the value of the railroad hospital in the sparsely settled portions of the West, the writer is of the opinion that, as cities grow up along the line of the railroad and develop the large general hospital, the railroad hospital must give way. The general hospital, with its large staff, particularly when there is a medical school associated with it, produces a degree of competition not known in the railroad hospital, and leads to the highest degree of hospital efficiency.

It is unfortunate that the railroads of America have been slow to recognize the importance of the medical service, with the result that each railroad has built up such a system as seemed to its management necessary for its requirements. Up to the present date there has been no effort at a standard method. This is the more remarkable when one realizes the number of existing organizations which have only one object in view, viz., that of producing standards which may be adopted by all railroads. Thus, we have associations of the following different officers: General Managers; Traffic Managers, covering freight and passenger services; Transportation Officers; Master Car Builders; Motive Power Superintendents; and Engineers of Maintenance of Way. As a result of the action of these various associations, specific rules have been formulated for the guidance of the employees of the various departments; and consequently, in changing from one railroad service to another, the employee takes up his work with a well-developed knowledge of his duties. This is not true, however, of the medical service of a railroad, and there can be little doubt that the best result will not be obtained until this state of affairs is changed.

Personnel of a Railroad Medical Organization.—The following brief outline may be given of the organization of medical officers in one large system, where a somewhat elaborate relief department is in operation. Executive control is vested in the Chief Surgeon, or—to give him a title more comprehensive of his various duties—the Chief Medical Officer. He is the adviser of the railroad executive on all matters of a medical nature. He recommends for appointment all medical officers associated with the railroad service. He acts as the medical head of the relief department, passing upon all matters of a medical nature. He keeps records of all reports from Local or Division Surgeons; certifies as to the fitness for employment of all permanent employees; passes upon all examinations in regard to vision, color sense, and hearing; reports upon all applications for retiring allowance on account of injury or sickness; reports upon the medical aspect of all claims for damage as a result of personal injury and determines the medical defence of all cases of personal-injury claims to be tried before the courts, discussing with the officers of the Legal Department in regard to the choice of medical experts. All expenditures of a medical nature are subject to his approval. He is responsible for the instructions or regulations under which the department is managed.

Under the Chief Surgeon are Division Surgeons in charge of one or more divisions. These officers reside in all cases at the Division Headquarters, where they are in close touch with the transportation and other divisional officers; and, while they report directly to the Chief Surgeon, they also report all matters coming under their observation to the Chief Divisional Officers.

The Division Surgeon has no direct control over the Local Surgeons except in one respect: in the event of a large number of persons being injured through a derailment or other accident to a passenger train, it is his duty to go immediately to the scene of the accident and take charge of the relief of the injured persons, arranging for their disposition by sending them to their homes or to convenient hospitals adjacent to the scene of the accident. Much responsibility devolves upon the Division Surgeon in distributing the local medical men called to the scene of the accident, and in arranging for proper emergency treatment and subsequent care.

To the Division Surgeon may be delegated, by the Chief Surgeon, such special duties as that of examining and reporting on special cases. He is paid a monthly salary for these various services.

The Local Surgeons or District Medical Officers are usually general practitioners appointed at towns and cities with regard to the train service, that they may be easily available in time of need. In some instances their duties cover the town and immediate neighborhood; in other cases the territory assigned to each officer represents a small district that extends ten or fifteen miles in each direction. The limits of each district within city, town, or country, are specially defined, in order that there may be no misunderstanding or delay in reaching the proper surgeon.

"Employees' Time Tables" have a complete list of all surgeons and their residences. In addition, notices are posted in stations, workshops, and other prominent places, giving their names, addresses, and office hours, that all employees may familiarize themselves with their names. Each Local Surgeon supplies the name of a substitute acceptable to the Chief Surgeon, and his name, address, and office hours are added to the notice. The District Medical Officer is appointed by, and is directly under the control of, the Chief Surgeon. The knowledge that the Local Surgeon is under the authority of the Chief Surgeon and has not received his appointment through any other means, tends to establish a better "esprit de corps," through which only the highest class of surgical service may be maintained.

Duties of the District Medical Officer.—The District Medical Officer may be summoned to render first aid to all persons, employee or otherwise, injured under any circumstances on the railroad property. He must then decide upon the disposition of the injured person. This is often a difficult matter to determine, much has to be left to the judgment of the medical officer. In the case of passengers, the decision rests with the injured passenger. Employees are forwarded, if able to travel, to their own homes, or to the nearest hospital. When it appears necessary, the District Medical Officer accompanies the injured person, the authority to do this being derived from the Chief Despatcher. The care of trespassers has always been a matter of difficulty. It is generally understood that municipal authorities are responsible for the homeless. In large cities no special difficulty is experienced, as a case can be referred to police authorities without delay; in small towns or country places, however, it is often necessary to carry an injured person out of one municipality into another, thus throwing the responsibility for future care on a municipality other than the one in which the injury took place. In practice it is customary to carry the injured man to the nearest hospital, the expectation being that the charitable management of the institution will continue the care of the case.

The District Medical Officer reports to the Chief Medical Officer on a printed form, forwarding the report by train mail. The following is a sample of the report:—

Name, Age, Occupation, Residence, and whether married or single. If an employee, state where and how employed.

Date and place of accident.

Amount of insurance, if any, carried by injured person, and name of company writing policy.

What evidence of old injury, as a crippled hand, loss of limb, or eye, or any evidence of disability, stated by patient or apparent to surgeon.

Patient's statement as to manner in which injury was caused.

Describe the injuries:—

 (a) Character and extent of wound.
 (b) Location of wound.
 (c) What complication, if any.
 (d) Condition of patient when first seen by surgeon. If any shock or hemorrhage, describe same.

What services were rendered, and by whom.

What disposition was made of patient.

Your opinion as to length of time patient will be disabled.

       (*Signed*)...................

Residence ....*Date*..............................

NOTE.—

When a surgeon is called, on account of this Company, to attend the injured, whether passengers, employees, or others, one of these reports must immediately be made out by the surgeon and sent by train mail to........................

This form, with slight modifications, is in very general use in all parts of America, and may be modified to meet special requirements.

The further attendance on the part of a Local Surgeon or District Medical Officer, is determined by the Chief Medical Officer, or by the regulations of the Relief Department, which govern attendance on medical cases where provision for such cases is made. When a case continues under the care of a Local Surgeon, further reports follow at intervals of two or three weeks until the patient has recovered, when there is forwarded to headquarters a report in which are given further details covering the final particulars of the case and the ultimate disposition of the patient.

First-Aid and Equipment.—Not the least important feature in accident surgery is the care and handling of the injured person before the arrival of the surgeon. With the introduction of Listerism first-aid dressings assumed much greater importance, although the importance of the early care of fractures, hemorrhages, and shock remained the same as formerly. As a result, instruction in first-aid became imperative.

Instruction in first-aid has been in common use in Europe for many years, especially in Germany and Great Britain, but has been introduced only to a limited extent in America.

The St. John Ambulance Association in Great Britain has done much to promote the dissemination of knowledge in British countries, with the result that most of the ambulance classes on British railroads are held under its auspices. The general plan is to give a series of from six to ten lectures and demonstrations based upon a syllabus published by the Association for distribution among pupils. At the end of the course, the class is examined by a medical man who is appointed by the local branch of the Association, and who makes his report direct to the Association. If the candidate is successful, he gets a certificate. A second and a third course are given during the two succeeding years, and, if all examinations are passed, a badge or a pin, which can be worn, is granted. The badge has become a very familiar object in Great Britain, and most of the London policemen wear it.

Though these classes, so far as railroad employees are concerned, are voluntary, they have been taken advantage of by very large numbers of men.*

In Germany, systematic instruction is compulsory for all employees engaged in the movement of trains, under authority of a decree issued by the Minister of State Railroads. This instruction is provided for in the somewhat elaborate and minute regulations in force for the guidance of employees in case of accidents. It might be well to enumerate briefly the more important features.

In the event of injury to passengers, as the result of an accident to a train, auxiliary trains have, as part of their equipment, special physicians' cars fully equipped. Certain of the employees are told off to aid the railroad surgeon, and part of their duty is to wash their hands and make ready during the journey to the scene of the accident. This train is also equipped with a portable telephone apparatus to be attached to the telegraph wires. Twice a year an emergency call is made, and all employees assigned to this service, including the railroad surgeon, have to respond. One call takes place at night, another in the daytime, once in winter and once in summer. The train has to depart within thirty minutes in daytime, and within forty-five minutes at night. Should some of the employees fail to arrive within the time specified, the senior official on duty determines whether or not the train will depart, to be followed later by another with the remaining members of the staff.

Two types of emergency chest are in use to meet the emergencies of an accident—a small box kept in the baggage-car of all trains, and a large box kept at every station and main workshop. The care of each box is under a specially designated employee. Special provision is made to have a sufficient supply at out-of-the-way stations, that there may be no want in the event of a number of persons being injured and of dressings being required which may not easily be obtained elsewhere. These boxes are kept locked, with the key fastened to the box and sealed through the cord. All employees at important points have received instruction in the use and contents of the box.

The boxes must be examined by the Local Surgeon at least once a year, and every three months by the senior official of the station. At these examina-

* "First-Aid to the Injured," published by the St. John Ambulance Association, had, in 1908, reached its eleventh edition, with a total of 480,000 books.

tions, all articles which are not serviceable must be withdrawn and replaced. Record of the examination is made in writing.

At the end of the pamphlet of instructions there are a number of illustrations depicting the application of various forms of bandages and splints, and the methods of practising artificial respiration.*

In America each railroad has been free to inaugurate what it deemed best. The Pennsylvania Railroad has led the way in giving systematic instruction

* It may be interesting to enumerate here the contents of the German emergency chests, as the necessity for so large and varied an equipment is not generally admitted in other countries.

The small emergency chest contains:—

1. Pair of scissors for cutting clothing.

2. Two strips of splinting, 60 cm. long, and 6 cm. wide.

3. Five metres of sublimate mull, each metre packed in a specially strong blue-paper wrapping, with the label: 1 metre sublimate mull.

4. Five metres of sublimate mull, cut in pieces 20 cm. long and 20 cm. wide, each metre being packed in a specially strong yellow paper wrapping with a label: 1 metre mull in small pieces.

5. One hundred grammes of absorbent cotten.

6. Twenty bandages of unstarched mull, 6 cm. wide and 5 metres long, wrapped in paper and provided each with a label.

7. One von Bardeleben bandage for burns.

8. Six triangular bandages, the shorter sides of which are each 90 cm. long.

9. One dozen of strong safety pins in a box.

10. One bottle containing 200 grammes of alcohol.

11. One tube of blue or brown glass, with tightly closing screw-cap, containing ether drops (50 grammes) with the inscription: "Ether Drops, liable to catch fire; for adults, up to 15 drops internally in fainting fits and weak conditions."

12. A drop bottle of opium drops (30 grammes), composed of opium tincture and valerianic drops (15 grammes of each) and bearing the inscription: "Opium Drops; for adults, up to 20 drops for diarrhœa and intestinal colic. Not to be given to small children."

13. Ten pieces of lump sugar in a glass bottle with label.

14. Two rolls of adhesive plaster.

15. A nail-brush wrapped in parchment paper.

16. A metal nail-cleaner.

17. A piece of good soap wrapped in silver paper.

18. A towel about one metre and a half long.

19. A wash basin of papier maché.

20. Ten sublimate tablets (as prepared by Prof. Angerer, of Munich), containing 1 gramme each, and packed in well-corked glass bottles bearing the inscription: "Poison." One tablet is sufficient for one litre of water.

21. Two elastic bandages 5 metres long and 6 cm. wide; one 3 metres long and 6 cm. wide.

22. One copy of the "Short Hints" fastened to the inside of the lid.

23. One list of the contents of the small emergency chest fastened to the inside of the lid.

The large emergency chest has two separate compartments (A and B). The compartment "A" is for the common use of the physician and the officials. Compartment "B" is for the exclusive use of the physician and is provided with an inscribed plate, on which this fact is stated.

Contents of Compartment "A":—

1. Two pairs of large clothing scissors.

2. Six splints of shoemaker's thin board, 75 cm. long and 6 cm. wide.

3. Six splints of shoemaker's thin board, 60 cm. long and 6 cm. wide.

4. Twelve cardboard splints, 60 cm. long and 6 cm. wide.

5. Sixty metres of sublimate mull, each metre wrapped separately in a specially strong blue-paper wrapping, with label: "One metre sublimate mull."

6. Sixty metres sublimate mull, cut into pieces 20 cm. x 20 cm., and packed in small bundles which are wrapped with a specially strong yellow paper. Each bundle contains a sufficient

to its employees. This consists in a simple lecture and a demonstration covering an hour and a half. It is given to all Agents, Sub-Agents, Track-Foremen, and men selected from all branches of the service. The official medical examiner of the Company is the lecturer. The head of a department arranges for the lecture, delegating certain employees to attend, usually to the number of thirty. The roll is called at the lecture, and all absentees must account to their chief for their absence. Arrangements are then made for them to attend

number of small pieces to make one square metre, and it bears the label: "One metre sublimate mull in small pieces."

7. Thirty small packages of pure antiseptic dressing gauze, of 100 grammes each, wrapped in a strong paper wrapping, and with the inscription: "Dressing Gauze."

8. Twelve plates of common glued wadding, wrapped in a strong paper wrapping, with label.

9. Six bandages of strong unstarched mull, three of which are 6 cm. wide and 5 metres long.

10. Thirty bandages of starched mull, 6 cm. wide and 5 metres long.

11. Twelve triangular bandages, the shorter sides of which are each 90 cm. long.

12. Four von Bardeleben bandages for burns.

13. One gross of strong safety pins in a box with label.

14. One bottle containing 500 grammes alcohol.

15. Two tubes of blue or brown glass (with tight-closing screw-cap) containing ether drops, with the label: "Ether Drops, liable to catch fire; for adults, up to 15 drops internally in fainting fits and weak conditions."

16. Ten pieces of lump sugar in a glass bottle with label.

17. Two nail-brushes wrapped separately in parchment paper.

18. Two metal nail-cleaners.

19. Two pieces of good soap wrapped separately in silver paper.

20. Two towels about one metre and a half long.

21. Three wash-basins of papier maché.

22. Twenty sublimate tablets (as prepared by Prof. Angerer, of Munich) of 1 gramme each, in well-corked glass, with the label "Poison." One tablet is sufficient for the contents of the litre-bottle. (See 23.)

23. A bottle of thick glass, having a capacity of 1 litre, and suitable for use as an irrigator It possesses the usual one above, and one at the side near the bottom, the latter so narrow that a common irrigator tube can be drawn over it. Both openings are closed with good corks. This bottle must always be kept filled with sublimate water. (For mode of preparing sublimate solution, see later.)

24. One box with two Berzelius tubes and cork stoppers. One stopper of each of the kinds in the large emergency chest.

25. One rubber tube for the irrigator—1 metre in length, fitting on the lower opening of the irrigator, and provided at one end with a small glass tube drawn out to a point (so-called Berzelius tube).

26. Four elastic bandages, 5 metres long and 6 cm. wide; two rubber bandages 3 metres long and 6 cm. wide.

27. One thick wax taper.

28. Two portable stretchers.

29. A small cooking apparatus with spirit lamp and soda tablets for the sterilizing of the instruments.

30. One copy of the directions ("Regulations for the First-Aid to the Injured").

31. One copy of the "Short Hints" on cardboard.

32. One list of the contents of the large emergency chest on cardboard.

33. One folding stretcher.

Compartment "B" contains:—

1. One canvas dressing case, in which are:—(a) 1 single-blade bistoury; (b) 1 pair scissors; (c) 1 common probe; (d) 1 director; (e) 1 needle holder; (f) 1 pair dissecting for-

a later lecture; and this is repeated till the required number of men are instructed.

This railroad has published a syllabus of the lecture for distribution among its employees. Inasmuch as this syllabus contains all the important essentials of first-aid lay instruction, it will perhaps be well to summarize it here. The syllabus opens with a short introduction, explaining the fact that persons have been instructed in giving first-aid to the injured and sick by all the armies and navies of the world, and by the police departments in municipalities, and that the wisdom of the plan has been more or less recognized by railroads and manufacturers employing large numbers of men. It points out that some employee should at once assume charge of an injured person. In train service this person is the conductor; in yards, shops, and stations the duty devolves upon employees especially designated for the purpose.

Upon the occurrence of an accident, the first available physician is summoned, others being called later if necessary. The character of the injury should, when possible, be mentioned in the summons. If an ambulance is available it should be sent for. If a train going to a point where a hospital is located is available the injured person should be forwarded at once in charge of an instructed person. Efforts should be made to quiet the injured person and to keep all who are present from getting excited.

When a train is wrecked, intelligent efforts should be made to extricate and remove all injured persons promptly. Rough handling is to be avoided. Especial promptness is called for in the presence of escaping steam or fire.

When means of transportation are required, the Company's standard stretcher, or, in its absence, a door or board, should be employed for the purpose. In addition, the car or caboose cushions should be utilized for making the injured person more comfortable. The method of placing a patient on a stretcher is referred to in these instructions, special regard being paid to the proper manner of lifting an injured limb. In carrying the patient on a stretcher the bearers should break step.

ceps; (g) 4 artery forceps; (h) 10 large bent needles; (i) 1 Deschamps needle; (k) 1 razor; (l) 1 metal catheter.

2. One subcutaneous syringe of non-rusting metal, with ground metal handle.

3. Sewing silk in three thicknesses on Ihle threadholders of non-rusting metal.

4. Four tubes of chloroform, of 50 grammes each, in a brown glass, with a tightly closing screw-cap.

5. One Esmarch chloroform mask.

6. Six closed glass tubes with points drawn out, which are each filled with one gramme of a two-per-cent solution of morphia hydrochlorate. In order to prevent the freezing of the contained solutions or the breaking of the tubes themselves, each of the latter is separately packed in wadding, to be kept in a cardboard box. A file for the filing through of the drawn-out points, together with directions, is to be added.

N. B. All bottles contained in the emergency chest must be provided with cork stoppers, which project over the edge of the bottle. The bottles must either be in a wooden casing or wooden box or packed in wadding in a tin box. All vessels must be provided with a plain inscription stating what their contents are, and, besides, the vessels containing poisonous substances must bear a label "To be used with care."

It is important to keep the crowd away. This allows air and prevents questions being asked of the injured person.

In the examination of an injured person, it is important to remove the clothing carefully. One should always resort to cutting rather than to the ordinary method of removing clothing, especially when the injury is a burn or scald.

Due stress is laid, in the instructions, upon the importance of cleanliness. Full details are given regarding the danger of introducing germs and the necessity of not directly touching the wound or of applying water or tobacco to it.

The proper manner of applying the contents of the First-Aid packet is plainly set forth. Instruction is also given as to the right way of applying bandages to different parts of the body, reference being made to the linen available in Pullman cars.

Warning is given that a wound should first be exposed and then the first-aid dressings applied without any attempt being made to cleanse the wound.

Advice is given as to the direct application of dressings and the making of pressure over the wound by bandages, in cases in which there is hemorrhage. The use of the tourniquet is taught and a warning given against the employment of too great force and against the too frequent use of the apparatus. Elevation of the part of the body which is bleeding is advised.

Fractures receive due consideration, and attention is called to the danger of unwise handling of the fractured limb. Full details are furnished with regard to the proper method of applying splints and dressings. Mention is also made of the various materials which may be utilized in improvising a splint.

Symptoms of the commoner fractures are described.

As regards the management of a case of burns, the warning is given that the burned spot must not be touched, that engine oil must not be applied to it, and that no attempt should be made to remove the loose skin which often covers the part. Instead, compresses moistened with warm water should be laid over the burned area, and, so far as may be possible, air should be excluded from the wound.

As regards the treatment of shock, advice is given against the use of drugs or stimulants, and in favor of hot drinks, such as coffee and milk. Attention is called to the necessity for warmth in cases of this nature and also in those of drowning; and a demonstration of the method of applying artificial respiration in the latter class of cases, as well as in those of electric shock and of the inhalation of a noxious gas, is furnished.

The four common types of sickness—viz., pain, unconsciousness, convulsions, and the effects of heat—are discussed in detail and methods are described for recognizing and treating these various conditions.

The instructions given above can scarcely fail, in the course of time, to increase greatly the effectiveness of the measures of relief employed in emergency conditions, and one cannot too strongly recommend the use of this or some similar method of first-aid instruction. Johnson's "First-Aid Manual" is in use on many railroads.

Closely following a consideration of first-aid are the questions of transportation and subsequent care of the injured. Where an ambulance is available, this should be made use of and the patient transferred to his home or to a hospital by this means. If transportation is to be by train, a stretcher, car cushions, or a berth may be used. As a rule, the patient may be carried into a baggage car and there made comfortable on a stretcher. In this way he can be transported for long distances with ease. It is important to the injured man, as well as to other passengers on the train, that he should not be brought in contact with the passengers.

The Hospital Car.—The hospital car (Figs. 399–402) is a car specially assigned for transportation of the injured, and, although it has been in use since the Baltimore & Ohio Railroad provided the first one in 1894, only a very few railroads have adopted it. The chief difficulty lies in the fact that, with the limited number of hospital cars so far provided by any one railroad, too much time is lost in getting the car to the scene of the accident. On one large system only two hospital cars have been provided—one in the eastern portion of the road,

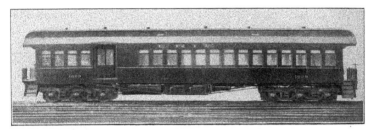

Fig. 399.—Exterior View of one of the Hospital Cars of the Erie Railroad, in Actual Use at the Present Time.

and the other four hundred miles distant, or about the centre of the extreme mileage between the east and the west. These cars are fully equipped with all necessary appliances and are despatched to the scene of the accident by special train, such surgeons as may be considered necessary being collected on the way. It has been claimed that, unless the accident occurs within a short distance of the point at which the car is usually stationed, patients can be given first-aid and transported to a hospital before the car is available.

If the economics of railroad management could provide such a car at all divisional headquarters, its use would become general and a great advance in the transportation of injured persons would result.

The hospital cars thus far provided in Great Britain have been for the transportation of passengers not necessarily injured on the railroad, rather than for the use of injured passengers and employees.

When an injured employee arrives at the end of the journey, should he be taken to his home, to a general hospital, or to a Company's hospital? As has already been pointed out, much difference of opinion exists in regard to the proper course to adopt.   There can be no doubt that, in all severe forms of injury, the hospital, as compared with the home, offers greater advantages; and, as a matter of fact, the hospital is being used with increasing frequency.

American Methods of Providing Relief for the Different Kinds of Railroad Injuries.—In America, as has already been pointed out, there is much variation in equipment.   Until standards, with special education in their use,

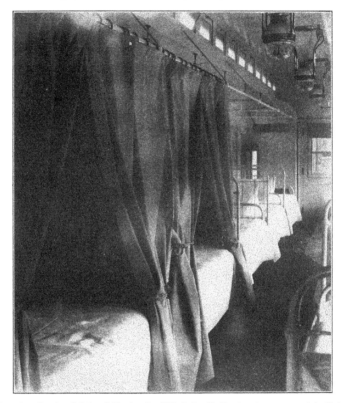

FIG. 400.—Interior of Railroad Hospital Car (Erie Railroad), Showing Arrangement of the Beds.

are systematically provided for, the fullest benefit will not be obtained.   As one might expect, the cost is considered an important factor in a problem of this nature.   Briefly, there are three separate conditions to be met:—

(a) Injuries occurring on passenger and freight trains.

(b) Injuries occurring on the railroad right-of-way, not associated with the operation of trains—for example, injuries to members of track- and bridge-repair gangs.

(c) Injuries occurring in shops, stations and freight sheds, and in the work of switching.

To meet the conditions of the first type, the tendency is to provide first-aid packages or boxes, as a part of the equipment of each train. Some railroads provide an emergency box for each dining car; others have the box placed in the baggage car. As a rule, only the more important through trains have been so provided; little or no provision has been made for trains running on branch lines. It is difficult to understand why this discrimination prevails, as not infrequently serious accidents occur on the branch lines.

In collisions on branch lines, the destruction is often relatively great, because

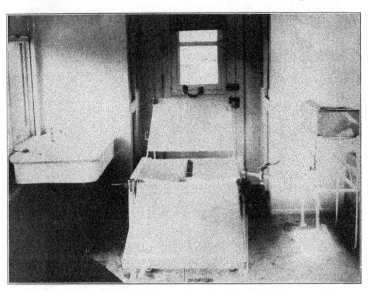

Fig. 401.—Operating Room of a Railroad Hospital Car.

it is on the branch line, and on the less important trains on the main line, that one finds the old rolling stock in use.

During the evolution in car building, the Pullman Company led the way in increasing the strength of the car. This added to the weight, with the result that, in time of collision, the central cars on the trains, between the heavy engine ahead, and the heavy Pullman in the rear, suffered great destruction, owing to the fact that they were structurally weaker. This state of affairs led to the construction of stronger passenger coaches, the last cars to be brought up to the new standard being baggage and express cars. At the present time important through trains are entirely made up of modern strong cars.

The emergency package containing only a simple dressing, with bandages and safety pins, is coming into general use in all departments of the railroad service. The packages are kept in convenient places in stations, workshops, and trains. Nussbaum's dictum "that the fate of the injured depends on the individual who makes the first dressing" has been followed by the further fact that unless a wound can be dressed by a surgeon under favorable conditions, it is safer to apply immediately to the wound a simple dressing.

The first-aid packages at present in use on trains are not intended to meet the needs of a large number of injured passengers, but rather for the isolated individual injury occurring from any cause on a moving train. To provide

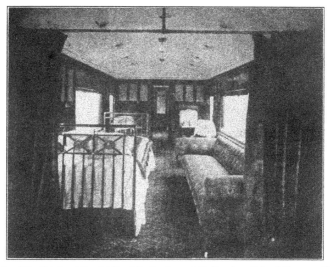

Fig. 402.—Interior of Hospital Car of the London and Northwestern Railroad Company, Great Britain.
Besides a bed, couch, and easy chairs, the compartment contains a lavatory with hot and cold water. The floor is covered with a thick Wilton pile carpet, which is laid on the thickest gray felt. This serves to deaden the sound and lessen the vibration, and makes the compartment very quiet and still while the car is running. The saloons are electrically lighted, the lights having opal-tinted shades; they are ventilated by extractors and are steam-heated, the temperature being controlled by the passengers themselves.

sufficient supplies for a large number of accidents, would involve a very great expense to the railroad.

For the second class of cases, no special provision has been made. On some railroads, however, first-aid packages, as above described, are kept in section houses and in the tool box on the sectionmen's hand-car.

First-Aid Package.—There are many different kinds in use, some made to the special order of the railroad, and many made by surgical supply houses. The standard package of the Pennsylvania Railroad, originally founded on the army package, is made up of the following items:—

A tin box, measuring 6¾ inches x 4½ inches x 2½ inches, and provided with a movable cover, is contained within a canvas case which is tied by tape. The seams of the case are covered by bright red binding, which gives a distinctive appearance to the case, thus rendering it easily recognizable. The cover of the tin box is made dust-proof by a strip of adhesive plaster covered by a stamp of sealing wax. Attached to the box is a tag with the following instructions:— "If the seal of the box is broken the box must be forwarded to the nearest shop to be replaced by one properly sealed, etc." The box contains a small card

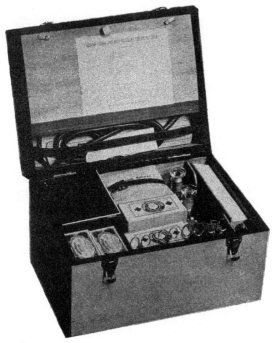

FIG. 403.—A Type of Accident Dressing Case for Use on Wrecking Trains and in Terminals.

giving "Hints on First-Aid to the Injured"; and six other cards on which are instructions as to details desired with regard to the injured person, number of train, name of conductor, etc. Each package contains:—

1. Antiseptic bandage of sublimate cambric, 6 inches x 3 inches.
2. Antiseptic compresses of sublimate gauze in oiled paper.
3. Triangular bandage and 2 safety pins.

These objects are encased in oiled paper, and the inner package is of thin waterproof material, completely sealed at one end. These packages are carried on all trains, and are placed in stations, in the company's shops, and in other convenient places.

Stretchers are also put in suitable places, including (on many railroads) one in each train.

Accident dressing cases of more or less elaborate designs are of value. The smaller type is for use on trains, the larger type is kept at terminals and on wrecking trains. These cases (Figs. 403 and 404) contain all the supplies that are to be found in the first-aid package, and, in addition, much that may be of

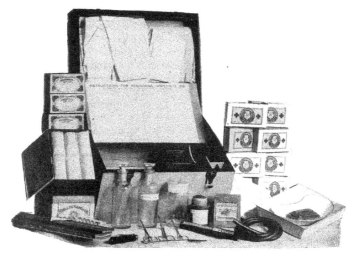

Fig. 404.—Accident Dressing Case Showing Contents Displayed.

use to the surgeon, especially should there be a number of persons injured. The one in use on the Grand Trunk Railroad is strongly made of wood (10¾ inches deep, 12¼ wide, and 16¼ long) and is divided into compartments. The edges of the opening of the lid are covered with baize to keep out dust.*

* In the box are the following contents:—
(1) ½ lb. bottle zinc ointment, with one per cent carbolic acid.
(2) ½ lb. bottle spirits sal volatile.
(3) ½ lb. bottle carbolic oil.
(4) 1 dressing basin.
(5) 1 kidney-shaped pan.
(6) 1 doz. roller bandages (cotton).
(7) 1 doz. plain gauze bandages.
(8) ½ doz. triangular bandages.
(9) ¼ doz. small packages absorbent cotton.
(10) ½ doz. small packages lint.
(11) 50 gauze dressing packages, in special envelopes.
(12) 1 cotton sheet.
(13) 1 towel.

The box is kept on auxiliary trains, at important stations, in the company's workshops, and at terminal points. Part of the contents, such as antiseptic packages, triangular and other bandages, clothing scissors, and simple board splints are intended for use by the employees. The remaining contents are intended for the use of the surgeons, and are only to take the place of, or to necessary to supplement, their own emergency kit.

Accompanying these first-aid boxes, it is customary to furnish a few instructions for the guidance of those who are called upon to give assistance. As these are very similar to those mentioned on pages 1044 and 1045, it will not be repeat them here.

The Care of Men Engaged in Railroad Construction Work.—As in other branches of railroad surgery, no standard method has yet been established for the care of men engaged in the construction of railroads. In the construction of the earlier railroads the lack of any special provision was especially noticeable. In the far West it was left to the railroad contractor to provide such medical services as he considered necessary, and this plan is followed to a large extent at the present time. The usual method is for the contractor to have associated with him a medical man who, for a consideration, undertakes to provide an adequate service. In this method there is a joint responsibility. Another common method is for the railroad contractor to sublet this service to a medical man who undertakes complete responsibility, financial and otherwise; the consideration being the payment of a certain sum which is to be collected monthly from the wages of the employees. In return for this, the medical contractor provides camp hospitals and field medical officers, distributing them over the work in proportion to the number of men employed, due regard being had for the difficulties of locomotion and the time of year. This method has many disadvantages, the most apparent being that, as the revenue depends on the number of men employed, the service must be regulated to meet this revenue,—that is, if a fair remuneration is to be paid for the medical work done. What is considered fair remuneration is left largely to the decision of the medical contractor. Another disadvantage is, that the medical contractor is largely dependent upon the fortunes of the railroad contractor, and, when work is not available for long periods, he must remain without income until another contract is available.

(14) 1 package safety pins.
(15) 1 package plain pins.
(16) 1 cake of soap.
(17) 1 roller rubber adhesive plaster.
(18) 1 rubber tourniquet.
(19) 1 pair clothing scissors.
(20) 1 pair surgical scissors.
(21) 1 jack knife.
(22) 1 razor.
(23) 3 pair artery forceps.
(24) 100 formalin tablets.
(25) splints.
"See instructions for use on the other side."

The tendency at the present time is for the company, when a new railroad is to be built, to become responsible for the medical service, which is supplied through a Medical Department. The advantage of such a service is that, while the employees still continue to pay for the service supplied in the form of monthly deductions, the revenue going directly to the company owning the railroad, the Medical Department has a freer hand and is therefore better able to supply an adequate service. This plan, it is true, may entail a slight financial loss upon the railroad company. Another advantage is to be found in the fact that the Medical Department, being a continuous service, independent of one contractor, can spread the revenue over the whole work and thus be able to retain, from year to year, the same group of field medical officers, who, by virtue of their continuous employment in this class of work, tend to become more efficient.

Recent legislation in Canada has made it compulsory to supply medical service under the supervision of a Government Inspector. No matter what methods obtain, there are many difficulties in providing a surgical service in the field. The work may be compared with that of an army under canvas. The most important difficulty is, that the management of the railroad is not prepared to provide the same proportion of money, in relation to the number of men employed, that an army medical service costs, although the demands on the railroad medical service are greater than the needs of an army in the field in time of peace. A few comparisons may not be without interest:—In the army all soldiers are subject to a rigid medical examination before taking the field, they are all vaccinated, there is careful supervision over the development of venereal disease, they are subject to discipline, and, by this training, are taught promptly to submit to physical examination. They are all of the same nationality, or at least speak the same language. A considerable portion of the army is engaged in fatigue work, including camp hygiene, especially the care of the water supply and latrines. The food supply is controlled by the authorities, and only such food as is considered beneficial to the soldiers is permitted to be served. In the army the sole object is to have the men efficient, healthy, and capable of performing work when called upon, rather than to do so many hours of work. Should infectious diseases break out, the camp is immediately divided without regard to cost or previous arrangements made. In a railroad camp practically the opposite to this obtains in every particular. The railroad and its construction contractor are only interested in the number of men it can employ for a certain number of hours a day. When labor is scarce, inducements are offered in many ways to attract workmen, and the railroad which can offer what the workman considers good food, and freedom from interference with what may be considered the right of the individual workman to live as he considers best, gets the largest number of men. The lack of physical examination permits a number of physically unfit men to enter the service, only too soon to become a charge on the Medical Department or the medical contractor. No adequate provision is made for a proper water supply, and, where this happens to be good, no proper provision is made to keep it free from contamination. The matter of camp hygiene is left largely to the care of the camp cook and the attendant at the horse tent. It is difficult to enforce the use of the latrines. The care of the bedding is largely left to the individual workman. The large number of different nationalities to be found in the ordinary railroad camp makes collective effort almost impossible. The desirability of having the conditions the same as those of an army camp is recognized in the abstract, but it is not feasible to secure these same conditions in the real work of railroad construction.

Public opinion or legislation is likely in time to bring about an important change. Much improvement has taken place in the past few years, and more attention is being given to the subject. An outbreak of infectious disease interferes with regular work and creates an unusual expense which is apparent

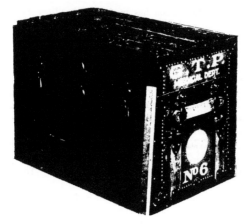

FIG. 405.—Railroad Construction Medical Chest, Containing Medical and Surgical Supplies.
Note: The rule leaning against the side of the chest has a length of 18 inches.

to all concerned, but there are many minor conditions which militate against efficient service, and which do not receive adequate recognition. For example, a thorough physical examination before engagement would exclude from the construction camp many who were physically unfit.

On one large railroad which is being constructed at the present time, the following method obtains:—The line of construction is divided into medical districts of from ten to forty miles in length, varying according to the character of the work and the number of men employed. A camp medical officer has charge of each district, with headquarters at a convenient point in the centre of the district. It is his duty to visit each camp at least once a week, but it is customary to visit the central camps twice a week. If he is adjacent to a general hospital, this is used as a base hospital and all important cases are forwarded there for treatment. Patients may be transported by wagon for a distance of as much as sixty miles without great discomfort. Rivers and lakes are taken advantage of for transportation by water. If, owing to the nature of the country, it is not practicable to use these means of transportation, field hospitals are established. They consist of tents in the summer time, and of rude wooden or log buildings during the winter season. The hospital accommodates from ten to thirty patients. The service of the hospital is supplied by orderlies, and in large camps engaged in rock excavation, where the same hospital may remain for a year or more and is accessible by existing railroads, trained female nurses are employed.

In small field hospitals it is more economical to have the diet supplied by

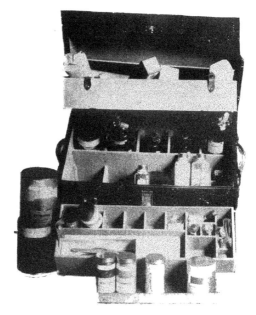

Fig. 406.—Railroad Construction Medical Chest, Contents Displayed.

a neighboring construction camp; in the larger hospitals, a complete kitchen service is maintained within the hospital.

For infectious diseases each medical district is supplied with special tents, and other things that may be necessary for securing complete isolation may be quickly arranged for.

When the laying of steel rails is done by a large gang using rail-laying machines, a medical officer accompanies the work, as the employees in such a work live in boarding cars which are moved forward every four or five days. A hospital car is supplied. This car is fitted up with six cots; it contains a medical chest and is supplied with facilities for boiling water. Minor injuries are cared for at the front. In the event of a serious injury or illness, this car is attached to the first returning supply train and the patient is forwarded in it to the base hospital.

In the large field hospitals of the more permanent character, provision is made for the performance of major operations. If a second medical officer is not attached to the hospital, the medical officers of the neighboring districts are called upon to assist.

As regards the needed surgical outfit, it has been found more satisfactory to have each medical officer supply his own instruments; the surgical dressings and drugs are supplied by the department.

A Division Surgeon supervises a series of medical districts. It is his duty to see that all cases forwarded to base hospitals are properly cared for; to visit the medical districts from time to time; to provide for immediate supply in the event of the withdrawal, for any reason, of a field medical officer; to see that the medical supplies are forwarded, to inspect the same before shipment, and to provide for any contingency which may arise.

The Medical Chest.—The medical chest (Figs. 405 and 406) consists of a strong trunk divided into compartments which are so arranged as to protect against breakage during transport. It contains a full assortment of drugs, supplies, and dressings.* Slight variations in the list of contents are made to

* MEDICAL CHEST AND LIST OF CONTENTS.

Drugs.

1.	¼ gal.	syrup white pine, with eucal. and honey.
2.	½ "	elix. antiseptic digestive co.
3.	½ "	hospital liniment.
4.	½ "	columbian spirits (alcohol).
5.	1 lb.	chloroform (Smith's).
6.	1 "	acid. carbolic. liq.
7.	1 "	tr. iodine (B. P.).
8.	4 ozs.	toothache drops.
9.	5 lbs.	ung. zinc. oxidi with ac. carb. (1 per cent).
10.	5 "	ung. sulphur.
11.	5 "	petrolatum.
12.	1 "	ung. gallæ with opium.
13.	1¾ "	ung. hydrarg. fort.
14.	5,000 tabs.	calomel 1 grain, soda 1 grain.
15.	5,000 "	lead 1 grain, opium ½ grain.
16.	800 "	salol and acid. boracic., āā gr. 5.
17.	800 "	phenacetin 5 gr., caffeine 1 grain.
18.	1,500 "	Dover powders, 5 gr.
19.	1,000 "	bronchial (Red Cross).
20.	1,000 "	throat mentholated.
21.	500 "	mercury bichlor. (Wilson).
22.	1,200 "	soda salicylate, 5 gr.
23.	1,000 "	quinine sulph., 2 gr.
24.	1,500 "	migraine (Red Cross).
25.	1,000 "	comp. digestive aromatic.
26.	200 "	cocaine mur. ¼ gr.. for hypod. use.
27.	200 "	morph. sulph. ¼ gr., for hypod. use.
28.	200 "	strych. sulph. ₃₀ gr., for hypod. use.

meet the individual tastes of the field medical officers. Renewals of contents are ordered by numbers.

Legislation.—The Interstate Commerce Commission has introduced a number of regulations covering safety appliances for the protection of passengers and employees. Some States have adopted measures obliging railroads to provide "First-Aid Packages" on passenger and freight trains.

Canada, through the operation of the "Public Works Health Act" of 1899, provides, among other things, that, in the construction of railroads, provision must be made for the care of the sick and injured. Government Inspectors are appointed whose duty it is to see that the provisions of the Act are lived up to.

Physical Examination of Employees.—It has been claimed that the greatest advantage which a railroad company enjoys through the operation of a relief department, is that obtained from the examination of applicants for employment. Originally started to protect the members of the relief department the measure has gradually been adopted by railroad companies which do not operate such a department.

29.	1	lb.	pil. cath. co., imp. sugar-coated.
30.	1	"	pil. Blaud 5 gr., pink.
31.	2½	"	sodium bicarbonate.
32.	1½	"	acid boric., pulv.
33.	6	"	magnes. sulphate, pulv.

Dressings, etc.

34.	1	jar	5 yds. iodoform gauze (10 per cent).
35.	2	lbs.	absorbent cotton.
36.	1	pk.	lint.
37.	1	"	5 yds. adhesive plaster (12 in.).
38.	1	"	5 yds. carton plain gauze.
39.	1	doz.	3 in. gauze bandage.
40.	½	"	coaptation blind splints.
41.	1		tourniquet (rubber).
42.	2		Lee's tank packages catgut—liq.
43.	1		card surgeon's silk, ass'd.
44.	2	bots.	drainage tubing, ass'd.

Containers, Extra Jars, Bottles, etc.

45.	1	pk.	nested chip boxes.
46.	1		H. R. iodoform duster.
47.	1	doz.	6 oz. bottles with corks.
48.	100		folding boxes, ass'd.
49.	1	bag	ass'd corks.
50.	4		glass-stoppered Winchester bottles.
51.	4		screw-stopped jars (5½ x 3 in.).
52.	11		screw-stopped bottles (7½ x 2¾ in.).
53.	3		5 lb. tins (5¼ x 7¼ in.).
54.	2		2 lb. tins (4¼ x 5½ in.).
55.	2		4 oz. glass-stop. bottles, N. M.
56.	2		6 oz. " " " N. M.
57.	2		2 oz. " " " W. M.
58.	1		6 in. spatula.
59.	1,000		blank labels, gummed.
60.	1		2 oz. graduate.

Only by means of a systematic examination of employees is it possible to exclude persons physically unfit for entering a railroad service. For employees whose duties are in train service, the examination should include that of the special senses. The advantage to the Company comes from having a good type of healthy employee, free from physical defects; the possibilities of accidents being thus lessened. In the event of an employee subsequently making claim for injury, a record of the physical examination will show whether there was any previous evidence of disability (such, for example, as a previously existing hernia). Great as the advantage of such an examination is to the railroad, there is, in addition, the protection afforded to the prospective employee against accident to himself or others through an epileptic attack or through some other constitutional defect, both of which conditions can be determined only by a rigid physical examination. An interesting fact relating to the question which we are here discussing, was ascertained in Great Britain as the result of the operation of the "Workingmen's Compensation Act," which was largely brought into force by the demands of the workingman. Under the operation of this "Act," it was found that claims for injury were so common that the employers were forced to introduce physical examination, with the result that a very large number of faithful employees of long standing were unable to pass and were thus thrown out of employment, creating much hardship. An age limit of not over thirty-five to forty-five years, for applicants for employment, together with a retiring limit at the age of from sixty to seventy years, is in common use on the larger railroad systems.

The examination of employees may be made by local surgeons; the examination of the special senses should be made by specially appointed medical men. Many railroads provide that the latter examination shall be made by officials of the Transportation and Motive Power Departments, the usual tests being employed. Should a candidate fail or pass a doubtful examination, he is referred to a specially designated medical man for final decision. Some companies employ a corps of medical men whose primary duty is to perform the examination. The latter includes not only a rigid physical examination, but also a testing of the vision, color sense, and hearing. Other duties have been added, such as conducting "First-Aid" classes, and the sanitary supervision of rolling stock and station property. These men are given the title of "Medical Examiners" and are not expected to treat the employees except in case of an emergency.

Medico-Legal Questions.—In recent years there has been a marked increase in the number of litigious claims for compensation for injury the result of accident. The machinery of the law courts is precarious and expensive, both for the employer and for the injured employee, and often unjust claims are unduly compensated while deserving cases receive either inadequate compensation or no compensation whatever. Such litigations are responsible for the variety of so-called expert medical evidence which casts such discredit on our profession. The problems involved are numerous and intricate, and only one country, Germany, has attempted to deal comprehensively with their manifold difficulties. In that country, workmen whose annual wages do not exceed 2,000 marks ($500), are, with some few exceptions, insured against the hazards of their various occupations. In case of accident the injured workman receives free surgical attendance and an indemnity graded in accordance with the disability. In case of death his widow receives the burial expenses and an indemnity for herself and children until the latter attain the age of fifteen years.

One of the wisest clauses of this German law, which was passed in 1884, provides that the indemnity allowance may be diminished or increased according to any important change which may take place in the indemnified person's condition. The picture, so often presented in our country, of a bedridden victim of a traumatic neurosis making a rapid recovery and continuing in full enjoyment of the extravagant indemnity granted by an indulgent and sympathetic jury, cannot exist under a system where such a rational and comprehensive act is in force.

The exact amount of indemnity in a given case is based upon a medical certificate from a regularly appointed official, and is graded in accordance with the scale fixed by law. Provision is made for appeal from a particular decision through one or more tribunals, where prompt decisions are returned at a minimum of cost to the parties involved in the claim.

The various workmen's compensation acts already introduced, or under consideration, may do much to mitigate the present difficulties on this continent.

The writer has recently been associated with a case where the parties concerned agreed to submit a claim to a board of three, one to be chosen from the senior surgeons of each of three large general hospitals. Such a board is better able to deal with the consideration of a surgical condition than is any committee or body of men selected in accordance with the method which obtains in our law courts.

Statistics.—The following brief summary, taken from the report of the Interstate Commerce Commission for the year ending June 30th, 1907, gives some idea of the numbers of fatal and other accidents to passengers, employees, and others, which result from operating our railroads:—

Miles of road	242,000
Passengers carried	738,804,667
Passengers carried one mile	23,800,149,436
Employees at the end of the year	1,672,074
Total persons killed	11,839
Total persons injured	111,016
Employees killed	4,534
Passengers killed	610
Persons other than employees and passengers killed	6,695

Of the persons injured 87,644 were employees, 13,041 passengers, and 10,331 other than employees and passengers. This represents an increase, in the number killed, of 11.50 per cent, and an increase, in the number injured, of 13.62 per cent over the casualties experienced in the previous year.

A number of railroads, through the operation of their respective relief organizations, are able to establish the exact percentage of injuries to total membership. The facts are as follows:—

The records of the Insurance and Provident Society of the Grand Trunk Railway for 1908 show:—

Number of accidents to total number of members................ 8.24 per cent
Number of fatal injuries to total number of members............. 0.29 per cent

Railroad Surgical Associations.—Many railroads have organized associations among the members of their surgical staff. Annual meetings are held at some convenient point. The meetings usually occupy two days and afford opportunity for the discussion of subjects of scientific interest bearing on surgery. Some part of the meeting is devoted to subjects pertaining to the relations of the staff, collectively and individually, to the Management of the Company. Such disputed subjects as the responsibilities of the Company for the care of injured trespassers and passengers injured by their own recklessness are considered. Much benefit is obtained from these associations, and in time they may assist in evolving a standard system applicable to all railroads and possessing sufficient elasticity to accommodate itself to the ever-changing necessities of surgery.

Bibliography.—Adams, Notes on Railroad Accidents, 1879.—Butler, Emergency Notes, 1889.—Fletcher, Railways in their Medical Aspects, 1867.—Golebiewski, Diseases Caused by Accident, 1900.—Herrick, Railway Surgery, 1896.—Interstate Commerce Commission, Annual Reports.—Mitchell, Reference Handbook of the Medical Sciences, Vol. VI., 1903.—Outten, Medical Jurisprudence, by Witthaus and Becker, Vol. II., 1907.—Page, Railway Injuries in their Medico-Legal and Clinical Aspects, 1891.—R. C. Richards, Railroad Accidents, 1906.—Lawson Roberts, Lecture on Ambulance Work, 1895.—Willoughby, Workingmen's Insurance, 1898.

APPENDIX.

THE RELATION OF BLOOD-PRESSURE TO SURGERY.

By J. E. SWEET, M.D., Philadelphia, Pa.

GENERAL CONSIDERATIONS.—The division of medicine into special branches is only an outgrowth of the demands of the practice of the profession. Even in practice an extreme subdivision does not necessarily make for the highest ideal; the best specialist is he who is the best physician. Now when we approach the consideration of any of the fundamental principles of medicine, we must bear in mind that the consideration of a principle cannot be undertaken from any special, limited, point of view, but must be looked upon, first, in all its breadth, as a principle; the specialist may then, perhaps, see certain phases of the subject which to him may be of greater interest than are others. But he must never forget that the phenomena of the branch depend upon the root, else he will fall into the fatal errors of the unbalanced judgment.

The relation of the blood-pressure to surgery is therefore, primarily, precisely the same relation as that which blood-pressure bears to physiology; secondarily, it is the same relation as that which exists toward pathology; the surgical relation is broader than either, because it must embrace both. Not only is the problem, therefore, a broad one, but its complexity must always be borne in mind; hardly a single factor can be considered alone, for each change of every factor reacts throughout the whole combination of factors.

Three elements are united in the expression "blood-pressure": (1) The pressure due to the specific gravity of the fluid itself,—hydrostatic pressure; (2) the pressure caused by force exerted upon this fluid by the vessel walls and other external factors, the fluid being contained in a closed system of elastic tubes,—hydraulic pressure; (3) The pressure due to movements of the fluid itself,—hydrodynamic pressure. Of these three elements, the third—hydrodynamic pressure—hardly enters into a consideration of what is ordinarily included under the term blood-pressure. It is of importance in the study of certain manifestations of the transmission of pressure, such as the study of the pulse wave. A discussion of the hydrodynamic pressure would therefore be more or less out of place within the limits of the present discussion.

HYDROSTATIC PRESSURE OF THE BLOOD.—A consideration of the hydrostatic pressure of the blood leads us at once to a realization of the complexity of the factors which govern the pressure of the fluid within the blood-vascular system. It is evident that the pressure of every layer of blood must be increased by the weight of that amount of blood which lies in vertical direction upon it, i.e., only the purely physical conditions should be considered, and all the other factors should be left entirely out of account. Thus the pressure of the blood in the arteries of the adult foot must be increased by the weight of a column of 165 cm. of blood (equal to 13 cm. of mercury), entirely apart from all other factors. The hydrostatic factor also enters into the distribution of the blood in the head and upper extremities, in fact, in all parts of the body, depending upon their position.

The blood, because of its weight, will naturally obey the laws of physics and seek the lowest level; nevertheless, changes of posture in the normal animal have but slight effect, because of the perfection of the compensating mechanism. The amount of blood flowing to a given part of the body can be varied by changes in the calibre of the arteries of that part, or by changes in the calibre of the arteries of other parts; furthermore, the total pressure of the blood can be changed by alterations in the frequency of the heart beat, or by changes in the strength of the individual systole. It is therefore impossible to consider the hydrostatic pressure in the normal animal apart from the hydraulic pressure; for the factor of hydrostatic pressure is a purely physical factor, and the phenomena of the vasomotor nerves change the purely physical conditions in a never-ending play.

As soon as we turn to a consideration of the abnormal, we find that the hydrostatic pressure alone may produce considerable and even fatal changes in the distribution of the blood throughout the body. These pathological conditions are such as influence the capacity of the blood-vessels, by affecting either the elasticity or the tone of the vessel walls, or even by removing the supporting action of the muscles of the body upon the vessels lying beneath them, as in the relaxation of deep anæsthesia. One of the most instructive examples of the effect of hydrostatic pressure acting alone is the experiment of Hill and Barnard (1*). If a tame rabbit be held in the vertical, head-up position, the blood will flow into the lower areas, especially the splanchnic area, and in a comparatively short time so much of the blood of the body may accumulate in the latter area as to cause the death of the animal. The rabbit has bled to death into the vessels of its own splanchnic area; yet we can hardly say that it died of "shock," for if the experiment be tried with a wild rabbit, whose abdominal muscles are strongly developed, or if the belly wall of the tame rabbit be supported by a bandage, the animal does not die. In this experiment it is therefore not a question of vasomotor innervation, nor of the peripheral blood-vessels, but simply a question of the hydrostatic pressure of the blood; a factor which is always present, but in this case is made into an active, positive factor by the failure of the muscles of the belly wall to give a normal support to the vessels of the splanchnic area.

An entirely comparable condition may exist in patients whose general muscular system is relaxed by long illness in bed, or by fainting, or by deep anæsthesia; or when the pressure exerted upon the blood-vessels of the splanchnic area by a distended urinary bladder, or a large cyst, is suddenly relieved.

* These numbers refer to the corresponding numbers in the list of bibliographical references at the end of the article.

The clinical usefulness, in such conditions of muscle relaxation, of a suitable posture, or of mechanical aids such as the pneumatic suit, or compression of the limbs by a roller bandage, becomes self-evident.   In analogy with the experiment cited above, it would be advantageous, especially in cases in which surgical shock is known frequently to occur, to support the abdominal wall by a strong bandage before beginning the anæsthesia; particularly when one operates in a position in which the head and shoulders of the patient are raised above the level of the abdomen.

HYDRAULIC PRESSURE OF THE BLOOD.—The hydraulic pressure of the blood is the resultant of a primary force, produced by the contraction of the heart, acting against a resistance produced by the friction of a viscid fluid, chiefly in the small vessels of the periphery.   What we commonly call "blood-pressure" is therefore the tension of the vessel wall, produced by the systole of the ventricle, and transmitted by an incompressible fluid.   This tension of the vessel wall will depend upon the elasticity of the wall and the force which stretches it.   The elasticity depends upon:

(1) the inherent elasticity, due to the presence of elastic membranes and fibres, and

(2) the "tone" of the involuntary muscle cells, which cells persist in the smaller arteries after the elastica has disappeared, and form the most important structural element in the vessel wall.   This tone depends not alone upon nerve impulses, but upon

(3) the presence, in the circulating blood, of the products of the internal secretion of certain glands.

The force acting to stretch the vessel wall will depend upon

(4) the amount of blood in the vessel, which is in turn dependent upon the relation of the inflow to the outflow.   The inflow will depend upon

(5) the volume of blood forced out of the heart at each systole, and

(6) the rate of the heart beat.   The outflow will depend upon the resistance, especially

(7) the resistance in the arterioles, and

(8) the consistency of the blood.   Under abnormal conditions we must also, as was just pointed out, consider the influence of

(9) the hydrostatic pressure.   In the background there is always the controlling activity of

(10) the vasomotor centres.

The blood-pressure may be considered fairly constant in the normal animal; but it is a constant resulting from the combination of ten variables, if such a combination can ever be said to result in a constant.   Further, the activity of one factor in one part of the body may be balanced by the activity of the same factor working in an opposite direction in another part of the body.   It is my purpose to take up the components of blood-pressure in the order in which they have just been mentioned, with the exception of the seventh,—the resistance in the arterioles,—a discussion of which is basic to the consideration of several of the others.

The Resistance in the Arterioles.—The whole question of blood-pressure may practically be referred to the arterial system, the pressure in the capillaries and veins being thus left out of account. The resistance encountered by the blood after it has passed the capillaries is negligible, because the current is constantly passing from small to larger vessels. If we start from the heart and follow the blood to the capillaries in a search for the point of greatest resistance to the blood stream, we find that the resistance does not materially increase until we have reached the arterioles. While physiologists for a long time seemed to find the greatest resistance in the capillaries, they are now generally agreed that the greatest resistance is in the last branchings of the arteries, or arterioles; there are very many more capillaries than arterioles, and the combined sectional area is much larger; therefore the rate of flow in the capillaries must be slower, and the resistance much less. In fact, the rate of flow in the capillaries is so slow that the resistance at this point becomes of slight practical importance (2). The endothelial cells which compose the walls of the capillaries have been shown to possess contractility, yet the capillaries are not otherwise supplied with a mechanism of sufficient power to influence the pressure or movement of the blood.

The mechanical construction, particularly of the smaller arteries, is described as follows (3): "Followed toward the capillaries, the coats of the artery gradually diminish in thickness, the endothelium resting directly upon the internal elastic membrane so long as the latter persists, and afterward upon the rapidly attenuating media. The elastica becomes progressively reduced until it entirely disappears from the middle coat, which then becomes a purely muscular tunic, and, before the capillary is reached, is reduced to a single layer of muscle cells. In the precapillary arterioles the muscle no longer forms a continuous layer, but is represented by groups of fibre cells that partially wrap around the vessel, and at last are replaced by isolated elements. After the disappearance of the muscle cells, the blood-vessel has become a true capillary." This, then, is the mechanism which supplies the resistance to the force generated by the heart, resulting in the tension of the vessel wall called "blood-pressure,"—a mechanism which must be borne in mind throughout the discussion of all the most important elements of the composite picture.

Inherent Elasticity.—The inherent elasticity of the arteries, while differing in different individuals, is a factor which is constant in a given individual during the space of time in which it would be of interest to the surgeon. It is further hardly separable, in the normal individual, from the elasticity due to the "tone" of the muscle cells. The function of an elastic vessel wall consists in affording the vascular system a mechanism by which the intermittent force imparted to the blood by the heart can be made practically continuous, and gradually transmitted throughout the entire system. To the elastic coats of the artery is due its great resistance to rupturing strain; under normal conditions the artery is able to withstand a pressure at least fifteen, and even as high as fifty, times in excess of the normal blood pressure. In pathological conditions, such as arteriosclerosis, the loss of elasticity can be of importance in two ways:

elasticity being lost, any slight increase of pressure due to changes in local conditions in some area of the body causes a disproportionate increase of general pressure, which increase may cause the rupture of the inelastic and often friable vessel wall. To the presence of the elastic membranes and fibres is due the safety of one of the most common surgical procedures—the ligation of vessels; the ligature neither cuts through the elastic membrane, nor does it slip off.

Tone of the Muscle Cells of the Arteries.—It is in a way a misfortune that the physiologists have found no other term to express what is known as "tone." The word savors too strongly of the condition so well known to the general praetitioner, when the system lacks "tone,"—*i.e.*, when something is evidently wrong, but the exact nature of the pathological condition is more or less obscure. But far from representing such an unfortunate condition of affairs in physiology, tone means a certain, definite condition, even though it must be added that the condition is not yet fully understood in all its details. By tone is meant a condition of semi-contraction in which the smooth muscle-cells are normally found; it is even thought by some that these cells maintain themselves in this condition of semi-contraction without the constant expenditure of energy, as would be the case with the voluntary muscle-cells. This condition of tone evidently serves two purposes: first, to aid in supplying elasticity to the vessel wall; and, second, by a simple relaxation of this state of semi-contraction the lumen of the vessel can be enlarged, there being no separate muscular arrangement for actively increasing the calibre of the vessel.

There appear to be four factors concerned in the maintenance of this condition of semi-contraction called tone. It seems, first, to be an inherent property of all smooth muscle tissue, a property termed myotatic irritability,—the responsivity to the mechanical stimulus of stretching. In the specific case of the smooth muscle tissue of the blood-vessel walls, this inherent tone has been demonstrated as follows:—If the vasomotor centres in the brain and the subsidiary centres are excluded by cutting all the nerves leading to a section of an artery, the artery will at first dilate; but, after a few days, it will be found again in a contracted state,—its tone has reappeared. This dilatation which immediately follows section of the nerves can also, in some cases at least, be still further increased. Thus, if the blood-vessels of the submaxillary gland be caused to dilate by section of all the vasoconstrictor nerves leading to the gland, a still greater dilatation of these vessels can be produced by stimulation of the chorda tympani. A further example of the independent tone of the arteries can be seen in any operation where the vessel is exposed to the air, as in the direct transfusion of blood, where the artery may contract until the lumen becomes hardly patent. John Hunter (4) records such an observation of the contraction of the posterior tibial artery on being exposed to the air for some time. It might seem that this contraction were due to a stimulation of the exposed nerves in the sheath of the artery by the drying influence of the air. The more logical deduction, nevertheless, is to interpret the contraction as due to the independent tone of the muscle cells, for MacWilliam (5), who has studied the question very completely, finds that the artery contracts after removal from the body and also several hours, or even days, after death. This contraction also occurs on cutting into the artery, which might also be considered a nerve reaction, were it not for the fact that this phenomenon of the arterial wall is greatly lessened by covering the vessel with olive oil, which would hardly prevent the irritation of the nerve produced by the cut. This action of oil in preventing the local contraction of an exposed vessel supplies a more logical reason for the use of an oil during a surgical operation upon the vessels themselves than the reason usually advanced,—*i.e.*, to prevent the coagulation of the blood.

A second factor in the maintenance of tone is the tension produced by the pressure of the blood itself. If a suitable preparation of involuntary muscle tissue, preferably from some of the lower animals, be stretched, it will be found on removing the tension that the preparation not only returns to its original length, but becomes even shorter, to return again after a time to its original length. Or, if the volume of a limb be passively increased by causing an increase of blood-pressure by stimulation of a sensory nerve, it will be found, as soon as the pressure returns to its former level, after cessation of the sensory stimulation which caused the increase of pressure, that the limb not only returns to its former volume, but becomes of less volume, and then gradually returns to its original state. The importance to surgery of the relation of blood-pressure to tone becomes evident in a condition of lowered pressure due to extensive hemorrhage. In addition to the fall of pressure due to the loss of blood, this very fall causes a still more pronounced fall of pressure because of the loss of the tonic reaction to the normal tension. What is therefore needed in such a condition is simply the addition of salt solution to the fluid in the blood-vessels, not only to increase the volume of fluid and facilitate the action and nourishment of the heart itself, but also to restore the tone which results from the stretching of the vessel wall.

The third factor in the maintenance of tone is the activity of the vasomotor nerve centres. Since the time of Claude Bernard it has been known that the cutting of a vasomotor nerve is followed by a dilatation of the vessels supplied by the cut nerve. It is therefore concluded that vasoconstrictor impulses are constantly being sent out from the centres to the musculature of the arteries, keeping them in the tonic semi-contracted state,—the nervous mechanism acting, of course, with the other factors concerned in the maintenance of tone. These impulses are thought by some to be reflexes from the sensory impulses which are constantly being sent to the centres from every portion of the body. Stimulation of all sensory nerves, with the exception of the depressor nerve, normally causes vasoconstriction. In deep anæsthesia this vasoconstrictor reflex is not always present, which has been ascribed to a lowering of the sensitiveness of the centres to the sensory stimuli. It is not here the place, in this discussion, to take up the vasomotor nerves, and I shall therefore merely mention their rôle in the preservation of tone, and return later to the vasomotor phenomena.

The Secretion of Certain Glands.—A fourth factor in this peculiar phenomenon of tone is the action, upon the muscle cell, of the products of certain of the ductless glands, or, as they are more broadly termed, the glands of internal secretion. The glands in question are grouped together as the "chromaffine" system, so named from the affinity possessed by certain cells of these organs for the salts of chromic acid. The chief representative of this group is the suprarenal gland, in the medulla of which are found these chromophile cells. Similar cells are also found in other glands, such as the hypophysis cerebri, and in the ganglia of the sympathetic nervous system. In fact, the entire chromaffine system is intimately connected embryologically with the sympathetic nervous system. The relation of the suprarenals to the tone of the skeletal muscles has been known since the time of Addison, one of the chief symptoms of the disease which bears his name being a pronounced asthenia. A low blood-pressure is a second characteristic symptom, a condition referable to the loss of tone, or the asthenia, of the musculature of the arteries.

The results obtained from studies of Addison's disease, in which the adrenals are destroyed by the pathological process, together with the experimental results found after the ablation of both adrenals, have led to extremely important findings in connection with the question of blood-pressure. The first of these is that the product of the adrenals is necessary to the maintenance of blood-vessel tone. It is not yet definitely settled how the adrenal secretion acts, whether upon the muscle substance itself, or upon the end-plates of the nerves within the cell wall,—a question, however, which makes little difference in the point of practical importance, which is that adrenalin does preserve the tone of the musculature of the arteries. A continuous tracing of the blood-pressure taken from an animal from which the adrenals have been removed shows the picture of typical shock,—a gradual, progressive fall of blood-pressure.

A study of the condition known as "status lymphaticus," in which condition accidents of narcosis are peculiarly liable to occur, led to the finding that the adrenals are marked in this disease by an extreme hypoplasia. The low blood-pressure in Addison's disease, and the progressive fall of pressure after the experimental removal of the adrenals, coupled with the occurrence of accidents of narcosis in the status lymphaticus and the finding of adrenal insufficiency in this condition, led to experimental studies of the second relation of the adrenals to blood-pressure,—the study of the effect of narcosis upon the adrenals (6). Without taking up the work here in detail, it will be sufficient to condense the results (7).

After a narcosis of sufficient duration with chloroform, ether, or Billroth's mixture, the adrenals are found to have lost either a great part or all of the chromaffine reaction of the cells of the medulla. These cells are supposed to contain the specific blood-pressure-raising substance of the glands, and the extent of the chromaffine reaction is taken as a measure of the functional condition of the gland. The various reactions for testing the presence of adrenalin in the blood serum give negative results at this stage of narcosis. At varying periods after the narcosis has ended and the animal has been allowed to recover, the chromophile reaction reappears. These experimental findings have been confirmed by some workers in studies of the adrenals in cases of death due to narcosis; others have failed to find a loss of chromaffine substance, in part because they have included in their studies cases of death under narcosis due to causes entirely apart from any lowering of the blood-pressure, such as fatty degeneration of the heart and eclampsia.

Our own work in the Laboratories of the University of Pennsylvania (8) has led me to the conviction that the idea that the chromaffine system is intimately connected with the preservation of blood-pressure is correct. A comparison of the record of the blood-pressure of an animal from which the adrenals have been removed, with the record of pressure of an animal which is solely under constant ether anæsthesia, shows that the two records are, with the exception of the time element, essentially alike; the only striking feature being the constant, progressive fall of blood-pressure in both records. If the secretory activity of the pancreas be also watched, it is found that the pancreas begins to secrete sooner or later after the removal of both adrenals, and continues to secrete actively, and even very actively, until death. . Such a flow of pancreatic juice never occurs in the normal animal, but there may occur, in the last minutes of life, a distinct secretory activity. The only explanation of this phenomenon, it would seem, is that the continued narcosis in the normal animal finally exhausts the adrenals, which organs normally exert some kind of control over the activity of the pancreas. Prolonged narcosis has therefore accomplished at last the same result as is found after operative removal of the adrenals.

The importance of this discovery to practical surgery is to be found in the demonstration of the fact that typical surgical shock, which finds its expression in a gradual but progressive fall of blood-pressure, can occur as a purely peripheral phenomenon, without any involvement of the vasomotor centres. This would seem the most conservative way of expressing the results, in view of certain conflicting statements. The conclusions of Hornowski (9), from his work along this line, are of great surgical interest, although, perhaps, his views may seem too enthusiastic. His most interesting conclusions are:

"Chloroform increases the need for tonic substance and at the same time causes an exhaustion of the chromaffine system, which may cause death." "Chloroform does not cause an immediate exhaustion of the tonic substance, but gradually, after several hours." "Chloroform may cause a sudden exhaustion of the chromaffine substance, if this be not present in abundance." "The resistance of the organism to surgical shock is expressed in the possibility of satisfying a greater need for tonic substance and in the ability of the organism to secrete it."

In view of the fact that a narcosis of from twelve to fifteen hours is required to produce a fatal effect upon the blood-pressure of a normal dog, it would seem that the question had little practical bearing. This would be true, indeed, if the chromaffine system were always normal; many observers have found that the chromaffine system is seriously impaired in various pathological conditions, notably in the toxic diseases. Bacteriologists have long been familiar with the almost specific effect of diphtheria toxin upon the adrenals. If, now, to such a condition of exhaustion, narcosis be added, an ordinarily harmless period of narcosis might prove serious, as, in fact, seems to be the case in the condition of status lymphaticus.

These findings in regard to the adrenals are of further fundamental importance, for if it be eventually confirmed that narcosis may cause a progressive exhaustion of the chromaffine system, which exhaustion may lead to a condition of shock, quite apart from the primary intervention of the vasomotor system, then the therapeutic use of adrenalin which has become so general since Crile's work (10), and which is considered a specific by many surgeons, will have received an actual basis of specificity, in addition to the pressure-raising action, because of which it was introduced and has been heretofore used.

It may not be out of place here to discuss the surgical use of adrenalin. One of the most striking results of the introduction of adrenalin into the blood stream is the apparently very fleeting nature of the rise in blood-pressure,—the extreme rise being attained in a very short time and continuing for less than a minute, depending on the dose used, after which a rapid fall to the normal level takes place. This might seem to indicate that adrenalin is quickly used up, or neutralized, but that, in any event, its action is too brief to be of any value. As a matter of fact, however, this apparent brief action is really due to a compensation by some factor or factors concerned in maintaining the normal level of pressure, for adrenalin also affects the skeletal muscles, and can be demonstrated in them long after the blood-pressure symptoms have disappeared. Further, in a dog in which, because of the removal of a large part of its chromaffine system, the pressure had fallen to nearly zero, an injection of adrenalin produced an effect visible on the continuous tracing for a little over thirty minutes. The destruction of the injected adrenalin is not due to oxidative processes in the blood, but occurs either in the muscles or in the liver. Others believe that the alkalinity of the blood is the element which neutralizes the adrenalin. The effect takes place more slowly and continues over a longer period if the adrenalin be injected subcutaneously (at least in rabbits; said not to be the case in the dog) or intramuscularly.

Aside from the use of adrenalin in local surgery, as in nose and throat work, or in ophthalmology, it is indicated in cardio-vascular conditions where there is evident dilatation of the blood-vessels, and where the heart muscle is in good condition. Such conditions are chloral poisoning, asphyxia, and shock. Good results have been reported in accidents due to overdoses of ether, while it is held to be of little value where the heart is paralyzed by chloroform. It has further been reported to be of value in preventing the recurrence of serous exudates in all cases in which the simple withdrawal of the fluid is without effect. Wiggers (11), in his studies of inaccessible hemorrhage, reaches the following general conclusions in regard to the use of adrenalin in intestinal hemorrhage:—

"(1) Large doses of adrenalin (0.05 to 0.1 mg.) cause a short preliminary increase of hemorrhage, followed quickly by a decrease or cessation of bleeding. On account of the great preliminary loss of blood they are always contraindicated.

"(2) Small doses of adrenalin (0.01 to 0.025 mg.) cause little or no preliminary increase, but shorten the course of hemorrhage. As they save the red blood cells in every way they are therapeutically desirable.

"(3) The method of introducing adrenalin determines the effect on blood-pressure and hemorrhage. No results are obtained by subcutaneous administration. By continuous intravenous injection of weak solutions a slight elevation of pressure can be maintained and hemorrhage simultaneously checked. This can also be accomplished by intramuscular injections.

"(4) Adrenalin is not indicated in all intestinal hemorrhages. The condition of the blood-pressure is the criterion for its use. In hemorrhages of short duration, when the pressure has not fallen to any extent, a judicious use of nitrites proves of more benefit than adrenalin. When the bleeding has been profuse, however, and a low pressure exists, it becomes vital that hemorrhage should be checked without further reduction of pressure. Adrenalin finds its use in this field.

"(5) The use of adrenalin should always be closely followed by blood-pressure observations. A dose sure to be below the safety limit should first be tried and the pressure carefully estimated. If no rise occurs, gradually increasing doses may be injected until a slight elevation of pressure is present, in which case we may be certain that enough has been introduced to affect hemorrhage, and at least no significant preliminary increase has resulted."

In a subsequent paper, Wiggers concludes that adrenalin is not efficacious in the treatment of hemorrhages from the lungs. The most interesting of the above-quoted conclusions, aside from the practical use of adrenalin in intestinal hemorrhage, is the suggestion as to the manner of introducing the adrenalin. It seems that the preferable method is to introduce small quantities continuously, by means of dilution in saline solution (in his experimental work Wiggers introduced at the rate of 0.007 to 0.01 mg. per minute), instead of the common method of injecting the entire dose with a syringe into the rubber tube close to the needle or cannula in the vein. This method of gradual and constant introduction in dilution is to be preferred for restoring a low blood-pressure, as well as in hemorrhage.

These conclusions recall the opinion expressed by Schaefer, that adrenalin, when given by the mouth, may control internal hemorrhages from the stomach, intestine, bladder, and uterus, even post-partum hemorrhage. Schaefer believes that the extract of the adrenals exhibits a greater effect upon the wounded than upon the normal vessels. When given by the mouth adrenalin is said not noticeably to increase the general blood-pressure.

The question of what to use for raising the blood-pressure by simply increasing the amount of fluid within the vessels, whether saline solution or some less simple mixture of salts, is one which can be definitely answered in so far as certain experimental phases of the matter are concerned. Ringer (12) found that the contractions of the heart quickly disappear when the heart is placed in pure physiological salt solution, but that the contractions reappear and increase in strength if a $CaCl_2$ solution be added. In such a mixture of Na and Ca salts the heart beats very powerfully, but inclines to tonic contraetions; to avoid this a suitable amount of a potassium salt must be added. In view of such results, Locke (13) states that the best solution for vertebrate hearts—a solution based upon analysis of serum—is composed of 0.9 to 1.0 per cent NaCl, 0.02 to 0.024 per cent CaCl$_2$, 0.02 to 0.042 per cent KCl, 0.01 to 0.03 per cent NaHCO$_3$ (not Na$_2$CO$_3$). Locke further calls attention to the fact that the distilled water used in making up this solution should be distilled from glass vessels, to avoid the disturbing effect of the salts of the heavy metals which might be present in water prepared in stills having metal parts. While such a solution might in some cases be of value, where so much fluid is used intravenously as materially to dilute the blood, I am not aware that any sufficiently extensive clinical comparison with the effects of salt solution has been made to warrant the drawing of any practical conclusions. It would certainly seem that Locke's solution should be at hand, and should be tried in those cases of extensive hemorrhage which do not react to salt solution, perhaps especially where the fluid rapidly leaks through the vessel walls, and the action of the heart is unsatisfactory.

The Amount of Fluid within the Blood-Vessels.—That the total amount of fluid within the vascular system must have a decisive influence upon the blood-pressure seems perfectly natural in view of the mechanical structure of the blood-vascular apparatus; if more fluid be forced into a closed elastic tube, the tension of the walls will naturally be greater. But the conditions in the living animal do not change as they should in simple accord with the mechanics of the elastic tube. Thus it has been shown that the loss of up to forty per cent of the total amount of blood does not produce any lasting effect upon the blood-pressure. This amount would be equal to nearly two litres in the human being, if the total amount of blood is reckoned as 7.7 per cent or one-thirteenth of the body weight; others (14), using a different method for the determination, reckon the amount of blood as 4.9 per cent, or a little more than one-twentieth of the body weight. The transfusion of one and one-half times the total amount of blood produces also no lasting effect upon the blood-pressure. The mechanism by which this regulation is carried out has been sought in different places; in the liver, which is said to take up a great part of the increased quantity of blood; by transudation into the thoracic and abdominal cavities, and into the subcutaneous connective tissue; by an increased action of the intestine and especially the kidneys; and by a dilatation of the blood-vessels. After hemorrhage essentially the reverse phenomena occur—gradual giving up by the liver of its reserve blood, passage of fluid from thorax and abdomen into the blood-vessels (hence the value of rectal injections of warm saline solution, or of other enemata), fall of the secretion of urine to the minimum, and contraction of the peripheral vessels.

The amount of fluid lost by hemorrhage is replaced in a short time (15) by the absorption, by the blood stream, of water from the tissues and the food. The formed elements and the other constituents of the blood are replaced by an increased activity of the sources of these elements, which restore the normal condition in the course of some weeks or months, depending upon various factors, such as the amount of blood lost, the patient's general condition, the circumstances of his life, etc. The proteins are resupplied most rapidly, often in a few days. The formation of red cells takes place rapidly, and more rapidly than the hæmoglobin; they are often smaller than normal, with some enlarged, and some containing nuclei. The leucocytes also increase markedly.

The results of the lowered pressure following loss of blood are such as constantly to make matters worse. If the hemorrhage has been so severe that the compensatory mechanism is unable to balance the loss, the lowered pressure becomes progressively lower, first, by removing the tone of the arteries which is caused by the pressure itself, then, since the heart can work best under a certain tension, which is that supplied by an approximately normal pressure, the effectiveness of the heart becomes disturbed, its own nourishment becomes poor (since the heart receives its nourishment essentially during the diastolic period, after the closure of the aortic valves, and low pressure would drive less blood into the coronary arteries), then the vasomotor centres become anæmic and unable to fulfil their normal function.

The Volume of Blood Forced out of the Heart at each Systole.—The systolic output of the heart is a factor of possibly little practical interest to surgery, except in so far as it is influenced by the amount of blood which flows into the heart in diastoles; no more can be pumped out during systoles than has run in during diastoles. It is further known that a muscle can reach its highest efficiency when under a certain tension. It is this mechanical upset due to the loss of blood that brings about death from acute hemorrhages; there is not enough blood present to fill the heart in the diastoles, which of course lessens the systolic output, and also unfavorably influences the tension of the heart musculature. Death occurs at a time when there is still enough blood left in the body to carry on all the vital functions of the blood, but when the volume of fluid is so small that the heart, as it has been expressed, cannot maintain its grip upon the column of fluid. It was the recognition of this fact by von Bergmann, together with the work of Landois upon hæmolysis, which, some thirty years ago, placed the practical value of the intravenous injection of salt solution above that of the direct transfusion of blood; a position in which it doubtless still stands, in spite of the recent revival of the ancient operation, except in those cases in which, because of an actual or functional anæmia, the red blood cells are insufficient numerically or in hæmoglobin to carry on the normal oxygenating functions of the blood, or in cases where, to stop further loss, the addition of active fibrin ferment may be indicated.

The Rate of the Heart Beat.—The rate of the heart beat, in its relation to blood-pressure, is of more theoretical than practical interest. If the heart were filled in each diastole, a rapid rate would of course result in an increased output,—provided the increased rate did not mean a weakened heart; but the weakened action as manifested in the rapid rate means not only that less blood flows into the ventricles, but also that the blood is driven out of the heart with less force. There would seem to be one condition encountered in practice in which the heart action alone is of interest. It can often be seen in the course of surgical operations that a spurt from a large artery will reduce the blood-pressure more than will the loss by oozing of a much greater amount of blood. In the case of the oozing, the loss occurs so slowly that the compensatory mechanisms have time to balance the loss. But the sudden loss must react in two ways upon the heart: the resistance being suddenly lowered lessens the effectiveness of the ventricles, because of the lowering of the normal tension of the ventricular wall; while at the same time it interferes with the supply of venous blood to the heart. Pressure falls, then, not only because of the loss of fluid, but because of the direct effect upon the compensating mechanisms; the output of the heart diminishes, because the inflow is decreased; with the fall of pressure occurs a loss of cardiac tension, accompanied by a loss of vagus tone, and the rate of the heart increases. The result is that the heart runs away with itself, like an engine suddenly relieved of its load.

The Consistency of the Blood.—The consistency of the blood is another factor which is not liable to any sudden change unless purposely altered by the surgeon. That the viscosity of the blood is of interest to the surgeon, is pointed out in a recent article by Mueller (16), on the viscosity of human blood, with especial consideration of its relation to surgical diseases. The interest centres here, however, in the question of diagnosis, and not in the relation to blood-pressure. At the same time, it would seem that the viscosity of the blood may be a subject of direct surgical interest, as, for example, in certain types of acute infection, where the peculiar viscous condition of the blood may oppose an insuperable obstacle to the circulation. It has been pointed out that salt solution may be even better than defibrinated blood for raising blood-pressure, for the reason that the salt solution, by decreasing the normal viscosity of the blood, decreases the resistance, and thus aids in another manner than by simply increasing the quantity of fluid within the vessels.

General Physiological Factors.—Various physiological factors of a general nature may exercise an effect upon blood-pressure. The position of the body is usually thought to have an influence, although this has often been denied. It is commonly accepted that the blood-pressure is highest in the horizontal position, lower in the sitting position, and lowest in the standing position. Broeking (17) concludes that the pressure is highest in the sitting posture, with the limbs extended horizontally, due to the pressure upon the abdomen. These considerations have little practical surgical value, except as they substantiate the value of the horizontal position to prevent fall of pressure during operation, with, if necessary, the compression of the abdomen.

Another general physiological factor is external temperature. Two factors enter into the effect of cold and heat upon the vessels—a direct action upon the vessels themselves, and an indirect action upon the vasomotor centres. The effect of temperature changes upon the vessel itself, separated from its nerves, and even removed from the body, was studied by MacWilliam (5). A section of a large artery, with one end closed, and the other end connected with a manometer, showed, at temperatures from about 25° C. to about 35° C., a decrease of the volume of fluid contained within it,—*i.e.*, a contraction, while, at temperatures of from about 35° C. to about 45° C., there occurred an increase of volume,—*i.e.*, a dilatation. Further lines of experimentation have confirmed the idea that the effect of heat is a direct one upon the vessel wall. The surgical application of this principle is seen in the use of heat to produce a local hyperæmia,—the hot poultice being one of the oldest therapeutic measures in surgery,—and in the use of cold packs to produce a local anæmia.

It would further seem, at first sight, that the dilatation of the vessels produced by heat would be a contraindication to the use of heat in cases of shock, because the local dilatation would but seem to aggravate the general vaso-dilatation. The fact that heat is positively indicated, however, seems to be clinically established; its experimental justification is perhaps found in the work of Kahn (18) who explains the beneficial effect of heat by the warming of the vasomotor centres. He observed that warming the carotid blood alone, thereby warming only the head, caused a considerable dilatation of the superficial vessels of the body; the blood-pressure did not sink, but rose somewhat, which must have been caused by contraction in some other region than the superficial parts. This contraction was found in the splanchnic area, since on cutting both splanchnics the blood-pressure fell on raising the temperature of the blood of the head. Kahn concludes that the result is due to direct stimulation of the vasomotor centres, and not to a temperature reflex from the skin of the head. While the results of Kahn's work may perhaps be taken as the reason for the use of heat in the treatment of shock, the reflex effects of variations in the temperature of the skin upon blood-pressure should be borne in mind. In both animals and man, local cooling is followed by a contraction, local warming by a dilatation, of the blood-vessels in remote parts of the body. If a rabbit be seated with its posterior extremities in warm water, the blood vessels of the ear dilate; if in cold water, the vessels contract. This reaction does not appear if the spinal cord is cut. The application of cold douches, or of ice, to the skin has been shown to affect not only the skin but the internal organs, to such an extent that the general blood-pressure is raised (19). In endeavoring to combat the "cold, clammy extremities," it may therefore be well to remember that we are dealing only with a symptom, which will disappear when the cause of the symptom is removed; no measure should be instituted to remove a symptom which can possibly have a deleterious effect upon the primary cause.

The Vasomotor Nerves and Centres.—In the foregoing pages I have purposely said practically nothing in regard to the vasomotor nerves and centres. The reason for this is not because I believe that the function of the nervous mechanism should be, or can be, disregarded, but because I am convinced that the most serious consequences of a fall of pressure may occur without the intervention of the nervous mechanism; in cases of failure of the adrenal function, I believe that a typical surgical shock, which is characterized by a constant, progressive fall of blood-pressure, may occur, not because of exhaustion of the nervous apparatus, but because of the failure of the peripheral apparatus to respond to the nervous impulses which may be normally endeavoring to counterbalance the fall of pressure; a legless man may desire to run, could run in so far as the brain and nerves are concerned, only he has nothing to run with.   Practically all the methods in vogue for restoring a fall of blood-pressure are further directed toward the mechanical equipment of the vascular system, except when stimulants are resorted to, in which case a stimulation of the heart—and wrongly, as we shall see later—is perhaps as often aimed at as is a stimulation of the nervous centres.   There can, no doubt, be no question of the action of anæmia upon the nerve centres, nor that a long-continued low pressure may result in irreparable injury to the centres; but in this regard it must be remembered that the vessels of large areas can be separated from the centres by total destruction of the spinal cord, without a fatal result, provided measures such as saline injections, etc., be instituted to keep the pressure up.   The least possible conclusion is that the vasomotor mechanism may, possibly most often does, primarily bring about a fall of blood-pressure; but that this is by no means necessarily the case. The practical surgeon must bear this in mind; for the lines of treatment to be followed in the case of a fall of pressure due to exhaustion of the vasomotor nerves or centres, in a fall of pressure due to the spurting of large vessels, in a fall of pressure due to loss of adrenal function, or in a fall of pressure combined with a pathological condition of the blood, are not necessarily the same.   In all, the immediate increase of pressure is desired, and can be accomplished by an intravenous injection of saline solution.   But, beyond this, vasomotor exhaustion due to fatigue of the centres caused by excessive irritation of the sensory nerves, would require vasomotor stimulation; a fall of pressure due to sudden loss of large amounts of blood, needs only a saline solution intravenously, possibly only a rectal injection of warm saline solution or of some other enema; the centres are not injured, they can and will balance the loss if given a sufficient volume of fluid to work on; a fall of pressure due to adrenal insufficiency needs long-continued, constant injection intravenously of small quantities of adrenalin in salt solution; a fall of pressure combined with a pathological blood condition, —a very low red-cell and hæmoglobin content before further loss by hemorrhage,—needs transfusion of blood.   On the other hand, in a fall of pressure due to a failing heart, the heart should not have a still greater burden thrust upon it.

It might be contended that such suggestions are actually carried out in practice; but a study of the literature, and the finding, for example, of cases of death due to narcosis which were studied from the standpoint of adrenal insufficiency, among which are included cases with an autopsy finding of fatty degeneration of the heart, and even of death during an operation in eclamptic coma, inclines one to the conviction that the term "shock" is to surgery what the term "rheumatism" is to medicine,—a convenient dressing-gown to cover a dreadful nakedness.   Whether the accurate diagnosis of the causes of a fall in pressure would make any great difference in the choice of the therapy or not, will certainly have to wait for an answer until such accurate diagnoses are made.

It is a very general law of physiology that the vital processes are accomplished by the proper balancing of two opposed forces, just as the movements of the eyes are effected by the action of antagonistic muscle groups. This same law also holds in regard to the vasomotor nerves; vasoconstriction and vasodilatation result in a proper balance. Inhibition of the vasoconstrictors and stimulation of the vasodilators give the same general result,—dilatation; and inhibition of the vasodilators and stimulation of the vasoconstrictors result in constriction. It is therefore not surprising that those who see a positive stimulus back of every vital function, should find their views criticised by those to whom inhibition spells the secret of life. The only practical result which can be translated out of the confusion of tongues which has arisen in consequence, is simply to state what is actually known, and to leave the explanation until the physiologists have found it.

The heart, with its automatic force-pump action, emptying into a system of elastic tubes, would be sufficient to maintain a uniform circulation of blood. But there would be no means of regulating the supply to different parts, such as the organs of digestion, to supply the varying demands during active digestion and in the intervals between the ingestion of food. The function of regulating the supply to the different parts of the body in accordance with functional demand is the normal physiological rôle of the vasomotor nerves. The energy generated in the centres and transmitted by the nerves, is transformed into work through the medium of the muscular coat of the arteries, and especially the musculature of the arterioles, as we have seen above. The term vasomotor nerve is the name commonly used in reference to the vasoconstrictors alone. The vasoconstrictors are nerves whose stimulation normally causes a contraction of the circular muscles, and therefore a constriction of the vessels. Their discovery, as well as the discovery of the vasodilators,—nerves the stimulation of which results in the dilatation of the arteries,—is due to Claude Bernard (20). Stimulation of the vasoconstrictors causes a contraction of the arterioles, the resistance to the blood stream is increased, the general pressure rises (if the constriction occurs in a sufficiently large area), less blood flows through the organs, and that which comes from the veins is more highly charged with the products of metabolism, is darker. Stimulation of the vasodilators has an opposite effect. Vasomotor nerves have also been demonstrated in the veins; the dilatation of the veins, especially of those in the enormous vascular area supplied by the splanchnic nerves, may therefore play an active part in the fall of blood-pressure.

The vasodilators can be stimulated by weaker electric currents than are required for the vasoconstrictors. If a nerve trunk containing both nerves be cut, it has been found that the dilators degenerate more slowly than the constrictors, and therefore retain their irritability longer. The centres of the vasoconstrictors are both cerebral and spinal; the existence of centres in the cord is doubted by some, who place the secondary centres below the medulla in the sympathetic ganglia. These secondary centres refer directly to certain parts or organs, and are subordinate to the centre in the medulla, which has control of all the regions of the body. After complete cross-section of the cerebral peduncle immediately behind the corpora quadrata, the blood-pressure is found to remain normal, except for a slight transitory change, and the normal reflexes can be obtained on irritation of sensory nerves. Section of the cervical cord is followed by a marked fall of pressure, and stimulation of the cervical cord causes a great rise of pressure. According to Ditmer (21), the more exact location of the vasoconstrictor centre in the rabbit is in the *formatio reticularis*, median of the exit of the facialis. The same author traced the vasomotors from this centre, by partial sections of the cord, into the lateral columns of the same side, although some fibres cross to the opposite side. The fall of pressure observed after section of the cervical cord is followed in a few days by a return to approximately the normal pressure, which is followed by a fall if the nerves leading to some important vasomotor area are cut, showing that there are present subsidiary centres which possess a tone of their own. The dilatation following section of the nerves again disappears, due to the peripheral tone of the vessels, as was pointed out above. The existence of centres subordinate to the chief centre in the medulla, was first proven by Goltz in the frog, in which animal destruction of the brain and medulla does not cause a fatal fall of pressure; but such fatal fall of pressure does follow the further destruction of the cord.

The subsidiary centres are stimulated by sensory impulses, especially after strychnine poisoning, and by asphyxia. They evidently begin in the thoracic region, opposite the first thoracic vertebra, and are thought by some to extend only to the region of the last thoracic vertebra. Whether vasodilator centres exist at all has not been definitely demonstrated.

The vasoconstrictors leave the cord in the anterior roots, going thence by way of the white *rami communicantes* of the spinal nerves into the sympathetic ganglia, ending there at ganglion cells, and, in part also, ending in the prevertebral ganglia. Because of the intimate connection of the vasomotors with the sympathetic ganglia these have been termed "vasomotor ganglia." The post-ganglionic fibres thence pass, in part, by way of the gray *rami communicantes* into the spinal nerves, and reach their peripheral distribution as part of the spinal nerves; in certain parts of the body, vasoconstrictor fibres are united to form separate nerves. The vasodilators leave the central system partly in the cerebral nerves, partly in the spinal nerves. Their ganglion cells are in the ganglia *spheno-palatinum, oticum,* and *submaxillare,* and in the sympathetic ganglia. From these ganglia they pass to the periphery in general with the vasoconstrictors. (But see Bayliss [22] who finds the vasodilators of certain regions in the posterior spinal roots, with their ganglion cells in the spinal ganglia. There also the detailed course of the vasomotor nerves is given.)

In actual surgical practice, the point to be remembered from this discussion of the vasomotor centres is that they are stimulated by irritation of the sensory nerves; normally this sensory irritation causes constrictor stimulation, but excessive sensory stimulation soon causes fatigue of the centres, with consequent fall of pressure. In deep anæsthesia this normal constrictor reflex is also not always present, due to a diminished sensitiveness of the sensory nerves to the stimuli. The means at hand for preventing a fall of pressure are two: first, carefully to avoid unnecessary sensory stimulation, and, second, to "block" the sensory nerves by intraneural injection of cocaine, or some allied drug, before cutting or otherwise stimulating them.

In addition to the stimulation of the vasomotor centres through the sensory nerves, two conditions very common in surgical practice exert a profound influence upon these centres. Asphyxia causes at first an enormous stimulation of the bulbar centre, and therefore a very marked increase of blood-pressure. Following the rise, the pressure falls, at first rapidly, later more slowly, the later slowing of the rate of fall being due to the stimulation of the subsidiary centres, which are more slowly affected by the asphyxia. Similar to the effect of asphyxia is that of anæmia of the brain, caused, for example, by the increase of intracranial pressure due to intracranial hemorrhage or the presence of a tumor (23). In the anæmia of the spinal cord which causes a loss of motor reflexes, the reflexes influencing blood-pressure remain for a time intact.

If, in the stage of asphyxia or anæmia, when the blood-pressure has fallen considerably, arterial blood be sent to the centres, there follows a marked post-dyspnœic or post-anæmic stimulation of the centres, which results in a considerable increase of blood-pressure (27). The constriction of the blood-vessels in asphyxia does not affect the vessels of the entire body, but the vessels of the entire intestine, the spleen, kidneys, and uterus contract, while the vessels of other internal organs (the adrenals [25], for example), and especially the vessels of the skin, muscles, and brain, dilate. The difference of reaction of the vessels of the skin, etc., seems to be due to the fact that the increase of pressure following the constriction of the splanchnic area causes a passive dilatation of the peripheral vessels, although they are also receiving constrictor impulses (26).

Action of Various Drugs upon the Vasomotor Centres.—In regard to the action of the various drugs which influence the vasomotor centres, we must turn to the pharmacologist. The literature and a general résumé of the pharmacological ideas can be found in the article by Gottlieb (27) upon which the following is based. Before instituting any therapeutic measures, it must be known exactly what conditions are present. The blood may be collected in the vessels of the splanchnic area because of paralysis of the splanchnics or of the vasomotor centre or it may be collected in the veins of the same region owing to a stagnation of the venous flow, because of insufficiency of the valves of the heart. The normal function of the vasomotors, as has been already pointed out, is to regulate the distribution of blood in such a way that the total cross-sectional area of the vascular system remains the same,—dilatation in one area is counterbalanced by contraction in other areas. When the vasomotors are paralyzed, the heart drives the blood into the regions where the vessels are most expansile, the tone of the smaller arteries is lost, the blood is not forced into the veins in sufficient quantity, too little blood is returned to the right heart and therefore to the left heart, the pressure in the aorta falls. The peripheral vessels are almost bloodless, the skin becomes pale and cold. The vessels of the brain likewise receive an insufficient amount of blood; the first symptoms of cerebral anæmia are seen in the effects upon the higher centres,—faintness, and then loss of consciousness. The pulse becomes rapid and small; it becomes rapid, because the lowering of the aortic pressure has lowered the tone of the vagus, or perhaps, too, because it is making a compensatory effort to increase the output by increasing its rate; the pulse is small, nevertheless, because the diastolic period is shortened, and the heart has less time in which to fill, and because, at best, the venous pressure is insufficient properly to fill the heart.

Heart stimulants are therefore not indicated,—the heart does not lack ability to work, but material to work with. The picture is purely one of collapse due to vasomotor paralysis. The same picture, I believe, can result from loss of function of the peripheral mechanism, as I have already sufficiently emphasized. It was also pointed out that the measures indicated are not the same as those needed in the conditions of intact peripheral mechanism, but in those of primary vasomotor failure, which we are now discussing. The only means of re-establishing the normal conditions in vasomotor paralysis is to cause a contraction of the dilated blood-vessels, primarily in the splanchnic area.

In addition to the mechanical aids already mentioned, such as posture and compression of the limbs and abdomen, the typical vasomotor drug is strychnia. In England and France it is, in fact, much used. Since, however, the blood-pressure-raising dose of strychnia lies close to the point at which convulsions result, Gottlieb considers it better to use caffeine, which acts as a vasomotor stimulant without causing convulsions; camphor is another vasoconstrictor drug which is practically applicable.

Just as the effect of a fall of pressure is to start a progression of unfavorable symptoms, so the successful stimulation with a vasoconstrictor drug lays the foundation for a progressive series of favorable reactions. The vessels in the splanchnic area contracting, there results a filling of the peripheral blood-vessels, either passively because of the increase of pressure, or because the splanchnic area, by virtue of some internal arrangement of the vasomotor centre itself, is normally in balance with the areas of the skin and brain (loi de balancement of Dastre and Morat [28]). The brain becomes demonstrably better supplied with blood (29), and this causes the post-anæmic reaction of the vasomotor centre, which raises the blood-pressure. The anæmia of the brain and heart being removed, the organism can again assume control of the circulation. Local irritation of the sensory nerves by cold applications to the skin is also said to act upon the splanchnics, increasing the blood-pressure and improving the circulation of the brain (30). In regard to the use of ether and alcohol, they are certainly not vasoconstrictor stimulants. Both act undoubtedly as dilators of the blood-vessels generally, and are therefore absolutely contra-indicated.

BIBLIOGRAPHICAL REFERENCES.—(1) Journ. of Phys., 1897, 21, 321.— (2) See Nicolai, in Nagel's Handbuch d. Phys., 1909, Bd. 1, Pt. 2, 760.—(3) Piersol, Human Anatomy, Philadelphia, 1907, 675.—(4) Works, London, 1837, 3, 157.—(5) Proc. Roy. Soc., 1902, 70, 109.—(6) Schur und Wiesel, Wien. klin. Wchschr., 1908, 21, 247. (7) Sweet, Annals of Surgery, Oct. 10, 1910. (8) Sweet and Pemberton, Arch. of Int. Med., vol. vi., 536, 1910; Stone, Univ. of Penn. Med. Bulletin, June, 1909.—(10) Blood-pressure in Surgery, 1903.—

(11) Arch. of Int. Med., 1909, 3, 139.—(12) Jour. of Phys., 6, 361.—(13) Central-blatt für Phys., 1900, 14, 672.—(14) Haldane and Smith, Journ. of Phys., 1899–1900, 25, 331.—(15) Krehl, Pathologische Physiologie, 1910, 138.—(16) Mitth. a. d. Grenzgeb. d. Med. u. Chir., 1910, 21, 377.—(17) Zeitschr. f. exp. Path., etc., 1907, 4, 220.—(18) Engelmann's Archiv, 1904, Suppl., 81.—(19) Wertheimer, Arch. de physiol., 1894, 308 and 732.—(20) Compt. r. de la Soc. de Biol., 1851, 163; Journ. de la Physiol., 1858, 1, 237.—(21) Ber. d. sächs. Ges. d. Wiss., 1873, 25, 448.—(22) Ergebnisse der Phys., 1906, 5, 319.—(23) Cushing, Mitth. a. d. Grenzgeb. d. Med. u. Chir., 1902, 9, 791.—(24) Mayer, Wien. Sitzungsber., 1880, 81, 130.—(25) Pflüger's Archiv, 1897, 67, 450.—(26) Bay-liss and Bradford, Journ. of Phys., 1894, 16, 20.—(27) Verh. d. 19ten Kong. f. inn. Med., Berlin, 1901, 21.—(28) Système nerveux vasomoteur, 1884.—(29) Gottlieb und Magnus, Arch. f. exp. Path., etc., 1902, 48, 270.—(30) Wertheimer, Arch. de Phys., 1893.

GENERAL INDEX

TO VOLUMES I.–VIII.

ABBE's method of treating stricture of œsophagus, vii. 435

Abbe and Hutchinson's modification of the intracranial operation on the trigeminal nerve, v. 400

Abdomen, anatomical landmarks, vii. 108
aponeuroses, vii. 109
inspection of, for diagnosis, i. 514
muscles, vii. 109
nerve supply, vii. 112
surface of, vii. 109
surgical landmarks, vii. 108
tumors of, diagnosis of, vii. 96
vascular supply, vii. 112

Abdominal aorta, diagnostic significance of pulsation in, i. 531

Abdominal cavity, drainage of, vii. 114
irrigation of, vii. 119
surgery of, i. 62

Abdominal distention, post-operative, treatment, iv. 155

Abdominal hernia, vii. 555

Abdominal operations, under local anæsthesia, iv. 251–256

Abdominal section, vii. 105
adhesions after, vii. 132
anatomical considerations, vii. 107
closure of incision, vii. 128
disinfection of abdomen, vii. 137
drainage, vii. 114
dressing the wound, vii. 140
hernia after, vii. 133
historical, vii. 105
incisions, vii. 123
irrigation in, vii. 119
linea alba, vii. 110
linea semilunaris, vii. 111
lineæ transversæ, vii. 111
muscles, vii. 109
nerve supply, vii. 112
operative technique, vii. 137
peritoneum, vii. 111
position of patient during operation, vii. 120
post-operative care, vii. 141
post-operative sequelæ, vii. 132

Abdominal wall, abscess of, vii. 78
actinomycosis of, vii. 89
adenoma of sebaceous glands of, vii. 86
anatomy of, vii. 75
angioma of, vii. 86
burns of, vii. 93
carcinoma of, vii. 87
contusions of, vii. 91
desmoid tumors of, vii. 83
embryology of, vii. 75

Abdominal wall, fibroma molluscum of, vii. 87
hydatid cysts of, vii. 89
incised wounds of, vii. 94
landmarks, vii. 107
lipoma of, vii. 87
lymphatics of, vii. 75
nerve supply of, vii. 77
phlegmon of, vii. 77
punctured wounds of, vii. 95
sarcoma of skin of, vii. 87
scalds of, vii. 93
surgical diseases of, vii. 75, 77
ulceration of, vii. 80
wounds of, vii. 75, 91

Abducens nerve, surgery of the, v. 380

Aberrant testis, vi. 660

Abscess, i. 128; ii. 143
absorption of, ii. 153
acute, i. 254; ii. 147, 456
auricular, v. 672
axillary, vii. 66
bone, in Pott's disease, iv. 935
burrowing, i. 141
by-results of, ii. 153
cerebellar, v. 256, 789
cerebral, v. 251, 789
diagnosed from cerebral tumor, v. 317
chronic, i. 141, 255; iii. 580, 644
circumtonsillar, v. 818
classification, ii. 143
clinical features of, ii. 147
cold, i. 141, 255; ii. 159; iii. 572
sterility of contents, ii. 78
surgical treatment, ii. 88, 161
congestive, i. 141
constitutional disturbance in, ii. 152
deep-lying, ii. 457
Dubois's, of thymus, vi. 398
dumb-bell, of brain, v. 252
eliminating, ii. 148
embolic, i. 128, 129
external discharge of dead material from, i. 233
extradural, v. 789, 793
gravitation, ii. 152, 160
healing of, i. 103
hemorrhagic, ii. 149
Hilton's method of opening, ii. 159 vi. 341
in Pott's disease, iv. 935, 947
intradural, v. 789, 794
intraglandular, vi. 512
intraperitoneal (and see Subphrenic abscess), vii. 494
ischio-rectal, vii. 811
mammary, vi. 511
mediastinal, iv. 981

Abscess, metastatic, i. 129; ii. 152
miliary, i. 129
palmar, ii. 157
deep, vii. 60
pelvirectal, vii. 811
perianal, vii. 810, 812
perirectal, vii. 810, 812
perisinous, v. 793
periumbilical, vii. 78
periurethral, vi. 752, 808
postmammary, vi. 512
psoas, in Pott's disease, iv. 950
retro-œsophageal, in Pott's disease, iv. 949
retroperitoneal (and see Subphrenic abscess), ii. 159; vii. 493
retropharyngeal, ii. 535, 536; v. 819; vi. 343
in Pott's disease, iv. 949
retrorectal, vii. 811
submammary, vi. 512
subphrenic (and see Subphrenic abscess), vii. 450, 478
treatment of, ii. 153, 156; iii. 677, 720
tropical, of liver, viii. 209
tuberculous, or "cold," iii. 572
general constitutional treatment of, ii. 163
of liver, viii. 224
treatment of, iv. 978
tubo-ovarian, viii. 409
union by second intention in, ii. 148

Abscission, Critchett's operation for, v. 618

Absorbable sutures, i. 728

Absorption, ulcerative or interstitial, the term defined, ii. 202

Acanthoma adenoides cysticum, ii. 349

Acanthosis nigricans, or dystrophia papillaris et pigmentosa, ii. 388

Accessory pancreatic bodies, viii. 161
sinuses, diseases of, x-ray in diagnosis of, vi. 209
exostoses of, iii. 410
tumors of, vi. 186, 200
thyroids, vi. 353, 366, 396

Accident (railroad) dressing cases, viii. 1050, 1051, 1054, 1055, 1056

Accidents, in naval service, viii. 972

A. C. E. mixture as an anæsthetic, iv. 202
or anesthol, or chloroform-ether sequence for anæsthesia, iv. 210

Acetabulum, in congenital dislocation of the hip, iv. 751

Acetonæmia, fatal, iv. 162

Acetone in the urine of diabetics an unfavorable prognostic sign, i. 794

Achillo-bursitis, iv. 889

Acid intoxication, post-operative and post-anæsthetic, iv. 162

Acidosis in diabetic patients, i. 794

Acinous carcinoma of breast, female, vi. 534

Acne, ii. 308
artificialis, ii. 308
cachecticorum, ii. 310
diabeticorum, ii. 308
indurata, ii. 310
keloid, ii. 310
punctata, ii. 310
rosacea, ii. 310, 315
of face, v. 478
tar, ii. 310
varioliformis, ii. 310
vulgaris, ii. 308

Acquired syphilis, bone lesions of, iii. 369–378

Acquired torticollis, iv. 781

Acromegaly, iii. 340–343, 397
and gigantism, resemblances and differences between them, iii. 342
possible relations between it and the genital glands, thyroid, thymus, pituitary, etc., iii. 343
relation of, to hypophyseal tumors, v. 26
x-ray features of, i. 685

Actinomycosis, ii. 55, 330; iii. 34
bovis, ii. 56
leads to ulceration, i. 227
maduræ, ii. 61
of abdominal wall, vii. 89
of brain, v. 302
of breast, female, vi. 519
of cæcum, vii. 725
of chest wall, vi. 410
of cranium, v. 47
of face, v. 458
of gall-bladder, viii. 233
of jaws, vi. 883
of liver, viii. 225
of lung, viii. 25
of neck, vi. 346
of peritoneum, vii. 752
of pharynx, v. 823
of rectum, vii. 800
of salivary glands, vi. 303
of spine, vi. 448
of thyroid, vi. 372
of tongue, vi. 242
of vermiform appendix, vii. 636

Actual cautery as a sterilizing agent, i. 710

Acupressure, control of hemorrhage by, vii. 243

Acupuncture, iv. 604

Adamantine epithelioma, iii. 474
of jaw, vi. 841

Adamantinoma, iii. 474

Adami, J. G., classification of tumors, i. 297

Adenectomy, v. 830

Adenitis, axillary, vii. 66

Adenoids, v. 825; vi. 860

Adeno-carcinoma, i. 346, 356

Adeno-carcinoma, of Bartholin's gland, vi. 570
of breast, female, vi. 536
of cervix of uterus, viii. 594
of rectum, vii. 899
of uterus, viii. 663
primary, in mice, i. 390

Adeno-cystoma, of breast, female, vi. 523

Adeno-fibroma, i. 304, 346
of breast, female, vi. 523

Adeno-papilloma of palate, hard vi. 863

Adeno-sarcoma, cystadeno-sarcoma, i. 348
of jaw, iii. 474
of kidney, viii. 137

Adenoma, i. 345
alveolar, i. 345
intranasal, vi. 195
its relations to glandular hyperplasia, i. 349
its transition to malignancy, i. 350
malignum or carcinomatosum, i. 350
papilliferous, i. 345
tubular, i. 345

Adenomyoma of uterus and accessory organs (and see Uterus, adenomyoma of), viii. 575

Adhesions, nasal, vi. 81
peritoneal, vii. 726

Adhesive plaster, i. 736
abdominal scultetus, iv. 594
after abdominal operations and for abdominal support, i. 737
in closure of wounds, i. 738

Adiaemorrhysis, definition of, v. 107

Adiposis dolorosa, i. 189

Administrative surgical work, viii. 823

Adrenalin in treatment of shock, i. 494, 495

Advancement, for strabismus, v. 640

After-cataract, v. 637

Age as a predisposing factor in tuberculous arthritis, iii. 567–569
as influencing diagnosis, i. 507
influence of, upon prognosis in surgical diseases, i. 772

Aged, operations upon the, i. 776

Agent, surgeon responsible for act of his, viii. 717

Agglutination thrombi, i. 85

Agglutinin and its action, i. 417

Agnew, D. Hayes, i. 19

Aikins' hoop-iron splint, iii. 306

Ainhum, ii. 389

Air as a source of infection, i. 698
collections in the scalp, v. 11
embolism, vi. 325
in veins of neck, vi. 325

Akoin as a local anæsthetic, iv. 233

Alæ of nose, restoration of, iv. 693

Albuminuria, i. 568
surgical importance of, when due to presence of blood in the urine, i. 569

Alcohol as an accessory hand disinfectant, i. 707

Aleppo boil, ii. 342

Alexander-Adams operation for shortening the round ligaments, viii. 471

Alexander's operation, Mayo's internal, vi. 615

Alexin, action of, i. 418

Alimentary tract, disorders of, in their relation to surgical prognosis, i. 790

Allen, Freeman, on anæsthetics and the production of general anæsthesia, iv. 169

Alligator forceps, vii. 771

Allis' inhaler, iv. 187
method for the reduction of backward dislocations of the hip, iv. 79
method of treatment of forward (thyroid) dislocations of the hip, iv. 82

Alveolar border, adamantine epithelioma of, vi. 843
diffuse hypertrophy of, in leukæmia, vi. 817
necrosis of, vi. 881
tumors of, primary, vi. 816
operations for, vi. 866

Alveolar periostitis, vi. 879

Amann's method in radical operations for carcinoma of uterus, viii. 638

Amazia, vi. 507

Ambulances, viii. 842

Ambulance cars, viii. 841

Ambulance companies in military service, viii. 954

Ambulatory dressings, iii. 207

American practice of surgery, characteristics of, i. 39

Ammonium excretion, total, determination of, in diabetic patients, i. 795

Ammunition, investigations as to its poisonous qualities, made by Major La Garde, iii. 36

Amœbic appendicitis, vii. 636

Amputating knives and scalpels, iv. 274
saws, varieties used, iv. 274

Amputations and disarticulations, iv. 263
mortality statistics of, iv. 360–363

Amputation above the shoulder joint, the interscapulo-thoracic method, iv. 308–311
the interscapulo-thoracic method as elaborated by Paul Berger, its successive steps, iv. 308
the interscapulo-thoracic method, Le Conte's modification in dealing with the clavicle, iv. 311
after-treatment, iv. 278
agents for the coaptation of flaps and for drainage, iv. 274
agents for controlling hemorrhage in, iv. 273

Amputation, choice of methods, iv. 272
circular method, two varieties of, iv. 270
classified as immediate, primary and secondary, iv. 276
drainage after, iv. 274
dressing of the stump, iv. 275
elliptical method, iv. 271
flap methods, divisions of, iv. 271
in shock, iv. 276
instruments and other agents needed for, iv. 273–276
manner of using the knife, iv. 275
modified circular method, iv. 271
mortality statistics of, iv. 360–363
neuroma, i. 289; iv. 268
oval or racquet method, iv. 271
question of, in simultaneous fractures of the tibia and fibula, iii. 201
racquet method, iv. 271
site of, iv. 276
special, iv. 278–360
the stump, iv. 268–270
carcinoma of, vii, 67
use of the saw in, iv. 276
Amussat's operation of atresia of rectum, vii. 775, 778
Amygdalectomy, v. 834, 836
after-treatment, v. 840
Amygdalitis, v. 813, 815
Amyloid, i. 194, 195
appearance of organs affected by, i. 196
diseases in which it is frequently found, i. 195
experimentally produced, i. 195
transformation, a result of prolonged suppuration, i. 255
tumors of tongue, vi. 254
views of von Recklinghausen and Czerny in regard to sources of, i. 195
Anæmia, i. 234, 238
choice of anæsthetics in, iv. 220
chronic splenic, viii. 71
circumscribed, i. 239
collateral, i. 239
from hemorrhage, i. 245
pernicious, blood-counts in, i. 241
primary, i. 240, 241
secondary, i. 240, 244
splenic, viii. 71
Anæmic necrosis or infarction, i. 239
Anæsthesia, i. 63
administration of stimulants preliminary to, iv. 175
after-effects of, management of patient after withdrawal of anæsthetic, iv. 198
by chloroform, dangers attending its use, iv. 198
by Cushing's "morphia-cocaine-chloroform" combination, iv. 238
by endoneural injection, as introduced by Crile, Cushing, and Matas, iv. 237

Anæsthesia, by ether, the close method, iv. 191
by mixtures of nitrous oxide and air or oxygen, its advantages and disadvantages, iv. 182
by nitrous oxide, iv. 178
by nitrous oxide and air with a Bennett's inhaler, iv. 182
by nitrous oxide and oxygen with a Hewitt's apparatus, iv. 183, 184
by nitrous oxide, signs of, iv. 181
by perineural injection, as proposed by Hulsted, iv. 236
choice of methods for different operations, iv. 215
contra-indications to use of, iv. 108
diseases and conditions requiring special methods of, iv. 220
first operation under, i. 63
general, conditions contra-indicating its use, iv. 108
local, by application or injection of drugs, iv. 232
by cold, iv. 232
by infiltration, as used by Reclus and Schleich and modified by Matas and Braun, iv. 236
by pressure, iv. 231
by surface application, iv. 236
constriction, cooling, and adrenalin as aids in its production, iv. 234
general considerations, iv. 231
general preparations and technique, iv. 238–240
indications and contra-indications, iv. 237
methods of application, iv. 236
mixed, iv. 173
advantages and disadvantages of, iv. 174
moral, i. 489
mouth-gags, tongue forceps, and various appliances that may be needed in, iv. 176–178
of larynx, v. 896
physical examination of patient preliminary to, iv. 175
preparation of the patient for, iv. 172
recovery period, iv. 172
relation to surgical shock, i. 479
spinal, iv. 256–262
drugs used in producing it, and their doses, iv. 258
extent of its influence, and on what dependent, iv. 257
in rectal surgery, iv. 250
indications and scope, iv. 260–262
unpleasant and dangerous symptoms connected with its use, iv. 257
used for diagnostic examination, i. 553

Anæsthesia, vomiting during or after, the management of, iv. 228
Anæsthesia dolorosa and its explanation, iv. 234
Anæsthetic agents and methods, choice of, iv. 211
mixtures, action and mode of administration of, iv. 203
safety of, iv. 202
Anæsthetics, administration of, iv. 178
in cerebral operations, v. 344
administration of; circumstances under which it is especially dangerous, i. 784
and the production of general anæsthesia, iv. 169
after-effects of, iv. 227
choice of, in operations, iv. 147
consent to use of, viii. 753
death from, medico-legal aspect of, viii. 753, 754, 755
historical sketch of their introduction and use in surgery, iv. 169–172
in naval service, viii. 984
in sequence, administration of, iv. 208
various forms of, iv. 209
irritant effects of, upon certain diseases, i. 786
Anæsthetist, preparation and equipment of the, iv. 175
Anæsthetization of aged patients, iv. 213
of infants and children, iv. 212
of patients having obstruction in the upper air passages, the use of tubes in, iv. 213, 214
of so-called "difficult subjects," iv. 213, 214
Anæsthetized patient, attentions demanded for his care and comfort, iv. 148
Anæsthol as an anæsthetic, iv. 202
introduced by Willy Meyer, iv. 172
Anal examinations, vii. 765
papillæ, hypertrophied, vii. 897
Anal-urinary fistula, vii. 828
Anasarca, definition of, i. 236
Anatomical appearances as diagnostic factors, i. 513
Anatomical tubercle, ii. 637
Andrews, E. Wyllys, on Abdominal Hernia, vii. 555–617
Andrews' operation for cure of inguinal hernia, vii. 577
stone searcher, vii. 309
Anel's method of ligating for aneurysm, vii. 278
Aneurysm, vii. 258, 261
and angioma of bone, their relation to sarcoma, iii. 439, 440
and atheroma, anæsthetics indicated in, iv. 221
and interstitial hemorrhage, treatment of, ii. 663
arterial varix, vii. 258
arterio-venous, vii. 288
by anastomosis, vii. 259
cirsoid, vii. 259

Aneurysm, congenital, vii. 263
  cylindrical, vii. 262
  dissecting, vii. 262
  embolic, vii. 186, 263
  false, vii. 261
  fusiform, vii. 261
  Hunter's principles of treatment of, i. 39
  idiopathic, vii. 263
  in mouth, vi. 248
  in neck, venous, vi. 338
  of aorta, diagnosed from Pott's disease, iv. 955
    Macewen's method of needling for, viii. 40
  of arteries in neck, vi. 331
  of common carotid artery, vi. 331
  of external carotid artery, vi. 335
  of eyelids, v. 552
  of face, v. 473, 475
  of gluteal artery (traumatic), vii. 25
  of innominate artery, vi. 336; viii. 42
  of internal carotid artery, vi. 336
  of internal pudic artery (traumatic), vii. 28
  of obturator artery, vii. 28
  of scalp, v. 23
    arterio-venous, v. 23
    cirsoid, v. 19
  of sciatic artery, traumatic, vii. 27
  of subclavian artery, vi. 337
  of thoracic aorta and branches, viii. 37
  of vertebral artery, vi. 337
  operations for, by Wright Post, i. 40
  racemose. See Cirsoid aneurysm
  saccular, vii. 262
  spontaneous, vii. 263
  traumatic, vii. 262
    after organization of clot, i. 288
  true, vii. 261
  tubular, vii. 261
Aneurysmal varix, vii. 289
  and varicose aneurysm, ii. 664
Angina, Ludwig's, ii. 536; v. 444; vi. 341
  of pharynx, v. 822
  Vincent's, v. 822
Angioma, i. 319
  arteriale racemosum, i. 321
  fissural, i. 321
  intranasal, vi. 195
  neuropathic, i. 321
  senile, i. 321
  simple hypertrophic, i. 320
  Thoma's views of its etiology, i. 322
  traumatism a cause of, i. 321
Angio-sarcoma, i. 320, 333, 338, 340, 344
  endothelial, i. 323, 340
  of skull, v. 32
  perithelial, i. 323, 340

Anglo-sarcoma, plexiform, i. 340
Angiosclerosis, vii. 204
Angular curvature of spine (and see Pott's disease), iv. 927
Aniridia, v. 613
Ankle, amputation for tuberculous disease of, iii. 720
  contusions of, iii. 758
  sprains of the, iii. 755
Ankle-clonus in diagnosis, i. 539
Ankle-joint, a frequent seat of chronic abscess (tuberculous), iii. 715
  congenital dislocation of, iv. 766
  disarticulation at (Syme's operation), surgical anatomy, iv. 329
  excision of, iv. 457–463
    for tuberculous disease, iii. 720
  incised wounds of, iii. 759
  Kocher's operation for excision of a tuberculous astragalus, iii. 719
  normal motion at, iv. 915
  radiographic study of epiphyseal development about it, i. 596
  tuberculous disease of, iii. 711, 712, 720
Ankyloglossia, vi. 226
Ankyloblepharon, v. 561
  operations for, v. 566
Ankylosis of the hip, arthroplastic operation by Murphy, iv. 376, 377
  of the knee, bony, as an indication for excision or arthroplasty, iv. 438
  of maxillary joint, vi. 889
  of spine, vi. 456
  of the shoulder as an indication for excision, iv. 395
  x-rays in diagnosis of, i. 687
Annam ulcer, i. 231
Annular pancreas, viii. 161
Annulus senilis, v. 603
Anomalies of Fallopian tube, viii. 397
  of ovary, viii. 397
  of pancreas, viii. 160
  of prostate, viii. 340
  of spleen, viii. 61
  of urinary bladder, viii. 282
Anophthalmos, v. 554
Anorchidia, vi. 659
Ano-rectal fistula, vii. 816
  syphiloma, of Fournier, vii. 800
Anteflexion of uterus (and see Uterus, anteflexion of), viii. 455, 456
Anteposition of uterus (and see Uterus, anteposition of), viii. 455
Anterior mediastinum, operations on, viii. 57
Anterior reposition, in congenital dislocation of the hip, iv. 762
Antero-posterior curvature of spine (and see Pott's disease), iv. 927
Anteversion of uterus (and see Uterus, anteversion of), viii. 455, 456
Anthracosis, i. 207

Anthrax, ii. 48; iii. 31
  bacteriological diagnosis, ii. 49, 52, 338
  external, ii. 335
  immediate causes of, ii. 335
  inoculation, ii. 335
  internal, ii. 335
  intestinal, ii. 52
  œdema, ii. 337; iii. 32
  of face, v. 436
  prophylactic vaccinations, ii. 53
  pulmonary, ii. 52
  Sclavo's anti-anthrax serum in treatment of, iii. 33
  treatment, ii. 53
Anthrax-œdema, ii. 337–339; iii. 32
Antisepsis, i. 66
Antiseptic and aseptic, as discriminated in surgery, i. 695
  irrigation in the treatment of compound fractures, iii. 205
  surgery, its meaning as used by Lister, i. 695
Antiseptics, definition of, i. 695
Antistreptococcic serum in the treatment of infectious polyarthritis, iii. 503
Antitoxin, its bactericidal action, i. 418
Antrum, absence of, vi. 148
  accessory ostia, vi. 156
  acute inflammation of, vi. 156
  anatomy of, vi. 148
  carcinoma of, vi. 169, 832
  catheterization of, vi. 160
  chronic inflammation of, vi. 159
  chronic suppuration of intranasal, operation for, vi. 163
  dentigerous cyst of, vi. 158, 830
  diseases of, vi. 148, 156
  fibrosarcoma of, vi. 830
  fibromyxosarcoma of, vi. 830
  foreign bodies in, vi. 158
  inflammation of, vi. 156, 159
  malignant disease of, vi. 169
  mucocele of, vi. 159
  pathology of, vi. 156
  sarcoma of, vi. 170
  transillumination of, vi. 207
  tuberculosis of, vi. 883
  tumors of, vi. 200, 830
    operations for, vi. 866
  wounds of, vi. 169
Antyllus' method of ligating for aneurysm, vii. 280
Anuria, in renal calculus, viii. 116
  treatment, viii. 120
Anus, abnormal narrowing of, vii. 775
  abnormalities of, vii. 785
  anatomy of, vii. 761
  artificial. See Colostomy
  atresia of, vii. 775
  examination of, vii. 765
  fissure of, vii. 801
  imperforate, vii. 775
  lymphatics of, vii. 763
  malformations of, vii. 774
  nerve supply of, vii. 763
  occlusion of, by membrane, vii. 781
  operations on, anæsthetics in, vii. 771

Anus, physiology of, vii. 761, 764
  surgical diseases of, vii. 761
  syphilis, congenital, of, vii. 800
  ulcer of, irritable, vii. 801
  wounds of, vii. 761
Aorta, abdominal, ligature of,
    transperitoneal and retroperi-
    toneal methods, iv. 506
  aneurysm of, Macewen's method
    of needling for, viii. 40
  distortion of, in Pott's disease,
    iv. 938
  gunshot wounds of, vii. 230
  thoracic, aneurysm of, viii. 37
Apoplectic pancreas, viii. 180
Apoplexy, late, v. 261
  late post-traumatic, v. 266
Appendicitis, acute, vii. 628
  abdominal distention in, vii.
    656
  abscesses in, vii. 642
  bacteria in, vii. 630
  blood count in, vii. 653
  catarrhal, vii. 632
  chronic, vii. 628
  exudative, vii. 633
  facial expression in, vii. 652
  fever in, vii. 651
  fulminating, vii. 647
• gangrenous, vii. 634
  intermittent, vii. 628
  interstitial, vii. 633
  jaundice in, vii. 657
  muscular rigidity in, vii. 650
  nausea in, vii. 649
  onset of, vii. 643
  operation for, vii 675
  pain in, vii. 648
  posture in, vii. 655
  pulse in, vii. 652
  question of operation in, vii.
    667
  secondary abscesses in, vii.
    642
  tenderness in, vii. 649
  tuberculous, vii. 628
  tumor in, vii. 655
  varieties of, vii. 627
  vomiting in, vii. 649
  perforative, vii. 628
  time when operative treatment
    was introduced, i. 58
Appendicostomy, vii. 696, 797
Appendicular colic, vii. 631
Appendix epididymidis, vi. 630
Appendix vermiformis, actinomy-
    cosis of, vii. 636
  amputation of, vii. 683
  anatomy of, vii. 618
  cancer of, vii. 625
  carcinoma of, vii. 625
  colic of, vii. 631
  congenital malformations of,
    vii. 624
  cysts of, vii. 624
  delivery of the, vii. 682
  development of, vii. 619
  diseases of, vii. 618
  endothelioma of, vii. 625
  fibro-myoma of, vii. 625
  fossæ of, vii. 621
  inflammation of (and see Ap-
    pendicitis), vii. 618, 632

Appendix vermiformis, intussus-
    ception of, vii. 624
  malformation of, congenital,
    vii. 624
  mesentery of, vii. 622
  nerve supply of, vii. 622
  papilloma of, vii. 625
  peritoneal folds of, vii. 621
  physiology of, vii. 623
  positions of, vii. 618, 619, 622
  removal of, by Thomas G.
    Morton, i. 58
  removal of, when not dis-
    eased, vii. 691
  sarcoma of, vii. 625
  search for the, vii. 681
  shape of, vii. 618
  statistics of diseases of, by
    George Lewis, i. 58
  tuberculosis of, vii. 636
  tumors of, vii. 624
Appliances, prosthetic, vi. 3
  dental, vi. 7
Aprosexia, v. 827
Arachnitis, localized traumatic
    serous, v. 182
Arachnoid cysts, v. 181
Archibald, Edward, on Surgical Af-
    fections and Wounds of the Head,
    v. 3–378
Arcus senilis, v. 603
Areola (of breast), affections of
    (and see Nipple), vi. 507
Argyria, i. 207
Argyrosis of conjunctiva, v. 582
Arlt's method of blepharoplasty, iv.
    675
  for epicanthus, v. 570
  for pterygium, v. 594
  operation for entropion, v. 563
  for symblepharon, v. 567
Arm, amputation of, by circular
    method, iv. 299
  by method in which anterior
    and posterior flaps are em-
    ployed, iv. 299
  methods of, iv. 299
  surgical anatomy, iv. 298
  through the surgical neck of
    the humerus, iv. 300
Arm, transverse section of, in the
    middle, iii. 237
Armstrong, George E., on surgical
    diseases and wounds of the mouth,
    tongue, and salivary glands, vi.
    221–312
Armstrong's method of excision of
    tongue, vi. 286
Army (and see Military organiza-
    tion of), viii. 896
  authorized strength of, viii. 897
  in time of war, viii. 923
  medical department, administra-
    tion of, viii. 944
Arsenical ostitis, of jaws, vi. 889
  periostitis, of jaws, vi. 889
Arterial hemorrhage, vii. 233
  varix, iv. 258
Arteries and veins, ligature of, in
    their continuity, iv. 468
Arteries, contusions of, vii. 208
  "end" or "terminal," their
    relation to infarctions, i. 239

Arteries, guides for incision and
    locating, iv. 469
  in neck, injuries of, vi. 323
  inflammation of (and see Ar-
    teritis), vii. 202
  ligature of individual, iv. 476
    in treatment of acute simple
    inflammation, i. 114
  of brain, v. 101
  rupture of, vii. 235
  suture of, control of hemor-
    rhage by, vii. 249
  temporary control of the circu-
    lation in, by ligature, iv. 475
  wounds of, vii. 222
Arteritis, vii. 202
Arteriocapillary fibrosis, vii. 204
Arterioliths, i. 200; vii. 180
Arteriorrhaphy, Brewer's method
    of, vii. 253
  Carrel's method of, vii. 252
  control of hemorrhage by, vii.
    249
  De Gaetano's method of, vii. 255
  Dorrance's method of, vii. 255
  Murphy's method of, vii. 250, 251
  Payr's method of, vii. 251
  technique of, vii. 257
Arteriosclerosis, vii. 204
Arteriosclerotic gangrene, vii. 207
Arteriothrombosis, vii. 181
Arterio-venous anastomosis, treat-
    ment of beginning arterio-
    sclerotic gangrene by, vii. 207
  aneurysm, vii. 288
Arterioversion, vii. 243
Arthrectomy, definition of term, iv.
    368
  in the treatment of tuberculous
    joint disease, iii. 590
Arthritis, atrophic, iii. 504
  chronic non-tuberculous, x-ray
    appearances of, i. 656
  chronic villous, iii. 528–530
  deformans, as distinguished
    from tuberculosis of the
    knee-joint, iii. 699
  of spine, vi. 454
  hypertrophic, iii. 513, 517, 520,
    525
  neuropathic, as a cause of path-
    ological dislocation, iv. 7
  rheumatoid, iii. 504
  suppurative, as a cause of path-
    ological dislocation, iv. 8
  of the shoulder joint as an
    indication for excision, iv.
    395
  tuberculous, iii. 565, 573
Arthrodesis at hip, for paralytic de-
    formities of the lower extrem-
    ities, iv. 869
  for acquired talipes, iv. 921, 923
  for infantile paralysis, iv. 843
Arthropathies, ii. 514
Arthroplastic operation for anky-
    losis of knee, report of case by
    Murphy, iv. 375
Arthroplasty, aims of the operation,
    iv. 372
  Murphy's studies on the restora-
    tion of mobility and function
    in a joint, iv. 373

Arthroplasty, principles involved in Murphy's operation for adhesive synovitis, iv. 373, 374

Artificial. See Prosthesis

Artificial anus. See Colostomy
  ears, iv. 728; vi. 27
  eyes, v. 657
  glottis, vi. 32
  larynx, v. 925; vi. 31
  lips, vi. 26
  nose, iv. 717; vi. 20
  palate, vi. 18
  tongue, vi. 29
    of Martin, vi. 29
    of Terrell, vi. 30
  velum, for cleft palate, vi. 12

Artillery, definition of the term, ii. 643

Ascent of great trochanter above Nélaton's line, iii. 161, 162

Ascites, definition of, i. 236
  differentiated from ovarian cyst, viii. 435
  in portal cirrhosis, viii. 227

Aseptic closed wounds, repair of, i. 261
  open wounds or ulcers, repair of, i. 268
  protection of the wound, i. 273
  surgery, the meaning of the term, i. 695
  thrombosis of the dural sinuses, v. 247

Asphyxiation, viii. 978

Aspiration apparatus of Dieulafoy and of Potain, iv. 601
  of chest, viii. 48
  suprapubic, viii. 321

Assistants in hospital, responsibility of surgeon for, viii. 719

Assisting in applying dressings constitutes relation of surgeon and patient, viii. 719

Association areas of cerebral cortex, v. 273

Asthma, anæsthetics indicated in, iv. 221
  thymic, vi. 398, 399

Astragalectomy, for talipes, iv. 909

Astragalo-calcaneoid joint, motion at, iv. 915

Astragalus, dislocations of, iv. 100
  excision of, iv. 464
  tuberculous disease of, iii. 721

Astrocytes, derivation of, i. 325

Ataxia, cerebellar, v. 325

Athelia, vi. 507

Atheroma, vii. 204
  of auricle, v. 674

Atlas, fracture of, vi. 430

Atresia of anus, viii. 775
  of external auditory canal, v. 679
  of hymen, vi. 573
  of vagina, acquired, vi. 573
    congenital, vi. 577

Atrophia lipomatosa, i. 166
  musculorum lipomatosa, i. 171
  pigmentosa, i. 165

Atrophic bone the habitat of tuberculosis, iii. 337

Atrophy, i. 163
  as it affects certain tissues and organs, i. 170

Atrophy, brown, i. 171
  caused by severance of nerve trunk, i. 178
  cranial, v. 25
  degenerative, i. 164
  discriminated from agenesia, aplasia, and hypoplasia, i. 164
  from impaired nutrition, i. 168
  from inactivity or disuse, i. 167
  from over-activity, i. 167
  from pressure, i. 168
  marantic, i. 168
  neurotrophic, i. 170
  nutritive disorders leading to, i. 165
  of kidney (one), viii. 88
  of limbs, causes of, classified, iii. 331
  of ovary, viii. 401
  of tongue, vi. 297
  pathological, i. 167
  physiological, i. 166
  with induration, cause of, i. 165

Auditory canal, external, atresia of, v. 679
  ceruminous concretions in, v. 683
  chondromata of, v. 681
  exostosis of, v. 680
  foreign bodies in, v. 682
  fracture of, v. 678
  furunculosis of, v. 683
  laminated epithelial plugs in, v. 685
  osteomata of, v. 680
  stenosis of, v. 679
  wounds of, v. 678

Auditory nerve, surgery of the, v. 412

Aural fistulæ, congenital, v. 661
  polypi, v. 710

Auricle, abscess of, v. 672
  absence of, v. 660
  angiomata of, v. 672
  atheromata of, v. 674
  blood tumor of (and see Othæmatoma), v. 666
  burns of, v. 665
  carcinoma of, v. 676
  cat's, v. 661, 662, 664
  congenital malformations of, v. 660, 662
  cutaneous horn of, v. 675
  cystomata of, v. 674
  deformities of, v. 660, 662
  epithelioma of, v. 676
  erysipelas of, v. 671
  fibromata of, v. 674
  frost-bite of, v. 665
  gangrene of the, v. 671
  hypertrophy of, v. 675
  incised wounds of, v. 666
  keloid of, v. 674
  lacerated wounds of, v. 666
  lupus of, v. 670, 676
  malignant tumors of, v. 676
  malposition of, v. 663, 664
  mole of, v. 675
  nævus of, v. 675
  noma of, v. 671
  ossification of cartilage of, v. 670
  othæmatoma of, v. 666, 668
  papillomata of, v. 675

Auricle, perichondritis of, v. 668
  tuberculous, v. 669
  pernio of, v. 665
  sarcoma of, v. 676
  scalds of, v. 665
  sebaceous cysts of, v. 674
  supernumerary appendages of, v. 661
  syphilis of, v. 671, 676
  tophi of, v. 675
  tumors of, benign, v. 672
  ulceration of. v. 670
  warts of, v. 675
  Wildermuth, v. 661
  wounds of, v. 666

Auriculo-temporal nerve, surgery of the, v. 391

Auto-intoxication exciting chronic inflammations, i. 139

Autopsies, consent to making of, viii. 753, 755

Award of damages, in surgical malpractice, viii. 807

Avicenna's method of reducing forward dislocations of the humerus, iv. 43

Avulsion of the tubercle of the tibia, iii. 194

Axial rotation of fragments in fracture of the femur, iii. 71

Axilla not a favorable seat for local anæsthesia, iv. 247

Axillary abscess, vii. 66
  adenitis, vii. 66
  lymph · nodes, arrangement of, vi. 506

Axis, fracture of, vi. 430

Axonal reaction of Nissl, after injury of peripheral nerve, i. 289

Azotorrhœa in pancreatic diseases, viii. 177

BABINSKI's reflex, diagnostic significance of, i. 540

Bacilli, various forms of, associated with osteomyelitis, iii. 273

Bacillus aërogenes capsulatus (Welch), ii. 459; iii. 30
  the cause of gas-forming inflammations, i. 131
  anthracis, characteristics and action, iii. 31
  lepræ, characteristics of, ii. 5
  mallei, bacteriology of, ii. 42
  of malignant œdema, its characteristics, iii. 30
  of tetanus, or of Nicolaier, iii. 22
  pestis, description and bacteriology of, ii. 28
  pyocyaneus, the cause of green or blue pus, i. 418

Back and neck, sprains and contusions of, iii. 734

Bacon, · Leonard Woolsey, Jr., on General Prognosis in Surgical Diseases, i. 771

Bacon's method of entero-anastomosis, vii. 854

Bacteria causing suppuration, ii. 144
  in appendicitis, vii. 630
  in the formation of pus, i. 253
  passage of, through sound mucous membranes, i. 416

Bacteria, their sources and portals of entrance in surgical infections, i. 697

Bacteriæmia, how produced, i 426 in inflammation, i. 96

Bacterial examination of blood, its utility and the necessary precautions, i. 559 infection as influenced by wound or operative conditions, i. 701 pathological changes following, i. 415 injury to tissues, how caused, i. 417 proteins and toxalbumins, their production, i. 417

Bactericidal agencies, sources of, i. 89

Bacteriolysin and its action, i. 417

Bacteriuria, viii. 320

Baker's method of trachelorrhaphy, vi. 592

Balanitis, vi. 669, 753

Balano-posthitis, vi. 753

Balch, Franklin G., on Surgical Diseases and Wounds of the Male Genital Organs, vi. 622–699

Ballance's method of forming meatal flap, v. 721

Ballance-Edmunds stay-knot described, iv. 473

Bandage-machines, iv. 543

Bandages, iv. 541
Barton's, iv. 550
caoutchouc, iv. 591
circular, iv. 547
classification of, iv. 542
compound, iv. 576
Desault, iv. 559
dimensions of, iv. 544
Esmarch's, iv. 596–600
figure-of-8, iv. 549
fixation, history of, iv. 581–583
four-tailed, iv. 579
fronto-occipital, iv. 549
gauntlet, iv. 563
Gibson's, iv. 551
manufacture of, iv. 543
Martin s India-rubber, iv. 596–600
materials, iv. 541
oblique, iv. 547
occipito-facial, iv. 552
of breast, double, iv. 567
of breast, single, iv. 566
of chest, anterior figure-of-8, iv. 565
of chest, posterior figure-of-8, iv. 565
of chest, spiral (two forms), iv. 566
of elbow, figure-of-8, iv. 560
of eye, one, iv. 554
of eyes, both, iv. 554
of finger, reversed, spiral, iv. 565
of finger, spiral (three forms), iv. 563–565
of foot and ankle, figure-of-8, iv. 573
of foot, recurrent, iv. 575
of foot, reversed spiral, iv. 573
of foot, serpentine, iv. 524

Bandages, of foot, spica, iv. 574
of foot, spiral, iv. 573
of forehead and chin, iv. 553
of forehead and neck, iv. 553
of forehead and upper lip, iv. 553
of great toe, serpentine, iv. 575
of great toe, spica, iv. 575
of groin, ascending single spica, iv. 568
of groin, descending single spica, iv. 569
of groins, both, ascending spica, iv. 509
of groins, both, descending spica, iv. 570
of hand and wrist (dorsal), figure-of-8, iv. 561
of hand and wrist (palmar), figure-of-8, iv. 561
of hand, demi-gauntlet dorsal, iv. 561
of hand, demi-gauntlet palmar, iv. 562
of head, iv. 549
of head, crossed, iv. 552
of head, oblique, iv. 549
of head, recurrent, iv. 550
of jaw, oblique, iv. 553
of knee, figure-of-8, iv. 571
of knees, both, figure-of-8, iv. 571
of leg, long figure-of-8, iv. 573
of leg, short figure-of-8, iv. 572
of lower extremity, reversed spiral, iv. 572
of neck and axilla, figure-of-8, iv. 555
of neck, combined, iv. 556
of shoulder, ascending spica, iv. 556
of shoulder, descending spica, iv. 557
of thumb, spica, iv. 563
of upper extremity, reversed spiral, iv. 561
paraffin, iv. 591
plaster-of-Paris, application of, iv. 586–588
manufacture of, iv. 584
precautions necessary during application of, iv. 584–586
removal of, iv. 588–590
pressure, iv. 596
recurrent, iv. 550
retractor, iv. 580
reversed spiral, iv. 548
scultetus, iv. 580
soluble-glass, iv. 590
spica, iv. 548
spiral, iv. 548
starch, application of, iv. 590
triangular, iv. 578
uses, iv. 541
Velpeau, iv. 557–559

Bandaging, iv 541–600
general rules for, iv. 545–547

Banden's modification of Lisfranc's operation, iv. 324
operation of disarticulation at the knee-joint. iv 345

Banti's disease, viii. 71

Bardenhauer's method of splenopexy, viii. 76

Bardenhauer and Schimmelbusch's operation for restoring the cheek, iv. 647

Barker's method of holding the fragments together in fracture of the patella, iii. 185

Bartholin's gland, adeno-carcinoma of, vi. 570
cysts of, vi. 565
inflammation of, vi. 560

Bartlett's method of repairing cheek, iv. 639

Barton's fracture, iii. 152

Base-ball fingers, vii. 72

Basedow's disease (and see Exophthalmic goitre), vi. 375

Bassini's operation for cure of inguinal hernia, vii. 573

Battle, duties of naval medical corps with reference to, vii. 986

Battleship, profile of, viii. 973
sick-bay on, viii. 982
space allotted to medical department on, viii. 981

Bavarian splint, iii. 204, 205

Bayer's operation for restoration of lower part of nose, iv. 702

Beck's method of treating tuberculous sinuses, vii. 553
operation for hypospadias, vi. 649

Bectercio's spinal rigidity, vi. 458

Bed-sores, ii. 297
treatment of, prophylactic measures, ii. 299, 300

Behla, bodies of, i. 388

Bell, James, on Surgical Diseases and Wounds of the Kidneys and Ureters, viii. 78–158

Bellevue hospital medical college, when organized, i. 30

Benign and malignant growths of epithelial and connective tissue, types of, i. 296

Benqué or "Narcotile" inhaler for ethyl chloride, iv. 205, 206

Bennett's closed ether inhaler, description and mode of use, iv. 192
combined nitrous-oxide and ether inhaler, iv. 172
fracture, iii. 153
gas and ether inhalation apparatus, iv. 209, 210
gas inhaler, its mechanism, and precautions in using it, iv. 180

Berg's operation for restoration of lower lip, iv. 659

Bergenhem's operation for ectopia vesicæ, viii. 285

Berger's method of rhinoplasty, iv. 686

Beriberi or kakke, ii. 500

Beta-oxybutyric acid in the urine of diabetics an unfavorable prognostic sign, i. 794

Beyea's operation for gastroptosis, vii. 390

Bichloride of mercury, its use and properties as a disinfectant of the hands, i. 706

Bier method of treating sinuses in Pott's disease, iv. 981
treatment of tuberculous joint disease, iii. 590
Bifid scrotum, vi. 658
Bigelow, Henry J., i. 20, 50, 53
Bigelow's evacuator, viii. 329
method for the reduction of backward dislocations of the hip, iv. 98
Bigerminal teratomata, vii. 16
Bilateral lithotomy, viii. 328
Bile-ducts (and see Biliary ducts), viii. 195
abnormalities of, viii. 205
carcinoma of, viii. 252
catarrhal inflammation of, viii. 230
echinococcus cysts of, viii. 252
inflammation of, viii. 229
operations on, viii. 256, 262
after-treatment, viii. 276
sequelæ and complications, treatment of, viii. 277
physiology of, viii. 203
sarcoma of, viii. 252
suppurative inflammation of, viii. 231
ulcerative inflammation of, viii. 232
Bile passages, anatomy of, viii. 195
Bilharzia appendicitis, vii. 636
Biliary duct (and see Bile-ducts), adenoma of, viii. 252
cysts of, viii. 252
papilloma of, viii. 252
tumors of, viii. 252
Biliary fistula, viii. 243, 278
Biliary passages, perforation of, viii. 277
surgery of, viii. 193, 256
Billroth's method of treating stricture of œsophagus, vii. 437
Binder, abdominal, iv. 578
Bircher's operation for stenosis of œsophagus, vii. 438
Birth-mark, i. 320
Birth-palsy, brachial, vii. 71
Biskra button, ii. 342
Bites of man and other animals not rabid, iii. 15
wounds by, viii. 974
Bladder, aspiration of, suprapubic, vi. 797, 805
contracture of neck of, vi. 771
diagnosis of rupture of, i. 550
tuberculosis of, viii. 122
Bladder, urinary (and see Urinary bladder), modes of diagnostic examination of, i. 551
Blake's method of treating fractures of the patella, iii. 190
Blank-cartridge wounds of feet, vii. 42
Blasius' method of rhinoplasty, iv. 683, 685
operation (blepharoplasty), iv. 673
for restoration of lower lip, iv. 658
Blastomata, i. 366
Blastomycosis, ii. 318, 327
Blear-eye, v. 549

Blebs, i. 116
purulent, definition of the term, i. 121
Bleeding from the ear in fracture of the skull, v. 73
in treatment of acute simple inflammation, i. 114
Blenorrhœa, definition of the term, i. 121
Blepharitis, ciliary, v. 549
marginalis, v. 549
Blepharo-adenitis, v. 549
Blepharophimosis, v. 561
Blepharoplasty, iv. 672; v. 570
Arlt's method, iv. 675
Blasius' operation, iv. 673
Burow's operation, iv. 677
Dieffenbach's method, iv. 674; v. 572
French method of, iv. 674
Fricke's operation, iv. 672; v. 570
Harlan's method of, iv. 675; v. 571, 572
Hasner's operation, iv. 673, 676; v. 574
Indian method of, iv. 672
Italian method of, iv. 678
Knapp's operation, iv. 677; v. 574
Landolt's operation, iv. 674
Le Fort's method of, v. 575
Monk's operation, iv. 674
Morax's method of, v. 575
von Siklossy's operation, iv. 675
Snydacker's method of, v. 575
Szymanowski's method, iv. 675; v. 574
Tagliacotian method of, the, v. 574
Blepharospasm, v. 555
Blisters, i. 116, 117
Blood, the, i. 240, 555
alterations of, i. 240
and its constituents as furnishing contra-indications to operating and to some anæsthetics, iv. 122
changes in, in chronic anæmia, i. 245
characteristics of, in secondary anæmias, i. 244
cryoscopy of, in investigating the kidney, viii. 84
diseases of, in their relation to surgical conditions, i. 791
hydraulic pressure of, viii. 1065
hydrostatic pressure of, viii. 1063
in the stools, its varied appearance and sources, i. 572
in the urine, its significance, i. 571
regeneration of, after hemor-.rhage, i. 245
simple tests of, as to clot-formation, fibrin formation, etc., i. 556
Blood-corpuscles, changes in, i. 240
Blood-cysts of neck, vi. 347
of tongue, vi. 244
Blood-examinations, i. 557
Blood-plates, their relation to surgical diseases, i. 559

Blood-pressure in relation to diagnosis, i. 533
in shock, i. 468
relation of, to surgery, viii. 1063
Blood-supply, regulation of, in wounds, i. 274
Blood-vessels, asepsis in lateral wounds of, i. 288
conditions modifying modes of repairing, i. 287
diagnostic significance of abnormalities in, i. 531
of the scalp, traumatic affections of the, v. 23
repair of, i. 287
surgery of, vii. 146
Bloodgood, Joseph C., i. 463
on Surgical Diseases and Wounds of the Jaws, vi. 813–890
Bloodless surgery, i. 750
"Blue ball," vi. 706
Body fluids in general surgical disease, with special reference to their diagnostic value, i. 555
Boils, i. 128, 129
of neck, vi. 339
Bond's splint, iii. 149
Bone, abscess of, differential diagnosis of, ii. 84
in Pott's disease, iv. 935
treated by trephining, i. 59
aneurysm and angioma of, ii. 439
atrophy, i. 172; iii. 264, 328
associated with increase of fatty tissue, iii. 330, 331
concentric and excentric, i. 173; iii. 328
in "calcareous diathesis," i. 174
marantic form of, i. 173
of disuse, iii. 329
pressure form of, giving "egg shell crackle," i. 174
x-ray diagnosis of, i. 687
blisters, Codman's, as seen by aid of x-rays, i. 665
caries of, i. 232
cavities, after removal of sequestra, the question of their healing, iii. 308–310
plastic and osteoplastic operative methods of treating, iii. 309, 310
Charpy's classification of, iii. 334
chronic (tuberculous) abscess in, iii. 582
cysts, iii. 430, 435
development of, i. 280
elongation of, after castration, i. 163
from lack of pressure (Haab), iii. 331
expansion of, iii. 266
extrinsic hypertrophy of, with increase in length from mechanical and chemical irritants, i. 161
formation of a sequestrum, iii. 576
furunculosis of, iii. 268

Bone, growth of, as influenced by the epiphyseal cartilage, iii. 561

gummata, as seen by aid of x-rays, i. 668

hypertrophy of, as shown in inequality of growth of the lower extremities, iii. 337

inflammatory affections of, iii. 252

limited or circumscribed hypertrophy of—osseous elephantiasis, iii. 343

mechanical structure of, iii. 323

membranous, i. 280

minute anatomy of, i. 279

necrosis, i. 220, 222

of hand, vii. 63

non-inflammatory affections of, iii. 323

Ollier's "atrophic elongation" of, iii. 329

parasitic tumors of, iii. 482

red or vascular, iii. 334

regeneration of, i. 285, 286

regenerative power of, iii. 324

results of pressure upon, iii. 333

sarcoma, frequency with which the various bones are attacked, iii. 442

softening and fragility, discussion of etiological, nutritional, and nerve conditions, iii. 358, 359

spontaneous adaptability of, to pathological conditions, iii. 333

tuberculous disease of, changes, iii. 558, 574-577

tumors of, iii. 394, 480

x-ray characteristics of, i. 673

typhus, iii. 268

white or consumptive, iii. 336

yellow or fatty, iii. 334

Bones and joints, excisions of, general considerations and definition, iv. 367

Bonnet's operation for restoration of alæ nasi, iv. 696

for ectropion, iv. 668

Bony callus formed via cartilage, i. 282

union, causes of failure to secure it, i. 284

Borden, Major William C., on Gunshot Wounds, vii. 642

Bougies-à-boule, vi. 784

Bougies, bulbous, vi. 784

filiform, vi. 783

for examining œsophagus, vii. 409

woven, vi. 784

Bouisson's method of restoring the alæ nasi, iv. 696

Bovée's method of uniting divided ureter, viii. 155

Bovine tuberculosis, the question of its transmissibility to man, ii. 80

Bowels, overloading of, in its relation to surgical prognosis, i. 790

obstruction of (and see Intestinal obstruction), vii. 727

Bow-leg (and see Genu varum), iv. 860

braces for, iv. 861

in rickets, iii. 350

operative treatment, iv. 862

treatment, iv. 861

Bowman's method of operation for stricture of the lachrymal duct, v. 595

race for bow-legs, iv. 861

Brachial plexus, injury to, vi. 330; vii. 69

birth-palsy, vii. 71

Brachiocephalism, iii. 327

Bradford frame for Pott's disease, iv. 961

Bradford-Goldthwait genuclast, iii. 512

Brain, v. 100

abscess of (and see Cerebral abscess), v. 251

cerebral, v. 789

cerebellar, v. 789

diagnosed from cerebral tumor, v. 317

extradural, v. 789

intradural, v. 789

relation of otitis to, v. 780

site of, in relation to ear disease, v. 780

surgery of, v. 801

actinomycosis of, v. 302

angioma of, v. 311

areas of localization, v. 270, 271

arteries of, v. 101

association areas of, v. 273

blood supply of, v. 101

carcinoma of, v. 310

changes in, in Jacksonian epilepsy, v. 293

cholesteatoma of, v. 312

circulation in, v. 105

hydrostatics and hydrodynamics of, v. 108

compensatory mechanism of, v. 108

commotion of, v. 145

compression of, v. 111

acme of manifest compression (Kocher), v. 127, 131

beginning stage of manifest compression (Kocher), v. 126, 129

circulatory changes in, v. 119

circulatory symptoms in, v. 131

Cushing's work on, v. 116

diagnosis of, v. 142

effect on vagus centre, v. 132, 134

experimental investigations, v. 112

from hemorrhage, coincident with concussion or contusion, v. 197

general, v. 119

Hill's work on, v. 116

historical, v. 112

Kocher's views on, v. 125

Leyden's work on, v. 113

local, v. 118

physiological considerations, v. 112

Brain, compression of, relation of Cheyne-Stokes respiration to, v. 124, 132

respiratory symptoms in, v. 132

stage of paralysis, v. 136

stage of compensation (Kocher), v. 126, 129

symptomatology, v. 128

treatment, v. 143

unconsciousness in, v. 135

use of manometer in, v. 132

vasomotor centers in, v. 138

von Bergmann's views on, v. 113

von Schulten's eye phenomenon in, v. 129

von Schulten's work on, v. 115

concussion of the, v. 145

Cannon's researches on, v. 159

cause of unconsciousness, v. 160, 164

coincidence of, with compression from hemorrhage, v. 197

correlation of physiological with clinical phenomena, v. 159

Duret's theory of, v. 153

Ferrari's experiments, v. 152

Fischer's theory of the pathogenesis of, v. 160

Horsley and Kramer's experiments, v. 155

Kocher's theory of the pathogenesis of, v. 163

Maasland and Saltikoff's investigation on, v. 157

modes of death in, v. 169

physiological effects of, as ascertained by experimental observations, v. 151

Polis' investigation on, v. 156, 162

relation to shock, v. 161

researches of Koch and Filehne, v. 153, 162

vital centres in, v. 167

contusion of, v. 172

coincidence of, with compression from hemorrhage, v. 197

cortical centres, v. 268

cranio-cerebral topography, v. 360

Kroenlein's method, v. 362

Taylor and Houghton's method, v. 363

cystic tumors of, v. 308

damage to, in gunshot wounds of skull, v. 92

decompression of, occipital operation for, v. 371

temporal operation for, v. 370

dermoids of, v. 312

disease of, occipital operation for, v. 312

disease, otitic, v. 779

displacement of the, v. 369

endothelioma of, v. 303

fibroma of, v. 311

frontal lobe, diagnosis of tumors in, v. 318

Brain, glanders of, v. 303
glioma of, v. 305
hemorrhages in substance of, v. 260
hernia of, v. 377
infectious granulomata of, v. 301
lateral ventricles, relation to cranium, v. 365
lesions due to otitis, diagnosis of, v. 787
symptoms of, v. 787
lesions of frontal lobe, symptoms of, v. 281
lesions of occipital lobe, symptoms of, v. 278
lesions of parietal lobe, symptoms of, v. 277
lesions of pre-central convolution, symptoms of, v. 275
lesions of post-central convolution, symptoms of, v. 276
lesions of temporal lobe, symptoms of, v. 280
lymphatics of, v. 105
meninges of, v. 100
molecular disturbance of, v. 145
motor areas of, v. 269
neuroglioma ganglionare of, v. 301
occipital lobe of, diagnosis of tumors in, v. 322
operations on, technique of (and see Cerebral operations, technique of), v. 340
parietal lobe, diagnosis of tumors in, v. 321
parieto-occipital fissure, line of, v. 362
physiological considerations, v. 105
psammoma of, i. 200; v. 311
pulsations of the, v. 106
pyogenic diseases of the, of otitic origin, v. 779
regulatory mechanisms of, v. 106
Rolandic area, diagnosis of tumors in, v. 321
Rolandic fissure, line of, v. 362, 363
sand or psammoma, i. 200
sarcoma of, v. 310
senile atrophy of, i. 177
sensory areas of, v. 270
substance, diseases and injuries of, v. 259
surgical procedures on, v. 801
Sylvian fissure, line of, v. 362, 363
syphilis of (and see Meningitis, syphilitic), v. 301
temporo-sphenoidal lobe, diagnosis of tumors in, v. 322
throwing or flinging movement of, v. 152
tuberculosis of, v. 301
tumors of, v. 300
vasomotor nerves in, v. 121
veins of, v. 101
ventricular puncture, location, v. 365
vibration of, v. 145, 146

Brain, water on the (and see Hydrocephalus), v. 220
Brain-squeezing, v. 153
Brainard, Daniel, i. 27
Branchial cysts, vi. 315
dermoids, vi. 315
fistula, vi. 313, 384
Branchiogenic multilocular cysts, vi. 317
treatment, vi. 317
Brandegee's adenoid forceps, v. 832
Brasdor's method of ligating for aneurysm, vii. 280
Brashear, Walter, i. 60
Bratz's retention splint for torticollis, iv. 785
Brauer apparatus, operating on chest with, viii. 44
Breast bandage, iv. 566, 567
binder, iv. 579
female, aberrant (supernumerary), vi. 508
abscess of, vi. 511
intraglandular, vi. 512
postmammary, vi. 512
submammary, vi. 512
absence of, vi. 507
acinous carcinoma of, vi. 534
actinomycosis of, vi. 519
adeno-carcinoma of, vi. 536
adeno-cystoma of, vi. 523
adeno-fibroma of, vi. 523
adenoma of, vi. 522
affections of nipple and areola, vi. 507
amputation of, during pregnancy, i. 779
anatomy of, vi. 502
angioma of, vi. 528
cancer en cuirasse, vi. 537
carcinoma of, vi. 531
cystadenoma of (and see Mastitis, chronic), vi 514, 524
cystic disease of (and see Mastitis, chronic), vi. 514
cysto-sarcoma, vi. 523
cysts of, vi. 526
diseases of, vi. 507
duct-cancer of, vi. 536
echinococcus cyst of, vi. 528
enchondroma of, vi. 529
fibro-adenoma of, vi. 520, 522
fibroma of, vi. 522
gumma of, vi. 519
hypertrophy of, vi. 508.
imperfect development of, vi. 507
inflammation of. See Mastitis
intracanalicular myxoma of, vi. 523
lenticular cancer of, vi 538
lipoma of, vi. 520, 528
lymphatics, vi. 504
malignant papillary dermatitis (and see Paget's disease of the nipple), vi. 556
medullary carcinoma of, vi. 535
method of examining, vi. 516, 541

Breast, female, myxoma of, vi. 529
nævus of, vi. 529
nerve supply, vi. 504
neuralgia of, vi. 509
neuroma of, vi. 529
neuroses of, vi. 509
operations not adapted to local anæsthesia, iv. 245
osteoma of, vi. 529
physiology of, vi. 502
sarcoma of, vi. 529
scirrhous, vi. 515
scirrhous carcinoma of, vi. 534
supernumerary, vi. 507
surgical diseases and wounds of, vi. 502
syphilis of, vi. 519
tuberculosis of, vi. 517
tumors of, vi. 520
benign, vi. 520
malignant, vi. 520
vascular supply, vi. 503
wounds of, vi. 507, 509
male, surgery of, vi. 420
pigeon, vi. 407
Brewer's method of arteriorrhaphy, vii. 253
Broad ligament of uterus, anatomy of, viii. 394
Brodie's abscess, iii. 259, 275, 314, 316
Bronchiectasis, viii. 23
Broncholiths, i. 200
Bronchitis, anæsthetics indicated in the presence of, iv. 221
Bronchocele (and see Goitre), viii. 358
Bronchoscopy, v. 905, 908, 910
Brophy's method of operating for cleft palate, v. 539
Brown induration resulting from passive congestion, i. 236
Brown's (Buckminster) splint for torticollis, iv. 788, 789
Bruns' (von) ambulant splint, iii. 207
Bryant, Joseph D., i. 501
Bryant's triangle, relation of the great trochanter to, in fracture of femur, iii. 162
Bubo, vi. 705
chancroidal, vi. 706
Buchanan's operation for restoration of lower lip, iv. 657
Buck, Gurdon, i. 52
Buck's extension apparatus, iii. 169, 171-173
Buck, Gurdon, operation for restoring upper lip, iv. 651
"Bucked shins," in young horses, iii. 255
Buckshot wounds, ii. 655
Bullæ, purulent, definition of the term, i. 121
Bullets, destructive effect of, increased in proportion to the shortness of range, ii. 652
effects of, on muscles and fasciæ, ii. 661
relatively to the part of the brain perforated or penetrated, ii. 703

Bullets, explosive effect of, ii. 652
  injuries of body tissues and
    structures, ii. 659
  nature of injury inflicted by, in
    gunshot wounds of the
    skull, v. 86
  effect on bone, v. 87
  effect on cranial contents, v.
    93
  varieties and qualities of, ii.
    644, 645
Bullet wounds as a cause of aneu-
    rysmal varix and varicose
    aneurysm, ii. 663
  of blood-vessels, ii. 662
  of entrance and of exit, ii.
    660
  of nerves, ii. 666
  of tendons, ii. 661
  of the skin, ii. 659
Bumm's operation for carcinoma of
  uterus, viii. 636
Bumstead, Freeman J., i. 37
Bunion, ii. 347, 444; iv. 894
Buphthalmos, v. 604
Burghard's method of prostatectomy, viii. 370
Buried sutures, the requirements
  answered by catgut, i. 730
Burns, ii. 581
  and effects of electric currents
    and lightning, ii. 581
  characteristics of the resulting
    cicatrices, ii. 582
  from electric currents, ii. 589
  from lightning stroke, ii. 590
  of first degree, causes of death
    from, ii. 584
  of second degree, local and gen-
    eral symptoms, ii. 584
  treatment, ii. 586
  of the third degree, ii. 585, 588
  of abdominal walls, vii. 93
  of auricle, v. 665
  of conjunctiva, v. 590
  of face, v. 428
  of larynx, v. 866
  of pharynx, v. 811
  of chest, vi. 404
  of male external genitals, vi. 666
  of tongue, vi. 232
  ulceration resulting from, ii. 583
  x-ray, vii. 39
Burow's method of flap formation in
    plastic operations, iv. 615
  operation (blepharoplasty), iv.
    677
Burrage needleholder, vi. 588
Bursa beneath the popliteus ten-
    don, ii. 442
  gluteal, inflammation of, ii. 443
  hæmatomata of, ii. 438
  hamstring, inflammation of, ii.
    442
  ilio-psoas, vii. 51, 52
  injuries and diseases of, ii. 438
  lying over the tuber ischii, ii. 443
  of the hand, ii. 445
  olecranon, inflammation of, ii.
    445
  over the head of the first meta-
    tarsal bone, inflammation of, i
    or bunion, ii. 444

Bursa, prepatellar, affections of, ii.
    441
  subdeltoid, inflammation of, ii.
    445
  subpatellar, inflammations of,
    ii. 442
  tumors of, ii. 445
  under the psoas tendon, disten-
    tion of, ii. 443
  under the tendo Achillis, in-
    flammation of, ii. 442
  various, about the hip, ii. 444
  wounds of, ii. 438
Bursal cysts of neck, vi. 348
Bursitis, acute, simple and suppura-
    tive, ii. 439
  chronic, ii. 439
  gouty, ii. 441
  ilio-psoas, vii. 51
  over head of first metatarsal
    bone, treatment of, ii. 444, 445
  pelvic, vii. 29
  subacromialis, vii. 44
  subiliac, vii. 51
  syphilitic, ii. 441
  tuberculous, ii. 440
Butlin's method of excision of
    tongue, vi. 285
Byrne's method of removing uterus
    and parametrium, by cautery,
    viii. 645

CABOT, HUGH, on chancroid, vi.
    700–714
  on gonorrhœal urethritis, vi.
    715–812
Cachexia thyreopriva, vi. 389
Cadaveric tubercle, ii. 325
Cæcum, actinomycosis of, vii. 725
  arteries of, vii. 623
  carcinoma of, vii. 724
  internal configuration of, vii.
    622
  tuberculosis of, vii. 724
Cæsarean section, and its substi-
    tutes, viii. 701
  Porro's operation, viii. 703
  pubiotomy, viii. 707, 709
  Saenger's operation, viii. 705
  symphyseotomy, viii. 707
  vaginal operation, viii. 705
Calcareous concretions of eyelids, v.
    559
  of Meibomian glands, v. 559
Calcareous matter, deposits of, seen
    by aid of x-rays, i. 687
Calcification and analogous con-
    ditions, i. 198
  and petrifaction contra-distin-
    guished from ossification, i.
    200
  chemico-vital theories as to its
    origin, i. 199
  of subdeltoid bursa, iii. 526
  of tunica vaginalis, vi. 696
  of urethra, vi. 695
  usually occurs in tissues already
    diseased or the seat of foreign
    bodies, i. 199
Calculi or concretions, i. 200
  cystic-oxide, viii. 113
  fecal, i. 203
  hepatic, i. 200

Calculi, lachrymal, v. 592
  mixed, viii. 113
  mulberry, viii. 113
  oxalate, viii. 113
  pancreatic, i. 203; viii. 190
  phosphatic, viii. 113
  in prostate, viii. 350
  renal, viii. 110
  salivary, i. 203; vi. 259
  ureteral, viii. 142
  uric-acid, viii. 112
  urinary, i. 200, 203; viii. 110
  vesical, viii. 306
  xanthin, viii. 113
Calculous anuria, treatment of, viii.
    120
Caliper splints, iii. 511
  in treatment of deformity from
    arthritis, iii. 501
Callositas, ii. 346
Callus, ii. 346
  disappearance of, i. 282
  external, as related to the posi-
    tion of the fractured ends
    of bone, i. 284
  its earliest stage, i. 281
  formation and functions of, after
    fractures, iii. 79
  intermediate, definitive or per-
    manent, iii. 79
  internal or myelogenous, i. 281
  proportioned to deformity, i.
    285
Calot's operation in Pott's disease,
    iv. 983
Cammidge reaction, viii. 175
Cancer (and see Carcinoma and
    Sarcoma)
  and the acute exanthemata, i.
    388, 389
  aigu du sein, vi. 539
  characteristics of the unknown
    stimulus in, i. 403
  diagnosis of, hæmolytic reaction
    in, vi. 543
  en cuirasse, of breast, female,
    vi. 537
  general arguments in favor of its
    infectious nature, i. 390
  hæmolytic reaction in diag-
    nosis of, vi. 543
  inclusions in, i. 387, 389
  in mice, evidence of an acquired
    immunity, i. 399
  its communicability, i. 391
  its spontaneous retrogres-
    sion, i. 398
  lenticular, of breast, female, vi.
    538
  of breast, female. See Carcino-
    ma
  of rectum, vii. 899
  of tongue (and see Tongue, car-
    cinoma of), vi. 263
  of uterus. See Uterus, carcino-
    ma of, and sarcoma of
  of vermiform appendix, vii. 625
  parasitical relations of, i. 387,
    411
  summary of arguments for its
    infectiousness, i. 409
  transplantation experiments, i.
    390

Cancer-cells, an infectious factor in them, i. 405
  bodies observed in them, i. 387
  non-chemical nature of their x-factor, i. 405
  their unlimited power of proliferation, i. 935
  transference of their infectious factor to normal epithelium, i. 393
Cancerous cachexia, i. 369
Cancroid body or papule, its characters, ii. 376
Cancrum oris, ii. 301; vi. 222
Canities of eyebrows and eyelashes, v. 550
Cannon, researches on cerebral concussion, v. 159
Canthoplasty, v. 562
Canthotomy, v. 561
Canthus, fissure of, v. 556
Cantlie's method of treating subphrenic abscess, vii. 491
Caoutchouc bandages, iv. 591
Caps for operative work, i. 721
Capsule of Tenon, inflammation of, v. 648
Caput obstipum (and see Torticollis), iv. 767
Carbolic acid, its use as a germicide, i. 706
Carbuncle, i. 128, 129, 130; ii. 157, 307
  choice of anæsthetics in treating, iv. 222
  of chest wall, vi. 408
  of face, v. 434
  of neck, vi. 339, 340
  staphylococci most commonly found in, i. 130
Carcinoma (and see Cancer), i. 361
  adenomatosum, i. 350
  alveolar, i. 361
  character of the stroma, i. 360
  colloid or gelatinous, i. 363
  cylindrical-celled, i. 360
  cylindromatosum, i. 363
  development from epithelial structures, i. 354, 355
  encephaloid or medullary, i. 361
  extension by dissemination, i. 364
    by implantation, i. 365
    by infiltration, i. 364
  histological classification, i. 358
    resemblances, i. 354
  influence of external traumatism with causation, i. 293
  intranasal, vi. 199, 857
  metastasis in, i. 364
  methods of extension and metastasis, i. 364
  mode of growth, i. 356
  myxomatodes, i. 363
  of abdominal wall, vii. 87
  of antrum, vi. 169, 832
  of auricle, v. 676
  of biliary ducts, viii. 252
  of brain, v. 310
  of breast, female, vi. 531
  of cæcum diagnosed from tuberculosis, vii. 724
  of chest wall, vi. 414

Carcinoma of ends of stumps, vii. 67
  of eyelids, v. 559
  of face, discoid, v. 489
  of gluteal region, vii. 31
  of intestine, vii. 740
  of jaw, secondary, vi. 849
    operations for, vi. 868
    secondary to mouth and gum, vi. 846
    operations for, vi. 868
  of kidney, viii. 134
  of larynx, v. 885
  of liver, viii. 220
  of lung, viii. 30
  of mediastinum, viii. 34
  of Meibomian glands, v. 559
  of mucous membrane, mouth, and gum, with secondary involvement of jaw, vi. 846
    operations for, vi. 868
  of nasopharynx, vi. 860
  of neck, vi. 351
  of œsophagus, vii. 413
  of orbit, vi. 854
  of ovary, viii. 426
  of pancreas, viii. 188
  of parotid gland, vi. 308
  of pelvic bones, vii. 14
  of penis, vi. 689
  of peritoneum, vii. 752
  of pharynx, v. 857
  of pleura, viii. 14
  of prostate, viii. 355
  of rectum, vii. 898
    colloid, vii. 900
  of salivary glands, vi. 308
  of scrotum, vi. 696
  of seminal vesicles, vi. 699
  of skull, v. 34
  of spine, diagnosed from Pott's disease, iv. 955
  of stomach, vii. 393
  of testis, vi. 698
  of thyroid, vi. 373
  of tongue, vi. 263
  of tonsil, vi. 863
  of umbilicus, scirrhous, vii. 90
  of urethra, vi. 695
  of urinary bladder, viii. 310
  of uterus (and see Uterus, carcinoma of), viii. 582
  of vermiform appendix, vii. 625
  of vulva, vi. 569
  round-celled, i. 359
  secondary changes in, i. 362
  scirrhous, its distinctive features, i. 361
  squamous-celled (epithelioma), i. 358-359
  umbilicated, i. 363
  whence arising, i. 354
Carcinoma-cells, characteristics of, i. 356
Carcinomatous growth, its atypical and aberrant character, i. 355
  transformation of adenoma, i. 355
Carden's operation, iv. 345
Cardiac dilatation, acute, postoperative treatment of, iv. 160

Cardiac diseases, a source of danger in administration of anæsthetics, i. 784
Cardiocentesis, vii. 175
Cardiolysis, vii. 159
Cardiorrhaphy, vii. 168
Cardiospasm, vii. 445, 446
Cargile membrane, uses of, i. 736
Caries, i. 210, 232; ii. 201, 202, 203
  Billroth's views of the process, i. 232
  necrotica, i. 232
  of orbital walls, v. 649
  of spine (and see Pott's disease), iv. 927
  or ulceration of bone, tuberculous, iii. 575
  sicca, i. 232; iii. 579, 604
  x-ray evidence of, i. 648
  von Volkmann's views of the process, i. 232
Carotid, common, ligature of, i. 60, 61
  sheaths, acute inflammations of, vi. 343
Carpus, congenital dislocation of, iv. 742
  dislocations of the second row and of individual bones of, iv. 65
  development studied by radiographs, i. 579
Carrel's method of arteriorrhaphy, vii. 252
"Carrying angle," definition of the term, iv. 51
  of forearm with arm, iii. 609
Carson, Joseph, i. 7, 17
Carson, Norman B., on Surgery of the Thorax and Spinal Column, vi. 401-501
Cartilage, tuberculous disease of, pathology, iii. 577
Cartilaginous exostosis, i. 315
Caruncle, of urethra, vi. 571
  urethral, vi. 571
Case, obturator-velum of, vi. 14
Caseation, i. 215
Castration, vi. 698
Casts in urine, their significance, i. 570
Cataract, after-, v. 637
  anterior polar, v. 625
  capsular, v. 625
    anterior central, v. 625
  congenital, v. 625
  cortical, v. 625
  diabetic, v. 625
  hypermature, v. 624
  Morgagnian, v. 624
  nuclear, v. 625
  operations for, v. 627
  polar, anterior, v. 625
    posterior, v. 625
  pyramidal, v. 625
  secondary, v. 625
  senile, v. 623
  soft, v. 626
  traumatic, v. 626
  treatment of, v. 626
  zonular, v. 625
Catarrh, chronic, i. 141
  desquamative, i. 116

Catarrh, mucous, i. 116
of lachrymal duct, v. 591
of lachrymal sac, v. 591
purulent, i. 121, 127
serous, i. 116
spring, v. 581
Catgut as suture material, i. 728, 753
Catheter holder, viii. 388
Catheterization of antrum, vi. 160
of frontal sinus, vi. 117
of sphenoidal sinus, vi. 175
precautions to be observed, iv. 158
Catheters, vi. 785
webbing, vi. 786
treatment, vi. 786
Cat's auricle, v. 661
treatment, v. 662, 664
Cauda equina, diseases of, vi. 501
injuries of, vi. 501
tumors of, vi. 500
Cauliflower growths, ii. 359
Cauterization of cornea, v. 617
Cautery, its uses and modern forms, i. 767
Cavernitis, vi. 669, 752
Cavernoma, i. 321
Cavernous sinus, v. 102
Cells, death of, necrosis and necrobiosis, i. 183
division, indirect, described, i. 257
multiplication and differentiation of, i. 147
proliferation after infliction of an injury, i. 76, 93
its protective and sometimes imperfect features, i. 94
Cellular and less cellular tumors, i. 295
Cellulitis, acute circumscribed, ii. 456
cervical, v. 444
diffuse, ii. 458
gaseous, ii. 459
of neck, diffuse, non-erysipelatous, vi. 344
orbital, v. 445, 647
treatment, v. 648
Cementoma of Bland-Sutton, iii. 476
Centipede, its sting and the treatment of it, iii. 5
Centres, cerebral, for association, v. 273
hearing, v. 272
motion, v. 269
sensation, v. 270
sight, v. 272
smell, v. 273
speech, v. 273
taste, v. 273
cortical, v. 268
Cephalhæmatoma, v. 9
Cephalocele, v. 213
Cerebellar abscess (and see Abscess, cerebellar), v. 256
relation of, to otitis, v. 781
fits, v. 284
influx, the, v. 284
Cerebellum, v. 282
dermoid cyst of, v. 312, 314

Cerebellum, functions of, v. 284
tuberculosis of, v. 301
tumors of, ataxia in, v. 325
diagnosis, v. 323, 330
disordered hearing in, v. 327
eye symptoms in, v. 327
involvement of facial nerve in, v. 327
motor symptoms in, v. 325
muscular atonia in, v. 328
nystagmus in, v. 328
paresis of homolateral muscles in, v. 328
sensory symptoms in, v. 329
vertigo in, v. 326
Cerebral abscess (and see Abscess, cerebral), v. 251
circulation, v. 105
compensatory mechanism of, v. 108
effect of gravity on, v. 108
hydrostatics and hydrodynamics of, v. 108
lesions, organic, symptoms of, v. 274
localization, v. 267
operations, anæsthetic in, v. 344
control of hemorrhage after v. 343
Cryer's spiral osteotome, v. 355
decompression of brain, v. 370
displacement of brain, v. 369
Doyen's burrs, v. 353
drainage after, v 342
faradization of the cortex during, v. 360
hernia cerebri following, v. 377
infection in, v. 340
influencing of the vital centres in, v. 347
instruments commonly used, v. 350
Kuester's craniotomy chisel, v. 357
Lane's rongeur forceps, v. 353
making of a permanent window, v. 352
osteoplastic flap, the, v. 353
prevention of shock after, v. 343
shaving the scalp, v. 340
special procedures, v. 366
Sudeck's fraise, v. 355
technique of, v. 340
trephining, v. 351
two-stage operations, v. 367
under local anæsthesia, v. 346
paralysis and its deformities, iv. 871
pressure gauge of Hill, v. 108
substance, escape of, in fracture of skull, v. 76
syphilis, v. 242
tumors (and see Brain, tumors of), v. 300
Cerebro-spinal fluid, v. 103
absorption of, v. 104

Cerebro-spinal fluid, as obtained by lumbar puncture, its diagnostic value, i. 560
circulation of, v. 219
escape of, diagnostic of cranial fractures, v. 75
meningitis, v. 231
Ceruminous concretions in external auditory canal, v. 683
symptoms, v. 683
treatment, v. 683
Cervical ribs, vi. 318, 408
vertebræ, treatment of dislocations of, iv. 24, 25
Cervix of uterus, adenocarcinoma of, viii. 594
amputation of, vi. 592
lacerated, repair of (and see Trachelorrhaphy), vi. 586
Chalazion, v. 558
Chalcosis, i. 207
Chancre, characteristics of, ii. 105
diagnostic tests of, ii. 106
differential diagnosis, ii. 108
hard, of female genitals, vi. 565
of conjunctiva, v. 582
of face, v. 457
of mouth, ii. 123
of pharynx, v. 843
of rectum, vii. 799
of tonsil, v. 843
soft, of female genitals, vi. 565
Chancroid, vi. 700
bubo complicating, vi. 705, 706
character of lesion, vi. 702
Ducrey-Unna bacillus, characteristics of, vi. 700
frequency of occurrence, vi 701
lesions of, vi. 701, 702
lymphadenitis complicating, vi. 705
lymphangitis complicating, vi. 705
mixed, vi. 703
of anus, vii. 798
of rectum, vii. 798
period of incubation, vi. 701
phagedena complicating, vi. 705
phimosis complicating, vi. 704
simultaneous infection with syphilis and, vi. 703
Chapel, of hospitals, viii. 879
Charbon, iii. 32
of face, v. 436
Charcot's disease, as distinguished from tuberculosis of the knee-joint, iii. 699
bone changes in, iii. 363
joint, iii. 536, 540
x-ray characteristics of, i. 668
knee-joint, its diagnosis, ii 122
Charley-bone, vii. 73
Charley-horse, vii. 73
Cheek, lupus of, v. 454
plastic repair of, vi. 223
plastic surgery of the, iv. 638–647
Bardenhauer and Schimmelbusch's operation, iv. 647
Bartlett's method, iv. 639
Czerny's operation, iv 643
Gersuny's operation, iv. 640

Cheek, plastic surgery of the, Gussenbauer's operation, iv. 642
　Hahn's operation, iv. 646
　Israel's operation, iv. 644
　Kraske's operation, iv. 642
　Monod and Van Vert's method, iv. 647
Chemical substances alone may excite purulent inflammation, i. 126
Chemosis, v. 584
　filtration, after cataract operations, v. 637, 639
Chemotaxis, a protective factor in inflammation, i. 84
Chest (and see Chest wall, Thoracic wall, Thorax)
　aspiration of, viii. 48
　burns of, vi. 404
　contused wounds of, vi. 403
　contusions of, vi. 402
　flat, vi. 406
　funnel, vi. 407
　incised wounds of, vi. 403
　lacerated wounds of, vi. 403
　non-penetrating wounds of, vi. 403
　operations on the, viii. 43
　punctured wounds of, vi. 403
　topography, diagnostic points in, 527
　uniformity of expansion, how interfered with, i. 528
　wounds of, vi. 403; viii. 16
Chest wall, abscess of (and see Chest, Thoracic wall, and Thorax), vi. 409
　actinomycosis of, vi. 410
　carbuncle of, vi. 408
　carcinoma of, vi. 414
　deformities of, vi. 406
　diseases of, vi. 408
　echinococcus of, vi. 411
　enchondroma of, vi. 413
　fibroma of, vi. 413
　fibroma molluscum of, vi. 413
　furuncle of, vi. 408
　hæmangioma of, viii. 15
　keloid of, vi. 414
　phlegmon of, vi. 409
　sarcoma of, vi. 414
　tumors of, vi. 411
　　benign, vi. 412
　　malignant, vi. 414
Chetwood's plastic operation for restoring functional activity of anus, vii. 827
Cheyne and Burghard's operation on external ear, iv. 722
Cheyne-Stokes respiration, relation of, to cerebral compression, v. 124, 133
Chilblains, ii. 268, 595, 599
　of face, v. 431
Chimney-sweep's disease, vi. 696
Chin, sinuses in, from alveolar periostitis, vi. 880
Chisel, craniotomy, Kuester's, v. 357
Chloroform (and see Anæsthetics) accidents and their treatment, iv. 201
　administration of, iv. 198–202

Chloroform and ether, their relative influence in producing shock, i. 479
　anæsthesia less dangerous in infants, i. 774
　anæsthesia, signs of complete, iv. 200
　signs of its being too deep, iv. 201
　signs of its being too light, iv. 201
　as an anæsthetic, its properties, and action when inhaled, iv. 197, 198
Chloroma, i. 342
Chlorosis, i. 241
Cholangitis, catarrhal, viii. 230
　suppurative, viii. 231
Cholecyst-duodenostomy, viii. 270
Cholecystectomy, viii. 264, 267
Cholecystendysis, viii. 268
Cholecystenterostomy, viii. 269
Cholecystitis, viii. 229
　catarrhal, viii. 230
　diagnosed from acute appendicitis, vii. 657
　membranous, viii. 233
　suppurative, viii. 230
Cholecystostomy, viii. 262, 267
Choledochenterostomy, viii. 275
Choledochotomy, viii. 271
　retroduodenal, viii. 272
　supraduodenal, viii. 271
　transduodenal, viii. 272
Choledochectomy, viii. 274
Choledochostomy, viii. 275
Cholelithiasis (and see Gall-stones), viii. 233
Cholesteatoma, i. 367
　of brain, v. 312
　of ear, v. 711
Cholesterin, i. 192
Chondral osteoma of metacarpal bone, iii. 423
Chondro-dystrophia, iii. 347, 414
Chondroma, i. 310, 313; iii. 418
　bones affected by, iii. 422
　changes due to place of origin, iii. 423
　degenerative changes in, iii. 424
　etiology of, iii. 419–422
　microscopical appearances of, iii. 424
　of external auditory canal, v. 681
　of finger, iii. 422
　of penis, vi. 687
　of pelvic bones, vii. 13
　of pelvis, iii. 428
　of pharynx, v. 854
　of sacrum, iii. 425
　of scapula, with statistics of operations, iii. 428
　of skull, iii. 429
　of tongue, vi. 256
　Virchow's division of them into ecchondromata and enchondromata, iii. 418, 419
Chondro-myxoma, i. 306
Chondro-myxo-sarcoma, i. 344
Chondro-sarcoma, i. 333, 344
Chopart's operation, procedure, and results, iv. 325

Chopart's operation for restoration of lower lip, iv. 660
　surgical anatomy, iv. 324, 352
Chordoma, i. 311; iii. 429
Chorio-epithelioma malignum, or deciduoma malignum, i. 368
　of uterus, viii. 674
Chromato-phoroma, i. 341
Chromidrosis, of eyelids, v. 550
Chylangiomata, i. 323
Cicatrices, Treves' classification of, iv. 268
　of face, v. 463
Cicatricial deformities, correction of. See Plastic surgery
Cicatricial tissue, formation of, i. 249, 252; ii. 166
　results of its contractility, ii. 167
Cicatrix, ii. 365
　conditions of, demanding treatment, ii. 366
Cigarette drains, iv. 539
Ciliary body, diseases of, v. 608
Circulation, cerebral, v. 105
　compensatory mechanism of, v. 108
　hydrostatics and hydrodynamics of, v 108
　disturbances of the, i 233
　mechanism of the, i. 233
Circulus articuli vasculosus, described, iii. 562
Circumcision, vi. 640
Circumtonsillar abscess, v. 818
Cirrhosis of liver, viii. 227
Cirsoid aneurysm, i. 321; vii. 259
Cittelli's bone punch, vi. 142
Civil obligation of surgeon and patient (and see Obligation, civil), viii. 713
Clamp and cautery operation for hemorrhoids, vii. 866
Clavicle and scapula, tuberculous disease of, iii. 601
Clavicle, deformities of, vi. 420
　diseases of, vi. 416
　dislocations of, iv. 31
　excision of, iv. 401, 402; vi. 417, 418
　habitual luxation of the inner end, iv. 33
　sarcoma of, iii. 459
　syphilis of, vi. 416
　tuberculosis of, vi. 416
　tumors of, vi. 416
　wiring of, under local anæsthesia, iv. 245
Clavus, ii. 346
　complicated with a synovial sac beneath, treatment of, ii. 348
　treatment, ii. 347, 348
Cleanliness, surgical, importance of, i. 272
Cleft palate, v. 500, 521
　acquired, v. 541
　age for operation, v 502, 521
　anatomical success after operation for, v. 529
　Brophy's method of operating for, v. 539
　chances of functional usefulness after operation for, v. 530

Cleft palate, control of hemorrhage in operation for, v 529
Davies-Colley's method of operation for, v. 532
Ferguson's operation for, v. 534
Fillebrown's method of operating for, v. 538
Lane's first operation for, v. 535
second operation for, v. 537, 538
Lannelongue's method of operating for, v. 532
mechanical appliances for, in new-born, vi. 19
Taylor's method, v. 538
use of obturators in, v. 531
Clergyman's sore throat, v. 815
Climacteric, the effect of, upon neoplasms, i. 780
Climate, influence of, upon results of surgical operations, i. 797
Clinical instruction, early efforts toward, i. 29
Clinocephalism, iii. 327
Cloudy swelling, i. 184
Clover's closed inhaler for ether, iv. 191
combined nitrous-oxide and ether inhaler, iv. 171
Club-foot (and see Talipes equinovarus), iv. 899
in infantile paralysis, iv. 815
Judson's modification of Taylor's brace for, iv. 910
Taylor's brace for, iv. 910
Taylor's shoe for, iv. 830, 831
Coal dust, cirrhosis anthracotica from inhaled, i. 208
Coal pigment, absence of, in lungs of infants, i. 208
Coaptation splints for fracture of the femur, iii. 170
Cobb's conclusions as to operative treatment of ununited fracture of the neck of the femur, iii. 177
Cocaine as used for local anæsthesia, iv. 232
as used for spinal anæsthesia, iv. 258
Coccygeal region, pendulous tumors of, vii. 15
Coccygodynia, iv. 28: vii. 31
Coccyx, dislocations of, iv. 28
excision of, vii. 33
Cochlea, surgical relations of, v. 773
Cœliotomy, vii. 106
Coffey, plication operation for shortening the round ligament, viii. 477
Cohnheim's development theory of tumor growth, i. 293
Coin-catcher, Graefe's, vii. 426
Cold, control of hemorrhage by, vii. 239
conditions influencing its effects upon the body, ii. 592
in treatment of simple inflammation, i. 113
Coley's fluid in malignant disease of pharynx, v. 860
Colic, appendicular, vii. 631
lead, diagnosed from acute appendicitis, vii. 661

College of Physicians and Surgeons, New York, when first organized, i. 11
Colles' law of syphilitic inheritance, ii. 96
or silver-fork fracture, iii. 149
Colliquative necrosis (red or yellow softening) of the brain, i. 239
Collodium as a dressing, iv. 537
Colloid struma, i. 347
Coloboma, v. 614
Colon, artificial distention of, in diagnosis of abdominal tumors, vii. 102
Color as furnishing diagnostic aid, i. 515
Colorectostomy, vii. 922
Colostomy, vii. 759, 855, 937
Colotomy, vii 106
Colporrhaphy, abdominal, Graves' method of, vi. 618
Colubrines, characterized, iii. 7
Compensatory hypertrophy of one limb with atrophic elongation of the bone in amputated stump of the other, iii. 338
Complexus muscle, anatomy of, iv. 788
Compound fractures, comparative mortality of, in civil and Spanish-American wars, ii. 743
of extremities, cases, operations, and deaths from, in Spanish-American war, ii 743
Compression, control of hemorrhage by, vii. 241
of brain (and see Brain, compression of), v. 111
in treatment of simple acute inflammation, i. 115
Concretions or calculi, i. 198
calcareous, of eyelids, v. 559
of Meibomian glands, v. 559
ceruminous, in external auditory canal. v. 683
Concussion of brain (and see Brain, concussion of the), v. 145
Condylomata, ii. 112
acuminata, i. 331: ii. 359
of vulva, vi. 568
as hyperplasiæ of connective tissue, i. 108
of the anus, ii. 360
of penis, vi. 688
syphilitic, of female genitals, vi. 565
Congelation or frost-bite, ii. 592
Congenital circumcision, vi. 686
cysts of pancreas, viii. 180
deformities, iv. 731
dislocations, iv. 731
genu recurvatum, iv. 765
malformations, x-ray appearances in, i. 686
torticollis, iv. 767
Congestion, passive, final results of, i. 236
gross appearances at seat of, i. 236
of ovary, viii. 401
Conical stump, iii. 332

Conjunctiva, argyrosis of, v. 582
burns of, treatment, v. 590
chancre of, v. 582
circumcorneal hypertrophy of, v. 581
cysticercus of, v. 584
cysts of, v. 584
dermoid tumor of, v. 584
ecchymosis of, v. 583
emphysema of, v. 584
essential atrophy of, v. 583
fibroma of, v. 584
foreign bodies in, v. 590
granulomata of, v. 584
hyperæmia of, v. 578
inflammation of (and see Conjunctivitis), v. 578
injuries of, v. 585
lipoma of, v. 584
treatment of, v. 590
lithiasis of, v. 584
lymphoma of, v. 581
œdema of, v. 584
operations upon, v. 594
osteoma of, v. 584
papillomata of, v. 584
pemphigus of, v. 583
sarcoma of, v. 584
tuberculosis of, v. 582
tumors of, v. 595
xerosis of, v. 583
Conjunctivitis (and see Ophthalmia)
acute contagious, v 578
catarrhal, v. 578
croupous, v. 581
diphtheritic, v. 581
exanthematous, v. 582
follicular, v. 580
granular v. 579
herpetic, v. 579
metastatic gonorrheal, v. 579
Parinaud's, v. 581
phlyctenular, v. 579
purulent, v. 579
syphilitic, v. 582
vernal, v. 581
vesicular, v. 579
Connective tissue, contusions of, ii. 455
Connell suture, vii. 736, 738, 754
gastro-enterostomy with, vii. 365
Consent of husband, wife, or parent, for operation, viii. 752, 753
of patient, necessary for operation, viii. 743. 747, 749
Conservatism in surgery, i. 692
Constipation, viii. 785
Consulting surgeon not in relation of surgeon and patient, viii. 716
Contagious diseases, hospitals for, viii. 892, 894
Contract between surgeon and patient, viii. 7-1
limited by public policy, viii. 722
to perform an impossible act, viii. 722
unaltered when services are gratuitous, viii. 723

Contract-surgeon in U. S. Army, viii. 904
Contracted foot, iv. 891
"Contre-coup" theory of cranial fractures, v. 64
Contusions of abdominal walls, vii. 91
  of arteries, vii. 208
  of brain, v. 172
  of chest, vi. 402
  of face, v. 423
  of joint, iii. 726, 758
  of liver, viii. 206
  of spine, vi. 422
  of veins, vii. 322
Conus medullaris, diseases and wounds of, vi. 501
Conus terminalis, diseases and wounds of, vi. 501
Convalescent camp, viii. 937
Cooper's (Sir Astley) method of reducing forward dislocations of the humerus, iv. 44
  method of treating dislocations backward of both bones at the elbow, iv. 55
Copperhead snake, iii. 9
Corectopia, v. 614
Corelysis, v. 621
Corn, ii. 346
Cornea, abrasions of, treatment of, v. 608
  cauterization of, v. 617
  congenital anomalies of, v. 604
  conical, v. 604
  dermoid cysts of, v. 604
  diseases of, v. 599
  fistula of, v. 606
  foreign bodies in, v. 608
  inflammation of (and see Keratitis), i. 76 v. 599
  injuries of, v. 599, 604
  maculæ of, v. 604, 605
  opacities of, v. 604
  operations upon, v. 616
  paracentesis of, v. 517
  perforating ulcers of, v. 619
  removal of foreign bodies from, v. 616
  staphyloma of, v. 604
  tattooing of, v. 619
  transplantation of, v. 619
  ulcer of, v. 599
  wound of, v. 604
Corneal wound, suppuration of, after cataract operations, v. 635
Cornification, i. 193
Cornu cutaneum, v. 485
Coronoid process of the ulna, fractures of, iii. 142
Corpus luteum, cysts of, viii. 403
Corsets, for Pott's disease, iv. 975
Corson's case of excessive bone atrophy, following fracture, iii. 213, 214
Cortex, excito-motor, v. 268
  motor, v. 269
  sensory, v. 270
Cortical areas, concerned with hearing, v .272
  smell, v. 273
  speech, v. 273
  taste, v. 273

Cortical areas, vision, v. 272
  centres, v. 268
Costo-transversectomy. vi. 449
Cotton as a dressing, i. 719
Couching, for cataract, v. 632
Councilman's experiments on the production of pus i. 253
Counter-irritants in treatment of acute simple inflammation, i. 114
Cowperitis, vi. 753
Cowper s glands, vi. 632
Coxa valga, iv. 857
Coxa vara iv. 848
  bilateral iv. 850, 851, 852
  cervical. iv. 849, 851
  epiphyseal, iv. 850
  in congenital dislocation of hip, iv. 751
  latent. iv. 849
  physical effects, iv. 850
  relation to rickets, iii. 350
Coxalgic pelvis, vii. 4
Cranial atrophy, v. 25
  bones, diffuse hypertrophy of (and see Leontiasis ossea), v. 26
  disturbances in the growth of, v. 25
  surgical affections of (and see Cranium, and Skull), v. 25
  syphilitic lesions of, iii. 367–375
  syphilitic necrosis of, v. 42
  defects, closure of, v. 366
  gumma, v. 40
  injuries, hyperalgesic zones in, v. 98
  late effects of, v. 285
  nerves, lesions of, in fractures of skull, v. 76
  surgery of the, v. 379
  soft parts (and see Scalp), v. 3
  gangrene of, v. 23
  infectious granulomata of, v. 24
  neuralgic affections of, v. 23
  tumors of, v. 11
  wounds of, v. 4
  syphilis. v. 36
Cranio-cerebral topography, v. 360
  Kroenlein's method, v. 362
  Taylor and Houghton's method, v. 363
  Rolandic fissure, v. 362, 363
  Sylvian fissure, v. 362, 363
  ventricular puncture, v. 365
Craniosclerosis, iii. 397
Cranio-tabes, iii. 349
  of rickets, v. 25
Cranium, actinomycosis of, v. 47
  diffuse hyperostosis of the bones of, v. 27
  effusions of blood within, v. 175
  glanders of, v. 47
  pneumatocele of, v. 11
  tuberculosis of, v. 44
Cretinism, vi. 392
  an imperfect growth from athyroidea, i. 163
  experimental, iii. 327, 328
  fœtal, iii. 349
  sporadic, vi. 392

Crile's pneumatic suit in treatment of surgical shock, i. 496
Criminal malpractice, viii. 763
Critchett's abscission operation, v. 618
Croft's method of flap transfer in p.astic surgery. iv. 619
  splints iii. 199–203
Crossed sciatic phenomenon, vii. 35
Crotalidæ or pit vipers, iii. 9
Crotaius adamanteus, the diamond rattler, iii. 9
  horridus the banded rattlesnake iii. 9
Crushes of ankle, iii. 758
  of penis, vi. 664
Cryer's spiral osteotome, v. 355
Cryoscopy of the blood, and the urine, in investigating the kidney, viii. 84
Cryptorchidia, vi. 660
Crystalline and amorphous urinary deposits, their relation to calculi, i. 571
Cuneiform bones, dislocations of, iv. 102
  osteotomy of, for talipes, iv. 94
Cupping, iv. 604
Curvature of legs, anterior, iv. 867
  of spine, angular (and see Pott's disease), iv. 927
Cushing, Harvey, work of, on cerebral compression, v. 116, 138
  method of exploring, for brain abscess, v. 804
  "morphia-cocaine-chloroform" combination for anæsthesia, iv. 238
  right-angle suture, vii. 738, 754
  technique for operations on inguinal hernia, iv. 255
  and Lexer's method of operation, intracranial, upon the trigeminal nerve, v. 397
Cutaneous gangrene, treatment of, ii. 270
  horn of auricle, v. 675
Cut-throat, v. 866; vi. 326
Cyclitis, v. 609
Cylindroma, sarcomatous, i. 340
Cyphose Hérédo-Traumatique, vi. 459
Cyst, or Cysts
  after herniotomy, vii. 592
  arachnoid, v. 181
  branchial, vi. 315
  branchiogenic, multilocular, vi. 317
  contents, microscopical and chemical examinations required for diagnosis, i. 576
  dentigerous, of antrum, vi. 158, 830
  of jaw, vi. 837
  operations for, vi. 867
  dental-root, of jaw, vi. 835
  operations for, vi. 867
  dermoid, lingual, vi. 396
  of mouth, vi. 261
  of neck, vi. 315
  of penis, vi. 637
  of prepuce, vi. 637
  of scrotum. vi. 658

Cyst, dermoid, of temporal fossa, vi. 865
of testis, vi. 697
of tongue, vi. 261
hydatid, of abdominal wall, vii. 89
of liver, viii. 214
of auricle, v. 674
of Bartholin's glands, vi. 565
of biliary ducts, viii. 252
of breast, female, vi. 526
of cerebellum, v. 312, 314
of conjunctiva, v. 584
of cornea, v. 604
of corpus luteum, viii. 403
of ethmoid sinus, vi. 851
of face, dermoid, v. 482
of face, echinococcus, v. 480
of face, mucous, v. 479
of face, sebaceous, v. 480
of face, sequestration, v. 482
of Graafian follicle, viii. 403
of hydatids of Morgagni, vi. 697
of iris, v. 613
of kidney, viii. 137
of lachrymal gland, v. 592
of liver, viii 219
multiple congenital, i. 253
of lower eyelid, with microphthalmos or anophthalmos, v. 554
of mesentery, vii. 751
of middle turbinated bone, vi. 859
of mouth, mucous, non-parasitic, vi. 243
of nasopharynx, vi. 860
of neck, vi. 347
of œsophagus, vii. 420
of omentum, vii. 748
of orbit, v. 651, 652
of organ of Giraldès, vi. 697
of ovary (and see Tumors of ovary), viii. 402, 423
of pancreas, viii. 180
of penis, sebaceous, vi. 687
of pharynx, v. 810
of prostate, viii. 367
of salivary glands, vi. 309
of scalp (and see Wens), v. 13, 14
of scrotum, vi. 695
of seminal vesicles, vi. 698
of skull, v. 28
of spleen, viii. 70
of testis, vi. 697
of thymus, vi. 398
of tongue, vi. 243
of urachus, vii. 80
of ureter, viii. 145
of urethra, vi. 695
of vas deferens, vi. 698
of vermiform appendix, vii. 624
of vulva, vi. 565, 566
parovarian, viii. 429
peri-pancreatic, viii. 181
sacro-coccygeal, vii. 20
spinal, vi. 500
subconjunctival, treatment of, v. 595
tooth, vi. 196
tubo-ovarian, viii. 409

Cystadenoma atheromatosum, i. 348
mucosum, i. 348
of female breast (and see Mastitis, chronic), vi. 514, 524
of jaw, iii. 474
of ovary, i. 352; viii. 423
Cystadeno-fibroma, i. 304
Cystic carcinoma, iii. 474
chondro-sarcoma of the femur, iii. 421
disease of female breast (and see Mastitis, chronic), vi. 514
duct, viii. 198
gall stones in, viii. 238
epithelial odontoma, section of wall of, iii. 475
follicles of ovary, viii. 402
kidney, congenital, viii. 137
middle turbinate, vi. 98
oxide calculi, viii. 113
tumors of brain, v. 308
of orbit, v. 651
Cysticercus telæ cellulosæ, ii. 396
bladders in the skin, diagnosis of, ii. 396
disease of bone, iii. 484
of conjunctiva, v. 584
of eyelids, v. 554
of iris, v. 613
of orbit, v. 652
Cystitis, viii. 292
diphtheritic, viii. 295
dolorosa, viii. 300
exfoliative, viii. 295
gangrenous, viii. 295
gonorrhœal, vi. 745
membranous, viii. 295
œdema bullosum, viii. 295
post-operative, iv. 159
septic, viii. 294
subacute catarrhal, viii. 294
suppurative, viii. 294
Cystocele, vi. 608
Cystoid cicatrix, after cataract operations, v. 636
Cystoids of pancreas, viii. 181
Cystomata, i. 350, 351
and cysts, the distinction between, i. 350
glandular type of, i. 451
of auricle, v. 674
of kidney, i. 353
of larynx, v. 881
of pharynx, v. 855
of rectum, vii. 896
ovarian, i. 351
papilliferous, i. 352, 451
Cysto-sarcoma of breast, female, vi. 523
Cystoscopy, viii. 330
combined with litholapaxy, viii. 335
Cystotomy, viii. 323
Czerny's operation for restoring the cheek, iv. 643
for saddle nose, iv. 710
suture, vii. 734
Czerny-Lembert enterorrhaphy, vii. 735
method of lateral anastomosis, vii. 749
Czerwinski's operation for saddle nose, iv. 715

DACRYOADENITIS, v. 592
Dacryocystitis, v. 592
Dacryoliths, v. 592
Dacryops, v 592
Dactylitis, strumous, iii. 579
syphilitic, x-ray features of, i. 670
Damages, award of, in surgical malpractice, viii. 807
Dark-room for developing x-ray photographs, i. 621
Darnall, Captain Carl R., on Simple and Infected Wounds of the Soft Parts by cutting and piercing instruments, ii. 605
Dartmouth College, Hanover, N. H., medical department of, organized, i. 21
Davidge, John B., i. 47
Davies-Colley's method of operating for cleft palate, v. 532
Deafness, viii. 979
Death of a limited part, the signs of, ii. 203
somatic, as distinguished from necrobiosis and necrosis, i. 209
Decinormal salt-solution in the treatment of septicæmia and pyæmia, i. 443
Decompression of brain, in cerebral tumors, v. 338, 339
occipital operation for, v. 371
temporal operation for, v. 370
Decortication, in empyema, viii. 11
pulmonary, viii. 53
Decubitus or bedsore, i. 137; ii. 180, 297
Defects, congenital, of face, v. 495
macrostoma, v. 495
microstoma, v. 495
nasal deformities, v. 496
unilateral hypertrophy, v. 497
cranial, closure of, v. 366
Wolff-Koenig method, v. 367
Deformities and disabilities of the lower extremities, iv 848-926
congenital, of sacro-coccygeal region, vii. 14
nasal, rare, v. 496
of chest wall, vi. 406
of clavicle, vi. 420
of jaws, vi. 890
of nose, vi. 67
of œsophagus, vii. 410
of pelvis, bony, vii. 3
of ribs, vii. 408
of stomach, due to dilatation, vii. 335
of thoracic wall, vi. 401
resulting from epiphysitis, operative treatment of, iii. 313
de Trey's somnoforme inhaler, iv. 207, 208
De Gaetano's method of arteriorrhaphy, vii. 255
Degeneration, i. 182
and infiltration, distinction between, i. 183
Warthin's classification of, i. 183
colloid, i 190

Degeneration, distinguished from atrophy, i. 182
glycogenous, i. 194
hydropic, i. 190
mucinous, i. 191, 192
physiological and pathological, i. 182
reaction of, i. 543
Degenerative and necrotic inflammations, acute, i. 134
Delair's artificial glottis, vi. 32
Delanger's method of prosthesis, iv. 625
Delayed union, after cataract operations, v. 636
Delhi sore, i. 231; ii. 342
DeLorme and Mignon's operation, pericardotomy, vii. 158
Delpech's method of rhinoplasty, iv. 683
Deltoid paralysis, iii. 735
Demon's method of repair of septum, iv. 704
de Nancrède, Charles G. B., on Surgical Diseases, certain Abnormities, and Wounds of the Face, v. 417-499
on influences and conditions which should be taken into account before one decides to operate, iv. 107
Denonvillier's operation for restoration of alæ, iv. 694
Dental corps, of U. S. Army, viii. 904
prosthesis, v. 5
-root cyst of jaw, vi. 835
Dentigerous cysts, iii. 476
of antrum, vi. 830
Dentures, artificial, vi. 8
restoration of function by, vi. 10
De Page's operation for saddle nose, iv. 709
Deposits, i. 184
Derbyshire neck (and see Goitre), vi. 358
Dermatitis, acute, as distinguished from erysipelas, i. 449
malignant papillary, of breast (and see Paget's disease of the nipple), vi. 556
papillaris capillitii, ii. 370
x-ray, chronic, vii. 39
Dermatolysis, explanation of the term, ii. 371
Dermoid cysts, i. 367, 368
of brain, v. 312
of cerebellum, v. 312, 314
of conjunctiva, v. 584
of cornea, v. 604
of mouth, vi. 261
of neck, vi. 315
of orbit, v. 651
of ovary, viii. 427
of penis, vi. 637
of prepuce, vi. 637
of pharynx, v. 810
of scalp, v. 14
of scrotum, vi. 658
of spleen, viii. 70
of temporal fossa, vi. 865
of testis, vi. 697
of tongue, vi. 261

Dermoids, branchial, vi. 315
extra-rectal, vii. 896
lingual, vi. 396
post-rectal, vii. 18
Desault's method of treating fractures of the femur, i. 51
operation for salivary fistula, v. 444
sign, iii. 162
Descemetitis, v. 603
Descensus of ovary, viii. 398
Desiccation, as associated with gangrene, ii. 204
Desmoid tumors, of abdominal wall, vii. 83
post-operative, complicating femoral hernia, vii. 591
Detmold, William, i. 55
De Vilbiss bone forceps, vi. 135
Diabetes, as influencing the choice of anæsthetics, iv. 222
effect of, upon surgical procedures and conditions, i. 794
Diabetic gangrene (and see also Gangrene), ii. 231
Diacetic acid in the urine of diabetics an unfavorable prognostic sign, i. 794
Diagnosis, general surgical, i. 501
Diapedesis in inflammation, i. 85
Diaphragm, anatomy of, vii. 450
congenital defects of, vii. 457
degeneration of, vii. 460
displacement of, vii. 460
eventration of, vii. 459
hernia of, vii. 458, 460, 612
infection of, modes of, vii. 451
lymphatics of, vii. 451
phenomenon, Litten's, i. 529; vii. 467
surgical diseases of, vii. 450
Diaphragmatic pleurisy, diagnosed from acute appendicitis, vii. 659
Diastasis, defined, iii. 65
of distal end of the fibula iv. 94
of head of the ulna, iv. 64
of lower epiphysis of the femur, iv. 88
Diathesis, influence of, upon surgical conditions, i. 781
Diday's operation for webbed fingers, iv. 635, 636
Didot's operation for webbed fingers, iv. 635
Dieffenbach's method of blepharoplasty, iv. 674; v. 572
of flap formation, in plastic operations, iv. 615
of repair of septum, iv. 704
of restoring the alæ, iv. 697
of rhinoplasty, iv. 681, 688
of treating saddle nose, iv. 707
operation for ectropion, iv 669, 670
for restoration of lower lip, iv. 654
for saddle nose, iv. 714
Digestive system, its diagnostic importance, i. 516
Digital compression to prevent hemorrhage, iv. 267

Dilatation, idiopathic, of œsophagus, vii. 444
of œsophagus, for strictures, vii. 430
for carcinoma, vii. 416
of stomach, deformity due to, vii. 335
of urethra, vi. 647
Dilators, urethral, vi. 787
Dimples, postanal, vii. 897
sacro-coccygeal, vii. 20
Diphtheritic inflammation, i. 118
Bacillus diphtheriæ a cause of, i. 135
epithelial, or superficial, i. 135
intestinal, i. 135
streptococcus as a cause of, i. 135
paralysis, diagnosed from infantile paralysis, iv. 824
Disarticulation at ankle-joint (Syme's operation), iv. 329
at hip-joint by antero-posterior flaps, cut by transfixion, iv. 353
Lister's procedure, iv. 357
Lloyd's method of controlling hemorrhage, iv. 351
McBurney's method of controlling hemorrhage, iv. 351
precautions against shock, iv. 351
Senn's bloodless method, iv. 355
surgical anatomy, iv. 350
through an anterior racquet incision, iv. 358
through an external racquet incision, iv. 356, 357
Trendelenburg's method of controlling hemorrhage, iv. 352
at knee-joint, by the elliptical method (Bauden's operation), iv. 345
by lateral flaps (Stephen Smith), iv. 344
by a long anterior flap (Pollock's operation), iv. 345
at medio-tarsal joint (Chopart's operation), iv. 324
at metacarpo-phalangeal joint, the oval method, the method by equal lateral flaps, iv. 283, 284
at wrist-joint, elliptical operation, iv. 288
long palmar flap, iv. 287
of anterior portion of foot at the tarso-metatarsal joint (Lisfranc's operation), iv. 320
of great toe at the metatarso-phalangeal joint, iv 314
terminal phalanx, iv. 313
together with its metatarsal bone, instruments needed, iv. 317
of little toe, together with its metatarsal bone, iv. 318

Disarticulation of phalangeal joints, exceptions as to removal of proximal phalanx, iv. 283
first (surgical), two methods, iv. 282
of toes at the metatarso-phalangeal joints, iv. 315
of second, third, or fourth toe, with its respective metatarsal bone, iv. 319
of two toes, together with their metatarsal bones, iv. 319
subastragaloid, surgical anatomy, iv. 326
with a heel flap, iv. 327
Discission, for cataract, v. 627
in empyema, viii. 13
Disinfectants, chemical, in skin disinfection, i. 705
Disinfection and sterilization, i. 701
Dislocations, i. 47
as distinguished from diastasis, iv 3
basis of Malgaigne's classification of, iv. 5
by Emmet Rexford, iv. 3
congenital (and see Congenital deformities), iv. 9, 731
congenital elevation of scapula, iv. 735
congenital genu recurvatum, iv. 765
etiology, iv. 731
obstetrical paralysis of shoulder, iv. 738
of ankle, iv. 766
of carpus, iv. 742
of elbow, iv. 741
of hip, iv. 746
of humerus, iv. 738
of patella, iv. 765
of shoulder, iv. 738
of trunk, iv. 735
of wrist, iv. 742
Kirmisson's theory of, iv. 734
Stimson's theory of, iv. 734
Young's theory of, iv. 734
definition of term, iv. 3
habitual, iv. 4
importance of x-ray examination in diagnosis of, iv. 16
of acromio-clavicular joint, pathology, iv. 34
of ankle, rotary, iv. 96, 97
of astragalus, treatment, iv 101
of atlas, treatment, iv. 24
of carpus, iv. 65
of clavicle, iv. 31-36
total, iv. 33
of coccyx, iv. 28
of cuneiform bones, iv. 102
of eyeball, v. 656
of elbow, iv. 50
operation devised by Murphy, of Chicago, to secure mobility, iv. 63
of fibula, upper end of the, iv. 88
of fingers, iv. 67-71
of foot, iv. 94
of hip, iv. 71-85
of humerus, iv. 36

Dislocations of individual joints, iv. 18
of knee-joint, iv. 85
of larynx, v. 864
of lens, v. 626
of lower jaw, iv. 29-31
of medio-tarsal joint (Chopart's), iv. 99
of metacarpal bones, iv. 67
of metatarsus and toes, iv. 103
of occipito-atlantal and atlanto-axial articulations, iv. 20-23
of occiput, treatment, iv. 24
of patella, iv. 91-94
of pelvis, iv. 27
of penis, vi. 665
of radio-ulnar joint, distal, iv. 64
of radius alone at the elbow, treatment, iv. 60
of ribs, iv. 28
of scaphoid, iv. 67 (navicular), iv. 102
of semilunar bone, iv. 66
of semilunar cartilages, iv. 89
of semilunar cartilages, treatment, iv. 90
of shoulder-joint, associated with fracture, operative treatment of, iv. 401
of spinal column, vi. 429
of sterno-clavicular joint, anatomical considerations, iv. 31, 32
(both), iv. 32
subastragaloid, treatment, iv. 99
of tarsal bones, individual, iv. 100
of tarsus, classification of, iv. 94
of thumb, iv. 68-71
of tibia backward, iv. 86
of vertebræ, iv. 18
of wrist, iv 64, 65
old, iv. 5
unreduced, as indications for excision of the elbow-joint, von Eiselberg's operation, iv. 410
Displacement of brain, v. 369
of Fallopian tube, viii. 398
of ovaries, viii. 398
of uterus, viii. 454
Distichiasis, v. 559
Distortions of spine, vi. 422
Diverticula, acquired (of intestines), vii. 703
of œsophagus, vii. 439
Diverticulitis, vii. 934
of sigmoid, vii. 703
Diverticulum ilei, vii. 701
Meckel's, vii. 701, 708
Dodd, Walter J., i. 599
Doellinger's statistical report on treatment of cases of old subcoracoid dislocation, iv. 48
Dolichocephalism, iii 327
Dorrance's method of arteriorrhaphy, vii. 255
Dorsey, John Syng, i. 17, 34, 45
"Elements of Surgery," by, i. 34
Double lip, v. 477
monsters, vii. 16
penis, vi. 637

Double ureters, viii. 89
urethra, vi. 648
vagina, vi. 579
Douglas, semilunar fold of, vii. 111
Dowd, Charles N., on Surgical Diseases and Wounds of Lymph Nodes and Vessels, ii. 525
Doyen's burrs, in cerebral operations, v. 353
panhysterectomy, viii. 565
Dracuncular ulcer, i. 231
Drainage by rubber tissue and tubes and by glass tubes, iv. 540
gastric, interference with, vii. 334
materials and methods of, now approved, i. 762
materials, their preparation, medication, and mode of employment, iv. 139, 142
objections to it, and conditions where indicated, i. 764
of urinary bladder, viii. 325, 326
secondary, i. 765
various methods employed and the results, i. 763
Drainage tubes, viii. 326
Draper, William H., i. 16
Dressing stations in military service, viii. 955, 957
Dressings, surgical, iv. 537
after closing a wound, i. 754
and their use at operations, iv. 142
Dry heat, the "baking" process, i. 767
Dubois's abscess of thymus, vi. 398
Ducrey-Unna bacillus, characteristics of, vi. 700
Duct cancer, of breast, female, vi. 536
Ductulus aberrans, vi. 630
Dudley, Benjamin W., i. 25
Duell's operation for malposition of auricle, v. 664
Dugas' posture test in the diagnosis between a fracture and a dislocation of the shoulder, iii. 127
Duodenal hernia, vii. 610
sphincter, the, vii. 392
Duodeno-choledochotomy, vii. 273
Duodenum, peptic ulcer of, vii. 713
perforation of, vii. 717
Duplay's method of operating upon displaced intermaxillary bone, v 520
Dupuytren's apparatus for fractures of the leg, iii. 198
method of restoring the alæ, iv. 697
operation for repair of septum, iv. 703
operation for shoulder joint amputation, iv. 307
suture, vii. 738
Dura mater, cerebral, anatomy of, v. 173
endothelioma of, v. 286
sinuses of, v. 174
Dural sinuses, thrombosis of the, v. 247
aseptic, v. 247

Dural sinuses, thrombosis of the, septic, v. 248
Durand's operation, pericardotomy, vii. 158
Duret's theory of concussion of the brain, v. 153
Dust, inhalation of, protection against, i. 208
Dusting powders as dressings, i. 722
Duval's supramalleolar amputation of the leg, iv. 335, 336
Dwarfing (general), micromanosomia, and cretinism, iii. 326
Dysdiæmorrhysis, definition of, v. 107
Dysentery, causing ulceration of rectum, vii. 794
Dyspnœa, the requirements of anæsthetics in, iv. 222
Dystrophy, muscular, diagnosed from infantile paralysis, iv. 826

Ear (and see Auditory canal, Aural, Auricle, Labyrinth, Mastoid, Membrana tympani, Ossiculectomy, Otitis, Sinus thrombosis, Synechtomy)
adherent lobule, iv. 721
angioma of, v. 672
artificial, iv. 728; vi. 27
bleeding from, in fracture of the skull, v. 73
brain disease following disease of, v. 779
Cheyne and Burghard's plastic operation on, iv. 722
cholesteatoma of, v. 711
cicatricial contraction of external, iv. 722
damage to, in naval service, viii. 979
deformities of, acquired and congenital, iv. 718
erysipelas of, v. 671
exostoses of auditory canal, iii. 404
gangrene of, v. 671
Gersuny's operation in external, iv. 724
hæmatoma of (and see Othæmatoma), v. 666
handle-shaped, v. 663
inflammation of. See Otitis
large, treatment of, v. 662
middle, v. 686
normal, iv. 717, 718
outstanding, iv. 721, 722
Parkhill's plastic operation on, iv. 722
plastic operations for formation of new lobule of, v. 677
Gavello's method, v. 677
Nélaton's method, v. 678
plastic surgery of, iv. 717
prominent, iv. 723, 725
pyogenic diseases of brain due to, v. 779
shape of, iv. 725, 727
surgical diseases and wounds of, v. 660
synechiæ of, v 714
wounds of, v 660, 666
Ear-protector, Elliott's, viii. 980, 981

Earle, Samuel T., and Tuttle, James P., on Surgical Diseases and Wounds of the Anus and Rectum, vii. 761–948
Earle's hemorrhoidal clamp, vii. 873
method of operating for hemorrhoids, vii. 872
rectal speculum, vii. 768
Eburnation, iii. 264, 266, 366
from tuberculous disease, iii. 579
Echinococcus disease of bones, iii. 482, 483
cysts of biliary ducts, viii. 252
of breast, female, vi. 528
of chest wall, vi. 411
of face, v. 480
of liver, viii. 214
of lung, viii. 27
of neck, vi. 348
of pelvic bones, vii. 13
of pleura, viii. 15
of prostate, viii. 367
of skin, ii. 397
of sternum, vi. 411
of thyroid, vi. 372
of tongue, vi. 243
Ecchondromata, i. 311; iii. 419
of larynx, iv. 881
Ecchondrosis physalifera, of Virchow, i. 311
Ecchondrosis prolifera (and see physalifera) (Virchow), iii. 429
Ecchymosis in nasopharynx, in fracture of skull, v. 72
of conjunctiva, v. 583
of eyelids, v. 557
Eckstein's method of prosthesis, iv 625
Ectopia testis, vii. 660
vesicæ, vi. 636; viii. 282
Ectopic gestation (and see Extrauterine pregnancy), viii. 690
Ectropion, v. 560
of the uvea, v. 614
operations for, v 565
senile, v. 560
spasmodic, v. 560
Eczema of eyelids, v. 548
of nipple, vii. 507
Edebohls' operation for fixation of kidney, viii. 154
Effusions into the body cavities, effects of, i. 238
Ejaculatory ducts, anatomy of, vi. 632
Elapidæ, Indian and American subfamilies, iii. 8
Elbow-joint, amputation by anterior elliptical flap, iv. 296
by large anterior flap, iv. 296
by large external flap, iv. 297
by posterior elliptical flap, iv. 297
lines of incision formerly proposed by Brasdor, iv. 297
surgical anatomy, iv. 294, 295
as affected by hypertrophic arthritis, iii. 525
congenital dislocation of, iv. 741
dislocations of, iv. 50

Elbow-joint, elliptical disarticulation of, iv. 271
erasion of, with report of an operation, iv. 417, 418
excision of, ii. 749; iv. 407–417
fractures of, iii. 132
infantile paralysis of, iv. 818
its development studied by radiographs, i. 582
penetrating wounds of, iii. 737
sprains of, iii. 737
tuberculous disease of, iii. 607
Elder, John M., on Surgical Diseases and Wounds of the Neck, vi. 313–352
Electric currents, effects of, ii. 588
Elephantiasis, i. 108, 305, 321
as caused by Filaria sanguinis hominis, ii. 576
mollis of scalp, v. 16
nervorum of scalp, v. 16
of eyelids, v. 554
of gluteal region, vii. 31
of penis, vi. 676
of scrotum, vi. 676
of vulva, vi. 563
Elevation, control of hemorrhage by, vii. 240
Elliott's ear protector, viii. 980, 981
position in abdominal surgery, vii. 122
Embolectomy, vii. 220
"Embolia insensibilis," vii. 191
Embolic aneurysm, vii. 186
Embolus, viii. 183
air, vii. 195
fat, vii. 199
pulmonary, vii. 190
seat of impaction of, vii. 184
source of, vii. 183
Embryoid tumors or embryomata, i. 366
Emergency chest (railroad), contents of, viii. 1042
Emmet's denuding scissors, vi. 588
operation for lacerated perineum, vi. 599
round-eyed, half-curved cervix needle, vii. 587
Emprosthotonus in tetanus, i. 457
Emphysema, of conjunctiva, v. 584
of eyelids, v. 557
of mediastinum, viii. 31
of orbit, v. 640
of penis, vi. 680
of scalp, v. 11
of scrotum, vi. 680
pulmonary, viii. 23, 24
Empyema, i. 128; viii. 6
as distinguished from abscess, ii. 143
combined, of accessory sinuses, vi. 87
decortication in, viii. 11, 53
thoracoplasty in, viii. 52
discission in, viii. 13
inveterata, viii. 11
necessitatis, viii. 7
Thiersch's method of drainage in, viii. 49
tuberculosum, iii. 573
vesical, viii. 230
Encephalitis, v. 250

Encephalitis, cortical, v. 794
Encephalocele, v. 213
Encephalo-cystocele, v. 213
Encephalo - cysto - meningocele, v. 213
Enchondroma, i. 311, 312; iii. 419
  of breast, female, vi. 529
  of chest wall, vi. 413
  of epididymis, vi. 696
  of rectum, vii. 891
  of scrotum, vi. 695
  of testis, vi. 696
  producing metastases, i. 312
Endarteritis, chronic, vii. 204
  progressive, of alcoholics, ii. 226
Endoaneurysmorrhaphy, vii. 281
Endocervicitis, gonorrhœal, vi. 561
Endostoma, iii. 405
Endothelial cells, active functions of, in inflammation, i. 86
Endothelioma, i. 338, 339, 340
  of bone, iii. 469-471
  of brain, v. 303
  of dura mater, v. 286
  of kidney, viii. 134
  of liver, viii. 219
  of mediastinum, viii. 14, 34
  of mouth, vi. 253
  of ovary, viii. 429
  of pleura, viii. 14
  of scalp, v. 18
  of tongue, vi. 253
  of urachus, vii. 81
  of uterus, viii. 674
  of vermiform appendix, vii. 625
Endothelium, vascular, its secretory powers important factors in the occurrence of œdemas, i. 236
Endurance, power of, greater in women, i. 777
Enophthalmos, v. 656
Enostoses, i. 314
Entero-anastomosis, Bacon's method of, vii. 854
Enteroclysis, in abdominal surgery, vii. 119
Enteroplasty, vii. 753, 757
Enterorrhaphy, vii. 755, 757
  Czerny-Lembert method, vii. 735
  Connell suture in, vii. 739
Enterostomy, vii. 758
Entodermal cysts, i. 367
Entropion, v. 560
  acute, v. 560
  cicatricial, v. 560
  senile, v. 560
  spasmodic, v. 560
Environment as furnishing contraindications to operating, iv. 108
  influence of, upon surgical prognosis, i. 795
Eosinophilia, i. 246
Eosinophilic marrow cells found in blood in myelocytic leukæmia, i. 243
Epiblastic structures, i. 299
Epicanthus, v 561
Epidermoid cysts, i. 367
  of bone, iii. 478
Epididymis, anatomy of, vi. 629
  enchondroma of, vi. 696

Epididymis, inflammation of, vi. 669
  syphilis of, ii. 126
  tuberculosis of, vi. 672
  tumors of, vi. 696
Epididymo-orchitis, tuberculous, vi. 672
Epiglottis (and see Pharynx)
  congenital deformities of, v. 811
  lupus of, v. 879
Epilepsy, v. 292
  classification, v. 292
  essential, v. 293
  idiopathic, v. 297
    excision of sympathetic ganglia for, v. 299
  Jacksonian, v. 293
  non-traumatic, v. 297
  reflex, treatment, v. 294
  traumatic, with generalized convulsions, v. 296
Epiphora, treatment of, v. 592
Epiphyseal fractures of the lower end of the femur, iii. 181
  injury of the elbow-joint as indication for excision, iv. 411
  irritation, for infantile paralysis, iv. 845
  separation of the trochanter major, iii. 165
Epiphyses, atavistic, iii. 562
  of new-born child invisible in radiograph, i. 579
  pressure, iii. 562
  radiographic interpretation of, i. 578
  traction, iii. 562
Epiphysitis, acute, iii. 277, 311
  as distinguished from tuberculous disease, iii. 699
  suppurative type, iii. 268
Epiplopexy, viii. 227
Episcleral tissue, diseases of the, v. 590
Episcleritis, v. 590
Epispadias, vi. 654
  Thiersch's operation for, vi. 656
  von Dieffenbach's operation for, vi. 655
  in female, vi. 579
Epistaxis, vi. 52
Epithelial cells in urine, i. 570
  defect in covering wounds, i. 274
  growths, atypical, i. 355
  pearls or cell-nests, i. 357
  plugs in external auditory canal, v. 685
  structures of typical growth, i. 354
  tumors of bone, iii. 478
    metastatic, iii. 479
    primary, iii. 478
    secondary, iii. 479
Epithelioma, ii. 373
  adamantine, of jaw, vi. 841
  adenoides cysticum, ii. 349
  basal cell, of gum, vi. 847
  deep-seated nodular, ii. 380
  malignant spinous-cell of gum, vi. 847
  metaplasia of, i. 358
  of auricle, v. 676

Epithelioma of conjunctiva, v. 584
  of eyelids, v. 551
  of face, v. 488, 490, 491
  of gluteal region, vii. 31
  of larynx, v. 886
  of orbit, v. 652
  of pharynx, v. 857
  of prostate, viii. 355
  of rectum, vii. 899
  of scalp, v. 21
  of tongue, vi. 263
  of umbilicus, vii. 90
  papillary, ii. 379
  spinocellulare malignum, of gum, vi. 847
  superficial, its mode of development, ii. 376
  transformed into sarcoma by transplantations, i. 397
Epitheliomatosis, senile multiple, ii. 380
Epitheliomatous transformation of chronic ulcers, i. 231
Epithelium, its power of regeneration, i. 257
Epulis, i. 336; iii. 457; vi. 816, 818
Equinia, ii. 332
Erasion or arthrectomy, in the treatment of tuberculous joint disease, iii. 590
  of elbow-joint, iv. 417, 418
  of knee-joint, iv. 453, 454
  term defined, iv. 368
Ericson's spine, vi. 422
Erysipelas, i. 445; iii. 15
  as related to pyæmia, i. 450
  bullosum, i. 130
  curative influence of, on other diseases, i. 453
  due to Streptococcus erysipelatis or Streptococcus pyogenes, iii. 16
  facial, iii. 19
  gangrenous, i. 449
  habitual, iii. 17
  infectiousness of, i. 446
  migrans or ambulans, i. 447
  neonatorum, iii. 20
  of auricle, v. 671
  of ear, v. 671
  of eyelids, v. 547
  of face, v. 448
  of larynx, v. 870
  of mucous membranes, iii. 20
  of neck, vi. 340
  phlegmonous, i. 447; iii. 19
  traumatic, special features of, i. 449
Erythema contusiformis, ii. 390
  gangrænosum, ii. 269
  induratum, ii. 323
  nodosum, ii. 389
  of eyelids, v. 547
  simulating an erysipelatous dermatitis, i. 449
Erythromelalgia, ii. 509
Eschricht and Berg's theory of origin of talipes, iv. 898
Esmarch's amputation at hip-joint, iv. 358
  bandage, i. 741
    application of, iv. 597

Esmarch's double-inclined plane in the treatment of fractures of the shaft of the femur, iii. 180

rubber bandage and elastic tourniquet to prevent hemorrhage, advantages and disadvantages, iv. 266

Estlander's operation for restoration of lower lip, iv. 663

thoracoplasty, viii 52 '

Ether, administration of, by open method, iv. 186

by semi-open method, details of the procedure, iv. 187-191

as an adjuvant in disinfection, i. 708

methods of administering, for anæsthesia, iv. 186

properties and effects of inhalation, iv. 184

per rectum, iv. 173

pneumonia, its prophylaxis and treatment, iv. 229, 230

Etherization, accidents, treatment by artificial respiration, iv. 196

by close method, advantages and disadvantages, iv. 193

Ethmoid sinus, cysts of, vi. 851

Ethmoidal cells, applied anatomy of, vi. 90

anterior ethmoidal cells, vi. 93

ethmoidal bulla, vi. 93

ethmoidal labyrinth, vi. 90

in middle turbinate, vi. 98

middle meatus of nose, vi. 92

opening of the naso-frontal duct, vi. 93

posterior ethmoidal cells, vi. 94

spheno-ethmoidal recess, the, vi. 95

diseases of, vi. 90

labyrinth, anatomy of, vi. 90

operations upon, vi. 103

anterior or external route, vi. 104

intranasal route, vi. 103

size of, vi. 96

tumors of, vi. 200

Ethyl-chloride as an anæsthetic, its properties, iv. 203, 204

safety, when inhaled, compared with other anæsthetics, iv. 204

signs of an overdose, iv. 206

signs of complete anæsthesia from it, iv. 205

spray as a local anæsthetic, iv. 232

-ether sequence for anæsthesia, iv. 210

Eucain, beta, as a local anæsthetic, iv. 233

Eudiæmorrhysis, definition of, v. 107

Eve, Duncan, on fractures, iii. 63

Eve, Paul F., i. 29

Eventration of diaphragm, vii. 459

Evidence, expert, and opinion, viii. 773

Ewin perineal sheet, vi. 581, 582, 583

Examination, general, of patient, i. 505, 507

of patient, without treatment, may establish relation of surgeon and patient, viii. 719

Excisions and resections, history of, iv. 367

arguments favoring its performance, iv. 368

complete and partial, objects of, respectively, iv. 372

instruments required in, iv. 369, 371

of ankle-joint, a form of plaster-of-Paris bandage for immobilization, and its advantages, iv. 458-460

Kocher's operation, iv. 462

method by two lateral incisions, iv. 458

modifications of the operation by two lateral incisions, iv. 460

objections to and indications for the operation, iv. 457

operation by anterior transverse incision, in cases of tuberculosis, iv. 461, 462

of astragalus, iv. 464

of bones and joints, iv. 367

of clavicle, iv. 401; vi. 417, 418

of coccyx, iv. 435; vii. 33

of elbow-joint, iv. 407, 417

of fibula, iv. 457

of hip, iv. 426-434

of innominate bone, iv. 434

of knee-joint, iv. 435-453

of lower jaw, iv. 385-390

of metatarso-phalangeal joint of the great toe, iv. 466, 467

of os calcis, iv. 465

of pylorus, with gastro-enterostomy, vii. 367

of radius, iv. 418

of scapula, total or partial, iv. 403

of shoulder-joint, iv. 392

of sternum, iv. 405

of superior maxilla, iv. 378-389

of temporo-maxillary articulation, iv. 391

of tibia for giant-celled sarcoma, iv. 456

of wrist, iv. 419-426

partial, defined, iv. 368, 372

process of repair after, iv. 369

special, iv. 378

Excito-motor cortex, v. 268

Excretions, i. 567

Exenteration of orbit, v. 653

Exercise bone, i. 315

Exhibitions in evidence before juries, viii. 790, 792, 793, 794

Exophthalmic goitre, vi. 375

acute, vi. 376

chronic, vi. 376

Crile's method of treatment, vi. 378

Exophthalmos in fracture of skull, v. 71

Exophthalmos of exophthalmic goitre, v. 650

Exophthalmos pulsans, v. 206

vascular non-pulsating, v. 651

Exostoses, i. 314; iii. 401

and osteophytes, iii. 344

beneath chronic ulcer of leg, iii. 344

cartilaginous, iii. 406-409

connective-tissue, i. 315

de croissance, iii. 414

disconnected, iii. 402

eburneous, most common seat of, iii. 402

fibrous, iii. 401, 404

intranasal, vi. 195

multiple cartilaginous, iii. 403, 414-418

of accessory nasal sinuses, iii. 410, 413

of external auditory canal, iii. 404; v. 680

of jaw, iii. 404; vi. 816

of orbit, treatment of, v. 655

of pelvic bones, vii. 13

or osteomata, and enchondromata, as interpreted by x-rays, i. 671

sometimes atavistic, as in the case of exostoses bursata, iii. 345

spongy, of the fibula, iii. 402

subungual, iii. 409, 410

Exstrophy, of urinary bladder, viii. 282

Extension apparatus in the treatment of fractures of the upper end of the femur, iii. 170, 179

Extraction, combined, for cataract, v. 631

of lens in its capsule, for cataracts, v. 631

simple, for cataract, v. 628

with iridectomy, for cataract, v. 631

Extradural abscess. See Abscess, extradural

Extra-rectal dermoids, vii. 896

Extra-uterine pregnancy, viii. 690

Extravasation, middle meningeal, v. 177

of urine, viii. 92

Extremities, minor disorders of, vii. 37

plastic surgery of, iv 627

Exudates, i. 574

inflammatory, differences between them and passive effusions, i. 247

removal of, i. 259

varieties of, and their characters, i. 237, 248, 416, 574

Eye. See Ciliary body, Conjunctiva, Cornea, Eyeball, Eyelids, Glaucoma, Iris, Lachrymal, Lens, Orbit, Sclerotic, Strabismus

Eyeball, dislocation of, v. 656

enucleation of, v. 645

evisceration of, v. 646

Mule's operation, v. 646

foreign bodies in, v. 644

glioma of, v. 644

Eyeball, muscles that move, diseases of the (and see Strabismus), v. 638
operations upon, v. 645
pseudo-glioma of, v. 644
sarcoma of, v. 644
tumors of, v. 644
Eyebrows, poliosis of, v. 550
Eyelashes, absence of, v. 550
canities of, v. 550
poliosis of, v. 550
Eyelids, abscess of, v. 547
adenoma of, v. 559
adhesion of edges of (and see Ankyloblepharon), v. 561
aneurysm by anastomosis, of Bell, of, v. 552
angioma of, v. 552
calcareous concretions of, v. 559
carcinoma of, v. 559
chromidrosis of, v. 550
cornua cutanea of, v. 551
cyst of lower lid, with microphthalmos or anophthalmos, v. 554
cysticercus cellulosæ of, v. 554
ecchymosis of, v. 557
eczema of, v. 548
elephantiasis of, v. 554
emphysema of, v. 557
epithelioma of, v. 551
erysipelas of, v. 547
erythema of, v. 547
eversion of margin of (and see Ectropion), v. 560
fibroma of, v. 553
furuncle of, v. 551
gangrene of, v. 554
granular, v. 579
herpes of, v. 551
horny growths of, v. 551
hyperæmia of, v. 549
injuries of, v. 558
inversion of margin of (and see Entropion), v. 560
lipoma of, v. 553
lupus of, v. 552
lymphangioma of, v. 554
malignant œdema of, v. 554
malignant pustule of, v. 550
milium of, v. 550
molluscum contagiosum of, v. 550
molluscum epitheliale of, v. 550
"mother's mark" on, v. 552
nævus maternus of, v. 552
neuroma of, v. 553
œdema of, v. 547
paralysis of, v. 550
plastic surgery of, iv. 667
blepharoplasty, iv. 672
ectropion, iv. 668
rhus poisoning of, v. 550
sarcoma of, v. 558
sympathetic spasm of, v. 556
syphilis of, v. 552
telangiectasis of, v. 552
warts of, v. 551
wounds of, v. 558
xanthelasma of, v. 550
Eyes, artificial (and see Artificial eyes), v. 657
VOL. VIII.—70

Eyes, blear, v. 549
hare-, v. 556
pink, v. 578
reformed, v. 658
surgical diseases and wounds of the, v. 547
Eyster, work of, on relation of Cheyne-Stokes respiration to cerebral compression, v. 124, 133

FABRIZI's operation for rhinoplasty, iv. 688
Face, abnormities of, v. 417
abscess of, v. 439
acne rosacea of, v. 478
actinomycosis of, v. 458
adenoma of, v. 486
aneurysms of, v. 475
anthrax of, v. 436
arterial varix of, v. 473
bones of, affected by tuberculosis, iii. 600
blood supply of, v. 417
burns and scalds of, v. 428
carbuncle of, v. 434
cavernous angiomata of, v. 472
chancre of, v. 457
charbon of, v. 436
chilblain of, v. 431
cicatrices of, v. 463
cirsoid aneurysm of, v. 473
congenital defects of, v. 495
connective-tissue tumors of, v. 467
contusions of, v. 423
dermoid cysts of, v. 482
diffuse hyperostosis of the bones of, v. 27
discoid carcinoma of, v. 489
echinococcus cysts of, v. 480
epithelioma of, v. 488, 490, 491
erysipelas of, v. 448
fibroma of, v. 467
fibroma molluscum of, v. 468
frost-bite of, v. 431
furunculosis of, v. 432
gangrene of, v. 436
glanders of, v. 464
gunshot wounds of, v. 426
hæmangiomata of, v. 470
hairy mole of, v. 467
incised wounds of, v. 424
infections of the, and their results, v. 432
injuries of, v. 423
inspection of, in diagnosis, i. 514
keloid of, v. 463
keratosis senilis of, v. 488
lacerated wounds of, v. 424
lipoma of, v. 466
lupus of (and see Tuberculosis), v. 452
lymphangioma of, v. 475
lymphatics of, v. 417, 420
malignant epithelial neoplasm of, v. 488
malignant pustule of, v. 436
mother's marks on, v. 470
mucous cysts of, v. 479
nævus of, v. 467
nævus araneus of, v. 470
nævus flammeus of, v. 470

Face, nævus mollusciformis seu lipomatodes of, v. 467
nævus sanguineus of, v. 470
neuroma of, v. 469
œdème charbonneux of, v. 438
pernio of, v. 431
pigmented nævi of, v. 467
plastic surgery of the, iv. 637
port-wine marks on, v. 470
prosthesis of, vi. 20
punctured wounds of, v. 425
restoration of parts of, vi. 28
rodent ulcer of, v. 489
sarcoma of, v. 486
scalds and burns of, v. 428
sebaceous cysts of, v. 480
sequestration dermoids of, v. 482
spider cancer of, v. 470
strawberry marks on, v. 470
surgical diseases of, v. 417
syphilis of, v. 457
telangiectasis of, v. 470
tuberculosis of (and see Lupus of face), v. 452
tumors of, v. 466
benign, v. 466
malignant, v. 486
unilateral hypertrophy of, v. 497
white mole of, v. 467
wounds of, v. 417
contused, v. 423
gunshot, v. 426
incised, v. 424
lacerated, v. 424
punctured, v. 425
Facial nerve, lesions of, in fractures of the skull, v. 77
paralysis of, v. 406
surgery of, v. 406
Facio-hypoglossal anastomosis, v. 410
Fæcal fistula, vii. 711
after operation for appendicitis, vii. 695
impaction, post-operative, iv. 166
Fæces, deductions to be drawn form their goss appearances, i. 571
value of bacterial examination of, i. 574
Faintness, or ischæmia of the brain, i. 239
Fajersztajn's sign, vii. 35
Fallopian tube, absence of, viii. 397
accessory, viii. 398
anatomy of, viii. 393
anomalies of, viii. 397
displacements of, viii. 398
embryology, viii. 391
hernia of, viii. 400
inflammation of. See Salpingitis
resection of, viii. 416
surgery of, viii. 391
tuberculosis of, viii. 420
tumors of, viii. 443
False passage in urethra, vi. 806
Farabeuf's method of amputating through the surgical neck of the humerus, iv. 300

Farabeuf's modification of Carsen's operation, iv. 346
  subastragaloid disarticulation, iv. 329
Farcy, ii. 332; iii. 33
Faradization of the cortex of the brain during operations, v. 360
Farlow's tonsil punch, v. 838
  tonsil snare, v. 837
Fasciæ, contractures of, ii. 446
  diseases and wounds of, ii. 446
  palmar, Dupuytren's contracture of, ii. 446
  tuberculosis of, ii. 449–454
Fat embolism, vii. 199
  necrosis, i. 216; ii. 271
    associated with pancreatic lesions, i. 217
    in pancreatic diseases, vii. 178
    microscopic characters of, i. 185
    researches of Hildebrand and Flexner, i. 217
Fatty degeneration, causes of, i. 185, 187
    gross appearances of, i. 189
    microscopical appearances of, i. 189
    presence or absence of ovaries or testes related to, i. 188
    rationale of fat accommodation, i. 188
    results of, i. 189
  infiltration, i. 187
Fauces, pillars of, slits in, v. 810
Fear of death as a contra-indication to operating, iv. 119
Fees, recovery of, and malpractice, viii. 814
Feet, as affected by hypertrophic arthritis, iii. 517
  blank-cartridge wounds of, vii. 42
  nails in, vii. 42
  open wounds of, iii. 760
  splinters in, vii. 42
  sprains and contusions of, iii. 760
Felon, i. 128, 130; ii. 157; vii. 57
Femoral artery, ligation of common, at base of Scarpa's triangle, iv. 517
  superficial, at apex of Scarpa's triangle, iv. 517
  in Hunter's canal, iv. 518
  surgical anatomy and relations of, iv. 516
Femoral hernia, vii. 584
  atypical forms of, vii. 587
  thrombo-phlebitis, post-operative, iv. 160, 161
Femur, acute osteomyelitis of, iii. 279
  depression of neck of (and see Coxa vara), iv. 848
  diastasis of, iv. 853
  of distal end of, iv. 88, 94
  elevation of neck of (and see Coxa valga), iv. 857
  fractures of. See under Fractures

Femur, fracture of neck, iv. 853
  its epiphyseal development as shown by radiography, i. 592
  ossification of, at different ages, iii. 163
  pseudarthrosis in, iii. 244
  sarcoma of, iii. 462
Ferguson, Alexander Hugh, on Surgical Diseases, Wounds, and Malformations of the Urinary Bladder, and the Prostate, viii. 279–390
Ferguson's method of treating saddle nose, iv. 707
  operation for cleft palate, v. 534
  operation for ectopia vesicæ, viii. 284
Ferguson-Gilliam operation for retroverted uterus, viii. 478
Ferrari, experiments of, in concussion of the brain, v. 152
Fever following operation, i. 535
  of suppuration, i. 535
Fibrin, its removal and changes, i. 260
Fibro-adenoma, i. 346
  of breast, female, vi. 520, 522
Fibro-angioma of pharynx, v. 853
Fibroids of nasopharynx, vi. 860
  of uterus (and see Uterus, fibroids of), i. 303; viii. 515
Fibro-lipoma, i. 307
  of gluteal region, vii. 31
  of kidney, viii. 133, 134
Fibroma, i. 301, 302; ii. 370
  cavernosum, i. 303
  diffusum, i. 304
  durum, i. 302, 305
  hard, ii. 370
  intracanalicular, i. 304
  intranasal, vi. 190
  lipomatodes, i. 303
  lymphangiectaticum, i. 303
  molle, i. 302
  molluscum, of abdominal wall, viii. 87
    of chest wall, vi. 413
    of face, v. 468
    of scalp, v. 16
  naso-pharyngeal, iii. 435
  nodular, i. 304
  of auricle, v. 674
  of bones, iii. 435
  of brain, v. 311
  of breast, i. 304; vi. 522
  of chest wall, vi. 413
  of conjunctiva, v. 584
  of eyelids, v. 553
  of face, v. 467
  of intestine, vii. 737
  of jaw, iii. 435, 476
  of kidney, viii. 133
  of larynx, v. 880
  of liver, viii. 219
  of neck, vi. 349
  of ovary, viii. 428
  of pelvic bones, vii. 13
  of penis, vi. 686
  of peripheral nerves, i. 305
  of pharynx, v. 853
  of prostate, viii. 354
  of rectum, vii. 891
  of scrotum, vi. 695

Fibroma of scalp, v. 16
  of testis, vi. 696
  of tongue, vi. 251
  of vault of pharynx, vi. 190
  of vulva, vi. 570
  ossificum, i. 303
  papillare, of nose, vi. 194
  papillary, of umbilicus, vii. 89
  pedunculated, i. 303
  pericanalicular, i. 304
  petrificum, i. 303
  plexiform (Ranken-neurom), i. 305
  retrogressive changes in, i. 303
  teleangiectatic, i. 303, 319
  soft, ii. 371
  tuberosum, i. 304
Fibromyoma of tongue, vi. 251
  of vermiform appendix, vii. 625
  uterine (and see Uterus, fibroids of), viii. 515
Fibro-myxoma, i. 306
Fibromyxosarcoma of antrum, vi. 830
  of jaw, periosteal, vi. 825
Fibro-sarcoma, i. 333, 335
  of antrum, vi. 830
  of jaw, periosteal, vi. 825
  of umbilicus, vii. 90
Fibrosis, arteriocapillary, vii. 204
Fibula, diastases of distal end of, iv. 94
  dislocations of upper end of, iv. 88
  sarcoma of, iii. 464
Field army, viii. 940
  chief surgeon, duties of, viii. 940
Filaria infection, ii. 577
  sanguinis hominis, ii. 575
Filehne and Koch, researches of, on cerebral concussion, v. 153, 162
Fillebrown's method of operating for cleft palate, v. 538
Filtration experiments, significance of, i. 406
Fingers, anatomy of, vii. 53
  and thumb, amputation of, details of surgical anatomy, iv. 279, 280
  base-ball, vii. 72
  dislocations of, iv. 67
  hypertrophic arthritis of, iii. 527
  infections of, vii. 53
  methods of using local anæsthesia and nerve blocking, iv. 247
  webbed, iv. 634
Finney's method of pyloroplasty, vii. 372
  method of rhinoplasty, iv. 691
Finney-Pancoast trunk for operations, iv. 145
Fire-arms and their classification, ii. 643
  explosives used with, ii. 647
First-aid equipment, in railroad surgery, viii. 1040, 1049
  naval, viii. 988
  packet, the materials supplied and objects sought to be accomplished by its use, ii. 692, 693

First-aid stations, in military service, viii. 950
First intention, healing by, i. 100, 249, 261, 265
Fischer, theory of pathogenesis of cerebral concussion, v. 160
Fish-bites, viii. 974
Fishbone catcher, Weiss', vii. 427
Fissure in ano, vii. 801
  of canthus, v. 556
  of nipple, vi. 507
Fistula, i. 133, 255
  anal-urinary, vii. 828
  ano-rectal, vii. 816
  aural, congenital, v. 661
  biliary, viii. 243, 278
  branchial, vi. 313, 394
  cervical, vi. 394
  congenital, of neck, vi. 313
  fæcal, vii. 711
    after operation for appendicitis, vii. 695
  following cysts of pancreas, viii. 187
  following deep-seated infection, i. 419
  in ano, vii. 815
  intestinal, vii. 711
  lachrymal, treatment of, v. 597
  of cornea, v. 606
  of lachrymal gland, v. 592
  of lip, v. 495
  of neck, vi. 394
    branchial, vi. 394
  of Stenson's duct, vi. 298
  of thyro-glossal duct, vi. 395
  perineal-urinary, vii. 828
  perineo-urethral, vii. 828, 829
  pharyngeal, v. 810
  postauricular, plastic operations for closing, v. 727
    Mosetig-Moorhof method, v. 729
    Passow-Trautmann method, v. 730
  rectal-urinary, vii. 828
  recto-genital, vii. 835
  recto-ureteral, vii. 828, 835
  recto-urethral, vii. 828, 829
  recto-uterine, vii. 835
  recto-vaginal, vii. 835
  recto-vesical, vii. 828, 833
  recto-vulvar, vii. 835
  resulting from suppuration, i. 121
  salivary, v. 440; vi. 298
  salivary-duct, v. 440
  vesico-vaginal, operations for, vi. 620
Fistulæ connecting with anus or rectum, vii. 815
Fitz, R. J., on perforative inflammation of the vermiform appendix, i 59
Fixation of wounded tissue, i 273
Flap, osteoplastic, in cerebral operations, v 353
"Flarebacks," viii. 976
Flat bones, fibrous osteomata of, iii. 404
  of skull, tuberculosis of, iii 599
  chest, vi. 406

Flat-foot (and see Weak foot), iv. 872
  in rickets, iii. 350
Flint, Carleton P., excision of knee without opening the joint, iv. 448
Floating cartilages, iii. 726
  goitre, vi. 365
  kidney, viii. 97
Fœtus, wounds of head of, v. 8
Folliculitis, vi. 751
Foot, amputation of, by Pirogoff's method, iv. 332
  contracted, iv. 891
  disabilities of, iv. 872
  dislocations of, iv. 94
  distortions of, iv. 896
  hollow, iv. 891
  infantile paralysis of, iv. 815
  osteoplastic resection of, by Wladimiroff-Mikulicz' method, iv. 334
  partial amputations of, iv. 317
  sprain of, chronic, iv. 880
  twisting, for flat foot, iv. 885
  weak (and see Weak foot), iv. 872
Foramen of Winslow, hernia at, vii. 609
Forbes' operation of disarticulating at the scapho-cuneiform joint, iv. 326
Forceps, alligator, vii. 771
  Lutter, vii. 424
  œsophageal, vii. 425
  pharyngeal, vii. 424
  rongeur, Lane's, v. 353
Forcipressure, control of hemorrhage by, vii. 243
Ford's experiments to prove the presence of bacteria in healthy tissues, i. 253
Forearm, amputation of, by circular method, iv. 290, 291
  by equal antero-posterior flaps, iv. 292
  by modified circular method, iv. 291
    advantages, iv. 293
  methods and instruments required, iv. 290
  partial, according to the double-flap method, iv. 293
  surgical anatomy, iv. 289
  pseudarthrosis in bones of, iii. 238
  transverse section of, at junction of the upper and middle thirds, iii. 243
Foreign bodies, disposal of, in healing, i. 105
  giant cells, i. 106
  in antrum, vi. 158
  in conjunctiva, treatment of, v. 590
  in cornea, removal of, v. 616
  in external auditory canal, v. 682
  in eyeball, v. 644
  in heart, vii. 164
  in intestines, vii. 705, 708
  ın joints, iii. 530
  in larynx, v 871

Foreign bodies in or on male genitals, vi. 663
  in œsophagus, vii. 422
  in orbit, v. 656
  in or on penis, vi. 663
  in pharynx, v. 811, 812
  - in rectum, vii. 946
  in sigmoid, vii. 946
  in tongue, vi. 232
  in trachea, v. 905
  in urethra, vi. 663
  left in wounds after operations, malpractice, viii. 760
Formative cells or fibroblasts, ii. 165
Fossa, ileo-appendical, vii. 620
  ileo-colic, vii. 620
  retro-cæcal, vii. 621
  subcæcal, vii. 621
Fourth tonsil, v. 841
Foveæ sacrales, vii. 20
  sacrococcygeal, vii. 20
Fowler, Russell S., on Minor Surgery, iv. 537
Fowler's position in abdominal surgery, vii. 119
Fracture, abnormal mobility as a sign, iii. 73
  beds, iii. 91
  box, or box-splint, for fractures of the leg, iii. 206
  "closed," Dr. James A. Kelley's operative treatment of, iii. 93
  complete, iii. 64
  complicated, iii. 65, 80
  complicated with dislocation, their management and sequelæ, iii. 82
  compound, after-treatment of, iii. 204
  crepitus as a sign of, iii. 74
  definition of term, iii. 63
  degree of displacement as a sign, iii. 73
  delayed union in, iii. 85
  depression of fragments in, iii. 72
  differential diagnosis from dislocation, iii. 76
  direct longitudinal displacement in, iii. 72
  displacements of the fragments after, iii. 71
  disturbance of function as a symptom of, iii. 75
  double, iii. 64
  ecchymosis as a sign of, iii. 74
  egg-shell, iii. 64
  epiphyseal, iii. 77, 182
  extracapsular, iii. 65
    of the neck of the femur, iii. 162-165
  fat embolism as a complication, iii. 84
  fissure of bone, iii. 64
  formation and changes of callus after, iii. 79
  frequency of, and the degree of liability of different bones, iii. 67
  green-stick, iii. 64
  gunshot, iii. 65, 67

Fracture, hickory-stick, iii. 64
immobilization essential in treatment of, i. 285
impacted, iii. 65, 71
incomplete, iii. 64
infection as a complication, iii. 83
injuries to blood-vessels and lymphatics, as complications of, iii. 80
injuries to nerves, complicating, iii. 81
injury of the soft parts in, iii. 72
intercondyloid, iii. 65
interstitial, iii. 64
intracapsular, iii. 65
of the upper end of the femur, iii. 159–162
intraperiosteal, iii. 64
intra-uterine, iii. 69
as related to fragilitas ossium, iii. 357
mixed, iii. 65
modifications of treatment required when the fracture extends into or close to a joint, iii. 95
modifications of treatment when the fragments are much displaced, iii. 92
multiple or comminuted, iii. 64
named from peculiarities of shape, iii. 66
named from surgeons who described them, iii. 66
new growth as a complication, iii. 85
non-union in, iii. 86
of astragalus, iii. 209
of atlas, vi. 430
of axis, vi. 430
of bones of the foot, iii. 208
of carpal bones, iii. 152
of clavicle, iii. 114
of costal cartilages, iii. 113
of different bones, iii.
of elbow-joint, iii. 138
of external auditory canal, v. 678
of femur, iii. 158
of fibula, iii. 196
of fingers, iii. 154
of forearm (both bones), iii. 138, 144
of frontal sinus, vi. 147
of hip-joint, iii. 159
of humerus, iii. 123
of hyoid bone, larynx, and trachea, iii. 107
of inferior maxilla, iii. 103
of larynx, v. 864
of leg, iii. 192, 200
of malar bone and zygomatic arch, iii. 101
of malleus, v. 686
of metacarpal bones, iii. 153
of metatarsal bones, iii. 211
of nasal bones, iii. 99; vi. 59
of olecranon process, iii. 139
of os calcis, iii. 208
of patella, iii. 182
of pelvis, iii. 155
of penis, vi. 664

Fracture of phalanges. iii. 154
of radius, iii. 141
of ribs, iii. 110
of scapula, iii. 121
of skull, v. 48
in children, v. 67
of spinal column, vi. 429
of sternum, iii. 108
of superior maxilla, iii. 102
of surgical neck of humerus with concomitant dislocation, iv. 46
of tarsal bones, iii. 210
of thumb, iii. 153
of tibia, iii. 193
of toes, iii. 211
of ulna, iii. 138, 168
of vertebræ, vi. 429
of walls of orbit, v. 655
of wrist, iii. 148, 152
overriding of fragments, iii. 71
pain as a symptom of, iii. 75
partial, iii. 64
pneumonia as a complication, iii. 85
predisposing causes of, iii. 69
processes of repair, iii. 78
punctured, iii. 65
question of amputation after, iii. 82
relations of spontaneous to cancer, iii. 357
repair of, i. 279, 280
serrated or toothed, iii. 65
"setting" of, and the requirements of retentive dressings, iii. 88, 89
signs and symptoms, iii. 73
simple, operative treatment of, iii. 91
simple or single, iii. 64
spontaneous, causation of, iii. 70
spontaneous, conditions leading to, iii. 65
subjective or rational symptoms of, iii. 75
time required for the repair of, iii. 80
transverse, oblique, and longitudinal, iii. 65
ulcerations, sloughing, and gangrene as complications of, iii. 83
value of anæsthesia in diagnosis of, iii. 76, 77
value of x-rays in diagnosis of, iii. 77, 78
varieties of, iii. 63
vicious union, iii. 87
x-ray diagnosis of, i. 643
Fracture-dislocation of spinal column, vi. 429
use of the term in cases of injury of dorsal and lumbar vertebræ, iv. 26
Fraenkel's laryngeal forceps, v. 873
Fragilitas ossium, iii. 356
idiopathic, v. 25
or periosteal dysplasia, and osteogenesis imperfecta, x-ray features of, i. 685
scorbutica, ii. 69
Fraise, Sudeck's, v 355

Framboesia or yaws, ii. 342
Frank's method of operation for femoral hernia, vii. 590
Frank and Ssbanajew's method of gastrostomy, vii. 405
Frazier, Charles H., on Surgery of the Cranial Nerves, v. 379–416
Frazier's method of operating on trigeminal nerve, v. 398, 402, 403
modification of Jones' method of treating fractures of the elbow-joint, iii. 138
Free bodies, sometimes wholly organic, i. 200
French method of blepharoplasty, iv. 674
of plastic operations, iv. 613, 614, 674, 684
of rhinoplasty, iv. 684
Freund's operation for prolapsed uterus, viii. 502
Fricke's method of blepharoplasty, v. 570
operation (blepharoplasty), iv. 672
Friedrich's multiple rib resection for treatment of unilateral pulmonary tuberculosis, viii. 54
Fritz's method of restoring the alæ, iv. 697
Frontal branch of trigeminal nerve, extracranial operations upon, v. 385
Frontal lobe of brain, diagnosis of tumors in, v. 318
lesions of, symptoms, v. 281
sinus, acute inflammation of, vi. 113
anatomy of, vi. 106
anterior wall, vi. 110
backward prolongation, vi. 108
dangerous area of, vi. 111
floor of, vi. 110
form, vi. 106
incomplete or partial septa, vi. 109
large sinus, vi. 107
mucous membrane, vi. 106
naso-frontal duct, vi. 112
outward prolongation, vi. 107
posterior or cranial wall, of, vi. 110
pulley of superior oblique muscle, vi. 113
size, vi. 106
small sinus, vi. 107
septum, vi. 108
vessels, vi. 106
catheterization of, vi. 117
chronic inflammation of, vi. 115
chronic suppuration of, treatment, by opening in anterior wall, vi. 120
by obliteration of the sinus, vi. 125
Killian's operation for obliteration of sinus, vi. 127

Frontal sinus, chronic suppuration of, Mosher's method of operation for, vi. 164
procedure for small sinuses, vi. 147
diseases of, vi. 113–147
enlarging duct of, from nose, vi. 122
fracture of, compound depressed, vi. 147
simple depressed, vi. 147
inflammation of, acute, vi. 113
chronic, vi. 115
irrigation of, vi. 121
obliteration of, vi. 125
Killian's operation for, vi. 127
osteoma of, v. 29
punctured wound of, vi. 147
radical operations on, vi. 125, 134
transillumination of, vi. 208
tumors of, vi. 200
Frost-bite of auricle, v. 665
of external genitals, male, vi. 666
of face, v. 431
Fulguration treatment of carcinoma of uterus, viii. 660
Fulminates, ii. 647
Functional activity of the kidneys, test of, viii. 83
joint disease, iii. 544–547
Fungous or exuberant ulcer, i. 229
Fungus, umbilical, vii. 89
Funnel chest, vi. 407
Furuncle, i. 128, 130; ii. 304
a result of bacterial inflammation, i. 418
of chest wall, vi. 408
of eyelids, v. 551
Furunculosis, ii. 156, 305
of external auditory canal, v. 683
of face, v. 432
of vestibule of nose, vi. 80
Fused kidney, viii. 85

Gaboon ulcer, i. 231
Gait, its diagnostic significance, i. 538
Galactocele, vi. 516
Galezowski's method of operation for pterygium, v. 594
Gall-bladder, abnormalities of, viii. 205
actinomycosis of, viii. 233
anatomy of, viii. 196
gangrenous inflammation of, viii. 232
gall stones in, viii. 237
inflammation of, viii. 229
operations on, viii. 256, 262
perforation of, viii. 242, 277
phlegmonous inflammation of, viii. 232
physiology of, viii. 204
suppurative inflammation of, viii. 230
surgery of, viii. 193, 256
tuberculous inflammation of, viii. 233

Gall-bladder, ulcerative inflammation of, viii. 232
Gall-stones, i. 201; viii. 233
in common duct, viii. 239
in cystic duct, viii. 238
in hepatic duct, viii. 241
in intrahepatic ducts, viii. 242
in pelvis of gall-bladder, viii. 237
influence of obstruction on, viii. 235
localization of, viii. 251
mode of formation of, viii. 233
Gallie tie-down, iv. 961, 962
Gallie's bed-splint, iii. 662
Ganglion, ii. 432
Gangrene, i. 136
acute, ii. 205
affections of the heart and blood-vessels leading to, ii. 208–210
after subcutaneous infusion of normal salt solution, cocaine, adrenalin, etc., ii. 269
amputation in, ii. 229
and gangrenous diseases, ii. 201
arteriosclerotic, vii. 207
as a complication of hæmophilia, ii. 246
as associated with intermittent claudication, ii. 215
as caused by aneurysm, ii. 218
by disease of the kidneys, ii. 222
by disorders of the nervous system, ii. 221
by laceration of vessels, ii. 217
by ligature of an artery, ii. 218
by periarteritis, ii. 219
by phlebitis, ii. 220
by rupture of the intima, ii. 219
by traumatism, ii. 222
by venous thrombosis, ii. 220
as distinguished from abrasion, ii. 201
from ulceration, ii. 201
as related to thrombosis of arteries, ii. 215
aseptic moist, ii. 205
associated with syphilis, ii. 245
atheroma and arterial sclerosis as causes of, ii. 212
black, i. 137
caused by phimosis, ii. 292
by senile tissue changes, ii. 223
circumscribed, i. 136
classification, ii. 204, 205
diabetic, i. 136; ii. 231
amputation in, ii. 239
varieties, ii. 232
definition, ii. 201
diffuse, i. 136
dry, i. 136, 137, 218; ii. 204
due to drugs, ii. 260
to ergot, ii. 261
to heat and to cold, ii. 268
to inadequate collateral blood supply, ii. 207
to mercury, ii. 261
to orthoform, ii. 262

Gangrene due to the effects of electricity, ii. 270
embolic, ii. 210
emphysematous, i. 137; ii. 223, 247
hospital, ii. 253
idiopathic, i. 136
in connection with intussusception, ii. 287
with paraphimosis, ii. 294
in phosphatic diabetes, ii. 240
infantile or juvenile, ii. 225
latent pulmonary, ii. 277
lithæmic, ii. 247
moist, i. 136, 137, 218
Murphy's rules for amputation in, ii. 230
neuropathic, i. 136
nosocomial, ii. 253
of appendix, ii. 288
of auricle, v. 671
of bladder, ii. 297
of bowel following operations, ii. 288
of ear, v. 671
of external genitals, ii. 295
of eyelids, ii. 269; v. 554
of face, v. 436
of gall-bladder, ii. 282
of genito-urinary system, ii. 292
of heart, ii. 272
of hollow viscera, ii. 285
of intestines, ii. 285–288
of kidneys, ii. 282
of liver and spleen, ii. 282
of lung, ii. 273, 280; viii. 19
of Meckel's diverticulum, ii. 288
of œsophagus, ii. 285
of pancreas, ii. 283
of penis, ii. 294; vi. 675
of scalp, v. 23
of scrotum, ii. 295; vi. 675
of solid viscera, ii. 272
of spermatic cord, ii. 295
of stomach, ii. 285
of testes, ii. 296
of thyroid gland, ii. 273
of tongue, ii. 284; vi. 241
of tonsils, ii. 284
of uterus, ii. 283
of uvula and pillars of the fauces, ii. 284
of vulva, ii. 295
phagedenic, i. 136
pleuro-pulmonary, following measles, ii. 277
presenile, ii. 225
primary cutaneous, including hysterical gangrene, ii. 269
puerperal, ii. 267
pulpy, ii. 253
rare forms of, ii. 271
secondary, ii. 265
senile, i. 136; ii. 204, 223–225
septic or putrid moist, ii. 205
spontaneous, ii. 266
spreading traumatic, ii. 205, 223, 247
thermal, i. 136
toxic, i. 136
traumatic, i. 136; ii. 205
white, i. 137
Gangrène foudroyante, i. 421; ii. 247

Gangrenous emphysema, ii. 247
  hernial sac, ii. 285
  inflammation, primary and sec-
    ondary, i. 136
  omentum, ii. 285
  pancreatitis, viii. 167
  phlegmon following sting of a
    spider, ii. 271
  stomatitis, ii. 301
  strangulated hernia, ii. 286
  urticaria, ii. 269
  zona, ii. 269
Garland, F. E., on Anæsthetics
  and the Production of General
  Anæsthesia, iv. 169
Garrow, Alexander Esslemont, on
  Surgery of the Spleen, viii. 59–77
Gas phlegmons and necrosis, classification proposed by Kropac, ii.
  251
Gaseous cellulitis, ii. 459
  œdema, iii. 30
Gases, irrespirable, viii. 976
Gasserian ganglion, operations on,
  v. 394
  physiological extirpation of,
    v. 398
Gastrectomy, dangers of, vii. 397
  partial, vii. 396
Gastric juice, importance of exam-
  ining it in diagnosis of
  carcinoma of the stomach,
    i. 562
  ulcer, and its sequelæ (and see
    Stomach, ulcer of), vii. 337
Gastro-duodenostomy, vii. 375
  Willard's method, vii. 376
  Kuemmel's method, vii. 377
Gastro-enteritis, diagnosed from
  acute appendicitis, vii. 660
Gastro-enterostomy, vii. 343
  McGraw's method, vii. 352
  Moynihan-Mayo method, vii.
    345
  posterior, vii. 359
  Rodman's method, vii. 367
  Roux's method, vii. 357
Gastro-gastrostomy, vii. 382
Gastro-intestinal apparatus, its
  bearing on the question of opera-
  tion, iv. 117
Gastro-mesenteric ileus, vii. 736
Gastroptosis, vii. 389
  Beyea's operation for, vii. 390
Gastrorrhaphy, vii. 106, 384
Gastrostomy, vii. 377, 398, 419
  Marwedel's method of, vii. 404
  Ssbanajew-Frank's method of,
    vii. 405
  Witzel's method of, vii. 402
Gastrotomy, vii. 105
  for removal of foreign body
    from œsophagus, vii. 427
Gauze as a dressing, i. 718; iv. 537
  as directly applied to sterile
    wounds, i. 755, 759
  bandages, i. 719
Gavello's method of forming a new
  lobule of, ear v. 677
Gaylord, Harvey R., i. 387
Genital tract, female, secretions of,
    i. 565
  male, secretions of, i. 566

Genitals, external, female (and see
    Vulva)
  abnormalities of, vi. 573
  chancre of, hard, vi. 565
    soft, vi. 565
  condyloma, syphilitic, vi.
    565
  diseases due to inflam-
    mation or circulatory
    disturbances, vi. 559
  elephantiasis, vi. 563
  gonorrhœa, vi. 559
  hypertrophic ulceration,
    vi. 564
  pruritus, vi. 561
  surgical diseases of, vi.
    559
  syphilitic condyloma, vi.
    565
  tuberculosis, vi. 565
  tumors of, vi. 565
  ulceration, hypertrophic,
    vi. 564
  ulcus rodens, vi. 564
  wounds of, vi. 559
  female, embryology of, viii. 391
    surgical anatomy of, viii. 393
  male, anatomy of, vi. 622
    burns of, vi. 666
    embryology of, vi. 634
    foreign bodies in or on, vi.
      663
    frost-bites of, vi. 666
    gangrene of, vi. 675
    herpes of, vi. 674
    inflammations of, vi. 668
    infections of, vi. 668
    injuries of, vi. 663
    malformations of, vi. 637
    skin diseases of, vi. 674
    surgical diseases of, vi. 622
    swellings which are neither
      inflammatory nor neo-
      plastic, vi. 678
    tuberculosis of, vi. 671
    tumors of, vi. 678, 686
    verruca acuminata, vi. 674
    warts, vi. 674
    wounds of, vi. 622
Genito-urinary apparatus, indications it may furnish against
  operations or administration
  of an anæsthetic, iv. 117–119
Genuclast, its use in deformities following atrophic arthritis, iii. 512
Genu recurvatum, congenital, iv.
    765
  in infantile paralysis, iv. 832
  valgum (and see Knock-knee),
    iv. 863
  varum (and see Bow leg), iv. 860
Gerontoxon, v. 603
Gersuny's method of prosthesis, iv.
    625
  operation for restoring the
    cheek, iv. 640
  operation on external ear, iv. 724
Giant cells, mononuclear, i. 88
Giant-cell sarcoma of bone, iii. 445
  of ulna, iii. 464
  (medullary) of ulna, iii. 453
Gibney, V. P., on Tuberculosis from
  a Surgical Standpoint, ii. 75

Gibney's method of strapping a
  sprained ankle, iii. 756
Gibson, William, i. 18, 34
Gibson's blood chart, vii. 654
  method of valvular colostomy,
    vii. 796
Gigantism or giant growth, iii. 340
  an example of intrinsic con-
    genital hypertrophy, i. 151
  of skull, v. 28
  partial, iii. 397
Gila monster, the bites of, iii. 5
Gingivitis, vi. 878, 879
Giraldès' operation for hare lip, v
    512
Girard's operation for diverticula of
  œsophagus, vii. 443
Glanders, ii. 41, 332; iii. 33
Glass arm, vii. 73
Glaucoma, v. 642
  acute, v. 642
  chronic, v. 643
  fulminans, v. 643
  hemorrhagic, v. 643
  infantile, v. 604
  primary, v. 642
  secondary, v. 642
Glioma, i. 324
  and sarcoma, their relationship,
    i. 326
  differentiation of various forms
    of, i. 325
  durum, i. 324
  ependymal (Flexner), i. 326, 327
  malignant, i. 327
  molle, i. 324
  of brain, v. 305
  of eyeball, v. 644
  of retina, v. 326
  teleangiectaticum, i. 324
Gliosis occurring with syringomyelia, i. 327
Globus major, vi. 629
  minor, vi. 630
Glossitis, vi. 233
  acute parenchymatous, vi. 240
  chronic superficial, vi. 235
  hemiglossitis, vi. 234
  mercurial, vi. 241
  phlegmonous, vi. 240
  superficial, vi. 234
Glossopharyngeal nerve, surgery of
  the, v. 413
Gluteal artery, aneurysm of, vii. 25,
    26
  injuries of, vii. 24
  ligation of, iv. 512; vii. 27
  region, abscess of, vii. 29
  angioma of, vii. 31
  carcinoma of, vii. 31
  elephantiasis of, vii. 31
  epithelioma of, vii. 31
  fibro-lipoma of, vii. 31
  incised wounds of, vii. 24
  lipoma of, vii. 31
  lymphangioma of, vii. 31
  neuralgia of, vii. 31
  sarcoma of, vii. 31
Glycosuria, its surgical significance,
    i. 569
Goitre, vi. 358
  abnormal, vi. 365

Goitre, circular, vi. 360, 365
colloid, i. 191
congenital, vi. 367
cystic, i. 347; vi. 369
cystico-colloid, vi. 369
cysto-colloid, vi. 360, 364, 365
endemic, vi. 358
epidemic, vi. 359
exophthalmic (and see Exophthalmic goitre), vi. 375
floating, vi. 365
hyperplastic, vi. 369
sporadic, vi. 359
tubular, vi. 365
vascular, vi. 369
wandering, vi. 359
Goldmann's operation for diverticula of œsophagus, vii. 443
Goldthwait and Osgood's sacral brace described, iii. 621
Goldthwait's genuclast for the forcible reduction of resistant deformities, iii. 705
operation for dislocation of the patella, iv. 766
Gonococcus, vi. 715
Gonorrhœa (and see Gonorrhœal urethritis), vi. 715
of external genitals, female, v. 560; vi. 560
Gonorrhœal cystitis, vi. 745
endocervicitis, vi. 561
proctitis, vii. 798
urethritis, vi. 715
Gooch's splinting, iii. 89
Gottstein's adenoid curette, v. 833
Gould's suture, vii. 736
Gout, x-ray characteristics of, i. 660
Gouty affections of joints, iii. 549
Graafian follicle cysts, viii. 403
Graefe's coin-catcher, vii. 426
Gram stain, vi. 716
Grandmont's operation for ptosis, v. 569
Grant's Dundas safety forceps, v. 883
Granular lids, v. 579
Granulating wounds, local infections of, i. 422
Granulation tissue, its character and conversion into scar tissue, i. 93, 251, 263
its constituents, ii. 165
Granulations as an element of pathological regeneration or reconstruction, ii. 164
Granuloma coccidioides, ii. 318, 328
infectious, as sequela of an infective inflammation, i. 108, 144
of brain, v. 301
of scalp, v. 24
of conjunctiva, v. 584
of umbilicus, vii. 89
Grattage, v. 588
Gratuitous services do not alter contract, viii. 723
Graves, William P., on Surgical Diseases and Wounds of the External Genitals and Vagina of the Female. vi. 559–621
Graves' disease (and see Exophthalmic goitre), vi. 375

Graves' disease, influence of, in surgical opertions, i. 791
acquired, vi. 379
pseudo-, vi. 379
method of abdominal colporrhaphy, vi. 618
operation for absence of vagina, vi. 578
for cystocele, vi. 609
Grawitz tumor, iii. 481
Great toe-joint, painful, iv. 896
Green's operation for entropion, v. 563
Greene's thermo-ether inhaler and the mode of using it, iv. 186, 187
Green-silk and rubber-tissue protective as a dressing, iv. 438
Griffith, J. D., on Surgical Diseases and Wounds of the Abdominal wall, vii. 75–95
Gritti's transcondyloid amputation through the knee-joint, iv. 346
Gross, Samuel D., i. 14, 27, 35
Growing pains, iii. 339
Guérin's operation for ectropion, iv. 668
Gumma, cranial, v. 40
of breast, female, vi. 519
of iris, v. 613
of larynx, ii. 125
of lip, ii. 124
of palate and of the nasal bones, ii. 124
of tongue, ii. 124; vi. 294
of rectum, vii. 800
of synovial membrane, iii. 538
of umbilicus, vii. 90
syphilitic, of bones, iii. 364
Gums, carcinoma of, with secondary involvement of jaw, vi. 846
epithelioma of, malignant spinous-cell, vi. 847
papilloma of, vi. 846
Gunn, Moses, i. 49
Gunpowder, its composition, ii. 647
smokeless, ii. 647
Gunshot wounds, ii. 642
according to regions, ii. 694
and injuries as indications for excision of the knee, iv. 439
by different weapons, frequency of, ii. 646
classes of, ii. 646
closure, aseptic, the first important step in treatment, ii. 690
first-aid packet, ii. 692
gauze for first dressing, ii. 691
infection of, ii. 683
as influenced by conditions due to the missile, ii. 684
as influenced by conditions of the clothing, ii. 685
by the tetanus bacillus, ii. 686
lodged missiles in, ii. 680
means to secure fixation of the injured part, ii. 693

Gunshot wounds, micrococci producing infection in them, ii. 685
objections to probing for bullets, ii. 681
of abdomen, ii. 725
of ankle-joint, ii. 763
of bladder, treatment of, ii. 739
of chest, ii. 719
of cranial region, ii. 696
of diaphysis of the femur, ii. 758
of different regions, relative fatality of, ii. 695
of elbow-joint, ii. 747
of extremities, frequency and fatality, ii. 740
of eye, ii. 711
of face, ii. 709
with fracture of the facial bones, ii. 709
of foot, ii. 764
of hip-joint, ii. 752
of joints, ii. 674
of kidney, ii. 736
of knee-joint, ii. 761
of larynx, v. 866
of larynx and trachea, treatment of, ii. 713
of liver, treatment of, ii. 736
of lower extremities, ii. 752
of lung, ii. 721
of neck, ii. 712
involving the nerves, ii. 713
of œsophagus, ii. 713
of pelvic region, ii. 737
of penis, ii. 665
of shoulder, ii. 745
of skull, v. 86
of solid viscera, ii. 736
of spine, vi. 423
of spine and spinal cord, ii. 714
of spleen, ii. 736; viii. 66
of stomach and intestines, character of, ii. 732, 733
of testicles, ii. 740
of trachea, v. 866
of upper extremities, ii. 744
of urethra, ii. 740
of urinary bladder, ii. 738
of wrist, ii. 750
penetrating, with intrathoracic injury, ii. 721
Gunstock deformity, the production of, in fractures of the lower end of the humerus, iii. 136
Gunther's modification of Pirogoff's amputation, iv. 334
Gussenbauer's clamp, iii. 92
operation, for restoring the cheek, iv. 642
Guthrie's amputation at hip-joint by antero-posterior flaps. cut from without inward, iv. 359
oval-flap method of amputating through surgical neck of the humerus, iv. 300
Guyon's supramalleolar amputation, iv. 271, 335

Gynæcology as a special branch of surgery, i. 56
Gynæcomastia, vi. 508

Habit torticollis, iv. 806
Habits as bearing on diagnosis, i. 509
Hæmangioma, i. 310, 321
arteriale, i. 320, 321
cavernosum, i. 320
of chest wall, viii. 15
of face, v. 470
of mouth, vi. 248
of parotid gland, vi. 307
simplex, i. 320
simplex, of scalp, v. 18
venosum, i. 321
Hæmatemesis, post-operative, iv. 153, 154
Hæmatocele, vi. 686
after herniotomy, vii. 592
Hæmatoidin, i. 203
Hæmatoma, ii. 456; v. 4, 5
fœtal, v. 9
of ear (and see Othæmatoma), v. 666
of ovary, viii. 401
of quadriceps extensor femoris, vii. 73
of vulva, vi. 572
pachymeningitic, diagnosed from middle meningeal hemorrhage, v. 189
Hæmaturia, essential, viii. 131
in renal calculus, viii. 116
Hæmochromatosis, i. 205
Hæmocytology in its relation to surgical prognosis, i. 791
Hæmofuscin, i. 194
Hæmoglobin, importance of knowing percentage of, in chlorotic anæmia, i. 556
Hæmoglobinæmia, i. 205
Hæmoglobinuria, i. 205
Hæmolytic reaction in the diagnosis of cancer, vi. 543
Hæmophilia as affecting the joints, iii. 553
hereditary, importance of, in surgical prognosis, i. 783, 792
Hæmophiliac as distinguished from tuberculous knee-joint, iii. 699
Hæmostasis, complete, a surgical principle, in treatment, i. 273
methods adapted to different needs in operation, i. 149
Hæmostatic forceps, i. 746
Hæmothorax, treatment of, ii. 724
Hagedorn's operation for double hare lip, v. 516
operation for hare lip, v. 513
Hahn's operation for restoring the cheek, iv. 646
Hajek's hook, vi. 104
Halisteresis, iii. 355
Hallux rigidus, iii. 518; iv. 896
valgus, ii. 444; iv. 894
varus, iv. 892
Halsted's method of operating for carcinoma of the breast, vi. 550
suture, vii. 736, 754
Hamilton, Frank H., i. 36

Hamilton's long side splint, with traction, iii. 170
Hammer-nose, v. 478
Hammer-toe, iv. 893
Hancock's operation, iv. 334
Hand, anatomy of, vii. 53
amputation of, at the wrist, iv. 286
blank-cartridge wounds of, vii. 42
bone necrosis of, vii. 63
fascial spaces of, vii. 56
infected wounds of, points where incisions should be made, as indicated by Kanavel's experiments, iii. 743
infections of, vii. 53, 60
nails in, vii. 42
penetrating wounds of the joints of, iii. 742–745
plastic surgery of the, iv. 630
sloughing tendon of, vii. 63
splinters in, vii. 42
sterilization, conclusions concerning, i. 703, 708
tendons of, vii. 54
Hardie's operation for rhinoplasty, iv. 690
Hare eye, v. 556
lip, v. 500, 501
Harlan, George C., on Surgical Diseases and Wounds of the Eye, v. 547–659
Harlan's method of blepharoplasty, iv. 675; v. 571, 572
operation for entropion, v. 563
Harrington's solution of bichloride of mercury for sterilizing the hands, i. 706
Harris, Malcolm La Salle, on the Diagnosis of Tumors of the Abdomen, vii. 96–104
Hartley, Frank, on Laryngectomy, v. 914–932
Harvard College, Cambridge, Mass., medical department of, organized, i. 10
Hasner's method of blepharoplasty, v. 574
operation (blepharoplasty), iv. 673, 676
Hayward, George, i. 20
Head, supports of, for Pott's disease, iv. 972
surgical affections and wounds of, v. 3
Headache, as a symptom of organic cerebral lesion, v. 274
Head-rest, for cerebral operations, v. 348, 349
Hearing, cortical area concerned with, v. 272
disturbances of, in fractures of skull, v. 78
sense of, and its defects, as concerned in diagnosis, i. 542
Heart, adherent, liberation of, vii. 159
affections of, contra-indicating general anæsthesia and certain operations, iv. 115, 116
atrophy of, i. 171

Heart, complications, post-operative, iv. 160
disease, choice of anæsthetics as indicated in, iv. 223
foreign bodies in, vii. 164
massage of, vii. 173
paracentesis of, vii. 175
penetrating wounds of, vii. 163
projection of, on thorax, vii. 149
repair of injury of, i. 287
structures covering, vii. 146
surgery of, vii. 146, 160
wounds of, vii. 160
Heat, a symptom of inflammation, i. 94
and cold, surgical uses of, i. 765, 766
in treatment of acute simple inflammation, i. 113
control of hemorrhage by, vii. 240
sense (thermo-æsthesia) in relation to diagnosis, i. 537
Hebb's hemorrhoidal clamp, vii. 874
scissors, vii. 874
modification of Earle's method of operating for hemorrhoids, vii. 872
Heberden's nodes, iii. 514, 527
in terminal phalanges, iii. 529
Heel, pain in, iv. 890
Heinecke-Mikulicz method of pyloroplasty, vii. 370
Helferich's method of ligating vertebral artery, vi. 338
of rhinoplasty, iv. 685
operation for saddle-nose, iv. 712
Helmet, plaster, retention dressing for torticollis, iv. 778
Hemianopsia, varieties, v. 279
Hemiglossitis, vi. 234
Hemilaryngectomy, v. 926
Hemorrhage, after operation for appendicitis, vii. 695
arterial, vii. 233
as influencing the choice of anæsthetics, iv. 224
cerebral, compression from, coincident with concussion or contusion, v. 197
control of, after cerebral operations, v. 343
epidural, v. 179
extradural, v. 177
from bullet wounds of bloodvessels, ii. 665
from nasal cavities (and see Epistaxis), vi. 52
in fractures of skull, v. 70
in orbit, v. 649
intracerebral, v. 260
intracranial, v. 175, 176, 179
intradural, v. 179
meningeal, at birth, v. 208
lumbar puncture in diagnosis of, v. 199
precautions in, v. 200
middle meningeal, v. 177
of veins of neck, vi. 325
orbital, in fracture of the skull, v. 71

Hemorrhage, recurrent, after bullet wounds of blood-vessels, ii. 665
repeated small, leading to chronic anæmia, i. 245
secondary, iv. 167
after gunshot wounds, ii. 666
subconjunctival, in fractures of the skull, v. 71
subdural, v. 179, 195
Hemorrhagic exudate, i. 416
Hemorrhoids, vii. 860
accidents and complications following operations for, vii. 873
after-treatment. vii. 873
treatment of internal and mixed, vii. 864
varicose, vii. 861
Hennequin and Wille's sutures for bone. iii. 92
Hepaptosis, viii. 229
Hepatic duct, viii. 196
gall stones in, viii. 241
operations on, viii. 275
Hepatic toxæmia, iv. 162
Hepaticostomy, viii. 275
Hepaticotomy, viii. 275
Hepato-cholangioenterostomy, vii. 276
Hepato-hepaticotomy, viii. 276
Hereditary syphilis, see under Syphilis
Heredity, influence of, upon surgical conditions, i. 782
predisposing influence of, in tuberculous arthritis, iii. 570
Hermaphroditism, vi. 635
Hernia (and see Abdominal hernia), vii. 555
as affected by parturition, i. 780
cerebri, v. 377
at foramen of Winslow, vii. 609
diaphragmatic, vii. 612
duodenal, vii. 610
femoral, vii. 584
inguinal, vii. 557
internal, vii. 609
intersigmoid, vii. 611
ischiatic, vii. 605
lumbar, vii. 607
obturator, vii. 603
of Fallopian tube, viii. 400
of ovary, viii. 400
of urinary bladder, viii. 312
perineal, vii. 606
sciatic, vii. 605
umbilical, vii. 594
ventral, vii. 599
Herniotomy, vii. 106
Herpes, inflamed, differential diagnosis of, ii. 107
of eyelids, v. 548
of pharynx, v. 824
of tongue, vi. 235
progenitalis, vi. 674
zoster ophthalmicus, v. 548, 601
treatment of, v. 607
Heryng's laryngeal knives and curettes, v. 878
Heurtaux's operation for restoration of lower lip, iv. 655
Hewitt's nitrous oxide and oxygen apparatus, iv. 183

Hey's modification of Lisfranc's operation, iv. 323
operation, amputation of leg, iv. 339
Hickey, Preston M., i. 578
Hill, Leonard, cerebral pressure gauge of, v. 108
work of, on cerebral compression, v. 116
Hilton's method of opening abscesses, vi. 341
Hip-joint, Alden March's treatment of disease of, by fixation and traction, i. 54
amputation at, i. 60
by Guthrie's method of antero-posterior flaps, cut from without inward, iv. 359
arthrodesis at, for paralytic deformities of the lower extremities, iv. 869
congenital dislocation of, iv. 746
development and relations of its capsule, iii. 625
disarticulation at, ii. 757; iv. 350-360
disease of, i. 54
dislocations of, i. 48; iv. 71-85
Esmarch's amputation at, iv. 358
excision of, iv. 426-434
the operation, iv. 429
functional disease of, iii. 547
hypertrophic arthritis of, iii. 520
infantile paralysis of, iv. 817
intermediary excision, ii. 756
Jordan Furneaux's amputation, iv. 357
penetrating wounds of, iii. 746
Physick's method of treating disease of, i. 54
Sayre's splint in treatment of disease of, i. 55
secondary excision, ii. 756
sprains and contusions of, iii. 745
tuberculous disease of, iii. 623
Hippus, v. 612
Hodgen's modification of Nathan R. Smith's anterior splint, iii. 175
Hoffa's classification of congenital deformities, iv. 733
method of treating congenital dislocation of the hip, iv. 758
Holden's operation for lacerated perineum, vi. 603
Hollow foot, v. 891
Holmes, Christian R., on Hospitals and Hospital Management, more particularly with reference to the Surgical Needs of these Institutions, viii. 823-894
Holtz's operation for symblepharon, v. 567
Holtz-Anagnostakis' operation for entropion, v. 563
Hordeolum, v. 551
Horns, cutaneous, ii. 345; v. 485
development of epithelioma in, ii. 345
of auricle, v. 675
of penis, vi. 687

Horns, cutaneous, on eyelids, v. 551
genital, ii. 345
Horsehair for sutures, i. 726
Horseshoe kidney, viii. 86
Horsley, J. Shelton, on Syphilitic Disease of the Bones, iii. 364
Horsley's antiseptic wax as a hæmostatic, iv. 273
Horsley and Kramer's experiment on cerebral concussion, v. 155
Hospital or hospitals (and see Army medical department), viii. 823
arrangement of, viii. 823
at Nuernberg, Germany, viii. 843
base, in military service, viii. 967
block, viii. 823
Boucicaut, at Paris, viii. 872, 873
car (railroad), viii. 1046, 1047, 1048, 1049
cars, Japanese, viii. 938
chapel of, viii. 879
corps, naval, viii. 1001
corps, of U. S. Army, viii. 903
corps pouch, naval, viii. 1000
evacuation, in military service, viii. 965
field, in military service, viii. 959
floating, on Tyne, England, viii. 828
for contagious diseases, viii. 892, 894
for contagious diseases, Philadelphia, viii. 892
heating of, viii. 855
in army medical service, viii. 935
isolation, viii. 892
Japanese military, viii. 934-967
kitchen, viii. 881
lighting of, viii. 850
Lying-in, New York, viii. 848
management, viii. 823, 881
Hospitalism, viii. 824, 826
operative treatment, vii. 380
Hour-glass stomach, vii. 379
Housemaid's knee, ii. 442
Houston, valves of, vii. 833
Howell, W. H., on the cause of shock, i. 464
Howship's lacunæ, in osteoporosis, iii. 262
Howship-Romberg sign in obturator hernia, vii. 604
Humerus, acute osteomyelitis of, iii. 305
congenital dislocation of, iv. 738
dislocations of, iv. 36
fractures of, iii. 123
sarcoma of, iii. 459
separation of the upper epiphysis of, iii. 125
ununited fractures in, iii. 236
Hunter's operation for aneurysm, vii. 278
Hutchison, James Alexander, on Administrative Railroad Surgery, viii. 1030-1060

Hutchison and Abbe's modification of the intracranial operation on the trigeminal nerve, v. 400

Hyalin, epithelial, i. 192
    resemblances and differences between it and amyloid, i. 197

Hydatid cysts of abdominal wall, vii. 89
    of liver, viii. 214
    of pancreas, viii. 181
    of prostate, viii. 367
    of spleen, viii. 70
    of tongue, vi. 243

Hydatidiform mole or myxoma chorii racemosum, i. 307

Hydatids of Morgagni, vi. 629
    cysts of, vi. 697

Hydræmia defined, i. 240

Hydrencephalocele, v. 213

Hydrocele, i. 236; vi. 680

Hydrocephalus, v. 218, 232
    acquired, v. 218, 225
    acute, v. 218
    chronic, v. 218, 239
    congenital, v. 218, 220
    diagnosed from cerebral tumor, v. 317
    external, definition of, i. 236
    externus, v. 218
    idiopathic, v. 218
    internal, definition of, i. 236
    internus, v. 218, 222

Hydronephrosis, viii. 100

Hydropericardium, definition of, i. 236

Hydrophidæ or water snakes, iii. 8

Hydrophis cyanocincta, iii. 9

Hydrophobia, iii. 38

Hydrophthalmos, v. 604

Hydrops vesicæ felleæ, viii. 237

Hydrosalpinx, viii. 407

Hydrothorax, definition of, i. 236

Hygroma colli congenitum, i. 323

Hylomata or pulp tumors, i. 298

Hymen, atresia of, vi. 573
    imperforate, vi. 573

Hyoid bone, chondroma of, iii. 429
    fractures of, iii. 107

Hyperacidity, in gastric ulcer, vii. 340

Hyperæmia or congestion, i. 234
    active, causes of, i. 234
    arterial, effects due to, i. 235
    artificially induced, in acute mastitis, vi. 514
    following infection, i. 415
    local, passive or venous, i. 234
    of conjunctiva, v. 578
    of eyelids, v. 549
    of ovary, viii. 401

Hyperæsthesia of larynx, v. 896
    of scalp, v. 23

Hyperalgesia due to gunshot wounds of the skull, v. 98

Hyperalgesic zones in cranial injuries, v. 98

Hyperaseptic operations, v. 240

Hyperdiæmorrhysis, definition of, v. 107

Hyperemesis, post-operative, iv. 153

Hyperkeratosis, ii. 344
    linguæ, vi. 239

Hypernephroma, viii. 135
    benign, i. 347
    metastatic, iii. 481

Hyperostosis, i. 314; iii. 340, 397
    diffuse, general, iii. 397
    diffuse, of the bones of the cranium and of the face, v. 27

Hyperplasia of the bone marrow, iii. 465

Hypertrichosis, treatment of, by electrolysis, ii. 391

Hypertrophic bone changes after typhoid, referred to irritation along epiphyseal junctions, iii. 338
    nodes on the tibia and tarsal bones, iii. 517

Hypertrophied tonsils, faucial, v. 834

Hypertrophy, i. 148
    circumcorneal of conjunctiva, v. 581
    compensatory, as when fibula is thickened on weakening of tibia, i. 156
    complemental, as between thyroid and pituitary body, i. 156
    cranial, v. 26
    diffuse, of alveolar border, in leukæmia, vi. 817
    of cranial bones (and see Leontiasis ossea), v. 26
    due to errors of metabolism, i. 162
    extrinsic, i. 153, 154, 155
    from chronic irritation, as intermittent pressure, i. 159
    from failure of involution, as sometimes occurs in the thymus gland or the uterus post partum, i. 157
    from increased nutrition, as by enlarged blood-vessels, i. 158
    from removal of pressure, as in a microcephalic skull when brain is undeveloped, i. 159
    from removal of pressure, as in the overgrowth of fat about a contracted kidney, i. 157
    influence of the ductless glands upon extrinsic, i. 162
    intrinsic, i. 151
    mutual relations between growth and development, i. 149
    neurotrophic, as in a hypertrophied bladder in children, i. 163
    numerical, or hyperplasia, i. 150
    of auricle, v. 675
    of bone, iii. 337
    of female breast, vi. 508
    of lachrymal gland, v. 592
    of lingual tonsil, v. 841
    of lip, v. 476
    of ovary, viii. 402
    of prostate, viii. 358
    of scrotum, vi. 658
    quantitative, or true hypertrophy, i. 150
    unilateral of face, v. 497

Hypoblastic structures, i. 299

Hypodermic injection, instruments and methods, iv. 602

Hypodermoclysis, iv. 609

Hypoglossal nerve, surgery of the, v. 416

Hypophysis, tumors of, v. 331
    relation of acromegaly to, v. 26

Hypopyon, v. 599

Hypospadias, vi. 635, 648
    in female, vi. 579
    penile, vi. 650
    perineal, vi. 654

Hysterectomy (and see Uterus, cancer of), viii. 418, 556
    abdominal, viii. 556
    and double salpingo-oöphorectomy, viii. 418
    supravaginal, viii. 558, 559, 564
    vaginal, viii. 647

Hysterical joint, iii. 726
    as distinguished from tuberculosis of the knee-joint, iii. 700
    spine, vi. 461

ICHOROUS pus defined, i. 253

Icterus or jaundice, causes of, i. 206

Ileus, dynamic, vñ. 727
    gastro-mesenteric, vii. 736
    mechanical, vii. 727
    obturation, iv. 156
    strangulation, iv. 155

Iliac, primitive, ligation of, i. 44
    vessels, injuries and diseases of, vii. 24

Ilio-psoas bursitis, vii. 51

Imperforate anus, vii. 775
    hymen, vi. 573

Implantation in mice, natural immunity to, i. 397

Inclusions in cancer, question of their parasitic nature, i. 388

Incontinence of urine, viii. 316
    false, viii. 316, 319
    in hypertrophied prostate, viii. 364

Index finger, amputation of, iv. 284

Indian method of blepharoplasty, iv. 672
    of plastic operations, iv. 613, 614, 672, 680
    of rhinoplasty, iv. 680

Indican, significance of, in urine, i. 569

Indigestion, acute, diagnosed from acute appendicitis, vii. 660

Infantile paralysis (and see Paralysis, infantile), iv. 807
    old or neglected, as an indication for excision of the knee, iv. 439
    or acute anterior poliomyelitis, ii. 483

Infarct, viii. 187
    anæmic or white, explanation of the term, i. 239
    red or hæmorrhagic, its origin, i. 239

Infected wounds, i. 271

Infected wounds of joints of the hand, points where incisions should be made, as indicated by Kanavel's experiments, iii. 743

Infection, i. 696
from the mouth and upper air passages, i. 699
of closed wounds, effects of, i. 271, 272
of fingers, vii. 53
of genitals, male, external, vi. 668
of hands, vii. 53
of healing wound, i. 418
of periurethral ducts, vi. 753
of the face, v. 432
of wounds, conditions favorable to the development of, i. 699
of wrist-joint, vii. 66
pelvic, viii. 403
resisted by granulation tissue, i. 274

Infectious arthritis, x-ray indications of, i. 659
bacilli, their presence in bone as related to previous or coexistent disease, iii. 274
diseases, acute, influence of, upon surgical conditions, i. 792
venereal granuloma of the dog. i. 407

Infective agents—the most important bacteria, i. 415
granulomata, distinctions between them and tumors, i. 291

Inferior dental nerve, surgery of the, v. 390
intrabuccal method of reaching, v. 390

Infiltration, i. 194
amyloid, etiologically connected with chronic cachexias, i. 195
anæsthesia, according to the methods of Matas and Braun, iv. 236
as practised by Schleich, iv. 236
glycogenous, i. 203
hyaline, exact nature of, undetermined, i. 197
of urine, vi. 807, 808
pigmentation, i. 203
purulent, i. 121
small-celled, i. 121

Inflammation, i. 71
a bodily function, fundamentally protective, with varying manifestations, i. 81
acute degenerative and necrotic, i. 134
acute fibrinous, i. 118
acute purulent, i. 121
acute serous, i. 115
adhesive, i. 104
aseptic, i. 110
Boerhave's conception of, i. 73
certain products of, i. 247
chronic atrophic, i. 144
chronic indurative, i. 145
chronic productive, i. 145
Cohnheim's conception of, i. 73

Inflammation, croupous, i. 118
diphtheritic, i. 135
fibrino-purulent, i. 122
fibrinous, i. 119
formative, i. 110
gangrenous, i. 137
healing of, i. 100
membranous, i. 118
of antrum (and see Antrum, inflammation of), vi. 156, 159
of Bartholin's glands, vi. 560
of bile-ducts, viii. 229
of breast, female. See Mastitis
of bursæ about the knee as distinguished from tuberculosis of the joint, iii. 699
of capsule of Tenon, v. 648
of carotid sheaths, acute, vi. 343
of conjunctiva (and see Conjunctivitis), v. 578
of cornea (and see Keratitis), v. 599
of ear. See Otitis
of epididymis. See Epididymitis
of Fallopian tube. See Salpingitis
of frontal sinus (and see Frontal sinus, inflammation of), vi. 113, 115
of gall bladder, viii. 229
of genitals, male, external, vi. 668
of jaws, and their soft parts, vi. 874
of kidney, suppurative, viii. 106
of lachrymal gland, v. 592
of larynx. See Laryngitis
of leptomeninges, v. 226
of lingual tonsil, v. 841
of mastoid process. See Mastoiditis
of mediastinum, viii. 32
of Meibomian glands, v. 558
of mouth (and see Stomatitis), vi. 221
of neck, vi. 339
of pancreas (and see Pancreatitis), viii. 162
of parotid gland, vi. 300, 301
of penis, vi. 669
of pharynx. See Pharyngitis
of prepuce, vi. 669
of prostate. See Prostatitis
of salivary glands, vi. 299, 301, 302
of seminal vesicles. See Vesiculitis
of Skene's glands, vi. 560
of sphenoidal sinus (and see Sphenoidal sinus, inflammation of), vi. 180, 181
of spine, chronic ankylosing, vi. 456
of submental connective tissue, v. 444
of testis. See Orchitis
of thyroid. See Thyroiditis and Strumitis
of tongue. See Glossitis
of tonsils. See Amygdalitis
of ureter, viii. 144·
of urethra. See Urethritis

Inflammation of urinary bladder. See Cystitis
of vas deferens. See Vesiculitis
phlegmonous, i. 131
purulent, i. 121
sero-purulent, i. 121

Infraorbital nerve, extracranial operations upon, v. 386

Infusion, intravenous, of a saline or an adrenalin solution, iv. 606

Ingrowing toe-nail, vii. 43

Inguinal canal, vii. 563
fossæ, v. 559
hernia, vii. 557

Injection, hypodermic, iv. 602

Injured person, duty of, to employ surgeon, viii. 735

Innominate artery, aneurysm of, vi. 336; viii. 41
ligature of, i. 42, 43
surgical anatomy, iv. 476–481

Insane, softening of bone in the, iii. 358

Insect bites and stings, iii. 3, 4

Insertions of muscles, exostoses at, iii. 405

Inspection, diagnostic data acquired by, i. 512

Instruments, i. 741
and suture material, their sterilization and preparation for use, iv. 136–138
used in excision and resections, iv. 369, 370

Intermaxillary bone, displaced, operation upon, v. 516
Duplay's method, v. 520
Kronlein's method, v. 520
Wyeth's method, v. 521

Intersigmoid hernia, vii. 611

Intestinal epithelium, regeneration of, i. 258
exclusion, vii. 758
fistula, vii. 711
intussusception, vii. 728, 730
obstruction, vii. 727
obturation, vii. 732
stenosis, chronic, vii. 732
strangulation, vii. 727
ulceration, diagnosed from acute appendicitis, vii. 661
ulcers, vii. 713

Intestines, adenoma of, vii. 737
adynamic paralysis of, postoperative, iv. 152, 155
anastomosis of, vii. 749
angioma of, vii. 737
anomalies of, congenital, vii. 700
carcinoma of, vii. 740
congenital anomalies of, vii. 700
development of, vii. 704
diverticula, acquired, vii. 703
examination of, and diagnostic data obtainable from, i. 524
fibroma of, vii. 737
foreign bodies in, vii. 705, 708
injuries of, vii. 705
lipoma of, vii. 737
myoma of, vii. 737
obstruction of (and see Intestinal obstruction), vii. 727

Intestines, operations on, vii. 754
　peritoneal adhesions, vii. 726
　perforation of, typhoid, vii. 720
　sarcoma of, vii. 738
　tumors of, vii. 737
　typhoid perforation of, vii. 720
　wounds of, i. 275, 276; vii. 698
Intra-articular ligaments, iii. 559,
　560
Intracapsular and extracapsular
　fractures of the upper end of the
　femur, iii. 159
Intracranial hemorrhages in the
　new born, v. 208
Intradural abscess.　See Abscess,
　intradural
　hemorrhage, v. 179
Intrahepatic ducts, gall-stones in,
　viii. 242
　operations on, viii. 275
Intranasal adenoma, vi. 195
　angioma, vi. 195
　carcinoma, vi. 199, 857
　diseases, operations for, vi. 873
　exostosis, vi. 195
　fibroma, vi. 190
　osteoma, vi. 195
　papilloma, vi. 194
　sarcoma, vi. 198, 857, 858
　tumors, vi. 855
Intra-ocular irrigation in cataract
　extractions, v. 632
Intraperitoneal abscess (and see
　Subphrenic abscess), vii. 494
Intrathoracic surgery (Heart and
　Œsophagus excluded), viii. 3–58
Intravascular antisepsis in the
　treatment of septicæmia, i. 444
Intubation of larynx, v. 890
Intussusception, intestinal, vii. 728,
　730
　of vermiform appendix, vii. 624
Inversion of uterus, viii. 510
Involucrum as a periosteal repro-
　duction, i. 286
Iodides, use of, in diagnosis of cere-
　bral tumors, v. 317
Iodine as a sterilizing agent, i. 707
Iodoform emulsion, its use in treat-
　ing cold abscesses, i. 723
　gauze, its uses and preparation,
　i. 723
　poisoning, post-operative, iv.
　165
　value of, as a dressing, i. 723
Iodophilia, inferences to be drawn
　from, i. 559
Iridectomy, v. 619
Irideremia, v. 613
Irido-cyclitis, v. 609
Iridodesis, v. 621
Iridodialysis, v. 612
Iridodonesis, v. 612
Iridonchisis, v. 621
Iridotomy, v. 622
Iris, absence of, v. 613
　bombé, v. 609
　congenital anomalies of, v. 613
　contusion of, v. 613
　crater-shaped, v. 609
　cysticercus of, v. 613
　cysts of, v. 613
　diseases of, v. 608

Iris, gumma of, v. 613
　inflammation of (and see Iritis),
　v. 608
　injuries of, v. 612
　operations upon, v. 616
　rupture of, v. 613
　sarcoma of, v. 613
　tubercle of, v. 613
　tumors of, v. 613
　vascular tumors of, v. 613
Iritis, v. 608
　diabetic, v. 610
　fibrinous, v. 611
　gelatinous, v. 611
　gonorrhœal, v. 610
　gouty, v. 610
　insidious, v. 611
　purulent, v. 611
　quiet, v. 611
　rheumatic, v. 610
　serous, v. 611
　spongy, v. 611
　syphilitic, v. 609
　traumatic, v. 611
　treatment of, v. 614
　tuberculous, v. 610
Irradiation theory of the causation
　of cranial fractures, v. 64
　Rawling's modifications of,
　v. 64
Irrespirable gases, viii. 976
Irrigation of abdominal cavity, vii.
　119
　peritoneal, in septic peritonitis,
　vii. 515
　when and how to be used, i.
　704
Irritants, reaction of cells to them
　in inflammation, i. 71
Ischæmia defined, i. 240
　and anæmia, distinction drawn
　between them, i. 238
Ischæmic myositis, vii. 37
Ischiatic hernia, vii. 605
Ischio-rectal abscess, vii. 811
Isodiametric cells, i. 359
Isolation hospital, viii. 892, 893
Israel's method of rhinoplasty, iv.
　689
　operation for restoring the
　cheek, iv. 644
　for saddle-nose, iv. 708, 713
Italian method of blepharoplasty,
　iv. 678
　of plastic operations, iv. 613,
　618, 678, 685
　of restoring lower part of
　nose, iv. 701
　of rhinoplasty, iv. 685
Ivory exostosis of frontal sinus, iii.
　411, 413

Jackson, Charles T., i. 66
Jackson, James, i. 11
Jacob's ulcer of face, v. 489
Jacobson, Nathan, on Tuberculous
　Peritonitis, vii. 527–554
Jaeger and Richet's operation for
　ectropion, iv. 669
Jaesche's method in plastic surgery,
　iv. 616
　operation for restoration of
　lower lip, iv. 654

Jalaquier-Kammerer incision, vii.
　124
Jameson, Horatio Gates, i. 45
Janet's method of treating acute
　urethritis by irrigation, vi. 735
Jansen's bayonet-shaped bone for-
　ceps, vi. 143
Japanese field sterilizer, viii. 954
Jarvis' adjuster for the reduction of
　dislocations of the humerus, iv.
　45
Jaundice, hæmo-hepatogenous, i.
　206
Jaw, lower (and see Jaws, and Man-
　dible)
　dislocation of, iv. 29
　fractures of, iii. 103
　giant-cell sarcoma of, vi. 828
　medullary tumors of body of,
　vi. 827
　tumors of, vi. 816
　upper (and see Jaws)
　fractures of, iii. 102
　Kocher's osteoplastic resec-
　tion of both halves of, vi.
　871
　tumors of, vi. 816
Jaws, actinomycosis of, vi. 883
　adamantine epithelioma of, vi.
　841
　cystic, vi. 844
　of the alveolar border, vi.
　843
　solid, vi. 844
　carcinoma of, secondary, vi. 849
　deformities of, vi. 890
　dental-root cyst of, vi. 835
　dentigerous cyst of, vi. 837
　epithelioma of, adamantine, vi.
　841
　cystic, vi. 844
　of the alveolar border, vi.
　843
　solid, vi. 844
　exostosis of, vi. 816
　fibroma of, iii. 435, 476
　fibromyxosarcoma, periosteal,
　of, vi. 825
　fibrosarcoma, periosteal, of, vi.
　825
　hemorrhagic periostitis of, vi.
　876
　infections of, through and about
　the teeth, vi. 877
　inflammation of, vi. 874
　ossifying periostitis of, vi. 816
　osteomata of, iii. 404
　osteomyelitis of, vi. 875, 879
　osteosarcoma of, vi. 816
　periosteal, vi. 824
　ostitis of, arsenical, vi. 889
　phosphorous, vi. 887
　periosteal fibromyxosarcoma of,
　vi. 825
　fibrosarcoma of, vi. 825
　osteosarcoma of, vi. 824
　sarcoma of, vi. 823
　spindle- and round-cell sar-
　coma of, vi. 826
　tumors of body of, vi. 821
　periostitis of, vi. 875, 879
　arsenical, vi. 889
　mother-of-pearl, vi. 889

Jaws, periostitis of, phosphorous, vi. 887
    vi. 887
    ossifying, vi. 816
    syphilitic, vi. 887
    resection of, ante-operative appliances, vi. 44
    immediate, vi. 42
    Martin's method, vi. 36, 40, 45
    permanent appliances, vi. 44
    post-operative treatment, vi. 44
    prosthesis after, vi. 35
    temporary appliances, vi. 43
    sarcoma of, iii. 456
    periosteal, vi. 823
    spindle- and round-cell, periosteal, vi. 826
    surgical diseases and wounds of, vi. 813
    syphilis of, vi. 886
    toxic inflammation with necrosis of, vi. 887
    tuberculosis of, vi. 881
    tumors of, vi. 813, 816, 817
    wounds of, vi. 813
Jefferson Medical College of Philadelphia, when founded, i. 26
Jejunum, peptic ulcer of, vii. 718
Joan Baptiste dos Santos, vii. 17
Johnston, George Ben, on the Preparation for an Operation, the operation itself, and the care of the patient during and immediately after the operation, iv. 126
Joints, atmospheric pressure as a factor in retaining their surfaces in contact, iii. 563
    atrophy, reflex, iii. 547
    blood-vascular supply of, iii. 562
    bloody effusions in, O'Conor's treatment of, by incision and drainage, iii. 733
    chronic non-tuberculous and non-traumatic inflammations of, iii. 487
    disease, tuberculous: constitutional measures of treatment, iii. 506
    factors on which their strength depends, iii. 563
    foreign bodies in, iii. 530, 531
    fringes, iii. 533–535
    gouty affections of, iii. 549
    hæmophilia as affecting, iii. 553
    hysterical, iii. 726
    "mice," iii. 419
    nerve supply of, iii. 562
    neuroses, hysterical joints, ii. 509
    pedunculated tumors in, iii. 530
    suppuration within, results of, i. 255
    syphilitic lesions of, iii. 536
    the degree of approximation of articular surfaces in, iii. 560
    their structure at different periods of childhood, as differing from that of adults, iii. 560
    tuberculous disease of, iii. 558
    wounds of, iii. 725
Jonas, August F., on abscesses, ii. 143

Jones, John, i. 8, 34
    twins, the, vii. 16, 17
Jones' (Wharton) operation for ectropion, iv. 668
Jordan's (Fourneaux) amputation at hip-joint, iv. 357
Joseph's operation for elongated nose, iv. 716
Judson's apparatus for deformities of foot, iv. 902
    brace for talipes calcaneus, iv. 920
    modification of Taylor's club-feet brace, vi. 910
Jugular vein, internal, resection of, in sinus thrombosis, v. 747
Jury mast for Pott's disease, iv. 972

KAMMERER-BATTLE incision, in operation for appendicitis, vii. 680
Kanavel's experiments with regard to the lymph spaces of the hand, iii. 743
Kangaroo tendon for buried sutures, i. 730
Karyokinesis, i. 257
Kaufmann's method of operating for salivary fistula, v. 443
Kaulyang splints, viii. 955
Keegan's method of rhinoplasty, iv. 685
Keen's operation for torticollis, iv. 802
Kelly, Howard A., i. 4
Kelly's cystoscope, viii. 331, 332
    method of hysterectomy, viii. 568
Keloid, ii. 368
    idiopathic or spontaneous, i. 365
    of auricle, v. 674
    of chest wall, vi. 414
    of face, v. 463
    of tongue, vi. 257
    secondary, scar, cicatricial, or spurious, i. 305
Keloidal acne, ii. 370
Keratitis, bullous, v. 600
    deep punctate, v. 603
    dendritic, v. 601
    fascicular, v. 600
    filamentous, v. 601
    gouty, treatment of, v. 607
    hypopyon, v. 599
    interstitial, v. 602
    malarial, v. 601
    neuroparalytic, v. 600
    "oyster-shucker's," v. 600
    parenchymatous, v. 602
    phlyctenular, v. 600
    punctate, v. 602, 611
    rheumatic, treatment of, v. 607
    ribbon-shaped, v. 601
    sclerosing, v. 603
    scrofulous, v. 603
    sloughing, v. 599
    striated, after cataract operations, v. 636
    striped, v. 603
    superficial, v. 599
    syphilitic, v. 602
    tuberculous, v. 603
    vascular, v. 599

Keratocele, v. 600
Kerato-conus, v. 604
Kerato-globus. v. 604
Keratomalacia. v. 607
Keratosis of pharynx, v. 821
    senilis of face, v. 488
Keratotomy, Sæmisch, v. 617
Keyes, Edward L., Jr., on Syphilis from a Surgical Standpoint, ii. 91
    John M., on Ligature of Arteries and Veins in their Continuity, iv. 468
Kidney, and see Renal
    abnormalities of, viii. 85
    absence of one, viii. 88
    adenoma of, viii. 133
    adenosarcoma of, viii. 137
    anatomy of, viii. 78
    angioma of, viii. 133
    atrophy of one, viii. 88
    carcinoma of, viii. 134
    cysts of, viii. 137
    development of, viii. 78
    diseases of, viii. 96
    a source of danger in administration of anæsthetics, i. 785, 787
    drainage of, viii. 152
    embryology of, viii. 78
    endothelioma of, viii. 134
    epithelium of, its limited power of repair, i. 258
    examination of, as to its mobility and pathological relations, i. 552
    fibro-lipoma of, viii. 133, 134
    fibroma of, viii. 133
    floating, viii. 97
    fused, viii. 85
    histology of, viii. 80
    horseshoe, viii. 86
    injury to, without wound, viii. 90
    laceration of, viii. 90
    lipoma of, viii. 133, 134
    misplaced, viii. 87
    movable, viii. 96
    myo-lipoma of, viii. 133, 134
    operations upon, viii. 146
    papilloma of, viii. 133
    perithelioma of, viii. 134, 135
    physiology of, viii. 81
    rupture of, viii. 93
    sarcoma of, viii. 134, 136
    separation of the urines of the two, viii. 83
    structure of, viii 78
    supernumerary, viii. 88
    suppurative inflammations of, viii. 106
    surgical, viii. 107
    surgical diseases of, viii 78
    test of the functional activity of, viii. 83
    tuberculosis of, viii. 121
    tumors of, viii. 132
    wounds of, viii. 78, 90, 96
Killian's bronchoscopy, v. 908
    operation for obliteration of frontal sinus, vi. 127
    periosteal elevator and eye-retractor, vi. 131

Killian's phantom for bronchoscopy, v. 912
tracheoscopy, v. 907
King's College, New York, medical department of, organized, i. 8.
Kingsley's splint, iii. 105
velum, vi. 12
Kirmisson's theory of congenital defects, iv. 734
dislocations, iv. 734
Kit for operations, portable, iv. 147
Knapp's method of blepharoplasty, iv. 677; v. 574
method of iridectomy, v. 622
method of operation for epicanthus, v. 570
method of operation for pterygium, v. 594
Knee-jerk, or patellar reflex, as a diagnostic factor, i. 539
loss of, in alcoholism, an unfavorable prognostic sign, i. 797
Knee-joint, amputation at, surgical anatomy, iv. 343
ankylosis following septic arthritis, iii. 753
as affected by hypertrophic arthritis, iii. 518
bursæ about it, iii. 688
contusions and sprains of, iii. 746–748
development of epiphyses about it, as shown by radiographs, i. 592
disarticulation at, by lateral flaps (Stephen Smith), iv. 344
dislocations of, iv, 85
efforts towards preventing readhesion of surfaces after treatment for ankylosis, iii. 754
excision of, iv. 435–453
functions of, as conditioned by its ligaments, iii. 747, 748
Gritti's transcondyloid amputation through, iv. 346
hypertrophic arthritis of, iii. 518
infantile paralysis of, iv. 816
infected, objections to posterior incisions, iii. 752
internal derangement of, iv. 89, 90
method of using local anæsthesia in exploration of, iv. 249
penetrating wounds of, iii. 749–754
septic arthritis and cellulitis; the question of amputation, iii. 753
special features of its synovial cavity, iii. 688
Stokes' supra-condyloid amputation through, iv. 347
tuberculous disease of, iii. 684
Knight, Charles H., on Surgical Diseases and Wounds of the Pharynx, v. 810-862
Jonathan, i. 22
Knight's adenoid forceps, v. 832
bow-legs brace, iv. 861
electric tonsil snare, v. 837

Knives, surgical, i. 743
Knock-knee (and see Genu valgum), iv. 863
etiology, iv. 864
in infantile paralysis, iv. 817, 824
in rickets, iii. 350
Thomas brace for, iv. 864, 865, 866
Knots used in the ligature of arteries, iv. 473
Koch and Filehne, researches of, on cerebral concussion, v. 153, 162
Kocher's enucleator, v. 922
forceps, for thyroid operations, vi. 384, 385
histotribe, v. 923
method of excision of tongue, vi. 281
method of ligating vertebral artery, vi. 337
method of operating on the mandibular division of the trigeminal nerve, v. 392
method of reducing forward dislocations of the humerus, iv. 45
method of treatment of forward (thyroid) dislocations of the hip, iv. 82
operation for arthrectomy of the elbow joint, iii. 611
operation for excision of a tuberculous astragalus, iii. 719
operation for excision of the shoulder joint by posterior incision, iv. 400
operation for extracranial division of the maxillary nerve, v. 387
operation for torticollis, iv. 800, 803
operation, intracranial, upon the trigeminal nerve, v. 396
osteoplastic resection of both halves of upper jaw, vi. 871
remarks on the surgical treatment of goitre, vi. 381
spoon, vi. 385
theory on pathogenesis of cerebral concussion, v. 163
transduodenal choledochotomy, viii. 273
views on compression of the brain, v. 125
views on vascular pressure in relation to thyroidectomy, iv. 116
Koelliker's chromatophores, i. 194
Koenig's method of rhinoplasty, iv. 684, 692
operation for hare lip, v. 514
Koerner's method of forming meatal flap, v. 722
Kollmann dilator, vi. 788
Kouwer's method of splenopexy, viii. 76
Kramer and Horsley's experiments on cerebral concussion, v. 155
Kraske's operation for restoring the cheek, iv. 642
parasacral method of resecting rectum, vii. 913

Kraurosis vulvæ, vi. 562
Kroenlein's method of cranio-cerebral topography, v. 362
method of operating upon displaced intermaxillary bone, v. 520
operation for tumor of optic nerve, v. 654
operation on the mandibular division of the trigeminal nerve, v. 391
Krohne's regulating chloroform inhaler, as modified from Junker's, iv. 199, 201
Kryoscopy of the blood and of the urine, i. 560
Kuemmel's method of gastro-duodenostomy, vii. 377
Kuester's craniotomy chisel, v. 357
method of rhinoplasty, iv. 689
Kuestner's operation for inverted uterus, viii. 515
Kussmaul's air hunger, iv. 162
Kyphosis (and see Pott's disease), iv. 927
Kyphotic pelvis, vii. 3

LABAT's method of rhinoplasty, iv. 681, 683
operation for repair of septum, iv. 705
Laboratories, pathological, of hospitals, viii. 879
Labyrinth, complete exenteration of, v. 756
indications for entering, v. 755
suppurative disease of, v. 731, 749
Lacerated perineum, operations for repair of (and see Perineum, lacerated, operations for repair), vi. 595
Laceration of kidney, viii. 90
of ligaments of the ankle, iii. 758
of penis, vi. 664
Lachrymal apparatus, disease of the, v. 591
operations upon the, v. 594
calculi, v. 592
duct, catarrh of, v. 591
stricture of, treatment, v. 595
Bowman's method, v. 595
fistula, treatment of, v. 597
gland, abscess of, treatment, v. 593
cyst of, v. 592
diseases of, v. 592
fistula of, v. 592
hypertrophy of, v. 592
inflammation of, v. 592
Mikulicz's disease, vi. 303
sarcoma of, v. 593
tumors of, v. 592
sac, catarrh of, v 591
Lactation, prolonged, effects of, i. 780
La Garde, Major Louis A., on Poisoned Wounds Inflicted by the Implements of Warfare, iii. 36, 37
Lagophthalmos, v. 556
Lagoria's sign, iii. 162

Laminectomy, for spinal tumors, vi. 498
Landau's operation for prolapsed uterus, viii. 506
Landing parties, viii. 1028
Landolt's operation (blepharoplasty), iv. 674
Landreau's method of rhinoplasty, iv. 681
Lane's methods of operation for cleft palate, v. 534
  first operation, v. 535
  modified operation, v. 536
  second operation, v. 537, 538
  operative method in treatment of simple fractures, iii. 91
  rongeur forceps, v. 353
Lange's method of tendon transplantation, iv. 836, 841
Langenbeck's method of restoring alæ, iv. 694
  method of rhinoplasty, iv. 683
  operation for restoration of lower lip, iv. 658, 663
  operations for saddle-nose, iv. 714
Lannelongue's method of operating for cleft palate, v. 532
Laparotomy, vii. 106
Larger's operation for restoration of lower lip, iv. 662
Larrey's operation for shoulder-joint amputation, iv. 306, 307
Laryngectomy, v. 914
  partial (and see Hemilaryngectomy), v. 926
  total, v. 918
Laryngitis, œdematous, v. 870
  phlegmonous, v. 870
  septic, v. 870
Laryngocele, v. 867
Laryngo-fissure (and see Thyrotomy), v. 889
Laryngo-œsophagectomy, v. 930
Laryngotomy, v. 904
Larynx, abscess of, v. 870
  adenoma of, v. 881
  anæsthesia of, v. 896
  angioma of, v. 881
  anomalies of, v. 863
  artificial, v. 925; vi. 31
  benign growths of, v. 880
  burns of, v. 866
  carcinoma of, v. 885
  cut-throat, v. 866
  cystoma of, v. 881
  deformities of, v. 863
  dislocations of, v. 864
  ecchondroma of, v. 881
  epithelioma of, v. 886
  erysipelas of, v. 870
  fibroma of, v. 880
  foreign bodies in, v. 871
  fractures of, iii. 107; v. 864
  gunshot wounds of, v. 866
  hyperæsthesia of, v 896
  inflammation of. See Laryngitis
  intubation of, v. 890
  lipoma of, v. 881
  local anæsthesia in, iv. 244
  lupus of, v. 879
  malformations of, v. 863
  malignant growths of, v. 884

Larnyx, membranous formations in, v. 863
  myxoma of, v. 881
  neuralgia of, v. 896
  neuroses of, v. 896
  papilloma of, v. 880
  paræsthesia of, v. 896
  paralysis of, v. 897
  persistent thyro-glossal duct, v. 869
  sarcoma of, v. 884
  scalds of, v. 866
  spasm of, v. 896·
  surgical diseases of, v. 863
  syphilis of, v. 874
  tuberculosis of, v. 875
  wounds of, v. 863
Lasègue's phenomenon, vii. 34
Lateral sinus, exploring of, v. 807
  lithotomy, viii. 328
Laudable pus, i. 125
Law, the, and surgery (and see Surgery and the law), viii. 713
Lead colic, diagnosed from acute appendicitis, vii. 661
Le Conte, Robert G., and Stewart, Francis T., on Surgery of the Pericardium, Heart, and Blood-Vessels, vii. 146–331
Le Dentu's operation for habitual dislocation of the patella, iv. 93
Lee's amputation of the leg by a large posterior flap, iv. 341
Leeches, employment of, iv. 605
Le Fort's method of blepharoplasty, v. 575
  modification of Pirogoff's amputation, iv. 333
Leg, amputation of, in lower third, iv. 334
  amputation of, in middle third, by long external flap, iv. 341
  amputation in middle third by a large posterior flap (Hey's operation), iv. 339
  amputation in upper third, by a large external flap, iv. 342
  anterior curvature of, iv. 867
  infantile paralysis of, iv. 815
  pseudarthrosis in bones of, iii. 249
  pseudarthrosis in bones of, transverse section of, in the middle, iii. 249
Leiomyoma (myoma lævicellulare), i. 316
  causing metastases, i. 319
Lembert suture, vii. 734, 754
Lens, and see Cataract
  diseases of, v. 623
  dislocated, after cataract operations, v. 637
  dislocation of, v. 626
  extraction of, in its capsule, for cataract, v. 631
  injuries of the, v. 623
Lentigines, definition of, ii. 355
Leontiasis, iii. 343, 346
  in leprosy, ii. 11
  ossea, iii. 397–401· v. 26
  an instance of localized intrinsic hypertrophy, i. 153
Lepers, syphilitic, ii. 13

Lepidomata or "rind" tumors, i. 297
Lepra bacillus, its diagnostic demonstration, ii. 17
  mutilans, ii. 13
Leproma, its characteristics, ii. 11
  "globi" found in, ii. 14
Leprosy, ii. 3
  anæsthetic or trophoneurotic, ii. 12
  geographical distribution, ii. 4
  inoculability, ii. 6
  mixed, ii. 13
  mode of invasion, ii. 10
  nerve (lepra nervosa), ii. 12
  nodular, ii. 11
  non-hereditary, ii. 5
  of tongue, vi. 243
Leprous infiltration of various organs, ii. 14
  laryngitis, ii. 18, 24
  orchitis, its diagnosis, ii. 18
  otitis media, ii. 18
Leptocephalism, iii. 327
Leptomeninges, inflammation of, v. 226
Leptomeningitis, diagnosis, v. 791
Lermoyez's method of prosthesis, iv. 625
Letenneur's operation in plastic surgery, iv. 616
Leucocytes, assemblage of, in vicinity of injury, i. 76
  diagnostic value of differential counts of, i. 558
  emigration of, i. 85
  marginal disposition of, in inflammation, i. 85
  removal of, by phagocytosis, i. 260
Leucocytosis, i. 240, 255
  degree of, important in surgical prognosis, i. 792
  diagnostic value of its presence and degree, i. 558
  in infancy, i. 246
  inflammatory, i. 246
  toxic, i. 246
Leucokeratosis (and see Leucoma), vi. 235
Leucoma, v. 605; vi. 235
Leucopenia defined, i. 240
Leucoplakia (and see Leucoma), ii. 125; vi. 235
Leucoplasia of the tongue and cheeks, ii. 374
Leukæmia, acute lymphatic, characteristic symptoms of the disease, i. 242
  acute lymphatic, or acute lymphocythæmia, i. 242
  chronic lymphatic, characteristic symptoms of the disease, i. 242
  lymphatic, features of the leucocytosis in this disease, i. 242
  myelocytic, course of the disease, i. 242
  myelocytic, diagnostic importance of the leucocytes in, i. 243
  myelocytic, features of the blood count in, i. 243

Leukæmia, myelocytic, types of myelocytes found in this disease, i. 243

myelogenous, characteristic changes in bone marrow in, i. 243

the blood picture of, modified by use of arsenic, i. 244

Levis' splint, iii. 148

Lewis, George, i. 58

Robert, Jr., on Surgical Diseases and Wounds of the Ear, v. 660–730

Lexer's operation for repair of septum of nose, iv. 704

study of the distribution of the arteries of the long bones in children, and its relation to the development of osteomyelitis, iii. 270–272

Lexer and Cushing's method of operation, intracranial, upon the trigeminal nerve, v. 397

Leyden, work of, on cerebral compression, v. 113

Leys, James Farquharson, on Leprosy, Plague, Glanders, Anthrax, Actinomycosis, Rhinopharyngitis mutilans, and Scurvy; with special reference to diagnosis and surgical treatment, ii. 3

Libraries, medical, in the United States, i. 38

"Ligamenta brevia" and "ligamenta longa," described, iv. 280

Ligaments, lacerated, iii. 726.

Ligamentum teres, function of, iii. 627

Ligation, control of hemorrhage by, vii. 244

Ligature of arteries and veins in their continuity, iv. 468: vi. 334; vii. 27· viii. 41, 544

Ligature operation for hemorrhoids, vii. 866

Ligature-carriers, i. 747

Ligatures and sutures, materials employed, i. 724

animal, suggested by Physick, i. 45

Lightning stroke, ii. 589

Limbs, artificial, general considerations, iv. 364–366

Linea alba, vii. 110

semilunaris, vii. 111

Lineæ transversæ, vii. 111

Linear extraction of cataract, v. 628

"Lingua plicata aut dissecata," vii. 229

Lingual artery, ligature of, iv. 487

dermoids, iii. 396

nerve, surgery of the, v. 391

tonsil, v. 841

abscess of, v. 841

excision of, v. 841

hypertrophy, v. 841

inflammation of, v. 841

varix of, v. 842

Linhart's method of rhinoplasty, iv. 683

Lipoma, i. 189, 307

myxomatous, i. 310

of abdominal wall, vii. 8

Lipoma of bone, iii. 436–439

of breast, female, vi. 520, 528

of conjunctiva, v. 584

of eyelids, v. 553

of face, v. 466

of gluteal region, vii. 31

of intestine, vii. 737

of kidney, viii. 133, 134

of larynx, v. 881

of mouth, vi. 251 ·

of neck, vi. 350

of parotid gland, vi. 307

of penis, vi. 686

of pharynx, v. 854

of rectum, vii. 891

of scalp, v. 15

of scrotum, vi. 695

of tongue, vi. 251

of vulva, vi. 571

retroperitoneal, i. 309

subconjunctival, v. 584

teleangiectatic, i. 319

Lipo-myxo-sarcoma, i. 344

Lipo-sarcoma, i. 333

Lipping of patella and articular surface of femur in hypertrophic arthritis, iii. 518

Lippitudo, v. 549

Lips, artificial, vi. 26

cancer of, operative procedure for removal of, ii. 562

double, v. 477

eversion of red border, correction of, iv. 667

fistula of, iv. 495

hare (and see Hare lip), v. 500

hypertrophy of, v. 476

lower, plastic surgery of the, iv. 652

Bey's operation, iv. 659

Blasius' operation, iv. 658

Buchanan's operation, iv. 657

Chopart's operation, iv. 660

Dieffenbach's operation, iv. 654

Estlander's operation, iv. 663

Heurtaux's operation, iv. 655

Jaesche's operation, iv. 654

Langenbeck's operations, iv. 658, 663

Larger's operation, iv 662

Malgaigne's operation, iv. 656

Mauclaire's operation, iv. 664

Post's (Alfred C.) operation, iv. 664

Sandelin's operation, iv. 660

Serre's operation, iv. 654

Syme's operation, iv. 657

Trélat's operation, iv. 658

von Bruns' operation, iv. 662

Watt's operation, iv. 664

Lips, lupus of, v. 453

lymphatics of, v. 421

"Lips" and osteophytes as formed about the acetabulum in hypertrophic arthritis, iii. 521, 522

Liquor puris, i. 252

Lisfranc's ligament, iv. 321

method of rhinoplasty, iv. 681, 683

operation, instruments required and the procedure, iv. 321–323

operation, surgical anatomy, iv. 320

operation, the coup de maître, iv. 321, 323

Lister, Joseph, i. 691

Lister's method of preventing hemorrhage, iv. 267

modification of Carden's operation, iv. 346

Liston's long splint, iii. 171

operation for excision of the elbow-joint, iv. 414

Lithiasis of conjunctiva, v. 584

Litholapaxy, viii. 329, 335

combined with cystoscopy, viii. 335

developed by Bigelow, i. 53

Lithotomy, i. 53

bilateral, viii. 328

lateral, viii. 328

median, viii. 325

suprapubic, viii. 328

Lithotrite and cystoscope, combined, viii. 336

Litigation spine, vi. 423

Litten's diaphragmatic phenomenon, vii. 467

Liver, abnormal relations of, and their diagnostic significance, i. 522, 790

abnormalities of, viii. 204

abscess of, viii. 208

actinomycosis of, viii. 225

adenoma of, viii. 219

anatomy of, viii. 193

angioma of, viii. 219

atrophy of, i. 181

carcinoma of, viii. 220

cirrhosis of, viii. 227

cysts of, viii. 214

echinococcus of, viii. 214

endothelioma of, viii. 219

epithelium of, its regeneration, i. 258

excretory ducts of, viii. 195

exposure of, viii. 212

fatty degeneration of, acute, following anæsthesia, iv. 162

fibroma of, viii. 219

hydatid cysts of, viii. 214

injuries of, viii. 206

lesions of, in their relations to surgical prognosis, i. 790

movable, viii. 229

multiple abscesses of, viii. 208

myoma of, viii. 219

physiology of, viii. 203

rupture of, viii. 206

sarcoma of, viii. 223

suppuration in, viii. 208

surgery of, viii. 193, 256

syphilis of, viii 226

Liver, traumatic affections of, viii. 206

tropical abscess of, viii. 209

tuberculosis of, viii. 223

tumors of, viii. 219

Locality, sense of, in relation to diagnosis, i. 537

Localization, cerebral, areas of, v. 267, 270, 271

spinal, vi. 492

Lock-jaw or trismus, iii. 24

Locomotor ataxia and paresis, their syphilitic relations, ii. 122

Long, Crawford W., i. 64

Long bones, central sarcoma of, iii. 446

of the extremities, tuberculosis of, iii. 724

traumatic exostoses of, iii. 404

Loose cartilage in the knee-joint as distinguished from tuberculosis of this joint, iii. 699

Lorenz's gypsbette, for Pott's disease, iv. 964

method of reducing talipes, iv. 906

method of treating congenital dislocations of the hip, iv. 757, 761

secondary operation, for hare lip, v. 544

Lorgnette nose, iv. 706

Louisiana, medical department of University of, organized, i. 28

Low-pressure sterilizers, i. 716

Ludwig's angina, v. 444; vi. 341

Lumbago and sciatica as symptoms of hypertrophic arthritis of the spine, iii. 524

Lumbar hernia, vii. 607

puncture, in cerebro-spinal meningitis, v. 234

in diagnosis of cerebral tumors, v. 318

in diagnosis of meningeal hemorrhage, v. 199

in treatment of intradural hemorrhage, v. 205

Lung, abscess of, viii. 19

actinomycosis of, viii. 25

atrophy of, i. 172

borders of, vii. 148

carcinoma of, viii. 30

echinococcus of, viii. 27

gangrene of, viii. 19

parasitic affections of, viii. 25

sarcoma of, viii. 30

sutures in, viii. 57

tuberculosis of, surgical treatment of, viii. 28

tumors of, viii. 30

wound in, viii. 57

Lupus erythematosus, ii. 325

exedens, v. 455

of auricle, v. 670, 676

of cheeks, v. 454

of epiglottis, v. 879

of eyelids, v. 552

of face (and see Tuberculosis), v. 452

of larynx, v. 879

of lip, v. 453

Lupus of nose, v. 453

of penis, vi. 671

of pharynx, v. 851

of scrotum, vi. 671

serpiginosus, ii. 318

verrucosus, ii. 318

vulgaris, ii. 317

Luschka's tonsil, v. 825

Lutter forceps, vii. 424

Luxatio obturatoria, iv. 80

Luxation and subluxation, the distinction between, iv. 3

Luxations. See Dislocations

Luxations, traumatic, in general, iv 9

Lymph, plastic or coagulable, distinctive character of, i. 247

organization of, in an incised wound, i. 248

channels, diffusion of inflammatory products by, i. 91

nodes, abdominal, cancerous disease of, ii. 567

acute inflammation of, ii. 530

axillary, arrangement of, vi. 506

tuberculous disease of, ii. 566

bronchial, ii 567

cervical, inflammations of, ii. 526, 533, 559

dual functions of, ii. 530

mesenteric, ii. 567

of mastoid group, v. 419

of neck, v. 417

parotid group, v. 419

retropharyngeal, suppuration of, ii, 535.

Ribbert's views regarding, i. 87

submaxillary group, v. 420

suboccipital group, v. 419

subparotid group, v. 420

Lymph - adenocele, diagnosis, ii 577

Lymphadenoma, iii. 465

of orbit, v. 652

of rectum, vii. 892

Lymphangiectases, etiology and pathology, ii. 574

Lymphangioma or angioma lymphaticum, i. 319, 322

cavernosum, i. 323

cystoides, i. 323

lymph-varices, lymphangiectases, and lymph-adenocele, ii. 573

of eyelids, v. 554

of face, v. 475

of gluteal region, vii. 31

of parotid gland, vi. 307

of tongue, vi. 244

Lymphangitis, i. 422; ii. 564

a frequent complication of felons, i. 131

ascending, i. 92

complicating chancroid, vi. 705

infective, treatment of, ii. 155

Lymphatic nodes, atrophy of, i. 180

system, part played by, in inflammation, i. 91

protective functions of, in inflammation, i. 92

Lymphatics and lymph nodes, Fischer's classification of diseases of, ii. 525

axillary, cancerous disease of, ii. 566

cervical, secondary cancerous involvement, ii. 561

lympho-sarcomata involving, ii. 560

occlusion of, as caused by filaria sanguinis hominis, ii. 575, 576

facial, v. 417, 420

of axilla and upper extremity, surgical diseases of, ii. 564

of brain, v. 105

of groin and lower extremity, surgical diseases of, ii. 568

of head and neck, anatomical arrangement, ii. 526

of lips, v. 421

of nose, v. 421

of thorax and abdomen, surgical diseases of, ii. 567

traumatisms of, ii. 563

Lymphatism, v. 826

Lymph gland, tonsillar, ii. 528

Lymphocytes, appearance and source of, in inflammation, i. 87

Lymphocytosis, i. 246

Lymphogenous metastasis in inflammation, i. 96

Lymphoma of conjunctiva, v. 581

Lympho-sarcoma, i. 334

Lymphosporidium trattæ, the relative sizes of its different forms, i. 406

Lymph-varices, definition of the term, ii. 574

Lynch, Frank W., and Murphy, John B., on Surgery of the Uterus and its Ligaments, viii. 444-969

Lynch, Major Charles, on Military Surgery, viii. 895-969

Lysol as a disinfectant, i. 707

Lyssa, explanation of the term, iii. 41

Lyssophobia, iii. 49

MAASLAND and Saltikoff, investigation of, on cerebral concussion, v. 157

Macewen's process of needling, viii. 40

Mackenrodt's operation for carcinoma of uterus, viii. 630

Mackenzie's tonsillotome, v. 839

Macrocheilia, i. 323; v. 477

Macroglossia, i. 317, 323

Macrostoma, v. 495

Madarosis, v. 550

Madelung's deformity or luxation, iv. 742, 743

Magnesium sulphate as a local anæsthetic, iv. 234

Maisonneuve's operation for absence of nose, iv. 717

urethrotome, vi. 789

Malar bone, osteomyelitis of the, v. 448

Malarial organisms, their presence as a contra-indication to operating, iv. 124

Malformations, congenital, of neck, vi. 313
　　of vermiform appendix, viii. 624
　　of anus, vii. 774
　　of male genitals, vi. 637
　　of œsophagus, vii. 410
　　of penis, vi. 637
　　of prostate, viii. 279
　　of rectum, vii. 774
　　of scrotum, vi. 657
　　of spleen, viii. 61
　　of testes, vi. 658
　　of urethra, vi. 646
　　of urinary bladder, viii. 279
　　of uterus, viii. 444, 453
Malgaigne's operation for restoration of lower lip, iv. 656
Malignant anthrax œdema, ii. 51, 247
　　callus-tumors, iii. 445
　　diseases, heredity of, i. 783
　　　recurring, under what conditions a contra-indication to operating, iv. 125
　　œdema, iii. 29
　　　bacillus of (Koch), i. 421
　　　bacteriology of, ii. 247–249
　　　differential diagnosis of, especially from infection due to Bacillus aërogenes capsulatus, iii. 29
　　　of the eyelids, v. 554
　　pustule, ii. 335; iii. 32
　　　of eyelids, v. 550
　　　of face, v. 436
　　　or anthrax carbuncle, ii. 50
Malleoderma, erysipeloid, ii. 333
　　furuncular, ii. 333
　　pustular, ii. 333
Malleus, ii. 332
　　fracture of, v. 686
Mal perforant du pied, ii. 189
Malpractice, viii. 756
　　action for, viii. 765
　　　extent of proof required from patients, viii. 765
　　　procedure in, viii. 765
　　　to whom it accrues, viii. 769
　　　when malpractice may be inferred, viii. 768
　　　　must be proved, viii. 767
　　and recovery of fees, viii. 814
　　and waiver of privilege, viii. 801
　　award of damages in, viii. 807
　　criminal, what constitutes, viii. 763
　　defined, viii. 756
　　degree and extent of proof required from patient in action for, viii. 765
　　from negligence, viii. 758
　　from want of learning, or of skill, viii. 757
　　liability for, may be a question for jury, viii. 768
　　question of, can be litigated but once, viii. 769
　　verification of charge of, viii. 765
　　when it may be inferred, viii. 768
Malum perforans, i. 137
Mamma. See Breast, female

Mamma, atrophy of, i. 182
Mammary gland. See Breast, female
　　male, surgery of the, vi. 420
　　secretion, i. 564
Mandible, fractured, splints for, vi. 48
　　resection of, prosthesis in, vi. 35, 44
Mandibular division of trigeminal nerve, intracranial operations on, v. 393
　　nerve, extracranial operations upon, v. 391
　　　Kocher's operation, v. 392
　　　Kroenlein's operation, v. 391
　　surgery of the, v. 390
　　　extracranial operations on, v. 391
　　　Kocher's method of operating on, v. 392
　　　Kroenlein's operation on, v. 391
Manipulation, avoidance of, a surgical principle, i. 273
　　reduction of dislocations of hip-joint by, i. 48
Manometer, use of, in cerebral compression, v. 132
March, Alden, i. 53
Marie's disease, iii. 360
Marrow cell of Cornil found in blood of myelocytic leukæmia, i. 243
Martin's artificial palate, vi. 19, 20
　　artificial tongue, vi. 29
　　method of prosthesis after resection of jaws, vi. 36, 40, 45
　　rubber bandages, i. 741; v. 599
Marwedel's method of gastrostomy, vii. 404
Marx's secondary operation for hare lip, v. 544
Masks for chloroform inhalation, Skinner's, Esmarch's, Schimmelbusch's, iv. 198–200
　　for operative work, i. 721
Mason, Major Charles Field, on Poisoned Wounds, including the Bites and Stings of Animals and Insects, iii. 3
Mason's pin, in fractures of the nasal bones, iii. 100
Massachusetts General Hospital ether cone, iv. 188, 189
Massage of heart, vii. 173
Mastin, William McDowell, on Abdominal Section, vii. 105–145
　　on ulcers and ulceration, ii. 164
Mastitis, vi. 510
　　carcinomatosa, vi. 539
　　cystic, vi. 514
　　interstitial, vi. 514
　　puerperalis, vi. 511
　　traumatica, vi. 511
Mastoid cells, indications for opening, v. 693
　　lymph nodes, v. 419
　　operation, in acute mastoiditis, v. 693

Mastoid operation in chronic purulent mastoiditis, v. 715
　　meato-mastoid operation, v. 725
　　radical operation, v. 715
　　Schwartze-Stacke operation, v. 715
　　Stacke operation, v. 727
Mastoidectomy, v. 803
Mastoiditis, acute, v. 690
　　chronic purulent, mastoid operations in, v. 715
Mastodynia, vi. 509
Matas' operation for aneurysm, vii. 281
Mathieu's snap guillotine, v. 882
　　tonsillotome, v. 839
Mattress sutures, vii. 736
Maturation, artificial, for cataract, v. 632
Mauclaire's operation for restoration of lower lip, iv. 664
Maxilla, inferior, fractures of, iii. 103
　　resections of, prosthesis in, vi. 35
　　　immediate, iii. 42
　　superior, excision of, iv. 378–389
　　　fractures of, iii. 102
Maxillary division of trigeminal nerve, extracranial operations upon, v. 386
　　joint, ankylosis of, vi. 889
　　　arthritis of, vi. 889
　　nerve, surgery of the, v. 386
　　　extracranial division of the, v. 387
　　　Kocher's operation, v. 387
Maxwell's method of treating fractures of the neck of the femur, iii. 177
Maydl's operation for ectopia vesicæ, viii. 285
Maydl-Reclus method of colostomy, vii. 940
Mayo's imbrication method in umbilical hernia, vii. 597
　　internal Alexander's operation, vi. 615
Mayo and Moynihan's method of gastro-enterostomy, vii. 345
McBurney, Charles, i. 59
McBurney's hooks, for skin grafting, iv. 621
　　gridiron incision, vii. 123, 126
　　operation, in appendicitis, vii. 679
　　point, vii. 650
McClellan, George, i. 26
McCosh, Andrew J., on Inflammatory and Other Diseases of the Vermiform Appendix, vii. 618–697
　　on Surgical Treatment of General Septic Peritonitis, vii. 505–526
McGraw, Theodore A., i. 370
McGraw's method of gastro-enterostomy, vii. 352
　　method of gastro-intestinal and entero-intestinal anastomosis, vii. 751

McMurtry, Lewis S., on Extra-uterine Pregnancy, viii. 690–700
on The Cæsarean Section and its Substitutes, viii. 701–710
Measurements for operating distances in the nose, vi. 203
Meato-mastoid operation, v. 725
Meatotomy, vi. 647
technique of, vi. 775
Meatus, of urethra, small, vi. 647
supernumerary, vi. 753
Meckel's diverticulum, vii. 701, 708
Median lithotomy, viii. 325
Mediastinal abscess, treatment, iv. 981
Mediastinitis, viii. 32
Mediastinum, anterior, conditions modifying relations of, vii. 150
operations on, viii. 57
posterior, operations on, viii. 58
carcinoma of, viii. 34
emphysema of, viii. 31
endothelioma of, viii. 14, 34
inflammation of, viii. 32
injuries of, viii. 31
sarcoma of, viii. 35
surgical affections of, viii. 31
tumors of, viii. 33
Medical Corps of U. S. Army, viii. 900
Medical officers, army, education and training of, viii. 914
Medical photography, viii. 877
Medical Reserve Corps of U. S. Army, viii. 902
Medicine, practice of, defined, viii. 715
Medico-legal considerations bearing upon the question of operation (and see Surgery and Law), iv. 112
questions in railroad surgery, viii. 1058
Medio-tarsal joint, motion at, iv. 915
Medullary carcinoma of breast, female, vi. 535
spindle-cell and giant-cell sarcomata of the femur, iii. 462, 463
Meibomian glands, adenoma of, v. 559
calcareous concretions of, v. 559
carcinoma of, v. 559
inflammation of, v. 558
sarcoma of, v. 559
Melanin, characteristics of, i. 342
Melano-carcinoma, i. 363
Melanoma, i. 341
Melano-sarcoma, i. 341
Meloplasty (and see Cheek, plastic surgery of the), iv. 638; vi. 223
Membrana tympani, rupture of, v. 685
Meningeal and cerebral syphilis, v. 242
artery, middle, extravasation, v. 177
topographical anatomy, of, v. 178

Meningeal infection, relation of cerebral abscess to, v. 254
syphilis, v. 242
Meninges, cerebral, v. 100
anatomical considerations, v. 173
injuries and diseases of, v. 173
Meningitis, amicrobic (and see Meningitis, serous), v. 236
cerebro-spinal, v. 231
epidemic, v. 226
posterior basal, of infants, v. 238
serosa, v. 236, 237
serous, v. 236
suppurative, v. 240
tuberculous, v. 227
Meningocele, v. 213; vi. 465
Menisci, or interarticular fibro-cartilages, iii. 560
Menstruation, influence of operations upon, i. 778
Mental disorders, after cataract operations, v. 637
effects of operations upon, i. 788
nerve, surgery of the, v. 391
torticollis, iv. 806
Mercurial stomatitis, vi. 889
Mesenchymal tissues, reproduction of, i. 258
Mesenteric vessels, embolism of, vii. 726
thrombosis of, vii. 726
Mesentery, cysts of, vii. 751
injuries of, vii. 750
surgical diseases of, vii. 698, 750
tumors of, vii. 751
wounds of, vii. 698, 750
Meso-appendix, vii. 622
Mesoblastic structures, i. 299
Mesodermal cysts, i. 367
Messerer and von Wahl's theory of the causation of cranial fractures, v. 53
Metacarpal bones, amputation through, iv. 286
chondral osteoma of, iii. 423
dislocations of, iv. 67
Metacarpals and phalanges, tuberculous disease of, iii. 616
Metastases of the liver in pyæmia, i. 437
of the lung in pyæmia, i. 437
of tumors, Virchow's views, i. 379
Metastatic calcification, or lime metastasis, i. 199
hypernephroma of bone, iii. 481
Metatarsal arch, depression of, iv. 886
weakness of, iv. 886
Metatarsalgia anterior, ii. 508; iv. 886
Metatarsals, tuberculous disease of, iii. 723
Metatarso-phalangeal joint of great toe, disarticulation of, by Farabeuf's method, iv. 314
Metatarsus, dislocations of, iv. 103, 104
Methæmoglobinuria, i. 205
Metritis dissecans, ii. 283

Miami Medical College, organization of, i. 23
Microcephalism, iii. 327
Microcornea, v. 604
Micrognathy, vi. 890
Micromonas Mesnili, relations of, to sheep-pox, i. 406
Micro-organisms, pyogenic, i. 125
Microphthalmos, v. 554
Microstoma, v. 495
Microtia, v. 661
Micturition, difficult, causes and relations of, i. 548
painful, causation and diagnostic importance, i. 549
urgent, its causative relations, i. 247
Mikulicz drain, iv. 537
Mikulicz's disease, vi. 303
method of ligating vertebral artery, vi. 337
method of treating intestinal carcinoma, vii. 744
operation for elongated nose, iv. 716
operation of complete tarsectomy, iii. 722
operation for saddle-nose, iv. 711
pad, how prepared, iv. 139
Mikulicz and Heinecke's method of pyloroplasty, vii. 370
Mikulicz-Stoerk tonsillar hæmostat, v. 840
Military policy for defence of the United States, viii. 898
surgery (and see Army), viii. 895
Militia, organized, viii. 905
Milium of eyelids, v. 550
Milliammeter, i. 616
Minerva jacket, for Pott's disease, iv. 950
Minor surgery, iv. 537
Mirault's operation for hare lip, v. 511
Misapplication of the terms "rheumatism" and "rheumatoid ostitis," iii. 339
Missiles, in naval surgery, viii. 991
lodged, the removal of, ii. 683
value of x-rays in locating, ii. 682
primary, definition of the term, ii. 642
secondary, definition of the term, ii. 642
Mitchell, James F., on the Production of local Anæsthesia for Surgical Purposes, iv. 231
Mitosis, i. 257
Mixed calculi, viii. 113
chancroid, vi. 703
infection in diseases of joints, ii. 80
Mixter's tube, vii. 756
Mixtures of chloroform and ether for anæsthesia, iv. 202
Mole, of auricle, v. 675
of face, hairy, v. 467
of face, white, v. 467
Molecular death defined, ii. 201
Mollities ossium or halisteresis, i. 174

Molluscum contagiosum, ii. 372
  of eyelids, v. 550
  epitheliale of eyelids, v. 550
  fibrosum, i. 305; ii. 371
Monks' operation (blepharoplasty), iv. 674
Monod's operation for restoring the cheek, iv. 647
Monorchidia, vi. 659
Monsters, double, vii. 16
Montgomery. Douglass W., on Surgery of the Diseases of the Skin, ii. 303
Moore, James E., i. 691
"Moral-anæsthetist," his functions, iv. 238
Morax's method of blepharoplasty, v. 575
Morbus coxæ senilis, iii. 520
Morgan, John, i. 7
Morgue, the, viii. 879
Moria, in cerebral tumors, v. 319
Morris' operation for fixation of kidney, viii. 154
  measurement, iii. 162
Mortification, ii. 201, 202
Morton, Thomas G., i. 58
Morton, W. T. G., i. 54
Morton's demonstration of the value of ether as an anæsthetic, iv. 169
  instruments for removing foreign bodies by direct bronchoscopy, v. 909
  toe, iv. 886
Mosher, Harris Peyton, on Surgical Diseases and Wounds of the Nasal Cavities and Accessory Sinuses, vi. 52–220
Mosher's cheek and lip retractor for exposing the canine fossa, vi. 166
  malleable eye retractor, vi. 140
  mask-splint for fracture of nasal bones, vi. 63
  method of operation for chronic suppuration of frontal sinus, vi. 134
  speculum for submucous resection of nasal septum, vi. 73
Mother's marks, i. 321; v. 470
  of eyelids, v. 552
Mother-of-pearl periostitis of jaws, vi. 889
Mothe's method of reducing forward dislocations of the humerus by traction vertically, iv. 44
Motion, its significance in diagnosis, i. 538
Motor area of brain, v. 269
  cortex of brain, v. 269
  tract, v. 276
Mott, Valentine, i. 5, 12, 13, 42, 44
Mouse tumors, histological characteristics of those retrograding, i. 399
  varying success in transplanting them, i. 394
Mouth (and see Tongue and Gums)
  aneurysm in, vi. 248
  blood expelled from the, its sources and diagnostic significance, i. 521

Mouth, carcinoma of, with secondary involvement of jaw, vi. 846
  cavernous tumors of, vi. 249
  congenital capillary nævi of, vi. 248
  cysts of, mucous, vi. 243
  dermoid cysts of, vi. 261
  diseases of, surgical, vi. 221
    cancrum oris, vi. 222
    stomatitis, vi. 221
  endothelioma of, vi. 253
  hæmangioma of, vi. 248
  inflammation of (and see Stomatitis), vi. 221
  lingual dermoids, vi. 396
  lipoma of, vi. 251
  mucous cysts of, vi. 243
  non-parasitic cysts of, vi. 243
  plastic surgery of the, iv. 665
    Serre's operation, iv. 667
  restoration of the, iv. 665
  telangiectasis of, vi. 248
  teratoid tumors of, vi. 262
  vascular tumors of, vi. 248
  wounds of, vi. 221
Movable kidney, viii. 96
  liver, viii. 229
  pancreas, viii. 190
Moynihan-Mayo's method of gastro-enterostomy, vii. 345
Mucocele of antrum, vi. 159
  of ethmoidal cells, vi. 98
  of sphenoidal sinus, vi. 181
Mucoid tissue, its character and relations, i. 306
Muco-pus, defined, i. 253
Mucous membranes, disinfection of, i. 708
  fibrinous exudate on, i. 118
  superficial exudative inflammation of, i. 250
  patch, ii. 111
    of pharynx, v. 844
Mucus in the stools, its significance, i. 573
Mudd, Harvey G., on Surgical Diseases and Wounds of the Female Breast, vii. 502–558
Mulberry calculus, viii. 113
Mules' operation for evisceration of eyeball, v. 646
Multilocular dentigerous cyst, iii. 474
Multiple abscesses of liver, viii. 208
  benign cystic epithelioma, ii. 349
  cartilaginous exostoses, iii. 415, 417
  myeloma, iii. 454
  neuritis, diagnosed from infantile paralysis, iv. 825
Mummification, ii. 202, 204
Mumps, vi. 300
Murphy, John B., and Lynch, Frank W., on Surgery of the Uterus and its Ligaments, viii. 444–689
Murphy button, gastro-enterostomy with, vii. 359
  method of securing mobility after old dislocation of elbow, iv. 63
  method of supravaginal hysterectomy, viii. 560

Murphy method of suturing arteries, vii. 250, 251
  method of treating fractures of the olecranon process, iii. 140
  operation for prolapsed uterus, viii. 500
Muscle, absence of regeneration in, i. 259
  animal parasites of, ii. 407
  as affected by atrophy, i. 170, 171
  contusions, sprains, and strains of, ii. 400
  cysticercus cellulosæ in, ii. 407
  echinococcus in, ii. 407–409
  hernia, ii. 402
  incised wounds of, their treatment, ii. 400
  inflammations, tumors, and parasites, ii. 403
  non-septic lacerated wounds of, their healing, ii. 400
  of head and neck, action of, iv. 788
  of neck, injuries to, vi. 331
  repair of, i. 287
  results of healing after complete transverse division, ii. 399
  rupture of, ii. 401
  spastic contraction of, as a cause of pathological dislocation, iv. 7
  teratomata of, ii. 406
  trichina spiralis in, ii. 407
  tuberculous infiltration of, ii. 405
  tumors of, ii. 406
  wounds and surgical diseases, ii. 399
Museums, pathological, value of, i. 33
Mussey, Reuben D., i. 23
Mutter's method of restoring the alæ nasi, iv. 697
Mycetoma, ii. 60, 329
Mycosis intestinalis, iii. 32
Mydriasis, v. 612
Myelocele, vi. 463
Myelogenous giant-cell sarcoma, iii 445
  pseudo-leukæmia, iii. 465
Myeloma, multiple, iii. 465–469
  of skull, v. 34
Myelomeningocele, vi. 464
Myles' lingual tonsillotome, v. 842
Myo-fibroma, i. 318
  telangiectatic and cavernous, i. 303
Myo-lipoma of kidney, viii. 133, 134
Myoma, i. 316
  of intestine, vii. 737
  of liver, viii. 219
  of œsophagus, vii. 420
  of rectum, vii. 892
  of testis, vi. 697
Myomectomy, viii. 548
  abdominal, viii. 548
  vaginal, viii. 550
Myopathy, primary, or progressive muscular dystrophy, i. 171
Myo-sarcoma or myoma sarcomatodes, i. 344
Myosis, v. 612

Myositis, acute suppurative, ii. 404
 chronic, ii. 405
 fibrosa, ii. 403
 ischæmic, vii. 37
 multiple purulent, associated with glanders, ii. 404
 ossifying, i. 315; vii. 38
 parasitic, ii. 405
 rheumatic, ii. 404
 simple acute traumatic, ii. 403
 syphilitic, ii. 405
Myringotomy, v. 688
Myxo-chondroma, i. 311
Myxœdema, acute, vi. 391
 influence of, in surgical conditions, i. 791
 post-operative, vi. 389
Myxo-lipoma, i. 307
Myxoma, i. 306
 intracanalicular, of breast, female, vi. 523
 lipomatodes, lipo-myxoma, i. 306
 of larynx, v. 881
 of mucous membranes, i. 307
 of rectum, vii. 892
 of testis, vi. 697
 teleangiectatic, i. 319
Myxo-sarcoma, i. 307, 333, 344

Nævus, ii. 354
 araneus, of face, v. 470
 capillary, of tongue, vi. 249
 flammeus, i. 320
 of face, v. 470
 lymphaticus, i. 323
 maternus, of eyelids, v. 552
 mollusciformis, ii. 355; v. 467
 of auricle, v. 675
 of breast, female, vi. 528
 of face, v. 467, 470
 pigmented, ii. 354
 pilosus, ii. 355
 prominens, i. 321
 Roentgen ray in the treatment of, ii. 357
 sanguineus, of face, v. 470
 trigeminal, v. 18
Nails in feet, vii. 42
 in hands, vii. 42
Napier's bow-legs brace, iv. 861
Narcosis, interrupted, as related to the production of shock, i. 475
Nasal adhesions, vi. 81
 bones, lateral deviation of, vi. 64
 fracture of, iii. 99; vi. 59
 branch of trigeminal nerve, extracranial operations upon, v. 386
 cavities, diseases of the, vi. 52
 deformities, rare, v. 496
 discharge, one-sided, vi. 85
 operations, adhesions after, vi. 81
 polypi, vi. 186
 pyorrhœa, vi. 85
 secretion, diagnostic data from cerebro-spinal fluid found in it, i. 563
 septum, abscess of, vi. 57
 blood supply of, vi 52
 deviations of, vi 70

Nasal septum, perforations of, vi. 79
 submucous resection of, vi. 70
Naso-frontal duct, anatomy of, vi. 112
 opening of the, vi. 93
Naso-pharyngeal fibroma, iii. 435
 tumors, vi. 859, 861
Nasopharynx, adenoids of, vi. 860
 benign tumors of, vi. 861
 carcinoma of, vi. 860 ·
 cysts of, vi. 860
 ecchymosis in, in fracture of the skull, v. 72
 fibroids of, vi. 860
 Payn's position for operations on, vi. 871
 sarcoma of, vi. 860
 teratoma of, vi. 861
 tumors of (and see Nasopharyngeal), vi. 859, 861
National Volunteer Aid Associations, viii. 905
Naval Medical corps, duties of, viii. 970
 surgery, viii. 970
Neck, abscess of, vi. 340
 Hilton's method of opening, vi. 341
 actinomycosis of, vi. 346
 aneurysms of, arterial, vi. 331
 angioma of, vi. 349
 as a field for the use of local anæsthesia, iv. 243
 blood cysts of, vi. 347
 boils of, vi. 339
 bursal cysts of, vi. 348
 carbuncles of, vi. 339, 340
 carcinoma of, vi. 351
 cellulitis of, v. 444; vi. 344
 congenital fistulæ of, vi. 313
 congenital malformations of, vi. 313
 cystic tumors of, vi. 347
 Derbyshire (and see Goitre), vi. 358
 dermoid cysts of, vi. 315
 diseases of blood-vessels of, vi. 331
 echinococcus cysts of, vi. 348
 erysipelas of, vi. 340
 fibroma of, vi. 349
 fistulæ of, vi. 394
 hydrocele of, vi. 315
 infection of, from alveolar periostitis, vi. 880
 inflammations of, vi. 339
 injuries of, vi. 323
 cut-throat, vi. 326
 inspection of, in diagnosis, i. 514
 lipoma of, vi. 350
 lymph nodes of, v. 417
 nerves of, injuries to, vi. 330
 neuroma of, vi. 350
 plastic surgery of, iv. 627
 sanguineous cysts of, vi. 395
 sarcoma of, vi. 351
 sebaceous cysts of, vi. 348
 sinuses in, from alveolar periostitis, vi. 880
 solid tumors of, vi. 349
 suppuration of, vi. 340

Neck, surgical diseases and wounds of, vi. 313
 syphilitic inflammations of, vi. 345
 triangles of, iv. 790
 tuberculous inflammations of, vi. 345
 tumors of, vi. 347
 venous aneurysms in, vi. 338
Necræmia, the term as used by Paget, ii. 203
Necrobiosis and necrosis, i. 208
Necrogenic wart, ii. 637
Necrosal fever, iii. 268
Necrosis, i. 213; ii. 201–203; iii. 315
 total, in osteomyelitis of the femur, iii. 302
 toxic agencies, causation of, i. 212
 traumatic insults causing, i. 210
 x-rays as a cause of, i. 211
Necrotic areas, healing of, i. 105
Needle, Emmet's, for cervix uteri, vi. 587
Needle-holder, Burrage, vi. 588
 requirements of, i. 745
Needling, Macewen's process of, viii. 40
Negri's bodies in rabies, iii. 44, 58
Negro, immunity of, in respect of certain diseases, i 784
Nélaton's line, as a basis of measurement in hip-joint disease, iii. 643, 647
 method of forming a new lobule of ear, v. 678
 method of rhinoplasty, iv. 684
 operation for hare lip, v. 511
 operation for webbed fingers, iv. 635
Nélaton's (A.) operation for restoration of alæ nasi, iv. 694
Nélaton's (Ch.) operation for repair of septum, iv. 705
 operation for restoration of lower part of nose, iv. 702
Nélaton and Ombrédanne's method of restoring the alæ nasi, iv. 698
 operation for saddle-nose, iv. 709
Neoplasms. See Tumors
 effect of the climacteric upon, i. 780
Nephrectomy, viii. 146
Nephritis, suppurative, viii. 106
Nephrolithiasis, viii. 110, 111
Nephrolithotomy, viii. 119, 152
Nephropexy, viii. 99, 154
Nephrorrhaphy, viii. 99, 154
Nephrotomy, viii. 151 ·
Nephrotriesis, viii. 152
Nerve and nerves
 anastomosis, ii. 473
 anterior crural, injuries of, ii. 481
 anterior tibial, surgical anatomy of, ii. 482
 blocking as a mode of anæsthesia, iv. 236
 brachial plexus of, injuries of, ii. 476
 circumflex, injuries of, ii. 478

Nerve, cranial, lesions of, in fractures of the skull, v. 76
surgery of the, v. 379
degeneration, i. 179; ii. 465
dislocation, ii. 498
external cutaneous, injuries of, ii. 481
genito-crural, injuries of, ii. 481
ilio-hypogastric, injuries of, ii. 481
ilio-inguinal, injuries of, ii. 481
implantation, ii. 473
injuries, joint conditions following, ii. 466
in fractures, iii. 81
internal saphenous, its anatomical relations, ii. 482
median, its injuries and surgical anatomy, ii. 479
musculo-cutaneous, injuries of, ii. 478
of leg, its surgical anatomy, ii. 483
musculo-spiral, anatomical details bearing upon treatment of, ii. 478, 479
injuries of, ii. 478
of neck, injuries to, vi. 330
optic, tumors of, v. 652
peripheral, degeneration associated with atrophy of, i. 178
injuries of, i. 289
peroneal, injuries of, ii. 482
phrenic, injuries of, ii. 474
pneumogastric, injuries of, ii. 474
posterior tibial, injuries and surgical anatomy of, ii. 483
rate of regeneration of, i. 290
recurrent laryngeal, injuries of, ii. 474
regeneration, ii. 465
sciatic, its injuries and their treatment, ii. 482
stretching in anæsthetic leprosy, ii. 25
supply of face and scalp from the cervical plexus and trigeminal nerve, iv. 242
surgical diseases and wounds of, ii. 463
suturing, technique of, ii. 472
sympathetic, injuries of, ii. 475
transplantation, for infantile paralysis, iv. 845
trunks of the upper extremity, points of injecting for local anæsthesia, iv. 245–247
ulnar, its injuries and their treatment, ii. 480
vasomotor, in brain, v. 121
wounds of, consideration of individual nerves, ii. 474
Nervous diseases, effect of, upon surgical prognosis, i. 788
system, as furnishing indications for or against operating, iv. 119
Neumann and Szymanowski's operation for saddle-nose, iv. 713
Neuralgia, ii. 503

Neuralgia, avulsion and excision of ganglia in treatment of, ii. 506
cataphoresis in treatment of, ii. 506
obturator, vii. 36
of female breast, vi. 509
of gluteal region, vii. 31
of internal pudic nerve, vii. 36
of larynx, v. 896
of pelvic region, vii. 31
of scalp, v. 23
of sciatic nerve. See Sciatica
of symphysis pubis, vii. 36
trigeminal, v. 381
unusual forms of, ii. 508
Neurasthenia, effect of, upon surgical conditions, i. 789
Neurexeresis, v. 384
Neuritis, ii. 498
Neuro-epitheliomata, i. 326
Neuro-fibroma, i. 305
Neuroglia, Weigert's views of the cells of, i. 325
Neuroglioma ganglionare, of brain, v. 301
Neurolysis, definition of the term, ii. 472
Neuroma, i. 328
cirsoid, of face, v. 469
ganglionic, i. 329
multiple cutaneous, i. 329
of breast, female, vi. 529
of central nervous system, i. 329
of eyelids, v. 553
of neck, vi. 350
plexiform, i. 329
plexiform, of face, v. 469
of scalp, v. 16
plexiform, reports of two cases, ii. 523, 524
Neuropathic atrophies, muscles involved in, i. 171
conditions in locomotor ataxia and syringomyelia, ii. 514
Neuroplastic operations, essentials of, ii. 473
Neuroses of female breast, vi. 509
of larynx, v. 896
traumatic, ii. 516, 517
Neurotic spine, vi. 461
diagnosed from Pott's disease, vi. 956
Neurotization of scar, i. 290
Neutrophilic marrow-cells (Ehrlich's Markzelle) found in blood of myelocytic leukæmia, i. 243
New-born, intracranial hemorrhages in, v. 208
Newcomb, James E., on Surgical Diseases and Wounds of the Larynx and Trachea, v. 863–913
New-growths. See Tumors
Nicholls, Albert G., i. 146, 291
Nichols, Edward H., i. 256
Nicoladoni's operation for replacing a lost thumb, iv. 633
Nicolaier, bacillus of, iii. 22
Nicoll's method of amputation of penis, vi. 691
Night cries as a symptom of tuberculous disease of the hip-joint, iii. 663
Nigrities linguæ, vi. 239

Nipple, affections of, vi. 507
Nitrous oxide, accidents which may occur from inhalation of, iv. 182
Nitrous-oxide-ether-chloroform sequence for anæsthesia, iv. 211
Nocardia, v. 459
Noma, i. 137, 220; ii. 301
of auricle, v. 671
Nose. See Nasal, Intranasal
absence of, iv. 717
artificial, iv. 717; vi. 20
deformities of, vi. 67
elongated, iv. 716
fibroma papillare of, vi. 194
furunculosis of vestibule of, vi. 80
hammer-, v. 478
hooked, vi. 67
increased size of, iv. 716
lorgnette, iv. 706
loss of, iv. 679
lupus of, v. 453
lymphatics of, v. 421
measurements for operating distances in the, vi. 203
middle meatus of, anatomy of, vi. 92
plastic surgery (and see Rhinoplasty), iv. 679
plugging the, in frontal sinus operations, vi. 120
polypi in middle meatus of, vi. 86
prosthesis, iv. 717
pus in middle meatus of, vi. 85
repair of lower part of septum of, iv. 703
replacement of, iv. 691
restoration of alæ of, iv. 693
restoration of lower part of, iv. 700
saddle-, iv. 625, 706; v. 458
saddle-back, vi. 68
tumors of (and see Nasal cavities), vi. 186
with drooping tip, vi. 69
Nose-bleed (and see Epistaxis), vi. 52
in fracture of the skull, v. 72
Nurse corps, of U. S. Army, viii. 904
Nurses, training school for, inaugurated in Bellevue Hospital, i. 32
Nursing department of hospital, viii. 889
Nutrition, disturbances of, in connection with surgical diseases and conditions, i. 146

Oakum as a dressing, iv. 537
Obesity, as influencing the choice of anæsthetics, iv. 224
Obligation, civil, of surgeon and patient, viii. 713, 723
Obliquus capitis inferior muscle, anatomy of, iv. 788
superior muscle, anatomy of, iv. 788
Obstetrical paralysis, diagnosed from infantile paralysis, iv. 824
Obstipation in its relation to surgical prognosis, i. 790

Obstruction, intestinal, diagnosed from acute appendicitis, vii. 660

pyloric (and see Pyloric stenosis), vii. 335

Obturation, intestinal, vii. 732

Obturator, for cleft palate, vi. 11
artery, injury of, vii. 28
ligation of, iv. 509, 510
traumatic aneurysm of, vii. 28
hernia, vii. 603
neuralgia, vii. 36

Obturators and vela, for cleft palate, relative advantages of, vi. 18

Occipital lobe of brain, diagnosis of tumors in, v. 322
lesions of, symptoms, v. 278

Occipital support, for Pott's disease, iv. 973

Occupation as related to diagnosis, i. 508
. palsies, prognosis and treatment of, ii 511
torticollis, iv. 783

Ochronosis, i. 194

Ochsner, Albert J., on Surgical Diseases and Wounds of the Stomach and Œsophagus, vii. 332–449
method of treating septic peritonitis, vii. 522
method of treating stricture of œsophagus, vii. 431

Ocular torticollis, iv. 806

Oculomotor nerve, surgery of the, v. 380

Odontoma, i. 314; iii. 471–478

O'Dwyer's intubation tubes, v. 891

Œdema or dropsy, i. 236
acute purulent, i. 420
factors determining the occurrence of, i. 236
inflammatory, i. 116, 236, 237
local, from passive congestion, i. 237
lymphatic, i. 236
of conjunctiva, v. 584
of eyelids, v. 547
of lungs, iv. 160
of penis, vi. 680
of scrotum, vi. 680

Œdematous tissues, microscopical features of, i. 238

Œdème charbonneux, of face, v. 425

Œsophageal forceps, vii. 425

Œsophagitis, vii. 411

Œsophago-jejuno-gastrostomie, vii. 438

Œsophagoscopy, vii. 410

Œsophagostomy, vii. 419

Œsophagotomy, vii. 426

Œsophagus, anatomy of, vii. 408
carcinoma of, vii. 413
cysts of, vii. 420
deformities of, vii. 410
dilatation of, for carcinoma, vii. 416
for strictures, vii. 430
diseases of, vii. 410
diverticula of, vii. 439
examination of, i. 518; vii. 409

Œsophagus, foreign bodies in, vii. 422
idiopathic dilatation of, vii. 444
injuries of, vii. 410, 421
involvement of, in laryngectomy, v. 930
malformations of, vii. 410
myoma of, vii. 420
papilloma of, vii. 420
phlegmon of, vii. 412
plastic operations on, after laryngo-œsophagectomy, v. 931
polypi of, vii. 420
resection of, vii. 417
sarcoma of, vii. 420
stricture of, vii. 428
surgery of, vii. 408
surgical diseases of, vii. 332
thrush of, vii. 411
tumors of, vii. 413
ulcer of, vii. 413
wounds of, vii. 332

Old people, operations upon, i. 776

Olecranon process, fractures of, iii. 139

Olfactory cortex, v. 273
nerve, surgery of the, v. 379

Oligæmia defined, i. 240

Oliver, John Chadwick, on Wounds of Joints, iii. 725

Ollier's bayonet-shaped incision for excision of the elbow-joint, iv. 415
method of rhinoplasty, iv. 692
operation, pericardotomy, vii. 157

Ombrédanne's method of rhinoplasty, iv. 684

Omental grafting, vii. 757

Omentum, accessory, vii. 748
anatomy of, vii. 745
surgical diseases of, vii. 698, 745
wounds of, vii. 698

Onyx, v. 599

Oophorectomy, viii. 439
for cancer of breast, vi. 555
performance of, during pregnancy, i. 779
results of, viii. 443

Oophoro-cystectomy, viii. 439

Oöspora bovis, ii. 56

Operating gowns, i. 721

Operating-room, its requirements and preparation, iv. 143–147

Operations, contra-indications to, iv. 108–125
details of local preparation of patient for, iv. 132
diseases which enhance the dangers of, i. 786
effect of, upon neurasthenia, i. 789
for diseased lymph nodes in the neck, choice of anæsthetic for, iv. 219
for establishment of a joint anterior to cicatricial bands fixing the lower jaw, iv. 390
influence of age upon, i. 772
of menstruation upon, i. 778
upon pregnancy, i. 778
rendered more dangerous by various diseases, i. 786

Operative facility, its dangers, i. 693
procedures in aid of diagnosis, i. 553

Ophidia, or snakes, divided into two sub-orders, iii. 7

Ophthalmia, gonorrhœal, v. 579
neonatorum, v. 579
nodosa, v. 582
phlyctenular, v. 579
scrofulous, v. 579
strumous, v. 579
sympathetic, v. 611

Opisthotonus in tetanus, i. 457

Opsonins and their relation to phagocytosis, iii. 593

Optic disc, in middle meningeal hemorrhage, v. 187
nerve, surgery of the, v. 379
tumors of, v. 652
neuritis, in cerebral tumors, v. 313
tract, lesions of, symptoms, v. 278

Orbicularis palpebrarum, paralysis of, v. 556

Orbit, abscess of, v. 446; vi. 852
angioma of, v. 651
carcinoma of, vi. 854
caries of walls of, v. 649
cellulitis of, v. 445, 647
contusions of, v. 655
cystic tumors of, v. 651
cysticercus cysts of, v. 652
dermoid cysts of, v. 651
diseases of, v. 647
emphysema of, v. 649
epithelioma of, v. 652
exenteration of, v. 653
exostoses of, treatment of, v. 655
foreign bodies in, v. 656
fracture of walls of, v. 655
hemorrhage in, v. 649
hemorrhage in neighborhood of, in fracture of the skull, v. 71
injuries of, v. 647, 655
lymphadenoma of, v. 652
necrosis of walls of, v. 649
osteoma of, v. 653
periostitis of walls of, v. 649
sarcoma of, v. 652
telangiectasis of, v. 651
tumors of, v. 651; vi. 850, 852
wounds of, v. 655

Orbital abscess, vi. 852
osteoma, iii. 404
tumors, vi. 850, 852

Orchidectomy, vi. 662, 698
bilateral, vi. 698

Orchidopexy, vi. 662

Orchitis, vi. 670
gummatous, ii. 126

Organ of Giraldès, vi. 630
cysts of, vi. 697

O'Reilly's method of treating fractures of the patella, iii. 185

Oriental boil, ii. 342

Oroya fever, ii. 344

Orthodiagraph, i. 630

Orthopedic surgery, i. 55; iv. 729

Os calcis, excision of, iv. 465
tuberculous disease of, operative treatment, iii. 721

Os innominatum acute osteomyelitis of, iii. 306
Osgood, Robert B., i. 599
Ossiculectomy, v. 712
Ossification, complete, of exuberant callus after fracture, iii. 397
of cartilage of auricle, v. 670
Ossifying myositis, vii. 38
Osteitis, i. 674; iii. 260–262; v. 27
deformans, iii. 344, 361
Osteo-arthritis, iii. 513
of spine, vi. 458
with true ankylosis of joints, iii. 362
Ostéoarthropathie hypertrophiante pneumique, i. 686; iii. 360, 396
Osteoblasts and osteoclasts, their action, i. 282
Osteo-chondroma, i. 311
Osteoclasis for knock‐knee, iv. 866
Osteoclasts, action of, in the separation of the sequestrum, iii. 283
as found in osteoporosis, iii. 262
Osteocopic pains, iii. 369
Osteogenesis imperfecta, v. 25
in chronic bone disease, i. 161
Osteogenetic extoses, iii. 414
tissues, their repair, i. 280
Osteoid chondroma (Virchow), iii. 426
development of, i. 281
tumors, distinguishing characteristics of, i. 315
Osteoma, i. 313, 314; iii. 394
of breast, female, vi. 529
of conjunctiva, v. 584
of external auditory canal, v. 680
of frontal sinus, v. 29
of orbit, v. 653
a misnomer, iii. 410
of penis, vi. 687
of pelvic bones, vii. 13
of skull, v. 28
of tongue, vi. 255
spongiosum or medullary osteoma, i. 313
spongy form of, iii. 395
types of, iii. 396
Osteomalacia, i. 174; iii. 355, 465
deformans, iii. 360
of skull, v. 26
of the adult, iii. 355
osteopsathyrosis, fragilitas ossium, osteoporosis, halisteresis, iii. 354
x-ray features of, i. 676
Osteomalacic pelvis, vii. 3
Osteomyelitis, iii. 267
of cranial bones, v. 34
of femur, iii. 301–303
of hip-joint, acute, iii. 307
of humerus, danger of suppurative arthritis of the elbow-joint, iii. 306
of jaw, vi. 875, 879
of malar bone, v. 448
of os innominatum, iii. 306
of pelvic bones, vii. 4
of radius and ulna, iii. 303
of ribs, vi. 409
of sternum, vi. 409

Osteomyelitis of tibia and fibula, danger of involvement of knee and ankle joints, iii. 304, 305
of Y-shaped cartilage of the acetabulum of the os innominatum, primary and secondary, iii. 308
Osteo-periostitis of acquired syphilis, iii. 378
Osteophytes, i. 314; iii. 396
Osteoplastic flap, the, in cerebral operations, v. 353
Osteoporosis, i. 165, 173
adiposa, iii. 335
or rarefying or rarefactive osteitis, iii. 262–264, 283
Osteopsathyrosis, iii. 357
or fragilitas ossium, i. 175
Osteo-sarcoma, i. 333, 344; iii. 444
of jaw, vi. 816
periosteal, vi. 824
of skull, v. 32
Osteosclerosis, i. 162
in fractures and other injuries, or absorption of provisional callus, iii. 266
in rheumatoid arthritis, iii. 266
or condensing osteitis, iii. 264–266
Osteotome, spiral, Cryer's, v. 355
Osteotomy, for infantile paralysis, iv. 845
Ostitis deformans, of spine, vi. 455
Ostitis of jaws, arsenical, vi. 889
phosphorous, vi. 887
Othæmatoma, v. 666
of auricle, v. 666
Otis urethrotome, vi. 789
Otitis, acute catarrhal, v. 686
acute purulent, v. 687
chronic purulent, v. 708
externa circumscripta, v. 683
externa diffusa, v. 684
media, purulent, intracranial complications of, summary of, v. 790
suppurative, intracranial complications of, diagnosis of v., 787
suppurative, intracranial complications of, symptomatology of, v. 787
relation of, to abscess of brain, v. 780
relation of brain affections to, v. 781
relation of cerebellar abscess to, v. 781 ;
Otoliths, i. 200
Ovariotomy, i. 61; viii. 439
Ovary, absence of, viii. 397
anatomy of, viii. 393
anomalies of, viii. 397
atrophy of, i. 181; viii. 401
carcinoma of, viii. 426
circulatory disturbances in, viii. 401
congestion of, viii. 401
cystadenoma of, viii. 423
cysts of (and see Ovary, tumors of), viii. 402, 423

Ovary, dermoid cysts of, viii. 427
descensus of, viii. 398
displacement of, viii. 398
embryology, viii. 391
endothelioma of, viii. 429
fibroma of, viii 428
hæmatoma of, viii. 401
hernia of, viii. 400
hyperæmia of, viii. 401
hypertrophy of, viii. 402
papilloma of, viii. 425
perithelioma of, viii. 429
pseudomucinous cyst of, viii. 423
reposition of, viii. 399
retention cysts of, viii. 402
sarcoma of, viii. 428
superfluous, viii. 398
surgery of, viii. 391
teratoma of, viii. 427
tuberculosis of, viii. 420
tumors of, viii. 422
Overgrowth of one bone, compensatory and physiological, because of weakness or loss of its companion, iii. 338
Overproduction of tissue as a sequela of inflammation, i. 108
Oviatt, Charles W., on Surgical Diseases and Wounds of the Intestines, Omentum, and Mesentery, vii. 698–760
Oxalate calculi, viii. 113
Oxycephalism, iii. 327

Pacchionian bodies, v. 104
Pachyakrie, iii. 340
Pachydermatocele, of scalp, v. 16
Pagenstecher's celluloid yarn, its preparation and uses in sutures, i. 727
operation of lens extraction for cataract, v. 631
Paget's disease, ii. 374
of bones, iii. 361, 362, 397
of nipple, vi. 556
Pain, i. 95
causes of, in a stump, iv. 268
differences in sense of, i. 537
seat of, as an element in diagnosis, i. 536, 537
Painter, Charles, F., on Chronic Non-Tuberculous and Non-Traumatic Inflammations of Joints, iii. 487
on congenital dislocations, iv. 731
on infantile paralysis, iv. 807
Palate, artificial, vi. 18
cleft (and see Cleft palate), vi. 521
hard, adenopapilloma of, vi. 863
tonsils, and pharynx, diagnostic indications furnished by, i. 517
tumors of, vi. 862
Palmar abscess, deep, vii. 60
fascia, vii. 55
Palpation, its use in diagnosis, i. 515
Palpebral commissure, contraction of, vi. 561
Palsy, cerebro-spastic, ii. 519
Pampiniform plexus, thrombosis of, vi. 666

Panaritium (and see Felon), i. 130; ii. 157
Pancreas, abscess of, viii. 171
　accessory, viii. 161
　adenoma of, i. 345
　anatomy of, viii. 159
　annular, viii. 161
　anomalies of, viii. 160
　apoplectic, viii. 180
　calculus in, viii. 190
　carcinoma of, viii. 188
　congenital cysts of, viii. 180
　cysts of, viii. 180
　cystoids of, viii. 181
　diseases of, Cammidge reaction in, viii. 175
　disturbances of external secretions in, viii. 176
　disturbances of internal secretions in, viii. 175
　hemorrhagic cysts of, viii. 180
　hydatid cysts of, viii. 181
　inflammation of (and see Pancreatitis), viii. 162
　Involvement of, in cholelithiasis, viii. 243
　movable, viii. 190
　physiology of, viii. 159
　proliferation cysts of, viii. 181
　pseudo-cysts of, viii. 181
　retention cysts of, viii. 180
　sarcoma of, viii. 189
　structure of, viii. 161
　surgery of the, viii. 159
　true cysts of, viii. 180
　tumors of, viii. 188
　wounds of, viii. 187
Pancreatic calculus, viii. 190
Pancreatico-lithiasis, viii. 190
Pancreatitis, viii. 162
　acute hemorrhagic parenchymatous, viii. 163
　catarrhal, viii. 163
　chronic interstitial, viii. 173
　diagnosed from appendicitis, vii. 659
　gangrenous, viii. 167
　subacute, viii. 171
Pancreoptosis, viii. 190
Pannus, treatment of, v. 588
Panse's method of forming meatal flap, v. 723
Papillary nævi, i. 329
Papilliferous cystadeno-fibroma, i. 304
Papilloma, i. 329; ii. 358
　intracanalicular, of the mamma, i. 351
　intranasal, vi. 194
　of auricle, v. 675
　of biliary ducts, viii. 252
　of bladder, i. 330
　of conjunctiva, v. 584
　of gums, vi. 846
　of kidney, viii. 133
　of larynx, v. 880
　of mouth, ii. 361
　of mucous surfaces, i. 329
　of œsophagus, vii. 420
　of ovary, viii. 425
　of penis, vi. 687
　of pharynx, v. 854
　of rectum, vii. 895

Papilloma, of scalp, v. 22
　of tongue, vi. 252
　of umbilicus, vii. 90
　of urethra, vi. 694
　of urinary bladder, viii. 310
　of vermiform appendix, vii. 625
Paracentesis abdominis, iv. 602
　of cornea, v. 617
　of heart, vii. 175
　pericardii, iv. 601; vii. 154
　thoracis, iv. 601
Paradidymis, vi. 630
Paraduodenal hernia, vii. 610
Paræsthesia of larynx, v. 896
Paraffin bandages, iv. 591
Paralysis, anæsthesia, ii. 496
　birth, ii. 498
　brachial, vii. 68
　cerebral, and its deformities, iv. 871
　crutch, ii. 497
　deltoid, ii. 497
　due to pressure from the callus of a fracture or from a dislocation, ii. 497
　facial, v. 406
　following application of an Esmarch bandage, ii. 497
　following injuries, ii. 496
　following parturition, ii. 497
　from ligation of a nerve, ii. 496
　infantile, iv. 807; vi. 810
Paralytic deformities of lower extremities, iv. 867
　degeneration of nerve, following injury, i. 289
　torticollis, iv. 804
Paramastitis, vi. 511
Paraphimosis, vi. 645
Paraplegia dolorosa, vi. 539
　in Pott's disease, treatment of, iv. 982
Parasites, animal, in tongue, vi. 243
　in pharynx, v. 813
　of skin that are sometimes surgically important, ii. 395
　to be sought for in the fæces, i. 573
Parasitic affections of the lungs, viii. 25
　tumors of the bones, iii. 482
Parasyphilides, ii. 93
Parathyroids, iv. 354, 400
　function of, vi. 357
Parietal lobe of brain, diagnosis of tumors in, v. 321
Parietal lobule, left inferior, lesions of, v. 278
　left superior, lesions of, v. 277
Parieto-occipital fissure, line of, v. 362
Parinaud's conjunctivitis, v. 581
Park, Roswell, on Non-inflammatory Affections of Bones, iii. 323
Parker, Willard, i. 15
Parkhill's operation on external ear, iv. 722
　plates and screws as used in ununited fractures, iii. 238
Paronychia, i. 418; vii. 57
Parosteal sarcoma, defined, iii. 442
Parostoma, definition of the term, iii. 395

Parotid gland, adenoma of, vi. 308
　angioma of, vi. 307
　carcinoma of, vi. 308
　extirpation of, vi. 310
　hæmangioma of, vi. 307
　inflammation of (and see Salivary glands), vi. 300, 301
　injuries of, vi. 297
　lipoma of, vi. 307
　lymphangioma of, vi. 307
　tumors of, vi. 303, 862
Parotid lymph nodes, v. 419
Parotitis (and see Salivary glands), vi. 301
　acute, post-operative, iv. 166
Parovarian cysts, viii. 429
Parrot's nodes, iii. 379
Parry's disease (and see Exophthalmic goitre), vi. 375
Partners, liability of, in practice of surgery, viii. 717
Parturition, effect of, upon surgical conditions, i. 780
Passow-Trautmann method of closing post-auricular fistulæ, v. 730
Patch, senile or seborrhœic, ii. 374, 377
Patella, congenital dislocation of, iv. 765
　　Goldthwait's operation for, iv. 766
　dislocations of, iv. 91–94
　pseudarthrosis of, iii. 247
　sawing through or removal of, in treatment of infected penetrating wound of knee-joint, iii. 752
　slipping, iv. 765, 766
Patellar reflex, absence of, in diabetes, an unfavorable prognostic sign, i. 793
Pathological laboratories of hospitals, viii. 879
Pathology, surgical, i. 69
Patient and surgeon (see Surgeon and patient), viii. 713
　civil obligation of, viii. 713
　consent of, to surgical operations, viii. 743, 747, 749
　contributory negligence of, viii. 736
　must co-operate with surgeon, viii. 734
　must give necessary information, viii. 732
　must give surgeon proper opportunity to treat him, viii. 735
　must procure assistance when directed, viii. 735
　must submit to treatment, viii. 733
　obligation of, to surgeon, viii. 732
　(or his parents) must obey directions of surgeon, viii. 734
　status of surgeon when services are refused by, viii. 720
Payr's method of arteriorrhaphy, vii. 251
　position for operations on nasopharynx, vi. 871

Peck, Charles H., on Surgical Diseases and Wounds of the Pelvic and Gluteal Regions, vii. 3–36
Pectus carinatum, vi. 407
  excavatum, vi. 407
Pelvic abscess, viii. 408
  bones, diseases of, vii. 4
  bursæ, diseases of, vii. 29
  colon, vii. 763
  infection, viii. 403
  region, surgical diseases of, vii. 3
  wounds of, vii. 3
Pelvi-rectal abscess, 811
Pelvis, chondroma of, iii. 428
  deformities of bony, vii. 3
  dislocations of, iv. 27
  kyphotic, vii. 3
  osteomalacic, vii. 3
  split, vii. 4
  sarcoma of, iii. 461
  spondylolisthetic, vii. 3
Pemphigus leprosus, ii. 12
  of conjunctiva, v. 583
  of pharynx, v. 824
Penis, absence of, vi. 637
  amputation of, vi. 690
  anatomy of, vi. 622
  crushing of, vi. 664
  dislocation of, vi. 665
  elephantiasis of, vi. 676
  emphysema of, vi. 680
  foreign bodies on or in, vi. 663
  fracture of, vi. 664
  gangrene of, vi. 675
  gunshot wounds of, vi. 665
  inflammation of, vi. 669
  injuries of, vi. 664
  laceration of, vi. 664
  lupus of, vi. 671
  malformations of, vi. 637
  skin diseases of, vi. 674
  stab-wounds of, vi. 665
  tuberculosis of, vi. 671
  tumors of, vi. 686
  varicosities of, vi. 678
Pennsylvania, University of, organization of medical department, i. 11
Peptic ulcer of duodenum, vii. 713
  of jejunum, vii. 718
Perforating ulcer of the foot, ii. 516
Perianal abscess, vii. 810, 812
Periarthritis of shoulder-joint, vii. 44
Pericardial effusion, effect of, on relations of anterior mediastinum, vii. 150
Pericarditis, vii. 152
  anæsthetics indicated in, iv. 224
Pericardium, anatomical considerations, vii. 146
  surgery of, vii. 146
Pericardotomy, vii. 156
Perichondritis of auricle, v. 668
  tuberculous, v. 669
Pericranial sinus, v. 12
Peridiverticulitis of sigmoid, vii. 703
Perimyositis crepitans, ii. 406
Perineal hernia, vii. 606
  position, the, vi. 581
  prostatectomy, viii. 378
  section, vi. 801
  sheet, Ewin, vi. 581, 582, 583

Perineal-urinary fistula, vii. 828
Perineum, its examination for diagnosis of urinary extravasation, i. 550
  lacerated, complete (through sphincter ani), repair of, vi. 605
  operations for repair of, vi. 595
Perinephritis, viii. 104
Periosteum and endosteum, their power to regenerate bone after death of a portion, i. 286
  inflammatory diseases of, iii. 254–260
  structure and character of, iii. 254, 255
Periostitis, acute or subacute, non-suppurative, iii. 255
  acute suppurative, iii. 258–260
  albuminous, of Ollier, iii. 255
  alveolar, vi. 879
  chronic or osteoplastic, iii. 256
  hemorrhagic, of jaws, vi. 876
  of jaw, vi. 816, 875, 879
  of orbital walls, v. 649
  of pelvic bones, vii. 4
Peri-pancreatic cysts, viii. 181
Periproctitis, diffuse septic, vii. 810
  idiopathic gangrenous, vii. 812
Perirectal abscess, vii. 810, 812
Perisigmoiditis, vii. 934
Persinous abscess, v. 793
Perithelioma, malignant, i. 340
  of kidney, viii. 134, 135
  of ovary, viii. 429
Peritoneal adhesions, vii. 726
  pouch, viii. 206
  tuberculosis, vii. 532
Peritoneum, vii. 111
  actinomycosis of, vii. 752
  carcinoma of, vii. 752
  operations involving, as practised under local anæsthesia, iv. 252
  relations of, to diaphragm, vii. 450
  tuberculosis of, vii. 533
Peritonitis and intestinal obstruction, precautions regarding anæsthesia in, iv. 225
  chronic, vii. 752
  complicating appendicitis, vii. 638
  pelvic, diagnosed from acute appendicitis, vii. 658
  post-operative, its treatment surgically and by Fowler's position, iv. 156
  sclerosing, vii. 753
  septic, after-treatment, vii. 525
  simple, development of, i. 249
  tuberculous, vii. 527
Periumbilical abscess, vii. 78
Periureteritis, viii. 144
Periurethral abscess, vii. 752, 808
  ducts, infection of, vi. 753
Periurethritis, vi. 808
Pernicious anæmia, characteristic changes in the blood, i. 241
Pernio, ii. 595
  of auricle, v. 665

Pernio of face, v. 431
Peroneal artery, ligation of, iv. 525, 526
Peroxide of hydrogen as a cleansing agent, i. 708
Perrin, Maurice, subastragaloid amputation of, iv. 328
Perthes' experiments with the x-ray on warts, i. 402
  report of operations for relief of habitual dislocation of the shoulder, iv. 50
Peruvian wart, ii. 344
Pes cavus, in infantile paralysis, iv. 816, 821, 822, 832
Pesquin's method of ligating for aneurysm, vii. 280
Pessaries, viii. 472
  fitting of, for retroplaced uterus, viii. 469
  in treatment of prolapsed uterus, viii. 496
Peters, George A., on Inflammatory Affections of Bone, iii. 252
Peters' bone forceps, iii. 93
  operation for ectopia vesicæ, viii. 286
  wrench for the forcible correction of deformity of the knee, iii. 705, 706
Petit's screw tourniquet to prevent hemorrhage, iv. 266
Petrifying infiltrations, i. 198
Phagedæna tropica, ii. 343, 344
Phagedena complicating chancroid, vi. 705
Phagedenism, tropical, ii. 270
Phagocytosis, a protective agency in inflammation, i. 74, 89
Phalanges of fingers, amputation of, iv. 281, 285
  of foot, tuberculous disease of, iii. 723
Pharyngeal forceps, vii. 424
  tonsil, v. 825
Pharyngitis, v. 813
Pharyngocele, v. 810, 867
Pharyngomycosis, v. 821
Pharyngotomy, v. 861
Pharynx (and see Nasopharyngeal)
  actinomycosis of, v. 823
  adenoids of, vi. 860
  anatomy, vi. 860
  angina of, v. 822
  anomalies of, v. 810
  burns of, v. 811
  chancre of, v. 843
  cyst of, v. 810
  deformities of, v. 810
  dermoid cyst of, v. 810
  diverticula of, v. 810
  fibroma of vault of, vi. 190
  fistula of, v. 810
  foreign bodies in, v. 811, 812
  glanders of, v. 824
  herpes of, v. 824
  keratosis of, v. 821
  lupus of, v. 851, 852
  malformations of, v. 810
  mucous patch of, v. 844
  parasites in, v. 813
  pemphigus of, v. 824, 825
  rhinoscleroma of, v. 824

Pharynx, scalds of, v. 811
surgical diseases of, v. 810
syphilis of, v. 842
teratoma of, v. 810
tuberculosis of, v. 847
tumors of, v. 853
ulcero-membranous angina of, v. 822
wounds of, v. 810, 811
Phelps' bed, for Pott's disease, iv. 964
operation for talipes, iv. 908
Philadelphia, College of, organization of medical department of, i. 7
Phimosis, vi. 638
complicating chancroid, vi. 704
Phlebectasia (and see Varicose veins), vii. 308
Phlebitis, vii. 297
after operation for appendicitis, vii. 692
Phleboliths, i. 200; vii. 180
Phlegmon of abdominal wall, vii. 77
of chest wall, vi. 409
of Heurtaux, vii. 77
of œsophagus, vii. 412
Phlegmonous inflammation, i. 121, 418, 420
septicæmia often present with, i. 131
periostitis, iii. 268
Phosphatic calculi, viii. 113
Phosphorus necrosis, ii. 263; iii. 315
ostitis of jaws, vi. 887
Photographs, admissibility of, in evidence, viii. 783
Photography, medical, viii. 877
Phrenoptosis, vii. 460
Phthiriasis ciliorum, v. 549
Physical examination, compulsory, of plaintiff, viii. 779, 782
Physician, definition of, viii. 715
Physick, Philip Syng, i. 16, 54
Pictures, admissibility of, in evidence, viii. 783
Pigeon breast, vi. 407
in rickets, iii. 349
Pigeon-toe, iv. 892
Pigment patches on the sclerotic, v. 591
Pigmentary deposit, biliary, i. 203
substances inhaled, chronic fibroid pneumonia from, i. 208
Pigmentation and cicatrices following syphilitic eruptions, ii. 116
by extraneous pigments, i. 193, 207
by way of the alimentary tract, by way of the lungs (pneumonokoniosis), i. 207
from cellular activity, i. 193
hæmatogenous, i. 203, 204
in chloroma, i. 194
in jaundice or icterus, i. 193
of organs in which pigment exists normally, i. 193
of the liver, i. 205
of the skin, by tattooing, i. 207
transference of, to spleen, from a sarcoma, i. 205

Pigments, autochthonous or metabolic, i. 193
Pilcher, Paul Monroe, i. 415
on congelation or frost-bite, ii. 592
Piles (and see Hemorrhoids), vii. 860
Pilo-nidal sinus, vii. 20
Pin callus, iii. 268
Pincus' weight-posture method, viii. 415
Pinguecula, v. 583
Pirogoff's amputation of the foot, iv. 332
form of immovable dressing, iii. 90
Pituitary body, tumors of, v. 331
Plagiocephalism, iii. 327
Plague, ii. 27
ambulant (pestis minor), ii. 38
pneumonic, ii. 36
the bubo, ii. 34
the doctrine of flea transference, ii. 31
Plaintiff, physical examination of, viii. 781
compulsory, viii. 779, 782
when a woman, viii. 781
Plasma cells, characteristics and source of, i. 88
Plasmodiophora brassicæ, i. 388
Plasmoma, iii. 465
Plaster, adhesive, as a dressing, iv. 537
corset, for Pott's disease, iv. 970
helmet, retention dressing for torticollis, iv. 778
Plaster-of-Paris, bandages, how prepared and used, i. 738
encasement in treatment of fractures of the upper end of the femur, iii. 170
jacket, for Pott's disease, iv. 964
Plastic and osteoplastic methods of healing bone cavities, iii. 309, 310
exudate, i. 248
operations (and see Plastic surgery), iv. 611
for closing postauricular fistulæ, v. 727
for formation of new lobule of ear, v. 677
in vagina (and see Vagina, plastic operations on), vi. 579
on cheek, iv. 638
on ears, iv. 718
on extremities, iv. 627
on eyelids, iv. 667
on face, iv. 637
on hands, iv. 630
on lips, iv. 648, 652
on mouth, iv. 665
on neck, iv. 627
on nose, iv. 679
on œsophagus, v. 931
on scalp, iv. 628
on trunk, iv. 627
skin-grafting, iv. 620
Platycephalism, iii. 327
Plethora, i. 234, 240

Pleura, carcinoma of the, viii. 14
echinococcus of, viii. 15
endothelioma of, viii. 14
neoplasms of, viii. 13
puncture of, by aid of local anæsthesia, iv. 245
reflection of, vii. 147
sarcoma of, viii. 14
surgical diseases of, viii. 3
Pleural effusion, effect of, on relations of anterior mediastinum, vii. 150
Pleurisy, after operation for appendicitis, vii. 693
diaphragmatic, diagnosed from acute appendicitis, vii. 659
purulent, anatomical changes in, i. 140
with effusion, viii. 5
Pleurocostomy, viii. 51
Pleurocele of cranium, v. 11
Plexiform angioma. See Cirsoid aneurysm
Plimmer's bodies, i. 381, 388
Plummer's olive-tipped bougie for diagnosing idiopathic dilatation of œsophagus, vii. 447
Pneumatic cabinet of Sauerbruch, vii. 418
for use in operations involving the pleural cavity, iii. 458; viii. 44
Pneumatocele of cranium, v. 11
Pneumectomy, viii. 55
Pneumogastric nerve, surgery of the, v. 414
Pneumonia as a complication of fracture, iii. 85
as influencing the use of anæsthesia, iv. 225
post-operative, iv. 157
Pneumothorax, viii. 3
prevention of, in thoracic surgery, by use of Brauer and Sauerbruch apparatus, viii. 44
Poisoned wounds as influenced by the character of the traumatism, iii. 37
in which the poison is bacterial. iii. 15
including the bites and stings of animals and insects, iii. 3
inflicted by the implements of warfare, iii. 35
Polioencephalitis, v. 250
Poliomyelitis, anterior (and see Paralysis, infantile), iv. 807, 867
Poliosis of eyebrows and eyelashes, v. 550
Polis, investigation of, on cerebral concussion, v. 156, 162
Pollock's operation of disarticulation at the knee-joint, iv. 345
Polyarthritis, 491–504
Polyarticular inflammation as distinguished from the monarticular type, iii. 491, 492
features of the infectious as distinguished from the atrophic type, iii. 490, 491
Polycoria, v. 614
Polycythæmia defined, i. 240

Polymastia, vi. 507
Polymazia, vi. 507
Polyorchidia, vi. 663
Polyotia, v. 661
Polypus, aural, v. 710
  bleeding, of septum of nose, vi.
    195
  in middle meatus of nose, vi. 86
  nasal, vi. 186
  of œsophagus, vii. 420
  of rectum, vii. 896
Polythelia, vi. 508
Poop, vii. 73
Pope, Charles A., i. 29
Popliteal artery, ligation from
  the inner side of the thigh, iv.
  521
Porencephaly, traumatic, v. 285
Poroplastic collar for Pott's disease,
  iv. 975
Porro's Cæsarean section, viii. 703
Portal cirrhosis, viii. 227
Port-wine marks, v. 470
  stain—nævus vinosus, i. 320
Porter, Charles A., and Quimby,
  William C., on Surgical Diseases
  of the Extremities, vii. 37–74
Post's (Alfred C.), operation for
  restoration of lower lip, iv. 664
Post, Wright, i. 12, 40
Postanal dimples, vii. 897
Postauricular fistulæ, plastic opera-
  tions for closing, v. 727
      Mosetig-Moorhof meth-
        od, v. 729
      Passow - T r a u t m a n n
        method, v. 730
Posterior basal meningitis of in-
  fants, v. 238
  mediastinum, operations on,
    viii. 58
Posthitis, vi. 669
Post-mortem pustule, ii. 342
Post-rectal dermoids, vii. 18
Postural drainage, vii. 118
Potassium permanganate and ox-
  alic acid or the Schatz method of
  sterilizing the hands, i. 707
Pott's disease, iv. 927
Pouch, peritoneal, viii. 206
Poultices, i. 759
Poupart's ligament, vii. 108, 110
Pourriture d'hôpital, ii. 253
Powder stains, ii. 394
Practice of medicine, defined, viii.
  715
  of surgery, defined, viii. 715
Precancerous diseases, ii. 374
Pre-central convolution, lesions of,
  symptoms, v. 275
Pregnancy and parturition, the
  choice of an anæsthetic in, iv.
  225
  appendicitis in, vii. 692
  complicating ovarian tumors,
    vii. 437
  considered as a contra-indica-
    tion to operating, iv. 125
  extra-uterine (and see Extra-
    uterine pregnancy), viii.
    690
      diagnosed from acute appen-
        dicitis, vii. 658

Pregnancy, influence of, upon
  neoplasms of the reproductive
  organs. i. 779
  influence of, upon operations, i.
    778
Pregnant uterus, retroversion of,
  viii. 463
Prepuce, anatomy of, vi. 624
  dermoid cysts of, vi. 637
  inflammation of, vi. 669
Pressure bandages, iv. 595–600
Prickle cells, i. 359
Primary cysts of bone, iii. 430
  splenomegaly, viii. 71
Primrose, Alexander, on Tubercu-
  lous Disease of the Bones and
  Joints, iii. 558
Prince's method of operation for
  pterygium, v. 594
Privileged communications, viii. 795
Procidentia of rectum (and see
  Rectum, prolapse of), vii. 875
  of uterus, viii. 487
Proctitis, gonorrhœal, vii. 798
  proliferating, vii. 800
  tuberculous, acute, vii. 793
Proctoplasty, vii. 854
Proctoscope, vii. 769
Proctotomy, vii. 851
Profunda femoris artery, ligation
  of, iv. 519
Prognosis, general, in surgical dis-
  eases, i. 771
Progressive muscular atrophy or
  wasting palsy, ii. 513
Projectiles, ballistics of, ii. 648
  resistance to deforming violence,
    ii. 651
Prolapse of rectum (and see Rectum, prolapse of), vii. 875
  of stomach (and see Gastrop-
    tosis), vii. 889
  of uterus, vi. 611, 614; viii. 487
Prolapsed mucous membrane of
  urethra, vi. 572
Proliferation cysts of pancreas, viii.
  181
  of epithelial and connective tis-
    sue cells, i. 262
Proptosis, in fracture of the skull,
  v. 72
Prosopectasis, iii. 340
Prostate, abscess of, vi. 744; viii. 343
  absence of, viii. 341
  anatomy of, viii. 337
  anomalies of, congenital, viii.
    340
  atrophy of, i. 181
  calculi in, viii. 350
  cysts of, viii. 367
  examination of, for diagnostic
    purposes, i. 550
  hypertrophy of, viii. 358
  injuries to, viii. 341
  malformations of, viii. 279
  surgical diseases of, viii. 279
  syphilis of, viii. 350
  tuberculosis of, viii. 347
  tumors of, viii. 354
  wounds of, viii. 279
Prostatectomy, viii. 370
  perineal, viii. 378
  suprapubic, viii. 370

Prostatic infections, viii. 344
  obstruction, viii. 365
  tractor, Syms', viii. 389
Prostatism, viii. 361
Prostatitis, viii. 341
  acute, vi. 741; viii. 341
    catarrhal, vi. 741
    follicular, vi. 741
    parenchymatous, vi. 742
  chronic, viii. 343
    parenchymatous, vi. 761
Prosthesis (and see Artificial), vi. 3
  conditions in which it is useful,
    vi. 4
  dental, vi. 5
  ears, vi. 27
  face, vi. 20, 28
  glottis, vi. 32
  in its relation to surgery of the
    face, mouth, jaws, and nasal
    and laryngeal cavities, vi. 3–
    51
  in plastic surgery, iv. 625–627
  jaws, vi. 35
  larynx, vi. 31
  lips, vi. 26
  nose, vi. 20
  teeth, vi. 5
  tongue, vi. 29
Prothesis oculi, v. 657
Proud flesh, i. 251
Pruritus ani, vii. 856
  vulvæ, vi. 561
Pryor's method of pan-hysterec-
  tomy, viii. 570
Psammoma, i. 340
  of the brain, v. 311
Pseudarthrosis, iii. 212
Pseudo-arthrosis defined, i. 284
Pseudo-chylous ascites, from obstruction of thoracic duct, i. 237
Pseudo-cysts of pancreas, viii. 181
Pseudo-glioma of eyeball, v. 644
Pseudo-hypertrophic muscular par-
  alysis, i. 171
Pseudo-leukæmia,   or   Hodgkin's
  disease, i. 244
  splenic, viii. 71
Pseudo-membrane in inflammation
  of mucous membranes, i. 250
Pseudomucinous cyst of ovary, viii.
  423
Pseudo-paralyses, diagnosed from
  infantile paralysis, iv. 825
Pseudo-tails, vii. 15
Psoas abscess, in Pott's disease, iv.
  950
Psoriasis of tongue (and see Leu-
  coma), vi. 235
Psychical torticollis, iv. 805
Pterygium, v. 583
Ptomaïns, how produced, i. 417
Ptosis, v. 556
  operations for, v. 568
Pubiotomy, viii. 707, 709
Puerperal septicæmia, local treatment of, i. 442
Pulmonary conditions as contra-
  indications to operating and
  to general anæsthesia, iv.
  120
  decortication, viii. 53
  emboli, vii. 190

Pulmonary embolism, post-operative, iv. 161, 162
emphysema, viii. 23, 24
thrombosis, after operation for appendicitis, vii. 693
tuberculosis, viii. 28
resection of ribs in, viii. 54
Pulpitis, vi. 879
Pulse as an aid in diagnosis, i. 533
Puncture, exploratory, in diagnosis of abdominal tumors, vii. 103
its objects and practice, iv. 600
lumbar, iv. 602
in diagnosis of cerebral tumors, v. 318
vaginal, vii. 414
Pupil, Argyll-Robertson, i. 540
Purmann's method of extirpating aneurysm, vii. 285
of treating fractures of the patella, iii. 185
Purse-string suture, vii. 748, 756
Purulent exudates, details of the examinations required, i. 576
removal of, i. 260
Pus, i. 121, 252
association with granulation tissue, i. 251
blue, i. 253
bonum vel laudabile, character and constituents of, i. 125, 252
cellular constituents of, i. 124
curdy, i. 253
entrance of, into the blood, i. 255
formation of, i. 416
in middle meatus of nose, vi. 85
in urine, its sources and significance, i. 571
its constituents and characters, ii. 146
physical characteristics of, i. 123
production of, a protective reaction to injury, i. 125
red, Ferchmin's description of, i. 254
sanious, i. 253
views regarding its origin, ii. 145
Pustule, i. 121, 129
malignant, of eyelids, v. 550
Putrefaction, as distinguished from mortification, ii. 203
Putrid degeneration, ii. 253
Pyæmia, i. 96, 433, 437
beginning of, in thrombi, i. 433
characteristic changes in temperature, i. 435
formation of metastatic abscesses, i. 434, 436
hemorrhagic icterus in, i. 436
Pyelitis, viii. 106
Pyelonephritis, viii. 106, 107
Pyelotomy, viii. 151, 152
Pylephlebitis complicating appendicitis, vii. 638
Pylorectomy, vii. 374
Pyloric obstruction (and see Pyloric stenosis), vii. 335
due to inflammatory adhesions, vii. 383
stenosis, vii. 335

Pyloric stenosis, pyloroplasty for (and see Pyloroplasty), vii. 370
Pyloroplasty, vii. 370
Finney's method, vii. 372
Heinecke-Mikulicz method of, vii. 370
Pylorus (and see Gastric, and Stomach)
excision of, with gastro-enterostomy, vii. 367
ulcer of, indurated, excision of, vii. 367
Pyogenetic membrane, i. 104, 255
micro-organisms, i. 125, 253
Pyonephrosis, viii. 102, 106
tuberculous, viii. 125
Pyorrhœa alveolaris, vi. 879
nasal, vi. 85
Pyosalpinx, viii. 408
Pyramidalis muscle, vii. 110

Quadratus lumborum muscle, vii. 110
Quadriceps extensor femoris, hæmatoma of, vii. 73
Quénu operation, modified, vii. 908
Questioning of patients, i. 502, 506
Quinby, William C., and Porter, Charles A., on Surgical Diseases of the Extremities, vii. 37–74

Rabic nodules, or Babès tubercles, iii. 40
virus, iii. 41
Rabies, iii. 38
Race, influence of, upon surgical conditions, i. 783
Racemose aneurysm. See Cirsoid aneurysm
Rachitic rosary, iii. 349
Rachitis (see also under Rickets), iii. 346–354
nodosa, iii. 414
Radiograph. See Roentgen rays, and X-rays
Radiographic localization of foreign bodies, i. 629
plates, method of examining them, i. 641
study of ossification, i. 579, 582, 598
technique, i. 599
tests, i. 612
value of x-ray tubes estimated by milliammeter, i. 616
Radiographs, admissibility of, in evidence, viii. 783, 785
interpretation of, i. 640
scheme of standards used in Massachusetts General Hospital in taking them, i. 626
Radiography in surgery, general considerations on, i. 599
Radioscopy, in diagnosis of œsophageal lesions, vii. 410
Radio-ulnar joint, distal, dislocation of, iv. 64
Radius and ulna, acute osteomyelitis of, iii. 303
sarcoma of, iii. 461
Radius, dislocation of, iv. 58
excision of, iv. 418

Rag-pickers' disease, iii. 32
Railroad employees, physical examination of, viii. 1057
injuries, viii. 1047
surgery, viii. 1030
Railway spine, iii. 735
diagnosed from Pott's disease, iv. 956
Rambaud, George Gibier, on Rabies, iii. 38
Ransohoff, J. Louis, and Joseph, on Intrathoracic Surgery (Heart and Œsophagus excluded), viii. 3–58
Ranula, vi. 257, 309
Raoult's operation for repair of septum, iv. 704
Rarefactive osteitis in acute inflammation of bone, iii. 262
in fractures and injuries to bones, iii. 263
in separation of necrosed bone, iii. 263
in syphilis, iii. 262
in tuberculous disease, iii. 262
Rattlesnakes, iii. 9, 11
Rawling's modifications of the irradiation theory of the causation of cranial fractures, v. 64
Ray fungus, ii. 56
Raynaud's disease, ii. 257
Reaction, Cammidge, viii. 175
Records, hospital, admissibility of, in evidence, viii. 783, 785, 786, 787
Recruits, naval, viii. 971
Rectal diseases diagnosticated, i. 525
examinations, vii. 765
Recto-genital fistula, vii. 835
Rectopexy, vii. 885
Recto-ureteral fistula, vii. 828, 835
Recto-urethral fistula, vii. 828, 829
Recto-uterine fistula, vii. 835
Recto-vaginal fistula, vii. 835
Recto-vesical fistula, vii. 828, 833
Recto-vulvar fistula, vii. 835
Rectum, abnormal opening of, treatment of, vii. 781
actinomycosis, vii. 800
anatomy of, vii. 761
atresia of, vii. 775
chancre of, vii. 799
communicating with uterus, treatment of, vii. 784
dermoids, extra-rectal, vii. 896
dilatation of, vii. 849
dimples, post-anal, vii. 897
drainage of pelvis through, vii. 118
examination of (and see Rectal examinations), vii. 765
excision of, vii. 853
extirpation of, vii. 908
fistula connecting with, vii. 815
foreign bodies in, vii. 946
gumma of, vii. 800
hemorrhoids (and see Hemorrhoids), vii. 860
hypertrophied anal papillæ, vii. 897

Rectum, lymphatics of, vii. 763
    malformations of, vii. 774
    physiology of, vii. 761, 764
    polypus of, vii. 896
    prolapse of, vii. 875
    rupture of, vii. 947
    stricture of, vii. 838
    surgery of, with local anæs-
        thesia, iv. 250–252
    surgical diseases of, vii. 761
    suspension of, from sacrum (and
        see Rectopexy), vii. 885
    syphilis, congenital, of, vii.
        800
    tumors of, benign, vii. 891
        malignant, vii. 898
    ulcers of, vii. 790
    vascular supply of, vii. 763
    verruca of, vii. 897
    wounds of, vii. 761, 947
Rectus abdominis muscle, vii. 110
    abscess of, vii. 78
    capitis anticus major muscle,
        anatomy of, iv. 788
        minor muscle, anatomy
            of, iv. 788
    lateralis muscle, anatomy of,
        iv. 788
    posticus major muscle, anat-
        omy of, iv. 788
        minor, iv. 788
Red blood cells, count of great
    prognostic importance in
    surgery, i. 791
    importance of studying them
        for diagnosis, i. 557
    their removal and changes, i.
        260
Red Cross, American National, viii.
    905
Redness, a symptom of inflamma-
    tion, i. 94
Reid, William W., i. 49
Reeve, J. Charles, Jr., on Surgical
    Diseases of the Diaphragm,
    and Subphrenic Abscess, vii.
    450–504
Referred pain, in Pott's disease, iv.
    944
Reflex joint atrophy, iii. 547
Reflexes, deep, in relation to diag-
    nosis, i. 539
    superficial, in relation to diag-
        nosis, i. 538, 539
Reformed eye, v. 658
Regeneration, i. 256
    after injury of peripheral nerve,
        i. 289
    comparative power of, in dif-
        ferent tissues, i. 257
    effected by cell proliferation, i.
        92
    factors influencing the power of,
        i. 256
Regions of the body as divided for
    surgical study, ii. 695
Reik, Henry Ottridge, on Pyogenic
    Diseases of the Brain, of Otitic
    Origin, v. 779–809
Renal (and see Kidney)
    arteries, abnormalities of, viii.
        89, 91, 92
    calculus, viii. 110

Renal complications, post-anæs-
    thetic, their prophylaxis, iv.
    230
    disease, as influencing the choice
        of anæsthetics, iv. 226
    in operations, i. 787
    source of danger in admin-
        istration of anæsthetics, i.
        785
Rendle's mask, iv. 187
Repair of skull fractures, v. 79
    the process of, i. 92, 256, 259,
        261
Reparative processes as they differ
    in experimental and complete
    fractures, i. 282
    surgery (and see Plastic sur-
        gery), iv. 610
Replacement of nose, iv. 691
Reposition of ovary, viii. 399
Resections and amputations, and
    deaths therefrom, in the Spanish-
    American War, ii. 742
Resection of acromial joint, iv. 402
    of clavicle, iv. 402
    of Fallopian tube, viii. 416
    of hip by anterior incision, as
        recommended by Hueter,
        Barker, Luecke, and Schede,
        iv. 432–434
    of hip, Kocher's method, iv. 432
    of hip, Langenbeck's incision, iv.
        431, 432
    of hip, Sprengel's incision, iv.
        432
    of hip, White's posterior incis-
        ion, iv. 430
    of internal jugular vein, in sinus
        thrombosis, v. 747
    of lower jaw, iv. 385
    of metacarpal and phalangeal
        bones and their joints, iv. 426
    of œsophagus, vii. 417
    of ribs, iv. 406; viii. 50
        Friedrich's, in pulmonary
            tuberculosis, viii. 54
    of sterno-clavicular articulation,
        iv. 402
    of tarsus, osteoplastic, iv. 463
    of temporo-maxillary articula-
        tion for the relief of fixation of
        the lower jaw, iv. 390
    of upper jaw, osteoplastic, with
        Langenbeck's incision, iv. 384,
        385
Resolution of inflammation, i. 98,
    99, 259
Respiratory acts, changes in them,
    and their diagnostic signifi-
    cance, i. 528
    disturbances, post-anæsthetic,
        the several affections em-
        braced in the name ether-
        pneumonia, iv. 229
    organs, diseases of, a source of
        danger in operations, i. 789
    system, diagnostic data ob-
        tained from, i. 527
Rest in treatment of acute, simple
    inflammation, i. 113
    of wounds, i. 754
"Rests" as related to neoplasms, i.
    293

Retention, chronic, in accessory
    sinuses, vi. 83
    of urine, iv. 158; viii. 318, 363
Retractor bandages, iv. 580
Retractors, i. 748
Retrobulbar tumors, vi. 850, 852
Retrocæcal hernia, vii. 611
Retrocollis, due to low dorsal Pott's
    disease, iv. 783
Retrodisplacements of uterus, viii.
    458
Retroduodenal   choledochotomy,
    viii. 273
Retroflexion of uterus, viii. 458
Retrograding mouse tumors, the
    immune factor in the blood, i.
    400
    tumors, action of x-ray and
        radium, i. 402
Retro-œsophageal abscess in Pott's
    disease, iv. 949
Retroperitoneal abscess (and see
    Subphrenic abscess), vii. 493
Retropharyngeal abscess, v. 819; vi.
    343
    in Pott's disease, iv. 949
    tumors, vi. 861
Retroversion of uterus, viii. 458
Reverdin method of skin-grafting,
    iv. 620
Rhabdomyoma, embryonic type of,
    i. 316
Rhabdomyo-sarcoma, i. 317
Rhachitic spine, the, vi. 450
    diagnosed from Pott's dis-
        ease, iv. 956
"Rheumatism" and "rheumatoid
    ostitis," misapplication of
    these terms, iii. 339
    as distinguished from tubercu-
        losis of the knee joint, iii.
        699
    diagnosed from infantile paral-
        ysis, iv. 826
Rhinoliths, i. 200
Rhino-pharyngitis mutilans, ii. 65
Rhino-pharynx, adenoids in, v. 825,
    826
Rhinophyma, v. 478
Rhinoplasty, iv. 679
Rhinoscleroma of pharynx, v. 824
Rhus poisoning of the eyelids, v. 550
Ribs, cervical, vi. 318, 408
    deformities of, iii. 110
    dislocations of, iv. 28
    fractures of, iii. 110
    osteomyelitis of, vi. 409
    resection of, iv. 245, 406; viii. 50
    sarcoma of, iii. 458
    syphilis of, vi. 410
    tuberculosis of, vi. 410
Rib-spreader, viii. 56
Richards, John D., on Sinus
    Thrombosis of Otitic Origin,
    and Suppurative Disease of the
    Labyrinth, v. 731–778
Richelot's method of operating for
    salivary fistula, v. 444
Richet's operation for ectropion,
    iv. 669, 670
Rickets, i. 677
    accompanying indications of, iii.
        350

Rickets and chondrodystrophia fœtalis, x-ray diagnosis between, i. 676
and osteomalacia not clearly distinguished, iii. 347
as affecting bones of the chest and spinal column, iii. 349
as affecting the bones of the head, iii. 349
as affecting the pelvic bones, iii. 349
as involving the bones of the lower extremities, ii. 349
as involving the bones of the upper extremity, iii. 349
chief pathological changes occurring in, iii. 347, 348
craniotabes of, v. 25
fractures of bones in, iii. 350
intra-uterine, iii. 347
Rider's bone, i. 315; ii. 404
Riedel's method of using lateral traction in reduction of forward dislocations of the humerus, iv. 43
Riedinger's classification of congenital deformities, iv. 733
Rifle, small-calibre, ballistic data of, ii. 645
the modern military, ii. 644
Rigg's disease, vi. 879
Rigidity, muscular, iv. 460
spinal, vi. 454
Risus sardonicus in tetanus, i. 457; iii. 24, 25
Rixford, Emmet, on Dislocations, iv. 3
Robert's operation for saddle-nose, iv. 715
Rochet's operation for hypospadias, vi. 651
Rodent ulcer, i. 359
of face, v. 489
Rodgers, John Kearney, i. 43, 44
Rodman, John Stewart, and William L., on Amputations and Disarticulations, iv. 263
Rodman's method of gastro-enterostomy, vii. 367
Roentgen-ray. See Radiographs, X-rays
Roentgen-ray department, of hospitals, viii. 879
Roentgen-rays, their divergence and its results in photographs, i. 578
Rolandic area of brain, diagnosis of tumors in, v. 321
fissure, line of, v. 362, 363
Roller bandages, varieties of, iv. 547–576
Rose corns, ii. 363
Rose's posture for extirpation of the tongue, iv. 217
Roser's method of treating dislocations backward of both bones at the elbow, iv. 55
Rotter's method of rhinoplasty, iv. 692
Rouge's method of restoring lower part of nose, iv. 703
Round ligament of uterus, anatomy of, viii. 395

Round ligament, hydrocele of, vi. 568
shortening of, viii. 471
Roux's disarticulation at the ankle-joint, iv. 332
method of gastro-enterostomy, vii. 357
nail operation for femoral hernia, vii. 590
Rubber drainage tubes, i. 740
gloves, their use and care, i. 709
tissue, how used, i. 741
Rudimentary tail-formation, vii. 14
Rumpel's test for idiopathic dilatation of œsophagus, vii. 448
Rupture of kidney, viii. 93
of liver, viii. 206
of membrana tympani, v. 685
of rectum, vii. 947
of spleen, viii. 64
of urethra, vi. 666
of urinary bladder, iii. 156; viii. 287
Rush Medical College, of Chicago, founded, i. 27
Rydygier's method of splenopexy, viii. 76

SABRE-BLADE deformity of leg in syphilitic osteitis, iii. 389
Sacro-coccygeal cysts, vii. 17, 20
dimples, vii. 20
foveæ, vii. 20
region, congenital deformities of, vii. 14
sinuses, vii. 20
tumors, vii. 17
Sacro-iliac articulation, as affected by hypertrophic arthritis, iii. 522
tuberculous disease of, iii. 618
synchondrosis, strain and partial dislocation of, iv. 28
tuberculosis of, vii. 8
Saddle-nose, iv. 625, 706; v. 458
Saemisch keratotomy, v. 617
Saenger's Cæsarean section, viii. 705
Saliva as a source of infection, i. 699
diagnostic data obtainable from its examination, i. 561
Salivary calculi, vi. 259
Salivary-duct fistula, v. 440
Salivary glands, absence of, congenital, vi. 312
actinomycosis of, vi. 303
anomalies of, vi. 312
diseases of, surgical, vi. 221
injuries of, vi. 297
Mikulicz's disease, vi. 303
syphilis of, vi. 303
tuberculosis of, vi. 303
tumors of, vi. 303
wounds of, vi. 221
Salpingectomy, viii. 416
Salpingitis, viii. 407
diagnosed from acute appendicitis, vii. 658
tuberculous and non-tuberculous, viii. 421
Salpingo-oöphorectomy, viii. 417, 543
Salt solution, normal or physiological, i. 704

Saltikoff and Maasland, investigation of, on cerebral concussion, v. 157
Salves and ointments, i. 759
Sampson of Albany, his method of controlling hemorrhage following pelvic operations, iv. 168
Sandelin's operation for restoration of lower lip, iv. 660
Sanies, a form of pus, i. 124
Sapræmia, i. 96, 423, 425
Sarcoma, as distinguished from tuberculosis of the knee-joint, iii. 700
alveolar, i. 334, 336
angiomatous, i. 338
atypical meso-hylomata, i. 331, 333
central, of the long bones, iii. 446
giant-celled, i. 335; iii. 445
gross appearances, i. 331
idiopathic multiple pigmented, ii. 387
in rats, transplantation of, i. 391
intranasal, vi. 198, 857, 858
large round-celled, i. 334
medullary, i. 332
melanotic, ii. 386
melanotic, spindle-celled and alveolar, i. 341, 342
mixed-celled, i. 335
myeloid, i. 335
of antrum, vi. 170
of auricle, v. 676
of biliary ducts, viii. 252
of bone, iii. 440–464
of brain, v. 310
of breast, female, iii. 529
of chest wall, vi. 414
of conjunctiva, v. 584
of eyeball, v. 644
of eyelids, v. 559
of face, v. 489
of femur, Budin's statistics of operative results, iii. 462
of fibula, iii. 464
of gluteal region, vii. 31
of humerus, iii. 459–461
of intestines, vii. 738
of iris, v. 613
of jaw, periosteal, vi. 823
of kidney, viii. 134, 136
of lachrymal gland, v. 593
of larynx, v. 884
of liver, viii. 223
of lung, viii. 30
of mediastinum, viii. 35
of Meibomian glands, v. 559
of mixed type, i. 343
of nasopharynx, vi. 860
of neck, vi. 351
of œsophagus, vii. 420
of orbit, v. 652
of ovary, viii. 428
of pancreas, viii. 189
of pelvic bones, vii. 13
of pelvis, vi. 461
of penis, vi. 688
of pharynx, v. 857
of pleura, viii. 14
of prostate, viii. 354
of radius and ulna, iii. 461

Sarcoma of rectum, vii. 903
  of salivary glands, vi. 304
  of scalp, v. 22
  of scrotum, vi. 695
  of seminal vesicles, vi. 699
  of skin, ii. 385
  of skin of abdominal wall, vii. 87
  of skull, v. 32
  of special bones, iii. 456
  of spine diagnosed from Pott's disease, iv. 955
  of spleen, viii. 69
  of testis, vi. 698
  of thyroid, vi. 372
  of tibia, iii. 463
  of tongue, vi. 291
  of urinary bladder, viii. 311
  of uterus (and see Uterus, sarcoma of), viii. 666
  of vermiform appendix, vii. 625
  of vulva, vi. 571
  periosteal, iii. 448
  perithelial, i. 338
  petrifying, i. 343
  Ziegler's classification of, i. 333
Sarcomatous osteitis, iii. 465
  transformation in other tumors, i. 333
Satellite veins, described, iv. 471
Sauerbruch's pneumatic cabinet, iii. 458; vii. 418; viii. 44
Sayre, Lewis A., i. 56
Sayre's (Lewis A.) apparatus for torticollis, iv. 779
Sayre's (Reginald) apparatus for torticollis, iv. 780
Scab, healing under a, i. 249
Scalds, viii. 975
  of abdominal wall, vii. 93
  of auricle, v. 665
  of face, v. 428
  of larynx, v. 866
  of pharynx, v. 811
  of tongue, vi. 232
Scalp, air collections in, v. 11
  anatomical peculiarities of, v. 3
  aneurysm of, v. 23
  blood-vessels of the, traumatic affections of the, v. 23
  cirsoid aneurysm of, v. 19
  dermoid cysts of, v. 14
  elephantiasis mollis of, v. 16
  elephantiasis nervorum of, v. 16
  emphysema of, v. 11
  gangrene of, v. 23
  hyperæsthesia of, v. 23
  infectious granulomata of, v. 24
  nævus vasculosus of, v. 18
  neuralgic affections of the, v. 23
  pachydermatocele of, v. 16
  plastic surgery of the. iv. 628
  Tillmanns' method of bridging a defect in, iv. 630
  post-zoster neuralgia of the, v. 24
  syphilis of, v. 24
  tumors of, v. 11
  wounds of, v. 4
Scalping, v. 7
Scaphoid, dislocations of, iv. 67
  (navicular), dislocations of, iv. 102

Scapula, chondroma of, iii. 428
  congenital elevation of, iv. 735
  excision of the glenoid angle of, iv. 405
  excision of entire, iv. 403–405
  fractures of, iii. 121, 122, 123
  partial excision of, iv. 405
  sarcoma of, iii. 459
Scarification, iv. 604
Scars, hypertrophic, ii. 366
Scar tissue, formation of, i. 263
Schaefer's method of treating fractures of the patella, iii. 191
Schede's operation (thoracoplasty), viii. 52
Schenck, Benjamin R., on Surgery of the Ovaries and Fallopian Tubes, viii. 391–443
Schimmelbusch's operation for restoring the cheek, iv. 647
  operation for saddle-nose, iv. 712
Schinzinger's method of reducing forward dislocations of the humerus by rotation, iv. 45
Schistosoma hæmatobium, causing ulcerations of rectum, vii. 794
Schleich's system of anæsthetic mixtures, iv. 171
Schools, medical, first organization of, in America, i. 3
Schools of medicine, not recognized, viii. 739
  practice must be in accordance with one to which surgeon belongs, viii. 738
Schreiber's ivory pins, iii. 92
Schroeder's method of trachelorrhaphy, vi. 592
Schroetter-Tuerck cannula forceps, v. 882
Schuetz's adenotome, v. 833
Schwartz's method of treating varicose veins, iii. 318
Schwartze-Stacke operation for mastoiditis, v. 715, 717, 756–758
Sciatic artery, injury of, vii. 27
  ligation of, iv. 510; vii. 28
  traumatic aneurysm of, vii. 27
  hernia, vii. 605
  nerve, stretching of, vii. 35
Sciatica, vii. 33
Scirrhous mamma, vi. 515
Scirrhus carcinoma of breast, female, vi. 534
Scissors, i. 744
  Emmet's denuding, vi. 588
Sclera, operations upon the, v. 616
Sclerosis, plastic peritoneal, vii. 753
Sclerotic, diseases of, v. 590
  wounds of, v. 591
Sclerotomy, anterior, v. 623
  posterior, v. 623
Scoliosis, vi. 470
Scopolamine-morphine anæsthesia, i. 480
Scorpion, its sting and the treatment of it, iii. 5
Scrofuloderma, ii. 323
Scrotum, absence of, vi. 657
  anatomy of, vi. 627
  bifid, vi. 658

Scrotum, cysts of, vi. 695
  emphysema of, vi. 680
  gangrene of, vi. 675
  hypertrophy of, vi. 658
  injuries of, vi. 665
  lupus of, vi. 671
  malformations of, vi. 657
  œdema of, vi. 680
  rudimentary, vi. 657
  skin diseases of, vi. 674
  tuberculosis of, vi. 671
  tumors of, vi. 695
  varicosities of, vi. 678
Scudder's method of treating fractures of the patella, iii. 186
Scultetus, abdominal, of adhesive plaster, iv. 594
Scurvy, ii. 68
Scurvy, ii. 68
Seaman, Valentine, i. 13
Seamen's skin, ii. 374
Seasoned tube, its radiographic value, indicated by milliammeter, i. 618
Sebaceous cyst, ii. 531
  of auricle, v. 674
  of neck, vi. 348
  of penis, vi. 687
  of scalp (and see Wens), v. 13
  glands, in abdominal wall, adenoma of, vii. 86
Second intention, healing by, i. 102, 268, 270
Secondary adhesion, healing by, i. 251, 252
Secretions, diagnostic value of, i. 561, 567
  from the female genital tract, bacterial examination of, i. 565
Sectio alta, vii. 105
Section, abdominal, vii. 105 .
  Cæsarean, vii. 105
  exploratory, vii. 113
Sédillot's method of repairing septum, iv. 705
  method of restoring the alæ nasi, iv. 697
  modification of Pirogoff's amputation, iv. 334
  operation for restoring upper lip, iv. 650
Sella turcica, tumors of region of, v. 331
Semilunar bone, dislocation of, iv. 66
  cartilages, dislocations of, iv. 89, 90
  fold of Douglas, vii. 111
Seminal secretion, diagnostic data obtained by examination of, i. 566
  vesicles, anatomy of, vi. 632
  cysts of, vi. 698
  tuberculosis of, vi. 674
  tumors of, vi. 698
  vesiculitis, chronic, vi. 763
Senn's and Watson's drainage tube, vii. 326
Senn's bloodless amputation at the hip-joint, iv. 355
  operation for excision of the shoulder joint, iv. 400

Senn's operation for restoring upper lip and face, iv. 651
plaster-of-Paris dressing in treatment of fractures of the neck of the femur, iii. 173
researches on the ligation of blood-vessels, i. 725
Sensory cortex, of brain, v 270
Sepsis, its surgical meaning, i. 695
Septicæmia, i. 96, 423
cryptogenetic, i. 430
due to mixed infection, i. 431
Septico-pyæmia, i. 439
as a result of diffuse suppuration, i. 255
Septum of nose, repair of lower part of, iv. 703
Sequestra, i. 223
their persistence, i. 286
Sequestrum, in cranial syphilis,v. 42
Sero-fibrinous catarrh, i. 116
Sero-purulent catarrh, i. 116
Sero-pus defined, i. 253
Serositis, multiple, vii. 753
Serous effusion in inflammation, i. 116
meningitis, v. 236
surfaces,fibrinous exudate upon, i. 119
Serre's operation for repair of septum, iv. 703
operation for restoration of lower lip, iv. 654
operation on mouth, iv. 667
Serum or agglutinative reactions, their surgical diagnostic value, i. 560
Serum therapy in septicæmia and pyæmia, i. 443
Sex as bearing on diagnosis, i. 508
relation of, to surgical prognosis, i. 777
Shepherd, Francis J., on Surgical Diseases and Wounds of the Thyroid and Thymus, vi. 353–400
Shippen, William, Jr., i. 7
Shock, i. 463, 464
alcoholism in relation to, i. 483
amputation during, i. 486
and collapse, differentiation between, i. 491
and hemorrhage, i. 485
blood-pressure to be watched as an index of, i. 490
choice and management of anæsthetics in, iv. 226
Crile's experimental work on, i. 468
diabetes as related to, i. 482
Howell's conclusions in regard to, i. 467
in abdominal operations, i. 475
in operations involving the diaphragm, i. 475
in operations on the head, i. 471
in operations on the neck, i. 472
in operations on the spleen, i. 476
in operations on the thorax, i. 473
infants less liable to, i. 774
influence of atmospheric pressure as a factor, i. 288

Shock, injuries of the skin in relation to, i. 469
nephritis in relation to, i. 482
operative details influencing, i. 469
pain as bearing on the production of, i. 469
relation of cerebral concussion to, v. 161
relation of, to fall in blood pressure, i. 465
relation of, to local infections, i. 483
relation of, to starvation, i. 484
relations of spinal anæsthesia to, i. 480
Shoes, proper, iv. 880
Shortening and rotation outward of the limb in fractures of the shaft of the femur, iii. 178
of the limb in hip-joint disease, means of ascertaining it, iii. 643
Shotgun wounds, ii. 655
Shoulder cap, in treatment of fractures of humerus, iii. 128
Shoulder-joint, amputation at, i. 59
congenital dislocation of, iv. 738
treatment, iv. 740
disarticulation by the racquet incision, iv. 309
disarticulation of arm and shoulder girdle, anterior incision, iv. 311
epiphyseal development as shown by radiography, i. 592
excision of, iv. 392–401
infantile paralysis of, iv. 818
obstetrical paralysis of, iv. 738
penetrating wounds of, iii. 736
periarthritis of, vii. 44
resection of, for unreduced dislocation, iv. 400, 401
sprains and contusions of, iii. 735
tuberculous disease of, iii. 601–607
Shrady's method of transferring flaps, iv. 618
Sialoadenitis acuta, vi. 299
Sialodochitis, vi. 302
Sialolithiasis, vi. 259
Sick-bay on battle-ship, viii. 982
Sickness, post-anæsthetic, its prophylaxis and management, iv. 228
Siderosis, i. 207
Sight, sense of, in relation to diagnosis, i. 540
Sigmoid flexure, vii. 763
diverticulitis of, vii. 703
drainage tube, viii. 326
foreign bodies in, vii. 947
peridiverticulitis of, vii. 703
Sigmoiditis, vii. 930
Sigmoidopexy, vii. 887
Silicosis, i. 207
Silk as used for sutures and ligatures, i. 725
Silkworm gut as material for sutures, i. 726
Silver wire as suture material, i. 727
in gynæcology, i. 57

Silver wire in treatment of fractures, i. 728
Simmons, Channing C., on tumors originating in bone, iii. 394
Simon's method of using lateral traction in reducing forward dislocations of the humerus, iv. 43
operation for hare lip, v. 513
Simpson as introducer of chloroform as an anæsthetic, iv. 169
Simpson's operation for retroverted uterus, viii. 479
Sims, J. Marion, i. 57
Sims' method of operation for vesico-vaginal fistula, vi. 621
position, vi. 582, 583
Sinkler's reflex, i. 540
Sinuses, accessory, of the nose, diseases of, in general, vi. 83–89
of antrum, vi. 156
of ethmoidal cells, vi. 90
of frontal sinus, vi. 113
of sphenoidal sinus, vi. 180
diseases of, vi. 83
pericranii, v. 12
pilo-nidal, vii. 20
sacro-coccygeal, vii. 20
sigmoid, septic thrombosis of, v. 249
superior longitudinal, septic thrombosis of, v. 249
tuberculous, Beck's method of treating, vii. 553
venous, injuries of the, v. 205
Sippy's œsophageal dilator, vii. 448
Skeleton, living, i. 171
use of, to illustrate testimony, viii. 791
Skene's glands, inflammation of, vi. 560
Skey's modification of Lisfranc's operation, iv. 324
Skin, atrophy of, i. 179
local anæsthetization of, iv. 240
methods of filling in gaps in the, iv. 614
sarcoma of, of abdominal wall, vii. 87
sterilization, i. 702, 708
Skin-grafting, iv. 620–624
after extensive burns, i. 252
for x-ray ulcers, vii. 40
Reverdin method, iv. 620
Thiersch method, iv. 620
Woelfe-Krause method, iv. 622
Skull, angiosarcoma of, v. 32
carcinoma of, v. 34
chondroma of, iii. 429
contusion of, by gunshot wound, v. 87
fractures of, v. 48
escape of cerebral substance in, v. 76
escape of cerebro-spinal fluid in, v. 75
gigantism of, v. 28
gunshot wounds of the, v. 86
gutter fracture of, ii. 702
new growths of, v. 28
osteomalacia of, v. 26
parasitic cysts of, v. 28

Skull, tænia echinococcus in, v. 28
　tuberculous disease in bones of,
　　iii. 599
　wounds of, v. 48, 95
Sling for lower extremity, iv. 577
　for upper extremity, iv. 576
Sloughing, i. 229; ii. 201, 202
　of the urethra, ii, 294
Small-arms, definition of the term,
　ii. 643
Smell, cortical area concerned with,
　v. 273
　sense of, its importance in diag-
　　nosis, i. 541
Smith, Alban G., i. 15
　Henry H., i. 19
　Joseph M., i. 14
　Nathan, i. 21
　Nathan R., i. 24, 48
Smith's (Nathan R.) apparatus for
　ununited fractures of the
　thigh, iii. 221, 224
　　anterior splint in the treat-
　　　ment of fractures of the
　　　neck of the femur, iii. 175
Smith's (Noble) operation for torti-
　collis, iv. 802
Smith's (R. W.) modification of Lis-
　franc's operation, iv. 324
Smith, Stephen, on Evolution of
　American Surgery, i. 3
　statistics of recovered am-
　　putations done in the pe-
　　riod of shock, iv. 278
Smith, Stephen, and Smith, Sidney,
　on the Civil Obligation of Sur-
　geon and Patient in the Practice
　of American Surgery, viii. 713–
　820
Smoker's patch, vi. 236
Smyth, A. W., i. 43
Snake-bites, iii. 6, 11
　poisoning by, Calmette's anti-
　　venene in treatment of, iii.
　　14
Snake-venom, its constituents and
　effects, iii. 9–11
Snakes, poisonous, peculiarities of
　teeth and fangs, iii. 7
Snydacker's method of blepharo-
　plasty, v. 575
Solarium, the, viii. 847
Soluble-glass bandages, iv. 590
Solutions of eucain B for local
　anæsthesia, iv. 235
　for local anæsthesia, Braun, iv.
　235
Somnoforme as an anæsthetic, iv.
　171, 207
Somnoforme-ether sequence for
　anæsthesia, iv. 210
Sonnenberg's operation for ectopia
　vesicæ, viii. 284
Sounds, urethral, vi. 786
　use of, in diagnosis of vesical cal-
　　culus, viii. 308
Space of Retzius, abscess of, vii. 78
Spanish windlass, iv. 263, 266
Spasm of larynx, v. 896
　spinal accessory, iv. 786
　sympathetic, of the eyelids, v.
　556
Spasmodic torticollis, iv. 767, 786

Spastic infantile paralysis, diag-
　nosed from infantile paralysis, iv.
　823
Spear's shell-wound packet, viii.
　999
Specialist, determination of fact
　whether surgeon is a, viii. 727
　standard of skill, etc., required
　　of, viii. 729, 740, 741
Speculum, Earle's rectal, vii. 768
Speech, cortical area concerned
　with, v. 273
Spence's operation for amputation
　at the shoulder-joint, advan-
　tages claimed for this method, iv.
　303–305
Spermaceti, in plastic operations, iv.
　625
Spermatic artery, thrombosis of, vi.
　666
　cord, anatomy of, vi. 630
　　injuries of, vi. 665
　　torsion of, causing strangula-
　　　tion of testis, vi. 667
　　tumors of, vi. 696
　　twisted, vi. 668
Spermatocele, vi. 685
Spermatocystitis, vi. 763
Spermatozoa, vi. 628
Sphacelus, ii. 201, 202
Spheno-ethmoidal recess, anatomy
　of the, vi. 95
Sphenoidal sinus, absence of, vi. 170
　acute inflammation of, vi.
　　180
　anatomy of, vi. 170
　catheterization of, vi. 175
　chronic inflammation of, vi.
　　181
　chronic suppuration of, vi.
　　181
　tumors of, vi. 200
Sphincterectomy, v. 620
Spider cancer, of face, v. 470
Spiller-Frazier method of operation,
　intracranial, upon the trigeminal
　nerve, v. 397
Spina bifida, vi. 462
　operative procedures, vi. 466
Spina bifida occulta, vi. 465
Spina ventosa, iii. 445, 616
　in the foot, iii. 723
Spinal accessory nerve, injury to, in
　neck, vi. 330
　operations on, iv. 800;
　　v. 415
　spasm, iv. 786
　anæsthesia, Bier's method of
　　injection, iv. 259, 260
　column, deformities of, vi. 462
　dislocation of, vi. 429
　fracture of, vi. 429
　fracture-dislocation of, vi.
　　429, 437
　surgery of, vi. 401
　tuberculous disease of, and
　　the deformities resulting
　　therefrom (and see Pott's
　　disease), vi. 927
　wounds of, vi. 421
　cord, atrophic diseases of, i. 178
　complete transverse injury
　　of, i. 543

Spinal cord, complete unilateral in-
　jury of, i. 543
　degeneration of (compres-
　　sion myelitis), i. 177
　diseases of cauda equina, vi.
　　501
　diseases of conus terminalis,
　　vi. 501
　injuries of cauda equina, vi.
　　501
　methods of exposing, vi. 498
　partial lesions of, i. 543
　tumors of cauda equina, vi.
　　501
　tumors of, relative frequency
　　of different varieties of,
　　vi. 489
　wounds of, vi. 421
　wounds of conus terminalis,
　　vi. 501
Spine, actinomycosis of, vi. 448
　anatomy of, iv. 927
　ankylosis of, vi. 456
　arthritis deformans, vi. 454
　arthritis of, infectious, vi. 451,
　　454
　attitude of, in stooping, iv. 941
　Becterew's disease of (spinal
　　rigidity), vi. 458
　caries of (and see Pott's dis-
　　ease), iv. 927
　chronic ankylosing inflamma-
　　tion of, vi. 456
　congenital scoliosis of, vi. 484
　contusions of, vi. 422
　curvature of, angular (and see
　　Pott's disease), iv. 927
　antero-posterior (and see
　　Pott's disease), iv. 927
　curves of, iv. 928
　cyphose hérédo-traumatique, vi.
　　459
　Ericson's, vi. 422
　fractures of, in general, patho-
　　logical changes, vi. 439
　gonorrhœal, vi. 452
　gunshot wounds of. vi. 423
　hysterical, vi. 461
　lateral curvature of (and see
　　Scoliosis), vi. 470
　litigation, vi. 423
　osteoarthritis of, vi. 458
　osteomyelitis of, acute, vi. 448
　ostitis deformans of, vi. 455
　rhachitic, the, vi. 450
　scoliosis, vi. 470, 484
　spondylitis deformans of, vi. 455
　spondylolisthesis, vi. 461
　spondylose rhizomélique, vi. 459
　stab-wounds of, vi. 423
　syphilis of, vi. 450
　tumors of, vi. 486
Spirochæta pallida, i. 566
Splay-foot (and see Weak foot), iv.
　872
Spleen, anomalies and diseases of,
　viii. 61
　surgery of the, viii. 59
　wounds of, viii. 66
Splenectomy, viii. 74
Splenic anæmia, viii. 71
Splenius muscle, anatomy of, iv. 787
Splenomegaly, primary, viii. 71

Splenopexy, viii. 76
Splenoptosis. viii. 61
Splenotomy. viii. 75
Splint, Bavarian, description of, iv. 583
  Brown's (Buckminster) for torticollis. iv. 788, 789
  dental, vi. 48
  in young horses. iii. 255
  Kaulyang, viii. 955
Splinters in hands and feet. vii. 42
Spondylitis deformans. vi. 455
Spondylolisthesis, iv. 956 vi. 461
Spondylolisthetic pelvis, vii. 3
Spondylose rhizomélique, vi. 459
Sponges or pads, i. 720. iv. 138
  left in wound after operation. malpractice, viii. 761
Sprains, iii. 725
  diagnosed from Pott's disease, iv. 956
Sputum, diagnostic importance of pathological findings therein, i. 563, 564
Squint (and see Strabismus), v. 638
Ssbanajew-Frank's method of gastrostomy, vii. 405
Stab-wound drain, vii. 117
  of penis, vi. 665
  of spine, vi. 423
  of spleen, viii. 66
Stacke's method of forming meatal flap, v. 723
  operation for mastoiditis, v. 727
Staphylococci and their effects. i. 417
Staphyloma, v. 605
Staphylorrhaphy, v. 524
Staphylotomy, v. 817
Starch bandages, iv. 590
Starr, Clarence L., on Tuberculous Disease of the Spinal Column and the deformities resulting therefrom, iv. 927
Status epilepticus, v. 300
  lymphaticus, vi. 397; viii. 34
  as related to rickets. iii. 351
Stay sutures, i. 752
Steam sterilizer, i. 714
Steatorrhœa, in pancreatic diseases. viii. 177
Steel brace, Taylor's (C. F.). iv. 971
Steinthal's operation for rhinoplasty, iv. 688
Stellwag's sign, v. 556
Stenosis, intestinal, chronic, vii. 732
  of external auditory canal, v. 679
  pyloric, vii. 335
Stenson's duct, fistula of, vi. 298
Stercoræmia in its relation to surgical prognosis, i. 790
Stereoscopic radiographs, how to take them, i. 636
Sterility, relation of uterine fibromyoma to, viii. 571
Sterilization of catgut, the Claudius or iodine method described, i. 731
  of dressings, i. 713
  of hands, i. 702
  of instruments, i. 711

Sterilization of nail brushes, i. 703
  of skin at seat of operation. i. 702
  of soap, i. 702
  of sutures and ligatures, i. 724
  of water, apparatus for, i. 712
Sterilizer, Japanese field, viii. 954
Sterilizing outfit, steam-pressure. viii. 987
Sterno-cleido-mastoid muscle, anatomy of, iv. 787, 788
  tenotomy of, for torticollis. iv. 774
Sternum, echinococcus of, vi. 411
  fractures of, iii. 108
  osteomyelitis of, vi. 409
  sarcoma of, iii. 458
  syphilis of, vi. 410
  tuberculosis of, vi. 410
Sternum and ribs, tuberculous disease of, iii. 617
Stevens, Alexander H., i. 14
Stewart, Francis T., and Le Conte, Robert G., on Surgery of the Pericardium, Heart, and Blood-vessels, vii. 146–331
Stewart, George David, on Surgery of the Liver, Gall-bladder, and Biliary Passages. viii. 193–278
  on Surgery of the Pancreas, viii. 159–192
Stewart, George D.. on Torticollis, iv. 767
Stewart, J. Clark, on Surgical Diseases and Wounds of Muscles, Tendons, Bursæ, etc., ii. 399
Stiff-neck, treatment of, iv. 785
Stimson, Lewis A., statistical tables of dislocations, quoted from, iv. 11–13
Stimson's method of reduction of backward dislocations of the hip, iv. 79
  method of treating fractures of the patella, iii. 185
  method of using lateral traction in reducing forward dislocations of the humerus, iv. 43, 44
  theory of congenital dislocations, iv. 734
Stings, viii. 974
  of bees and wasps on tongue, vi. 232
Stitch abscesses, i. 753
St. Louis Medical College, i. 29
Stokes, Surgeon-General Charles Francis, on Naval Surgery. viii. 970–1029
Stokes' apparatus for transferring wounded at sea, viii. 1023
  shell-wound packet, viii. 998
  splint stretcher, viii. 1008, 1009
  supracondyloid amputation at the knee-joint, iv. 347
Stomach, acute dilatation of, postoperative, iv. 154
  as a machine for digesting food, vii. 333
  atrophy of, i. 181
  hour-glass, vii. 379
  perforation of, vii. 341
  prolapse of (and see Gastroptosis), vii. 389

Stomach, surgical diseases of, i. 519; vii. 332
  wounds of, vii. 332
Stomatitis, vi. 221, 878
Stone, James S., on Hare Lip and Cleft Palate, v. 500–546
  on Plastic Surgery, iv. 610
Stone, Warren, i. 28
Stone in the urinary bladder, viii. 306
Stools, diagnostic examination of, i. 525
Stooping, attitude of spine in, iv. 941
Storp's suspension cuff, iii. 151
Stovaine as a local anæsthetic, iv. 233
Strabismus, v. 638
Strangulation, vii. 727
  of testis, from torsion of cord, vi. 667
Strawberry marks, v. 470
Streptococci and their effects, i. 417
Streptothrix maduræ, ii. 61
Stretching of sciatic nerve, vii. 35
Stricture of lachrymal duct, treatment of, v. 595
  of œsophagus, vii. 428
  of rectum (and see Rectum, stricture of), vii. 838
  of urethra (and see Urethra, stricture of), vi. 773
Struma Gravesiana colloides, vi. 379
  lingualis, vi. 256
  lipomatodes aberrata renis, viii. 135
Strumitis, vi. 365, 370
Stumps, amputation, iv. 268; vii. 67
Stye, v. 551
Styloid process of ulna or radius, fractures of, iii. 148
Styptics, control of hemorrhage by, vii. 240
Subastragaloid amputation by Farabeuf's method, iv. 329
  dislocation (luxatio sub talo), iv. 98
Subclavian artery, aneurysm of, vi. 337
  left. ligation of, within the scaleni, i. 43
  ligature of, iv. 493–495; viii. 41
Subdiaphragmatic abscess, i. 128
Subiliac bursitis, vii. 51
Submaxillary gland (and see Salivary glands), vi. 298
Submental connective tissue, inflammation of, v. 444
Suboccipital lymph nodes, v. 419
Subparotid lymph nodes, v. 420
Subperiosteal tuberculous disease of bone, iii. 579
Subphrenic abscess, vii. 450, 478
Substitutes for cocaine as local anæsthetics, iv. 233
Subungual exostoses, iii. 409, 410
Sudeck's fraise, v. 355
Suppuration, i. 121, 250
Suppurative meningitis, v. 240
Supraduodenal choledochotomy, viii. 272

Suprapubic aspiration, vi. 797, 805; viii. 321
lithotomy, viii. 328
prostatectomy, viii. 370
Surgeon and patient, civil obligation of, viii. 713
Sutures and other foreign bodies, i. 274
Connell, vii. 736, 738, 754
Cushing's right-angle, vii. 754
Czerny, vii. 734
Czerny-Lembert, vii. 734, 754
Dupuytren, vii. 738
Gould's, vii. 736
Halsted's, vii. 736, 754
in lung, viii. 57
insoluble, i. 275
intercuticular, vii. 129
intracuticular, vii. 129
Lembert, vii. 734, 754
materials, i. 274
mattress, vii. 736
of arteries, control of hemorrhage by, vii. 249
purse-string, vii. 748, 756
soluble, how disposed of, i. 275
subcuticular, ii. 613
Suturing of intestinal wounds, histology of the healing process, i. 276
of wounds; tier sutures and stay sutures, i. 752
Sweat, sterile and otherwise, i. 698
Sweet, J. E., on the Relation of Blood-Pressure to Surgery, viii. 1063–1082
Sylvester's method of artificial respiration, iv. 196
Sylvian fissure, line of, v. 362, 363
Symblepharon, operations for, v. 567
Syms' prostatic tractor, viii. 389
Syme's amputation, iv. 271
horse-shoe splint, iii. 206
modification of the circular amputation of the thigh, iv. 349
operation for disarticulation at the ankle-joint, iv. 329–332
operation, instruments required and details of the procedure, iv. 330
operation for restoration of lower lip, iv. 657
Sympathetic ganglia, removal of, for idiopathic epilepsy, v. 299
nerve, injury to, in neck, vi. 330
Symphyseotomy, viii. 707
Symphysis pubis, neuralgia of, vii. 36
tuberculosis of, iii. 622; vii. 11
Syndactylism, iv. 634
Syndesmosis defined, i. 284
Synechiæ, v. 609
after cataract operations, v. 635
anterior, separation of, v. 619
of ear, v. 714
Synechtomy, v. 714, 715
Synechtotomy, v. 621
Synostosis defined, i. 284
Synovial membranes described, iii. 559

Synovial membranes, gummatous deposits on, iii. 538
villi described, iii. 559
Synovitis, as distinguished from tuberculosis of the knee-joint, iii. 698
Syphilides, secondary, ii. 110
serpiginous ulcerative, ii. 114
Syphilis a cause of ulceration, i. 226
as a cause of pathological dislocation, iv. 8
as affecting the mucous membranes, ii. 111
as affecting the nails, ii. 112
cerebral, v. 242
congenital, of anus, vii. 800
of rectum, vii. 800
cranial, v. 36
hereditary, certain phases of, iii. 382
meningeal and cerebral, v. 242
methods of administering mercury other than hypodermic, ii. 138
mixed treatment in, ii. 139
not a bar to operative measures, i. 792
of accessory sinuses, vi. 85
of auricle, v. 671, 676
of blood-vessels, ii. 120
of bone, ii. 128
of brain (and see Meningitis, syphilitic), v. 301
of breast, female, vi. 519
of bursæ and tendon sheaths, ii. 128
of clavicle, vi. 416
of eye and ear, ii. 116
of eyelids, v. 552
of face, v. 457
of jaws, vi. 886
of joints, iii. 536
of kidney, ii. 119
of larynx, vi. 874
of liver, ii. 117 viii. 226
of lymph nodes, gummatous, ii. 128
of muscles, ii. 128
of nervous system, ii. 121
of pelvic bones, vii. 12
of pharynx, v. 842
of prostate, viii. 350
of rectum, ii. 121
of ribs, vi. 410
of salivary glands, vi. 303
of scalp, v. 24
of spine, vi. 450
of sternum, vi. 410
of testicle, ii. 126
of thyroid, vi. 372
of tongue, ii. 293
of upper air passages, ii. 123
of viscera, ii. 116
Syphilitic affections of bone, iii. 376, 387
alopecia, ii. 111
cachexia, ii. 101
caries, iii. 373–375
condylomata of female genitals, vi. 565
dactylitis, iii. 384
gumma, ii. 100
hyperostosis of the tibia, iii. 388

Syphilitic joint disease, its differentiation from tuberculosis, iii. 537, 699
necrosis, peculiarities of, iii. 376
nodes, their characters and significance, ii. 105
osteitis, showing sabre-blade deformity of leg, iii. 389
osteomyelitis, iii. 366–371
periostitis, iii. 365
rupia, ii. 114
skin lesions, their general characteristics, ii. 114
ulceration of rectum, vii. 799
ulcers, deep, i. 230
of leg, ii. 113
superficial, i. 230
Syphiloma, ano-rectal, of Fournier, vii. 800
Syringes and needles, for injections for spinal anæsthesia, iv 258, 259
Syringomyelia, bone changes in, iii. 363
Syringomyelocele, vi. 464
Szokalski's method of operation for pterygium, v. 594
Szymanowski's method of blepharoplasty, iv. 675; v. 572
method of closing artificial anus, vii. 943
method of restoring lower part of nose, iv. 703
operation for ectropion, iv 670
operation for making an external ear, iv. 719
operation for saddle-nose, iv. 713, 715

Tabes, bone changes in, iii. 363
Tænia echinococcus in skull, v. 28
Tagliacotian method of blepharoplasty, the, v. 574
Tagliacozzi's method of plastic surgery (and see Italian method), iv. 613
Tails, in human beings, vii. 14
Talipes, iv. 896
Tamponades and drains, iv. 539–542
Tansley's operation for ptosis, v. 569
Tarantula, its sting and the treatment of it, iii. 5
Tarsal bones, dislocations of individual ones, iv. 100
fractures of, iii. 210
tuberculous disease of, iii. 720, 722
Tarsitis, v. 558
Tarso-metatarsal articulations as grouped by Henry Morris, into three joints, iv. 321
Tarsorrhaphy, v. 566
Tarsus, resection of, iv. 463
Taste, cortical areas concerned with, v. 273
sense of, its alterations as influencing diagnosis, i. 542
Tattooing of cornea, v. 619
Tattoo marks, ii. 393
methods of removal, ii. 394
Tavel's modification of Kroenlein's operation for orbital tumors, vi. 869

Taxis, in strangulated inguinal hernia, vii. 569
Taylor chin cup, for Pott's disease, iv. 973, 977
    club-foot brace, iv. 910
    club-foot shoe, iv. 830, 831
    method of operating for cleft palate, v. 538
    steel brace, iv. 971
Taylor and Houghton's method of cranio-cerebral topography, v. 363
T-bandage, abdominal, or abdominal binder, iv. 578
    of chest, iv. 578
    single and double, iv. 577
Teale's amputation of the leg, with a large anterior flap, iv. 337
    suction operation for cataract, v. 628
Teeth, diagnostic data supplied by them, i. 517
    disorders resulting from loss of, vi. 5
    Hutchinson, v. 602
    infection of jaw through, vi 877
    non-erupted, vi. 878
Teething paralysis, iv. 807
Teleangiectasis, ii. 356
    of eyelids, v. 552
    of face, v. 470
    of mouth, vi. 248
    of orbit, v. 651
Temperament, influence of, upon surgical conditions, i. 781
Temporal fossa, dermoid cyst of, vi. 865
    tumors of, vi. 865
    lobe, lesions of, symptoms, v. 280
Temporo-maxillary articulation, excision of, iv. 391
    tuberculous disease of, iii. 600
Temporo-sphenoidal lobe of brain, diagnosis of tumors in, v. 302
Tendons and their sheaths, surgical diseases and wounds, ii. 409
Tendo-synovitis, ii. 427
Tendo-vaginitis, ii. 427
Tenonitis, v. 648
Teno-synovitis, acute, ii. 428
Tenotomy, for infantile paralysis, iv. 834
    Willett's method, iv. 835
    for strabismus, v. 640
    open method, ii. 416
    subcutaneous method, ii. 415
Teratoid tumors or cysts, simple or complex, i. 366, 367, 368
    of mouth, vi. 263
Teratomata, bigerminal, i. 366; vii. 16
    malignant, i. 366, 368
    monogerminal, endogenous or autochthonous, i. 366
    of nasopharynx, vi. 861
    of ovary, vii. 427
    of pharynx, v. 810
    of testis, vi. 697
    Warthin's classification of, i. 367
Terrell, artificial tongue of, vi. 30
Testis, aberrant, vi. 660

Testis, anatomy of, vi. 627
    atrophy of, i. 181
    inflammation of. See Orchitis
    injuries of, vi. 665
    malformations of, vi. 658
    malposition of, vi. 659
    strangulation of, from torsion of cord, vi. 667
    supernumerary, vi. 663
    teratoma of, vi. 697
    tuberculosis of, vi. 672
    tumors of, vi. 696
    undescended, vi. 659
Tetania thyreopriva, vi. 391
Tetanus, i. 453; iii. 26
Tetany, iii. 26
    post-operative, vi. 391
Thanatophidia, or death snakes, iii. 7
Thecitis, ii. 427
Thiersch's method of drainage in empyema, viii. 49
    method of rhinoplasty, iv. 685
    method of skin-grafting, i. 258; iv. 620
    operation, avulsion of trigeminal nerve, v. 384
    operation for epispadias, vi. 656
Thigh, amputation of, by equal antero-posterior flaps, iv. 349
    by equal lateral flaps (Vermale), iv. 349
    by long anterior and short posterior flaps (Farabeuf), iv. 349
    circular, iv. 347
    immediately above the knee-joint, iv. 345
    Syme's modification of the circular method, iv. 349
    hyperextension of, normal, iv. 952
    transverse section of, in the middle, iii. 246
Third intention, repair by, i. 271
Thomas, T. Turner, on pseudarthrosis, iii. 212
Thomas' brace for knock-knee, iv. 864, 865, 866
    collar for Pott's disease, iv. 974
    "heel," the, described, iii. 535
    splint for fractures of the neck of the femur, iii. 174
    wrench, for talipes, iv. 907
Thompson's lithotrite, viii. 337
    operation for restoration of alæ, iv. 695
    sound, viii. 309
Thoracic aorta and branches, aneurysm of, viii. 37
    cavity and its contents, wounds of, viii. 16
    duct obstruction, causing pseudo-chylous ascites, i. 237
Thoracoplasty, viii. 52
Thoracotomy, viii. 49
Thorax, inspection of, as furnishing diagnostic data, i. 514
    surgery of, vi. 401
Thrombectomy, vii. 220

Thrombo-phlebitis, infective, v. 732
    treated by ligature, i. 441
Thrombosis (and see Thrombus), vii. 175
    and embolism, post-operative, iv. 160
Thrombus, arterial, vii. 181
    autochthonous, vii. 179
    ball, vii. 179
    capillary, vii. 182
    cardiac, vii. 181
    changes undergone by, vii. 180
    combined, vii. 179
    fibrinous, vii. 179
    healing of, i. 105
    hyaline, vii. 179
    leucocytic, vii. 179
    localization of, vii. 181
    mixed, vii. 179
    mural, vii. 179
    obstructing, vii. 179
    of arterioles, vii. 181
    parietal, vii. 179
    primary, vii. 179
    propagated, vii. 179
    red, vii. 179
    secondary, vii. 179
    stages of, i. 288
    valvular, vii. 179
    venous, vii. 181
    white, vii. 179
Thrush of œsophagus, vii. 411
Thumb, amputations and disarticulations of, iv. 285
    dorsal dislocation of, iv. 68, 69
    fractures of, iii. 153
    Nicoladoni's operation for replacing lost, iv. 633
    simple and complicated dislocations of, treatment, iv. 68, 71
Thymic asthma, vi. 398, 399
Thymus, abscess of, vi. 398
    surgery of the, vi. 399
    surgical diseases of, vi. 353, 397
    wounds of, vi. 353
Thyro-glossal duct, fistulæ of, vi. 395
    persistent, v. 869
Thyroid, accessory, vi. 353, 366, 396
    actinomycosis of, vi. 372
    adenoma of, vi. 368
    anatomy of, vi. 353
    benign tumors of, vi. 372
    carcinoma of, vi. 373
    diseases of, vi. 358
    supernumerary, vi. 257
    surgical diseases of, vi. 353, 358
    syphilis of, vi. 372
    tuberculosis of, vi. 371
    tumors of, benign, vi. 372
    malignant, vi. 372
    wounds of, vi. 353
Thyroidectomy, choice of anæsthetic for, iv. 218
    partial, vi. 383, 386, 400
Thyroidism, acute post-operative, vi. 377, 389
Thyroiditis, vi. 365, 370
Thyroptosis, vi. 365
Thyrotomy, v. 873, 916
Tibia, dislocations of, iv. 85
    excisions of, iv. 455

Tibia, fractures of, iii. 193
　　osteoplastic operations on, iv. 457
　　sarcoma of, iii. 463
Tier sutures, i. 752
Tillmann's method of bridging a defect in the scalp, iv. 630
Tilton, Benjamin T., on Burns and the Effects of Electricity and of Lightning, ii. 581
Tobold's laryngeal lancet, v. 877
Toe, Morton's, iv. 886
Toe-nail, ingrowing, vii. 43
Toes, amputations of, iv. 312–316
　　dislocations of, iv. 104
　　fractures of, iii. 211
Tongue (and see Mouth)
　　abnormal mobility, acquired, \ i. 228
　　abnormalities of, vi. 226
　　abscess of, chronic, vi. 244
　　absence of, vi. 226
　　actinomycosis of, vi. 242
　　adherent, vi. 226
　　anatomical considerations, vi. 225
　　animal parasites in, vi. 243
　　artificial, vi. 29
　　　of Martin, vi. 29
　　　of Terrell, vi. 30
　　atrophy of, vi. 297
　　avulsion of, vi. 231
　　Bartlett's use of, in repairing the cheek, iv. 639
　　bifid, vi. 228
　　bites of serpents on, vi. 232
　　burns and scalds of, vi. 232
　　congenital defects of, vi. 226
　　echinococcus cysts of, vi. 243
　　enlargement of, vi. 248
　　excision of (and see Tongue, removal of), vi. 279
　　foreign bodies in, vi. 232
　　gangrene of, vi. 241
　　geographical, vi. 234
　　hairy black, vi. 239
　　herpes of, vi. 235
　　hyperkeratosis of, vi. 239
　　inflammation of (and see Glossitis), vi. 233
　　keloid of, vi. 257
　　leprosy of, vi. 243
　　mutilation of, vi. 229
　　nævi of, vi. 249
　　psoriasis of (and see Leucoma), vi. 235
　　ranula, vi. 257
　　removal of, vi. 280
　　scalds of, vi. 232
　　split, vi. 228
　　stings of bees and wasps on, vi. 232
　　syphilis of, vi. 293
　　trichina spiralis in, vi. 243
　　tuberculosis of, vi. 295
　　tumors of,. vi. 251
　　wounds of, vi. 229
Tongue-swallowing, vi. 228
Tongue-tie, vi. 226
Tonsil, carcinoma of, vi. 863
　　chancre of, v. 843
　　faucial, hypertrophied, v. 834
　　fourth, v. 841

Tonsil, inflammation of. See Amygdalitis
　　lingual, v. 841
　　Luschka's, v. 825
　　pharyngeal, v. 825
　　third, v. 825
　　tumors of, vi. 862
Tooth cysts, vi. 196
Tophi of the auricle, v. 675
Tornwaldt's disease, v. 855
Torsion, control of hemorrhage by, vi. 244
　　of omentum, vii. 748
Torticollis, iv. 767
Touch, sense of, in relation to diagnosis, i. 535
Tourniquet, India-rubber, its application, v. 596
Towels, as used in operations, i. 720
Toxic ulceration from drugs, i. 227
Toxinæmia, defined, i. 426
　　in inflammation, i. 96
Trabeculæ, their development, i. 281
Trachea, cut-throat, v. 866
　　foreign bodies in, v. 905
　　fractures of, iii. 107
　　gunshot wounds of, v. 866
　　malformations of, v. 898
　　surgical diseases of, v. 863
　　tumors in, v. 899
　　wounds of, v. 863, 899
Trachelo-mastoid muscle, anatomy of, iv. 787
Trachelorrhaphy, vi. 586
Tracheocele, v. 867
Tracheoscopy, v. 905
Tracheotomy and allied operations, v. 902
　　by local anæsthesia, iv. 244
　　choice of anæsthetic for, iv. 218
Trachoma, v. 580
Trained nurse and her duties, i. 722
Training-school for nurses inaugurated in Bellevue Hospital, i. 32
Transduodenal choledochotomy, viii. 273
Transfusion of blood, direct, Crile's method of, iv. 607–609
Transillumination of the antrum, vi. 207
　　of the frontal sinus, vi. 208
Translucency as an aid in diagnosis, i. 515
Transplantable mouse tumors, their characteristics, i. 394
Transplantation of cornea, v. 619
Transudates, i. 237, 574
Transversalis muscle of abdomen, vii. 110
Transverse myelitis, diagnosed from infantile paralysis, iv. 824
Transylvania University, medical department of, founded, i. 25
Trapezius muscle, anatomy of, iv. 787
Trauma. See Injury
Trélat's operation for restoration of lower lip, iv. 658
Trendelenburg fixtures, portable, iv. 146
Trendelenburg's operation for saddle-nose, iv. 712

Trendelenburg's position, in abdominal surgery, vii. 120, 121
Trephining, v. 351
Triangles of neck, iv. 790
Trichiasis, v. 559
Trichina spiralis in tongue, vi. 243
Trigeminal nerve, extra-cranial operations upon, v. 384
　　intracranial operations on, v. 393
Trigonum vesicæ, viii. 281
"Trinity of Pott's disease," iv. 951
Tripier's operation with section of the calcaneus, iv. 326
Trocar puncture of urinary bladder, viii. 322
Trochanter major, fractures through, iii. 165
　　minor, fractures of, iii. 165
Trochanteric bursa, cold abscess of, iii. 628
Trochlear nerve, surgery of the, v. 380
Trochocephalism, iii. 327
Tropical abscess of liver, viii. 209
Tropococain as a local anæsthetic, iv. 233
Trunk, congenital dislocations of, iv. 735
　　plastic surgery of, iv. 627
Trusses, vii. 599, 602
Trypsin treatment for carcinoma of uterus, viii. 661
Tubby's classification of congenital deformities, iv. 733
Tubercle, iii. 571
Tubercula dolorosa, i. 319, 328
Tuberculin as a diagnostic test, ii. 86
　　in Pott's disease, iv. 959
　　the opsonic index and its significance, iii. 594
　　Wright's technique, iii. 594
Tuberculo-gangrenous syphilide, ii. 245
Tuberculosis (and see Lupus)
　　analogous features in pulmonary and joint invasions, ii. 76
　　affecting the abdominal organs, ii. 82
　　as a cause of pathological luxation, its treatment, iv. 8
　　as an indication for excision of the elbow-joint, statistics of Kœnig and Kocher, iv. 407
　　conditions affecting its development, iii. 584, 585
　　of accessory sinuses, vi. 85
　　of antrum, vi. 883
　　of bladder, viii. 122
　　of bone, 644, 645
　　of brain, v. 301
　　of cerebellum, v. 301
　　of clavicle, vi. 416
　　of conjunctiva, v. 582
　　of cranium, v. 44
　　of epididymis vi. 672
　　of face, v. 452
　　of Fallopian tube, viii. 420
　　of female breast, vi. 517
　　of genitals, female, vi. 565
　　of genitals, male, external, vi. 671

Tuberculosis of individual bones and joints, iii. 599
of iris, v. 613
of jaws, vi. 881
of joints, infrequency of mixed infection, ii. 78
of kidney, viii. 121
of knee, iv. 437
of larynx, v. 875
of liver, viii. 223
of long bones of the extremities, iii. 724
of lymphatics and lymph nodes, relative frequency of, ii. 80
of metacarpo-phalangeal and of the interphalangeal joints, iii. 617
of ovary, viii. 420
of pelvic bones, vii. 7
of penis, vi. 671
of peritoneum, vii. 533
of pharynx, v. 847
of prostate, viii. 347
of ribs, vi. 410
of sacro-iliac synchondrosis, vii. 8
of salivary glands, vi. 303
of scrotum, vi. 671
of seminal vesicles, vi. 674
of sheaths of tendons, ii. 85
of shoulder-joint, iv. 395
of spleen, viii. 68
of sternum, vi. 410
of symphysis pubis, vii. 11
of testis, vi. 672
of thyroid, vi. 371
of tongue, vi. 295
of urethra, vi. 671
of urinary bladder, viii. 304
of vas deferens, vi. 674
of vermiform appendix, vii. 636
pulmonary, iii. 28
Tuberculous abscess, iii. 580; iv. 978; viii. 224
arthritis, tuberculin treatment in, iii. 592-599
bone disease, ii. 84
of clavicle and scapula, iii. 109
of elbow-joint, iii. 607-609
of hip-joint, iii. 623-684
of knee-joint, iii. 684-711
of metacarpals and phalanges, iii. 616
of metatarsals, iii. 723
of sacro-iliac joint, iii. 618-622
of shoulder-joint, iii. 601-607
of skull, iii. 599
of spinal column, ii. 84; iv. 927
of sternum and ribs, iii. 617, 618
of symphysis pubis, iii. 622
of tarsal bones, iii. 720-722
of temporo-maxillary joint, iii. 600
of wrist-joint, iii. 613-616
Tuberous potassium-iodide eruption, ii. 392
Tubes, Fallopian. See Fallopian tubes
Tubo-ovarian abscess, viii. 409

Tumors (or neoplasms), defined, i. 291, 292, 370
classification of, i. 294, 296
Tunica albuginea, vi. 628
vaginalis, vi. 631
vasculosa, vi. 628
Turbinate, inferior, removal of anterior part of, in chronic ethmoidal suppuration, vi. 103
trimming of, in chronic ethmoidal suppuration, vi. 101
middle, cystic, vi. 98, 859
Turner, Charles R., on Prosthesis in its Relation to Surgery of the Face, Mouth, Jaws, and Nasal and Laryngeal Cavities, vi. 3-51
Tuttle, James P., and Earle, Samuel T., on Surgical Diseases and Wounds of the Anus and Rectum, vii. 761-948
Tuttle's hemorrhoidal clamp, vii. 867
forceps, vii. 867
method of appendicostomy, vii. 797
method of closing artificial anus, vii. 942
modification of Whitehead's operation for hemorrhoids, vii. 870
operation for recto-urethral fistula, vii. 831
pneumatic protoscope, vii. 769
Twins, joined, vii. 16
the Jones, vii. 16, 17
Twisting the foot, for flat foot, iv. 885
Two-glass test, for gonorrhœal urethritis, vi. 727
Tyloma, ii. 346
Tylosis, ii. 346
Typhoid appendicitis, vii. 636
fever, diagnosed from acute appendicitis, vii. 659
spine, diagnosed from Pott's disease, iv. 955
Typhus, traumatic, ii. 253

ULCER (or Ulcers), i. 131, 132, 418
acute, ii. 175
annular, i. 142
eczematous, i. 230
erethistic, painful or irritable, ii. 183
fissured, ii. 174
fistulous, ii. 174
fungating, i. 132
fungous or fungoid, ii. 181
gangrenous, phagedenic, or diphtheritic, ii. 181
gastric, and its sequelæ (and see Stomach, ulcer of), vii. 337
gouty, i. 143, 230
hemorrhagic, i. 132; ii. 183
indolent, i. 132, 142; ii. 174
inflammatory, ii. 178
intestinal, vii. 713
irritable or painful, i. 143
irritable, of anus, vii. 801
local treatment of, ii. 188
malignant, i. 131, 132

Ulcer, œdematous, i. 142
of auricle, v. 670
of cornea, v. 599
of face, Jacob's, v. 489
rodent, v. 489
of stomach, its rupture into the lung, ii. 276
of tongue, tuberculous, vi. 296
of urinary bladder, viii. 300
peptic, of duodenum, vii. 713
perforating, i. 142
phagedenic, i. 132
pressure (decubitus), i. 133; ii. 179
progressive, ii. 174
raw, i. 142
rodent, ii. 377
scirrhous, i. 132
scorbutic, i. 230
serpiginous, i. 132, 142; ii. 182
simple, ii. 177
sloughing, i. 132; ii. 181
spreading, i. 132
syphilitic, i. 131, 133, 143
the infective class, ii. 171
the non-infective class, ii. 168
Thiersch's method of skin-grafting in treatment of, ii. 198
traumatic, i. 133
tuberculous, i. 144
varicose, i. 133, 144; ii. 178
weak, torpid or anæmic, ii. 181
Ulcus elevatum hypertrophicum, i. 142; ii. 181
rodens of vulva, vi. 564
serpens of Saemisch, v. 599
Ulna and radius, special fractures of the ends of, iii. 138
diastasis of the head of, iv. 64
isolated dislocation of, at the elbow, iv. 58
Umbilical fungus, vii. 89
hernia, vii. 594
Umbilicus, tumors of, vii. 89
Umbrella tampon, iv. 539
Unconsciousness, in cerebral compression, v. 135
Undescended testis, vi. 659
Ununited fracture of femur, iii. 245
of head of radius, iii. 241
of shaft of radius, iii. 242
Urachus, cysts of, vii. 80
endothelioma of, vii. 81
patent, vii. 81
Uranoplasty, v. 524
Urates, calculi of, viii. 112
Ureter, abnormalities of, viii. 85, 88
anatomy of, viii. 81
double, viii. 89
implantation of, viii. 155
inflammation of, viii. 144
tumors of, viii. 144
wounds of, viii. 78, 90, 141
Ureteral calculus, viii. 142
Ureterectomy, viii. 155, 156
Ureteritis, viii. 144
Uretero-lithotomy, viii. 155, 156
Uretero-plasty, viii. 155
Uretero-ureteral anastomosis, viii. 155
Urethra, absence of, vi. 646
anatomy of, vi. 632
caruncle of, vi. 571

Urethra, closure of, vi. 646
　dilatation of, vi. 647
　double, vi. 648
　false passage in, vi. 806
　foreign bodies in, vi. 663
　malformations of, vi. 646
　rupture of, vi. 666
　stricture of, vi. 773
　tuberculosis of, vi. 671
　tumors of, vi. 694
Urethral caruncle, vi. 571
　secretions, data obtainable by
　　examining them, i. 566
Urethritis, vi. 669
　acute posterior, differentiated
　　from prostatitis, viii. 342
　gonorrhœal (and (see Gonor-
　　rhœal urethritis), vi. 715
　female, vi. 559
Urethrometer, vi. 785, 789
Urethroscopy, vi. 759
Urethrotomes, vi. 788
Urethrotomy, external, vi. 801
　internal, vi. 799
Uric-acid calculi, viii. 112
　deposits in gout, i. 200
Urinary bladder, absence of, viii.
　282
　anatomy of, viii. 279
　aspiration of, viii. 321
　drainage of, viii. 325, 326
　exstrophy of, viii. 282
　hernia of, viii. 312
　injuries of, viii. 279, 286
　malformations of, viii. 279
　puncture of, by trocar, viii.
　　322
　rupture of, viii. 287
　stone in, viii. 306
　tuberculosis of, viii. 304
　tumors of, viii. 309
　ulcer of, viii. 300
Urination, diagnostic features of
　modifications in the manner
　and frequency of the act, i.
　546
　force of the stream, its varia-
　　tions, i. 549
Urine, cryoscopy of, in investigat-
　ing the kidney, i. 568; viii. 85
　extravasation of, viii. 92
　incontinence of, i. 548; viii. 316,
　　319
　infiltration of, vi. 807, 808
　overflow of, i. 547; viii. 316
　retention of, viii. 318
Urines, separation of, of the two
　kidneys, viii. 83
Urogenital tract, female, develop-
　ment of, viii. 445
Uronephrosis, viii. 100
Utero-sacral ligaments, shortening
　of, viii. 485
Utero-suspension, viii. 482
Uterus, absence of, viii. 446
　anteflexion of, viii. 455, 456
　anteposition of, viii. 455
　anteversion of, viii. 455, 456
　arcuatus, viii. 446
　bicornis, viii. 445, 450
　bilocularis, viii. 445
　didelphys, viii. 446
　displacements of, viii. 454

Uterus, double, viii. 449
　embryogenesis of, viii. 444
　fœtal, viii. 452
　incudiformis, viii. 445
　infantile, viii. 452, 453
　inversion of, viii. 510
　lateral flexions of, viii. 457
　lateral versions of, viii. 457
　malformations of, viii. 444, 453
　pregnant, retroversion of, viii.
　　463
　prolapse of, vi. 611; viii. 487
　pubescent, viii. 452
　radical operations on, results of,
　　viii. 683
　rectum communicating with,
　　treatment of, vii. 784
　retrodisplacements of, viii. 458
　retroflexion of, viii. 458
　retroversion of, viii. 458
　rudimentary, viii. 446
　septus, viii. 449
　septus duplex, viii. 445
　subseptus, viii. 445, 449
　surgery of, viii. 444
　tumors of, viii. 663
　unicornis, viii. 447
　vaginal fixation of, viii. 485
Utricle, cystic dilatation of, viii.
　367
Uvea, ectropion of the, v. 614
Uvula, bifida, v. 810
　elongated, v. 817

Vaccination, iv. 603
Vagina, absence of, vi. 577
　atresia of, acquired, vi. 573
　　congenital, vi. 577
　double, vi. 579
　drainage of pelvis through, vii.
　　118
　plastic operations in, vi. 579
　surgical diseases of, vi. 559
　wounds of, vi. 559
Vaginal hysterectomy, viii. 647
　puncture, viii. 414
　secretions, parasites to be found
　　therein, i. 566
Vaginapexy, vi. 617
Vaginitis, gonorrhœal, vi. 560
Vagus centres, effect of cerebral
　compression on, v. 132, 134
　nerve, injury to, in neck, vi. 330
Valves of Houston, vii. 761
Van Hook's operation on ureter,
　viii. 155
Van Leyden's bird's-eye inclusions,
　i. 388
Van Vert's operation for restoring
　the cheek, iv. 647
Varicocele, vi. 678
　after herniotomy, vii. 592
Varicose veins, vii. 308
Varicosities of penis, vi. 678
　of scrotum, vi. 678
Varix, vii. 308
　aneurysmal, vii. 289
　arterial, vii. 258
　of face, arterial, v. 473
　of lingual tonsil, v. 842
Vas aberrans of Haller, vi. 630,
　deferens, vi. 630
　　tuberculosis of, vi. 674

Vaseline, use of, in plastic opera-
　tions, iv. 625
Vasomotor nerves, in brain, v. 121
　paralysis, diagnostic features,
　　i. 544
Veins, anastomosing, vii. 310.
Veins in neck, injuries of, vi. 325
　air embolism, vi. 325
　hemorrhage, vi. 325
　inflammation of. See Phlebitis
　injuries of, vii. 322
　ligation of, iv. 528; vii. 327
　of brain, v. 101
　of Galen, v. 102
　perforating, vii. 310
　repair of injury to, i. 288
　temporary ligation of, and liga-
　　tion of veins en masse, iv. 536
　varicose, vii. 308
　wounds of, vii. 323
Vela and obturators, for cleft pal-
　ate, relative advantages of, vi.
　18
Veldt sores, i. 230
Velum, artificial, for cleft palate,
　vi. 12
Venesection, iv. 605, 606
Venom apparatus of the cobra, iii. 8
Venomous marine snakes, viii.
　974
Venous obstruction, sequence of
　pathological changes from, i. 235,
　532
Ventral fixation of uterus, vi. 616
　by means of utero-sacral
　　ligaments, vi. 617
　hernia, vii. 599
Ventral suspension of uterus, viii.
　482
Ventricular puncture, location, v.
　365
Ventrotomy, vii. 106
Vermiform appendix. See Appen-
　dix, vermiform
　perforative inflammation of;
　　report by R. J. Fitz, i. 59
Verneuil's method of rhinoplasty,
　iv. 685
　operation of substragaloid am-
　　putation, iv. 328
Verruca, ii. 361
　acuminata, vi. 674
　necrogenica, ii. 325
　of rectum, vii. 897
Verruga peruana, ii. 344
Vertebræ, anatomy of, iv. 929, 931
　caseation of, in Pott's disease,
　　iv. 932
　diastasis of, iv. 19
　dislocations of the, iv. 18
　fracture of laminæ of, vi. 429
　fractures of spinous processes of,
　　vi. 429
　fractures of transverse processes
　　of, vi. 429
　injuries of, partial, vi. 429
　　total, vi. 429
　isolated fracture of, vi. 435
Vertebral artery, aneurysm of, vi.
　337
　ligation of, iv. 495, 496; vi.
　　337
　column, anatomy of, iv. 927

Vesico-vaginal fistula, operations for, vi. 620
Vesiculitis, vi 670
Vincent's angina, v. 822
"Vincula accessoria" defined, iv. 280
Viperidæ. or true vipers, iii. 8
Viperines, usually poisonous, iii. 7
Vision, cortical area concerned with, v. 272
Vital centres, in cerebral operations, v. 347
Vitreous body, hemorrhage in, during cataract operations, v. 634
prolapse of, during cataract operations, v. 634
Volkmann block, how used, iv. 546
Volkmann's contracture. iii. 148; vii. 37
Voluntary-habit torticollis, iv. 783
Volvulus, vii. 728
Vomiting, as a symptom of organic cerebral lesion, v. 275
Von Ammon's method of operation for epicanthus, v. 570
Von Bergmann, views of, on cerebral compression, v. 113
Von Bruns' modification of Pirogoff's amputation, iv. 334
operation in plastic surgery, iv. 617
operation for restoration of lower lip, iv. 662
Von Dieffenbach's operation for epispadias, iv. 655
Von Graefe's method of rhinoplasty, iv. 683, 688
operation for ectropion iv. 670
symptom, v. 556
Von Hacker's method of rhinoplasty, iv. 692
Von Mangold's operation for saddle nose, iv. 708
Von Mosetig-Moorhof, bone plug, its preparation and use, i. 724
Von Recklinghausen's disease, v. 16
Von Schulten's eye-phenomenon, in cerebral compression, v. 129
work of, on cerebral compression, v. 115
Von Siklossy's operation (blepharoplasty), iv. 675
Vredena's method of rhinoplasty, iv. 690
Vulpius' method of tendon transplantation, iv. 836, 837, 838, 839
Vulva (and see Genitals, external, female)
carcinoma of, vi. 569
condylomata acuminata of, vi. 568
cysts of, vi. 565, 566
elephantiasis of, vi. 563
fibroma of, vi. 570
hæmatoma of, vi. 572
hypertrophic ulceration of, vi. 564
kraurosis of, vi. 562
lipoma of, vi. 571
pruritus of, vi. 561
sarcoma of, vi. 571

Vulva, ulcus rodens of, vi. 564
Vulvitis pruriginosa, vi. 561

WAIVER of privilege, viii. 798
Waldstein's and 'Werner postulates concerning cancer statistics, viii. 679
Walker's combined lithotrite and cystoscope, viii. 336
Walking, attitudes in, iv. 874
Wallerian degeneration, i. 178
"Wandering" acetabulum, iii. 308
spleen, viii. 61
Wardrop's method of ligating for aneurysm, vii. 280
Ware's .ethyl-chloride inhaler, iv. 205
Warfare, surgery of (and see Military surgery and Naval surgery), viii. 970
Warren, John, i. 10
Warren, John C., i. 19
Warren, Joseph, Gen., i. 10
Warthin, Aldred Scott, i. 71
Warts, divided into the true, and the flat or juvenile, ii. 361
of auricle, v. 675
of eyelids, v. 551
significance of Perthes' experiments with the x-ray on, i. 402
that occur under hard, horny epithelium, ii. 363
their contagiousness, ii. 362
venereal, vi. 674
Water canker of the earlier writers, ii. 301
Water-snakes, poisonous, iii. 8
Watkins' operation for prolapsed uterus, vii. 502
Watson's drainage tube, viii. 326
Watts' operation for restoration of lower lip, iv. 664
Weak-foot, iv. 872, 875
Webbed fingers, iv. 634
Weber's method of restoring the alæ nasi, iv. 697
operation for flap formation, in plastic surgery, iv. 618
Webster's operation for retroverted uterus, viii. 480
Wecker's method of operation for epicanthus, v. 570
Wehnelt's electrolytic interrupter, i. 603
Weir's modification of operation for rectal extirpation, vii. 925
operations of appendicostomy, vii. 797
fishbone catcher, vii. 427
Welch's Bacillus aërogenes capsulatus, ii. 459
Wells, Horace, i. 64
Wen (and see Goitre), ii. 351; v. 13; vi. 358
Werder's method of hysterectomy, by cautery, viii. 646
Wertheim's operation for prolapsed uterus, viii. 502
radical operation for carcinoma of uterus, viii. 622
Whitacre, Horace J., on Excisions of Bones and Joints, iv. 367

White gangrene from x-rays, ii. 169
scar tissue, an eligible seat for skin grafts, i. 270
swelling of the knee-joint, iii. ·689, 692
White's plate for fixation of ununited fracture after resection, iii. 230
Whitehead's method of excision of tongue, vi. 280
operation for hemorrhoids, vii. 868
Whitlow, i. 128; ii. 157; vii. 57
Whitman (Royal) on Deformities and Disabilities of the Lower Extremities, iv. 848
Whitman's brace for weak-foot, iv. 883
frame for Pott's disease, iv. 962
method for overcoming flexion deformity, iv. 452
method of treating fractures of the neck of the femur, iii. 175
operation for talipes calcaneus, iv. 924
Wildermuth auricle, v. 661
Willard, De Forest, on Surgical Diseases and Wounds of Nerves, ii. 463
Willard's method of gastro-duodenostomy, vii. 376
Willett's method of tendon-lengthening, iv. 835
Winter's postulates concerning cancer statistics, viii. 681
Wire cuirass for Pott's disease, iv. 964
Witness, expert, viii. 771, 773, 776, 777
matters for, viii. 775
qualifications of, viii. 774
ordinary, viii. 771, 773
surgeon as a, viii. 770, 774
Witzel's method of gastrostomy, vii. 402
Wladimiroff-Mikulicz osteoplastic resection of the foot, iv. 334
of the tarsus, results, iv. 464
Wolf's law of the transformation of bone, iii. 324
Wolfe graft, v. 431
Wolfe-Krause method of skin-grafting, iv. 622
Wolff-Koenig method of closing cranial defects, v. 367
Women, greater power of endurance in, i. 777
Wood, Alfred C., on Gangrene and Gangrenous Diseases, ii. 201
Wood, James R., i. 31
Wood ticks, or ixodidæ, ii. 395
Wool-sorters' disease, iii. 32
Wounds, accidental, arrest of hemorrhage, ii. 616
chemical agents used to secure asepsis, ii. 622
cleansing of, ii. 620
closure of, ii. 621
treatment of, ii. 616
arrow, ii. 635

Wounds, aseptic or septic, these terms defined, ii. 605
aseptic, surgical principles associated with them, i. 751
bayonet, ii. 633
blank cartridge, of feet, vii. 42
of hands, vii. 42
by shell fragments, ii. 657
by solid shot, ii. 608, 656
contused and lacerated, i. 756
diphtheritis of, i. 135
dissection and post-mortem, ii. 637
from explosions, their characteristics, ii. 647
gunshot. See Gunshot wounds
in naval surgery, viii. 972
incised, ii. 605
infections of, i. 415, 418, 757
inflicted by agricultural implements, ii. 635
by the bolo and other knives of the East Indian Archipelago, ii. 630
loss or impairment of function as a symptom, ii. 608
machete, ii. 632
made by cutting and piercing instruments, classification of, ii. 605
multiple, from jacketed bullets, ii. 660

Wright's tuberculin treatment, iii. 594
Wrist, congenital dislocation of, iv. 742
crushes of, iii. 740–742
disarticulations at, iv. 287
dislocations of, iv. 64
excision of, ii. 752; iv. 419–426
fractures of the bones of the, iii. 148, 152
incised and punctured wounds of, iii. 742
infections in, vii. 66
infantile paralysis of, iv. 818
laceration of ligaments of, iii. 739
Madelung's deformity of, iv. 742, 743
sprains of, iii. 738
tuberculous disease of, iii. 613
Wry-neck (and see Torticollis), iv. 767
diagnosed from Pott's disease, iv. 956
Wyeth's method of hæmostasis as applied to amputation at the hip-joint, iv. 352
as applied to an amputation at the shoulder-joint, iv. 302
of operating upon displaced intermaxillary bone, v. 521

XANTHELASMA of eyelids, v. 550
Xanthin calculi, viii. 113
Xanthoma, ii. 353
Xeroderma pigmentosum, ii. 374, 384
Xerophthalmia, v. 583
Xerosis of conjunctiva, v. 583
X-ray (and see Radiograph, Roentgen rays)
anatomy, its special features, i. 642
appearance of different types of ostemyelitis, i. 650
of late hereditary and tertiary bone syphilis, i. 665
of subperiosteal bone deposit compared with those of osteomyelitis and periostitis albumosa, i. 667
burns, i. 638; vii. 39
harmful effects of, i. 636
tubes, i. 608, 609

YOUNG'S theory of congenital deformities, iv. 734
of congenital dislocation, iv. 734

ZIEGLER'S method of iridotomy, v. 622
Zuckergussleber, i. 140

Lightning Source UK Ltd.
Milton Keynes UK
UKHW041356041218
333025UK00023B/958/P